*We
appreciate
this opportunity to be
of service to you and
your specialty of
dermatology.*

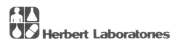

Herbert Laboratories

Providing today's therapy.
Pursuing tomorrow's promise.

Textbook of Dermatology

Textbook of Dermatology

EDITED BY

ARTHUR ROOK
MA, MD, FRCP
Honorary Consulting Dermatologist
Addenbrooke's Hospital,
Cambridge

D. S. WILKINSON
MD, FRCP
Formerly Consultant Dermatologist
Aylesbury and High Wycombe
Hospital Group

F. J. G. EBLING
DSc, PhD, CBiol
Emeritus Professor of Zoology
University of Sheffield

R. H. CHAMPION
MA, MB, FRCP
Consultant Dermatologist
Addenbrooke's Hospital,
Cambridge

J. L. BURTON
BSc, MD, FRCP
Reader in Dermatology, University of Bristol
Consultant Dermatologist
Bristol Royal Infirmary

IN THREE VOLUMES
VOLUME 3

FOURTH EDITION

BLACKWELL SCIENTIFIC PUBLICATIONS
OXFORD LONDON EDINBURGH
BOSTON PALO ALTO MELBOURNE

© 1968, 1972, 1979, 1986 by
Blackwell Scientific Publications
Editorial offices:
Osney Mead, Oxford, OX2 0EL
8 John Street, London, WC1N 2ES
23 Ainslie Place, Edinburgh, EH3 6AJ
3 Cambridge Center, Suite 208
Cambridge, Massachusetts 02142, USA
667 Lytton Avenue, Palo Alto
California 94301, USA
107 Barry Street, Carlton
Victoria 3053, Australia

First published 1968
Reprinted 1969
Second edition 1972
Reprinted 1975
Third edition 1979
Reprinted 1982, 1984
Fourth edition 1986
Reprinted 1988

Set, printed and bound in Great Britain by
Butler & Tanner Ltd, Frome and London

DISTRIBUTORS

USA
  Year Book Medical Publishers
  200 North LaSalle Street
  Chicago, Illinois 60601

Canada
  The C.V. Mosby Company
  5240 Finch Avenue East
  Scarborough, Ontario

Australia
  Blackwell Scientific Publications
  (Australia) Pty Ltd
  107 Barry Street
  Carlton, Victoria 3053

British Library
Cataloguing in Publication Data

Textbook of dermatology.——4th ed.
  1. Dermatology
  I. Rook, Arthur
  616.5   RL71

  ISBN 0–632–00949–7

For
F.J.E.R.
J.B.W.
E.E.
P.L.C.
P.A.B.

Contents

Contributors

David Atherton
MA, MB, BChir, MRCP(UK)
Hospital for Sick Children, London; Queen Elizabeth Hospital, London;
Consultant Paediatric Dermatologist, St John's Hospital for Diseases of the Skin, London
Co-Author: *Naevi and Other Developmental Defects; The New Born*

Harvey Baker
MD(Leeds), FRCP(London)
Consultant Dermatologist, The London Hospital, London
Author: *The Skin as a Barrier; Drug Reactions; Psoriasis; Reiter's Disease*

Robert Baran
MD(Paris)
Head of Dermatological Unit, Cannes General Hospital
Co-Author: *The Nails*

Martin Black
MD(Newcastle), FRCP(London)
Consultant Physician to the Skin Department, St Thomas' Hospital, London
Author: *Lichen Planus and Lichenoid Eruptions*
Co-Author: *Metabolic and Nutritional Disorders*

Stanley Sholam Bleehen
BA, MB, BChir(Cantab), FRCP(London)
Consultant Dermatologist, Sheffield Health Authority;
The Royal Hallamshire Hospital; The Childrens Hospital, Sheffield
Co-Author: *Disorders of Skin Colour*

John Lloyd Burton
BSc, MD(Manc), FRCP(London)
Reader in Dermatology, University of Bristol;
Consultant Dermatologist, Bristol Royal Infirmary, Bristol
EDITOR
Co-Author: *Genetics in Dermatology; The Ages of Man and their Dermatoses; Eczema, Lichen Simplex and Prurigo; Disorders of Keratinization; Disorders of Connective Tissue; The Subcutaneous Fat; The Breast*

Robert Harold Champion
MA, MB, BChir(Cantab), FRCP(London)
Consultant Dermatologist Addenbrooke's Hospital, Cambridge and Hospitals of the East Anglian Regional Authority
EDITOR
Author: *Cutaneous Reactions to Cold; Disorders Affecting Small Blood Vessels; Urticaria; Purpura; Disorders of Sweat Glands*
Co-Author: *Principles of Diagnosis; Atopic Dermatitis; Disorders of Lymphatic Vessels; General Aspects of Treatment; Systemic Therapy*

William James Cunliffe
BSc, MD(Manc), FRCP(London)
Consultant Dermatologist, Skin Department, Leeds General Infirmary
Author: *Necrobiotic Disorders*
Co-Author: *The Subcutaneous Fat; The Sebaceous Glands; The Skin and the Nervous System.*

Rodney Peter Richard Dawber
MA, MB, ChB(Sheffield), FRCP(London)
Consultant Dermatologist, John Radcliffe and Slade Hospitals, Oxford.
Clinical Lecturer in Dermatology, University of Oxford
Co-Author: *The Hair; The Nails; Physical and Surgical Procedures*

Robin Anthony Jeffrey Eady
MB, BS(London), FRCP
Senior Lecturer and Head, Department of Electron Microscopy and Cell Pathology, Institute of Dermatology, University of London.
Consultant Dermatologist, St John's Hospital for Diseases of the Skin, London.
Co-Author: *Genetics in Dermatology*

Francis John Govier Ebling
DSc, PhD(Bristol), C.Biol.
Emeritus Professor of Zoology, University of Sheffield
Independent Research Worker in Dermatology, Academic Division of Medicine, Royal Hallamshire Hospital, Sheffield.
EDITOR
Author: *The Normal Skin*
Co-Author: *Parasitic Worms and Protozoa; Disorders of Keratinization; Disorders of Skin Colour; Disorders of Connective Tissue; The Sebaceous Glands; The Hair*

ix

Malcolm Greaves
MD, PhD(London), FRCP(London)
Professor of Dermatology, Institute of Dermatology, University of London.
Director, Wellcome Skin Pharmacology Laboratories, Institute of Dermatology
Consultant Dermatologist, St John's Hospital for Diseases of the Skin, London
Honorary Senior Lecturer in Pharmacology, University College, London
Author: *Histiocytic Proliferative Disorders; Benign Lymphoplasias of the Skin; Mastocytoses*

William Andrew David Griffiths
MA, MD(Cantab), FRCP
Consultant Dermatologist, St John's Hospital for Diseases of the Skin, London
Honorary Senior Lecturer and Vice Dean, Institute of Dermatology
Co-Author: *Disorders of Keratinization; Topical Therapy*

Roger Richard Martin Harman
MB, BS(London), FRCP(London)
Consultant Dermatologist, Bristol Royal Infirmary
Co-Author: *Leprosy; Parasitic Worms and Protozoa*

Allan Stewart Highet
BSc, MB, ChB(Glasgow), MRCP(U.K.)
Consultant Dermatologist, York District Hospital
Co-Author: *Virus and Related Infections; Bacterial Infections*

Francis Adrian Ive
MBBS, FRCP
Consultant Dermatologist, Durham Hospital
Honorary Consulting Dermatologist, Royal Victoria Infirmary, Newcastle
Co-Author: *Diseases of the Umbilical, Perianal and Genital Regions; Topical Therapy*

William Henry Jopling
FRCP(Edin), FRCP(London), DTM & H(Eng)
Honorary Consulting Physician, Hospital for Tropical Diseases, London, and to St John's Hospital for Diseases of the Skin, London
Co-Author: *Leprosy*

Francisco Kerdel Vegas
Hon CBE, MD(Caracas), MSc(N.Y.), Hon DSc(California College of Pediatric Medicine)
Lecturer in Dermatology, Colombia University, New York, U.S.A.
Visiting Professor of Dermatology, Thomas Jefferson University, U.S.A.
Former Professor of Dermatology, Vargas Medical School, Universidad Central de Venezuela; Former Attending Dermatologist to the Vargas Hospital, Caracas
Author: *Rhinoscleroma; American Trypanosomiasis; Erythema Dyschromicum Perstans; Yaws; Pinta*

Donald William Ross Mackenzie
BSc, PhD
Director of the Public Health Laboratory Service Mycological Reference Laboratory, Colindale
Professor of Medical Mycology, London School of Hygiene and Tropical Medicine
Co-Author: *Mycology*

Rona McLeod Mackie
MD, FRCP, FRCPath, FRS(E)
Professor of Dermatology, University of Glasgow
Consultant Dermatologist, Greater Glasgow Health Board
Author: *Dermatological Aspects of the Leukaemias and Lymphomas; Tumours of the Skin*

Ronald Marks
BSc(Hons), DTM & H, FRCP, MBBS, MRCPath
Professor of Dermatology, University of Wales, College of Medicine, Cardiff
Honorary Consultant in Dermatology, University Hospital of Wales, Cardiff
Co-Author: *Disorders of Keratinization; Rosacea and Perioral Dermatitis*

Robert Steel Morton
MBE, MD, FRCP(Edinburgh)
Honorary Lecturer, History of Medicine, University of Sheffield
Formerly Consultant Venerologist, Sheffield Hospitals and University
Visiting Venereologist, Govt. Western Australia 1977–78.
Visiting Scientist, Centre for Disease Control, Atlanta U.S.A.
Occasional Consultant World Health Organization 1968–83
Author: *The Treponematoses*

Jack Nagington
MB, ChB, MD(Manchester), Dip. Bact.
Honorary Consulting Virologist, East Anglian Regional Health Authority and Cambridge Health Authority
Formerly Consultant Virologist, Public Health Laboratory Service, Addenbrooke's Hospital, Cambridge
Co-Author: *Virus and Related Infections*

William Everett Parish
MA, PhD(Cantab), B.V.Sc(Liv), MRCVS, FRCPath
Head of Environmental Safety Laboratory and Head of Toxicology, Unilever Research, Colworth, Beds
Author: *Inflammation; Clinical Immunology and Allergy; Immunofluorescence; Immuno-enzymes; Autoradiography*
Co-Author: *Atopic Dermatitis*

Jens Jørgen Pindborg
DDS, Dr Odont, FRCPath, Hon FDSRCS(London)
Professor of Oral Pathology, Royal Dental College and Director, Dental Department, University Hospital, Copenhagen
Author: *Disorders of the Oral Cavity and Lips*

Richard James Pye

MA, MD(London), MRCP(U.K.)

Consultant Dermatologist, Addenbrooke's Hospital, Cambridge and Hospitals of the East Anglian Regional Health Authority

Author: *Bullous Eruptions*

Co-Author: *Metabolic and Nutritional Disorders; Systemic Therapy*

Colin Andrew Ramsay

MD(London), FRCP(London), FRCP(C), DCH

Professor of Dermatology, University of Toronto

Director, Division of Dermatology, Department of Medicine, University of Toronto

Head, Division of Dermatology, Toronto General Hospital

Co-Author: *Cutaneous Reactions to Actinic and Ionizing Radiations*

Stephen Owen Bellamy Roberts

MA, MBBChir(Cantab), FRCP(London)

Consultant Dermatologist, Addenbrooke's Hospital, Cambridge, and Hospitals of the East Anglian Regional Health Authority

Co-Author: *Bacterial Infections; Mycology; The Skin in Systemic Disease; Systemic Therapy*

Arthur James Rook

MA, MD(Cantab), FRCP(London)

Honorary Consulting Dermatologist, Addenbrooke's Hospital, Cambridge

EDITOR

Author: *Dermatology; Skin Diseases caused by Arthropods and other Venomous or Noxious Animals; The Skin and the Eyes*

Co-Author: *The Prevalence, Incidence and Ecology of Diseases of the Skin; The Principles of Diagnosis; Genetics in Dermatology; Naevi and other Developmental Defects; The Newborn; The Ages of Man and their Dermatoses; Eczema, Lichen Simplex and Prurigo; Virus and Related Infections; Disorders of Keratinization; The Hair; The Breast; Psychocutaneous Disorders.*

Graham Arthur William Rook

MD, MB, BChir

Senior Lecturer & Honorary Consultant in Microbiology, Middlesex Hospital Medical School, London

Co-Author: *Mycobacterial Infections*

Neville Robinson Rowell

MD(Newcastle), FRCP(London), DCH

Consultant Physician, Department of Dermatology, General Infirmary at Leeds

Honorary Reader in Dermatology, University of Leeds

Consultant Advisor to the Department of Health and Social Security

Author: *Lupus Erythematosus, Scleroderma and Dermatomyositis—The 'Collagen' or 'Connective Tissue' Diseases*

Terence John Ryan

DM, MA(Oxon), BMSCh(London)

Consultant Dermatologist. Department of Dermatology, John Radcliffe & Slade Hospitals, Oxford

Clinical Lecturer in Dermatology, Oxford University

Co-Author: *Cutaneous Vasculitis—'Angiitis'; Diseases of Arteries and Veins—Leg Ulcers; Disorders of Lymphatic Vessels*

Richard John Graham Rycroft

MD, MRCP, MFOM, DIH

Consultant Dermatologist, St John's Hospital for Diseases of the Skin, London

Senior Employment Medical Officer (Dermatology) Medical Division, Health and Safety Executive

Author: *Occupational Dermatology*

Co-Author: *Contact Dermatitis; The Principal Irritants and Sensitizers*

John Andrew Savin

MA, MD(Cantab), FRCP(London), FRCP(Edinburgh), DIH

Consultant Dermatologist, The Royal Infirmary of Edinburgh

Part-time Lecturer in Dermatology, The University of Edinburgh

Co-Author: *The Prevalence, Incidence and Ecology of Diseases of the Skin; Mycobacterial infections including Tuberculosis; Sarcoidosis; The Skin and the Nervous System; Psychocutaneous Disorders*

Margaret Flora Spittle

MB, BS, MSc(London), DMRT, FRCP

Consultant Radiotherapist, St John's Hospital for Diseases of the Skin, London, and the Meyerstein Institute of Radiotherapy, Middlesex Hospital

Co-Author: *Cutaneous Reactions to Actinic and Ionizing Radiations*

Kaare Weismann

MD(Copenhagen)

Consultant Dermatologist, Bispebjerg Hospital, Copenhagen

Co-Author: *Metabolic and Nutritional Disorders; The Skin in Systemic Disease*

Darrell Sheldon Wilkinson

MD(London), FRCP(London)

Formerly Consultant Dermatologist, Aylesbury and Wycombe Hospitals

EDITOR

Author: *Formulary of Local Applications*

Co-Author: *The Prevalence, Incidence and Ecology of Diseases of the Skin; The Principles of Diagnosis; Eczema, Lichen Simplex and Prurigo; Cutaneous Reactions to Mechanical and Thermal Injury; Mycobacterial infections including Tuberculosis; Cutaneous Vasculitis: 'Angiitis'; Diseases of Arteries and Veins—Leg Ulcers; Rosacea and Perioral Dermatitis; Sarcoidosis; Diseases of the Umbilical, Perianal and Genital Regions; Psychocutaneous Disorders; General Aspects of Treatment*

John Darrell Wilkinson

MB, BS (London), MRCP (UK)

Consultant Dermatologist, Wycombe General Hospital

Honorary Clinical Tutor, University of London

Author: *Diseases of the External Ear*

Co-Author: *Contact Dermatitis; The Principal Irritants and Sensitizers; Topical Therapy; Physical and Surgical Procedures*

Preface to Fourth Edition

The success enjoyed by the first three editions of this book has clearly demonstrated that it has filled a gap in the dermatological literature.

Our general policy remains unchanged. We aim to provide a comprehensive and readable account of clinical dermatology, introducing each chapter by an up to date review of the relevant basic physiopathology.

Some contributors to the earlier editions have retired and to replace them we have chosen colleagues who have taken a special research interest in their subject for many years. We have left it to these members of the team to re-write the chapter completely or to revise the existing text. Whichever course they have chosen to follow they have sought to provide a comprehensive, clinically-orientated account.

We have also added to the editorial team so that continuity will be maintained when the senior editors retire after the present edition.

We are grateful to the large number of readers who sent us comments and suggestions, many of which have been incorporated in the text.

A.J.R.
D.S.W.
F.J.G.E.
R.H.C.
J.L.B.

Acknowledgements

The revision of this textbook would have been impossible without the willing cooperation of a great many colleagues. Several chapters have been submitted to the criticism of various members of our team, and this mutual assistance has been greatly appreciated. Some contributors have sought the advice of other authorities on technical or specialized aspects of their chapters. We should like to express our gratitude to all those who have helped in this way.

The source of almost every photograph or diagram is acknowledged in the legend which accompanies it. We are grateful to the publishers who have given us permission to reproduce those few illustrations which are not original.

Preface to First Edition

No comprehensive reference book on dermatology has been published in the English language for ten years and none in England for over a quarter of a century. The recent literature of dermatology is rich in shorter texts and in specialist monographs but the English-speaking dermatologist has long felt the need for a substantial text for regular reference and as a guide to the immense monographic and periodical literature. The editors have therefore planned the present volume primarily for the dermatologist in practice or in training, but have also considered the requirements of the specialist in other fields of medicine and of the many research workers interested in the skin in relation to toxicology or cosmetic science.

An attempt has been made throughout the book to integrate our growing knowledge of the biology of skin and of fundamental pathological processes with practical clinical problems. Often the gap is still very wide but the trends of basic research at least indicate how it may eventually be bridged. In a clinical textbook the space devoted to the basic sciences must necessarily be restricted but a special effort has been made to ensure that the short accounts which open many chapters are easily understood by the physician whose interests and experience are exclusively clinical.

For the benefit of the student we have encouraged our contributors to make each chapter readable as an independent entity, and have accepted that this must involve the repetition of some material.

The classification employed is conventional and pragmatic. Until our knowledge of the mechanisms of disease is more profound no truly scientific classification is possible. In so many clinical syndromes multiple aetiological factors are implicated. To emphasize one at the expense of others is often misleading. Most diseases are to some extent influenced by genetic factors and a large proportion of common skin reactions are modified by the emotional state of the patient. Our knowledge is in no way advanced by classifying hundreds of diseases as genodermatoses and dozens as psychosomatic.

The true prevalence of a disease may throw light on its aetiology but reported incidence figures are often unreliable and incorrectly interpreted. The scientific approach to the evaluation of racial and environmental factors has therefore been considered in some detail.

The effectiveness of any physician in practice must ultimately depend on his ability to make an accurate clinical diagnosis. Clinical descriptions are detailed and differential diagnosis is fully discussed. Histopathology is here considered mainly as an aid to diagnosis but references to fuller accounts are provided.

The approach to treatment is critical but practical. Many empirical measures are of proven value and should not be abandoned merely because their efficacy cannot yet be scientifically explained. However, many familiar remedies old and new have been omitted either because properly controlled clinical trials have shown them to be of no value or because they have been supplanted by more effective and safer preparations.

There are over nine hundred photographs but no attempt has been made to provide an illustration of every disease. To have done so would have increased the bulk and price of the book without increasing proportionately its practical value. The conditions selected for illustrations are those in which a photograph significantly enhances the verbal description. There are a few conditions we wished to illustrate, but of which we could not obtain unpublished photographs of satisfactory quality.

The lists of references have been selected to provide a guide to the literature. Important articles now of largely historical interest have usually been omitted, except where a knowledge of the history of a disease simplifies the understanding of present concepts and terminology. Books and articles provided with substantial bibliography are marked with an asterisk.

Many of the chapters have been read and criticized by several members of the team and by other colleagues. Professor Wilson Jones, Dr. R. S. Wells and Dr W. E. Parish have given valuable assistance with histopathological, genetic and immunological problems respectively. Many advisers, whose services are acknowledged in the following pages, have helped us with individual chapters. Any errors which have not been eliminated are, however, the responsibility of the editors and authors.

The editors hope that this book will prove of value to all those who are interested in the skin either as physicians or as research workers. They will welcome readers' criticisms and suggestions which may help them to make the second edition the book they hope to produce.

CHAPTER 47

Dermatological Aspects of the Leukaemias and Lymphomas

RONA M. MacKIE

INTRODUCTION

In the past decade morphological and functional studies of the lymphoid system and its development have enabled a number of methods of classification of lymphoid disease to be made. Cell markers are now available so that even the most morphologically primitive and relatively non-differentiated cell types can usually be assigned to the myeloid, monocyte, B-lymphoid or T-lymphoid series. The origin of the diagnostic cell of Hodgkin's disease is still debated as it appears to carry markers of both the B-lymphoid and the macrophage series.

T- (for thymus) and B- (for bursa or bone marrow) derived lymphocytes, although morphologically similar, differ in a variety of ways. They arise in different primary lymphoid organs and have an array of distinct surface antigens and markers. They colonize separate areas of the secondary lymphoid tissues and are responsible for different lymphocyte-mediated responses. T-cells control the cell-mediated immune responses such as graft rejection and delayed hypersensitivity, whereas B cells are the direct precursors of mature antibody secreting cells.

Cutaneous involvement in the leukaemias generally occurs as an 'overspill' or secondary phenomenon and appears to be commoner with a characteristic clinical expression in T-lymphocytic leukaemia than in the other leukaemias. Although primary Hodgkin's disease of the skin has been reported, it is so rare that the existence of such an entity is still debated. In the non-Hodgkin's lymphomas, malignancies both of the B- and T- cell series, frequently involve the skin. Common characteristics of cutaneous involvement with B lymphocyte-derived lymphoma are reported to include prior or concomitant nodal involvement and the development of multiple deep-seated cutaneous nodules. In other words, it appears to be relatively less common for B-cell lymphomas than T-cell lymphomas to originate or first declare themselves in the skin.

T-cell lymphomas, on the other hand, frequently appear to involve the skin prior to invasion of other organs and the classic example of this is of course mycosis fungoides (MF). Lymph node involvement occurs relatively late in the disease, and the marrow is commonly spared. The term 'cutaneous T-cell lymphoma' (CTCL) has become popular in North America as a label embracing mycosis fungoides, the Sézary syndrome, chronic T-cell leukaemia and other even rarer T-cell disorders. European dermatologists tend, however, to keep these entities separate and this policy will be followed in this chapter.

Classification of the non-Hodgkin's lymphomas. Classification of these entities until recently has been primarily based on morphological study of cellular characteristics and two of the best known, the Lukes and Collins [3] and the Kiel [2] classifications, are outlined in Table 47.1. Other similar classifications have been offered by Rappaport [4], W.H.O. and The British Lymphoma Group [1]. These attempts at logical groupings all predate the recent extensive and exciting use of monoclonal antibodies directed against the surface markers of both immature and mature lymphoid cell subsets on tissue sections of cutaneous lymphomas. It will be of interest to see if these marker studies correlate with the older morphological criteria, or if yet another classification will emerge.

REFERENCES

1 BENNETT M.H., et al (1974) Lancet ii, 405.
2 LENNERT K. (1978) In Handbuch der Speziellen Pathologischen Anatomie und Histologie 1/3B. Berlin, Springer Verlag, p. 92.
3 LUKES R.D. & COLLINS R.D. (1975) In The Reticuloendothelial System. I.A.D. Monograph 16. Eds. Rebuch J., Berard C.W. & Abell M.R. Baltimore, Williams & Williams, p. 213.
4 RAPPAPORT H. (1966) In Atlas of Tumour Pathology. Fascicle 8, Section III. Washington, D.C., Armed Forces Institute of Pathology, p. 97.

TABLE 47.1.   A comparison of the terminology used in the Kiel, Lukes and Collins, and Rappaport Classifications of lymphomas

Kiel	Lukes and Collins	Rappaport
Low grade malignant lymphoma	B-cell type	Well-differentiated lymphocytic
Lymphocytic	Small lymphocyte	
Lymphoplasmacytoid	Plasmacytoid lymphocyte	Poorly differentiated lymphocytic
Centrocytic	Follicular centre cell	
Centroblastic/centrocytic	(large or small,	Mixed histiocytic and lymphocytic
Follicular	cleaved or non-cleaved)	
Follicular and diffuse	Immunoblastic B-cell	Histiocytic
Diffuse	'sarcoma'	
High grade malignant lymphoma	T-cell type	Undifferentiated
Centroblastic	Small lymphocyte	
Lymphoblastic	Convoluted lymphocyte	
Burkitt type	Immunoblastic T-cell sarcoma	
Convoluted cell type	Mycosis fungoides	
Immunoblastic	Sézary syndrome	
	Histiocytic	
	Undefined	

Aetiology. Although the lymphomas and leukaemias are classed among the malignant neoplasms, they differ in several ways from most other malignant conditions and are usually considered as a separate group both pathologically and, more significantly, from an aetiological standpoint.

In aetiology the following factors should be considered:
1. Heredity
2. Chromosomal abnormalities
3. Ionizing radiation
4. Infective agents
5. Immunological factors
6. Other factors

1. *Heredity.* Although less important than external factors, heredity does play some part. Rigby *et al* [7] investigated 92 families where one member was known to have either leukaemia or lymphoma, and 69 control families. The incidence of reticuloses in other members of the family was 2·5 times as great in the leukaemia-lymphoma groups as in the controls. More impressive is the fact that identical twins of children with leukaemia have a one-in-five chance of developing leukaemia within weeks or months of the first child falling ill. This group of children represents one of the high-risk leukaemia groups reviewed by Miller [6].

2. *Chromosomal abnormalities* [2]. The connection between the Philadelphia chromosome and chronic myelogenous leukaemia was first noted in 1960 [7] and later interpreted as a deletion of one of the small acrocentric chromosomes of the group No. 21 or 22 of the Denver classification [4]. It is rarely found in relation to other reticuloses; 90–95% of typical cases show the abnormal chromosome. This is not an inborn change but an induced abnormality found only in the neoplastic haemopoietic cells. Late in the disease other chromosomal abnormalities may be found. Some cases of acute leukaemia show no chromosomal abnormalities, whilst others show minor changes of various types. Other reticuloses almost all show some chromosomal abnormalities but of non-specific type. Miller's other high-risk leukaemia groups [6], all of which have some chromosomal abnormalities, are as follows:

Radiation-treated polycythaemia vera—1 in 6 in 10–15 years.

Bloom's syndrome—1 in 8 up to 26 years of age.

Atomic bomb survivors who had been within 1,000 metres of hypocentre in Hiroshima or Nagasaki—1 in 60 in 12 years.

Children with Down's syndrome—1 in 95 under 10 years of age.

An important addition to the list of chromosomal abnormalities and malignancy is the confirmation of translocations of chromosomes 8, 14 and 22 in Burkitt's lymphoma. This appears to be a frequent finding in Burkitt's lymphoma from different geographical areas [3].

3. *Ionizing radiation.* Since 1911, when radiation was first suspected as a cause of leukaemia, the dangers of excess radiation have often been confirmed. Certain groups of people have been specially

liable to leukaemia including radiologists, adults irradiated for spondylitis, Japanese atom-bomb survivors, adults treated with radium or thorotrast, children irradiated for enlarged thymus and children irradiated before birth [5]. The liability to leukaemia is greater than to lymphoma [1]. Among experimental animals the mouse is especially sensitive to irradiation.

REFERENCES

1 ANDERSON R.E. & ISHIDA K. (1964) *Ann Intern Med* **61**, 853.
2 BAILIE A.G. (1966) *Acta Haematol* **36**, 157.
3 Denver Classification Report (1960) *Lancet* **i**, 1063.
4 GRAHAM S., *et al* (1966) *Preconception, Intrauterine and Postnatal Radiation as related to Leukaemia.* National Cancer Institute Monograph No. 23, Washington, D.C.
5 MILLER R.W. (1967) *Cancer Res* **27**, 2420.
6 NOWELL P.G. & HUNGERFORD D.A. (1960) *Science* **132**, 1497.
7 RIGBY F.G., *et al* (1966) *JAMA* **197**, 25.

4. *Infective agents.* Cell-free transmission of mouse leukaemia was demonstrated by Gross in 1951 [6] and later confirmed as due to a virus [7]. In 1957 [3] virus-like particles were found in human biopsy specimens from a lymph node of a patient with acute lymphatic leukaemia. The particles were similar to murine leukaemia virus. The viruses most suspect are the DNA herpes viruses including the Epstein–Barr virus. Although they have not yet been proven to cause leukaemia or lymphoma in humans they are known to do so in some non-human primate species [2]. There is very strong circumstantial evidence that the EB virus is involved in the aetiology of Burkitt's lymphoma (see p. 1735).

The recent reports of Gallo's group [5] of the isolation and characterization of a virus from a group of patients with a severe virulent form of T-cell leukaemia/lymphoma have raised considerable interest in the extent of viral involvement in the aetiology of T-cell lymphomas. For many years it has been recognized that Marek's disease, which causes B-cell lymphoma in chickens, is caused by a virus [11], and more recently the virus responsible for feline leukaemia has been identified [4, 8]. The human T-cell leukaemia virus (HTLV-1) has to date been identified in North American blacks with severe and fatal disease and in Japanese sufferers from T-cell leukaemia. A disturbing factor has been the detection of antibodies to this virus in two household contacts of patients with mycosis fungoides [17]. The virus is a retrovirus and carefully controlled growth conditions are necessary for its identification. The availability of T-cell growth factor or interleukin 2 on a commercial scale will be of assistance in clarifying the extent of HTLV involvement in T-cell malignancies. At the time of writing it has only rarely been identified in patients studied with classic MF.

5. *Immunological factors.* It was first postulated by Kaplan and Smithers [9, 16] that some of the symptoms, including some of the skin manifestations, of the lymphomas and leukaemia, especially those of Hodgkin's disease, might be the result of an autoimmune process. They suggested that lymphoid tumour cells may become immunologically differentiated from the cells of the host, possibly by antigenic depletion, but retain their ability to make antibodies. The tumour cells could thus acquire the ability to react against and destroy the patient's normal lymphoid and haemopoietic cells and produce the three cardinal symptoms—anaemia, wasting and lymphoid depletion—of 'runting' disease or graft-versus-host reaction.

The spontaneous development of lymphoma following an autoimmune process which has resulted from the injection of parental (inborn) spleen cells into mature F_1 hybrid mice shows that immunological factors certainly play a part in some mammalian neoplasms of reticular tissue [14]. An increased incidence of lymphoreticular malignancies is a recognized part of a number of immunological deficiency diseases (see Chapter 63) and there is a significant increase in the number of lymphomas which develop both as a second malignancy in patients in cytotoxic drug therapy for malignant disease [12] and also in patients on long-term immunosuppression following renal allografts [15]. Another type of malignancy which is increased in this situation is squamous cell carcinoma [1].

6. *Other factors.* There may be many other factors and their interaction is probably important. The entry of a virus into a cell may so alter the character of the cell that it induces autoimmune phenomena progressing to runting. Radiation and possibly chemical agents may have the same effect or they may induce chromosomal damage and eventually alter the metabolism of the cell. Chronic lymphoid stimulation as in chronic malaria is thought to be of importance, possibly by allowing a latent virus (e.g. EB virus in Burkitt's lymphoma) to become active [10, 13].

REFERENCES

1 CHATTERJEE S.N. (1982) *Organ Transplantation.* Bristol, John Wright & Sons, p. 208.

2 DEINHARDT F. (1975) *Br J Cancer* **31** (Suppl. ii), 140.
3 DOMOCHOWSKI L. & GREY C.E. (1957) *Texas Rep Biol Med* **15**, 256.
4 ESSEX M., *et al* (1975) *Adv Cancer Res* **21**, 175.
5 GALLO R. & WONG-STAAL F. (1982) *Blood* **60**, 545.
6 GROSS L. (1951) *Proc Soc Exp Biol Med* **76**, 27.
7 GROSS L. (1961) *Oncogenic Viruses*. Oxford, Pergamon.
8 JARRETT W.F.H., *et al* (1964) *Nature* **202**, 567.
9 KAPLAN H.S. & SMITHERS D.W. (1959) *Lancet* ii, 1.
10 Leading article (1970) *Lancet* ii, 1121.
11 NAZERIAN K., *et al* (1980) *Int J Cancer* **29**, 63.
12 PENN I. (1981) *Clin Exp Immunol* **146**, 459.
13 SCHWARTZ R.S. (1972) *Lancet* i, 1266.
14 SCHWARTZ R.S., *et al* (1966) *Ann NY Acad Sci* **129**, 804.
15 SLOAN G., *et al* (1977) *Transplant Proc* **9**, 1129.
16 SMITHERS D.W. (1967) *Br Med J* i, 263 & 337.
17 WONG-STAAL F., *et al* (1983) *Nature* **302**, 626.

Incidence of leukaemia and lymphoma [3]. These diseases are all rare. The leukaemia mortality [5] for 24 countries with a total population of about 582 million (20%) of the world's population) in 1960 was 33,682, a death rate of 5·8 per 100,000. The incidence of lymphomas is probably a little greater. Together, the two conditions represent only about 10% of all cancer deaths, and only 1·5% of deaths from all causes. The total for India is much lower, only 2·34% of all cancer cases being due to malignant lymphoma [2]. The age distribution is very uneven. In children, almost half of all cancer deaths are due to leukaemia, and one in nine to lymphoma. In the elderly the corresponding figures are 1 in 25 for each.

The incidence of mycosis fungoides has been estimated by Clendenning [1] at two new cases per million of the population per year in North America, and the Scandinavian [6] mycosis fungoides group report similar figures. In Scotland the incidence would appear to be somewhat less, with a figure of one new case per million of the population per year for the years 1972–77 [4].

REFERENCES

1 CLENDENNING W.E. (1977) *Bull du Cancer* **64**, 167.
2 DESAI P.B., *et al* (1965) *Cancer (NY)* **18**, 25.
3 GUNZ F.W. (1968) In *International Conference on Leukaemia-Lymphoma*. Ed. Zarafonetis C.J.D. Philadelphia, Lea & Febiger.
4 Scottish Dermatological Society Mycosis Fungoides Study Group (1983).
5 SEGI M. & KURIHARA M. (1964) In *Cancer Morbidity for Selected Sites in 24 Countries* (1960–61). Tohoku Sendai University School of Medicine, Sendai, Japan, Department of Public Health.
6 THOMSEN K. (1977) *Bull du Cancer* **64**, 287.

Cutaneous involvement in lymphomas and leukaemia. Skin lesions develop in the lymphomas either as a direct result of invasion of the skin by neoplastic cells or as a secondary 'non-specific' effect. Occasionally, in the latter group there is histological evidence of the disease at the site of the reaction, when it represents a true 'ide' reaction analogous to a tuberculide, but more often it is entirely non-specific.

Leukaemia or lymphoma cell infiltrates may be papular, nodular, tumorous or ulcerative, and are rare in the leukaemias and Hodgkin's disease, more common in the non-Hodgkin's lymphomas, and essential for the diagnosis in mycosis fungoides. Although the lesions are described as 'specific', it is often not possible to make a definite diagnosis from the histology of the skin lesions alone; a full blood count and lymph node biopsy and marrow examination are generally required. The lesions are not static, but may wax and wane with or without treatment.

'Non-specific' reactions are very varied, and include purpura, pigmentation, pruritus, prurigo, ichthyosiform atrophy, alopecia, exfoliative dermatitis (Fig. 47.1) and herpes zoster. Many other

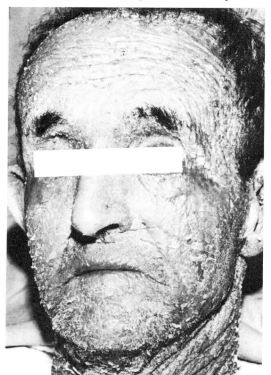

FIG. 47.1. Patient with exfoliative dermatitis and chronic lymphatic leukaemia.

diosensitive and will fade with a dose of 2–3 Gy. It is however better to give about 20 Gy in fractionated doses at 60–120 kV in an attempt to eradicate the disease. Recurrences may occur and are treated similarly.

In the large cell forms, treatment must be related to the degree of systemic involvement and will usually require polychemotherapy.

REFERENCES

1 Braun-Falco O., *et al* (1981) *Clin Exp Dermatol* **6**, 89.
2 Graham Brown R.A.C. & Calnan C.D. (1981) *Clin Exp Dermatol* **6**, 439.
3 Long J.C., *et al* (1976) *Cancer* **38**, 1282.
4 Saxe N., *et al* (1977) *J Cutan Pathol* **4**, 111.
5 Shelley W.B., *et al* (1981) *Arch Dermatol* **117**, 500.

AFRICAN LYMPHOMA
SYN. BURKITT'S TUMOUR; CENTRAL AFRICAN LYMPHOMA; LYMPHOBLASTIC LYMPHOMA

Although the skin is rarely involved [10], this disease makes such an important contribution to our knowledge of lymphomas in general that a short account of it is included here. It is characterized by tumours, especially in the jaws, ovaries and coeliac lymph nodes, and has a distinctive geographical distribution.

Aetiology. Davis [7] first noted the high incidence of malignant tumours of the reticulo-endothelial system in African children, and Burkitt [2] observed the clinical and geographical aspects of this tumour. It was soon realized that the distribution depended largely on temperature and humidity and that an infective agent might be incriminated, possibly with an insect vector [5]. The disease is commonest in childhood, and jaw involvement is most frequent in young children, occurring in 100% of African cases below the age of 3, and falling off thereafter [6]. The infective agent is thought to be the Epstein–Barr virus [8], and most persons exposed to it develop immunity. The disease occurs mainly in Africa, though it also has a high incidence in New Guinea [1] and has been reported from elsewhere. Epstein–Barr virus (EBV) is also the cause of infectous mononucleosis. It is unlikely that the EBV can produce Burkitt's lymphoma without some other factor, and it has been suggested that previous sustained lymphoreticular stimulation is needed, and that this may be the result of endemic malaria [4].

An important observation in Burkitt's lymphoma is the frequent translocation of the long arms of chromosomes 8, 14 and 22 [2]. There is currently great interest in the exact chromosomal location of cellular oncogenes such as c-myc found in a variety of human tumours [11]. This translocation appears in some Burkitt's cell lines to transpose c-myc to chromosome 14.

Histology. This is characteristic. Sheets of small, darkly staining round cells occupy the bulk of the soft tumour masses, which often contain areas of haemorrhage and necrosis. There are many clear spaces which usually contain one or more pale cells with a vesicular nucleus and large nucleoli. These give a 'water pot' or 'starry sky' appearance. The cells are small non-cleaved follicular centre cells [9]. It is, however, highly malignant.

Clinical characteristics. The condition is responsible for 50% of malignant tumours of African children under the age of 15 in Uganda, and in half the cases the jaw bones are involved. It is often bilateral and affects both maxillae and mandibles. Other organs frequently involved are the ovaries, kidneys and adrenals, again often bilaterally. The coeliac lymph nodes, liver and retroperitoneal tissues are often involved, and the stomach, intestines, testes and spleen may be affected also. The lungs, long bones and brain are usually spared, and involvement of lymph nodes other than coeliac is exceptional. There is usually no leukaemic process and no abnormalities of blood or urine. The tumours develop with great rapidity.

Prognosis and treatment. Patients have recovered after surprisingly small doses of cytotoxic drugs [3], suggesting that immunity to the tumour may develop and aid in its elimination.

REFERENCES

1 Booth K., *et al* (1967) *Br J Cancer* **21**, 687.
2 Burkitt D.P. (1958) *Br J Surg* **46**, 218.
3 Burkitt D.P. (1967) In *Conference on the Chemotherapy of Burkitt's Tumours*. Eds. Burshanel J. & Burkitt D.P. Berlin and New York, Springer–Verlag, Heidelberg.
4 Burkitt D.P. (1969) *J Natl Cancer Inst* **42**, 19.
5 Burkitt D.P. & Davies J.N.P. (1961) *Med Press* **245**, 367.
6 Burkitt D.P. & Wright D. (1966) *Br Med J* i, 569.
7 Davies J.N.P. (1948) *E Afr Med J* **25**, 1127.
8 Epstein M.A., *et al* (1967) *Br Med J* ii, 290.
9 Lukes R.J. & Collins R.D. (1975) *Br J Cancer* **31** (Suppl. II), 1.
10 Rogge T. (1975) *Hautarzt* **26**, 379.
11 Rowley J.D. (1983) *Nature* **301**, 200.
12 Zech L., *et al* (1976) *Int J Cancer* **17**, 47.

T-CELL LYMPHOMAS

Introduction. Recent immunological studies have further subdivided the T-lymphocyte subset into cells with a 'helper' function and those with cytotoxic and/or suppressor functions. The former are important in 'help' to B lymphocytes in antibody production while suppressor cells act as 'control' cells in terminating or reducing such interactions. The full extent of this helper/suppressor network and the feedback controls involved is not yet completely understood, but the recent availability of monoclonal antibodies raised against these helper and suppressor subsets has advanced our knowledge of the distribution of cells with these membrane markers in disease states. Whether or not the functional capacity associated with these markers is still present in pathological states remains to be fully established.

There has been recent recognition that not all malignant T-cell infiltrates of the skin are of the mycosis fungoides type. Newly recognized and described entities include adult T-cell leukaemia in the south islands of Japan [2], a rapidly progressive and fatal type of T-cell leukaemia with very frequent cutaneous involvement. The recent reports of the presence of the human T-cell leukaemia virus I (HTLV-I) in these patients suggests aetiological features in common with the other T-cell disorders in which HTLV has been identified (p. 1729).

A second recently recognized T-cell lymphoma with frequent cutaneous involvement is the Pinkus tumour [1, 3]. These lymphomas are composed of cells with large, grossly multilobular nuclei, having a 'clover leaf' pattern. In three of the four first reported cases massive cutaneous involvement was reported and recent membrane marker studies suggest that the cells have the markers of immature cortical thymocytes.

It has been suggested recently that the Pinkus tumour and Crosti's lymphoma (p. 1752) are the same entity. Further evidence is needed to confirm this suggestion.

REFERENCES

1 PINKUS G.S., *et al* (1979) *Am J Clin Pathol* **72**, 540.
2 SHAMOTO M., *et al* (1981) *Cancer* **47**, 1804.
3 VAN DER PUTTE S.C.J., *et al* (1982) *Br J Dermatol* **107**, 293.

MYCOSIS FUNGOIDES

Mycosis fungoides (MF) is a condition characterized by the infiltration of the skin with plaques and nodules composed of T lymphocytes. Marker studies have indicated that the majority of these cells have the membrane marker characteristics of the T helper subset—cells committed to helping B lymphocytes in immunoglobulin production and other functions. The characteristic slow evolution of MF over many years has given rise to two schools of thought concerning its classification. The first regards it *ab initio* as a T-cell malignancy and cites as evidence work suggesting monoclonality of the cells comprising separate lesions in three patients with untreated nodular disease [1]. This observation has not been confirmed and a more recent study reports polyclonality among the cells from patients with early multiple plaque lesions [4]. The second view is that initially MF is a reactive process, perhaps of chronic antigen stimulation [3] and that in only a proportion of cases does true malignancy supervene [2]. This pattern of events would correlate rather better with the observed variable rate of progression of the disease in individual patients.

REFERENCES

1 EDELSON R.L., *et al* (1979) *J Invest Dermatol* **73**, 548.
2 MACKIE R.M. (1981) *Lancet* **ii**, 283.
3 TAN R.S.-H., *et al* (1974) *Bri J Dermatol* **91**, 607.
4 WHANG PENG J., *et al* (1982) *Cancer* **50**, 1539.

Historical note. Mycosis fungoides has attracted the attention and imagination of dermatologists for nearly two centuries. The classic plaque form of MF was first described by Alibert [1] in 1806 and clinical progression through patch, plaque and tumour stages was described by Bazin in 1870 [2]. The so-called *d'emblée* variant was first reported by Vidal and Brocq in 1885 [8] and in 1892 the concept of erythrodermic MF was first clinically described by Besnier and Hallopeau [3]. Half a century later, in 1938, Sézary and Bouvrain [7] described the clinical features of what is now known as the Sézary syndrome.

Bringing history up to the present day, the careful and painstaking observation and recording of Samman [6] over several decades have given considerable insight into the natural history of MF. The work of Lutzner [5] in first describing the mycosis cell, and of Edelson [4] in establishing the T-lymphocyte lineage of this cell are also important landmarks in our understanding of this disease.

REFERENCES

1 ALIBERT J.L.M. (1806) *Tableau du Plan Fongoide. Description des Maladies de la peau observées à L'Hôpital St Louis.* Paris, Barrois l'Aîné et Fils, p. 157.

2 BAZIN P.A.E. (1870) *Leçons Sur Le Traitement des Maladies Chroniques.* Paris, Adrian De La Haye, p. 425.
3 BESNIER E. & HALLOPEAU H. (1892) *Ann Dermatol Syphiligr (Paris)* 3, 987.
4 EDELSON R.L., *et al* (1973) *J Invest Dermatol* 61, 82.
5 LUTZNER M.A., *et al* (1971) *Arch Dermatol* 103, 375.
6 SAMMAN P.D. (1976) *Clin Exp Dermatol* 1, 197.
7 SÉZARY A. & BOUVRAIN Y. (1938) *Bull Soc Fr Dermatol Syphiligr* 45, 254.
8 VIDAL E. & BROCQ L. (1885) *Fr Med* 2, 946, 967, 969, 983, 993, 1005, 1019.

Aetiology. This is at present not known. If initially the disease is one of antigen persistence, the antigen [3] remains to be identified. The recent work on human T-cell leukaemia viruses (HTLV) [1, 9], a C type retrovirus, requires extension to patients with earlier stages of classic MF, but preliminary results would not suggest that HTLV-1 is identifiable in the lesions of patients so far studied with early classic plaque stage MF [9]. Epidemiological observations from North America suggest that MF patients have a high incidence of allergies and of fungal and viral infections compared with controls, and that many of them are employed in petrochemical, textile, metal and machine industries. This observation covers a wide range of possible aetiological factors and requires both confirmation and more detailed study [2].

Histology. The histological picture of fully developed MF is that of a dense lymphocytic infiltrate which occupies the papillary dermis and extends up into the epidermis (Fig. 47.3). This feature of apparent affinity of these T lymphocytes for the epidermis is known as 'epidermotropism'. Lymphocytic cells may invade the epidermis either singly or in a group—these forming Pautrier microabscesses (Figs 47.4 & 47.5). The basal layer of the epidermis may be effaced, resulting in a somewhat lichenoid picture, and there is no area of normal papillary dermis (Grenz zone) between epidermis and dermal infiltrate. This is the so-called T-zone pattern of a lymphocytic infiltrate. As the disease progresses and lesions change from plaques to nodules to ulcerated tumours there is a tendency for the epidermotropic quality of the infiltrate to become less marked.

The early stages of MF, particularly the stage at which the patient has only one or two mildly pruritic small plaques, do not usually have such a characteristic histological pattern. Once again, however, the bulk of the infiltrate is gathered in the papillary dermis (Fig. 47.6), and occasional lymphocytes will be seen within the epidermis. There is a positive absence of spongiosis around the epidermal keratinocytes adjacent to these lymphocytes, and this helps

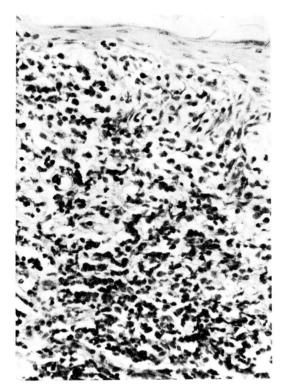

FIG. 47.3. Photomicrograph of mycosis fungoides showing a dense lymphocytic infiltrate occupying the upper zone of the dermis and invading the epidermis forming a Pautrier microabscess. Note the complete effacement of the basal of layer of the epidermis and the lack of any Grenz zone.

in the differentiation from a dermatitis reaction. There are frequently large numbers of lymphocytes adjacent to the basal layer in the papillary dermis, and they may give the appearance of a linear band. Although a few eosinophils may be admixed with these lymphocytes, large numbers are not commonly seen in MF and if present suggest alternative diagnoses such as a persistent insect bite or lymphomatoid drug reaction.

At higher power the lymphocytes will be seen to have heavily stained nuclei with a characteristic convoluted appearance. These are the so-called MF or Lutzner cells [4] (Fig. 47.5) and they can be visualized very much more clearly if the sections are cut at 1 µm after embedding the tissue in plastic or resin. This 'thin section' technique is of great value in examining nuclear detail and is particularly useful in the lymphomas.

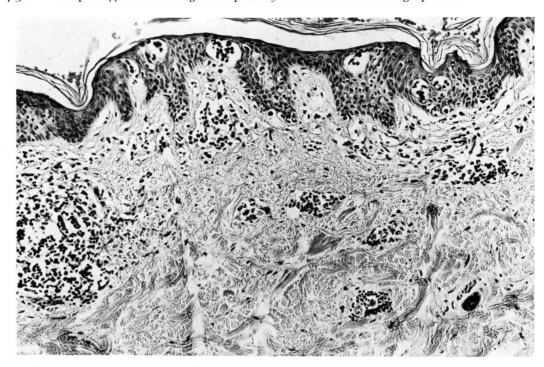

FIG. 47.4. Photomicrograph of early mycosis fungoides showing striking Pautrier microabscesses scattered at intervals in the epidermis.

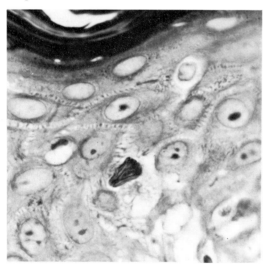

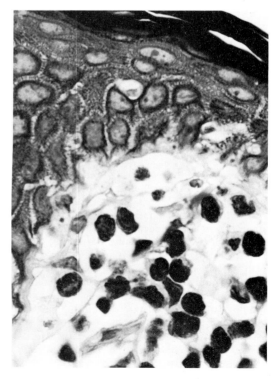

FIG. 47.5. High power thin section of mycosis fungoides to show one atypical lymphoid cell with a cerebriform nucleus situated in the mid-epidermal area.

FIG. 47.6. High power thin section (1 μm) of mycosis fungoides to show a cluster of lymphoid cells with atypical cerebriform nuclei situated in the papillary dermal area.

Surface membrane marker studies. Monoclonal antibodies raised against T-cell subsets and other cell types such as the epidermal Langerhans cells have been used extensively as a research tool in the past 3 years and their use is now a routine procedure in some larger centres. Frozen sections are cut from the lesion and the immunofluorescence or immunoperoxidase technique utilized. These methods have clearly demonstrated that the bulk of the lymphocytes in the majority of MF infiltrates have the surface markers of T helper lymphocytes and that lymphocytes with the T suppressor/cytotoxic phenotype are relatively few in number and tend to be distributed around the periphery of the lesions [8].

Several workers have shown both by immunological and ultrastructural techniques that Langerhans cells are present in these infiltrates in increased numbers, and that they are frequently in contact with T helper lymphocytes [5]. The significance of these observations is not yet clear but lends some support to an aetiological theory suggesting initial abnormalities of antigen presentation as at present the Langerhans cell is considered to be the epidermal cell responsible for this function.

Other diagnostic techniques. Two other aids to early diagnosis which are at present available only in specialized centres are *DNA cytophotometry* and measurement of the *nuclear contour index (NCI)*. The former depends on the fact that malignant cells have a hypertetraploid DNA content, whereas reactive cells will not have such a marked increase of nuclear DNA [7]. Quantification of the nuclear contour index is a method of measuring the degree of nuclear indentation. The perimeter of the nucleus is measured and related to the nuclear area. Once again, early results suggest that the method does have value in discriminating between reactive and malignant cells [6]. Problems relating to cell sampling exist and availability of the expensive and sophisticated technology required for DNA cytophotometry is limited.

Pathological differential diagnosis. The differential diagnosis of early MF from conditions such as contact dermatitis, arthropod bites and lymphomatous drug eruptions can be difficult and good clinico-pathological liaison is essential. In general, contact dermatitis reactions will show a greater degree of spongiosis, reactions to arthropod bites tend to show a higher proportion of eosinophils, and the disposition of the infiltrate in lymphomatous drug reactions will be perivascular rather than epidermotropic. In a proportion of cases, however, the diagnosis is suspected on clinical grounds but cannot confidently be made with certainty on histological examination. In these cases sequential biopsies at 3–6 month intervals will clarify the nature of the disease process. Until curative rather than palliative therapy is available, it is as well to remember the dictum of Pinkus—'Do not say 'Can I diagnose MF?'—rather say 'Must I diagnose MF?' "

REFERENCES

1 GALLO R. & WONG-STAAL F. (1982) *Blood* **60**, 545.
2 GREENE M.H., *et al* (1979) *Cancer Treatment Rep* **63**, 597.
3 HASHIMOTO K. & IWAHARA K. (1983) *Am J Dermatopathol* **5**, 29.
4 LUTZNER M.A. (1973) *Am J Clin Pathol* **59**, 887.
5 MACKIE R.M. & TURBITT M.L. (1982) *Br J Dermatol* **106**, 379.
6 MEIJER C., *et al* (1980) *Cancer* **45**, 2864.
7 VAN VLOTEN W.A., *et al* (1974) *Br J Dermatol* **91**, 365.
8 WILLEMZE R., *et al* (1983) *J Invest Dermatol* **80**, 60.
9 WONG-STAAL F., *et al* (1983) *Nature* **302**, 626.

Pathological diagnosis of extracutaneous spread. The normal pattern of extracutaneous spread in MF is via lymph nodes to other organs. Biopsy of palpable lymph nodes may yield clear evidence of MF cells replacing and effacing the normal nodal architecture, or, if in the earlier stages of disease, a pattern described as *dermatopathic lymphadenopathy*. This term describes enlargement of the paracortical area of the lymph node due to the presence of large numbers of macrophages and pale-staining cells of the reticulum series. Within the macrophages are aggregates both of melanin and lipid material, giving rise to the older term 'lipomelanic reticulosis' which was used for this pattern. Immunological analysis of these cells shows large numbers of Ia (immune-associated) antigen bearing dendritic cells in this infiltrate. These cells are thought to be involved in regulation of T-lymphocyte function [1, 2].

REFERENCES

1 LAMPERT I.A., *et al* (1980) *J Pathol* **131**, 145.
2 BURKE J.S. & COLBY T.V. (1981) *Am J Surg Pathol* **5**, 343.

'Staging systems' and clinical features. There is as yet no universal agreement concerning staging systems for use in MF. This is in contrast to other lymphomas where clear staging criteria exist. The TNM classification and the staging system

TABLE 47.2.   TNM classification of mycosis fungoides

Cutaneous involvement (T)
T_0: Lesions clinically and/or histologically suspicious but not diagnostic
T_1: Plaques involving less than 10% of skin
T_2: Plaques involving more than 10% of skin
T_3: Tumours present
T_4: Erythroderma

Lymph nodes (N)
N_0: Clinically and pathologically normal
N_1: Palpable. Pathologically not involved
N_2: Clinically non-palpable, pathologically MF
N_3: Clinically enlarged, pathologically MF

Viscera (M)
M_0: No visceral spread
M_1: Visceral spread present

Peripheral blood (B)
B_0 No atypical circulating cells
B_1: Atypical circulating cells present

TABLE 47.3.   A staging system for mycosis fungoides related to TNM classification

	T	N	M
IA	T_1	N_0	o
IB	T_2	N_0	o
IIA	T_{1-2}	N_1	o
IIB	T_3	N_{0-1}	o
III	T_4	N_{0-1}	o
IVA	T_{1-4}	N_{2-3}	o
IVB	T_{1-4}	N_{0-3}	M+

suggested by the North American MF Cooperative Group [1] is given in Tables 47.2 and 47.3. Many workers, however, prefer to give a clinical description of the lesions.

The usual progression of the disease is from small, limited, plaque stage disease, to large plaques, to nodules, ulcerated tumours and, in some cases, disseminated disease. The proportion of patients who reach end-stage disseminated disease appears to be variable in different parts of the world. In North America a high proportion of patients in three large series [2, 3, 4] were found on careful examination of material from peripheral blood and lymph nodes to have evidence of involvement outside the skin. This has not in general been the European experience [5], and it remains to be seen whether or not this reflects true differences in disease virulence, changes in the disease pattern secondary to cytotoxic therapy which is more commonly used in North America, or is a reflection of greater transatlantic thoroughness in seeking out extracutaneous involvement.

REFERENCES

1 BUNN P.A. & LAMBERG S.I. (1979) *Cancer Treatment Rep* **63**, 725.
2 BUNN P.A., *et al* (1980) *Ann Intern Med* **93**, 223.
3 EPSTEIN E.H., *et al* (1972) *Medicine (Baltimore)* **15**, 61.
4 FUKS Z.Y., *et al* (1973) *Cancer* **32**, 1385.
5 HAMMINGA L., *et al* (1982) *Br J Dermatol* **107**, 145.

Clinical features

Plaque stage MF. This develops insidiously on covered sites (Fig. 47.7), frequently first affecting the buttocks. The areas may be pruritic before definitive plaques are visible. These are oval or circular, finely scaling and erythematous. Some degree of epidermal atrophy is common. They may persist and slowly enlarge, or involute spontaneously in the early stages of the disease. Some plaques may only partially involute, leaving striking circinate lesions which may merge to give polycyclic patterns on the skin (Fig. 47.8).

Over a very variable period of time these lesions may slowly expand to form large plaques covering over 10% of the body surface (Fig. 47.9). Pruritus is common and no site is spared although the trunk is the commonest site. Rarely the clinical features of the lesions may be atypical and the initial appearance has been reported in individual cases as being acneiform [4], bullous [5], papillomatous [3], hypopigmented [1] and hyperkeratotic [6]. In general, however, the clinical appearance of the lesions is strongly suggestive of the diagnosis, even at a time when the definitive histological picture has not yet developed.

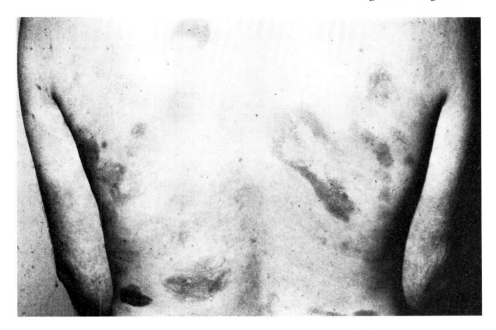

FIG. 47.7. Early mycosis fungoides. Clinical illustration of well-defined plaques on the back.

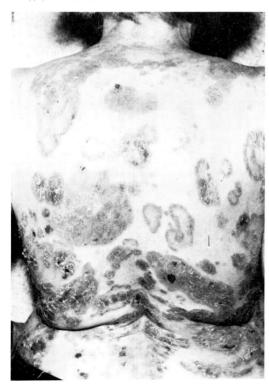

FIG. 47.8. Later plaque stage mycosis fungoides. In this patient approximately 30% of the cutaneous surface is replaced by MF plaque.

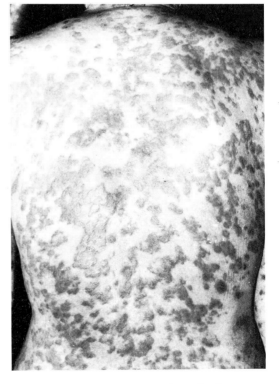

FIG. 47.9. Advanced stage mycosis fungoides showing gross replacement of epidermal surface with multiple plaques, some of which are merging into the early nodular stage of MF.

Many patients never progress beyond plaque stage MF, but a number develop indurated *nodules* and *ulceration* on their plaques (Figs 47.10 and 47.11). Such lesions may be painful and secondary infection is common.

A *tumeur d'emblée* form of MF in which patients rapidly developed large nodules without the prior presence of plaques has been described. Recent work on surface markers suggests that some of these lesions may be B-cell lymphomas rather than true MF.

The *erythrodermic* presentation of MF is unusual and current studies may result in its reclassification to another variant of T-cell lymphoma. Patients develop rapid-onset erythroderma and tend to progress to lymphadenopathy and peripheral blood involvement. This pattern may be related more closely to T-cell leukaemia than to true MF.

Poikilodermatous MF. A small proportion of MF patients develop clinical lesions characterized by widespread poikiloderma rather than frank plaques and nodules. The trunk is usually involved and the

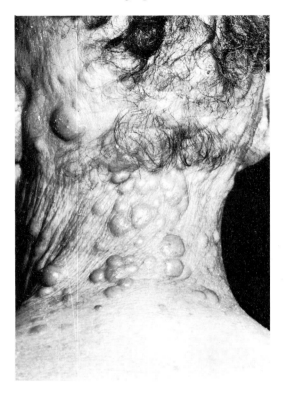

FIG. 47.10. Nodular state MF showing development of nodules on the scalp and neck. This picture has evolved in a patient who 10 years previously had follicular mucinosis involving the head and neck area.

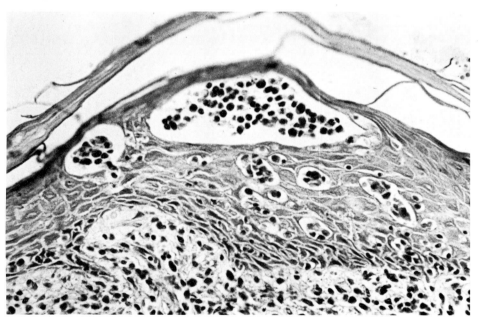

FIG. 47.11. Histopathology of patient illustrated in Fig. 47.10. Gross epidermotropism and large Pautrier abscesses are clearly seen in the epidermis.

breasts and buttocks may be particularly severely affected (Fig. 47.12). Alternating increase and decrease of pigmentation is seen and striking atrophy may be present. This clinical variant of MF develops subsequent to pre-reticulotic poikiloderma. A burning sensation rather than itch may be the most demanding symptom.

Recent studies from the American MF Cooperative Group suggest that the clinical variety of MF does not carry prognostic significance once correction is made for the TNM stage of the disease [2]. This contrasts with previous reports that both erythrodermic and poikilodermatous MF carry different prognoses.

Pruritus is the usual symptom, irrespective of the type of MF. This may be initially mild and easily controlled but frequently becomes very severe and demanding in more long-standing disease. Some patients experience frank pain and burning, but this is unusual. In advanced systematized disease, fever, lassitude and weight loss are all common and distressing symptoms.

REFERENCES

1 BREATHNACH S.M., *et al* (1982) *Br J Dermatol* **106**, 643.
2 GREENE S.B., *et al* (1981) *Cancer* **47**, 2671.
3 KANITAKIS C. & TSOITIS G. (1977) *Dermatologica* **155**, 268.
4 PIPER H.G. (1960) *Hautarzt* **11**, 462.
5 ROENIGK H.H. JR & CASTROVINCI A.J. (1971) *Arch Dermatol* **104**, 402.
6 STASKO T. (1982) *J Am Acad Dermatol* **7**, 792.

Follicular mucinosis (alopecia mucinosa) [1, 2, 3]. A boggy cutaneous plaque with histological evidence of mucinous degeneration of hair follicles, associated in some cases with MF (see also p. 2297).

There appear to be two distinct forms of follicular mucinosis, one associated with MF and an entirely separate form with no such disease association. MF-associated follicular mucinosis may develop on any site including the face and scalp, and may precede frank MF by many years. Boggy swellings develop and a sticky discharge may be seen from hair follicles (Fig. 47.13). Significant hair loss may be present, and the histological picture is that of degeneration of the hair follicle with striking

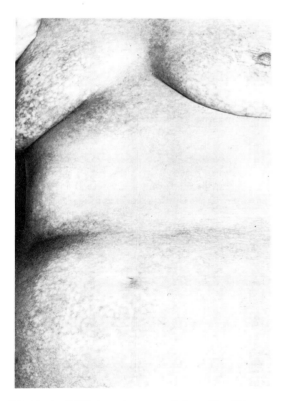

FIG. 47.12. Poikilodermatous mycosis fungoides. This patient has gross poikiloderma involving mainly the breast, abdomen and buttock area.

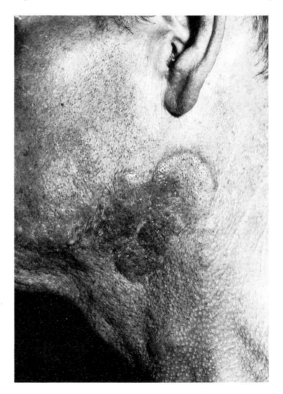

FIG. 47.13. Follicular mucinosis. This patient has boggy plaques on the cheeks and neck.

deposits of mucin seen on Alcian blue stains (Fig. 47.14).

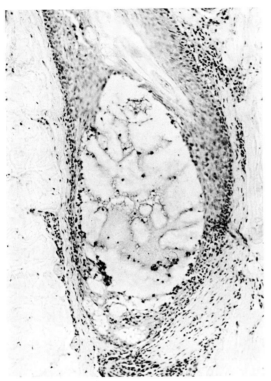

FIG. 47.14. Pathology of lesions depicted in 47.13. The degeneration of the hair bulb area is clearly shown. Specific stains for mucin in this area are strongly positive.

REFERENCES

1 BINNICK A.N., *et al* (1978) *Arch Dermatol* 114, 791.
2 COSKEY R.J. & MEHREGAN A.H. (1970) *Arch Dermatol* 102, 193.
3 EMMERSON R.W. (1969) *Br J Dermatol* 81, 395.

Differential diagnosis. In the early stages of plaque MF the clinical differential diagnosis may include such diverse conditions as allergic contact dermatitis and fungal infection. Any patient with persistent pruritic plaques, particularly on covered skin, should have a biopsy and histological confirmation of the disease. If this shows a significant degree of spongiosis, a dermatitis reaction should be considered. Fungal infection can be easily excluded by the clinical use of Wood's light, direct and indirect mycological examination, and staining of the biopsy with PAS stain to reveal fungal hyphae. The benign plaque dermatoses and *non*-prereticulotic poikilodermas are discussed further on p. 1747.

Staging procedures [1]. All patients with MF should have a full clinical examination, skin biopsy and examination of the peripheral blood for atypical mononuclear cells. Routine biochemical investigation and chest X-ray should be performed. Enlarged lymph nodes should be biopsied, but the practice of 'blind' lymph node biopsy of non-enlarged nodes is of little benefit. Lymphangiography is likewise of doubtful value [2, 3]. Non-invasive techniques such as liver and spleen ultrasound isotope scans and CAT scans may be of value in patients in whom extracutaneous disease is suspected. Sternal marrow aspiration will usually yield negative results. Cytogenetic analysis and electron microscopy will be done at more specialized centres.

REFERENCES

1 BUNN P.A., *et al* (1980) *Ann Intern Med* 93, 223.
2 CASTELLINO R.A., *et al* (1979) *Cancer Treatment Rep* 63, 581.
3 FUKS Z.Y., *et al* (1974) *Cancer* 34, 106.

Immunological assessment. A very large number of studies in the past decade have attempted to delineate the immunological abnormalities, if any, present in patients with early MF and to relate these to aetiology, prognosis or response to therapy. The great majority shows no significant degree of immunosuppression in patients who have plaque MF who have not received immunosuppressive therapy. Quantification of T and B lymphocytes in the peripheral blood have in general shown no consistent and confirmed increase or decrease of either lymphocyte subset. Several studies show elevation of serum IgE levels in around 20% of MF patients and elevated IgA levels in a smaller percentage. Serum levels of other immunoglobulins are unchanged. Reports of defects in mononuclear cell chemotaxis have not as yet been confirmed and it is difficult to attribute confidently some of the other minor reported immunological abnormalities to the disease process rather than to its therapy. More recent studies using monoclonal antibodies to T helper and suppressor subsets have likewise shown no consistent abnormality on examination of the peripheral blood lymphocytes in contrast to the cutaneous findings. This is also in contrast with the Sézary syndrome (p. 1748) in which there is a proliferation of T helper lymphocytes in the peripheral blood.

Treatment. In general, therapy is aimed at palliation and symptom relief rather than a more aggressive approach aimed at cure with total eradication of all abnormal cells. A few North American studies have recently adopted the latter approach to management and it will be of interest to compare disease-free interval and survival time in this group with patients treated by more conservative regimes.

In the early plaque stage MF symptomatic relief may be achieved by the use of either topical corticosteroids or UVB. At this stage in the disease the condition may remit spontaneously and very small quantities of a moderately potent steroid may be adequate. In more advanced plaque stage MF more potent steroids may be required. If this is not adequate, either PUVA or topical nitrogen mustard should be considered.

Photochemotherapy (PUVA). The great majority of studies using PUVA for control of symptoms in MF report excellent symptomatic and clinical response [1, 3]. Histological monitoring of the disease does show, however, that some atypical T lymphocytes persist in the deeper parts of the dermis [2], indicating that maintenance therapy is required if the lesions are not to recur. MF lesions tend to persist or develop in protected or 'sanctuary' sites—the goggle area around the eyes, the natal cleft and

genital regions. Relatively low doses of only 20 J/cm² may be adequate for clearance and only 2–4 J/cm²/week for maintenance (Figs 47.3 & 47.15) illustrates just how striking this depletion in cell numbers may be.

REFERENCES

1 GILCHREST B.A., *et al* (1976) *Cancer* **38**, 683.
2 MACKIE R.M., *et al* (1980) *Clin Exp Dermatol* **5**, 405.
3 ROENIGK H.H. (1977) *Arch Dermatol* **113**, 1047.

Topical nitrogen mustard (mechlorethamine). The use of topical nitrogen mustard has been pioneered by Van Scott and colleagues [3] who report good results in patients treated for many years. The drug is dissolved in water and painted over the entire body surface once or twice weekly. Sensitization [4] is a problem in some cases but desensitization regimes can overcome this. There are, however, a few recent reports of squamous carcinoma developing on nitrogen mustard-treated skin [2] on covered body sites [1]. Maintenance treatment is required.

REFERENCES

1 DU VIVIER A., *et al* (1978) *Br J Dermatol* **99**, 61.
2 KRAVITZ D.A. & MCDONALD C.J. (1978) *Acta Derm Venereol (Stockh)* **58**, 421.

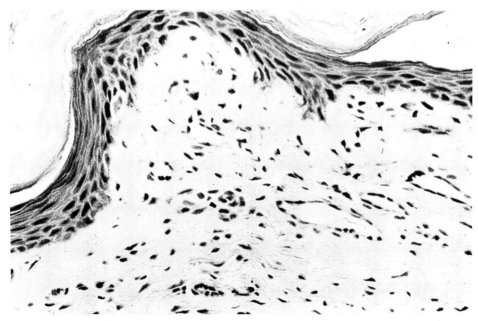

FIG. 47.15. Photomicrograph of biopsy from same area in patient illustrated in 47.3 6 weeks after commencing PUVA therapy. Note complete disappearance of lymphoid cells from the epidermis but the persistence of a few scattered atypical lymphoid cells in the dermis. Note hyperkeratosis which normally accompanies PUVA therapy.

3 VAN SCOTT E.J. & KALMANSON J.D. (1973) *Cancer* 32, 18.
4 VONDERHEID E.C., *et al* (1979) *Cancer Treatment Rep* 63, 681.

Electron beam therapy. In later stage disease the use of electron beam therapy or electrons from a strontium source also gives good symptomatic relief. The usual dose administered to the total body over a period of 4–6 weeks is 20–30 Gy. Temporary loss of hair and nails may occur and at higher doses some permanent telangiectasia may develop [1, 3]. Despite these problems, good long-term remissions lasting years rather than months may be achieved [4]. Early reports from the Stanford group [2] suggesting cure rather than palliation of MF using a higher radiation dose of 35 Gy have not been confirmed.

REFERENCES

1 HAMMINGA B., *et al* (1982) *Arch Dermatol* 118, 150.
2 HOPPE R.T., *et al* (1979) *Cancer Treatment Rep* 63, 625.
3 PRICE N.M. (1978) *Arch Dermatol* 114, 63.
4 SPITTLE M.F. (1979) *Cancer Treatment Rep* 63, 639.

Other forms of radiotherapy [1]. Conventional X-rays are of value in two situations in MF. The first is in the use of low dose superficial X-rays in patients with extensive large plaque disease in a centre where neither electron beam nor PUVA is available. Low doses using 55 kV X-rays may be adequate. The second situation in which X-rays are of value is in tumour doses to individual nodular lesions.

REFERENCE

1 LE BOURGEOIS J.O., *et al* (1979) *Bull du Cancer* 64, 313.

Combination therapy. It must be remembered that combination therapy is frequently useful in the management of the MF patient [1]. Regimes such as treating plaques with PUVA and giving additional X-ray therapy to the few tumours present or using PUVA and topical steroids alternately may be of value. Treatment should always be carefully tailored to the individual's needs and symptoms with regular and careful review, preferably accompanied by total body photography to chart disease spread, and biopsy at regular intervals.

REFERENCE

1 DU VIVIER A. & VOLLUM D.I. (1980) *Br J Dermatol* 102, 319.

Management of extracutaneous MF. The treatment of MF once there is histological evidence of nodal involvement or spread to other organs is unsatisfactory. Many chemotherapeutic regimes including such cytotoxic combinations as CHOP, COP, VP16 and bleomycin have been used, but results are in general very disappointing [1, 4]. A common course of events is for the patient to develop severe secondary immunosuppression following such chemotherapy and then to contract a fatal opportunistic infection. There are, however, early reports of successful use of the retinoids in extracutaneous MF and the new specific anti-T-cell drug deoxycoformycin offers hope for this group of patients. This drug acts by selectively inhibiting the enzyme adenosine deaminase which is present in large quantities in rapidly dividing T cells [2, 5]. The use of murine monoclonal antibodies against T lymphocytes is at present at the experimental stage, but development of antibodies to murine material is a limiting factor [3].

REFERENCES

1 GROZEE P.N., *et al* (1979) *Cancer Treatment Rep* 63, 647.
2 KUFE D., *et al* (1980) *Proc Am Assoc Cancer Res* 21, 328.
3 MILLER R.A. & LEVY R. (1981) *Lancet* ii, 226.
4 MOLIN L., *et al* (1980) *Acta Derm Venereol (Stockh)* 60, 542.
5 SCHNEIDER R., *et al* (1980) *Proc Am Assoc Cancer Res* 21, 185.

Prognosis. The prognosis for MF depends on accurate staging. Patients with limited plaque stage MF and no evidence of disseminated disease may live for many years with only minor discomfort and eventually die of other causes. Patients with widespread cutaneous disease have a poorer prognosis and may die of MF within 2–3 years of presentation [2]. For patients with extracutaneous disease the outlook is poor and few survive more than a few months irrespective of therapy [1].

Two groups have recently reported a high incidence of second malignancies in MF patients and also of malignancies, mainly lymphomas and leukaemias, in their relatives [3]. These observations suggest a general defect predisposing to malignant change in more than one cell type.

REFERENCES

1 BUNN P.A., *et al* (1979) *Cancer Treatment Rep* 63, 713.
2 EPSTEIN E.H., *et al* (1972) *Medicine (Baltimore)* 15, 61.
3 GREENE M.H., *et al* (1982) *Cancer* 49, 737.

'PREMYCOTIC' ERUPTIONS

The terminology surrounding these eruptions is antiquated and confusing. Two clinical presentations are included—plaques and poikiloderma—and the rationale for calling them 'premycotic' is that if followed sequentially over a period of years a proportion have been observed to progress to frank MF. As there is at present no way of differentiating this group prior to progression or, more important, offering preventive or curative therapy at this stage, the value to the patient of such a diagnosis is questionable.

The second problem that has arisen in the area of so-called 'premycotic' eruptions is the confusion between totally benign chronic dermatoses with persistent plaques and in the poikilodermatous area between 'pre-reticulotic' poikiloderma and poikiloderma totally unrelated to MF found in association with lupus erythematosus, dermatomyositis and drug eruptions.

It is recommended that the use of the term 'parapsoriasis' be discontinued. The early, possibly plaque stage of MF when the histology is not (yet) confirmatory can be designated ?MF stage T_0. This eliminates the need for the term 'parapsoriasis en plaque'. The term 'parapsoriasis variegata', previously used to describe pre-reticulotic poikiloderma, can also be abandoned. In practice patients with poikiloderma who do not have lupus erythematosus, dermatomyositis or a drug eruption generally have a histological picture diagnostic of MF and should be labelled poikilodermatous MF—MF T_1 or stage IA. The term 'poikiloderma atrophicans vasculare' is also better abandoned as the name can be used to describe both MF associated poikiloderma and non-MF associated poikiloderma.

BENIGN PLAQUE DERMATOSES WITH NO ASSOCIATION WITH SUBSEQUENT DEVELOPMENT OF MF

Logically this group of disorders should be included in the section devoted to dermatitis (p. 388), but a short section is included here to clarify terminology. The term recommended by Samman for this group of disorders is *persistent superficial dermatitis*. This should therefore render obsolete the terms 'chronic superficial dermatitis', 'digitate dermatosis' and 'xanthoerythroderma perstans'.

The condition is characterized by the presence of multiple superficial plaques on the trunk and limbs. They are usually asymptomatic and may be red or yellowish in colour and exhibit fine superficial scaling. The cause is unknown. Mild atrophy may develop (Fig. 47.16) and some are elongated and 'digitate' in shape. The histological picture is of a mild dermatitis with epidermal spongiosis, mild dermal oedema, and a sparse lymphoid infiltrate. There is no gross epidermotropism and Pautrier abscesses are not seen. This picture may persist unchanged for many years and does not progress to MF.

If therapy is required, ultraviolet light (UVB) and simple emollients may be of benefit.

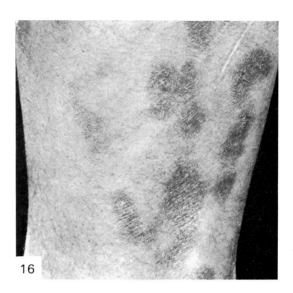

16

FIG. 47.16. Lesion of persistent superficial dermatitis demonstrating atrophy and fine scaling. This picture may persist unchanged for many years.

PAGETOID RETICULOSIS
(WORINGER–KOLOPP DISEASE; EPIDERMOTROPIC LYMPHOBLASTOMA)

This entity was described in 1939 [7] and has until recently been considered a variant of MF. The condition is rare but appears to affect young adults. An isolated plaque appears, commonly on the distal part of the lower limb (Fig. 47.17). The lesion may be asymptomatic and slowly expands, but no further plaques develop on other body sites. Biopsy shows very striking colonization of an acanthotic epidermis [4] by two populations of cells. One of these is small lymphocytes. Recently some cases have been shown to bear the surface membrane markers of T suppressor cells [6] and others of the T helper subset [3]. The second cell type is a larger, paler cell. There is controversy over whether these cells are related to histiocytes [1], Langerhans cells

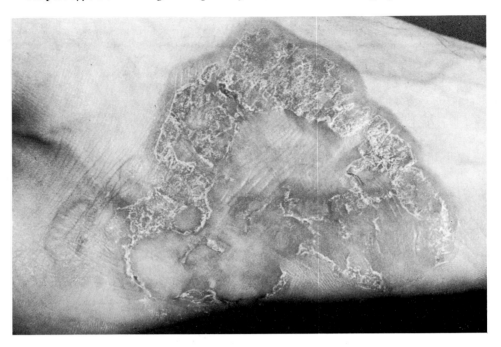

Fig. 47.17. Pagetoid reticulosis. Typical lesion on the dorsum of the foot showing the slowly advancing edge with central clearing of the lesion. (Photograph by courtesy of Dr R. Chapman, Stobhill Hospital.)

[4] or Merkel cells [2]. Personal observation would favour histiocytes due to the strong positive staining for lysozyme.

The natural history of this lesion is very slow local extension. Successful therapy has been reported with both surgical excision and low dose radiotherapy.

REFERENCES

1 CHU A.C. & MACDONALD D.M. (1980) *Br J Dermatol* **103**, 147.
2 DEGREEF H., *et al* (1976) *Cancer* **38**, 2154.
3 GEERTS M.L., *et al* (1982) *Dermatologica* **164**, 15.
4 DENEAU J.G., *et al* (1984) *Arch Dermatol* **120**, 1045.
5 HANEKE E., *et al* (1977) *Arch Dermatol Res* **258**, 265.
6 MACKIE R.M. & TURBITT M.L. (1984) *Br J Dermatol* **110**, 89.
7 WORINGER F. & KOLOPP P. (1939) *Ann Dermatol Syphiligr* **10**, 945.

THE SÉZARY SYNDROME

Diagnosis of the Sézary syndrome requires the presence of the triad of erythroderma, lymphadenopathy and 10% or more of mononuclear cells in the peripheral blood being atypical [9]. The presence of atypical mononuclear cells has also been reported in a variety of conditions including actinic reticuloid [6] (p. 647) and erythroderma due to a variety of causes, but in general the percentage of atypical cells in such situations is smaller than in the Sézary syndrome where 10% or more of the total lymphocyte count is composed of atypical cells. It is, however, important to realize that the total lymphocyte count does not have to be raised for the diagnosis to be made, and the presence of a normal total white cell count without careful morphological examination of the 'tail' of a blood smear or of a buffy coat preparation may mask this diagnosis.

The majority of patients are elderly males and may develop the syndrome either *ab initio* or following lesions considered to be histopathologically classical MF [11]. The former pattern appears to be commoner in the U.K. Skin biopsy shows large numbers of atypical mononuclear cells in the dermis but usually less epidermotropism than is typical of MF per se. Laboratory studies have suggested that the atypical cells in the peripheral blood are an 'overspill' phenomenon, and that the cells are in fact actively dividing in the dermis [8]. The accompanying erythroderma is presumed to be due to the presence of vasoactive lymphokines released by these cells. The presence of macrophage inhibiting factor (MIF) has been reported in the peripheral blood of Sézary syndrome patients [12]. Lymph node biopsy will reveal the presence of similar lymphocytes with convoluted nuclei in the nodes.

Studies of the function of the atypical circulating lymphocytes in the Sézary syndrome have indicated that these cells have the functional capacity to 'help' [1] other lymphocytes in their role of immunoglobulin production, and more recently these cells have been identified as bearing the membrane marker of the T helper cell (OKT4 positive) [3].

In the past it has been suggested that at the ultrastructural level there is both a large and a small cell variant of the Sézary cell [5], but careful functional and clinical studies are awaited to establish the clinical significance of these differing cell types. Cytogenetic studies reveal hyperdiploid cells with marker chromosomes in some cases and multiple translocations. DNA cytophotometry has shown an abnormal DNA content in the great majority of cases [10].

Treatment. Therapy in the Sézary syndrome is directed mainly at reducing the number of atypical circulating lymphocytes, as treatment directed mainly at the skin (e.g. PUVA) appears to be ineffectual. Chemotherapy with chlorambucil [4] and low doses of systemic corticosteroid has been reported to be of value in controlling the disease. Reports of leucapheresis are conflicting, with encouraging positive reports from North America [2] and less encouraging negative results from other centres. The use of specific anti-T-cell antibody has resulted in a temporary drop in the circulating white cell count but little lasting benefit to the patient [7].

Prognosis. In general the prognosis for patients with the Sézary syndrome is poor and the majority succumb to opportunistic infection within months of developing the disease.

REFERENCES

1 BRODER S., *et al* (1976) *J Clin Invest* **58**, 1297.
2 EDELSON R., *et al* (1980) *J Am Acad Dermatol* **2**, 89.
3 HAMMINGA L., *et al* (1979) *Br J Dermatol* **100**, 291.
4 KNOWLES E.M. & HARPER J.P. (1982) *Am J Pathol* **106**, 187.
5 LUTZNER M., *et al* (1975) *Ann Intern Med* **83**, 534.
6 MEIJER C.J.L.M., *et al* (1977) *Virchows Arch B* **25**, 95.
7 MILLER R.A. & LEWY R. (1981) *Lancet* **ii**, 226.
8 SAGLIER GUEDON L., *et al* (1977) *Bull du Cancer* **64**, 259.
9 SÉZARY A. & BOUVRAIN Y. (1938) *Bull Soc Fr Dermatol Syphiligr* **45**, 254.
10 VAN VLOTEN W., *et al* (1977) *Bull du Cancer* **64**, 249.
11 WINKELMANN R.K. (1974) *Symposium on Sézary Cell. Mayo Clin Proc* **49**, No. 8.
12 YOSHIDA T., *et al* (1975) *J Immunol* **114**, 915.

LYMPHOMATOID PAPULOSIS, LYMPHOMATOID PITYRIASIS LICHENOIDES, ACTINIC RETICULOID AND LYMPHOMATOID GRANULOMATOSIS

General introduction. The feature common to these four conditions and the reason for their brief inclusion in this chapter is the fact that although the first three mentioned were all originally reported as benign entities with histological features suggesting a more aggressive process than the subsequently observed natural course of the disease, they have all now been reported to occur in association with MF. Whether or not there are two distinct types of any of these disorders, one with and one without an association with MF, remains to be established. Lymphomatoid granulomatosis deserves inclusion in this section as on occasion it may cause histological confusion with the dermal component of MF.

Lymphomatoid papulosis. This term was first used in 1968 by Macaulay [1] for what he described as 'a self-healing rhythmical paradoxical eruption, histologically malignant but clinically benign'.

Affected patients have recurrent crops of papular lesions predominantly affecting the trunk [2] (Fig. 47.18). These lesions may grow rapidly over a few days and develop ulcerated necrotic centres. Healing occurs slowly with fine atrophic circular scars, and within a few months the cycle will recur. The lesions generally occur first in adult life and may recur in crops for up to 40 years. The histological features of the papules are a relative lack of epidermotropism and Pautrier abscesses, but the presence in the dermis of a mixed infiltrate composed of atypical lymphocytes with large nuclei and frequent abnormal mitoses, eosinophils, neutrophils, free red cells and large histiocytic cells [4]. The epidermis may be ulcerated and the infiltrate may extend deeply into the reticular dermis. True vasculitis is rarely seen.

The original description of lymphomatoid papulosis suggested a totally benign and non-premalignant chronic pattern of the disease, but since 1968 there have been several reports both of patients with lymphomatoid papulosis developing MF and patients with pre-existing MF developing lesions in-

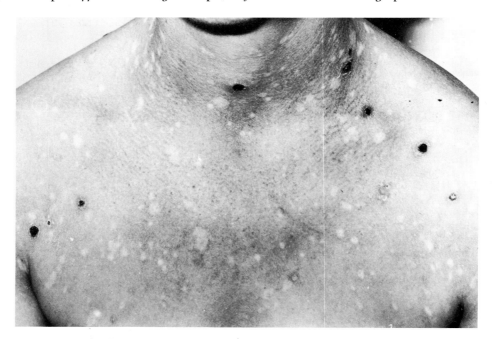

FIG. 47.18. Lymphomatoid papulosis. Typical lesions on the upper chest area showing scars of older lesions together with a fresh crop of necrotic lesions.

distinguishable from those of lymphomatoid papulosis. A follicular variant of the condition has also been described [3]. Recently it has been suggested that he condition can be divided on histological grounds into A and B subgroups [5]. In the A subgroup there appears to be a predominance of large cells related to the Langerhans cell series, while in the B subgroup atypical T lymphocytes with convoluted nuclei predominate. As both types of lesion may be seen in the same patient, it may be that these histological patterns are related to age of the lesion.

Approximately 10% of patients with lymphomatoid papulosis subsequently develop MF but good predictive markers for this 'at risk' group are lacking.

Treatment may be directed either symptomatically at the developed lesions or towards prevention of a fresh crop. Topical steroid therapy is of some value for the former while PUVA or electron beam therapy do appear to be of some value in the latter although this is difficult to quantify in the individual patient. There are isolated unconfirmed reports of the value of low dose cyclophosphamide, chlorambucil or dapsone in prevention of recurrent crops of lesions.

Careful long-term follow-up is obviously mandatory in all cases.

REFERENCES

1 MACAULAY W.L. (1968) *Arch Dermatol* **97**, 23.
2 MACAULAY W.L. (1978) *Int J Dermatol* **17**, 204.
3 PIERARD G.E., *et al* (1980) *Am J Dermatopathol* **2**, 173.
4 WEISSMAN V.F. & ACKERMANN A.B. (1981) *Am J Dermatopathol* **3**, 129.
5 WILLEMZE R., *et al* (1982) *Br J Dermatol* **107**, 131.

Lymphomatoid Pityriasis Lichenoides. This entity was first described by Verallo and Haserick [2] in 1966 and further discussed by Black and Wilson Jones [1] in 1972. The term describes patients with lesions thought to be pityriasis lichenoides on clinical grounds but with the histological appearance of atypical lymphocytes with a high nuclear/cytoplasmic ratio and abnormal mitoses.

The clinical picture in this condition is similar to that of 'classic' pityriasis lichenoides (p. 1181) with plaques of erythema and oedema in which papules and purpura may be present. There are several features of this condition in common with the 'small cell' or B type variant of lymphomatoid papulosis. A small proportion of affected patients proceed to frank MF.

The disease tends to be chronic but symptomatic relief can be obtained with topical steroids, UVB and, in some cases, PUVA.

REFERENCES

1 BLACK M.M. & WILSON JONES E. (1972) *Br J Dermatol* **86**, 329.
2 VERALLO V.M. & HASERICK J.R. (1966) *Arch Dermatol* **94**, 295.

Actinic reticuloid. This condition was first described by Ive *et al* in 1969 [1]. The original description was of a group of elderly, exclusively male patients who developed a severe and very disabling photosensitivity involving reaction to light throughout the UVB, UVA and visible part of the spectrum. A number of these patients had a past history of contact dermatitis and a milder form of photosensitivity ('persistent light reactors') but the true relationship between contact dermatitis, particularly to plants of the compositae family, persistent light reactors, and actinic reticuloid is not established. The photosensitivity is very severe, and the histological picture is that of an intense superficial and deep lymphocytic infiltrate extending from the papillary dermis deep into the reticular dermis. Signs of actinic damage to collagen are present and some of the lymphocytic cells are large and atypical, hence the term 'reticuloid'.

The clinical features are the symptoms of severe

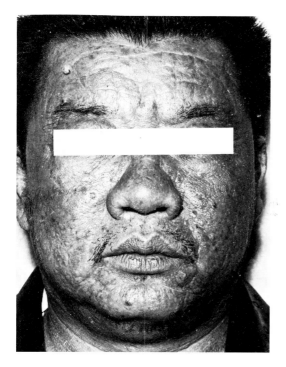

FIG. 47.19. Actinic reticuloid. Patient showing classic thickening of the skin of light-exposed sites.

and persistent photosensitivity with erythema, oedema, and striking 'leonine' thickening of the light-exposed skin of the face, neck and hands [3] (Fig. 47.19). Treatment is based on light avoidance and the use of both the titanium dioxide-containing physical light barrier creams and the newer, more effective chemical UVA and UVB blockers. A few patients find low dose systemic steroid therapy or systemic azathioprine of value.

The prognosis for recovery is poor and the majority of patients tend to have persistent light sensitivity problems for the remainder of their lives. Cases have been reported in association with MF [2] and therefore careful follow-up is once again necessary.

REFERENCES

1 IVE F.A., *et al* (1969) *Br J Dermatol* **81**, 469.
2 JENSEN N.E. & SNEDDON I.B. (1970) *Br J Dermatol* **82**, 287.
3 JOHNSON S.C., *et al* (1979) *Arch Dermatol* **115**, 1078.

Lymphomatoid granulomatosis. This was first described in 1972 by Liebow, Carrington and Friedman [3]. The cases discussed had severe involvement, predominantly of lungs, kidneys and central nervous system, with a granulomatous infiltrate centred around blood vessels and causing severe vascular destruction. The cells within this granulomatous infiltrate contained a high proportion of atypical lymphocytes, and the interest for the dermatologist or dermatopathologist was that at least 50% of patients had cutaneous lesions. Early reports suggested that the condition was reactive rather than malignant, but more recently this view has been revised as a high proportion of patients die of a form of lymphoma [1]. At least one patient has also developed Hodgkin's disease [4].

The cutaneous lesions described have been diffuse erythematous plaques with epidermal atrophy and purpura [5]. The striking feature on histological examination of these lesions is the angiocentricity of the infiltrate and the gross vessel destruction which is visible. A second important pathological feature is the apparent hyperplasia and involvement of the eccrine sweat glands [2].

The disease responds poorly to any form of therapy with 70% of cases being dead within 5 years of diagnosis. There are reports of cyclophosphamide being of some benefit in a few cases.

REFERENCES

1 KATZENSTEIN A.L., *et al* (1979) *Cancer* **43**, 360.
2 KESSLER S., *et al* (1981) *Am J Dermatopathol* **3**, 115.

3 Liebow A.A., *et al* (1972) *Human athol* 3, 457.
4 Macdonald D.M. & Sarkany I. (1976) *Clin Exp Dermatol* 1, 163.
5 Miners N., *et al* (1975) *Arch Dermatol* 111, 493.

HISTIOCYTIC MEDULLARY RETICULOSIS
[1, 2, 6]
SYN. MALIGNANT HISTIOCYTOSIS

This condition was first described by Scott and Robb-Smith [5]. Over 300 cases are now recorded [4]. It affects about two males to one female and presents a picture of asthenia, emaciation and profound general intoxication with high, and sometimes relapsing, pyrexia. The age of onset is very varied and several cases have been recorded in the first decade of life. The lymph nodes, liver and spleen are usually enlarged. Many patients later develop jaundice and purpura. In 13% of recorded cases the skin is involved, and a case [3] is described which presented with three purple-coloured nodules on the forehead, each 2 cm across. These enlarged and coalesced; similar lesions developed on the scalp, extremities and back. They were tender and slightly purpuric.

The blood picture is one of anaemia, usually normocytic, the severity depending on the duration of the disease. In addition, there may be leukopenia and thrombocytopenia or occasionally leukocytosis.

Histology. This is similar in all involved areas and consists of a systematic neoplastic proliferation of histiocytes and their precursors. In the lymph nodes there is a proliferation of cytologically identifiable histiocytes within the subcapsilar or medullary sinuses or within the lymphoid parenchyma. Some of the histiocytes are atypical and some of the abnormal as well as some of the normal are phagocytic either of red cells, white cells, lipid material or cell debris.

Prognosis. The condition is rapidly fatal, death usually occurring within 6 months. Very few cases survive 1 year from the time of diagnosis.

REFERENCES

1 Bryne G.E. Jr & Rappaport H. (1973) *Gans Monogr Cancer Res* 15, 145.
2 Ducatman B.S. *et al* (1984) *Human Pathology* 15, 368
3 Friedman R.M. & Steigrigel N.H. (1965) *Am J Med* 38, 130.
4 Marshall M.E., *et al* (1981) *Arch Dermatol* 117, 278.
5 Scott R.B. & Robb-Smith A.H.T. (1939) *Lancet* ii, 194.
6 Warnke R.A., *et al* (1975) *Cancer* 35, 215.

CROSTI'S LYMPHOMA

This entity was first described in 1951 by Crosti [1] in the Italian literature. He described middle-aged males with slowly developing indolent lesions on the trunk. The prognosis appeared to be good and the lesions responded well to radiotherapy. There appeared to be some confusion in the literature over the cell of origin of the lesion. The condition is well recognized in the French literature and referred to as 'reticulo-histiocytome du dos de l'adulte' [2, 3].

Recent studies of this condition using modern methods of cellular identification have shown that those cells which on conventional histological examination were thought to be histiocytic in origin bear the surface markers of immature T lymphocytes [6]. It has been suggested that the multilobulated T-cell lymphoma of Pinkus is synonymous with Crosti's lymphoma [5].

Clinical features. The condition is commonest in males over the age of 50 years and presents as a slowly expanding reddish nodule on the back. There is one recent report of an association with persistent superficial dermatitis [4].

Histology [6]. In contrast to MF, the epidermis appears to be spared and the lymphoid infiltrate occupies the mid-dermis, concentrating around the blood vessels. Two cell types are seen on light microscopy, one a small dark lymphocyte, and the other a larger paler-staining cell. These two cell types have been described as forming an 'inverted lymphoid follicle' arrangement with the dark cells situated centrally and the paler cells forming a 'cuff' around them.

Marker studies on two cases [7] show in one case that the lymphoid cells have the surface membrane characteristics of mature T-helper lymphocytes and in the second case that the markers are those of the less mature cortical thymocytes. Clearly further studies and sequential biopsies are needed to clarify these findings and establish the place of this condition in the spectrum of T-cell lymphoproliferative disorders.

Treatment. The lesions have been reported to respond well to radiotherapy at doses of 20–25 Gy. Local recurrences have been seen but appear to remain radiosensitive.

The prognosis appears to be good, with long remissions and eventual death from unrelated causes.

REFERENCES

1 Crosti A. (1951) *Minerva Dermatol* 26, 3.
2 Forestier J.Y., *et al* (1980) *Ann Dermatol Vénéréol* 107, 7.

3 Laugier P., *et al* (1974) *Dermatologica* **149**, 350.
4 Rowland Payne C.M.E., *et al* (1984) *Clin Exp Dermatol* **9**, 303.
5 Toonstra J., *et al* (1983) *Dermatologica* **166**, 128.
6 van der Putte S.C.J., *et al* (1982) *Histopathology* **6**, 35.
7 van der Putte S.C.J., *et al* (1982) *Br J Dermatol* **107**, 293.

CUTANEOUS PLASMACYTOMA [2, 3]

Extra-osseous lesions in association with multiple myeloma are not uncommon, and the skin is infiltrated in a fair number (9 of 88 in one series) [1]. Primary involvement of the skin without evidence of bone involvement is, however, extremely rare. The lesions present as small tumours of a red colour, which enlarge and may metastasize. Histologically they consist of a mass of plasma cells, mainly normal but with some abnormal forms. Treatment is by excision with or without radiotherapy.

REFERENCES

1 Bluefarb S.M. (1955) *Arch Dermatol* **72**, 506.
2 Johnson W.H. & Taylor R.G. (1970) *Cancer* **26**, 65.
3 Mikhail G.R., *et al* (1970) *Arch Dermatol* **101**, 59.

HISTIOCYTIC LYMPHOMAS

As with the T-cell disorders, terminology here is confused and made more so by the relative lack of precision with which histiocytes can be identified on light microscopy. The use, however, of immunological methods using antibodies raised against lysozyme (muramidase), α_1-antitrypsin and α_1-antichymotrypsin [2,3] is an important advance in the identification of histiocytic cells as all should demonstrate positivity to these three reagents. As the material labelled is intracytoplasmic rather than on the cell membrane, formalin-fixed and paraffin-processed material can be used, allowing retrospective identification.

Recent observations on large cell lymphoma—formerly called reticulum cell sarcoma—are divided as to the true frequency of histiocytic tumours in the skin. Many lesions previously designated reticulum cell sarcoma have now been identified as of B-cell lineage [1]. It would appear, however, that in other series up to 67% of tumours of the large cell lymphoma type are in fact of histiocytic origin [4].

Clinical features. The majority of affected patients are in the seventh decade or older and present with multiple, rapidly enlarging and metasazizing nodular lesions. Rapid metastasis to lymph nodes and viscera is common and the majority of patients are dead within 2 years of presentation.

The majority of reported cases have been treated with either radiotherapy or surgery with only temporary remission of disease spread, but it is suggested that the prognosis for these true histiocytic lesions is better than for the B-lymphocyte derived tumours [4].

REFERENCES

1 Burg G. & Braun-Falco O. (1977) *Bull du Cancer* **64**, 225.
2 Isaacson P., *et al* (1979) *Cancer* **43**, 1805.
3 Meister P., *et al* (1980) *Virchows Arch A* **385**, 233.
4 Willemze R., *et al* (1982) *Cancer* **50**, 1367.

CUTANEOUS INVOLVEMENT WITH LENNERT'S LYMPHOMA

In 1968 Lennert described an entity involving lymph nodes as 'Hodgkin's disease with a high content of epithelioid cells' [2]. These tumours also contained giant cells and atypical lymphocytes, but few mitoses.

The exact nosology of this entity and its place in lymphoma classification is problematical. Cutaneous involvement [1] is not common, but if present the histology of the cutaneous lesions mirrors that in the nodes. Elderly females are most commonly affected and the disease may first declare itself with gross lymphadenopathy of the cervical glands. The differential diagnosis may include Hodgkin's disease, angioimmunoblastic lymphadenopathy and toxoplasmosis.

The condition may respond to combination chemotherapy [3].

REFERENCES

1 Kim H., *et al* (1978) *Cancer* **41**, 620.
2 Lennert K. & Messdagh J. (1968) *Virchows Arch A* **344**, 1.
3 Roundtree J.M., *et al* (1980) *Arch Dermatol* **116**, 1291.

CHAPTER 48

Sarcoidosis

J.A. SAVIN & D.S. WILKINSON

Definition. There is no universally accepted definition of the disease [12]. Many attempts have been made but often these contain too many permissive clauses or too loose a construction. As long as the cause of the disease remains unknown, definition must be empirical and may also be inaccurate. However, it should studiously avoid aetiological implications and the illogicalities that may result from these. Scadding, after a full discussion of the difficulties, suggests the following [11]:

'Sarcoidosis is a disease characterized by the formation in all of several affected organs or tissues of epithelioid-cell tubercles, without caseation, though fibrinoid necrosis may be present at the centre of a few proceeding either to resolution or to conversion of the epithelioid cell tubercles into hyaline fibrous tissue.'

The characteristic histology should be present in all affected tissue and similar in all parts of it. This excludes the sarcoid-like histology found in tuberculosis, brucellosis, leprosy, etc. It is characterized by the presence of non-caseating epithelioid-cell granulomas.

The important features of sarcoidosis are:

1. The disease process is generalized. The term is not applicable to a localized granulomatous reaction with similar histological findings.
2. All the organs affected conform to a similar histological pattern. Other changes present to a varying and inconstant degree include suppression or weakening of tuberculin and other intradermal responses, an increase in the serum γ-globulins and a raised serum calcium level.
3. The Kveim reaction is positive in most active cases.
4. Tubercle bacilli are not found and there is no evidence of active tuberculous infection.
5. The clinical manifestations are protean, the disease process usually widespread, the course protracted and usually benign, though sometimes with dangerous and disabling sequelae and complications.

This systemic granulomatous disease may affect any organ of the body (the adrenal gland possibly excluded). The lymph nodes, lungs, liver, spleen, skin, eyes, small bones of hands and feet and salivary glands are most frequently involved.

History [11, 12]. A recent critical re-examination [12] suggests that the grounds for regarding the report by Hutchinson in 1878 [4] as the earliest description of a case that would now be categorized as sarcoidosis are tenuous. This honour should probably pass to Besnier's report in 1889 [1] of an association between reddish-blue lesions of the face and nose with swellings of the fingers; the name 'lupus pernio' reflected his view that this might be a variant of lupus vulgaris. Tenneson in 1892 added the histological description [15]. In 1898 Hutchinson described two more cases of a skin eruption, probably sarcoidosis, to which he gave the name 'Mortimer's malady' after one of his patients [5]. Boeck in 1899 [2] recorded his 'multiple benign sarkoid of the skin', and the current term 'sarcoidosis' stems from his misinterpretation of the histological changes. However, it was Boeck who first developed the concept of a disease involving both the skin and internal organs—a concept taken further by Schaumann [13, 14], who again emphasized the generalized nature of the disease and showed that skin changes were not a necessary feature of it. The disease was further expanded by the inclusion of 'osteitis tuberculosa multiplex cystica' [7], uveoparotid fever [3], pulmonary and other manifestations [9, 10]. The introduction of mass radiography led to the recognition of hilar lymphadenopathy, with or without erythema nodosum, as an early benign form [6, 8] and this has altered the whole concept of the disease which is now seen more frequently by chest and general physicians than by dermatologists.

REFERENCES*

1 BESNIER E. (1889) *Ann Dermatol Syphiligr* **10**, 333.
2 BOECK C. (1899) *J Cutan Genito-urin Dis* **17**, 333.

3 HEERFORDT C.F. (1909) *Albrecht v Gräfes Arch Ophthal*
70, 254.

4 HUTCHINSON J. (1878) *Illustrations of Clinical Surgery.*
London, Churchill, Vol. 1, p. 42.

5 HUTCHINSON J. (1898) *Arch Surg* 9, 307.

6 JAMES D.G. (1959) *Q J Med* 28, 109.

7 JUNGLING O. (1920–21) *Fortschr Röntgenstr* 27, 375.

8 KERLEY P. (1942) *Br J Radiol* 15, 155.

9 KUSNITSKY E. & BITTORD A. (1915) *Münch Med Wochenschr* 62, 1349.

10 LEITNER S.J. (1949) *Der Morbus Besnier–Boeck–Schaumann.* Basel, Schwabe, p. 6.

11 SCADDING J.G. & MITCHELL D.N. (1985) *Sarcoidosis.* 2nd
ed. London, Chapman & Hall, pp 1–12.

12 SCADDING J.G. (1981) *J R Soc Med* 74, 147.

13 SCHAUMANN J. (1914) *Mem présenté à la Societé Fr dermatol
pour le prix Zambaco,* Stockholm.

14 SCHAUMANN J. (1917) *Ann Dermatol Syphiligr* 6, 357.

15 TENNESON M. (1892) *Bull Soc Fr Dermatol Syphiligr* 3,
417.

*References to various international conferences on sar-
coidosis and other granulomatous disorders are quoted in
the text. The proceedings are published either in book
form or as a special issue of a journal. To save space,
references to recent conferences will be referred to as
follows.

The VIIth International Symposium, Tokyo, 1979. Eds.
Mikami R. & Hodosa Y. Univ. Tokyo Press, 1981.
    Author (1981) *Proc Int Symp Sarc, 1979.* Tokyo,
Univ. Tokyo Press, p. . . . .
    The VIIIth International Conference, Cardiff, 1980.
Eds. Jones Williams W. & Davies B.H. Cardiff, Alpha
    Omega:
    Author (1980) *VIIIth Int Conf Sarc.* Cardiff, Alpha
    Omega, p. . . . .
The IXth International Conference, Paris, 1981, has
been published (1983) as:
Sarcoidosis and other Granulomatous Disorders. Ninth
International Conference, Paris, 1981. Eds. Chretien
J., Marsac J. & Saltiel J.C. Paris, Oxford, New York,
Pergamon.
    Author (1983) *IXth Int Conf Sarc.* Paris, 1981. Paris,
Oxford, New York, Pergamon, p. . . . .

AETIOLOGY [10, 20]

Despite a mass of collected data and intensive investigations, the cause of sarcoidosis remains unknown. Many of the earlier theories have been discarded; others have remained unproven. Evidence
derived from genetic and environmental sources
has been inconclusive and immunological studies
have, perhaps, raised more questions than they
have solved. The current views are summarized
below.

Genetic predisposition. Concordance in identical
twins and the high incidence among Puerto Ricans
in New York and among Irish and West Indians in

London, have suggested a genetic factor [22]. However, this may amount to no more than a predisposition to an infective agent or a mode of response
to this.

Studies of HLA antigens have given conflicting
results. Earlier findings of an association with HLA
B7 [7, 13] have not been confirmed [2], though
differences between black and white subjects have
obscured the issue. There is some evidence that
patients with this histocompatibility antigen are
more likely to become tuberculin sensitive and to
have symptoms [18]. In London, Caucasians with
HLA B8 were more likely to have arthritis and/or
erythema nodosum [17]. Among black patients in
the U.S.A., sarcoidosis occurred significantly more
frequently in individuals with BW15; but so does
tuberculosis [1]. At present, the most one can say
is that a particular HLA type may tend to influence
the pattern of the disease, rather than determine its
occurrence [24]. Further studies on larger numbers
are awaited.

Infectious agents. Many infective agents have been
postulated as causes of sarcoidosis, but cultures
have always been negative and the response to
appropriate treatment has not supported these beliefs. However, it remains quite possible that the
disease represents an unusual host reaction to an
as yet unknown infective agent—or perhaps to
more than one.

Mycobacteria. Similarities to tuberculosis, particularly primary tuberculosis [10], and understandable diagnostic confusion between the two diseases,
led to speculation that *M. tuberculosis* might be responsible, perhaps in some transmuted form, for the
symptom complex of sarcoidosis. However, while
tuberculosis has declined rapidly over much of the
world, sarcoidosis has remained steady or become
more prevalent [22]. The tuberculin test is frequently negative in sarcoidosis and the Kveim test
usually negative in tuberculosis and other granulomatous diseases [23]. Angiotensin-converting enzyme (ACE) is raised in only very few patients with
tuberculosis.

The possibility of a role for other mycobacteria
continues to command support, especially for *M.
kansasii* and *M. avium-intracellulare.* Neither has
consistently been detected in or cultured from sarcoid tissue; when they have been found [5], the
patients have usually been naturally or therapeutically immunosuppressed. Raised antibody titres
against such mycobacteria [4, 19] are probably a
non-specific manifestation of the disease rather than
an indication of its cause. The finding that patients

with sarcoidosis lack mycobacteriophage antibodies [12] suggested a bacterial lysis, but this was not sustained by later studies [3]. So the trail ends, at any rate for the present.

Other organisms. As histoplasmosis and other fungi can produce granulomas exactly mimicking sarcoidosis, they have been suspected as possible causes, but their geographical limitations rule them out of court. Aspergillus and Nocardia [25] are recognized as secondary invaders only. So, almost certainly, are ubiquitous organisms such as Gram-negative bacteria, *P. acnes*, mycoplasma [6], and Yersinia [9]. Protozoa, metazoa and toxoplasmosis can probably also be excluded.

Viruses. It is always tempting to suspect a viral cause for an obscure disease and it is natural that these elusive organisms should have been considered as possible causes of an elusive condition. Again, raised levels of Epstein–Barr virus antibodies [11] are common to many infective and neoplastic diseases and though a viral cause cannot be ruled out, there is no evidence so far to advance this beyond mere speculation.

The transmissible agent of Mitchell and Rees. The original findings of a transmissible agent (passing a $0\cdot2$ μm filter) from mouse, or Crohn's sarcoid tissue homogenate [14, 15] have been established in sequential passage experiments [16]. The significance of these studies awaits further evaluation.

Immunological concepts. The occasional coexistence of collagen-vascular and autoimmune diseases and the immunological changes, have suggested an autoimmune basis for sarcoidosis [26], but most observers consider the immune system abnormalities to be secondary. Further investigations with monoclonal antibodies and new methods of cell isolation [10] may be rewarding.

Other agents. The similarities between sarcoidosis, chronic beryllium granulomatous disease and extrinsic allergic alveolitis, have led to speculation about environmental [8] and occupational factors. These cannot be dismissed. We know little enough about our environment and, although the pine pollen theory of the cause of sarcoidosis has been rejected, we must always consider very carefully the occupational and environmental history [22] of patients presenting with this disease. Scadding's view of 15 years ago [20, 21] is still apt—that sarcoidosis is a syndrome resulting from either one or many as yet unidentified causes. These may be mi-

crobiological or chemical and may affect subjects with a 'special sort of alteration of reactivity'. We can still go no further than this.

REFERENCES

1 AL-ARIF L., *et al* (1977) *Clin Res* **25**, 321.
2 AL-ARIF L., *et al* (1980) *VIIIth Int Conf Sarc.* Cardiff, Alpha Omega, p. 206.
3 BOWMAN B.U., *et al* (1972) *Am Rev Respir Dis* **105**, 85.
4 CHAPMAN J. & SPEIGHT M. (1964) *Acta Med Scand* **176** (Suppl. **425**), 61.
5 GRICE K. (1983) *Clin Exp Dermatol* **8**, 323.
6 HANNUKSELA M. & JANSSON E. (1974) *Proc VIth Int Conf Sarc. Tokyo,* Univ. Tokyo Press, p. 4.
7 HEDFORS E. & MOLLER E. (1977) *Tissue Antigens* **3**, 95.
8 HOSADA Y., *et al* (1976) *Ann NY Acad Sci* **278**, 355.
9 ITO Y., *et al* (1980) *VIIIth Int Conf Sarc.* Cardiff, Alpha Omega, p. 142.
10 JONES WILLIAMS W. (1982) *Pathol Res Pract* **175**, 1.
11 KATAOKA T., *et al* (1974) *Proc VIth Int Conf Sarc.* Eds. Iwai K. & Hosada Y. Tokyo, Univ. Tokyo Press, p. 231.
12 MANKIEWICZ E. (1964) *Acta Med Scand* **176** (Suppl. **425**), 7, 68.
13 McINTYRE J.A., *et al* (1977) *Transpl Proc* **9** (Suppl. 1), 173.
14 MITCHELL D.N. & REES R.S.W. (1969) *Lancet* ii, 81.
15 MITCHELL D.N. & REES R.J.W. (1976) *Ann NY Acad Sci* **278**, 233.
16 MITCHELL D.N. & REES R.J.W. (1983) *IXth Int Conf Sarc,* Paris, 1981. Paris, Oxford, New York, Pergamon, p. 132.
17 NEVILLE E., *et al* (1980) *VIIIth Int Conf Sarc.* Cardiff, Alpha Omega, p. 201.
18 PERSSON I., *et al* (1975) *Tissue Antigens* **6**, 50.
19 REID J.D. & WOLINSKY E. (1971) *Proc Vth Int Conf Sarc, Prague.* Univ. Karlova, p. 85.
20 *SCADDING J.G. & MITCHELL D.N. (1985) 2nd ed. *Sarcoidosis.* London, Chapman & Hall.
21 SCADDING J.G. (1970) *Postgrad Med J* **46**, 465.
22 *SILTZBACH L.E. (1969) *Practitioner* **202**, 613.
23 SILTZBACH L.E., *et al* (1980) *VIIIth Int Conf Sarc.* Cardiff, Alpha Omega, p. 679.
24 TURTON C.W.G., *et al* (1980) *VIIIth Int Conf Sarc.* Cardiff, Alpha Omega, p. 195.
25 UESAKA I., *et al* (1974) *Proc VIth Int Conf. Sarc.* Tokyo, Univ. Tokyo, p. 3.
26 WEISEN-HUTTER C.W. & SHARMA O.P. (1979) *Semin Arthr Rheum* **9**, 124.

Angiotensin-converting enzyme (ACE) [2]. The observation by Lieberman [3] in 1974 that serum levels of angiotensin-I-converting enzyme were elevated in sarcoidosis led to hopes that this might serve as a simple diagnostic test for the disease. Further experience has modified this view since abnormally high levels have only been found by other workers in one-half or less of patients with active untreated disease [1, 7, 9], though higher figures have been noted in young subjects, in males rather than females, and in Blacks [5]. Moreover, ACE is raised in a number of other conditions, including leprosy, berylliosis, silicosis, *M. avium-intracellulare* infections [1, 4, 5] and sometimes in tuberculosis. Nevertheless, in general it is reasonable to use ACE levels as a supporting diagnostic aid [8] and to distinguish between stable and progressive disease [9]. The value of ACE may rather lie in assessing the effect of treatment, high values indicating continuing disease activity or impending relapse [6].

REFERENCES

1 GRONHAGEN-RISKA C., *et al* (1979) *Scand J Respir Dis* **60**, 94.
2 Leading Article (1980) *Lancet* **i**, 804.
3 LIEBERMAN J. (1974) *Am Rev Respir Dis* **109**, 743.
4 LIEBERMAN J. (1976) *Ann NY Acad Sci* **278**, 488.
5 LIEBERMAN J., *et al* (1979) *Am Rev Respir Dis* **120**, 329.
6 SILTZBACH L.E. (1979) *Ann Intern Med* **91**, 501.
7 SILVERSTEIN E. & FRIEDLAND J. (1979) *Lancet* **i**, 382.
8 STUDDY P., *et al* (1978) *Lancet* **ii**, 1331.
9 TURTON C.M.G., *et al* (1979) *Thorax* **34**, 57.

Prevalence and incidence [1, 5, 9, 12, 16]. The increase in reported cases of sarcoidosis during the last 40 years has undoubtedly been partly due to increased recognition, especially by mass radiography, and with the decline of tuberculosis more cases of pulmonary disease have been uncovered [10]. However, even in countries with compulsory notification of the disease, there are bound to be many cases in the early asymptomatic stage that remain undetected—Røhmer's iceberg [12]. The assumption that the disease is extremely rare in parts of Asia, Africa and South America may not, therefore, be entirely valid, especially where leprosy and cutaneous tuberculosis are still common [14]. A recent study from South Africa [2] suggests that it may not have been uncommon in the Black and Coloured races, who had a higher prevalence of cutaneous lesions than the White population studied. Though figures from Korea [10] and Thailand [4] failed to show more than a handful of cases, a continuing survey from Japan [7, 8] shows a geometrical rise in recent years. The highest figures are found in the colder northern islands of Japan, notably Hokkaido, but the authors of this computer-based analysis of nearly 5,000 cases [8] believe that environmental as well as climatic factors may be important. Though it is more frequent in the north than in the south of Italy [3], it is 10 times more frequent in Sweden than in Finland [17], and is rare indeed in Greenland and Iceland where the racial strain is that of Norway and Iceland, countries in which there is a high prevalence. Sarcoidosis has long been known to be more common in American Negroes than in white inhabitants of the same area [15]. The prevalence in Jamaica could not be determined [11], but of 100 cases analysed recently, there was an unusual predominance of older males, differing considerably from the 4:1 female predominance among blacks and Puerto Ricans in New York [19].

The survey by James *et al* [9] of the world-wide distribution of sarcoidosis has recently been expanded to include six European cities [6]. The considerable variation in the incidence of skin lesions remains unexplained. A very useful survey of 401 consecutive patients presenting to a district general hospital in the U.K. [13] gives a representative view of the ethnic representation. Irish and West Indian patients appeared to be disproportionately common in the material, but no attempt was made to assess the incidence or prevalence in the population covered. Erythema nodosum was particularly common in the British and Irish; other skin manifestations occurred in 30 patients, 80% of whom were under 45 years of age.

Despite the voluminous data available, it is obvious that the factors influencing the prevalence (unknown) and the incidence (possibly undetected) of sarcoidosis remain obscure. Occupational [8] and socio-economic factors [18] may be more important than have so far been recognized.

An approximate indication of the prevalence is given in Table 48.1. More detailed figures are given by Hosoda [7, 8], Levinsky [12] and others.

REFERENCES

1 BAUER H.J. & LOFGREN S. (1964) *Acta Med Scand* (Suppl.), **425**, 103.
2 BENATAR S.R. (1980) *Prov VIIIth Int Conf Sarc.* Cardiff, Alpha Omega, p. 508.
3 BLASI A., *et al* (1974) *Proc VIth Int Conf Sarc.* Tokyo, Univ. Tokyo Press, p. 317.
4 BOVORNKITTI S. (1974) *Proc VIth Int Conf Sarc.* Tokyo, Univ. Tokyo Press, p. 311.
5 CALANDRA P. & STOCCHI F. (1982) *La Malattia di Besnier–Boeck–Schaumann. Ann Ital Derm Clin Exp* **36**, 114.
6 DJURIC B., *et al* (1980) *VIIIth Int Conf Sarc.* Cardiff, Alpha Omega, p. 527.
7 HOSODA Y., *et al* (1976) *Ann NY Acad Sci* **278**, 347.
8 HOSODA K., *et al* (1980) *VIIIth Int Conf Sarc.* Cardiff, Alpha Omega, p. 519.
9 JAMES D.G., *et al* (1976) *Ann NY Acad Sci* **278**, 321.
10 LEE J.Q. & LEE W.K. (1974) *Proc VIth Int Conf Sarc.* Tokyo, Univ. Tokyo Press, p. 311.
11 LOWE M.V. (1980) *VIIIth Int Conf Sarc.* Cardiff, Alpha Omega, p. 514.

TABLE 48.1. Reported prevalence of sarcoidosis

Vey low prevalence (< 1 per 100,000)
Spain	Most countries of Far East
Portugal	Indian sub-continent
Egypt	South America
China	

Low prevalence (1–2 per 100,000)
Israel
Southern Italy
Argentina

Moderate prevalence (2–10 per 100,000)
Czechoslovakia	Australia
Finland	France
Hungary	Yugoslavia
Japan	U.S.S.R.

High prevalence (> 10 per 100,000)
Sweden	Germany	Switzerland
Norway	Holland	Northern Italy
Great Britain	Poland	New Zealand
Eire	Canada	U.S.A. (variable)

Modified from various authors (refs. [1] and [4] and from the Proceedings of the VIth and VIIth International Conference on Sarcoidosis).

12 LEVINSKY L., *et al* (1976) *Ann NY Acad Sci* **278**, 335.
13 MIKHAIL J.R., *et al* (1980) *VIIIth Int Conf Sarc.* Cardiff, Alpha Omega, p. 532.
14 MORRISON J.G.L. (1974) *Br J Dermatol* **90**, 649.
15 SARTWELL P.E. (1976) *Ann NY Acad Sci* **278**, 368.
16 SCADDING J.G. & MITCHELL D.N. (1985) *Sarcoidosis.* 2nd ed. London, Chapman & Hall, pp. 43–71
17 SELROOS·O. (1974) *Proc VIth Int Conf Sarc.* Tokyo, Univ. Tokyo Press, p. 319.
18 SILTZBACH L.E. & JABELMAN M. (1981) In *La Sarcoidosi.* Scena, Centro stampa Univ., p. 189.
19 TIERSTEIN A.S., *et al* (1976) *Ann NY Acad Sci* **278**, 371.

Familial sarcoidosis. This is well recognized but rare. It usually involves genetically-related individuals, particularly females [6]. A British survey revealed 62 cases [1]; a further 174 were found in the world literature. Among 645 cases of the disease, 26 cases were found in 12 families in another survey [7]. Mother–child or brother–sister relationships predominate [6, 7], whereas a father–child relationship is exceedingly rare. We have seen it in mother and daughter and in sisters. When it occurs, it tends to do so at similar ages and with similar features. Cases in husband and wife are of obvious interest with reference to a possible transmissible agent. Thirteen cases are known to have occurred [2, 5].

Sarcoidosis and Crohn's disease have also been reported in four out of five members of one family; HLA typing revealed B8/DR3 in all those affected [3]. However, HLA typing in 59 members of 14 families with sarcoidosis did not support an association between HLA and the development of the disease [8], though it did not exclude an influence on the pattern of its development. Further studies may show whether environmental [4] rather than genetic factors are responsible for these familial cases.

REFERENCES

1 BRITISH THORACIC AND TUBERCULOSIS ASSOCIATION REPORT (1973) *Tubercle* London **54**, 87.
2 GANGE R.W. (1979) *Clin Exp Dermatol* **4**, 107.
3 GRÖNHAGEN-RISKA C., *et al* (1983) *Lancet* i, 1982.
4 HOSODA Y., *et al* (1980) *VIIIth Int Conf Sarc.* Cardiff, Alpha Omega, p. 519.
5 RENNER R.R., *et al* (1977) *NY State J Med* **77**, 118.
6 SHARMA O.P., *et al* (1976) *Ann NY Acad Sci* **278**, 356.
7 TURIAF J., *et al* (1978) *Nouv Presse Méd* **7**, 913.
8 TURTON C.W.G., *et al* (1980) *VIIIth Int Conf Sarc.* Cardiff, Alpha Omega, p. 195.

Histopathology [3, 10, 13]. The histological changes are consistent in all organs affected and are remarkably constant. The essential feature is a

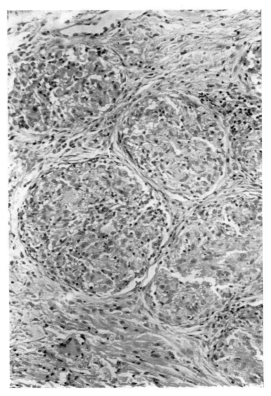

FIG. 48.1. Sarcoidosis. Typical appearance of well-defined non-caseating granulomas. H & E, × 100 (Professor E. Wilson Jones).

monotonous repetition of aggregates of epithelioid cells with pale-staining nuclei which form the characteristic discrete sarcoidal granulomas (Fig. 48.1). Multinucleate giant cells are usually, but not invariably, present. An inconstant and variable rim of lymphoid cells surrounds the granuloma but this is never well developed—hence the term 'naked tubercle'. Caseation is absent, though an inconspicuous focus of fibrinoid necrosis or coagulation may occur within the granuloma. A fine reticulin network encircles the granuloma and may penetrate it (Fig. 48.2). The infiltrate tends to occur lower in the dermis than that of lupus vulgaris, and in erythrodermic sarcoidosis the granulomas are looser and less well defined.

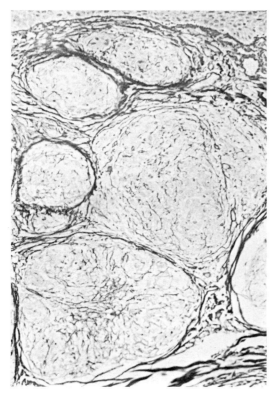

FIG. 48.2. Sarcoidosis showing reticulin fibres encircling the granulomas. Sparse fibres are also seen within the granulomas. Reticulin stain, × 100 (Professor E. Wilson Jones).

Development of the granuloma [4, 13]. The probable mode of evolution has been studied by utilizing the Kveim test [14]. Both the lymphoid cells at the periphery of the granuloma and the darkly-staining mononuclear cells within it have been shown to be derived from blood monocytes [2, 6, 11]. These loosely packed epithelioid cells of the early stage become more numerous and compact, and giant cells appear by their fusion. Reticulum develops and hyalinization becomes progressively more apparent as fibrosis gradually obliterates the characteristic features of the granuloma, and is the cause of the irreversible tissue scarring of the late stage of the disease.

Inclusion bodies. These are found inconstantly in the giant cells in sarcoidosis and other sarcoidal granulomas but are not specific. The following types are recognized [12, 13, 16]:

(a) *Schaumann (conchoid) bodies.* They consist of concentric lamellar structures 100 μm in diameter, probably derived from lysosomes [10].

(b) *Asteroid (stellate) bodies* (Fig. 48.3). Between 10 and 15 μm in size, they have a central core surrounded by radiating spicules (the

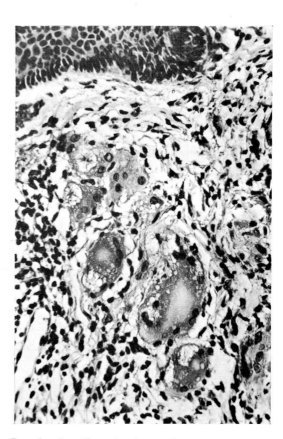

FIG. 48.3. Sarcoid reaction (in necrobiosis) showing centrosomes and asteroid bodies in giant cells. H & E, × 250 (Professor E. Wilson Jones).

'open umbrella frame') [16]. They consist of collagen [1] and are not specific for sarcoidosis [4].

Histochemical studies [7, 8] suggest that two types of epithelioid cells are involved, one being predominant in tuberculous and the other in sarcoidal granulomas and the Kveim reaction. It is suggested that an intermediate type of mononuclear cell, on stimulation by the 'sarcoidal agent', becomes a cell of the first type and, after a phagocytic life, changes to the second type which then secretes a substance which stimulates further mononuclear cell production.

Electron microscopic studies of the sarcoid granuloma have been reported by several authors [5, 9, 15, 17]. These have thrown considerable light on the formation of granulomas but little of direct interest to the clinician. The peripheral zone is the site of activity and cellular exchange [13] and ultrastructural differences may exist among the epithelioid cells [5].

As involution occurs, fibrosis extends from the periphery to the centre of the granulomas.

Differential diagnosis. Typical tuberculosis is usually distinguishable by its more diffuse histology, the presence of caseation and, occasionally, by the finding of bacilli (Table 48.2). Lupus vulgaris may present difficulties, especially if lymphocytes are more abundant than usual. In tuberculoid leprosy epithelioid cells surround and follow the nerves and there is more central necrosis [11]. The arrectores pili may be destroyed.

Lupoid leishmaniasis, granulomatosis disciformis and the rosaceas may also pose difficulties [3].

The histology of true sarcoidosis cannot be distinguished from that of sarcoidal granulomas of other causes. Plasma cells and coagulation necrosis are features of syphilis. The granulomas of cat-scratch disease are said to be larger than those of sarcoidosis [14]. Talc may be recognized by its refractile nature. An indistinguishable histology may sometimes be seen in Hodgkin's disease. The key to the diagnosis of sarcoidosis lies in the uniformity of the histological changes in all affected organs and in the reproduction of the epithelioid cell granuloma by the Kveim antigen.

REFERENCES

1 AZAR H.A. & LUNARDELLI C. (1969) *Am J Pathol* **57**, 81.
2 BJERKE J.R., *et al* (1981) *Acta Derm Venereol (Stockh)* **61**, 371.
3 CIVATTE J. (1982) *Histopathologie cutanée.* 2nd ed. Paris, Flammarion, pp. 105–107.
4 CUNNINGHAM J.A. (1967) *Sarcoidosis.* In *Pathology Annals.* Vol. 2,. Ed. Sommers S.G. New York, Appleton, p. 31.
5 FUSE Y. & HIRAGA Y. (1974) *Proc VIth Int Conf Sarc.* Tokyo, Univ. Tokyo Press, p. 269.
6 HUNDEKER M. (1960) *Hautartz* **20**, 164.
7 JONES WILLIAMS W., *et al* (1967) *J Chem Pathol* **20**, 574.
8 JONES WILLIAMS W., *et al* (1969) *J Pathol Bacteriol* **97**, 805.
9 JONES WILLIAMS W., *et al* (1971) *Proc Vth Int Conf Sarc.* Prague, Univ. Karlova, p. 115.
10 *LEVER W.F. & SCHAUMBERG-LEVER G. (1983) *Histopathology of the Skin.* 6th ed. Philadelphia, Lippincott, pp. 229–243.
11 MUSTAKALLIO K.K. & NIEMI M. (1966) *Dermatol Wochenschr* **151**, 1454.
12 *SCADDING J.G. & MITCHELL D.N. (1985) *Sarcoidosis.* 2nd ed. London, Chapman & Hall, pp 13–35.

TABLE 48.2. Main histological features of sarcoidosis and tuberculosis.

Feature	Sarcoidosis	Tuberculosis
General structure	Monomorphic tubercles	Caseating tubercles
Form	Discrete, sharply defined 'naked tubercles'	Confluent, diffuse
Epithelioid-cell	Large, grouped, predominant	Massed, irregular or at margin of caseation
		Less than 50%
Giant cells	Large, usually sparse Langhans' and foreign body	More numerous, Langhans' predominate
Lymphocytes	Sparse cuffing	More numerous and scattered
Inclusion bodies	Frequent	Occasional
Blood vessels	Usually normal or dilated	May show fibrinoid changes
Reticulin	Fine and abundant around tubercles	Destroyed
Caseation	No	Yes (but not lupus vulgaris)
Fibrinoid	Sometimes at centre of tubercle	Vascular and perivascular (late)
Healing process	Progressive hyalinization from periphery. Gradual dissolution	Dense collagen mesh. Retraction, fibrosis, calcifi cation

13 SHARMA O.P. (1975) *Sarcoidosis. A Clinical Approach.* Springfield, Thomas, pp. 14–22.
14 *SILTZBACH L.E. (1964) *Acta Med Scand* (Suppl.) **425**, 74.
15 SOLER P., *et al* (1976) *Ann NY Acad Sci* **278**, 147.
16 *UEHLINGER E. (1964) *Acta Med Scand* (Suppl.) **425**, 7.
17 WANSTRUP J. & CHRISTENSEN H.E. (1966) *Acta Pathol Microbiol Scand* **66**, 169.

IMMUNOLOGICAL ASPECTS [6]

Important advances have been made in the immunology of sarcoidosis in recent years. These have been well summarized by James and Williams [6], who see the sarcoid granuloma as a battleground between an invading but unknown antigen and the resilient defences of the body. The paradox of the disease lies in the evolution of a cell-mediated granuloma in a condition showing reduced cell-mediated immunity.

Cell-mediated immunity. Depression of cell-mediated immunity is the hallmark of sarcoidosis: indeed the first immunological defect to be demonstrated was lack of reactivity to tuberculin. Sensitivity to tuberculin is depressed to a variable degree and becomes negative in about two-thirds of patients [11]. However, there is no absolute correlation between reactivity and the state of the disease, and a relative or absolute failure of immunological response may persist despite apparent clinical resolution.

Later, this anergy was shown to extend to other intradermal allergens such as candida, pertussis, trichophytin and mumps antigens. Candida antigen (oidomycin) is frequently used in this country and tests to it are negative in about half of sarcoidosis patients. The combination of a depressed reaction to mumps antigen, with normal circulatory antibody responses, is characteristic of but not specific for sarcoidosis. The response to DNCB is also defective [12].

Recent studies of T-cell subsets, using monoclonal antibody techniques, have begun to shed light on the mechanisms involved. In pulmonary sarcoidosis at least, an excess of helper T-lymphocyte activity is present at the disease sites [4, 10]. The cutaneous and *in vitro* anergy which is characteristic of sarcoidosis may be partially explained by this movement of activated helper cells to the sites of disease activity, leaving in the circulation an excess of anergic suppressor cells [6]. Activity of killer and natural killer lymphocytes is higher in patients with sarcoidosis than in controls, and K-cell activity correlates with elevated serum angiotension-converting enzyme and lysozyme activity [5].

Humoral immunity. All classes of serum immunoglobulins are increased. Increased kappa and lambda chains reflect B-cell overactivity [8] and are found in more than three-quarters of patients with active sarcoidosis of more than 2 years' duration, and in only 1% of patients with healed inactive sarcoidosis. Significantly raised levels of circulating antibodies may be found to rubella, measles, herpes simplex, the Epstein–Barr virus and cytomegalovirus [1, 3]. The incidence of asthma, eczema and hay fever in patients with sarcoidosis is unaltered [9].

Immune complexes are present in more than 50% of sarcoid patients [2] and are manifested clinically by erythema nodosum, polyarthritis, uveitis and a raised ESR. There is some evidence that those with a particular HLA type are especially likely to express their sarcoidosis in this way [7].

REFERENCES

1 BYRNE E.B., *et al* (1973) *Am J Epidemiol* **97**, 355.
2 GUPTA R.C., *et al* (1977) *Am Rev Respir Dis* **116**, 261.
3 HIRSHAUT Y., *et al* (1970) *N Engl J Med* **283**, 502.
4 HUNNINGHAKE G.W. & CRYSTAL R.G. (1981) *N Engl J Med* **305**, 429.
5 INA Y., *et al* (1983) *IXth Int Conf Sarc.* Paris, 1981. Paris, Oxford, New York, Pergamon, p. 168
6 *JAMES D.G. & WILLIAMS W.J. (1982) *Am J Med* **72**, 5.
7 NEVILLE E., *et al* (1980) *VIIIth Int Conf Sarc.* Cardiff, Alpha Omega, p. 201.
8 RØMER F.K., *et al* (1983) *IXth Int. Conf Sarc.* Paris, 1981. Paris, Oxford, New York, Pergamon, p. 178
9 SCADDING J.G. & MITCHELL D.N. (1985) *Sarcoidosis.* 2nd ed. London, Chapman & Hall, pp. 414–443
10 SEMENZATO G., *et al* (1980) *J Clin Lab Immunol* **4**, 95.
11 SILTZBACH L.E., *et al* (1974) *Am J Med* **57**, 847.
12 VERRIER-JONES J. & PEARSON J.E.G. (1971) *Vth Int Conf Sarc.* Prague, Universita Karlova, p. 160.

THE KVEIM TEST

The Kveim reaction remains something of an immunological puzzle. A suspension of sarcoid tissue is injected intradermally and the area is excised for histological examination 4 to 6 weeks later. Epithelioid-cell granuloma formation is found in a high proportion of patients with active disease, though positive results become less frequent as the disease becomes chronic.

An adequate Kveim antigen must satisfy the criteria laid down by Siltzbach in 1976 [6]. It must be sensitive enough to detect at least 60% of cases of active sarcoidosis, and specific enough to exclude all but 2–3% of non-sarcoid cases. To achieve this the antigen must have been validated by extensive tests both on normal subjects and on patients with other conditions, such as Crohn's disease, in which false-positive reactions are known to occur [2].

Kveim material is heat stable, and was long thought to be extremely stable on storage, though some loss of sensitivity and specificity may occur over a period of years [1]. The active material is particulate [5], and probably lies within the membrane containing elements of the sarcoidal tissue [4], though its exact constitution has not yet been established.

The technique used for the test is important. An easily relocated or marked site, usually on the forearm, is injected with 0·1 to 0·2 ml of shaken antigen using a 26-gauge needle with a Huber point, the bevel of which must be uppermost to ensure deposition high in the dermis. A papule appears in 2 to 3 weeks and slowly increases in size. It is best excised in 6 weeks, and even if no papule can be found the area should still be removed for histology. Corticosteroid therapy may inhibit the reaction [3].

A positive result is the unequivocal presence of an epithelioid-cell granuloma, exactly mimicking the natural disease, though usually less profuse. Isolated epithelioid cells are acceptable only if present in groups. Langhans giant cells are seen in two-thirds of cases. Birefringent bodies occur only rarely, and may be unrelated. A minor degree of fibrosis may occur but may also be seen in negative tests. False-positive foreign body-type reactions are discarded, but equivocal results will occur in about 5% of tests.

REFERENCES

1 HURLEY T.H., *et al* (1975) *Lancet* i, 494.
2 JAMES D.G. (1975) *N Engl J Med* **292**, 859.
3 JONES WILLIAMS W., *et al* (1976) *Ann NY Acad Sci* **278**, 687.
4 MIDDLETON W.G. & DOUGLAS A.C. (1980) *Proc VIIIth Int Conf Sarc.* Cardiff, Alpha Omega, p. 655.
5 RIPE E., *et al* (1973) *Scand J Respir Dis* **54**, 111.
6 SILTZBACH L.E. (1976) *Ann NY Acad Sci* **278**, 665.

GENERAL MANIFESTATIONS OF SARCOIDOSIS [1, 4, 12, 15, 21, 22, 23]

There is no disease with more varied manifestations. Its course is unpredictable. Several years may separate one manifestation, e.g. lupus pernio, from another. A full history must include details of race, area of residence, details of any previous tuberculin test, BCG vaccination, industrial exposure to beryllium and any previous disease, such as erythema nodosum, that may be related, even distantly.

Any organ of the body may be involved—locally, sporadically or generally. Symptoms result from invasion and replacement, pressure, toxicity, anaemia, hypercalcaemia or pulmonary fibrosis. Pulmonary sarcoidosis has, by international convention, three stages:

Stage I. Bilateral hilar lymphadenopathy (BHL) alone (present in 51% of 3,676 subjects in a world-wide survey).

Stage II. BHL with parenchymal lung involvement of fine 'fluffy' or coarse type.

Stage III. The late stage of pulmonary infiltration with fibrosis and evidence of physiological pulmonary insufficiency.

The extra-pulmonary manifestations of sarcoidosis cannot be staged in this way, though some generalizations are possible. Erythema nodosum, *par excellence*, is an early feature, occurring in Stage I and carrying a good prognosis. Iridocyclitis and anterior uveitis are usually associated with the later stages and more persistent forms of the disease. The

TABLE 48.3. Involvement of various organs in sarcoidosis
(Adapted from James D.G., *et al* (1976) *Ann NY Acad Sci* **278**, 327)

Centre	No. in series	Organs affected (%)						
		Skin*	Eyes	Parotid glands	Lymph nodes	Spleen	CNS
London	537	25	27	6	29	12	7
Reading	425	13	16	5	27	3	9
Edinburgh	502	7	11	5	33	6	3
New York	311	19	20	8	37	18	4
Paris	350	12	11	6	23	9	4
Tokyo	282	12	32	5	23	1	4
Novi Sad	285	4	15	2·5	12	2·5	1·4
Geneva	121	6	12	2	11	6	1

*Excluding erythema nodosum.

best the dermatologist can do is to assess carefully the extent of the involvement of organs other than the skin and to classify as 'early' (e.g. erythema nodosum and BHL), 'intermediate' (e.g. papular and nodular forms), or 'late' (e.g. plaque, subcutaneous or lupus pernio forms). However, the prognosis and need for treatment will always depend on the functional and destructive effect of the disease in other organs and these may not always be clinically apparent until treatment is too late to be effective. Of this disease it has been aptly said, 'one of its most singular details ... is the frequency of its clinical silence'.

The extent of extrapulmonary involvement varies greatly from country to country and even within the same country.

General symptoms. The onset is frequently marked by lethargy, loss of weight and general malaise; but it may be symptomless. A dry cough, dyspnoea and chest pain are present in half the patients.

Reticulo-endothelial system. The lymphatic glands are involved in one-fifth to one-third of all cases; higher figures have been reported, especially in Negroes [18, 21]. The accessible right scalene node may be palpable [21]. Enlargement of the liver and spleen is present at some stage in 5–40% of patients [21].

Pulmonary changes [12, 21, 32]. These dominate the second and third stages of the disease, and progressive diminution of respiratory function is the most common cause of incapacity and morbidity. There is now a considerable literature covering all aspects of pulmonary sarcoidosis and the reader is referred to the proceedings of the recent international symposia for details, which lie outside the scope of this chapter. All patients who show clinical or radiographic evidence of pulmonary involvement should be referred to a chest physician who will have to make a vital decision on the need for and timing of treatment. The transition from Stage II to Stage III of pulmonary sarcoidosis is often imperceptible unless repeated studies of respiratory function are carried out. The diffuse parenchymal involvement that occurs in a minority of patients with the BHL-EN syndrome may often resolve but always demands careful follow-up. Progressive fibrosis is first shown by coarse strands in the middle zones. Emphysema and cor pulmonale occur in the late stages. Symptoms may at first be trivial and dyspnoea on exertion may be a late sign of irreversible damage. Lupus pernio is particularly likely to have associated lung changes [13].

Nervous system [6, 14, 21]. This was involved in 4% of 3,676 patients [5], but in only 5 of 401 patients seen in a general hospital in the U.K. [19]. A wide variety of syndromes may result [21], including meningo-encephalitis or multiple sclerosis-like changes. The *VIIth* nerve is frequently affected [24], with or without Heerfordt's syndrome. Involvement of the hypothalamus is rare but important [4]. It presents as diabetes insipidus, hypopituitarism, ocular nerve involvement [29] or other hypothalamic syndromes [5, 6, 30] or endocrine abnormalities [31]. The prolactin level may be elevated. Liver biopsies are useful in diagnosis. Corticosteroids are variable in their effect.

Bone changes [10, 11, 20, 27]. Being symptomless, these are seldom found unless specifically sought [4]. They were reported in only 3% of 3,676 cases in the literature [15] but were found in 8·5% of 260 patients routinely examined radiologically [19]. Classically, they involve the small bones of the hands and feet in middle-aged females with lupus pernio [20]. The most common change is lysis with bone cysts; other destructive lesions are less common. The nasal bones (p. 1773), and occasionally the calvarium, are involved, mimicking metastases [2, 33]. The bone marrow has also been affected [15, 21].

Joints [1, 9, 16, 26]. These are affected more frequently than the literature suggests. An acute polyarthralgia accompanies, or may precede the onset of erythema nodosum and is seldom reported though it may be severe enough to suggest rheumatic fever. A less widespread chronic polyarthritis appears later in the disease, chiefly in blacks. Epithelioid granulomas are found on synovial biopsy [1, 25]. An unusual tenosynovitis has been reported [3].

Skeletal muscles [3, 32]. Clinical involvement is rarely detected. The proximal limb muscles are chiefly affected and, if there are no other signs of sarcoidosis, a diagnosis of dermatomyositis or muscular dystrophy may be made. Deep subcutaneous granulomas have been described [8] and may be more common if sought; they are usually asymptomatic.

Cardiac involvement. The importance of myocardial sarcoidosis lies in its capacity to cause heart block and arrhythmias or even sudden death. The patients are often young. It may be clinically silent and only revealed at post-mortem. Other signs of sarcoidosis may be minimal but it is more common than was previously believed [28], and particularly so in the Japanese, though an abnormal ECG was found in 14% of 401 patients examined routinely in the U.K. [19]. Matsui [17] analysed 42 fatal cases. In a recent study of 128 cases of myocardial sarcoidosis [7], there was no sex predominance and most patients were white. Over half had heart block of some degree and 20 had died suddenly before diagnosis. The lungs were involved in 45 cases, the skin in 29. The diagnosis should be suspected in any unusual heart disease and a careful cardiac examination should be a routine procedure in all cases of established sarcoidosis.

Other organs. Lesions of the stomach and larynx have been reported. It is evident that no organ is exempt from the occasional deposit of sarcoidal granuloma and the dermatologist, as much as the general physician, should attempt to delineate the full extent of the disease in all patients under his care. In no disease is it more important to look continuously 'under the skin' for other signs.

REFERENCES

1 BIANCHI F.A. & KEECH M.K. (1964) *Ann Rheum Dis* **23**, 463.
2 BODIE B.F., *et al* (1980) *J Am Acad Dermatol* **3**, 401.
3 BURNS D.A. & SARKANY I. (1978) *Clin Exp Dermatol* **3**, 439.
4 CALANDRA P. & STOCCHI F. (1982) *La Malattia di Besnier–Boeck–Schaumann. Ann Ital Derm Clin Sper* **36**, 111–200.
5 CAMPBELL I.W., *et al* (1980) *VIIIth Int Conf Sarc*. Cardiff, Alpha Omega, p. 579.
6 DELANEY P. (1977) *Ann Intern Med* **87**, 336.
7 FLEMING H.A. (1980) *VIIIth Int Conf Sarc*. Cardiff, Alpha Omega, p. 493.
8 GROSS M.D., *et al* (1977) *Arch Dermatol* **113**, 1442.
9 GUMPEL J.M., *et al* (1967) *Ann Rheum Dis* **26**, 194.
10 HOLT J.A. & OWENS W.I. (1949) *Radiology* **53**, 11.
11 ISRAEL H.L. & SONES M. (1956) *Arch Intern Med* **102**, 766.
12 *JAMES D.G. (1959) *Q J Med* **28**, 109.
13 JAMES D.G. (1977) *Rec Progr Med* **63**, 181.
14 JAMES D.G. & SHARMA O.P. (1967) *Proc R Soc Med* **60**, 1169.
15 *JAMES D.G., *et al* (1976) *Ann NY Acad Sci* **278**, 327.
16 KAPLAN H. (1963) *Arch Intern Med* **112**, 924.
17 MATSUI Y., *et al* (1976) *Ann NY Acad Sci* **278**, 455.
18 *MAYOCK R.L., *et al* (1963) *Am J Med* **35**, 67.
19 MICKHAIL J.R. (1980) *VIIIth Int Conf Sarc*. Cardiff, Alpha Omega, p. 532.
20 NEVILLE E., *et al* (1976) *Ann NY Acad Sci* **278**, 475.
21 SCADDING J.G. & MITCHELL D.N. (1985) *Sarcoidosis*. 2nd ed. London, Chapman & Hall
22 *SHARMA O.P. (1975) *Sarcoidosis*, Springfield, Thomas.
23 SILVERSTEIN A. & SILTZBACH L.E. (1969) *Arch Neurol (Chicago)* **21**, 235.
24 SILVERSTEIN A., *et al* (1965) *Arch Neurol (Chicago)* **12**, 1.
25 SOKOLOFF L. & BUNIM J.J. (1959) *N Engl J Med* **260**, 841.
26 SPILBERG I., *et al* (1969) *Arth Rheum* **12**, 126.
27 STEIN G.N., *et al* (1956) *Arch Intern Med* **97**, 532.
28 STEIN E., *et al* (1976) *Ann NY Acad Sci* **278**, 470.
29 STUART G.A., *et al* (1978) *Ann Intern Med* **88**, 589.
30 VESELEY D.L., *et al* (1977) *Am J Med* **62**, 425.
31 WINNAKER J.L., *et al* (1968) *N Engl J Med* **278**, 48.
32 *WURM VON K., *et al* (1983) *Sarkodoise*, Stuttgart, G. Thieme.
33 ZIMMERMANN R. & LEEDS N. (1976) *Radiology* **119**, 384.

Ocular involvement [2, 3, 4, 13, 14]. The eyes are involved in 10–25% of patients with sarcoidosis [2, 9]. Some figures are higher, especially for London and Tokyo, where ocular lesions are particularly common [7, 12] and a major cause of uveitis [11]. In 278 out of 401 patients examined ophthalmologically in a U.K. general hospital, 41 had ocular involvement [8]. The very high figures in one series [7] included a number of peripheral fundal changes that might normally be disregarded. In 147 patients with ocular sarcoidosis, James [4] found intrathoracic lesions in 75% and erythema nodosum in 26%. Skin plaques were present in one-third. Three-quarters of the patients had acute or chronic anterior uveitis and 23% had conjunctival involvement.

Though anterior uveitis is the best known form of ocular sarcoidosis, any part of the visual system may be involved before, during or after other manifestations of the disease, of which it is sometimes the only manifestation. Symptomless lachrymal gland involvement is common and underdiagnosed [3]. Lachrymal gland biopsies are frequently diagnositic. Black races are more often affected.

The main types of ocular involvement are:

(a) *Uveitis.* Anterior and posterior uveitis are the most important and serious manifestations. Acute and chronic forms occur. *Anterior uveitis*, usually bilateral, and more prevalent in females, was found in 20% of cases of sarcoidosis in one series [9] and in 7.8% in another [6]. Though often seen in young adults, it can occur in infancy and old age, when the correct diagnosis is frequently overlooked [3].

Chronic uveitis more commonly affects older women and has a chronic and insidious course. Granulomatous nodules occur on the iris, and synechiae and lens opacities form and, if untreated, glaucoma, cataracts and blindness may ensue.

(b) *Retinochoroiditis* usually occurs with chronic uveitis [6, 8].

(c) *Conjunctivitis.* Conjunctival nodules are common and should be biopsied [6, 8]. Even 'blind' biopsies may reveal the disease. 'Millet seed' nodules may involve the eyelid margins.

(d) *Dacryostenosis* occurred in only 2% of 281 patients [6].

(e) *Keratoconjunctivitis sicca.* Diminished lachrymal gland secretion was present in 38% tested in one series [7].

(f) *Calcium deposits* with hypercalcaemia [9].

(g) *Optic nerve lesions* [5, 10]. These occur either as part of a widespread involvement of the CNS or as unilateral retrobulbar disease. Papilloedema, retrobulbar neuritis and optic atrophy may result. Eyelid swelling is probably due to lymphatic involvement [1].

(h) *Tumours.* Sarcoidosis is a rare cause of orbital tumours in elderly women [6, 9].

Ocular syndromes

(i) Erythema nodosum, bilateral hilar lymphadenopathy and acute iridocyclitis.

(ii) Lupus pernio, chronic iridocyclitis, bone cysts and pulmonary fibrosis.

(iii) Keratoconjunctivitis sicca with parotid and lachrymal gland enlargement (Sjögren's syndrome without arthritis).

(iv) Bell's palsy, parotitis and anterior uveitis (*Heerfordt's syndrome*, see below).

REFERENCES

1 DIESTELMEIER M.R., *et al* (1982) *Arch Dermatol* **118**, 356.
2 JAMES D.G. (1974) *J R Coll Phys* **9**, 63.
3 JAMES D.G., *et al* (1964) *Br J Ophthalmol* **48**, 461.
4 JAMES D.G., *et al* (1976) *Ann NY Acad Sci* **278**, 321.
5 JAMPOL L.M., *et al* (1972) *Arch Ophthalmol* **87**, 355.
6 KARMA A. (1979) *Acta Ophthalmol* (Suppl.) **141**, 1.
7 KOBAYASHI F. (1974) *Proc VIIIth Conf Sarc.* Tokyo, Univ. Tokyo Press, p. 349.
8 NIKHAIL J.R. (1980) *VIIIth Int Conf Carc.* Cardiff, Alpha Omega, p. 532.
9 OBENAUF C.D., *et al* (1978) *Am J Ophthalmol*
10 SCADDING J.G. & MITCHELL D.N. (1985) *Sarcoidosis.* 2nd ed. London, Chapman & Hall, pp 207–226.
11 URICH H. (1976) *Ann NY Acad Sci* **278**, 406.
12 UYAMA M. (1971) *Jpn J Clin Ophthalmol* **25**, 1513.
13 UYAMA M. (1974) *Proc VIth Int Conf Sarc.* Tokyo, Univ. Tokyo Press, p. 354.
14 WURM VON K. (1983) *Sarkoidose.* Stuttgart, G. Thieme, p. 173.

Parotid gland involvement [1, 7]. Clinically obvious parotid gland sarcoidosis is relatively uncommon [3, 6] but subclinical and histological involvement is more frequent. Xerostomia may accompany it.

The affected glands fluctuate in size from day to day but eventually subside. Mikulicz's syndrome probably includes a number of aetiological entities but the oculosalivary syndrome of sarcoidosis has an obvious affinity with Sjögren's syndrome in its sex and age incidence and its behaviour.

Heerfordt's syndrome [2, 5]. Uveo-parotid fever is a rare manifestation of sarcoidosis, chiefly affecting young adults and occurring as a presenting or subsequent granulomatous involvement of the uveal tract with parotid gland enlargement, fever and facial and other cranial nerve palsies. The last two features were present in only 50% of 15 cases observed in Northern Sweden [5]. Hilar lymphadenopathy or other organ involvement [4] was present in almost every case. Aptyalism has been reported [3] and sialometry may be of help in diagnosis [5]. Tissue biopsies will confirm sarcoidosis.

REFERENCES

1 *COWDELL R.H. (1954) *Q J Med* **23**, 29.
2 GARLAND H.G. & THOMPSON J.G. (1933) *Q J Med* **2**, 157.
3 GREENBERG G., *et al* (1964) *Br Med J* ii, 861.
4 ROSS J.A. (1955) *Br Med J* ii, 593.
5 *STJERNBERG N. & WIMAN L.G. (1974) *Proc VIth Int Conf Sarc.* Tokyo, Univ. Tokyo Press, p. 331.
6 TURIAF J., (1975) *Rev Fr Tuberc Mal Respir* **3**, 271.
7 TURIAF J. & BATTESTI J.P. (1976) *Ann NY Acad Sci* **278**, 401.

Renal involvement [2, 3, 5]. Clinical symptoms are rare but renal involvement can be more commonly found if looked for. Proliferative or membranous nephritis may occur [3, 6]. Renal failure may be caused by hypercalcaemia nephropathy or by direct granulomatous invasion [1, 4]. Renal involvement with hypercalcaemia is an indication for aggressive therapy [6].

REFERENCES

1 COBURN J.W., *et al* (1967) *Am J Med* **42**, 273.
2 *LEBACQ E., *et al* (1970) *Postgrad Med J* **46**, 526.
3 MIKAMI R., *et al* (1979) *Proc Int Symp Sarc.* Tokyo, Univ. Tokyo Press, p. 109.
4 OGILVIE R.L., *et al* (1964) *Ann Intern Med* **61**, 711.
5 SCADDING J.G. & MITCHELL D.N. (1985) *Sarcoidosis.* 2nd ed. London, Chapman & Hall, pp 390–413.
6 TEILUM G. (1964) *Acta Med Scand* (Suppl.) **425**, 14.

Hypercalcaemia and hypercalciuria. The frequency of hypercalcaemia varies greatly in different series; figures of 2–40% are quoted [2, 5, 6], but usually in the middle range of these extremes [1]. It appears to be more frequent in the U.S.A. than in the U.K.

[9]. It is less common than hypercalciuria, which may be found in 30–60% of patients at some stage of the disease [7, 8], but only in 7.5% of 56 patients in one British series [3]. It is usually a later finding and a more significant one. Hypercalciuria may be due to increased intestinal absorption, resorption from bone or a 'renal leak' in tubular reabsorption [8]. The basic defect causing hypercalcaemia may be a hypersensitivity to low doses of vitamin D with hyperabsorption of intestinal calcium. It is aggravated following exposure to UVR by conversion of the provitamin 7-dehydrocholesterol into vitamin D_3. Other possible mechanisms have been postulated [1]. Difficulties in assessing levels of hypercalciuria are partly due to the problems of imposing a suitable diet.

Persistent hypercalcaemia can result in nephrocalcinosis and renal failure. It has been suggested [4] that it may correlate closely with disease activity. Clinically, it is manifested by polyuria, nocturia or polydipsia in the absence of hypertension or overt signs of renal damage. Corticosteroids reduce the level to normal. Parathyroid values are usually normal [3].

REFERENCES

1 FALK E.S. & VIK T. (1980) *Acta Derm Venereol (Stockh)* **60**, 179.
2 GOLDSTEIN R.A., *et al* (1971) *Am J Med* **51**, 21.
3 HANDSLIP P.D., *et al* (1976) *Proc VIIIth Int Conf Sarc.* Cardiff, Alpha Omega, p. 225.
4 JAMES D.G., *et al* (1976) *Semin Arth Rheum* **6**, 53.
5 JAMES D.G., *et al* (1976) *Ann NY Acad Sci* **278**, 321.
6 JAMES D.G. & CARSTAIRS L.S. (1982) *Hospital Update*, **8**, 1022.
7 LEBACQ E.G., *et al* (1970) *Postgrad Med J* **46**, 526.
8 LEBACQ E.G., *et al* (1980) *Proc VIIIth Int Conf Sarc.* Cardiff, Alpha Omega, p. 215.
9 SCADDING J.G. (1976) *Ann NY Acad Sci* **278**, 488.

Sarcoidosis in children. The disease is uncommon in children and rare in young children [3, 7, 8, 9]. Out of more than 3,000 cases of sarcoidosis in the literature, only 104 patients were under 15 years of age; only 19 of these were younger than 6 years [7]. Over a 20-year period, only 117 cases were reported in children in the U.S.A. [2]. Most of those affected were from 9 to 15 years old. However, symptomless cases may not, as in adults, be revealed by routine radiography [6].

The early manifestations of sarcoidosis in children are diverse and the cause of considerable diagnostic difficulty; much depends on clinical acumen and the diagnostic facilities available. The most common presentation is one of general malaise and lethargy [5]. In a recent survey [2], different patterns were apparent in the young and in the older children. A characteristic trend was for skin lesions, uveitis and arthritis to predominate in the former [4, 8], whereas lung and lymph node involvement were more common in the latter. Uveitis and keratitis were common in both groups. Hypercalcaemia and hypercalciuria are also common [1] in older children.

REFERENCES

1 APPLEYARD W.J. (1976) *Proc R Soc Med* **69**, 345.
2 HETHERINGTON S. (1982) *Am J Dis Child* **136**, 13.
3 KENDIG E.L. JR (1974) *Pediatrics* **54**, 289.
4 KENDIG E.L. JR (1982) *Am J Dis Child* **136**, 11.
5 KENDIG E.L. JR & BRUMMER D.L. (1976) *Chest* **70**, 351.
6 Leading Article (1977) *Lancet* i, 737.
7 McGOVERN J.P. & MERRITT D.H. (1956) *Adv Pediatr* **8**, 97.
8 RASMUSSEN J.E. (1981) *J Am Acad Dermatol* **5**, 566.
9 SILTZBACH L.E. & GREENBERG G.M. (1968) *N Engl J Med* **279**, 1239.

Recurrent sarcoidosis. While relapse on reduction of steroid therapy is well recognized, recurrence after spontaneous healing is very rare [1, 3]. In a unique case [2] three separate episodes of erythema nodosum and pulmonary sarcoidosis occurred.

REFERENCES

1 LIM K.H. (1961) *Tubercle* **42**, 350.
2 MACFARLANE J.T. (1981) *Postgrad Med J* **57**, 525.
3 SYMMONS D.P.M. & WOODS K.L. (1980) *Thorax* **35**, 879.

ASSOCIATED DISEASES

A number of diseases have been reported in association with sarcoidosis. Some are understandable against the background of depressed immunological responses; some are due to simple blocking of the activity of an organ by granulomatous infiltration; and others are uncommon associations, doubtless published for their interest and rarity. In a disease as common as sarcoidosis a coincidental association can be expected to occur from time to time.

Infections. A critical review of previous reports of invasive fungal infections such as cryptococcosis [23] has suggested that in many of these the entire cause of the granulomatous illness was infectious, rather than sarcoidosis with complicating infection. In the series which accompanied the review 122 patients with sarcoidosis were found to be remarkably free of infections: three had aspergillus mycetomata in cystic areas in the lung, and another also had pulmonary tuberculosis, but the only extrathoracic infection was in one patient who had disseminated zoster [23]. Patients with sarcoidosis, however, do seem liable to extensive and stubborn wart virus infections, despite an unusually high prevalence of circulating antibodies to wart antigen [19].

Immunologically mediated conditions. Thyroid disorders have frequently been reported but only some of these have been immunological [10]. In a series of 190 female patients with sarcoidosis, four had hyperthyroidism and four had Hashimoto's thyroiditis with antibodies [11]. Another patient in the same series had myxoedema and Addison's disease. We have also seen sarcoidosis associated with vitiligo on three occasions but it has not been established that the relationship is other than coincidental. Sarcoidosis also developed in a 56-year-old woman 9 months after the onset of mixed connective tissue disease. Chronic urticaria was found [6] to be more frequent than expected but our own experience does not support this.

The effects of infiltration. Granulomas, especially in the pituitary or thyroid, may cause endocrine disease which obscures the primary cause. Thus invasion of the thyroid may be without effect or, if massive, can cause hypothyroidism [4, 11]. Cushing's syndrome and diabetes insipidus, secondary to involvement of the pituitary, have been reported [5, 16]. The list of such cases may be extended to cover most endocrine diseases.

Malignancy. Of 2,544 patients with respiratory sarcoidosis studied in Denmark [3], 48 developed a malignant tumour, one-third more than the expected rate, including a higher number of cases of lung cancer and of malignant lymphoma (11 cases). There have also been isolated reports of an association with mycosis fungoides [13, 17].

Granuloma annulare and necrobiosis lipoidica. Granuloma annulare is important in the differential diagnosis of sarcoidosis; the two diseases coexisted in five patients [21]. We have seen this association in one of two sisters with familial sarcoidosis [22]. However, patients with granuloma annulare have negative Kveim tests [9, 20]. Lesions resembling necrobiosis of the scalp have been reported in systemic sarcoidosis [1], but this may have been coincidental. We have also seen proven sarcoidosis with persistent necrobiosis lipoidica of the legs.

Other associations. Associations with thrombocytopenia [8], psoriasis and gout [7] and secondary syphilis [14] have been reported but seem likely to have been coincidental. An acquired ichthyosis has been noted [2]. Two Kveim-positive patients were found to have primary biliary cirrhosis [12] Two cases of porphyria cutanea tarda have also been reported [15, 18]; one had a positive Kveim test and improved with prednisolone [18].

REFERENCES

1 Anderson K.E. (1977) *Acta Derm Venereol (Stockh)* **57**, 367.
2 Braverman I.M. (1970) *Skin Signs of Systemic Diseases.* Philadelphia, Saunders, p. 279.
3 Brincker H. & Wilbeck E. (1974) *Br J Cancer* **29**, 247.
4 Cohen J.D. (1974) *Proc R Soc Med* **70**, 897.
5 Cowdell R.D. (1954) *Q J Med* **23**, 29.
6 Doeglas H.M.G. (1975) *Chronic Urticaria.* Thesis, Groningen, Druk Rijkstr. Niemager, p. 86.
7 Ecks L. (1975) *Hautarzt* **26**, 357.
8 Edwards M.H., *et al* (1952) *Ann Intern Med* **37**, 803.
9 Harrison P. & Shuster S. (1979) *Br J Dermatol* **100**, 231.
10 Karlish A.J. (1972) *La Sarcoidose.* Ed. Gallopin Y. Geneva, Hallow, pp. 147–150.
11 Karlish A.J. & MacGregor G.A. (1970) *Lancet* ii, 330.
12 Karlish A.J., *et al* (1969) *Lancet* ii, 599.
13 Kaugh Y., *et al* (1977) *Arch Dermatol* **113**, 1138.
14 Laughier P. (1976) *Arch Dermatol* **112**, 261.
15 Lockman D.S. (1980) *J Am Acad Dermatol* **2**, 62.
16 McDaniel W.E., *et al* (1970) *Arch Dermatol* **101**, 356.
17 McFarland J.P., *et al* (1978) *Arch Dermatol* **114**, 912.
18 Mann R.J. & Harman R.R.M. (1982) *Clin Exp Dermatol* **7**, 619.
19 Morison W.L. (1975) *Br J Dermatol* **93**, 717.
20 Rhodes E.L. (1979) *Br J Dermatol* **100**, 23.
21 Umbert P. & Winkelmann R.K. (1977) *Br J Dermatol* **97**, 48.
22 Wilkinson J.D. (1983) Personal communication.
23 Winterbauer R.H. & Kraemer K.G. (1976) *Arch Intern Med* **136**, 356.

Vasculitis with sarcoidosis. There have been occasional but well-authenticated reports of cutaneous vasculitis occurring in the course of sarcoidosis, usually early in the disease. Erythema nodosum itself may, of course, be regarded as a form of vasculitis. We have seen purpura of the legs and symptoms of Sjögren's syndrome precede scar infiltration and hilar lymphadenopathy in a 56-year-old woman. Macular erythematous lesions also preceded uveitis, parotitis and early pulmonary fibrosis in another Kveim-positive case [4]. Foci of epithelioid cell granulomas were centred on damaged dermal vessels which showed fibrinoid necrosis and deposition of C3. Another case presented with erythroderma and ulceration [6]. An apparently unique case of leukocytoclastic vasculitis associated with epithelioid cell granulomas has also been described [2]. There are several other reports of fibrinoid necrosis and hyaline degeneration of the capillaries, but not all patients have been investigated immunologically. Annular forms have also been recorded [1, 5].

The occurrence of vasculitis supports the view that circulating immune complexes may be found in the early stages of sarcoidosis, especially when the ESR is considerably raised [3, 7].

REFERENCES

1 BRANFORD W.A., *et al* (1982) *Br J Dermatol* **106**, 713.
2 CHOUVET B., *et al* (1980) *Ann Derm Vénéréol* (Paris) **107**, 279.
3 JOHNSON N.McI., *et al* (1980) *Thorax* **35**, 286.
4 KENNEDY C. (1979) *Br J Dermatol* **101** (Suppl. 17), 47.
5 MILLER J.A. & JOHNSON N.McI. (1983) *Br J Dermatol* **108**, 123.
6 SIMPSON J.R. (1963) *Br J Dermatol* **75**, 193.
7 VERRIER JONES J., *et al* (1976) *Ann NY Acad Sci* **278**, 212.

SARCOIDOSIS OF THE SKIN
[4, 8, 10, 12]

Between 20% and 35% of patients with systemic sarcoidosis have skin lesions [8]. With the exception of erythema nodosum the skin tends to be involved later than the other organs. However, cutaneous sarcoidosis can also occur without systemic abnormalities: in 6 of 13 patients, with cutaneous sarcoidosis but without a past history of sarcoidosis, no other systemic signs of the disease were detected during prolonged follow-up [9]. The cutaneous forms of sarcoidosis predominantly affect females [10], and the average age of onset is in the fourth to fifth decades.

Classification. The classification of cutaneous sarcoidosis has been distorted by eponyms that are no longer appropriate, and a simpler morphological classification should be adopted (Table 48.4). More than one type of lesion may exist at the same time, the differences between the main patterns lying in the manner and extent of the involvement of the skin or subcutaneous tissues. Erythema nodosum and lupus pernio have a special significance and should be retained as entities.

Clinical features. The features of the cutaneous lesions arise from the dense accumulation of epithelioid-cell granulomas in the dermis. In the

TABLE 48.4. Classification of sarcoidosis of the skin

Type of cutaneous lesions	Stage of disease
Erythema nodosum	Acute ('benign')
Erythematous and erythemato-papular	Acute and subacute
'Scar sarcoidosis'	Acute and subacute
Papular ('small nodular') (Boeck) Lichenoid variety	Acute and subacute
Erythrodermic (Schaumann)	Subacute and chronic
Nodular	Subacute and chronic
Annular (or circinate)	
Angiolupoid (Brocq–Pautrier)	
Subcutaneous	
Plaque	Chronic
Lupus pernio	
Miscellaneous	Usually chronic
Ulcerative, psoriasiform, palmo-plantar, ungual, mucosal, etc.	
Sarcoidosis of American Negro	

deep nodular and infiltrative types the subcutaneous tissue is involved by extension. The lesions are generally recognizable as firm soft nodules or plaques with a greater degree of infiltration than would be expected from their surface appearance. The colour ranges from yellow ochre to a livid violaceous hue which is most marked in lupus pernio. On diascopy a pale yellowish-grey colour remains; sometimes individual nodules are apparent. There is a tendency to form annular lesions. The epidermis is rarely affected, except for a light scaling, but some degree of vascular dilatation is frequent, especially in angio-lupoid. Scarring is unusual except in the papular and annular forms.

There is no characteristic distribution, though the small nodular type tends to involve the extensor aspects of the limbs, and rarely the trunk, while the large nodular type affects predominantly the face, hands and trunk. There appear to be differences in the manifestations of the disease in different countries: mucosal involvement, for instance, is rare in France but common in Scandinavia.

Erythema nodosum (p. 1156). The early stage of sarcoidosis is frequently associated with erythema nodosum, especially in young females. Of 200 patients with sarcoidosis, 31% had erythema nodosum and 33% other cutaneous forms of the disease [10]. Other authors give higher [11] or lower [15] figures, no doubt depending on their selection of racial material. In a series in south-east England, 35% of cases of erythema nodosum seen in 2 years were found to have sarcoidosis [17]. The prognosis is good, most cases resolving completely within 2 years.

'Scar sarcoidosis' (Fig. 48.4). Sarcoidosis appearing in scars may be the only cutaneous sign and is therefore of diagnostic value. It must be separated from local sarcoid granuloma formation in the absence of disease elsewhere. Long-standing scars, usually on the knees, become inflamed and infiltrated, giving rise to typical purplish-red lesions which turn brown as they fade. There is some resemblance to a cheloid but the lesions do not itch and the infiltrate is smoother and more regular. This form of sarcoidosis is as common in men as in women [13].

Scar sarcoidosis occurs in three situations:

1. In the acute eruptive phase, following erythema nodosum, or in the scars of biopsies taken at this time.
2. At any later stage of the disease; it was the only cutaneous sign in 6/23 patients [10]. In three, exacerbation of the disease was always preceded by this warning sign.

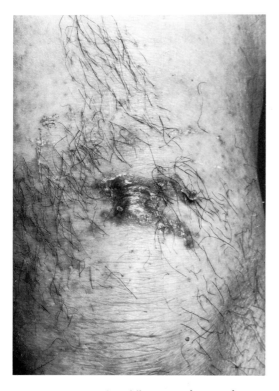

Fig. 48.4. Scar sarcoidosis following erythema nodosum (Wycombe General Hospital).

3. At inoculation sites, e.g. BCG or tuberculin tests. We have also seen it at venepuncture sites.

The histology is typical. Confirmatory evidence of sarcoidosis should be sought by chest X-rays, and other organ biopsy or the Kveim test.

Papular (small nodular type) [1, 2] (Figs 48.5 and 48.6). The papules are hemispherical and vary in size from a pinhead to a pea. Orange or yellowish-brown at first, they later become brownish-red or violaceous, indolent, painless and torpid. Only a few or several hundred lesions may appear, arising in crops but eventually becoming stationary. They particularly affect the face, especially in the Negro, and extensor aspects of the limbs, but rarely the trunk or mucous membranes.

On vitropression the lupoid grains are of a more opaque appearance and colour than those of lupus, resembling grains of sand. If probed with a needle they feel firm. When the lesions disappear they often leave a pale, yellowish-white or telangiectatic scar. Occasionally they become confluent, merging into an erythematous plaque. A ringed nummular configuration was present in the second of Schaumann's four cases [14].

Widely disseminated, hard, shotty subcutaneous papules can occur with the granulomas lying in the deep subcutaneous tissues and fascial planes. A lichenoid variety [1, 16], consisting of pinhead-sized yellowish lesions closely grouped in round or oval clusters and showing slight scaling, is discussed separately below. (It resembles lichen planus or lichen scrofulosorum, but the tuberculin test is negative, the course indolent and the histology characteristic. See lichenoid tuberculide p. 817.)

In general the papular type carries a more favourable prognosis than that of other types of infiltration. Confirmatory biopsy of other organs, or a Kveim test, should be carried out though this form may occur without other manifestations of the disease.

Histopathology. The infiltrate is in the high and mid-dermis. It may be hard to distinguish from acne agminata in which, however, caseation can be seen.

Differential diagnosis. The term 'disseminate miliary lupoid' emphasizes its resemblance to 'miliary tuberculosis of the face' which is no longer regarded in England as a tuberculide. The distribution, lack of necrosis, torpidity and persistence of papular sarcoidosis distinguishes it. Lupus erythematosus can be mimicked if the lesions become annular. Papular

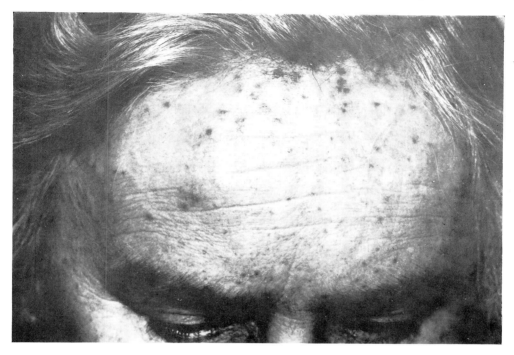

FIG. 48.5. Sarcoidosis. Multiple papules of the forehead (Addenbrooke's Hospital).

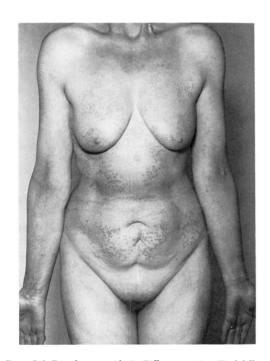

FIG. 48.6. Papular sarcoidosis. Diffuse eruption (Radcliffe Hospital).

forms of secondary syphilis are distinguished by the course and associated features of this disease.

Nodular forms (Fig. 48.7). Here the lesions are larger than a pea, usually single or relatively few, and remain circumscribed. Red or yellowish-red at first, but becoming violaceous or purplish-brown later, they are soft, or firm, round tumours affecting chiefly the proximal parts of the limbs, trunk and face. Dilated vessels may be seen on the surface of the lesions, which are extremely indolent. As they involute the centre may become depressed, and the lesions are eventually replaced by brownish telangiectatic marks, or yellowish-white atrophic and fibrotic patches. It is a rare presentation of the disease [3, 7].

Annular forms (Fig. 48.8). These are formed by peripheral evolution and central clearing. They occur particularly on the forehead, face and neck. The central area is depigmented and may be scarred. Ulceration is rare. The lesions may resemble annular necrobiosis of the scalp [6] but can be differentiated histologically. Diffuse papular forms may also show an annular configuration [12].

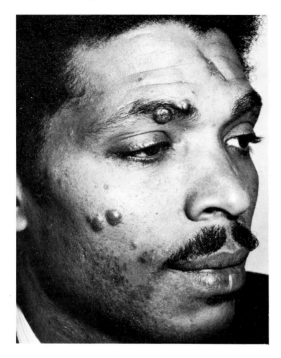

FIG. 48.7. Nodular sarcoidosis in a West Indian patient (Wycombe General Hospital).

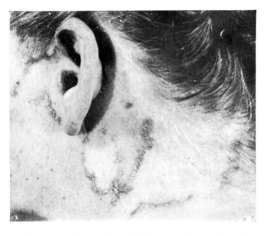

FIG. 48.8. Sarcoidosis. Annular lesions of the neck and cheek (Addenbrooke's Hospital).

Angiolupoid [2]. A rare but characteristic variety. It affects women predominantly, almost always occurring at the side of the bridge of the nose towards the corner of the eye, below the inner edge of the eyebrow, or on the adjacent area of the cheek. There are seldom more than two tumours.

They are soft and hemispherical, with a well-marked orange-red or reddish-brown colour and of a more livid hue than other forms. This is due to the marked telangiectatic vascular component which alters the normal grey-yellow appearance on diascopy. There is little tendency to spontaneous resolution.

Subcutaneous nodular sarcoidosis. This variety has been confused with other subcutaneous lesions showing a tuberculoid histology, particularly on the legs ('Darier—Roussy sarcoid' [5]). As long as the word 'sarcoid' is used morphologically, such difficulties will exist. But a true form of subcutaneous sarcoidosis occurs [13], and other signs of the disease are present. Lesions referred to as 'Darier–Roussy sarcoid' have shown a non-specific epithelioid-cell reaction in the subcutis for which other causes should be sought. The diagnosis of sarcoidosis depends on finding confirmatory evidence. This eponymous term should be abandoned.

Nodular subcutaneous infiltrations can occur with, or following, erythema nodosum [13]. These are fairly short-lived. Rarely, a profuse and much more indolent crop of lesions occurs later in the disease. The overlying skin is often normal [11].

Histopathology. The infiltrate is naturally greater than in nodular lesions but remains circumscribed. In the deep form it involves the subcutaneous tissue. In angiolupoid, vascular dilatation is prominent.

Differential diagnosis. The Spiegler–Fendt lymphoma and lymphocytoma cutis are separated by their histology. Four diseases cause particular difficulty in diagnosis and serial sectioning and cultures of biopsy material may be necessary. These are:

1. *Tuberculoid leprosy.* Distinguished by loss of thermal appreciation and of the histamine flare, a positive Mitsuda test and invasion of nerves.
2. *Lupus vulgaris.* In its exuberant form it can scarcely be distinguished. Vitropression is said to reveal more translucent nodules of an 'apple-jelly' rather than a greyish-yellow colour. Ulceration and scarring ultimately occur. Histology helps but does not decide: a therapeutic test does.
3. *Lupoid leishmaniasis.* The same difficulties exist clinically and histologically. Leishman–Donovan bodies are rarely found. The Kveim test is negative.
4. *Local sarcoid reaction.* By definition this is confined to local areas or sites of trauma. There

are no other signs of sarcoidosis and the Kveim test is negative.

REFERENCES

1 BOECK C. (1899) *J Cutan Genito-urin Dis* 17, 543.
2 BROCQ L. & PAUTRIER L.M. (1913) *Ann Dermatol Syphiligr* 4, 1.
3 CLAYTON R. & WOOD D. (1974) *Dermatologica* 149, 51.
4 CRONIN E. (1970) *Postgrad Med J* 46, 507.
5 DARIER J. & ROUSSY G. (1906) *Ann Med Exp* 18, 1.
6 DOWLING G.B. & WILSON JONES E. (1967) *Dermatologica* 135, 11.
7 GROSS M.D., *et al* (1977) *Arch Dermatol* 113, 1442.
8 HANNO R. & CALLEN J.P. (1980) *Med Clin North Am* 64, 847.
9 HANNO R., *et al* (1981) *Arch Dermatol* 117, 203.
10 *JAMES D.G. (1959) *Q J Med* 28, 109.
11 MARTEN R.H. & WARNER J. (1967) *Trans St John's Hosp Dermatol Soc* 53, 160.
12 RUSTIN M.H.A. (1984) Personal communication.
13 SCADDING J.G. & MITCHELL D.N. (1985) *Sarcoidosis*. 2nd ed. London, Chapman & Hall, pp 181–206.
14 SCHAUMANN J. (1936) *Br J Dermatol* 48, 399.
15 SONES M. & ISRAEL H.L. (1960) *Q J Med* 29, 84.
16 THAL M. (1955) *Dermatologica* 111, 87.
17 TURNER T.W. & WILKINSON D.S. (1971) Unpublished data.

The plaque form (diffuse sarcoidosis of the skin) (Fig. 48.9). It is convenient to keep this form distinct. It involves chiefly the limbs, shoulders, buttocks and thighs. The lesions are characteristically diffuse and extend farther than is apparent on the surface. They may form placards of an irregular shape with more superficial nodules superimposed, sometimes having a crescentic or serpiginous outline resembling tertiary lues. On the legs they may closely resemble necrobiosis lipoidica (Fig. 48.10). They are very persistent [2].

Lupus pernio [4, 10]. Large, soft, bluish-red and dusky violaceous, infiltrated nodules and plaques occur more or less symmetrically on the nose, cheeks, ears, fingers and hands (Fig. 48.11). Women, usually young or middle-aged, are affected six times as often as men [4]. The lesions feel soft, doughy or indurated. Discrete nodules, with the typical appearance on diascopy, may sometimes be found at the edge. The surface is often glistening, and the epidermis stretched, with large pilosebaceous follicles. Nasal involvement is associated with swelling, ulceration or crusting of the nasal vestibule and the patient may present with difficulty in breathing [6]. Ulceration rarely occurs in the skin; gross mutilation, as in lupus vulgaris, never. Involvement of the earlobes may be massive ('turkey-ears'). Scarring alopecia occurs on the scalp [2, 9]. Bone cysts and fusiform swellings of the fingers are present in 10–20% of patients [10], and the nails of affected fingers may become dystrophic [7].

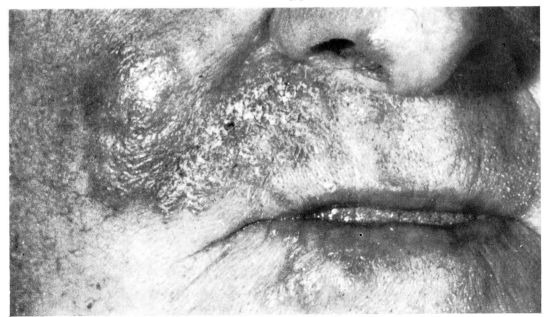

FIG. 48.9. Sarcoidosis—lesions of the plaque type.

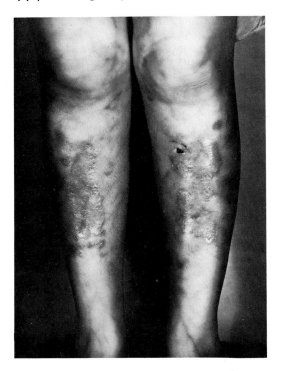

FIG. 48.10. Necrobiosis lipoidica-like lesions in a woman with parotitis and a positive Kveim test (Stoke Mandeville Hospital).

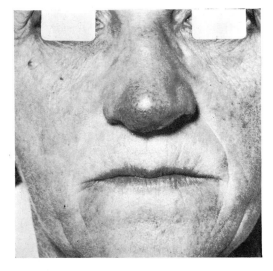

FIG. 48.11. Sarcoidosis: early lupus pernio of the nose. The nasal bones were eroded (Addenbrooke's Hospital).

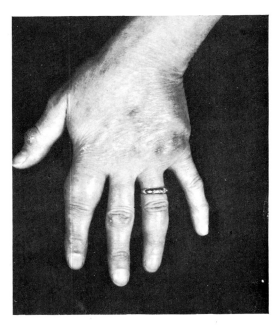

FIG. 48.12. Sarcoidosis. Typical fusiform appearance of the fingers from bone involvement (Dr H.R. Vickers, Radcliffe Infirmary).

Lupus pernio occurs in the chronic stage of sarcoidosis and is protracted, though the lesions occasionally resolve, sometimes with atrophy [3]. Despite the apparent predilection for the areas most susceptible to cold, there is no seasonal variation [6]. It is in this form of sarcoidosis that hyperglobulinaemia and hypercalcaemia may especially be found. Patients with lupus pernio often have sarcoidosis of the upper respiratory tract (SURT) though the two can exist separately: one-third of patients with lupus pernio have associated SURT, and SURT carries a 50% risk of developing lupus pernio [8]. Pulmonary infiltration is common. Iritis or posterior uveitis leading to blindness, or death from pulmonary or cardiac complications, may occur at any time.

Histopathology. This is typical. Nasal biopsies give the same information.

Differential diagnosis of nodular and plaque forms. The reticuloses, especially reticulosarcomas, may be indistinguishable. Granuloma faciale and granuloma annulare may be confused. The histology of the lesion and of other organs may be necessary to establish the diagnosis. Tertiary syphilis and lupus erythematosus (especially 'profundus') can cause difficulty. Lepromatous leprosy is more diffuse and symmetrical; eye changes are less frequent, and neural invasion is characteristic. The histopathology differs in detail.

Lupus pernio restricted to the nose and cheeks may be mistaken for rosacea but keratitis is not present and rosacea is seldom as fixed and infiltrated. 'Chilblain lupus' is also less infiltrated and shows scarring and telangiectasia: its colour is pinker. Lupus vulgaris is not symmetrical, usually less tumid, and more inclined to ulcerate and scar. The other manifestations of sarcoidosis are absent.

Maculopapular and erythematous forms. The papular form has been described above. Transient 'prodromal' maculopapular eruptions were noted in the early stages of sarcoidosis in no less than 8 of 33 patients who showed cutaneous signs of the disease [6] and are apparently seen more commonly by chest and general physicians. Diffuse forms of papular sarcoidosis do occur but in our experience are uncommon. Even less common are ill-defined patches of a lavender colour, sometimes slightly scaly or lightly infiltrated [3]. On the face, these simulate rosacea. Sand-like lupoid grains are sometimes seen on diascopy, but more frequently there is a diffuse yellow colouration. One such patient, a man of 39, also showed transient parotid swellings and hepatosplenomegaly [1]. Such cases pursue a long course, fluctuating in severity. Pruritic maculopapular lesions have been described [5, 10].

REFERENCES

1 BARNES H.M. & CALNAN C.D. (1975) *Proc R Soc Med* **68**, 651.
2 BLEEHEN S.S. (1969) *Proc R Soc Med* **62**, 348.
3 DEGOS R. (1981) *Dermatologie*. Paris, Flammaron.
4 Editorial (1977) *Br Med J* i, 930.
5 FONG Y.W. & SHARMA O.M. (1975) *Arch Dermatol* **111**, 362.
6 JAMES D.G. (1959) *Q J Med* **28**, 109.
7 MANN R.J. & ALLEN B.R. (1981) *Br J Dermatol* **105**, 599.
8 NEVILLE E., *et al* (1976) *Thorax* **31**, 660.
9 SCADDING J.G. & MITCHELL D.N. (1985) *Sarcoidosis*. 2nd ed. London, Chapman & Hall, pp. 194–195
10 SHARMA O.P. (1975) *Sarcoidosis. A Clinical Approach*. Springfield, Thomas.

UNUSUAL AND ATYPICAL FORMS

In addition to the 'classical forms' of the disease described above, a wide variety of unusual forms have been recorded, particularly in Negroes.

Erythrodermic sarcoidosis. This is extremely rare. Red scaling patches extend and merge into slightly infiltrated brownish-red sheets. Lymphadenopathy is usually pronounced. During resolution, typical papules and nodules may separate from the plaque, which gradually loses its infiltration and disappears. A reticulate yellowish stippling may be seen as it resolves.

A unique case was associated with periarteritis and ulceration [24]. A case resembling pityriasis rubra pilaris, with spiny follicular keratoses, micropapule formation, and generalized erythroderma, has been seen in a 6-year-old boy [18].

Ichthyosiform sarcoidosis. An ichthyosiform eruption has rarely been associated with sarcoidosis [6, 9, 13, 14]. Epithelioid cell granulomas are present in the dermis but the relation between the two conditions is unknown.

Atrophic and ulcerative forms. These are rare except in Negroes [12, 15, 21]. The nose and ears may be affected [20, 22]. An atrophic form resembling Pick–Herxheimer disease has been reported [3, 17]. Scarring alopecia [1, 4] is a rare consequence of scalp lesions, mostly in Negro women [10]. Atrophic and ulcerative forms have occurred together [2]. Ulceration has occurred on the fingers [5] but usually involves the legs [7, 11, 20]. Twenty-three cases were reviewed in 1977 [8] but other cases have occurred since [16, 21] and many are probably not reported. A remarkable case with widespread ulcerative lesions has recently been reported [19] (Fig. 48.13). The granuloma may be of necrotizing type [15], with caseation or minimal fibrinoid necrosis [11]. True primary vasculitic changes are usually absent but secondary vascular damage may be present. The ulcer usually occurs late in the disease and often in association with nodular or verrucous lesions [21].

Verrucous forms [23]. Papular lesions may progress to crusted verrucous and, sometimes, ulcerative lesions [11] which may mimic halogen eruptions, fungal infections or tuberculosis.

REFERENCES

1 BAKER H. (1965) *Proc R Soc Med* **58**, 243.
2 BAZEX A. (1970) *Br J Dermatol* **83**, 255.
3 BAZEX A. (1971) *Ann Soc Fr Dermatol Syphiligr* **98**, 401.
4 BLEEHEN S.S. (1969) *Proc R Soc Med* **62**, 348.
5 BOYD R.E. & ANDREWS B.S. (1981) *J Rheumatol* **8**, 311.
6 BRAVERMAN I.M. (1970) *Signs of Systemic Disease*. Philadelphia, W.B. Saunders, pp. 274–285.
7 BROOKIN R.H. (1969) *Acta Derm Venereol (Stockh)* **49**, 584.

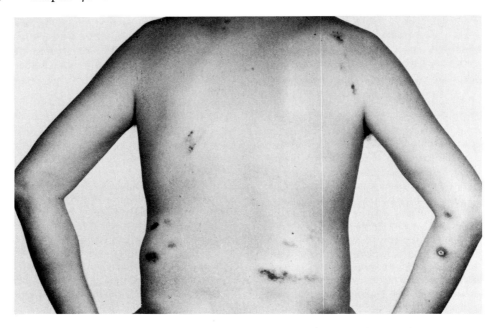

FIG. 48.13. Ulcerative sarcoidosis. Note surrounding hypopigmentation (St Bartholomew's Hospital).

8 CHEVRANT-BRETON J., *et al* (1977) *Ann Dermatol Vénéréol (Paris)* **104,** 805.
9 ELGART M.L. (1965) *Cutis* **1,** 283.
10 GOLITZ L.E., *et al* (1973) *Arch Dermatol* **107,** 758.
11 HERZLINGER D.C. (1979) *Cutis* **23,** 569.
12 IRGANG S. (1955) *Br J Dermatol* **67,** 255.
13 KAUH Y.C., *et al* (1978) *Ann Dermatol* **114,** 100.
14 KELLY A.P. (1978) *Arch Dermatol* **114,** 1551.
15 KLAUDER J.V. & WEIDMAN R.D. (1935) *Arch Dermatol* **31,** 421.
16 MEYERS M. & BARSKY S. (1978) *Arch Dermatol* **114,** 447.
17 MICHEL P.J., *et al* (1968) *Lyon Méd* **220,** 533.
18 MORRISON J.G.L. (1976) *Br J Dermatol* **95,** 93.
19 RUSTIN M.H.R. (1984) Personal communication.
20 SCHNIFFER J. & SHARMA O.P. (1977) *Arch Dermatol* **112,** 676.
21 SCHWARTZ R.A., *et al* (1982) *Arch Dermatol* **118,** 931.
22 *SHARMA O.P. (1975) *Sarcoidosis. A Clinical Approach.* Springfield, Thomas.
23 SHMUNES J. & SHARMA O.P. (1970) *Arch Dermatol* **102,** 665.
24 SIMPSON J.R. (1963) *Br J Dermatol* **75,** 193.

Lichenoid forms (Fig. 48.14). These are said to constitute 1–2% of skin sarcoidosis [4] and may pose difficulties in diagnosis [10]. Though more common in females, an eruptive form of sudden onset, consisting of closely-set shiny lichenoid papules, confluent in places, was described in two middle-aged males with no radiological evidence of pulmonary disease [5]. The appearances resembled those of

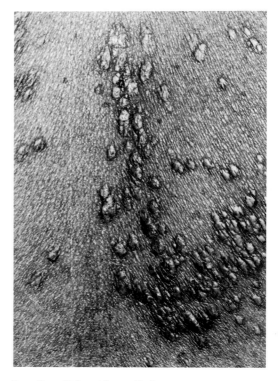

FIG. 48.14. Lichenoid sarcoidosis.

lichen scrofulosorum [14] and corresponded with Pautrier's 'sarcoides á petits nodules' [9].

The exact position of these lichenoid forms remains unclear. Arguments have been adduced [12] in favour of a tuberculous (or, at least a myco-bacterial) cause, because of atypical features which are sometimes present.

Miscellaneous forms. Among the many described one can include pseudotumoural [1], psoriasiform [2, 6] and pruriginous varieties [3]; lupus erythematosus-like and lupoid forms; a bizarre po-lymorphous light-eruption type; perifollicular pus-tules and papules widely scattered over the body; and keratotic lesions of the palms simulating pso-riasis or syphilis [13]. Hyperpigmentation may occur, particularly in the Negro [8]. One case presented only with a longstanding lymphoedema [11]. Calcinosis with subcutaneous plaques was an unusual feature [7]. Pain after alcohol or showering has also been described.

REFERENCES

1 BELAÏCH S., *et al* (1982) *Ann Derm Vénéréol (Paris)* 109, 741.
2 BURGOYNE J.S. & WOOD M.G. (1972) *Arch Dermatol* 106, 896.
3 DEGOS R. (1981) *Dermatologie*. Paris, Flammaron.
4 FEINSILBER D.G. & SCHROH P.G. (1983) *Rev Arg Dermatol* 64, 111.
5 GANGE R.W., *et al* (1978) *Clin Exp Dermatol* 3, 299.
6 IRGANG S. (1955) *Br J Dermatol* 67, 255.
7 KRULL J.J., *et al* (1972) *Arch Dermatol* 106, 894.
8 MAYOCK R.L., *et al* (1963) *Am J Med* 35, 67.
9 PAUTRIER L.M. (1940) *La Maladie de Besnier–Boeck–Schaumann*. Paris, Masson, pp. 39–44.
10 PINKUS H. (1977) *Cutis* 20, 651.
11 RAVINDA NATHAN M.P., *et al* (1974) *Arch Dermatol* 109, 543.
12 RIDGWAY H.A. & RYAN T.J. (1981) *J R Soc Med* 74, 140.
13 SCADDING J.G. & MITCHELL D.N. (1985) *Sarcoidosis*. 2nd ed. London, Chapman & Hall, pp. 195–6.
14 SMITH N.P., *et al* (1976) *Br J Dermatol* 94, 39.

Hypopigmentation. Macular hypopigmentation or hypopigmented areas around a central indurated lesion were first recorded in 8 of 145 patients (mostly Negroes) with sarcoidosis [4]. There have been several subsequent reports [1, 3, 6, 7]. The lesions are from 0·2 to 1 cm in diameter and occur predominantly on the limbs [7]. They may be ten-der but are not anaesthetic. They may be a present-ing sign of the disease [5].

Histologically, epithelioid cell granulomas are usually present in the dermis but occasionally the changes are non-specific [1, 5]. The melanocytes show degenerative changes but EM studies have not been helpful [1]. The differential diagnosis includes leprosy, post-inflammatory hypopigmentation, idio-pathic guttate hypomelanosis [2] and pityriasis lichenoides chronica [2]. The condition does not respond to corticosteroids [1] but has repigmented after prolonged PUVA therapy [5].

REFERENCES

1 CLAYTON R., *et al* (1977) *Br J Dermatol* 96, 119.
2 CLAYTON R. & WARIN A. (1979) *Br J Dermatol* 100, 297.
3 CORNELIUS C.E., *et al* (1973) *Arch Dermatol* 108, 249.
4 MAYOCK R.L., *et al* (1963) *Am J Med* 35, 67.
5 PATTERSON J.W. & FITZWATER J.E. (1978) *J Tennessee Med Assoc* 71, 662.
6 SHAW M. (1982) *Clin Exp Dermatol* 7, 115.
7 THOMAS M.R.H., *et al* (1981) *J R Soc Med* 74, 921.

Nail involvement. This is rare. Thickening, ridging or fragility of the nail plate may occur in association with lupus pernio affecting a finger [2]. In one case, lichen planus-like atrophic changes occurred with-out involvement of the affected digits [1]. Sarcoidal granulomas were found in the dermis beneath the nail bed.

REFERENCES

1 MANN R.J. & ALLEN B.R. (1981) *Br J Dermatol* 105, 599.
2 SAMMAN P.D. (1978) *The Nails in Disease*. 3rd ed. Lon-don, Heinemann, p. 80.

Alopecia. Alopecia of the scalp due to sarcoidosis is well recognized [1, 2]. Alopecia of the shin has been a presenting sign of the disease [3]. Sarcoidal gran-ulomas were found on histology and the Kveim test was positive.

REFERENCES

1 BAKER H. (1965) *Proc R Soc Med* 58, 243.
2 BLEEHEN S.S. (1969) *Proc R Soc Med* 62, 348.
3 FELIX R.H. (1983) *Br J Dermatol* 109 (Suppl. 24), 66.

Mucosal involvement. Buccal lesions are more fre-quently found when sought. They appear to be common in Scandinavia and rare in France and England. The nasal mucosa is often affected in lupus pernio [4, 6] and serves as a convenient biopsy site. Difficulty in breathing, or a purulent catarrh may be the presenting symptom [3, 5]. Yellowish-brown nodules or a diffuse infiltration with crusting occur [2]. The nasal bones may be involved; or the nasal cartilage may collapse [1]. Nodules with a hyper-pigmented halo, diffuse pale yellow plaques, or ulceration may be found on the buccal mucosa, palate, larynx or tongue.

REFERENCES

1 ALLEN B.R. (1978) *Br J Dermatol* **99** (Suppl. **16**), 54.
2 DEGOS R. (1981) *Dermatologie*. Paris, Flammarion.
3 DOWNIE L.N. (1964) *J Laryngol Otol* **78**, 931.
4 HOLMES R. & BLACK M.M. (1981) *Br J Derm.* **105** (Suppl **19**), 35.
5 JAMES D.G. (1954) *Q J Med* **28**, 109.
6 NEVILLE E., *et al* (1976) *Thorax* **31**, 660.

Sarcoidosis in the American Negro [6, 7, 9] (Fig. 48.15). The lesions are often exuberant and bizarre and the skin is especially affected, though erythema nodosum is uncommon [6]. Psoriasiform or lupus erythematosus-like lesions [4], verrucous and cheloid-like forms [2, 8], 'atypical' plaques or nodules [1], ulcerative lesions resembling papulonecrotic tuberculides [3], giant nodular forms and other atypical lesions occur with typical manifestations elsewhere. Shiny waxy papules are a particular presentation [6]. The histological features may be equivocal and tuberculosis is a common cause of death. When the lesions are annular, histoplasmosis must be excluded [5].

Small ulcerating nodules, sometimes associated with deep, softer non-ulcerative lesions, have been described [3]; the histology is that of sarcoidosis but the infiltrate is diffuse, fibroblasts are numerous and the vessel walls in the subcutis are thickened.

REFERENCES

1 CRONIN E. (1970) *Postgrad Med J* **46**, 507.
2 IRGANG S. (1950) *Arch Dermatol Syphil* **62**, 105.
3 IRGANG S. (1955) *Br J Dermatol* **67**, 255.
4 KLAUDER J.V. & WEIDMAN F.D. (1926) *Arch Dermatol Syphil* **13**, 675.
5 LUCAS O.A. (1970) *Br J Dermatol* **82**, 1.
6 MINUS H.R. & GRIMES P.E. (1983) *Cutis* **32**, 361.
7 ROSEN T. & MARTINS S. (1981) *Atlas of Black Dermatology*. Boston, Little & Brown, p. 40.
8 SHMUNES E., *et al* (1970) *Arch Dermatol* **102**, 665.
9 SONES M. & ISRAEL H.L. (1960) *Q J Med* **29**, 84.

Skin lesions in children. The general manifestations of sarcoidosis have been dealt with on p. 1767. In one series of 28 children [2], nine had skin lesions and three developed serious eye or joint symptoms. Erythema nodosum is a very rare presentation in children; we have never seen it in this age group. Though papular forms of skin sarcoidosis are seen in older children, younger ones may present with uveitis or keratitis, progressive joint disease and skin

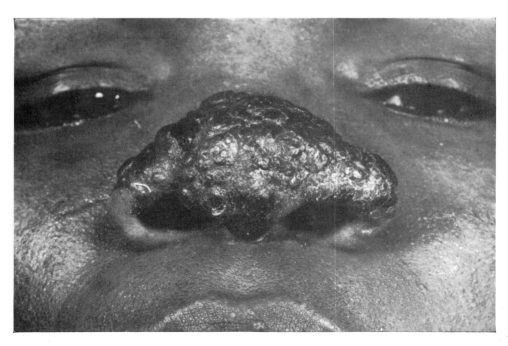

FIG. 48.15. Sarcoidosis. Atypical lesions in a Negro (St John's Hospital).

lesions consisting of papules, reddish-brown confluent plaques or eczema-like lesions [5, 6]. Other reported cases have shown unusual features: follicular [1], miliary [7] or erythrodermic lesions with keratotic pitting [4]. The chest X-ray is often normal [5]. The severity of the eye or joint involvement may justify corticosteroid therapy, often for several years [3] despite the risks at this early age.

REFERENCES

1 Appleyard W.J. (1970) *Proc R Soc Med* **69**, 345.
2 Kendig E.L. Jr (1974) *Pediatrics* **54**, 289.
3 Kendig E.L. Jr & Brummer D.L. (1976) *Chest* **70**, 351.
4 Morrison J.G.L. (1970) *Br J Dermatol* **95**, 93.
5 North P.A., *et al* (1970) *Am J Med* **48**, 449.
6 Rasmussen J.E. (1981) *J Am Acad Dermatol* **5**, 566.
7 Siltzbach L.E., *et al* (1974) *Am J Med* **57**, 847.

INVESTIGATIVE PROCEDURES [3]

The most important single criterion for the diagnosis of sarcoidosis is the finding of typical granulomas histologically, but the need for histological support varies with the pattern of clinical features. For example, in the U.K., patients with erythema nodosum and bilateral hilar gland enlargement may not require formal biopsy although this is necessary in other forms of the disease. Other investigations may add weight to the diagnosis, and may be useful in monitoring the activity of the disease.

Biopsy. A Kveim test, if a potent antigen is available, will often render the more traumatic forms of biopsy unnecessary; otherwise the involvement of several organs will allow the clinician to select the biopsy site best suited to his patient. The dermatologist has the advantage of dealing with a site easily accessible for biopsy, but it may still be necessary to confirm the presence of *sarcoidosis* as opposed to a *sarcoid reaction*, and biopsies from other organs or a Kveim test are then needed. Indeed, in one series [1] involving 292 biopsies from 10 sites, 87% were positive but biopsies from the skin proved less reliable than those from lymph nodes, parotid gland, or nasal mucosa. Scars that become infiltrated in the course of the disease provide acceptable histological evidence of sarcoidosis. A mucosal biopsy is an alternative to skin biopsy in lupus pernio.

A range of techniques is now available to obtain biopsy material from other areas. These include the removal of epitrochlear or scalene lymph nodes, mediastinoscopy with mediastinal node biopsy, liver biopsy, fine-needle splenic aspiration [4], and transbronchial lung biopsy through a flexible fibrescope [5]. The latter may be the most helpful and least disturbing for patients with suspected systemic sarcoidosis and intrathoracic manifestations.

Other investigations. A chest X-ray should be taken in all cases no matter what the clinical presentation. Hand X-rays show cystic changes only in chronic disease and usually only when there are clinical abnormalities in the fingers. Sputum should be examined and cultured for acid-fast bacilli, and a weak or negative tuberculin response may add weight to the diagnosis.

The erythrocyte sedimentation rate is usually raised in active phases but may at other times be normal. A rise in the ESR 6 to 8 weeks after the onset of erythema nodosum may indicate lung involvement [6]. Slight anaemia, neutropenia or lymphopenia are often noted, but these changes, and the hypergammaglobulinaemia which occurs in over half of the chronic cases, are not of proven diagnostic or prognostic significance.

The frequency of hypercalcaemia varies greatly in different series, being higher in the U.S.A. than in Europe. It was found in 17% of one series of 509 patients [2]. Although it may occur in all stages, it is most frequent in chronic or generalized forms of the disease. Hypercalcaemia and hypercalciuria may be due to increased intestinal absorption and are associated with increased sensitivity to vitamin D. Their presence may cause metastatic calcification, nephrocalcinosis or renal failure and investigations to exclude hyperparathyroidism may be required.

Three further recent techniques may be of value in monitoring the progress and activity of the disease [3]. Serum angiotensin-converting enzyme activity is usually raised in active sarcoidosis, but this is not a constant finding and activity may be increased in other conditions such as silicosis. Serial analysis of bronchoalveolar lavage fluid for T-lymphocyte numbers gives some guide to the intensity of alveolitis. Radioactive gallium-67 uptake occurs in some pulmonary infections and neoplasms as well as in sarcoidosis, but if these can be excluded it provides a way of separating active from fibrotic pulmonary disease.

REFERENCES

1 Israel H.L. Sones M. (1964) *Arch Intern Med* **113**, 255.
2 Mayock R.L., *et al* (1963) *Am J Med* **35**, 67.
3 Poole G.W. (1982) *Br Med J* **285**, 321.
4 Selroos O. (1976) *Ann NY Acad Sci* **278**, 517.
5 Tierstein A.D., *et al* (1976) *Ann NY Acad Sci* **278**, 522.
6 Vesey C.M.R. & Wilkinson D.S. (1959) *Br J Dermatol* **71**, 139.

Course and prognosis (Table 48.5) [2,7,8,11,12]. The prognosis of sarcoidosis is difficult to assess because of its frequent 'clinical silence' and the uncertainty of its onset [10]. Several attempts have been made to list favourable and unfavourable factors [2,11,12]. Most have been mentioned elsewhere in this Chapter. The prognosis is generally better in females, in those with less severe pulmonary disease at the onset and in patients with a positive tuberculin test and normal globulin levels [11].

Most cutaneous sarcoidosis occurs in the subacute and chronic stages, and its course is usually prolonged. Papules and nodules tend to resolve in 6 months to 3 years or longer, but plaques are more resistant. Lupus pernio is exceedingly persistent and often accompanied by other organ involvement that modifies the prognosis. In the American Negro, the course may be fulminant. Rapid disappearance of lesions may herald the onset of tuberculosis.

It has been suggested that patients with pulmonary sarcoidosis have a higher risk of developing

TABLE 48.5. The course of sarcoidosis

Favourable prognosis	Stage	Cardinal features	Unfavourable events
?Abortive cases or may be absent	*Prodromal* ↓	Malaise, fatigue, fever, depression, polyarthralgia	—
60%+ subside in 6–18 months	*Acute* ↓	*Erythema nodosum scar sarcoidosis, erythematopapular rashes,* polyarthralgia, iridocyclitis, lymphadenopathy	?Sudden cardiac death
	Subacute	*Papular, nodular, scar, etc.* pulmonary changes,	
Prolonged intermission or resolution	Intermittent	lymphadenopathy, recurrent iritis, parotitis,	May be cardiac death
	Chronic	spleen, liver, etc.	
Gradual, often slow	Progressive	*Lupus pernio erythrodermic* bone cysts, cataracts hypersplenism	Blindness
Irreversible but often extremely slow and patient survives, though disabled	Stage of fibrotic regression	Progressive pulmonary fibrosis nephritis, nephrosis, cataracts, glaucoma	Blindness, death
	Stage of functional failure	Emphysema, cor pulmonale nephrolithiasis, renal failure, tuberculosis	Death

About 60% of patients with Stage I disease will have recovered within 2 years [4,7]; those presenting with erythema nodosum did not do better than those presenting in other ways, or who were asymptomatic [9]. In the classic forms the prognosis is quite different; only about 12% of those in Stage II resolve [7]. Morbidity from blindness, pulmonary disease, renal failure and the cosmetic and social effects of a disfiguring skin lesion are the not inconsiderable burdens of a disease that follows a relentless course of smouldering activity [3]. Despite corticosteroid therapy, half the patients may continue to have abnormal respiratory function. Only about 12% of those in Stage III resolve [7]. SACE estimations may be a helpful guide to activity.

lung cancer [1]. However, this was not confirmed in a recent study [6].

Pregnancy. Sarcoidosis is not a contra-indication to pregnancy; in fact, most patients improve. Relapses may occur in the first 6 months after parturition [5].

Causes of death. The mortality has been estimated at 3–6% [7,11]. However, this may ignore undiagnosed deaths from cardiac involvement. Such deaths may occur late in the disease or from conduction failures in younger patients. Renal involvement is also a potential cause of death, though pulmonary disease itself is so less frequently.

REFERENCES

1 BRINKNER H. & WILLEK E. (1974) *Br J Cancer* **29**, 247.
2 DEREMEE A. & ZINSMEISTER A.R. (1983) *IXth Int Conf Sarc.* Paris 1981. Paris, Oxford, New York, Pergamon, p.457.
3 HANNO R. & CALLEN J.P. (1980) *Med Clin North Am* **64**, 847.
4 JAMES D.G. (1958) *Postgrad Med J* **34**, 240.
5 JAMES D.G. (1969) *Practitioner* **202**, 624.
6 RØMER F.F. (1980) *Proc VIIIth Int Conf Sarc.* Cardiff, Alpha Omega, p. 567.
7 SILTZBACH L.E., et al (1974) *Am J Med* **57**, 847.
8 STORK W.J., et al (1974) *Proc IVth Int Conf Sarc.* Tokyo, Univ. Tokyo Press, p.456.
9 TACHIBANA T., et al (1980) *Proc VIIIth Int Conf Sarc.* Cardiff, Alpha Omega, p.547.
10 TURIAF J., et al (1974) *Proc IVth Int Conf Sarc.* Tokyo, Univ. Tokyo Press, p.456.
11 WURM K. VON & ROSNER R. (1976) *Ann NY Acad Sci* **278**, 732.
12 WURM K. VON (1983) *Sarkoidose.* Stuttgart, G. Thieme, p.228.

THE TREATMENT OF SARCOIDOSIS [7, 11]

It is unjustifiable to expose the patient to the hazards of long-term immunosuppressive therapy if the manifestations of the disease are confined to the skin and lymphatic glands. At any time the pattern of the disease and the indications for treatment may change, but an expectant policy is often best if the course is not progressive and if vital structures are not involved.

The indications for treatment have been succinctly presented by several authors [6, 11]. Absolute indications include progressive, but not late, obstructive lung disease, posterior uveitis, cardiac, renal, endocrine or neurological involvement and hypercalcaemia [9] (but not hypercalciuria alone). Though corticosteroids may suppress granuloma formation, opinions differ about their effect on the course of pulmonary disease [4, 10]. If given, a course should last at least 6 months [6]. Treatment must be based, in any case, on an assessment of the site, stage and extent of involvement, and of the organ involved. The skill lies in choosing between early and sustained or unnecessary treatment with a powerful drug; timing is all-important. Stage I ('acute benign') sarcoidosis tends to clear without therapy [5, 6] though it has been suggested [4] that small doses of corticosteroids may minimize the chance of dissemination. Careful pulmonary function studies are essential to detect the early signs of progressive lung involvement. When symptoms, e.g. breathlessness, occur, it is too late for treatment to be effective. In any case, such a patient should be under the care of a chest physician, who can monitor progress regularly and efficiently. The SACE levels may be helpful in this.

Prolonged immunosuppressive treatment and sarcoidal anergy were believed to be responsible for the emergence of opportunistic mycobacterial infection [3] and for a gross proliferation of viral warts [8].

Hypercalcaemia and hypercalciuria may also be corrected by a low-calcium diet and oral phosphates or sodium phosphate [4].

The response of the patient with unsightly skin lesions [6], e.g. lupus pernio, is less predictable and in our opinion poor. In other cutaneous forms of sarcoidosis, intralesional therapy may be appropriate. Likewise, anterior uveitis may require treatment with topical or sub-conjunctival corticosteroids.

Other forms of therapy. Erythema nodosum, if severe and accompanied by arthralgia, sometimes requires a non-steroidal anti-inflammatory drug such as indomethacin [2]. Milder cases may respond adequately – if less dramatically – to aspirin and bed rest.

Methotrexate and chlorambucil have been used with success [4]. In a series treated with the former, over a mean period of 23 months, the skin lesions cleared in 12 out of 15 patients and uveitis in three out of four [13]. Pulmonary lesions and adenopathy were unchanged. *Azathioprine* improved 10 'hardcore' cases [6] resistant to other measures. However, aggressive immunosuppressive therapy may allow the emergence of opportunistic organisms [3] or a gross proliferation of viral warts [3]. *Chloroquine* and other antimalarials have undoubtedly been effective in some skin and mucosal lesions [6, 11] but carry their own hazards (Chapter 66). *Levamisole* was ineffective in 16 patients [12]. Etretinate was used with success in a patient with multiple warts [1].

REFERENCES

1 BOYLE J., et al (1983) *Clin Exp Dermatol* **8**, 33.
2 DEREMEE R.A. (1977) *Chest* **71**, 388.
3 GRICE K. (1983) *Clin Exp Dermatol* **8**, 323.
4 *ISRAEL H.L. (1970) *Postgrad Med J* **46**, 537.
5 JAMES D.G. (1969) *Practitioner* **202**, 624.
6 JAMES D.G. (1972) *Proc VIth Int Conf Sarc.* Tokyo, Univ. Tokyo Press, p.644.
7 *JAMES D.G. (1978) *Curr Prescr* Vol. **57**.
8 MACKIE R.M. (1972) *Br J Dermatol* **107** (Suppl. **22**), 97.
9 SCADDING J.G. & MITCHELL D.N. (1985) *Sarcoidosis.* 2nd ed. London, Chapman & Hall, pp. 570–598

10 SHARMA O.P., et al (1966) *Am J Med* **41**, 541.
11 *TURIAF J., et al (1976) *Ann NY Acad Sci* **278**, 743.
12 VEIEN N.K. (1977) *Dermatologica* **154**, 185.
13 VEIEN N.K. & BRODTHAGEN H. (1977) *Br J Dermatol* **97**, 213.

DIFFUSE SARCOIDAL REACTIONS (THE SYSTEMIC SARCOID TISSUE RESPONSE [1, 4, 6])

A number of infections and chemicals may cause sarcoid-like granulomas [10] though the features are usually not as clear-cut histologically [12] as in sarcoidosis. These reactions differ from sarcoidosis in several important respects (Table 48.6):

1. They involve only those organs normally affected by the disease in question or by the route of absorption or deposition of the chemical.
2. The Kveim test is negative.
3. The tuberculin reaction is usually not depressed.

consistent. Biopsies from other organs, the course of the disease and the response to treatment separate the two. Leprosy can also prove a particularly difficult problem clinically and histologically. Syphilis, brucellosis, fungus infections and some viral or bacterial diseases may also produce a sarcoidal type of tissue response but the clinical resemblance is usually superficial.

Silica, if inhaled, may induce pulmonary fibrosis but is otherwise localized to the skin, gut or wounds. 'Farmers' lung' [7, 8], caused by inhalation of mouldy hay, produces slowly developing, sarcoid-type granulomas around the air passages and runs a course not unlike that of pulmonary sarcoidosis. Titanium may also cause pulmonary granulomata [11].

Epithelioid-cell granulomas may occur in giant-cell [6] and other forms of arteritis, and isolated histological reports may be misleading. Ulcerating sarcoidosis of the leg with secondary arteritis may produce confusion with this type.

TABLE 48.6. Differentiation of sarcoidal tissue reactions

	Sarcoid granuloma confined to skin	Sarcoidal granulomatosis	Sarcoidosis
Pathogenesis	Silica, beryllium, mercury, zirconium	Inhalation of beryllium; viral, bacterial, fungal, parasitic disease	Unknown
Relevant history	Often occupational	Sometimes geographical	Occasionally familial
Skin	Nodules confined to inoculation site	Widespread lesions	Widespread lesions
Systemic involvement	None	Localization determined by source and spread of responsible agent	BHL*, liver, spleen, eyes, lymph nodes
Investigations			
Chest X-ray	Normal	May be abnormal	BHL*, pulmonary infiltration
Blood changes	None	May be hypergamma-globulinaemia; calcium normal	Usually hypergamma-globulinaemia; calcium often increased
Tuberculin reaction	Normal	Normal	Depressed or negative
Kveim reaction	Negative	Negative	Positive
Patch test	Often positive 4–6 weeks	Often positive 48 hours	Negative to many antigens
Intradermal test	Often positive	Positive in leprosy and zirconium	Negative
Treatment	Remove cause Intralesional steroids	Specific chemotherapy Steroids contraindicated	Steroids sometimes indicated

* BHL: Bilateral hilar lymphadenopathy.
HALL-SMITH P. & CAIRNS R.J. (1983) *Dermatology: Current Concepts and Practice*. London, Butterworths, p. 203.

Tuberculosis may exactly mimic sarcoidosis, but while the pure epithelioid-cell granuloma and its evocation by Kveim antigen are the hallmarks of sarcoidosis, the histopathology of tuberculosis is less

Beryllium disease [4, 9, 10, 12, 13]. Though now rarely seen [2, 13], occupational exposure to beryllium may cause pulmonary and cutaneous lesions closely resembling those of sarcoidosis, though uveitis and bone cysts have not been reported [12]. Workers in the electronic and neon tube industries are chiefly at risk, though cases have also occurred in a ceramics factory [3]. Inhalation of beryllium dust provides the usual source though spread to the lungs has been reported following accidental cutaneous implantation [5]. The tuberculin test and the Kveim test are negative but patch tests to beryllium are usually strongly positive [3]. Contact-sensitized patients show classical epithelioid-cell reactions to beryllium.

REFERENCES

1 HALL-SMITH P. & CAIRNS R.J. (1983) *Dermatology.* 3rd edition London, Staples, p. 203.
2 HASAN F.M. & KAZEMI H. (1974) *Chest* **65**, 289.
3 IZUMI T. & KOBARA Y. (1976) *Ann NY Acad Sci* **278**, 636.
4 JAMES D.G. (1974) *Proc VIth Int Conf Sarc.* Tokyo, Univ. Tokyo Press, p. 141.
5 JONES WILLIAMS W. & KILPATRICK G.S. (1974) *Proc. VIth Int Cong Sarc.* Tokyo, Univ. Tokyo Press, p. 141.
6 KINMONT P.D.C. & MacCALLUM D.I. (1964) *Br J Dermatol* **76**, 299.
7 PARISH W.E. (1963) *Thorax* **18**, 83.
8 RANKIN J., *et al* (1962) *Ann Intern Med* **57**, 606.
9 SCADDING J.G. & MITCHELL D.N. (1985) *Sarcoidosis.* 2nd ed. London, Chapman & Hall, pp. 482–497
10 *SHELLEY W.B. & HURLEY H.J. (1958) *Br J Dermatol* **70**, 75.
11 SHIGERMATSU N., *et al* (1980) *VIIIth Int Conf Sarc.* Cardiff, Alpha Omega, p. 728.
12 *SPRINCE N.L., *et al* (1976) *Ann NY Acad Sci* **276**, 654.
13 U.S. Dept. Health, Education & Welfare (1972) *Occupational Exposure to Beryllium* **72**, 10268.

Crohn's disease. The close similarity between the histological and immunological features of Crohn's disease and sarcoidosis have led to speculation about a common aetiology. The rarity of sarcoidosis of the intestine makes a direct relationship unlikely; but different modes of reaction, perhaps genetically determined, to a common causative agent have continued to aroused interest.

The reported prevalence of granulomas found in affected intestinal tissue has varied greatly. In a recent study of 79 patients [2], the highest number were found in anal and rectal tissue and in patients who had had no recurrences of the disease for 10 years. The authors felt that the granuloma formation might be an effective method of localizing and eliminating a poorly soluble antigen.

A transmissible agent has been shown to be present in sarcoid and Crohn's disease tissue [4, 6, 7] but the significance of delayed granuloma formation in mouse foot pads [4, 5] has been dis-

puted [9]. Earlier reports of positive Kveim tests in patients with Crohn's disease [3] or in inoculated mice [5] have not been fully substantiated [8]. Research continues.

Whipple's disease. Sarcoid-like changes have occurred in the skin and lymphatic glands [1]. The histopathological changes may also resemble those of sarcoidosis. However, jejunal biopsy confirms the correct diagnosis. Diarrhoea is an important distinguishing clinical feature.

REFERENCES

1 BEYLOT C., *et al* (1978) *Ann Dermatol Vénéréol* (Paris) **105**, 235.
2 CHAMBERS T.J. & MORSON B.C. (1980) *VIIIth Int Conf Sarc.* Cardiff, Alpha Omega, p. 750.
3 KARLISH A.J., *et al* (1972) *Lancet* i, 438.
4 MITCHELL D.N. & REES R.J.W. (1970) *Lancet* ii, 168.
5 MITCHELL D.N. & REES R.J.W. (1976) *Ann NY Acad Sci* **278**, 546.
6 MITCHELL D.N., *et al* (1976) *Lancet* ii, 761.
7 MITCHELL D.N. & REES R.J.W. (1980) *VIIIth Int Conf Sarc.* Cardiff, Alpha Omega, p. 121.
8 MIDDLETON W.G. & DOUGLAS A.C. (1980) *VIIIth Int Conf Sarc.* Cardiff, Alpha Omega, p. 655.
9 TAUB R.N., *et al* (1970) *Ann NY Acad Sci* **278**, 560.

Epidermolysis bullosa acquisita and bowel disease [4]. A connection has been recognized in recent years between EB acquisita and inflammatory bowel disease. There have been several reports of association with Crohn's disease [1, 2, 3] and we have been able to confirm this.

REFERENCES

1 CHOUVET B., *et al* (1982) *Ann Dermatol Vénéréol* (Paris) **100**, 53.
2 LIVDEN J.K., *et al* (1978) *Acta Derm Venereol* (Stockh) **58**, 241.
3 PECUM J.S. & WRIGHT J.T. (1973) *Proc R Soc Med* **66**, 234.
4 RAY T.L., *et al* (1982) *J Am Acad Dermatol* **6**, 242.

LOCAL SARCOID GRANULOMAS

Definition. Epithelioid-cell granulomas occurring locally without clinical or immunological evidence of sarcoidosis.

Pathogenesis. These are to be found in relation to:
  1. Tumours, lymphomas, necrobiosis lipoidica, fungal infections, granuloma inguinale, cat-scratch disease, etc.

2. Silica and silicaceous matter in wounds.
3. Certain metals such as mercury, zirconium, beryllium.
4. Foreign body reactions to lipids (fat granulomas, sebaceous cysts) naevi, gunpowder and foreign vegetable, mineral and chemical matter.
5. Sea-urchin spines (see below).
6. Aspiration pneumonia [14], coccidioidomycosis and hair sprayers (thesaurosis) [2].
7. In leprous patients, non-specific material such as normal tissue or injected milk.
8. In some conditions of unknown origin and significance, e.g. granulomatous cheilitis [12], rosaceous tuberculides and perioral eruptions [5].
9. After injection of local anaesthetics containing traces of silicon dioxide or beryllium from sterilized glassware [11].

1. Hodgkin's disease may cause especial difficulties [8]. A sarcoid-like histology may occur in other lymphomas [5, 9]. Such cases are rare and call for repeated and special organ biopsies.

2. Silica occurs in many forms: as talc (magnesium silicate), kaolin (aluminium silicate) and quartz, and as a constituent of slate, brick, gravel and coal. Silicosis from inhalation of silica dust is an important industrial hazard but wounds containing crystals of silica normally remain unchanged indefinitely. Talc was commonly the cause of such granulomas in surgical wounds when used as a glove powder. The long delay between the implantation of silica and the appearance of the granuloma suggests that the silica is not the immediate cause of the reaction. Though this may be a local manifestation of sarcoidosis [7, 14] the silica may also excite granuloma formation in response to a hypersensitivity state or by slow release in colloidal form. In one case a silica granuloma progressed to scar sarcoidosis [13]. The granulomas are associated with doubly refractile crystalline material with the characteristics of quartz or talc. Unlike Schaumann bodies, the crystalline material is spiculated but non-lamellated. X-ray diffraction spectroscopy confirms the presence of silica.

3. *Zirconium* [15] established the importance of immunological mechanisms. This specific hypersensitivity is reproducible by intradermal injection of the substance in high dilutions ($10^{-4}–10^{-6}$). 0.2 μg of sodium zirconium lactate was sufficient to produce a visible lesion in one patient tested. Zirconium is not doubly refractile.

4. The reactions to *stearates* [15], sebum and other lipid and non-lipid extraneous matter are variable. The granulomas are often less regular. Lipid crystals, soluble in hydrochloric acid, may be present. Giant cells are usually numerous.

5. *Sea urchin granulomas* [1, 4]. Foreign-body or sarcoidal granulomas may occur as a delayed reaction to sea urchin spine injury [1, 10, 17]. The exact cause of the reaction is unknown. Intralesional triamcinolone may help speed resolution, if excision is not practicable [17].

6. *Thesaurosis* [3, 6], a pulmonary infiltration occurring in those heavily exposed to polyvinyl-pyrrolidine hair-sprays in hairdressing procedures.

7. Patients with *tuberculoid leprosy* react more readily to non-specific agents than patients with sarcoidosis. This has led to difficulties in the interpretation of the Kveim test.

8. Epithelioid-cell granulomas may be a feature of the histology of the rosaceous tuberculides, and even of rosacea itself.

The comparative rarity of these granulomas, their inconstant appearance after a long period of dormancy, and their simultaneous eruption in several areas suggest a hypersensitivity mechanism. The reaction in scars in sarcoidosis itself is not constant and may add some weight to the view that the silica must be in a 'prepared' state, i.e. of suitable crystal size, or in a colloidal state [16]. The evocation of the granuloma by injection of minute amounts of zirconium suggested that a delayed hypersensitivity must be responsible.

The continued presence of silica is compatible with resolution of the granulomata. As the abnormal reactivity of the patient declines, a chronic stage of 'balance' may occur in which neither spread nor regression takes place.

Clinical features. The lesions are indistinguishable from those of sarcoidosis. Rarely, the granulomas are found unexpectedly on histological examination of quite different types of lesion [(iv) above].

Silica or beryllium granulomas develop in scars or at sites of trauma after an unpredictable, and long latent period. The scar becomes infiltrated and livid, fading to a brownish-orange colour after a few weeks. Dull grey or yellow 'grains' are visible on diascopy.

Diagnosis. The site of the lesions is helpful, e.g. the zirconium deodorant granulomata of the axillae [14], as are a history of a car accident, gravel wounds, or injections of foreign bodies. The Kveim test is negative but intradermal tests of the suspected substances to which hypersensitivity is assumed are often positive in high dilutions. Patch tests inconstantly produce a delayed granulomatous response. The tuberculin response is unaltered. The identification of crystalline material in section is not difficult with modern techniques.

Treatment. The lesions usually remain unchanged for months or years but then resolve spontaneously. Intralesional corticosteroids may speed resolution.

REFERENCES

1 BEECHING N.H., *et al* (1982) *Practitioner* **226**, 1567.
2 CARES R.M. (1965) *Arch Environ Health* **11**, 80.
3 DUPRÉ A., *et al* (1975) *Bull Soc Fr Dermatol Syphiligr* **82**, 162.
4 FISHER A.A. (1978) *Atlas of Aquatic Dermatology*. New York, Grune & Stratton, pp. 27–31.
5 GEORGOURAS K. & KOCSARD E. (1978) *Acta Derm Venereol (Stockh)* **58**, 433.
6 HERRERO E.U., *et al* (1965) *Am Rev Respir Dis* **92**, 280.
7 JAMES D.G. (1959) *Q J Med* **28**, 109.
8 JONES-WILLIAMS W., *et al* (1980) *VIIIth Int Conf Sarc.* Cardiff, Alpha Omega, p. 758.
9 KAHN L.B., *et al* (1974) *Cancer* **33**, 1117.
10 KINMONT P.D.C. (1965) *Br J Dermatol* **77**, 335.
11 KREBS VON A. & ANDRES H.V. (1967) *Dermatologica* **134**, 262.
12 RHODES E.L. & STIRLING G.A. (1965) *Arch Dermatol* **92**, 40.
13 ROWLAND PAYNE C.M.E., *et al* (1983) *Clin Exp Dermatol* **8**, 171.
14 SCADDING J.G. & MITCHELL D.N. (1985) *Sarcoidosis.* 2nd ed. London, Chapman & Hall, pp. 33–35
15 SHELLEY W.B. & HURLEY H.J. (1958) *Br J Dermatol* **70**, 75.
16 SHELLEY W.B. & HURLEY H.J. (1960) *J Invest Dermatol* **34**, 107.
17 WARIN A.P. (1977) *Clin Exp Dermatol* **2**, 405.

Sarcoid reactions in tattoos. A granulomatous dermal infiltrate may accompany sensitization reactions to any colour of the tattoo or may occur alone. Less commonly, a pure sarcoidal reaction is present [3], presenting as an indolent lump within the tattooed area. Patch and intradermal tests are usually negative. However, such lesions may be accompanied by other signs of sarcoidosis or a positive Kveim test [2, 3, 5] and are occasionally the only skin manifestation of the disease [1]. The association of a sarcoidal reaction in a cobalt tattoo with uveitis in three cases and with erythema nodosum in one [4] may represent an intermediate situation [2] and emphasizes the need for a thorough investigation of all cases showing a sarcoidal type of infiltrate.

REFERENCES

1 DICKINSON J.A. (1969) *Arch Dermatol* **100**, 315.
2 KENNEDY C. (1976) *Clin Exp Dermatol* **1**, 395.
3 MADDEN J.F. (1939) *Arch Dermatol* **40**, 256.
4 RORSMAN H., *et al* (1969) *Lancet* **ii**, 27.
5 WEIDMAN A.I., *et al* (1966) *Arch Dermatol* **94**, 320.

Sarcoid reactions to synthetic fibres. A sarcoid-like granulomatous reaction has been reported from exposure to acrylic or nylon fibres, either as dust or from walking on acrylic carpets [1]. The fibres were identified within the granulomatous cells by histochemical techniques.

REFERENCE

1 CORTEZ PIMENTEL J. (1977) *Br J Dermatol* **96**, 673.

Other sarcoid-like reactions. An epithelioid-cell granuloma histology is found in granulomatous cheilitis and the Melkersson–Rosenthal syndrome (p. 2127).

Annular lesions of the scalp with a serpiginous outline and well-marked border, resembling sarcoidosis, are now regarded as necrobiotic [1, 2, 3].

REFERENCES

1 DOWLING G.B. & WILSON JONES E. (1967) *Dermatologica* **135**, 11.
2 LAYMON C.W. (1961) *Arch Dermatol* **83**, 112.
3 RHODES E.L. & STIRLING G.A. (1965) *Arch Dermatol* **92**, 40.

CHAPTER 49

Disorders of Connective Tissue

J. L. BURTON & F. J. G. EBLING

THE DERMIS

The dermis [2, 3, 4, 9, 10], which is bounded distally by its junction with the epidermis and proximally by the subcutaneous fat, contributes 15–20% of the total weight of the human body. It varies in thickness from about 1 mm on the face to 4 mm on the back and thigh. It is a tough and resilient tissue which provides nutriment to the epidermis and cutaneous appendages and cushions the body against mechanical injury.

The basis of the dermis is a supporting matrix or ground substance in which polysaccharides and protein are linked to produce macromolecules with a remarkable capacity for holding water in their domain. Within and associated with this matrix are two kinds of protein fibre: collagen, which has great tensile strength, and elastin, which has considerable elasticity.

Collagen (see below) represents 75% of the dry weight and 18–30% of the volume of dermis. The embryonic dermis consists of a fine three-dimensional network of collagen fibres with abundant ground substance in between, but in the adult the collagen becomes greatly increased at the expense of the extrafibrillar space (Fig. 49.1). According to the size and arrangement of the collagen fibres two main regions can be distinguished in the human dermis. A thin, superficial papillary dermis interdigitates with the ridged underside of the epidermis, and its elements are continuous with the periadnexal dermis which forms sheaths around the hair follicles, sebaceous glands and sweat glands [9]. The underlying layer, nine-tenths of the total, is called the reticular dermis; it blends with the subcutaneous fat [9]. In some regions of the body, such as the nipple, the penis, the scrotum and the perineum, oriented smooth muscle fibres occur in the reticular layer.

The name reticulin was originally applied to fine branching fibres which, in contrast with collagen, stained black with ammoniacal silver nitrate and were especially abundant in the basement membrane and the midcortical layer of the kidney. Notwithstanding debate about their nature [5, 8], electron microscopy revealed an axial periodicity identical with that of collagen.

Elastic fibres (see below) form a very extensive network, even though they make up only 4% of the dry weight and 1% of the volume. Mature elastic fibres are restricted to the reticular dermis. Two structures regarded as immature elastic fibres have been described. Oxytalin is believed to anchor the basal lamina, from which it extends as little bundles of microfibrils into the papillary dermis [1, 9]. Oxytalin fibres also branch and form a horizontal plexus in the upper reticular layer. Small amounts of stainable elastic matrix become secreted onto this to give so-called elaunin fibres [1, 9].

The name fibronectin [6, 7] has been given to a glycoprotein which is found at cell surfaces and in the body fluids as well as in connective tissue. It is composed of two identical, or nearly identical, disulphide-linked polypeptides with a combined molecular weight of about 450,000. It appears to be involved in adhesion and interaction of cells and may be important in cell replication, mobility and differentiation. The polypeptide has been shown to interact with many other macromolecules, including collagens, glycosaminoglycans, fibrinogen, fibrin and actin. It seems that the domain of the large molecule embraces three separate binding sites for gelatin, cell attachment and heparin, respectively, and it has been postulated that fibronectin may act as an anchor for cells in the extracellular matrix.

The dermis contains few cells: most are fibroblasts (see Figs 49.5 and 49.11) which secrete the dermal constituents; others are mast cells, histiocytes or macrophages, lymphocytes or other leukocytes, and melanocytes. The dermis also has vascular beds at various levels, lymphatics, nerves and various kinds of nerve endings. (See also Chapter 2).

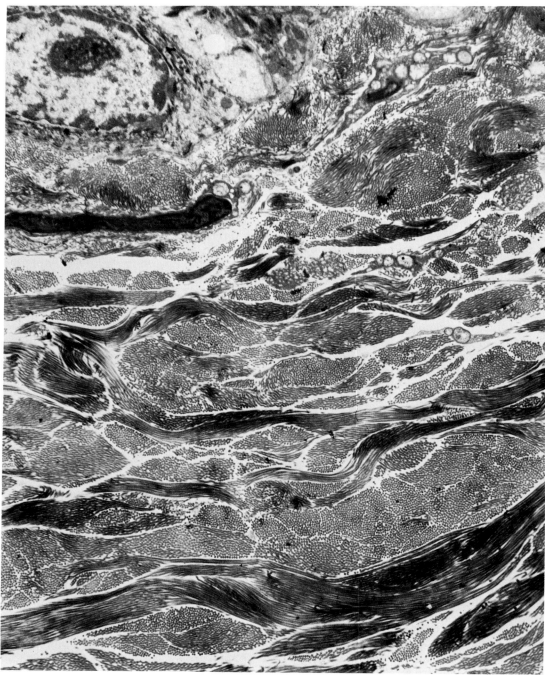

FIG. 49.1. Transmission electron micrograph of a section of dermis from the human forearm. A basal epidermal cell with underlying basement membrane is visible in the upper left-hand corner. The dermis is packed with bundles of collagen fibres sectioned both transversely and longitudinally. (Professor A. S. Breathnach; × 4,900.)

REFERENCES

1 COTTA-PEREIRA G., *et al* (1976) *J Invest Dermatol* **66**, 143.
2 JARRETT A. (Ed.) (1974) *The Physiology and Pathophysiology of the Skin.* Vol. III. *The Dermis and Dendrocytes.* London, Academic Press.
3 MONTAGNA W. & PARAKKAL P.F. (1974) *The Structure and Function of Skin.* 3rd ed. New York, Academic Press.
4 MONTAGNA W., *et al* (Eds.) (1970) *Advances in the Biology of Skin.* Vol. 10. *The Dermis.* New York, Appleton–Century–Crofts.
5 ROBB-SMITH A.H.T. (1958) In *Recent Advances in Gelatin and Glue Research.* Ed. Stainsby G. Oxford, Pergamon, p. 38.
6 RUOSLAHTI E., *et al* (1981) *Coll Res* **1**, 95.
7 RUOSLAHTI E., *et al* (1982) *J Invest Dermatol* **79**, 65s.
8 SMITH J.G., *et al* (1966) In *Modern Trends in Dermatology.* Ed. MacKenna R.M.B. London, Butterworths, Vol. 3, p. 110.
9 SMITH L.T., *et al* (1982) *J Invest Dermatol* **79**, 93s.
10 WUEPPER K.D., *et al* (Eds.) (1982) *J Invest Dermatol* **79** (Suppl. 1).

GROUND SUBSTANCE

Composition of ground substance [1, 2, 5–13]. The important components of the amorphous ground substance of the dermis are polysaccharides known as glycosaminoglycans. The chains are in general covalently linked to protein and may contain varying amounts of sulphate causing a strong negative charge. The resulting material is known as a proteoglycan. The historical term 'mucopolysaccharide' is loosely used to describe either kind of molecule. The proteoglycan molecule is capable of holding 1,000 times its own volume of water in its domain and plays the major role in the supporting matrix of the connective tissue.

The main glycosaminoglycans in skin are hyaluronic acid, chondroitin, dermatan sulphate (chondroitin sulphate B) and, in lesser amounts, chondroitin-6-sulphate (chondroitin sulphate C) and chondroitin-4-sulphate (chondroitin sulphate A). Heparin, normally remaining within the mast cells which produce it, and heparan sulphate fall into the same class.

Glycosaminoglycans are macromolecules made up of two different saccharide units which alternate regularly. They may be thus considered as a series of disaccharide units, each comprising a hexosamine linked either with uronic acid or, in one known case, with a hexose. The amino group of the hexosamine is always either acetylated or sulphated. In hyaluronic acid, for example, each unit consists of D-gluconuric acid linked by an ether

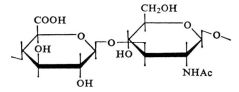

FIG 49.2. Repeating unit of hyaluronic acid.

bond at the C_1 position to the C_3 of D-glucosamine. The amino group of the hexosamine is acetylated. The D-glucosamine is in turn linked by an ether bond at C_1 to D-gluconuric acid at C_4 (Fig. 49.2). The regular alternation of C_1 to C_3 to C_1 to C_4 links is another general characteristic of glycosaminoglycans. Dermatan sulphate (chondroitin sulphate B) has a unit consisting of L-iduronic acid (the C_5 epimer of glucuronic acid) and D-galactosamine, which is the C_4 epimer of glucosamine (Fig. 49.3).

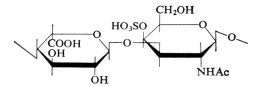

FIG. 49.3. Repeating unit of dermatan sulphate.

The proleoglycan structure has only been described for cartilage although skin is probably similar [4]. Hyaluronic acid does not link with protein. Dermatan sulphate and chondroitin-6-sulphate are each connected at their reducing ends to a trisaccharide consisting of galactosyl-galactosyl-xylose. The xylose is glysosidically linked to the

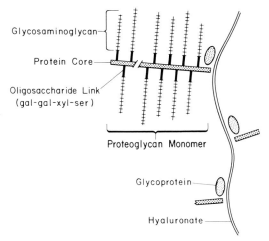

FIG. 49.4. Proteoglycan monomer and aggregate. Reproduced by permission of Dr J.E. Silbert.

hydroxyl of serine in the protein chain, a so-called oligosaccharide linkage [5]. The proteoglycan core is a molecule of molecular weight $(1-2) \times 10^5$ and this may have 50 or more similar glycosaminoglycans attached to it in a configuration like a bottle brush (Fig. 49.4), with a molecular weight of more than 10^6. Finally, as many as 100 individual proteoglycan monomers can be attached around a core hyaluronic acid to form aggregates with molecular weights of $(100-150) \times 10^6$ [3, 4].

REFERENCES

1 DAVIDSON E. A. (1965) In *Advances in Biology of Skin*. Vol. VI. *Ageing*. Ed. Montagna W. Oxford, Pergamon, p. 255.
2 DORFMAN A. (1963) *J Histochem Cytochem* **11**, 2.
3 HARDINGHAM T. E. & MUIR H. (1972) *Biochim Biophys Acta* **279**, 401.
4 HASCALL V. C. (1977) *J Supramol Struct* **7**, 101.
5 LINDAHL U. & RODEN L. (1972) In *Glycoproteins*. Ed. Gottschalk A. Amsterdam, Elsevier, p. 491.
6 MUIR H. (1961) In *The Biochemistry of Mucopolysaccharides of Connective Tissue*. Eds. Clark F. & Grant J. K. Cambridge, Cambridge University Press, p. 4.
7 MUIR H. (1964) In *Progress in the Biological Sciences in Relation to Dermatology*. Eds. Rook A. & Champion R. H. Cambridge, Cambridge University Press, Vol. II, p. 25.
8 MUIR H. (1964) In *International Review of Connective Tissue Research*. Ed. Hall D. A. New York, Academic Press, Vol. II, p. 101.
9 PEARCE R. H. & GRIMMER B. J. (1970) In *Advances in Biology of Skin*. Vol. X. *The Dermis*. Eds. Montagna W., *et al*. New York, Appleton–Century–Crofts, p. 89.
10 ROGERS H. J. (1961) In *The Biochemistry of Mucopolysaccharides of Connective Tissue*. Eds. Clark F & Grant J. K. Cambridge, Cambridge University Press, p. 51.
11 SCHUBERT M. (1964) *Biophys J* **4** (Suppl.), 119.
12 SILBERT J. E. (1982) *J Invest Dermatol* **79**, 31s.
13 SMITH J. G., *et al* (1965) In *Advances in Biology of Skin*. Vol. VI. *Ageing*. Ed. Montagna W. Oxford, Pergamon, p. 211.

Biosynthesis and metabolism of cutaneous glycosaminoglycans and proteoglycans. From studies on streptococci and from animal experiments using isotopically labelled D-glucose, it appears that glucose is the precursor of both the hexosamine and the uronic acid parts of the hyaluronic acid molecule. The process involves uridine nucleotides which function as glycosyl donors; for details of the biosynthesis of hyaluronic acid and of the sulphated polysaccharides reference should be made to reviews by Davidson [4], Dorfman [5, 6], Kent [11], Muir [13] and Silbert [15].

Enzymes which can degrade glycosaminoglycans or proteoglycans have been prepared from several sources, notably from testis, snake venom, bacteria and leeches. Testicular hyaluronidase, the originally described intradermal 'spreading factor' [9], splits hyaluronic acid into a series of oligosaccharides by attacking the β-linked N-acetyl-glucosaminyl groups within the chain [17]. Chondroitin-4-sulphate and chondroitin-6-sulphate are similarly degraded, but less rapidly [10, 12]; dermatan sulphate is unaffected [16]. Hyaluronidase from snake venom is identical, but bacterial enzymes appear to differ. No hyaluronidase could be detected in cultures of human skin fibroblasts [14] but an enzyme has been found in rat skin [2]. A series of other degradative enzymes of relevance to glycosaminoglycan storage diseases has been described [8].

The possible influences of hormones [1, 3, 7] on the ground substance is of importance in understanding cutaneous changes in endocrine disorder. Such effects have been experimentally investigated in several ways, including measurement of the spreading of fluids, chemical analysis of the dermis, and studies on the incorporation of isotopically labelled sulphate or D-glucose. In summarizing these facts three difficulties arise. Firstly, any change in the amount of glycosaminoglycans in the dermis must be interpreted in relation to the balance between synthesis and catabolism: an increased concentration can result from either increased synthesis or reduced degradation. Secondly, hyaluronic acid may be altered without any effect on dermatan sulphate, or vice versa. Thirdly, not all sites may show the same response; results demonstrated in cartilage, for example, may not apply to dermis.

Cortisone and cortisol reduce the spreading capacity of hyaluronidase, the concentration of dermal polysaccharides and their synthesis and breakdown as measured in uptake studies. Androgens such as testosterone greatly increase the concentration of hyaluronic acid without much affecting the sulphated polysaccharides; the effect may be due to an inhibition of degradation. Oestradiol, on the other hand, appears to have a specific inhibitory effect on the synthesis of dermatan sulphate.

After hypophysectomy the turnover of both hyaluronic acid and dermatan sulphate is decreased. Growth hormone exerts an anabolic effect; in cartilage, at least, the turnover of chondroitin sulphate is increased, but not that of hyaluronic acid. In hypothyroid animals both synthesis and breakdown are depressed; thyroxine increases turnover, though this generally leads to a reduction in concentrations. It must be recognized, however, that exophthalmos, occurring in hyperthyroidism, is associated with increased hyaluronic acid. The effect of parathyroid hormone may differ throughout the body. In some connective tissues synthesis of sulphated polysaccharides may be increased; in others their catabolism may be accelerated. In diabetes the turnover of proteoglycans is reduced.

REFERENCES

1 Asboe-Hansen G. (1963) In *International Review of Connective Tissue Research*. Ed. Hall D. A. New York, Academic Press, Vol. I, p. 29.
2 Cashman D. C., et al (1969) *Arch Biochem Biophys* **135**, 387.
3 Davidson E. A. (1964) *Proc 2nd Int Congr Endocrinol*. Amsterdam, Excerpta Medica, p. 398.
4 Davidson E. A. (1965) In *Advances in Biology of Skin*. Vol. VI. *Ageing*. Ed. Montagna W. Oxford, Pergamon, p. 255.
5 Dorfman A. (1964) *Biophys J* **4** (Suppl.), 155.
6 Dorfman A. (1970) In *Advances in Biology of Skin*. Vol. X. *The Dermis*. Eds. Montagna W., et al. New York, Appleton–Century–Crofts, p. 123.
7 Dziewiatowski D. D. (1964) *Biophys J* **4** (Suppl.), 215.
8 Hall C. W., et al (1978) *Methods Enzymol* **50**, 439.
9 Hoffman D. C. & Duran-Reynals F. (1931) *J Exp Med* **53**, 387.
10 Hoffman P., et al (1956) *J Biol Chem* **219**, 653.
11 Kent P. W. (1961) In *The Biochemistry of Mucopolysaccharides of Connective Tissue*. Eds. Clark F. & Grant J. K. Cambridge, Cambridge University Press, p. 90.
12 Meyer K. & Rapport M. M. (1950) *Arch Biochem* **27**, 287.
13 Muir H. (1964) In *Progress in the Biological Sciences in Relation to Dermatology*. Eds. Rook A. & Champion R. H. Cambridge, Cambridge University Press, Vol. II, p. 25.
14 Orkin R. W. & Toole B. P. (1980) *J Biol Chem* **255**, 1036.
15 Silbert J. E. (1982) *J Invest Dermatol* **79**, 31s.
16 Walker P. G. (1961) In *The Biochemistry of Mucopolysaccharides of Connective Tissue*. Eds. Clark F. & Grant J. K. Cambridge, Cambridge University Press, p. 109.
17 Weissman B. (1955) *J Biol Chem* **216**, 783.

Histology of the ground substance. The proteoglycans of the ground substance correspond closely to the mucins of the histologists, for which empirical staining methods have been available long in advance of the elucidation of their chemical structure.

Methods of fixation, staining and processing have been comprehensively and critically reviewed by Curran [1], Szirmai [7] and Fullmer [2]. Many traditional fixatives remove or denature ground substance, and formalin, freeze-drying or the use of frozen sections of fresh tissue are therefore recommended. The principal staining methods fall into three groups: the production of metachromasia, colloidal iron and Alcian blue. In addition, the periodic acid–Schiff (PAS) technique has often been used, but it appears useless for glycosaminoglycans, though it may stain other associated materials. The ground substance of normal human skin has been shown to react positively to the first three methods while PAS is negative [4].

Metachromasia means the production in the tissue of a colour which differs from that of the dye used. The phenomenon appears to depend on the availability of regularly spaced anionic groups and thus indicates sulphate, carboxyl and probably phosphoric acid esters. Toluidine blue O and azure A are the stains most frequently used.

The colloidal iron method depends on binding colloidal iron, from dialysed iron hydroxide, to the sulphate groups of glycosaminoglycans or the uronic acid of hyaluronic acid, and its subsequent coloration to Prussian blue with acidified ferrocyanide [3].

Alcian blue [6] is an empirical method which gives results in parallel with those obtained by colloidal iron or with metachromasia, and it has been shown to stain substances which are removable by hyaluronidase.

The PAS method [5] involves the oxidation of sections in 0·5% periodic acid followed by treatment with Schiff's reagent, when compounds containing —CH(OH)·CH(OH)— or CH(OH)CO— groups (the hydroxyl groups may be replaced by amino or alkylamine groups) give a purplish-red colour. In theory, glycogen, glycosaminoglycans, glycoproteins, glycolipids and glycolipoproteins should be demonstrable, but in practice pure hyaluronic acid and chondroitin sulphate do not appear to stain.

REFERENCES

1 Curran R. C. (1961) In *Biochemistry of Mucopolysaccharides of Connective Tissue*. Eds. Clark F. & Grant J. K. Cambridge, Cambridge University Press, p. 324.
2 Fullmer H. M. (1965) In *International Review of Connective Tissue Research*. Ed. Hall D. A. New York, Academic Press, p. 1.
3 Hale C. W. (1946) *Nature* **157**, 802.
4 Johnson W. C. & Helwig E. B. (1964) *J Invest Dermatol* **42**, 81.
5 McManus J. F. A. (1946) *Nature* **158**, 202.
6 Steedman H. F. (1950) *Q J Microsc Sci* **91**, 477.
7 Szirmai J. A. (1963) *J Histochem Cytochem* **11**, 24.

COLLAGEN

Structure, composition and types of collagen [1–3, 8–11, 13, 14, 24, 29, 32, 37, 42, 44, 46]. Collagen is the generic name for a family of proteins

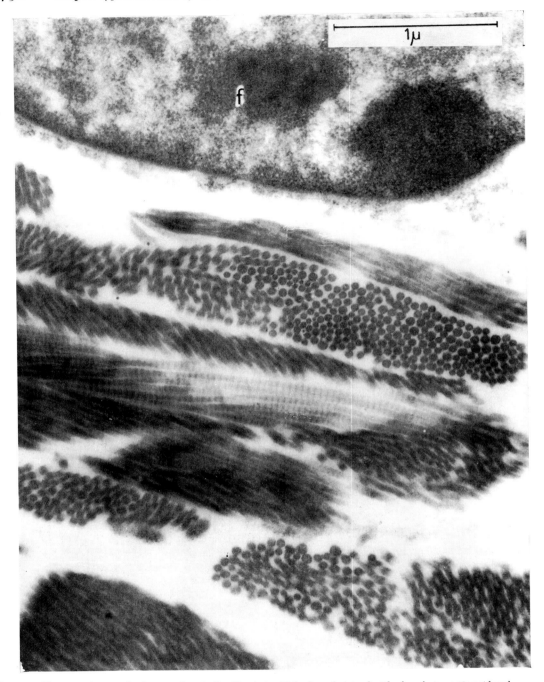

FIG. 49.5. Electron micrograph of mouse dermis, fixed in glutaraldehyde and stained with phosphotungstic acid and uranyl sulphate, showing part of a fibroblast (f) and collagen fibres (Dr G. A. Meek).

which are the major fibrous constituents of skin, tendon, ligament, cartilage and bone and account for one-third of the total human protein.

Under the ordinary light microscope collagen fibres appear as colourless branching wavy bands about 15 μm in width, with faint longitudinal striations. Using dark field it becomes evident that each fibre is a bundle of parallel, unbranching fibrils. In the electron microscope the fibrils appear to be about 100 nm (1,000 Å) wide and to be characteristically cross-striated, with a periodicity of about 60–70 nm (Figs 49.5–49.8). When collagen fibres are placed in 0·01% acetic acid they disintegrate into solution; in this form collagen has a molecular weight of 300,000–360,000 [21] and the molecules are about 280 nm long by 1·5 nm in diameter.

This basic molecule of structural collagens, originally known as tropocollagen [40, 49], consists of three polypeptide chains, so-called alpha subunits, which are coiled around one another in a triple helix. Collagen, however, is secreted by the fibroblast as a larger molecule (Fig. 49.9) which contains, in addition to the basic helical domain, a globular domain at each end [3]. The amino N-terminal domain may in some cases contain a short region of triple helix, and the carboxy-terminal domain contains both interchain and intrachain disulphide bonds. In structural collagens there are short regions of non-triple helix at either end of the triple helical domain which survive the extracellular removal of the globular domains.

When acid solutions of collagen are neutralized they are reconstructed in the native form with the 64 nm periodicity. Different precipitating agents produce various kinds of artificial collagen. Thus ATP induces so called 'segment long spacing' collagen, in which the tropocollagen units are packed in perfect register as polar units. Glycoprotein produces 'fibrous long spacing' collagen, with a period of 280 nm and a random positioning of heads and

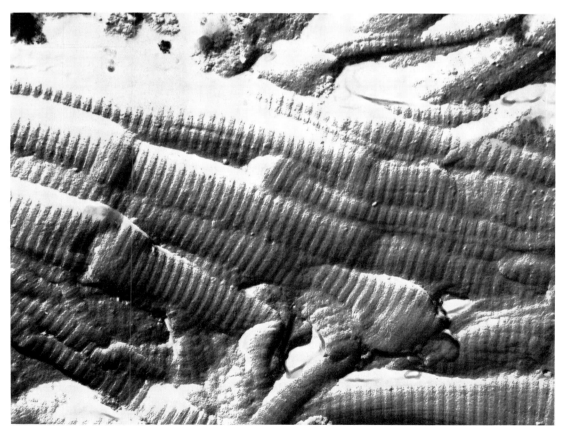

FIG. 49.6. Transmission electron micrograph of shadowed replica of unfixed, rapidly frozen and surface sublimated rat tail tendon showing stepped banding of collagen fibres (× 40,500).

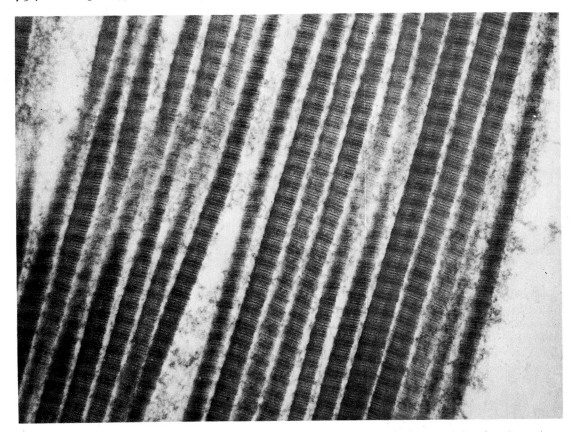

FIG. 49.7. Transmission electron micrograph of collagen fibres in human dermis (Professor A. S. Breathnach; × 82,500).

tails of adjacent molecules. The periodicity of native collagen has been explained on the hypothesis that molecules of tropocollagen become associated side by side with a regular overlap of about a quarter of their length [6, 12, 18].

Four major classes of vertebrate collagens, subdivided into a number of types, differing in their distribution, molecular structure and amino acid composition have been identified [3].

The first class contains the major elements which contribute to connective tissues and includes the three types which form the classically described banded structures resulting from cross-link-stabilized side-by-side interactions of the helical domains. In each of these collagens, the polypeptide chains are characterized by repeating triplets of amino acids in which glycine occupies every third place and proline and hydroxyproline, respectively, are the most frequent occupants of the first and second places. It is the placement of the glycine and hydroxyproline residues which specifies and stabilizes the helix of each alpha subunit, allows their

association into the triple conformation and thus accounts for the relative inflexibility of the fibre and its resistance to non-collagen-specific proteases. It may be added that hydroxyproline occurs in no other mammalian protein except elastin, and there only in small amounts, so that collagen can be quantified by hydrolyzing it and estimating this amino acid [20, 22, 28].

Type I collagen, the commonest, is found in the reticular dermis and in tendon and bone; it has two similar $[\alpha_1(I)]_2$ chains and one (α_2) which is different [1, 30, 45]. A type I trimer $[\alpha_1(I)]_3$ has also been discovered [15]. Type II collagen, largely restricted to cartilage, has three identical chains and is subdivided into a major $[\alpha_1 (IIM)]_3$ form [23] and a minor $[\alpha_1 (IIm)]_3$ form [4]. Type III is found particularly in developing tissues and seems to be associated with smaller fibre diameters and increased tissue extensibility. In skin it is localized in the papillary and periadnexal dermis. It is a trimer $[\alpha_1 (III)]_3$ [25, 26].

The second class comprises the type IV or base-

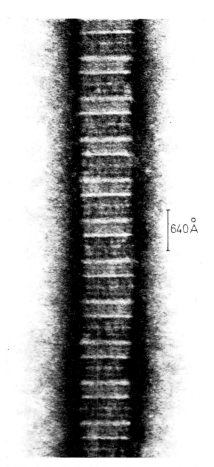

640 Å

FIG. 49.8. Single fibril of rat tail collagen, negatively stained with sodium phosphotungstate. One complete period of length 64 nm (640 Å) comprises a light D zone and a dark F zone with a number of interbands. (Electron micrograph by Dr G. A. Meek.)

ment membrane collagens [39, 43]. These are unable to associate into compact banded fibres but form open structures which are stabilized with disulphide bonds by end-to-end interactions at the non-helical amino and carboxy-terminal regions. It is probable that the molecules are composed of two similar α_1 (IV) chains and a second alpha chain, the α_2 (IV). Class 3 includes the pericellular collagens, so-called type V, which have been isolated from chorioamniotic membranes and a number of tissues, including skin [3]. Class 4 collagens have only recently been detected and are characterized by discontinuities in the triple helix which render the molecule susceptible to proteases [3].

Synthesis of collagens. Collagen is manufactured by the fibroblasts of the dermis or, in the other connective tissues, by the related cells such as chondrocytes and osteocytes [2, 7, 10, 17, 19, 29, 34–36]. The synthesis of type I collagen, as of any extracellular protein, occurs in a number of steps, and the analysis at the molecular level may prove highly relevant to the understanding of collagen disorders. The events will be summarized.

1. *Turning on of genes for pro-α_1 (I) and pro-α_2 (I).* Little is known about this first step, although the human pro-α_2(I) gene is known to be located on chromosome 7 [16, 34].

2. *Transcription of genes into hn RNAs.* The pro-α_2(I) human gene and the initial hn RNA transcript consist of about 40,000 bases, eight times the number necessary to code for the protein [27, 34]. This is accounted for by the presence of about 50 intervening sequences, which divide the central region of the gene into short coding sequences of 54 or 108 bases, each of which codes for 18 or 36 amino acid sequences with the structure $(Gly–x–y)_6$ or $(Gly–X–Y)_{12}$.

3. *Formation of mRNAs.* The processing of the hn RNAs to functional mRNAs requires over 50 enzyme steps, because of the 50 intervening sequences [34].

4. *Translation of mRNAs to prepro-α_1 (I) and prepro-α_2 (I) chains.* The amino terminal ends of the newly synthesized polypeptides contain a 'signal sequence' (Fig. 49.9) of hydrophobic amino acids which direct binding of the ribosome to the membranes of the rough endoplasmic reticulum [34].

5. *Processing of the prepro-α_1 (I) and prepro-α_2 (I) chains to pro-α chains.* The signal peptides are removed and the pro-α chains are processed to triple helical procollagen [17, 29, 34]. At least eight separate enzymes are involved in these post-translational modifications.

(a) *Synthesis of hydroxyproline.* Hydroxylation of proline is carried out by the enzyme prolyl hydroxylase which recognizes only the proline residues present in the Y position of the X–Y–Gly triplet [5, 48]. The enzyme requires molecular oxygen, ferrous iron, α-ketoglutarate and a reducing agent such as ascorbate as cofactors and cosubstrates.

It seems probable that the decreased formation of collagen fibres in scurvy results from a fault in the hydroxylation of proline due to ascorbic acid deficiency [38].

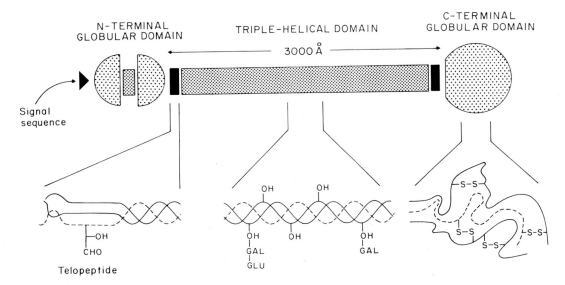

FIG. 49.9. The structure of collagens. Each has three major domains. The triple-helical domain is approximately 3,000 Å in length in the major structural and the pericellular collagens. The C-terminal domain contains both interchain and intrachain disulphide bonds. The short 'signal' sequence at the N-terminal directs the molecule into the secretory pathway and is removed intracellularly. After Burgeson [3].

(b) *Synthesis of hydroxylysine.* Hydroxylation of the lysine in the Y position of amino acid triplets is catalyzed by the enzyme lysyl hydroxylase which, like prolyl hydroxylase, requires molecular oxygen, ferrous iron, α-ketoglutarate and ascorbate [46]. The extent of such hydroxylation varies with the type of collagen.

(c) *Glycosylation.* Galactosyl residues are attached by O-glycosidic bonds through the hydroxyl groups of hydroxylysine by the enzyme collagen galactosyl transferase [33, 35]. A glucose molecule is then attached to each galactosyl residue by the enzyme collagen glucosyl transferase. Both enzymes utilize UPD-sugars as a source of carbohydrate and require manganous ions as a cofactor.

6. *Conversion of procollagen to collagen fibres.* This final stage involves at least two separate proteinases, namely procollagen amino-proteinase and procollagen carboxy-proteinase, which together remove about one-third of the procollagen molecule from the two ends of the three pro- α chains. The collagen then spontaneously assembles into fibres [34, 35, 47]. Their tensile strength is achieved by cross-linking with specific covalent bonds. The most common links are ones derived from lysine or hydroxylysine. First, aldehyde derivatives are formed by removal of amino groups from some of the resi-

dues [16, 31, 41]. Then either the aldehyde forms a Schiff base type of covalent link with an amino group in an unmodified lysine or hydroxylysine residue, or two aldehyde groups undergo an aldol condensation. Other more complex cross-links can also be formed. The initial de-amination of lysyl and hydroxylysyl residues can be catalysed by a single enzyme, lysyl oxidase [41], though two separate enzymes may perhaps be required. The enzyme requires copper as a cofactor and its activity is readily inhibited by nitriles. This explains why ingestion of β-aminoproprionitrile glutamate, which occurs in sweet peas, causes a condition known as lathyrism in which defective alpha chains do not adequately cross-link [38].

REFERENCES

1 BORNSTEIN P. & SAGE H. (1980) *Ann Rev Biochem* **49**, 957.
2 BORNSTEIN P. & TRAUB W. (1979) In *The proteins* IV Eds Neurath H. *et al* New York, Academic Press, p. 411.
3 BURGESON R. E. (1982) *J Invest Dermatol* **79**, 25s.
4 BUTLER W. T., *et al* (1977) *J Biol Chem* **252**, 639.
5 CARDINALE G. J. & UDENFRIEND S. (1974) *Adv Enzymol* **41**, 245.
6 CASSEL J. M. (1971) In *Biophysical Properties of the Skin.* Ed. Elden H. R. New York, Wiley Interscience, p. 63.

7 FESSLER J. H. & FESSLER L. I. (1978) *Ann Rev Biochem* **47,** 129.

8 GROSS J. (1964) *Biophys J* **4,** (Suppl.), 63.

9 GROSS J. (1974) *Harvey Lect* **68,** 351.

10 GROSS J. (1980) In *Gene Families of Collagen and Other Proteins.* Eds. Prockop D. J. & Champe P. C. New York, North-Holland, p. 5.

11 HARKNESS R. D. (1961) *Biol Rev* **36,** 399.

12 HODGE A. J. (1960) *Proc 4th Int Conf Electron Microsc* **2,** 119.

13 JACKSON D. S. (1970) In *Advances in Biology of Skin.* Vol. X. *The Dermis.* Eds. Montagna W., *et al.* New York, Appleton–Century–Crofts, p. 39.

14 JARRETT A. (1974) In *The Physiology and Pathophysiology of the Skin.* Ed. Jarrett A. London, Academic Press, Vol. III, p. 809.

15 JIMINEZ S. A., *et al* (1977) *Biochem Biophys Res Commun* **78,** 1354.

16 KANG A. J., *et al* (1966) *Biochemistry (NY)* **5,** 509.

17 KIVIRIKKO K. I. (1980) In *Gene Families of Collagen and Other Proteins.* Eds. Prockop D. J. & Champe P. C. New York, North-Holland, p. 107.

18 KUHN K. (1962) *Leder* **13,** 73.

19 LAYMAN D. L., *et al* (1971) *Proc Nat Acad Sci USA* **68,** 454.

20 LEACH A. A. (1960) *Biochem J* **74,** 70.

21 LEWIS M. S. & PIEZ K. A. (1963) *Proc Am Chem Soc New York Meeting, 9–13th September.*

22 MARTIN C. J. & AXELROD A. E. (1953) *Proc Soc Exp Biol Med* **83,** 461.

23 MILLER E. J. & MATUKAS V. J. (1969) *Proc Nat Acad Sci USA* **65,** 1264.

24 MILLER E. J. & MATUKAS V. J. (1974) *Fed Proc* **33,** 1197.

25 MILLER E. J., *et al* (1971) *Biochem Biophys Res Commun* **42,** 1024.

26 MILLER E. J., *et al* (1976) *Arch Biochem Biophys* **173,** 631.

27 MYERS J. C., *et al* (1981) *Proc Natl Acad Sci USA* **78,** 3516.

28 NEUMAN R. E. & LOGAN M. A. (1950) *J Biol Chem* **184,** 299.

29 PIEZ K. A. (1980) In *Gene Families of Collagen and Other Proteins.* Eds. Prockop D. J. & Champe P. C. New York, North-Holland, p. 143.

30 PIEZ K. A., *et al* (1963) *Biochemistry* **2,** 58.

31 PINNELL S. R. & MARTIN G. R. (1968) *Proc Natl Acad Sci USA* **61,** 708.

32 PINNELL S. R. & MURAD S. (1983) In *Biochemistry and Physiology of the Skin.* Ed. Goldsmith L. A. Oxford, Clarendon, p. 385

33 PROCKOP D. J. (1970) In *Chemistry and Molecular Biology of the Intracellular Matrix.* Ed. Balazs E. A. New York, Academic Press, Vol. 1, p. 335.

34 PROCKOP D. J. (1982) *J Invest Dermatol* **79,** 3s.

35 PROCKOP D. J., *et al* (1975) In *Biochemistry of Collagen.* Eds. Ramachandran G. N. & Reddi A. H. New York, Plenum.

36 PROCKOP D. J., *et al* (1979) *N Engl J Med* **301,** 13, 77.

37 RAMACHANDRAN G. N. & GOULD B. S. (Eds.) (1967, 1968) *Treatise on Collagen.* London, Academic Press, Vols I and II.

38 ROBERTSON W. VAN B. (1964) *Biophys J* **4** (Suppl.), 93.

39 SAGE H. (1982) *J Invest Dermatol* **79,** 51s.

40 SCHMITT F. O., et al (1955) *Symp Soc Exp Biol* **9,** 148.

41 SIEGEL R. C. (1974) *Proc Nat Acad Sci USA* **71,** 4826.

42 SMITH J. G., *et al* (1966) In *Modern Trends in Dermatology.* Ed. MacKenna R. M. B. London, Butterworth, Vol. III, p. 110.

43 STANLEY J. R., *et al* (1982) *J Invest Dermatol* **79,** 69s.

44 SZIRMAI J. A. (1970) In *Advances in Biology of Skin.* Vol. X. *The Dermis.* Eds. Montagna W., *et al.* New York, Appleton–Century–Crofts. p. 1

45 TOLSTOSHEV P. & CRYSTAL R. G. (1982) *J Invest Dermatol* **79,** 605

46 UITTO J. & LICHTENSTEIN J. R. (1976) *J Invest Dermatol* **66,** 59.

47 UITTO J. & PROCKOP D. J. (1973) *Biochem Biophys Res Commun* **55,** 904.

48 UITTO J. & PROCKOP D. J. (1974) *Arch Biochem Biophys* **164,** 210.

49 WOOD G. C. (1964) In *International Review of Connective Tissue Research.* Ed. Hall D. A. New York, Academic Press, Vol. II, p. 1.

Metabolism of collagen: collagenases [1, 11, 13, 17, 19, 25, 30]. Experiments using labelled amino acids suggest that collagen is relatively inert metabolically, and that once laid down it persists for long periods [8]. However, in some tissues and in some pathological states it is rapidly turned over. In the post partum uterus half the collagen can be absorbed in a day [12] and a high rate of resorption is known to occur from granuloma tissue [14]. In the skin of rodents, a fluctuation during the moult cycle is superimposed on the gradual increase with body growth; the concentration appears to fall sharply prior to and during the early phase of activity of the hair follicles [3]. The possible mechanisms of resorption are not the same for the different collagen types and are subject to specific tissue regulation [17].

Native collagen, whether fibrillar or in solution, is extremely resistant to degradation by proteolytic enzymes. The collagen must therefore be specifically attacked by a collagenase capable of acting at physiological levels of pH, temperature and salt concentration. Enzymes which can break down the triple helical structure at neutral pH were first described from culture filtrates of the bacterium *Clostridium histolyticum* [2, 18, 23, 26].

The existence of vertebrate collagenases was initially demonstrated in tadpoles. When explants of bullfrog tadpole tail, a tissue in which connective tissue is resorbed during metamorphosis, were cultured on a reconstituted native fibrous collagen substrate, the gel of the surrounding medium was digested [5, 10, 24]. By separating the epidermis from the underlying dermis, it was possible to show that the epidermis alone was responsible for collagenase production [5, 24].

Using a tissue culture technique similar to that employed with tadpole tail, it was shown that human skin cells can produce collagenase [5, 20]. The main source appears to be in the papillary dermis; no enzyme is produced by the lower dermis [4, 20], nor has it been collected from normal epidermis, though it is produced by proliferating epidermis in wound healing [9]. Collagenase is also produced by skin fibroblasts in culture [1], by granulocytes [21, 22] and by macrophages when activated by phlogistic stimuli [29].

It seems likely that fibroblasts are the primary *in vivo* source. Skin fibroblast collagenase appears to be identical with that derived from whole human skin in terms of collagen cleavage products, pH optimum and metal requirements [1, 27]. The enzyme makes a single cleavage across all three chains of the collagen molecule at a point about three-quarters of the distance from the NH_2 terminal, without disrupting the helical configuration of either fragment [6].

Skin collagenase appears to be similar to other collagenase by reason of its immunological cross-reactivity, but with the somewhat larger molecular weight of 60,000 daltons [31]. There is evidence that collagenase exists in a latent form, since overt collagenase activity is not detectable in fibroblast culture medium unless it has been pre-incubated with trypsin [7, 27, 28]. Moreover, gel electrophoresis of culture medium has revealed two protein bands with molecular weights of about 60,000 and 55,000. After trypsin activation, the weight of each procollagenase is reduced by 10,000 daltons; both have identical activities [1, 28].

The estimation of urinary hydroxyproline has proved of some value in the study of collagen metabolism [25]. It is higher during body growth than in the adult. More hydroxyproline appears to be excreted when collagen is synthesized or catabolized at an increased rate, as for example in hyperparathyroidism [15], some bone diseases and acromegaly, or after severe skin burns [16].

REFERENCES

1 BAUER E. A., *et al* (1983) In *Biochemistry and Physiology of the Skin*. Ed. Goldsmith L. A. New York, Oxford University Press, p. 411.
2 BORNSTEIN P. (1967) *Biochemistry* **6**, 3082.
3 EBLING F. J. & HALE P. A. (1966) *J Endocrinol* **36**, 177.
4 EISEN A. Z. (1969) *J Invest Dermatol* **52**, 442.
5 EISEN A. Z. & CROSS J. (1965) *Dev Biol* **12**, 408.
6 EISEN A. Z., *et al* (1968) *Biochim Biophys Acta* **151**, 637.
7 FIEDLER-NAGY C., *et al* (1977) *Eur J Biochem* **76**, 291.
8 GERBER G., *et al* (1960) *J Biol Chem* **235**, 2653.
9 GRILLO H. C. & GROSS J. (1967) *Dev Biol* **15**, 300.
10 GROSS J. & LAPIÈRE C. M. (1962) *Proc Natl Acad Sci USA* **48**, 1014.
11 GROSS J., *et al* (1980) In *Collagenase in Normal and Pathological Connective Tissues*. Eds. Woolley D. E. & Evanson J. M. Chichester, Wiley, p. 11.
12 HARKNESS M. L. R. & HARKNESS R. D. (1954) *J Physiol (Lond)* **123**, 492.
13 HARRIS E. D. & KRANE S. M. (1974) *N Eng J Med* **291**, 557, 605, 652.
14 JACKSON D. S. (1957) *Biochem J* **65**, 277.
15 KLEIN L., *et al* (1962) *Metabolism* **ii**, 1023.
16 KLEIN L., *et al* (1962) *Surg Forum* **13**, 459.
17 KRANE S. M. (1982) *J Invest Dermatol* **79**, 83s.
18 KUHN K. & EGGL M. (1966) *Biochem Z* **346**, 197.
19 LAPIÈRE C. H. (1980) In *Collagenase in Normal and Pathological Connective Tissues*. Eds. Woolley D. E. & Evanson J. M. Chichester, Wiley, p. 175.
20 LAZARUS G. S. & FULLMER H. M. (1969) *J Invest Dermatol* **52**, 545.
21 LAZARUS G. S., *et al* (1968) *Science* **159**, 1483.
22 LAZARUS G. S., *et al* (1968) *J Clin Invest* **47**, 2622.
23 MANDL I. (1961) *Adv Enzymol* **23**, 174.
24 NAGAI Y., *et al* (1966) *Biochemistry* **5**, 3123.
25 SMILEY J. D. & ZIFF M. (1964) *Physiol Rev* **44**, 30.
26 STARK M. & KUHN K. (1968) *Eur J Biochem* **6**, 534.
27 STRICKLIN G. P., *et al* (1977) *Biochemistry* **16**, 1607.
28 STRICKLIN G. P., *et al* (1978) *Biochemistry* **17**, 2331.
29 WAHL L. M., *et al* (1974) *Proc Natl Acad Sci USA* **71**, 3598.
30 WEISS J. B. (1976) *Int Rev Connect Tissue Res* **7**, 102.
31 WOOLLEY D. E., *et al* (1978) *Biochem J* **169**, 265.

Changes with ageing [7]. Collagen changes both qualitatively and quantitatively throughout life. The qualitative changes are reflected in decreasing solubility and an alteration in various physical properties [2, 16, 17]. For example, in strips of dermis the temperature at which rapid shrinkage begins and the tension developed in isometric contraction both rise with age [12]. Collagen becomes more stable with age. One hypothetical scheme for such ageing is that a progressive transesterification takes place in which intra-strand links are changed first into inter-strand links and ultimately into intermolecular links, without any increase in the total of ester bonds [3].

As observations on animals have been made mainly during their growth phase and those on man mainly during adulthood and senescence, there has been some confusion about how the concentration of collagen changes. As might be expected, since the skin increases in area and thickness as an animal grows, the collagen content of a complete skin and the amount of collagen per unit area are correlated with body weight [16]. In addition there is ample evidence, for example from rats [1, 4, 5, 8, 9, 16, 18], rabbits [11] and cattle [15], that the actual concentration of total collagen per unit weight of skin increases from birth to adulthood, when it remains stationary [10]. It seems likely that in man, also, the concentration of insoluble collagen in the skin increases from infant to adult [13]. From early adulthood onwards, however, there appears to be a gradual decrease in the absolute amount of collagen per unit area of skin, and this correlates with the clinical appearance of the skin during ageing. It occurs more rapidly in women than in men [14].

REFERENCES

1 CADAVID N. G., *et al* (1963) *Lab Invest* **12**, 598.
2 ELDEN H. R. (1968) In *Advances in Biology of Skin* Vol. X. *The Dermis*. Eds. Montagna W., *et al*. New York, Appleton-Century–Crofts, p. 231.
3 GALLOP P. M. (1964) *Biophys J* **4** (Suppl.), 79.
4 HOUCK J. C. & JACOB R. A. (1958) *Proc Soc Exp Biol Med* **97**, 604.
5 HOUCK J. C., *et al* (1961) *Proc Soc Exp Biol Med* **107**, 280.
6 JACKSON D. S. (1965) In *Advances in Biology of Skin*. Vol. VI. *Ageing*. Ed. Montagna W. Oxford, Pergamon, p. 219.
7 JARRETT A. (1974) In *The Physiology and Pathophysiology of the Skin*. Vol. III. *The Dermis and the Dendrocytes* Ed. Jarrett A. London, New York, Academic Press, p. 911.
8 KAO K-Y. T. & McGAVACK T. H. (1959) *Proc Soc Exp Biol Med* **101**, 153.
9 KAO K-Y. T., *et al* (1960) *Proc Soc Exp Biol Med* **104**, 359.
10 MURRAY D. H., *et al* (1961) *J Gerontol* **16**, 17.
11 NIMNI M. E., *et al* (1965) *Nature* **207**, 865.
12 RASMUSSEN D. M., *et al* (1965) In *Advances in Biology of Skin*. Vol. VI. *Ageing*. Ed. Montagna W. Oxford, Pergamon, p. 151.
13 SAMS W. M., JR & SMITH J. G., JR. (1965) In *Advances in Biology of Skin*. Vol. VI. *Ageing*. Ed. Montagna W. Oxford, Pergamon, p. 199.
14 SHUSTER S. & BOTTOMS E. (1963) *Clin Sci* **25**, 487.
15 SMITS G. (1957) *Biochim Biophys Acta* **25**, 543.
16 SOBEL H., *et al* (1953) *Arch Biochem Biophys* **46**, 221.
17 VERZAR F. (1964) In *International Review of Connective Tissue Research*. Ed. Hall D. A. New York, Academic Press, Vol. 2, p. 244.
18 WIRTSCHAFTER Z. T. & BENTLEY J. P. (1962) *Lab Invest* **ii**, 316.

ELASTIC FIBRES

Structure, composition and synthesis of elastic fibres. The characteristic property of elastic fibres [3, 13–15, 20, 21, 24, 30, 31] is that they can be stretched by 100% or more and still return to their original dimensions; they rebound rapidly when the extending stress is removed. They consist of delicate, straight, freely branching fibres which can be selectively stained with orcein, Weigert's resorcin, fuchsin, aldehyde fuchsin, Verhoeff's and orcinol new fuchsin stains, though these methods are not specific. The fibres fluoresce brilliantly, partly due to an amino acid known as desmosine [33] which is unique to elastin.

Ultrastructural examination has revealed that elastin fibres have two components. The central amorphous core of elastin is surrounded by microfibrils 10–12 nm in diameter which are composed of so-called elastic tissue fibrillar protein [6, 9, 11, 12, 17, 26, 27, 35, 36]. The relative amounts of these components change during development: the newly developed embryonic fibres are almost all microfibrillar protein, whereas the mature fibrils are 90% elastin [27, 36].

The chemistry of the microfibrillar component is not well known, but elastin is well characterized. Its molecular structure was opened to investigation by the isolation of a soluble protein named tropoelastin from pigs in which copper deficiency had caused inactivation of the lysyloxidase necessary for cross-linking [28, 29, 31, 32]. Tropoelastin is a single polypeptide chain of about 800 amino acid residues. Glycine, contributing 245 residues, is the commonest, but proline, alanine, valine, phenylalanine, isoleucine and leucine are also major constituents [30, 31]. All these are non-polar; in contrast, polar amino acids such as aspartate, glutamate, lysine and arginine account for less than 5% of the total. Unique to elastin are the amino acids desmosine and isodesmosine (Fig. 49.10,G), which account for about two out of each 1,000 residues [21, 30].

Several models have been proposed for the elastic molecule, and their validity has been provocatively debated by Rosenbloom [24]. One favoured hypothesis is based on a view that the polypeptide chain, before cross-linking, has two distinct areas [30, 31]. One is hydrophobic and stretchable. It is composed of the dominant amino acids glycine, proline, valine, phenylalanine and leucine (Fig. 49.10,A, large loops), frequently in a repeating pentapeptide sequence of pro–gly–val–gly–val. Further, the chain is folded back on itself to create an antiparallel arrangement of neighbouring lengths. This unique

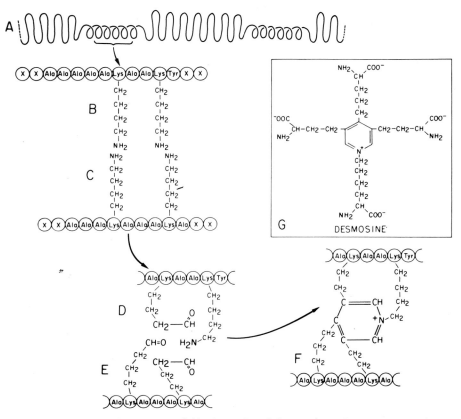

FIG. 49.10. Cross-linking of soluble elastin into insoluble elastin. Part G shows a desmosine molecule free from peptide linkages to the elastin polypeptide chains. With isodesmosine, the lysine-derived side chain opposite the nitrogen (*para*) is moved to the ortho # position. Adapted from Sandberg *et al* [30] with permission of the authors and publisher.

structure is known as a beta-spiral and possesses elastometric properties. In between are other areas, probably alpha-helical, which contain lysine residues separated by two or three alanine residues (Fig. 49.10,B and C). During cross-linking, chains with two alanines between two lysines (B) align in precise apposition to chains having three alanines between the lysines (C). This spatial relationship allows the lysyloxidase to convert three of their epsilon-amino groups to aldehydes, named allysines, (Fig. 49.10,D and E), leaving one of the residues with the epsilon-amino group intact. Condensation to form the stable desmosine cross-link (Fig. 49.10,F), by fusion of these three allysines and the unmodified residue, then occurs [19, 30, 31, 35].

Elastin is produced by fibroblasts in the dermis, but elsewhere it is synthesized by smooth muscle cells [1, 7], endothelial cells [8] and chondroblasts [22]. Its production follows the general pattern for proteins. The translation of messenger-RNA coding

for elastin polypeptides takes place on the polyribosomes of rough endoplasmic reticulum and the nascent chains are released into the cisternae [31, 35]. The Golgi vacuoles may be involved in its secretion into the extracellular space [34]. It seems that, in contrast with collagen, the molecules of newly synthesized and extracellular elastin are of similar size [25].

Metabolism of elastin. The metabolic turnover of mature elastin is normally slow, though some degradation occurs during growth, wound healing, tissue remodelling and pregnancy [38], and destructive changes occur in a number of chronic diseases. Newly synthesized elastin, however, is susceptible to degradation by a number of proteins [18], as are the microfibrillar components of the fibres.

Elastases were first described from bacteria [19] and their activity may contribute to the virulence of pathogens [38]. They are also produced by fungi, including those capable of infecting hair, nails and epidermis [23], and by the cercaria larvae of blood flukes, which penetrate human skin [10]. They have been identified amongst the proteinases of snake venoms [5]. In mammals elastases from pancreas [4], granulocytes [4] and macrophages [2] have been characterized and the degradation of elastin by implanting embryos [37] and by tumour cells [16] has been demonstrated.

REFERENCES

1 ABRAHAM P. A., *et al* (1977) *Adv Exp Med Biol* **79**, 397.

2 BANDA M. J. & WERB Z. (1980) *Fed Proc* **39**, 799.

3 BANGA I. (1966) *Structure and Function of Elastin and Collagen*. Budapest, Akademiao Kaido.

4 BARRETT A. J. & MCDONALD J. K. (1980) *Mammalian Proteases, a Glossary and Bibliography*. Vol. 1. *Endopeptidases*. New York, Academic Press.

5 BERNICK J. J. & SIMPSON J. W. (1976) *Comp Biochem Physiol* [13] **54**, 51.

6 BODLEY H. D. & WOOD R. L. (1972) *Anat Rec* **172**, 71.

7 BURKE J. M. & ROSS R. (1979) *Int Rev Connect Tissue Res* **8**, 119.

8 CARNES W. H., *et al* (1979) *Biochem Biophys Res Commun* **90**, 1393.

9 CLEARY E. G. & CLIFF W. J. (1978) *Exp Mol Pathol* **28**, 227.

10 GRAZINELLI G., *et al* (1966) *Comp Biochem Physiol* **18**, 689.

11 GOTTE L., *et al* (1972) *Connective Tissue Res* **1**, 61.

12 GOTTE L., *et al* (1974) *J Ultrastruct Res* **46**, 23.

13 HALL D. A. (1971) In *Biophysical Properties of the Skin*. Ed. Elden H. R. New York, Wiley Interscience, p. 187.

14 HASHIMOTO K. & DIBELLA R. J. (1967) *J Invest Dermatol* **48**, 405.

15 JARRETT A. (1974) In *The Physiology of the Skin*. Ed. Jarrett A. London, Academic Press, p. 847.

16 JONES P. A. & DECLERK Y. A. (1980) *Cancer Res* **40**, 3222.

17 KOBAYASI T. (1968) *Acta Derm Venereol (Stockh)* **48**, 303.

18 MECHAM R. P. & FOSTER J. A. (1977) *Biochemistry* **16**, 3825.

19 OAKLEY C. L. & BONERJEE N. G. (1963) *J Pathol Bacteriol* **85**, 489.

20 PARTRIDGE S. M. (1962) *Adv Protein Chem* **17**, 227.

21 PARTRIDGE S. M. (1970) In *Advances in Biology of Skin*. Vol. X. *The Dermis*. Eds. Montagna W., *et al*. New York, Appleton–Century–Crofts, p. 69.

22 QUINTARELLI G., *et al* (1979) *Connect Tissue Res* **7**, 1.

23 RIPPON J. W. & VARADI D. P. (1968) *J Invest Dermatol* **50**, 54.

24 ROSENBLOOM J. (1982) *Connective Tissue Res* **10**, 73.

25 ROSENBLOOM J., *et al* (1980) *J Biol Chem* **255**, 100.

26 ROSS R. & BORNSTEIN P. (1969) *J Cell Biol* **40**, 366.

27 ROSS R., *et al* (1977) *Adv Exp Biol Med* **79**, 7.

28 SANDBERG L. B. (1976) *Int Rev Connect Tissue Res* **7**, 159.

29 SANDBERG L. B., *et al* (1969) *Biochemistry* **8**, 2940.

30 SANDBERG L. B., *et al* (1981) *N Engl J Med* **304**, 566.

31 SANDBERG L. B., *et al* (1982) *J Invest Dermatol* **79**, 128s.

32 SMITH D. W., *et al* (1968) *Biochem Biophys Res Commun* **31**, 309.

33 THOMAS J., *et al* (1963) *Nature* **200**, 651.

34 VITTO J., *et al* (1976) *Arch Biochem Biophys* **173**, 187.

35 UITTO J., *et al* (1982) *J Invest Dermatol* **79**, 160s.

36 VARADI D. P. (1976) *J Invest Dermatol* **66**, 59.

37 WERB Z., *et al* (1980) *J Cell Biol* **87**, 138a.

38 WERB Z., *et al* (1980) *J Cell Biol* **79**, 154s.

THE FIBROBLAST [4, 7, 11]

Fibroblasts are the most numerous of the cells found in loose connective tissue. The term *fibroblast* should, historically, designate a cell at an early stage of differentiation and *fibrocyte* one which is fully differentiated [16], but in practice many researchers use fibroblast for an actively secreting cell and fibrocyte for an inactive one [7]. Fibroblasts are developed from the mesenchyme which also gives rise to chondroblasts and osteoblasts. It has been suggested that they may also originate from other mesenchymal elements, such as the vascular endothelium or by transformation of macrophages, and it is possible that differentiated fibroblasts can themselves transform into osteoblasts. Electron microscopy reveals that the fibroblast of developing (as distinct from mature) connective tissue has an abundant cytoplasm with a well-developed endoplasmic reticulum and prominent ribosomes attached to the membrane surfaces. The Golgi membranes are clearly seen. Such features are characteristic of cells which are engaged in active synthesis and secretion. In studies of the fate of tritiated proline by autoradiography [12], it has been shown that material is first synthesized in the cisternae of the endoplasmic reticulum and subsequently transferred to the Golgi region after which it passes out of the fibroblast. Though, historically, the issue has been debated, it now seems generally accepted that fibroblasts are responsible for the manufacture of all the dermal connective-tissue elements or their precursors.

Most researchers have been in agreement with Gersh and Catchpole [5] that fibroblasts are the source of the ground substance, notwithstanding the view of Asboe-Hansen [1] that the mast cell was implicated, on the grounds that it was the only connective-tissue cell shown to contain acid mucopolysaccharide. There is evidence, however, from autoradiographic studies that ^{35}S is incorporated into sulphated mucopolysaccharides in the Golgi complex of fibroblasts, and that such substances are secreted [4, 11]. The sulphated mucopolysaccharide

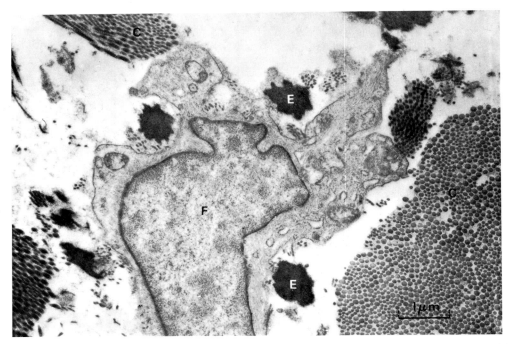

FIG. 49.11. Fibroblast (F) with elastic fibres (E) and collagen fibres (C) in transverse section. Electron micrograph of the forearm skin from an adult male, stained *PTA*, by Professor A. S. Breathnach.

produced by mast cells, however, is stored within the cell and is mainly heparin.

Human fibroblasts can be shown to produce collagen *in vitro* and there is no doubt that they are the source of the precursor of collagen [3, 10]. While the source of elastin is less obvious, it has been clear that elastic tissue never occurs except in the presence of collagen, and in electron micrographs is seen always in the vicinity of fibroblasts [2]. It is now established that tropoelastin, containing a leader sequence of about 25 residues which are ultimately lost, is synthesized on the rough endoplasmic reticulum in a similar fashion to collagen [15]. The existence of specific elastoblasts has been proposed but never demonstrated [2].

These considerations leave open the question of whether all fibroblasts are identical. Differences between papillary and reticular fibroblasts have been proposed [17], and fibroblasts from human gingiva have been shown to consist of two subpopulations differing in their response to prostaglandin E_2 [9].

Variants from scar tissue have been described. Knapp *et al* [8] found two types from normal skin and mature scars, one small and spindle shaped (S cell) and one larger, flatter and amoeboid in appearance (A cell). In fibroblast populations derived from keloids, A cells were predominant, and keloid out-growths often produced a third type, designated the K cell. Other researchers [13] were unable to detect differences in appearance or size distribution between fibroblasts cultured from normal skin and from keloids, though there were differences in response to hydrocortisone [14]. It has been suggested that keloid fibroblasts lack the normal ability to respond to the stresses imposed by wounding and thus produce badly aligned collagen fibrils [6].

REFERENCES

1 Asboe-Hansen G. (1957) In *Connective Tissue*. Ed. Tunbridge R. E. Oxford, Blackwell, p. 30.
2 Ayer J. P. (1964) In *International Review of Connective Tissue Research*. Ed. Hall D. A. New York, Academic Press, Vol. II, p. 33.
3 Bellamy G. & Bornstein P. (1971) *Proc Nat Acad Sci USA* **68**, 1138.
4 Branwood A. W. (1963) In *International Review of Connective Tissue Research*. Ed. Hall D. A. New York, Academic Press, Vol. 1, p. 1.
5 Gersh L. & Catchpole H. R. (1949) *Am J Anat* **85**, 457.
6 Hunter J. A. A. & Finlay J. B. (1976) *Br J Surg* **63**, 826.
7 Jarrett A. (Ed.) (1974) *The Physiology and Pathophysiology of the Skin*. Vol. III. *The Dermis and the Dendrocytes*. London, New York, Academic Press.

8 KNAPP T. R., *et al* (1977) *Am J Pathol* **86**, 47.

9 KO S. D., *et al* (1977) *Proc Natl Acad Sci USA* **74**, 3429.

10 LAYMAN D. L., *et al* (1971) *Proc Natl Acad Sci USA* **68**, 454.

11 PORTER K. R. (1964) *Biophys J* **4**, (Suppl.), 167.

12 ROSS R. & BENDITT E. P. (1965) *J Cell Biol* **27**, 83.

13 RUSSELL J. D. & WITT W. S. (1976) *Plast Reconstr Surg* **57**, 207.

14 RUSSELL J. D., *et al* (1978) *J Cell Physiol* **97**, 221.

15 SANDBERG L. B., *et al* (1982) *J Invest Dermatol* **79**, 1283.

16 SZIRMAI J. A. (1970) In *Advances in Biology of Skin*. Vol. X. *The Dermis*. Eds. Montagna W., *et al*. New York, Appleton–Century–Crofts.

17 TAJIMA S. & PINNELL S. R. (1981) *J Invest Dermatol* **77**, 410.

THE NATURE OF CONNECTIVE-TISSUE DISORDER

Connective-tissue diseases can, with some overlap, be put into four main groups. First are acquired metabolic disorders, such as scurvy, which is caused by a deficiency of vitamin C in the diet (see p. 2329). Secondly are those disorders of undoubted genetic determination, of which the range of mucopolysaccharidoses loosely described as gargoylism, pseudoxanthoma elasticum and cutis hyperelastica (Ehlers–Danlos syndrome) are good examples. Thirdly are those acquired conditions which appear to involve immunological reactions to autogenous antigens, such as systemic lupus erythematosus, rheumatic fever, systemic sclerosis (diffuse scleroderma) and dermatomyositis. Genetic factors may play some part in these. Lastly are degenerative conditions of ageing, such as osteoarthrosis and osteoporosis, which affect bone, and senile elastosis of skin. In senile elastosis, however, environmental exposure to sunlight, as well as age, play a very significant part.

The attempt to classify the pathological changes according to whether ground substance, collagen, elastin or cellular components are mainly or wholly involved is not always easy and may, historically, have been inaccurate. Clearly myxoedema and gargoylism can be quoted as conditions in which ground substance is affected and scurvy as one that involves collagen deficiency. However, to take only one example, the traditional designation of Ehlers–Danlos syndrome as an elastosis in which the elastic fibres are increased in number [2, 16] is misleading. The most obvious characteristics of the syndrome are hyperelasticity of the skin and hyperextensibility of the joints, which could not occur unless there were a decrease in the restraints to deformation imposed by collagen.

The problem was initially complicated by the questionable specificity of the histological methods employed for staining elastic tissue. Thus it was suggested that the apparent increase in elastic fibres in Ehlers–Danlos syndrome could be an artefact due to polymerization of a precursor by acid orcein stain [16]. It was also proposed that, abnormally, collagen could change into a material, given the name 'collastin', which took elastic tissue stains. Smith *et al* [25], having reviewed the evidence, sensibly considered this view to be untenable.

By chemical and ultrastructural analysis of the defective components, combined with assay of the enzyme activity of fibroblasts cultured *in vitro*, considerable progress has been made in identifying the biochemical faults in heritable connective-tissue diseases [14, 22, 26, 27].

Thus eight conditions [10, 21, 22], characterized by skeletal, connective-tissue and intellectual defects and involving faulty degradation of glycosaminoglycans, have been identified (see Chapter 62). Similarly, Ehlers–Danlos syndrome has been divided into eleven types, [23, 24] according to the nature of the collagen faults (see p. 1837), and a number of conditions involving elastin abnormalities [27] such as, for example, pseudoxanthoma elasticum, cutis laxa and Marfan syndrome have received some biochemical as well as histopathological characterization (see p. 1834).

It is less easy to define changes in connective tissue in such conditions as lupus erythematosus, scleroderma and dermatomyositis (Chapter 35) which are frequently described as 'collagen' or 'connective-tissue' diseases. The concept of 'collagen' disease stems historically from study of the pathology of systemic lupus erythematosus and rheumatic fever [12]. In systemic lupus erythematosus there is a swelling and blurring of the fibrillar structure and an increased tendency to stain with acidic dyes, a change described as fibrinoid necrosis [15]. An alteration in the dermal barrier is indicated by the demonstration that the spread of an indicator takes longer to reconstitute following the intradermal injection of hyaluronidase. The connective tissue is similarly involved in rheumatic fever; even apparently healthy areas of skin in this condition do not blister in response to irritation as readily as normal skin because permeability of the dermis is increased.

The discovery that human skin cells can produce collagenase [18, 19] has thrown new light on the pathogenesis of dystrophic epidermolysis bullosa [3–5]. This blistering disease (see p. 1625) is characterized by collagen destruction in the papillary layer of the dermis [1, 11]. Increased synthesis of collagenase [4–6, 18] has been demonstrated both *in vivo* and by fibroblasts *in vitro*. Furthermore, partially purified preparations of the collagenase appeared to show marked thermal stability and diminished affinity for Ca^{2+}, a cofactor, suggesting that the condition arises from a mutant enzyme [4].

Collagenase is also implicated in inflammatory conditions such as rheumatoid arthritis [7–9, 13, 20]. It appears that monocyte macrophages produce a stimulatory factor which increases the synthesis by fibroblasts of both collagenase and prostaglandin E_2 [17].

The rest of this chapter deals with a wide range of disorders, hereditary and acquired, in which collagen, elastic tissue or cartilage are conspicuously involved, but specifically excluding tumours and the so called collagen vascular diseases.

REFERENCES

1 ANTON-LAMPRECHT I., *et al* (1981) *Lancet* **ii**, 1077.
2 AYER J. P. (1964) In *International Review of Connective Tissue Research*. Ed. Hall D. A. New York, Academic Press, Vol. II, p. 33.
3 BAUER E. A. (1977) *Proc Natl Acad Sci USA* **74**, 4646.
4 BAUER E. A. (1982) *J Invest Dermatol* **79**, 105s.
5 BAUER E. A., *et al* (1977) *J Invest Dermatol* **68**, 119.
6 EIZEN A. Z. (1969) *J Invest Dermatol* **52**, 449.
7 EVANSON J. M. (1971) In *Tissue Proteinases*. Eds. Barrett A. J. & Dingle D. T. Amsterdam, North-Holland, p.327.
8 EVANSON J. M., *et al* (1967) *Science* **158**, 499.
9 EVANSON J. M., *et al* (1968) *J Clin Invest* **47**, 2639.
10 FLUHARTY A. L. (1982) *J Invest Dermatol* **79**, 38s.
11 GEDDE-DAHL T. (1971) *Epidermolysis Bullosa. A Clinical, Genetic and Epidemiological Study*. Baltimore, Johns Hopkins Press.
12 GLYNN L. E. (1964) In *International Review of Connective Tissue Research*. Ed. Hall D. A. New York, Academic Press, Vol. II, p. 214.
13 HARRIS E. D., JR, *et al* (1970) *Arthritis Rheum* **13**, 83.
14 HOLBROOK K. A. & BYERS P. H. (1982) *J Invest Dermatol* **79**, 7s.
15 JARRETT A. (1974) In *Physiology and Pathophysiology of the Skin*. Ed. Jarrett A. London, Academic Press, Vol. III, p. 937.
16 JARRETT A. (1974) In *Physiology and Pathophysiology of the Skin*. Ed. Jarrett A. London, Academic Press, Vol. III, p. 973.
17 KRANE S. M. (1982) *J Invest Dermatol* **79**, 83s.
18 LAZARUS G. S. (1971) *Clin Res* **19**, 362.
19 LAZARUS G. S. (1972) *Br J Dermatol* **86**, 193.
20 LAZARUS G. S., *et al* (1968) *N Engl J Med* **279**, 914.
21 LINKER A. (1970) In *Advances in the Biology of Skin* Vol. X. *The Dermis*. Eds. Montagna W., *et al*. New York, Appleton–Century–Crofts, p. 163.
22 MCKUSICK V. A. (1972) *Heritable Disorders of Connective Tissue*. 4th ed. St Louis, Mosby.
23 PINNELL S. R. (1982) *J Invest Dermatol* **79**, 83s.
24 PINNELL S. R., *et al* (1972) *N Engl J Med* **286**, 1013.
25 SMITH J. G., JR, *et al* (1966) In *Modern Trends in Dermatology*. Ed. MacKenna R. M. B. London, Butterworth, Vol. III, p. 110.
26 UITTO J. & LICHTENSTEIN J. R. (1976) *J Invest Dermatol* **66**, 59.
27 UITTO J., *et al* (1982) *J Invest Dermatol* **79**, 160s.

ATROPHY

Atrophy of the skin is a term which is usually applied to the clinical changes produced by a decrease in the dermal connective tissue. It is characterized by thinning and loss of elasticity. The skin usually appears smooth and finely wrinkled, and it feels soft and dry. Veins or other subcutaneous structures may be unduly conspicuous. There is often associated loss of hair follicles, and telangiectasia and irregular macular pigmentation are frequently present. The term *poikiloderma* is applied to the combination of cutaneous atrophy associated with conspicuous telangiectasis and prominent finely reticulate pigmentation (p. 1812).

Atrophy of the skin occurs in varying degree in a large number of skin conditions, and the underlying histological changes are also variable, since the several components of the connective tissue may be involved to a different degree, and there may or not be atrophy of the epidermis. Atrophy which includes subcutaneous tissue or even deeper structures is referred to as *panatrophy*.

The term *cicatricial atrophy* has been applied to the association of atrophy with sclerosis, as may occur in cicatricial alopecia, but there is usually little loss of substance and this confusing term should perhaps be abandoned.

The following classification is provisional, as our knowledge of many of these disorders is far from complete:

1. Scars
2. Macular atrophy (anetoderma)
   Primary
       (i) Anetoderma of Jadassohn–Pellizari
       (ii) Anetoderma of Schweninger–Buzzi
   Secondary to another inflammatory disease
3. Chronic atrophic acrodermatitis
4. Varioliform atrophy
5. Follicular atrophoderma
6. Vermiculate atrophoderma
7. Atrophoderma of Pasini and Pierini
8. Atrophic naevi
9. Panatrophy
       (i) Local panatrophy
       (ii) Facial hemiatrophy
10. Poikiloderma

11. Scleroatrophic syndrome of Huriez
12. Rheumatoid atrophy
13. Glucocorticosteroid-induced atrophy

ATROPHIC SCARS

Atrophy may result from the destruction of connective tissue by trauma or by inflammatory changes induced by known or by poorly understood disease processes. The distribution and character of the atrophic lesions may be so distinctive as to betray their origin, and are sometimes of considerable importance in diagnosis. The scars left by tertiary syphilis, certain tuberculides and some deep mycoses, especially sporotrichosis, are usually completely atrophic. Lupus erythematosus may also leave atrophy without clinical evidence of sclerosis. Lupus vulgaris and the chronic follicular pyodermas and some cases of lupus erythematosus leave a combination of atrophy and sclerosis, in which the latter predominates.

Exposure to ionizing radiations gives rise to a very striking combination of atrophy, pigmentation and telangiectasis (p. 654).

The wide atrophic scars which follow injuries in the Ehlers–Danlos syndrome (p. 1837) emphasize the importance of constitutional factors in determining the pattern of dermal response to a known external injury.

The lesions of mastocytosis may also become atrophic, presumably as a result of a pharmacological effect [1].

REFERENCE

1 THIVOLET J., *et al* (1981) *Ann Dermatol Vénéréol* 108, 259.

Stellate and discoid pseudoscars [1–4]. Stellate pseudoscars are white, irregular or 'star-shaped' atrophic scars. They are common on light-exposed skin, particularly on the extensor aspects of the forearms, often in association with senile purpura. These are seen in 20% of patients aged 70–90 yr, and a much less common pre-senile form occasionally occurs before the age of 50 yr. They have also developed after prolonged topical corticosteroid therapy. It has been demonstrated that these pseudoscars are secondary to trauma and are probably always preceded by haemorrhage with or without epidermal erosion.

REFERENCES

1 BRAUN-FALCO O. & BALDA B. R. (1970) *Hautarzt* 21, 509.
2 CHRISTIANSEN H. B. & MITCHELL W. T. (1969) *Arch Dermatol* 100, 703.
3 COLOMB D. (1972) *Arch Dermatol* 105, 551.
4 ZAK F. G., *et al* (1968) *Arch Dermatol* 98, 499.

ANETODERMA
SYN. MACULAR ATROPHY

Definition and nomenclature. The term anetoderma refers to a circumscribed area of slack skin associated with a loss of dermal substance on palpation and a loss of elastic tissue on histological examination [15, 16]. The term 'macular atrophy' has been used synonymously, but this term is less desirable as it has also been applied to other types of focal dermal atrophy. 'Primary' anetoderma implies that there is no associated underlying disease, whereas 'secondary' anetoderma can be attributed to some associated condition.

The term anetoderma was first used by Jadassohn in 1891 (*anetos* = slack), and since then several hundred cases have been reported under a variety of different names such as idiopathic macular atrophy, dermatitis atrophicans maculosa, etc. In the past, cases of primary anetoderma have been divided into the Jadassohn–Pellizari type, in which the lesions are preceded by erythema or urticaria, and the Schweninger–Buzzi type, in which there are no preceding inflammatory lesions [4, 5]. A recent review of 16 cases showed that the same patient may show some lesions that have, and some that have not, had an inflammatory onset. It also showed that the presence or absence of clinical inflammatory lesions at the onset does not affect the prognosis [6]. It was therefore suggested that the clinical classification based on the presence or absence of inflammation is of historical interest only.

Primary anetoderma
Aetiology. The cause is unknown, but some cases appear to have an infective origin, since they respond to penicillin [12]. The distinction between these cases and chronic atrophic acrodermatitis is unclear [13].

The histology of anetoderma suggests that the basic abnormality is focal elastolysis. This may be secondary to the release of elastase from the inflammatory cells which are probably always present in the early stages [15].

Pathology [15]. During the early stages the dermis is oedematous and a lymphocytic infiltrate surrounds the blood vessels and appendages. Plasma cells and histiocytes with some granuloma formation may also be seen. Later the oedema and perivascular infiltrate subside and elastic fibres become scanty. The persistence of fine, irregular or twisted elastic fibres is common. The dermal collagen may also be diminished, but the fragmentation and disappearance of elastic tissue is the essential change, beginning superficially in the subpapillary zone and extending downwards.

In one patient immunofluorescence testing showed IgM in a segmental granular pattern at the basement membrane zone, with granular C3 deposition. Electron microscopy showed dendritic extensions of macrophages which were intimately associated with fragmented elastic fibres. It was suggested that elastolysis due to release of cytoplasmic lysosomal contents had been mediated by immune events [10].

Clinical features [2, 3, 8, 9, 11, 14, 16]. This rare disorder occurs mainly in women aged 20–40 but is occasionally reported in younger and older patients of both sexes. It is perhaps more frequent in central Europe than elsewhere. In the most usual form, crops of round or oval pink macules 0·5–1 cm in diameter develop on the trunk, thighs and upper arms, less commonly on the neck and face, and rarely elsewhere. The scalp, palms and soles are usually spared. Each macule extends for a week or two to reach a size of 2–3 cm. Sometimes, there are larger plaques of erythema, and nodules have also been reported as a primary feature [7]. Slowly each lesion fades and flattens from the centre outwards, to leave a macule of wrinkled, atrophic skin which yields on pressure, admitting the finger through the surrounding ring of normal skin. The colour varies

from skin-colour to grey, white or blue. The number of lesions varies widely, from less than 5 to 100 or more. The lesions remain unchanged throughout life, and new lesions often continue to develop for many years. If the lesions coalesce they form large atrophic areas which are indistinguishable from acquired cutis laxa.

In some cases (the Pellizari form) the lesions are initially urticarial weals which, after a succession of exacerbation and remission, perhaps continuing for many weeks, are succeeded by atrophy. They may become confluent to cover large areas especially at the roots of the limbs and on the neck. Variants are described in which the lesions are initially bullous [6] or involve unusual sites such as the forehead, scalp, ear lobes or feet.

Diagnosis. The white cicatricial lesions of 'white spot disease' (p. 1368) around the base of the neck and shoulders should not be confused with anetoderma. Histological examination establishes the diagnosis. Focal dermal hypoplasia and atrophic scars following lichen planus must also be considered.

Acquired cutis laxa is probably a variant of anetoderma.

The diagnosis of 'primary' anetoderma can be established only by excluding the presence of any of the diseases known to be associated with 'secondary' atrophy.

Treatment. Penicillin has been advocated in the inflammatory stage [7], but too few cases have been treated for a reliable assessment of its efficacy. In the atrophic stage there is no effective treatment.

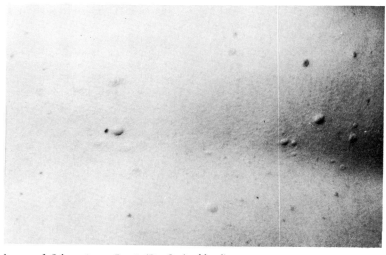

FIG. 49.12. Anetoderma of Schweninger–Buzzi (Dr G. Auckland).

REFERENCES

1 BECHELLI L. M., *et al* (1967) *Dermatologica* **135**, 329.
2 BONELLI U. (1968) *Ann Ital Dermatol* **35**, 177.
3 CHARGIN L. & SILVER H. (1931) *Arch Dermatol Syphil* **24**, 614.
4 CORNEJO A. & ABULAFIA J. (1955) *Arch Argent Dermatol* **5**, 335.
5 FELDMAN S. (1938) *Arch Dermatol Syphil* **38**, 107.
6 GREENBAUM S. S. (1921) *Arch Dermatol Syphil* **3**, 209.
7 INDIANER L. (1970) *Arch Dermatol* **102**, 697.
8 JOULIA P. & LE COULANT P. (1944) *Ann Dermatol Syphiligr* **4**, 238.
9 KORTING G. W., *et al* (1964) *Arch Klin Exp Dermatol* **218**, 374.
10 KOSSARD S., *et al* (1979) *J Am Acad Dermatol* **1**, 325.
11 PANCONESI E. (1955) *Rass Dermatol Sifilogr* **8**, 1.
12 STEPPERT A. (1956) *Dermatol Wochenschr* **133**, 213.
13 SWITZER S. E. & MAYMON C. W. (1935) *Arch Dermatol Syphil* **31**, 196.
14 TOURAINE A. (1941) *Bull Soc Fr Dermatol Syphiligr* **48**, 602.
15 VENENCIE P. Y. & WINKELMANN R. K. (1984) *Arch Dermatol* **120**, 1040.
16 VENENCIE P. Y., *et al* (1984) *Arch Dermatol* **120**, 1032.

Secondary anetoderma. This arises in association with another identifiable disease, but the atrophic areas do not always develop at the sites of the known inflammatory lesions. They are soft, round or oval areas which occur mainly on the trunk.

Perifollicular macular atrophy [4, 10]. Elastase-producing strains of *Staphylococcus epidermis* have been held responsible for perifollicular macular atrophy reported in women aged 30–40. There are greyish white, finely wrinkled, round or oval lesions on the ear lobes, neck, arms and upper trunk.

Syphilis. The lesions occur in association with secondary, latent, congenital or tertiary syphilis, but even where cutaneous syphilitic lesions are present the atrophy develops independently on the trunk, and not at the sites of the lesions. It has also occurred in patients with positive serology but without cutaneous lesions of syphilis.

Lupus erythematosus. Macular atrophy has occurred in association with systemic or chronic discoid lupus erythematosus, not in relation to the lesions. It has also occurred in association with lupus profundus [7] and in discoid lupus with hereditary complement (C2) deficiency [3]. Biopsy shows a focal loss of elastic tissue and a perivascular infiltrate with prominent plasma cells [11].

Urticaria pigmentosa. Anetoderma has been reported in the site of the lesions [9].

Leprosy. Leprosy has also been reported to cause anetoderma [1].

Other diseases [6, 11]. Some of the many other reported associations may be coincidental, but it is probable that many inflammatory diseases may occasionally be complicated by macular atrophy. An apparently valid association with severe dental sepsis has been observed [5]. Penicillamine-induced anetoderma has also been reported [2]. The post-inflammatory elastolysis and cutis laxa described in African children may be a reaction to arthropod bites [12].

REFERENCES

1 BECHELLI L. M., *et al* (1967) *Dermatologica* **135**, 329.
2 DAVIS W. (1977) *Arch Dermatol* **113**, 976.
3 DE BRACCO M. M., *et al* (1979) *Int J Dermatol* **18**, 713.
4 DICK G. F., *et al* (1976) *Acta Derm Venereol (Stockh)* **56**, 279.
5 FERRARA R. J. (1957) *Arch Dermatol* **79**, 516.
6 OPPENHEIMER M. (1931) *Handbuch der Haut und Geschlechtskrankheiten.* Berlin, Springer, Vol. 8, p. 617.
7 RYLL-NARDZEWSKI C., *et al* (1960) *Ann Dermatol Syphiligr* **87**, 627.
8 SCULL R. H. & NOMLAND R. (1937) *Arch Dermatol Syphil* **36**, 809.
9 THIVOLET J., *et al* (1981) *Ann Dermatol Vénéréol* **108**, 259.
10 VARADI D. P. & SAQUERON A. C. (1970) *Br J Dermatol* **83**, 143.
11 VENENCIE P. Y. & WINKELMANN R. K. (1984) *Arch Dermatol* **120**, 1032.
12 VERHAGEN A. R. & WOERDEMAN M. J. (1975) *Br J Dermatol* **92**, 183.

CHRONIC ATROPHIC ACRODERMATITIS
SYN. ACRODERMATITIS CHRONICA ATROPHICANS

Definition. This is a syndrome characterized by the insidious onset of painless dull-red nodules or plaques on the extremities which slowly extend centrifugally for several months, leaving central areas of atrophy. The histology in the early stages is nonspecific, but the later stage shows a dense band-like infiltrate beneath a subepidermal zone of degenerate connective tissue.

Aetiology. The cause is unknown, although the successful inoculation of human volunteers [8, 15] incriminates an infective agent. It has been suggested that this may be transmitted by the tick *Ixodes ricinus*, and in some areas the prevalence of the disease correlates with the density of the tick population

[10]. The disease occurs mainly in northern or central Europe, Italy and the Iberian Peninsula. Occasional cases occur in other parts of Europe and Africa, but it is very rare in America, Australia and Asia.

The condition bears some resemblance to Lyme disease, which is due·to a spirochaete borne by the tick *Ixodes dammini* (p. 1090).

Pathology [9, 13]. During the early stages there is dermal oedema with perivascular inflammatory infiltration. Subsequently, the epidermis becomes atrophic and the epidermal appendages are destroyed. Beneath a subepidermal zone of degenerate connective tissue lies a dense band-like infiltrate consisting predominantly of lymphocytes, histiocytes and plasma cells. Ultimately, the infiltrate is reduced to narrow bands between collagen fibres. Electron microscopy shows swelling of the endothelial cells of the dermal vessels, with abnormal material in the subendothelial area and in the layers in the perivascular region [1]. The lymph nodes may show sinus hyperplasia and plasma cell proliferation and plasma cells may be increased in the bone marrow. There are no constant cellular changes in the peripheral blood but hyperglobulinaemia is frequent [9] and monoclonal gammopathies are recorded [11].

Clinical features [3, 12, 14]. Most cases occur in country dwellers between the ages of 30 and 60 but onset in childhood or old age has been reported [5]. The onset is usually insidious and constitutional symptoms at any stage are exceptional. Painless, dull-red nodules or plaques, more or less infiltrated, develop on the feet or legs, less often on the forearms and hands. Extension to the trunk and to the greater part of the body, including the face, is sometimes seen. Single or multiple lesions may be present. They slowly extend centrifugally, the active inflammatory stage persisting for months or years. Marginal extension may continue whilst the central areas have already entered the atrophic stage, in which the skin is smooth, hairless and tissue-paper like, dull-red, pigmented or poikilodermatous. Subcutaneous nodules may develop around the knees and elbows and fibrous bands along the ulnar margins of the forearms. Gaiter-like sclerosis of the lower third of the legs, often accompanied by ulceration, is a further frequent complication. In some cases involvement of the joint capsules in the inflammatory process results in limitation of movement of the joints of the hands and feet or of the shoulders. Peripheral neuropathy is common [10].

Very rarely, squamous carcinoma has developed in the atrophic skin, and lymphoma has also been reported in the non-affected skin [2, 6].

Diagnosis. During the early stage, erythema chronicum migrans—possibly a related disease (p. 1090)—must be considered. The evolution of the annular lesions establishes the differentiation. In the atrophic stage the diagnosis is usually readily made and can be confirmed histologically.

Treatment. Penicillin for 10–14 days gives good results in the early inflammatory stages, but there is little or no response once atrophy has supervened. The improvement occurs gradually, several weeks after the course of treatment.

REFERENCES

1 BIAGINI G., *et al* (1976) *J Cutan Pathol* **3**, 199.
2 BRAUN-FALCO O. & PUPPIM D. (1971) *Dermatol Monatschr* **157**, 740.
3 BURGDORF W. H. C., *et al* (1979) *Int J Dermatol* **18**, 595.
4 DANDA J. (1963) *Hautarzt* **14**, 337.
5 GOOR W. & SCHWARZ-SPECK M. (1972) *Dermatologica* **145**, 287.
6 GOOS M. (1971) *Acta Derm Venereol (Stockh)* **51**, 457.
7 GOOS M., *et al* (1971) *Arch Dermatol Forsch* **241**, 122.
8 GOETZ H. (1954) *Hautarzt* **5**, 491.
9 HAUSER W. (1955) *Hautarzt* **6**, 77.
10 HOPF H. C. (1975) *J Neurol Neurosurg Psychiatry* **38**, 452.
11 KRAUS S., *et al* (1961) *Acta Derm Venereol (Stockh)* **43**, 163.
12 MARSHALL J. (1958) *S Afr Med J* **32**, 853.
13 MONTGOMERY H. & SULLIVAN R. R. (1954) *Arch Dermatol Syphil* **51**, 32.
14 THYRESSON N. (1949) *Acta Derm Venereol (Stockh)* **29**, 572.
15 ZMEGAC Z. (1966) *Hautarzt* **17**, 294.

VARIOLIFORM ATROPHY

This syndrome has been reported only in young adults. Varioliform pits, sometimes preceded by slight erythema and scaling, developed spontaneously on the face, mainly on the lower cheeks and chin. No causative factor could be incriminated in these otherwise healthy patients.

REFERENCES

1 HEIDINGSFELD M. L. (1918) *J Cutan Genito-urin Dis* **36**, 285.
2 McCORRISTON L. R. & ROYS H. C. (1951) *Arch Dermatol Syphil* **64**, 59.
3 SENEAR F. E. (1923) *Arch Dermatol Syphil* **7**, 405.

FOLLICULAR ATROPHODERMA

In this distinctive syndrome dimple-like follicular depressions at the follicular orifices are present from birth or early life, usually on the backs of hands and feet and sometimes in the elbow region [1].

It appears to be due to a variety of genetic defects, and it may be associated with the following conditions [2]:

(i) the Conradi syndrome (p. 163)
(ii) the Bazex syndrome (p. 129)
(iii) hyperkeratosis palmoplantaris with hyperhidrosis

It may also occur as an isolated defect of limited extent [3].

REFERENCES

1 BRAUN-FALCO O. & MARGHESCU S. (1967) *Hautarzt* **18**, 13.
2 CURTH H. O. (1978) *Arch Dermatol* **114**, 1479.
3 STREITMANN R. (1966) *Hautarzt* **17**, 274.

VERMICULATE ATROPHODERMA

See p. 1437.

ATROPHODERMA OF PASINI AND PIERINI

Definition. This condition appears to be an atrophic variant of morphoea (p. 1334) in which one or more

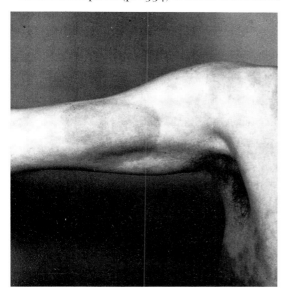

FIG. 49.13. Atrophoderma of Pasini and Pierini (Dr A. Ive).

patches of skin become bluish and sharply depressed, with no surrounding erythema [8, 11].

Aetiology. The cause is unknown. No genetic factor has been reliably incriminated, though familial cases have been reported [1, 12], and morphoea and atrophoderma of Pasini have occurred in siblings with phenylketonuria [7].

Pathology. The histological changes are slight. During the earlier stages the collagen in the lower dermis may be oedematous and elastic tissue clumped and scanty. Later, the oedema subsides and there is some reduction in the total thickness of the dermis. Eventually there may also be some epidermal atrophy.

Clinical features [3–6, 10]. The lesions, which may be single or multiple, range in size from 2 cm to many centimetres in diameter and are round or oval in shape, but may become confluent to form irregular patches. They are smooth, slate coloured or violet brown and are slightly depressed below the level of the entirely normal surrounding skin. The back is almost always involved, the chest and abdomen frequently and the proximal extremities occasionally. The patches extend very slowly, increase in number for 10 yr or more and then usually persist unchanged. The eventual development of sclerodermatous changes within the patch has been observed, as has the presence in the same patient of lesions typical of atrophoderma and of morphoea [2, 5, 9].

Diagnosis. Clinical differentiation from morphoea, possibly an academic exercise, is based on the ivory-white indurated plaque with an oedematous iliac ring so characteristic of the latter. Histologically, sclerosis may be prominent in morphoea and is usually absent in atrophoderma.

REFERENCES

1 BARSKY S. (1970) *Arch Dermatol* **101**, 374.
2 CABRE J. (1967) *Actas Dermosifilogr* **58**, 183.
3 CANIZARES O., *et al* (1958) *Arch Dermatol* **77**, 42.
4 JABLONSKA S. (1975) *Scleroderma and Pseudoscleroderma*. 2nd ed. Warsaw, Polish Medical Publishers.
5 JABLONSKA S. & SZCZEPANSKI A. (1962) *Dermatologica* **125**, 236.
6 KEE C. E., *et al* (1960) *Arch Dermatol* **82**, 154.
7 LASSER A. E., *et al* (1978) *Arch Dermatol* **114**, 1215.
8 MILLER R. F. (1965) *Arch Dermatol* **92**, 653.
9 PIERINI L. & PIERINI D. (1952) *Arch Argent Dermatol* **2**, 243.
10 PIERINI L., *et al* (1970) *Ann Dermatol Syphiligr* **97**, 391.

11 POCHÉ G. W. (1980) *Cutis* **25**, 503.
12 WEINER M. A. & GANT J. Q. (1959) *Arch Dermatol* **80**, 195.

ATROPHIC NAEVI

Congenital cutis laxa may rarely be confined to an area such as the abdomen. There may be other associated defects, e.g. dysplasia of the abdominal muscles, deformity of the thorax or mediastinal hernia. This condition must be distinguished from centrifugal abdominal lipodystrophy (p. 1873) and the prune-belly syndrome, which is associated with malformation of the urogenital tract [1, 2].

REFERENCES

1 BURKE E. C. (1969) *Am J Dis Child* **117**, 668.
2 WELLING P., *et al* (1975) *Z Kinderheilkd* **118**, 315.

LOCAL PANATROPHY

Definition and aetiology. Local panatrophy is a rare disorder involving partial or total loss of subcutaneous fat and atrophy of overlying skin, sometimes associated with atrophy or impaired growth of muscle or bone. A primary neurogenic disturbance has been postulated but not proved. The syndrome may represent the end result of more than one pathological process.

Two groups of cases can be differentiated:

(a) *Panatrophy of Gowers* [1]: no scleroderma or other sclerotic process accompanies or follows the loss of subcutaneous tissue. Most cases have occurred in women, usually in the second to fourth decades.
(b) *Sclerotic panatrophy*: either typical morphoea or similar sclerotic change in dermal collagen precedes the atrophy.

Clinical features
Panatrophy of Gowers [2, 4, 5, 8]. Sharply defined areas of atrophy, irregular in size, shape and distribution, develop over a period of a few weeks, without preceding inflammatory stages. In each affected area the subcutaneous tissue disappears and the overlying skin appears atrophic but is otherwise normal. There may be a single area of atrophy or two or more. In size they range from 2 to 20 cm in diameter, and in shape they are very variable but are sometimes triangular or quadrangular. Most lesions have occurred on the back, buttocks, thighs or arms, but some have involved forearms or lower legs. The atrophy reaches its maximum extent within a few months and then remains unchanged indefinitely.

Sclerotic panatrophy. Atrophy of subcutis, and sometimes of underlying muscle and bone, may follow clinically and histologically typical morphoea, especially when the process begins in childhood and involves a limb [6, 7] (see p. 1337).

Sclerotic panatrophy may also occur in the absence of morphoea. The sclerosis involves subcutaneous tissue and muscle, and dense sclerotic scar-like linear bands develop along a limb [9], or encircle the trunk in a metameric distribution or encircle a limb [3]. These lesions have also usually occurred in childhood. They cease to progress after a few months and, although new areas may be involved, most lesions have been solitary.

In the differential diagnosis of panatrophy the various forms of panniculitis must be excluded (Chapter 50). The preceding inflammatory changes are the single most distinctive feature.

REFERENCES

1 BARNES S. (1939) *Br J Dermatol* **51**, 377.
2 BETTLEY F. R. (1953) *Proc 10th Int Derm Congr, London*, p. 467.
3 BRUINSMA W. (1967) *Dermatologica* **134**, 107.
4 JAEGER H., *et al* (1955) *Dermatologica* **110**, 384.
5 KLUCKEN N. & GEIB K. H. (1965) *Hautarzt* **16**, 422.
6 KRESBACH H. (1959) *Z Haut GeschlKrankh* **27**, 343.
7 SCHNYDER U. W. (1956) *Dermatologica* **112**, 444.
8 SCHULFZ W. & KNUNZE E. (1958) *Dermatol Wochenschr* **138**, 865.
9 WITHAM M. (1958) *Br J Dermatol* **70**, 379.

FACIAL HEMIATROPHY
SYN ROMBERG'S SYNDROME

Definition and aetiology [1, 3]. Facial hematrophy is an atrophic dysplasia of the superficial facial tissues, but the underlying muscles, cartilage and bone may also be affected. The cause is unknown, but it may be a disorder of the sympathetic nervous system.

There is no evidence that it is usually genetically determined but it appears to be hereditary in a few pedigrees. Some cases have been associated with syringomyelia, epilepsy or cerebro vascular disease, but in 90% of cases no such association is demonstrable. The sexes are equally affected.

Clinical features [3, 8–12]. This rare disease usually starts within the first two decades. The first manifestation is usually increased or decreased pigmentation in irregular patches on cheeks, forehead or lower jaw. Occasionally there may be premonitory muscle spasms or neuralgia. Progressive atrophy gradually develops in the affected sites, involving skin, subcutis, muscle and bone, and may extend in area—and sometimes in depth—for months or years with temporary remissions. The skin becomes dry, thin and atrophic, but may be scar-like and adherent in some areas. When the atrophy is fully developed the contrast between the sunken haggard pigmented affected half of the face and the un-affected half is dramatic. The hair may be lost in the frontoparietal region on the affected side but is often normal; occasionally, localized canities in an early change. A variety of neurological signs have been reported, of which Horner's syndrome is the most frequent. Heterochromia of the iris [6] has developed at the same time as the facial atrophy in about 5% of cases, and other ocular changes may also be present [5].

The atrophy may remain limited both in extent and depth. It may be confined to the distribution of one division of the trigeminal nerve or involve the whole of the side of the face, sharply demarcated at the midline. Rarely, it may be bilateral and very rarely may involve half the body, usually on the same side as the face but exceptionally the opposite side—crossed hemiatrophy. The atrophy may, in such cases, begin on the trunk or a limb and only later involve the face [2].

The degree of bone atrophy as established radio-logically is usually much less than the clinical appearance suggests and is severe only in some cases of early onset. In such cases the cerebral cortex may also be affected, and contralateral epilepsy may result.

Scleroderma of the 'sabre-cut' paramedian form may be associated with some degree of facial hemiatrophy, especially if it begins early in life. However, it is a more superficial process than progressive facial hemiatrophy. The skin in scleroderma is bound down and adherent, and loss of hair and pigmentary changes are conspicuous. In progressive facial hemiatrophy the skin may remain mobile and grossly normal. The two processes have been confused frequently in the literature [9, 12] and may in fact be closely related [7].

Diagnosis [3]. When the cutaneous involvement is early and conspicuous the diagnosis presents few difficulties. Hypoplasia following radiotherapy given in infancy, perhaps in treatment of a naevus in the region of the temporomandibular joint, could cause confusion. If the skin changes are slight, or of later onset, physiological asymmetry, unilateral mandibular agenesis, hemihypertrophy and atrophy secondary to facial paralysis must be excluded. Hemihypertrophy is always congenital. When the limbs are involved, infantile hemiplegia and lipodystrophy must also be considered.

Treatment [4, 7, 10]. Plastic surgery using large buried pediculated flaps of dermis and fat or silicone implants offer some cosmetic benefit.

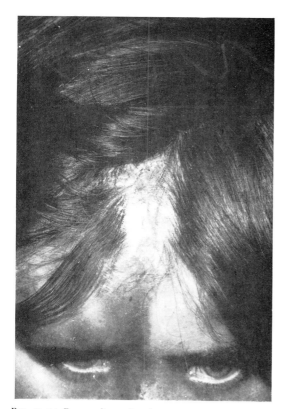

FIG. 49.14. Paramedian scleroderma associated with a moderate degree of facial hemiatrophy (Addenbrooke's Hospital).

REFERENCES

1 BLATT N., et al (1960) *Rev Otoneuroophthalmol* **32**, 1.
2 BRAMLEY P. & FORBES A. (1960) *Br Med J* i, 1476.
3 DECHAUME M., et al (1954) *Rev Stomatol* **55**, 12.
4 DEDO D. D. (1978) *Arch Laryngol* **104**, 538.
5 FRANCESCHETTI A. & KOENIG H. (1952) *J Genet Hum* **1**, 27.
6 FRANCESCHETTI A. & MAEDER G. (1958) *J Genet Hum* **7**, 116.
7 FRIES R. (1964) *Klin Med* **2**, 70.
8 HERRMANN W. P. (1960) *Z Haut GeschlKrankh* **28**, 319.
9 JABLONSKA S. (1975) *Scleroderma and Pseudoscleroderma.* 2nd ed. Warsaw, Polish Medical Publishers.

10 NEUMANN C. G. (1953) *J Plast Reconstr Surg* 11, 315.
11 ROGERS B. D. (1963) *Progressive Facial Hemiatrophy, A Review of 772 Cases.* Washington, Excerpta Medica, pp. 681.
12 SINGH G. & BAJPAI H. S. (1969) *Dermatologica* 138, 288.

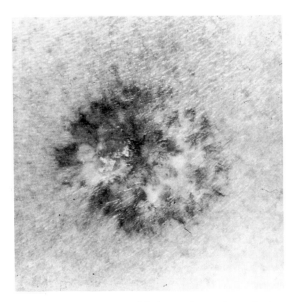

FIG. 49.15. Acquired poikiloderma due to X-irradiation (Bristol Royal Infirmary).

POIKILODERMA

Poikiloderma is a descriptive term, often somewhat loosely applied. Atrophy, macular or reticulate pigmentation and telangiectasia are the essential features. Depigmentation, miliary lichenoid papules, fine scaling and small petechial haemorrhages are less constantly present.

Congenital poikiloderma. Poikiloderma may occur as an apparently primary abnormality in certain genetically determined syndromes, including the Rothmund–Thomson syndrome (p. 150), dyskeratosis congenita (p. 148) and the Mendes da Costa syndrome (p. 1431).

Several other syndromes have been described in which poikiloderma is a prominent feature.

Hereditary sclerosing poikiloderma of Weary [11]. This rare autosomal dominant syndrome was described in a large Negro family. Generalized poikiloderma, which developed in early childhood, was accompanied by sclerosis of the palms and soles, and linear hyperkeratotic and sclerotic bands developed in the flexures of the arms and legs.

Hereditary acrokeratotic poikiloderma of Weary [12]. This autosomal dominant condition produces vesicopustules of the hands and feet which start at the age of 1–3 months and resolve in childhood. There is also a widespread eczema, and the gradual appearance of poikiloderma which persists into adult life. Keratotic papules develop in childhood on the hands, feet, knees and elbows, and these also persist indefinitely [6, 10, 12].

Kindler's syndrome [1–4, 8]. This is probably a variant of hereditary acrokeratotic poikiloderma, in which the poikiloderma is preceded by a tendency to blistering following mild trauma. The relationship of this syndrome to epidermolysis bullosa is uncertain. The skin in these patients is thin, wrinkled and devoid of surface marking. Colloid bodies which show IgM deposition on direct immunofluorescence have been described [7]. Other cases have been reported which do not fit clearly into either of the above syndromes. The nosological status of the Weary–Kindler syndrome has been recently reviewed [7].

Diffuse and macular atrophic dermatosis [5, 9]. This rare condition is characterized by the presence from birth of generalized poikilodermatous changes which give the appearance of prematurely sundamaged skin. The facies, hair and skeleton are normal. Biopsy shows thinning of the epidermis, with large hyaline bodies in the superficial dermal collagen, and these stain positively with PAS and elastin stains. Electron microscopy shows that these globular structures consist of microfibrillar material, and the adjacent fibroblasts may be degenerative.

Acquired poikiloderma. Poikiloderma may occur as a pattern of cutaneous response to injury by cold, heat or ionizing radiation. Poikiloderma of Civatte (p. 1579) is a similar reaction mediated by photosensitizing chemicals in cosmetics. Some inflammatory dermatoses, such as lichen planus, may also give rise to poikilodermatous changes.

Poikiloderma is also a feature of some 'collagen diseases' and is particularly characteristic of dermatomyositis. It is also seen in lupus erythematosus and rarely in systemic sclerosis. Poikiloderma occurs as a manifestation of some reticuloses, especially mycosis fungoides (p. 1736).

REFERENCES

1 ALPER J. C., *et al* (1978) *Arch Dermatol* **114**, 457.
2 BORDAS X., *et al* (1982) *J Am Acad Dermatol* **6**, 263.
3 DRAZNIN M. B., *et al* (1978) *Arch Dermatol* **114**, 1207.
4 KINDLER T. (1954) *Br J Dermatol* **66**, 104.
5 KIRBY J. D. (1980) *Clin Exp Dermatol* **5**, 57.
6 LARRÈGUE M., *et al* (1981) *Ann Dermatol Vénéréol* **108**, 69.
7 MALEVILLE J., *et al* (1982) *Acta Derm Venereol (Stockh)* **109**, 949.
8 PERSON J. R. & PERRY H. O. (1979) *Acta Derm Venereol (Stockh)* **59**, 347.
9 STEVANOVIC D. V. (1975) *Dermatol Monatsschr* **161**, 831.
10 WALLACH D., *et al* (1981) *Ann Dermatol Vénéréol* **108**, 79.
11 WEARY P. E., *et al* (1969) *Arch Dermatol* **100**, 313.
12 WEARY P. E., *et al* (1971) *Arch Dermatol* **103**, 409.

THE SCLEROATROPHIC SYNDROME OF HURIEZ

This syndrome has been identified in 42 of 132 members of two families. It is determined by an autosomal dominant gene. The changes are present at birth and progress throughout childhood. The essential features are (1) diffuse scleroatrophy of the hands, in plaques or as sclerodactyly but without Raynaud's syndrome, (2) ridging or aplasia of the nails, and (3) lamellar keratoderma of the palms and, to a lesser extent, of the soles. Aggressive squamous carcinoma in the atrophic skin is common.

REFERENCE

HURIEZ C., *et al* (1969) *Ann Dermatol Syphiligr* **96**, 135.

Systematized mesodermal dysplasia. An apparently distinct syndrome has been described, characterized by diffuse dermal sclerosis, contractures of limb joints, osteolysis of phalanges, multiple subcutaneous nodules, stunted growth and recurrent sepsis.

REFERENCE

PURETIC S., *et al* (1962) *Br J Dermatol* **74**, 8.

ATROPHIC SKIN WITH RHEUMATOID DISEASE

In rheumatoid patients over the age of 60, and in women more often than men, the skin on the backs of the hands may become thin, loose, smooth, inelastic and transparent, so that the details of veins and tendons are clearly seen. The change is generalized but is seldom conspicuous except on the

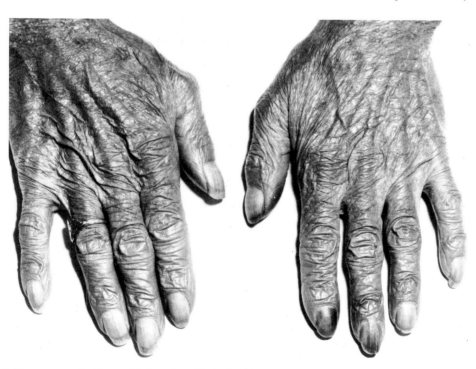

FIG. 49.16. 'Transparent skin' in an elderly patient (Dr A. Rook).

hands and forearms. Histologically the dermis is thinned but shows no distinctive changes.

There is a significant association between transparent skin, rheumatoid arthritis and osteoporosis, and it is assumed to form part of a general connective-tissue defect. Steroid therapy is not a factor but will potentiate the problem.

REFERENCES

1 McConkey B., *et al* (1963) *Lancet* i, 693.
2 McConkey B., *et al* (1965) *Ann Rheum Dis* **24**, 219.
3 Ryckewaert A., *et al* (1966) *Rev Fr. Etud Clin Biol* **11**, 838.
4 Shuster S., *et al* (1967) *Lancet* i, 525.

GLUCOCORTICOSTEROID-INDUCED ATROPHY

Both systemic and topical glucocorticoid therapy can produce cutaneous atrophy by a dose-related pharmacological effect. The effect is more severe with the more potent steroids (as assessed by the vasoconstrictor assay test) but both fluorinated and non-fluorinated topical steroids can cause atrophy. The effect is most marked when potent steroids are applied topically under an occlusive dressing. The skin becomes thin, fragile and transparent, and striae may develop [10].

The earliest histological change is marked thinning of the epidermis, with flattening of the rete ridges and decreased corneocyte size [1, 4]. This is followed a few weeks later by thinning of the dermis, which can be measured either by skinfold calipers or by a radiographic technique [37].

The epidermal thinning probably results from a reduction of mitotic activity in the germinal layer [9], but the mechanism by which dermal thinning is produced is uncertain. Topical steroids inhibit the activity of enzymes involved in collagen biosynthesis [11, 13] and they have been shown to depress collagen synthesis both *in vivo* and in fibroblast cultures [12]. They can also depress collagenase production and collagen breakdown [8] and the rate of collagen turnover is probably decreased. Even a weak steroid, such as hydrocortisone, can suppress the stimulatory effect of cyclic nucleotides on collagenase production [2]. There is a decreased thickness of collagen fibrils, with a decrease in the number of fibroblasts [6]. Many microfibrils form globular microfibrillar bodies, although the changes are not specific for steroid atrophy [6]. These ultrastructural changes can develop in the early stages before there is clinical or histological evidence of atrophy. Digestion of collagen fibrils in the endocytic vesicles of fibroblasts may be involved in the production of steroid-induced atrophy [8, 15].

Capillaroscopic studies have shown that steroid-induced vasoconstriction involves the superficial capillary network, and prolonged superficial ischaemia could also play a role in producing atrophy [14].

REFERENCES

1 Burton J. L. & Winter G.D. (1976) *Br J Dermatol* **94**, (suppl 12), 107
2 Cartwright E. C. & Reynolds J. J. (1976) *Arch Int Physiol Biochim* **84** (Suppl. 3), Abstract 80.
3 Dykes P. J. & Marks R. (1977) *J Invest Dermatol* **69**, 275.
4 Groniowska J, *et al* (1976) *Dermatologica* **152** (Suppl. 1), 147.
5 Holze E. & Plewig G. (1977) *J Invest Dermatol* **68**, 350.
6 Jablonska S., *et al* (1979) *Br J Dermatol* **100**, 193.
7 James M. P., *et al* (1977) *Br J Dermatol* **96**, 303.
8 Koob T. J., *et al* (1974) *Biochem Biophys Res Commun* **61**, 1083.
9 Marks R., *et al* (1971) *J Invest Dermatol* **56**, 470.
10 Meara R. H. (1964) *Br J Dermatol* **76**, 481.
11 Oikarinen A., *et al* (1982) *Br J Dermatol* **106**, 257.
12 Ponec M., *et al* (1977) *Arch Dermatol Res* **259**, 125.
13 Risteli J. (1977) *Biochem Pharmacol* **26**, 1295.
14 Stuttgen G. (1976) *Dermatologica* **152**, 91.
15 Ten Cate A. R. & Deporter D. A. (1975) *Anat Rec* **185**, 1.

STRIAE
SYN. STRIAE ATROPHICAE; STRIAE DISTENSAE; 'STRETCH MARKS'

Definition. Striae are the visible results of limited intradermal rupture beneath an intact epidermis. They are produced by stretching the skin.

Aetiology. The factors which govern the development of striae are poorly understood. It has been suggested that they develop more easily in skin which has a critical proportion of rigid cross-linked collagen, as occurs in early adult life [15]. They are common during adolescence [10, 16] and they seem to be associated with rapid increase in size of a particular region. They are very common over the abdomen and breasts in pregnancy, and they may develop on the shoulders in young male weight lifters when their muscle mass rapidly increases. They are a feature of Cushing's disease, and they may be induced by ACTH or corticosteroids [7]. A high incidence has been noted in debilitating disease, particularly tuberculosis [11].

Investigations in pregnant women [114] and in

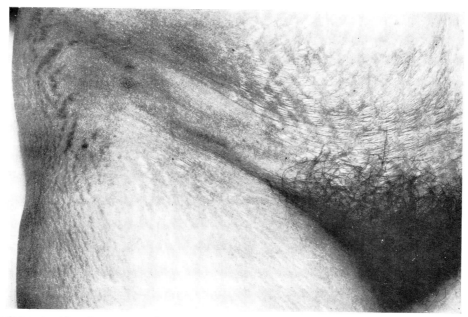

Fig. 49.17. Striae atrophicae. In pregnancy the striae may involve most or all of the pubertal sites as well as the abdominal wall (Addenbrooke's Hospital).

patients with Cushing's syndrome [9] suggest that the development of striae is related to excessive adrenocortical activity. In young obese adults with striae a small increase in the secretion rate of cortisol has been found [8]. The topical application of the more potent steroids, particularly if applied under occlusive dressings, may result in the formation of striae [5, 17, 19]. Linear atrophy has been described following intralesional steroid injections [2, 11, 17]. This has been assumed to be due to the tracking of the steroid along the lymph vessels. The effect of the steroids is to reduce collagen fibre formation, probably by an incomplete inhibition of fibroblasts [18]. The importance of genetic factors in determining susceptibility of connective tissue is emphasized by the absence of striae in pregnancy in the Ehlers–Danlos syndrome.

Pathology. In the early stages inflammatory changes may be conspicuous, the dermis is oedematous and perivascular lymphocytic cuffing is present.

In the later stages the epidermis is thin and flattened. The dermal collagen is layered and oriented in the direction of the presumed stress. Scanning electron microscopy shows amorphous sheet-like structures [1]. The elastin is scanty and fragmented, but newly synthesized elastin is also present [3, 13].

Clinical features [4, 12, 14, 16]. Adolescent striae may first develop soon after the appearance of pubic hair. The commonest sites are the outer aspect of the thighs and the lumbosacral region in boys and the thighs, buttocks and breasts in girls, but there is considerable variation and other sites including the outer aspect of the upper arm are sometimes affected. Early lesions may be raised and irritable, but they soon become flat, smooth and livid red or bluish in colour. Their surface may be finely wrinkled. They are commonly irregularly linear, several centimetres long and 1–10 mm wide. After some years they fade and become inconspicuous.

The striae in Cushing's syndrome or those induced by steroid therapy may be larger and more widely distributed and involve other regions, including sometimes the face. In pregnancy the striae appear first and are most conspicuous on the abdominal wall, and later on the breasts, but may involve most or all of the pubertal sites.

The striae induced by topical steroid therapy [6] have been observed particularly in the inguinal flexures but may appear in other sites if occlusive plastic films increase absorption. They may disappear or become less conspicuous when treatment is stopped.

Striae usually are only a cosmetic problem but occasionally, if extensive, they may ulcerate or tear easily should the patient be involved in an accident.

Diagnosis. The diagnosis of striae is usually simple. In the absence of an obvious cause careful endocrine investigation is advisable to exclude the possibility of Cushing's syndrome.

Treatment. None is available. In the case of common adolescent striae the patient may be reassured that in time they will become less conspicuous.

REFERENCES

1 AREM A.J. & KISCHER C.W. (1980) *Plas Reconstr Surg* **65**, 22.
2 AYRES S., JR (1964) *Arch Dermatol* **90**, 242.
3 BHANGOO K.S., *et al* (1976) *Plast Reconstr Surg* **57**, 308.
4 CARR R.D. & HAMILTON J.F. (1969) *Arch Dermatol* **99**, 26.
5 CHERNOVSKY M.E. & KNOX J.M. (1964) *Arch Dermatol* **90**, 15.
6 EPSTEIN N.N., *et al* (1963) *Arch Dermatol* **98**, 450.
7 FOLDVARI F., *et al* (1962) *Dermatologica* **125**, 93.
8 GOGATE A.N. & PRUNTY F.T.G. (1963) *J Clin Endocrinol Metab* **23**, 747.
9 HAUSER W. (1958) *Dermatol Wochenschr* **138**, 1291.
10 HERXHEIMER J. (1953) *Lancet* ii, 204.
11 KIKUCHI I. & HORIKAWA S. (1974) *Arch Dermatol* **109**, 558.
12 MACRAE-GIBSON N.K. (1952) *Br J Dermatol* **64**, 315.
13 PINKUS H., *et al* (1966) *J Invest Dermatol* **46**, 283.
14 POIDEVIN L.O.S. (1959) *Lancet* ii, 436.
15 SHUSTER S. (1979) *Acta Derm Venereol (Stockh)* **59** (Suppl. **85**), 161.
16 SISSON W.R. (1954) *J Pediatr* **45**, 520.
17 STEIGLEDER G.K. (1973) *Hautarzt* **24**, 261.
18 STEVANOVIC D.V. (1972) *Br J Dermatol* **87**, 548.
19 THIESS H., *et al* (1969) *Ann Dermatol Syphiligr* **96**, 29.

PREMATURE AGEING SYNDROMES

Increasing age appears to cause many anatomical and functional changes in human skin, but some of these may be the result of cumulative damage due to sun exposure, etc. To date, no disease has been found to cause a true acceleration of the rate of ageing in all tissues. More than 150 diseases manifest one or more features of apparent premature ageing, but there are discrepancies between this process and true ageing [4]. All the premature ageing syndromes are probably inherited, though the defect may not be obvious in the first few years of life. Cutaneous changes which may be a sign of a premature ageing syndrome include atrophy (p. 1804), loss of cutaneous fat, wrinkling, canities,

hair loss, nail dystrophy, defective pigmentation, poikiloderma, sclerosis or ulceration.

The following conditions are associated with cutaneous signs of premature ageing [1–3].

Pangeria (Werner's syndrome)
Progeria (Hutchinson–Gilford syndrome)
Acrogeria
Metageria
Familial mandibulo-acral dysplasia
Neonatal progeroid syndrome of Wiedemann–
    Rautenstrauch
Osteodysplastic geroderma
Poikiloderma congenitale (p. 150)
Cockayne's syndrome (p. 148)
Generalized lipodystrophy (p. 1873)
Trisomy 21 (Down's syndrome) (p. 114)
Diabetes mellitus
Prolidase deficiency

REFERENCES

1 GILCHRIST B. (1981) *Birth Defects* **xvii** (2), 227.
2 GILKES J.H.H., *et al* (1974) *Br J Dermatol* **91**, 243.
3 GOLDSTEIN S. (1971) *N Engl J Med* **285**, 1120.
4 MARTIN G.M. (1978) In *Genetic Effects of Ageing*. Eds. Bergsma D. & Harrison D.E. New York, Alan R. Liss for the National Foundation March of Dimes, BD: DAS XIV, p. 5–63.

PANGERIA
SYN. WERNER'S SYNDROME [12, 20]

Definition. An inherited disorder characterized by short stature, senile appearance, cataracts, joint contractures, early menopause, various skin changes including premature canities, baldness and ulceration, and an increased risk of malignancy.

Aetiology. The syndrome may be due to an autosomal recessive gene, with a calculated gene frequency of 1 to 5 per 1,000 population [4]. Another possibility is that there may be chromosomal instability, with deletion of one or more genes [2]. Fibroblast growth in tissue culture is impaired [17, 19] and clones of pseudodiploid cells with variegated translocation mosaicism have been described [14, 15]. Glycosaminoglycan metabolism is abnormal. The synthesis is increased in the sclerodermatous skin [5] but decreased in the normal-looking skin [2]. The urinary excretion of acidic glycosaminoglycans is increased [10].

Pathology [5, 11, 18]. Many tissues show premature ageing, but the changes are not uniform. Microsplanchnia and generalized atheroma are usually present. The epidermis is atrophic and skin appendages are sparse. The dermis is probably thickened, with replacement of subcutaneous fat by hyalinized collagen, increased glycosaminoglycans and vessel changes in the dermis which resemble those seen in diabetes mellitus [5].

Clinical features [3, 4, 8, 9, 11, 16, 22]. The earliest manifestation of the syndrome is greying at the temples which usually develops between the ages of 14 and 18 but may rarely be present as early as 8. The greying rapidly becomes uniform and is soon associated with progressive alopecia. The first skin changes are usually noticed between 18 and 30 but may begin earlier. The lower legs and feet, forearms and hands are most severely involved, the face and neck less so; the skin is tense, shining and adherent, the joints become fixed and there may be sclerodactyly and acral gangrene. Mottled or diffuse pigmentation and telangiectasia are often conspicuous on the limbs, face and neck. Keratoses over pressure points on the feet and ankles separate to leave indolent ulcers. The loss of subcutaneous tissue results in a bird-like facies and thin spindly legs, which contrast with the normal or obese trunk. The voice may be high pitched and hoarse from thinning of the cords and fixation of the epiglottis. Intelligence is usually normal.

Most patients are of small stature and hypogonadal, with sparse or absent pubic and axillary hair, but some achieve normal stature and successful pregnancies. Other endocrine deficiencies are sometimes present: frank diabetes mellitus in at least 30% and abnormal glucose tolerance in many others. The diabetes is characterized by relatively low blood glucose levels and peripheral resistance to insulin [16].

Cataracts develop between the ages of 20 and 35 in most cases and are usually posterior and subcapsular. Other ocular defects may occur [16].

The incidence of malignancy is high, especially fibrosarcomas which occur in 10% of patients [2]. Carcinoma has developed in a chronic leg ulcer [6] but skin cancer is relatively rare. Generalized atheroma develops early. Abnormalities of lipid metabolism are sometimes present but are of no uniform type [16]. Death usually occurs in the fourth to sixth decade, due to myocardial infarction or malignancy.

The radiological changes [1, 7, 22] are often striking. There may be calcification of arteries, ligaments, tendons and subcutaneous tissue with osteoporosis of the extremities, especially the legs.

Diagnosis. The prematurely aged appearance, the physical immaturity, the scleroderma-like changes and the cataracts, in combination, are unmistakable. In the Rothmund and Thomson syndromes, erythema which is of early onset is followed by poikilodermatous changes and although the facies may be superficially similar there is no sclerosis. In systemic sclerosis the hands are involved more than the feet and there is no premature ageing; in some advanced cases confusion is possible but can be resolved by biopsy.

Huriez' syndrome may require exclusion (p. 1813). The differentiation from some of the other ageing syndrome is indicated in Table 49.1.

Treatment. Only symptomatic measures are available. The management of the recurrent painful ulceration of the feet and legs is difficult and amputation may be needed. Cataract surgery should be undertaken with special caution for it is often complicated by severe degenerative changes of the cornea.

REFERENCES

1 ALBERTI K.G., *et al* (1974) *Proc R Soc Med* **67**, 36.
2 BJORNBERG A. (1976) *Acta Derm Venereol* **56**, 149.
3 BOATWRIGHT H., *et al* (1952) *Arch Intern Med* **90**, 243.
4 EPSTEIN C.J., *et al* (1966) *Medicine* **45**, 1977.
5 FLEISCHMAJER R. & NEDWICH A. (1973) *Am J Med* **54**, 11.
6 GERTLER H. (1964) *Dermatol Wochenschr* **150**, 606.
7 HARLONSKA S. & SEGAL P. (1959) *Minerva Dermatol* **34**, 259.
8 KNOTH W., *et al* (1963) *Hautarzt* **14**, 145.
9 MILLER L. & ANDERSON B. (1953) *Acta Med Scanda* [*Suppl*] **146**, 284.
10 MURATTA K. (1982) *Experientia* **38**, 313.
11 REED R., *et al* (1953) *Br J Dermatol* **65**, 165.
12 SALK D. (1982) *Hum Genet* **62**, 1.
13 SALK D., *et al* (1981) *Hum Genet* **58**, 310.
14 SALK D., *et al* (1981) *Cytogenet Cell Genet* **30**, 92.
15 SCAPPATICCI S., *et al* (1982) *Hum Genet* **62**, 16.
16 SCHUMACHER K., *et al* (1969) *Arch Klin Med* **216**, 116.
17 SHANNON-DANES B. (1971) *J Clin Invest* **50**, 2000.
18 TAO L.C., *et al* (1971) *Can Med Assoc J* **105**, 971.
19 THOMPSON K.V.A. & HALLIDAY R. (1983) *Gerontology* **29**, 73.
20 WERNER O. (1904) Uber Katarakt in Verbindung mit Sclerodermie. *Doctoral Dissertation*, Kiel University, Kiel.
21 ZALLA J.A. (1980) *Cutis* **25**, 275.
22 ZUCKER F.D., *et al* (1968) *Geriatrics* **23**, 124.

PROGERIA
SYN. HUTCHINSON–GILFORD SYNDROME [5, 8]

Definition. This is a disorder characterized by retarded development, an abnormal facies (see below),

TABLE 49.1. Clinical features of the premature ageing syndromes

	Metageria	Pangeria (Werner's syndrome)	Acrogeria	Progeria	Total lipodystrophy
Stature	Tall and thin	Small stature. Cessation of growth at 12 yr	Normal	Dwarf	90th percentile, increased growth rate
Facies	Bird-like facies, pinched face, beaked nose	Beaked nose. Skin of ears atrophic and tightly bound down	Micrognathia. Atrophy of skin on tip of nose	Mid-facial cyanosis. Bird-like facies. Glyphic nasal tip. Prominent frontal tuberosities and scalp veins. Chin recessed	Pinched face with absent buccal pad of fat
Skin	Atrophic—most marked on limbs. Mottled hyperpigmentation. Telangiectasia	Dry atrophic skin. Mottled hyperpigmentation. Telangiectasia	Atrophic with telangiectasia and mottled hyperpigmentation on extremities	Dry, thin and wrinkled with mottled pigmentation. May present with scleroderma-like changes on limbs	Coarse dry skin. Patchy hyperpigmentation. Hypertrichosis. Normal skin elasticity
Scalp hair	Fine and thin	Premature greying 20 yr. Loss of hair 20–25 yr	Normal	Hair lost in first 2 yr of life	Abundant and curly
Eyes	Prominent eyes. No true exophthalmos	Bilateral juvenile cataracts (20–30 yr). Keratopathy. Glaucoma	Normal	Prominent eyes; otherwise normal	Small punctate corneal opacities
Nails	Normal	Normal	Dystrophic or thickened	Thin and brittle	Normal
Limbs	Generalized loss of subcutaneous fat. Ischaemic leg ulcers (one case)	Lower limb ulcers. Hyperkeratosis over bony prominences. Generalized loss of subcutaneous fat	Atrophy of skin most marked on extremities. No leg ulcers	Prominent joints. Coxa valga. Generalized subcutaneous fat loss. Poorly developed muscular system. No acrosclerosis or Raynaud's phenomenon	Apparent muscular hypertrophy due to loss of subcutaneous fat

skeletal abnormalities and the onset in early childhood of progressive senile degeneration [6].

Aetiology. It is probably due to an autosomal recessive gene, though most cases are sporadic. Consanguinity was present in three of 19 pedigrees, and affected families have a high incidence of spontaneous abortion. The incidence is around 1 in 8 million live births [3] and 60% of cases are male.

Pathology [4]. The skin shows atrophy of epidermis and dermis. There may be progressive hyalinization of dermal collagen and loss of subcutaneous fat. Scanning electron microscopy of hairs from one patient showed unusual longitudinal depressions with minor cuticular defects [4].

The cardiovascular system shows extensive atheroma, and there may be extensive myocardial fibrosis, with extensive lipofuscin ('age pigment') deposition characteristic of elderly adults [10].

In tissue culture, progeria fibroblasts have a decreased survival time [2].

Clinical features [3, 4, 11]. Affected children usually appear normal at birth, and growth may be only slightly retarded in the first year, but during the second year there is profound growth failure with reduced subcutaneous fat on the face and limbs [1]. The facial appearance is reminiscent of a fledgling bird, with a disproportionately large cranium with patent fontanelles and frontal bossing, prominent eyes and scalp veins, very sparse downy scalp hair, sparse or absent eyebrows and eyelashes, centrofacial cyanosis, micrognathia, thin lips and a 'beaked' nose [3]. By the second year, the skin has become thin, taut and shiny in some areas but lax and finely wrinkled in others. Eccrine sweating is decreased. The veins are prominent and there may be easy bruising. After several years, progressive mottled hyperpigmentation develops, most marked on exposed sites, but there is no photosensitivity. Thickened sclerotic areas may be present on the lower trunk or thighs. The nails are usually small, thin and dystrophic, and koilonychia and onychogryphosis may occur. Generalized alopecia often begins in the first year of life and the few remaining hairs are pale, fine and 'fuzzy'. The nipples may be hypoplastic.

The dentition is abnormal and delayed, and there may be skeletal abnormalities such as dystrophic clavicles and coxa vulga, with joint contractures and a 'horse-riding' stance. Progressive bone resorption may lead to frequent fractures [9]. Ocular defects, especially microphthalmos, may occur [7].

Sexual maturation is absent but intelligence is normal.

Death usually occurs in the second decade as a result of severe generalized atheroma.

Diagnosis. The large bald head with conspicuous veins, the bird-like facies and the well-proportioned little body are distinctive. Bird-headed dwarfism (p. 161) is distinguished by the absence of skin atrophy.

Cockayne's syndrome may cause confusion, but progeria is distinguished by the loss of hair, the lack of photosensitivity and the absence of disproportionately large extremities.

In metageria, sexual maturation and somatic growth are normal.

REFERENCES

1 COOKE J.V. (1953) *J Pediatr* **42**, 26.
2 DANES B.S. (1971) *J Clin Invest* **50**, 2000.
3 DE BUSK F.L. (1972) *J Pediatr* **80**, 697.
4 FLEISCHMAJER R. & NEDWICH A. (1973) *Arch Dermatol* **107**, 253.
5 GILFORD H. (1904) *Practitioner* **73**, 188.
6 GILKES J.J.H., *et al* (1974) *Br J Dermatol* **91**, 243.
7 GREGERSEN E. (1956) *Acta Ophthalmol (Kbh)* **34**, 347.
8 HUTCHINSON J. (1886) *Med Chir Trans* **69**, 473.
9 OZONOFF M.B. & CLEMETT A.R. (1967) *Am J Roentgenol* **100**, 75.
10 REICHEL W., *et al* (1970) *Am J Clin Pathol* **53**, 243.
11 THOMSON J. & FORFAR J.O. (1950) *Arch Dis Child* **25**, 224.

ACROGERIA
SYN. GOTTRON'S SYNDROME [3]

Definition. This disorder begins at birth or soon afterwards and is characterized by cutaneous atrophy and loss of subcutaneous fat, particularly over the distal extremities, but with no tendency to atheroma, diabetes mellitus or decreased life expectancy. The term 'acrogeria' refers to premature ageing of the extremities.

Aetiology. Some cases have occurred in siblings, and it is presumed to be inherited as an autosomal recessive disorder. Most patients have been female. Some patients with this syndrome may have Ehlers–Danlos syndrome, type IV.

Pathology. The subcutaneous fat is absent in the most severely affected regions. The dermis is atrophic, with sparse thin collagen bundles, but there is abundant elastin which appears clumped due to the deficiency of collagen.

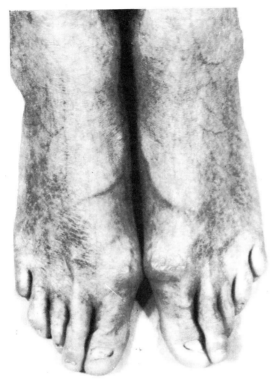

FIG. 49.18. Acrogeria. The skin of the hands and feet of this young woman is thin and transparent. (Dr H. T. Calvert.)

Clinical features. The changes develop at or soon after birth. The skin becomes dry, thin, transparent and wrinkled, especially over the hands and feet, though the trunk and face may be affected to a lesser extent. The veins are prominent, and there may be easy bruising, poikiloderma and telangiectasia. The nails may be atrophic or thickened. The face appears 'pinched' and micrognathism may be present. The lack of subcutaneous fat accentuates the appearance of premature senility. Some patients have low birthweight and persistent short stature, but the general health and life expectancy are normal. The hands and feet may be very small [1, 7].

Diagnosis. The normal hair and eyes help to distinguish the condition from progeria and pangeria (Table 49.1).

REFERENCES

1 BATSCHVAROFF B., *et al* (1961) *Dermatol Wochenschr* **143**, 59.
2 BAZEX A. & DUPRE A. (1955) *Ann Dermatol Syphiligr,* **82**, 604.
3 GOTTRON H. (1941) *Arch Dermatol Syphatol* **181**, 571.
4 GRUNBERG T. (1960) *Arch Klin Exp Dermatol* **210**, 409.
5 HJURTSKOJ A.R. & NEYDENRICH G. (1977) *Dermatologica,* **154**, 355.
6 LAMY M., *et al* (1961) *Arch fr Pediat* **18**, 18.
7 LEVI L., *et al G Ital Dermatol* **45**, 645.

METAGERIA

The two reported cases of this condition were tall and thin, with very sparse subcutaneous fat and a thin face with a beaked nose. At puberty diffuse mottled hyperpigmentation developed accompanied in one case by very poor peripheral circulation with vasospasm which produced ulceration and gangrene. The skin was soft and atrophic, and the hair was fine but normal in amount and colour. Both patients developed diabetes mellitus during the second decade.

REFERENCE

GILKES J.J.H., *et al* (1974) *Br J Dermatol* **91**, 243.

FAMILIAL MANDIBULO-ACRAL DYSPLASIA

The main features of this rare syndrome are mandibular hypoplasia, delayed cranial suture closure, dysplastic clavicles, abbreviated club-shaped terminal phalanges associated with acro-osteolysis and atrophy of the skin over the hands and feet [5]. Other characteristics may include short stature, multiple wormian bones, prominent eyes and a sharp nose [2, 4]. In one family the condition was also associated with the loss of the lower teeth and alopecia [6]. The condition appears to be inherited as an autosomal recessive trait.

The cutaneous changes resemble those of a premature ageing syndrome, and some cases have been mistakenly diagnosed in the past as acrogeria [3] or Werner's syndrome [1].

REFERENCES

1 COHEN L.K., *et al* (1973) *Cutis* **12**, 76.
2 DANKS D.M., *et al* (1974) *Birth Defects* **x** (12), 99.
3 LEVI L., *et al* (1970) *G Ital Dermatol* **iii**, 645.
4 WELSH O. (1975) *Birth Defects* **xi**, (5), 25.
5 YOUNG L.W., *et al* (1971) *Birth Defects* **7**, 291.
6 ZINA A.M. (1981) *Br J Dermatol* **105**, 719.

NEONATAL PROGEROID SYNDROME OF WIEDEMANN–RAUTENSTRAUCH [1–3]

This rare autosomal recessive condition is characterized by mental and physical retardation and frontal and lateral bossing of the skull, with small facial bones, a small beak-shaped nose, low set ears and small mouth with dysodontia. The scalp hair is long and sparse, the extremities are thin, and the hands are large with long fingers and atrophic nails. The subcutaneous fat is decreased, the skin is thin and wrinkled and the veins are prominent. The long-term prognosis is unknown.

REFERENCES

1 Devos E.A., *et al* (1981) *Eur J Pediatr* **136**, 245.
2 Snigula F. & Rautenstrauch T. (1981) *Eur J Pediatr* **136**, 325.
3 Wiedemann H.R. (1979) *Eur J Pediatr* **130**, 65.

OSTEODYSPLASTIC GERODERMA [1–3]

This syndrome has been reported in at least 14 patients. In the full syndrome, stunting of growth from early childhood is associated with senile changes in the skin, with normal scalp hair, generalized osteoporosis, multiple fractures and skeletal malformations. The face appears sad, with drooping eyelids and jowls. Relatives presenting partial forms of the syndrome showed geroderma and osteodysplasia without dwarfism. Skin biopsy may show fragmented elastic fibres [4].

REFERENCES

1 Bammer F., *et al* (1950) *Ann Pediatr* **174**, 126.
2 Boreux G. (1969) *J Genet Hum* **17**, 137.
3 Hunter A.G.W., *et al* (1978) *Hum Genet* **40**, 311.
4 Lisker R., *et al* (1979) *Am J Med Genet* **3**, 389.

POIKILODERMA CONGENITALE
SYN. ROTHMUND–THOMSON SYNDROME

This condition is fully described on p. 150. It may be considered as a premature ageing syndrome because of the atrophic hyperpigmented skin, the early onset of cataracts and the premature greying and loss of hair.

COCKAYNE'S SYNDROME (p. 148)

The atrophic skin with mottled pigmentation and loss of subcutaneous fat on the face produce an appearance of premature senility.

GENERALIZED LIPOATROPHY (p. 1875)

The absence of subcutaneous fat may give an aged appearance in affected children, but the associated cutaneous features of coarse dry skin, hypertrichosis and acanthosis nigricans are not those of premature ageing.

REFERENCE

Senior B. & Gellis S.S. (1964) *Pediatrics* **33**, 593.

TRISOMY 21
DOWN'S SYNDROME (p. 114)

This disorder shows more features of true ageing than the classical premature ageing syndromes [2]. These features include progressive dementia with the neurofibrillary tangle seen in senile dementia, amyloid and lipofucsin deposition in many organs, diabetes mellitus, cataracts, cardiovascular disease, increased incidence of autoimmune disease and malignancy and a decreased life expectancy [1].

The cutaneous features include dry lax skin, premature greying, and loss of hair [1].

REFERENCES

1 Goldstein S. (1978) In *The Genetics of Ageing*. Ed. Schneider E.L. New York, Plenum, p. 171.
2 Martin G.M. (1978) In *Genetic Effects of Ageing*. Eds. Bergsma D. & Harrison D.E.. New York, Alan R. Liss for the National Foundation March of Dimes, p. 5.

DIABETES MELLITUS

Diabetes may be classified as a premature ageing syndrome because of the predisposition to cataracts and atheroma and the reduced life expectancy [2]. Some patients with insulin-dependent diabetes mellitus have thick, tight, waxy skin and limited joint mobility [3], and these patients have an increased risk of retinal and renal disease due to microvascular damage [5]. This increased risk is probably due to thickening of the capillary basement membrane secondary to changes in collagen. Enzymatic digestion of tendon collagen from young patients dying from diabetes showed that their collagen behaved as if it were from patients who were 50–65 yr older than their actual age [4]. The chemical changes in the collagen of diabetic subjects have been discussed elsewhere [1].

REFERENCES

1 BURTON J.L. (1982) *Br J Dermatol* **106**, 369.
2 GOLDSTEIN S. (1978) In *The Genetics of Ageing*. Ed. Schneider E.L. New York, Plenum, p. 171.
3 GRGIC A., *et al* (1976) *J Pediatr* **88**, 584.
4 HAMLIN C.R., *et al* (1975) *Diabetes* **24**, 4.
5 ROSENBLOOM A.L., *et al* (1981) *N Engl J Med* **305**, 191.

PROLIDASE DEFICIENCY

Definition and aetiology. Deficiency of prolidase (peptidase D) is a rare inborn error of collagen metabolism which is usually associated clinically with chronic skin ulceration and mental retardation. It is probably inherited as an autosomal recessive [5].

Pathology. There is little abnormality to be seen on light or electron microscopy of the skin, but large amounts of imidodipeptides are excreted in the urine [1, 6], and the proline:hydroxyproline ratio in collagen is increased. Prolidase deficiency is assumed to be the cause of the clinical features, but the role of prolidase in normal physiology is obscure and some siblings of patients have the enzyme deficiency with no clinical manifestations [3].

Clinical features [2, 4, 5]. Most patients are mentally defective with abnormal facies, though with no characteristic or consistent pattern. Splenomegaly, recurrent infections and obesity or a protuberant abdomen occur in about 30% of cases. Skin changes occur in about 85% of cases, and these include skin fragility, ulceration and scarring (usually on the lower extremity), photosensitivity, telangiectasia, purpura, premature greying and lymphoedema.

Diagnosis. The diagnosis is confirmed by the finding of massive imidodipeptiduria with prolidase deficiency in the red cells, white cells or cultured fibroblasts [4].

Treatment. Only symptomatic treatment is available.

REFERENCES

1 ARATA J., *et al* (1979) *Arch Dermatol* **114**, 62.
2 GOODMAN S.I., *et al* (1968) *Am J Med* **45**, 152.
3 ISEMURA M., *et al* (1979) *Clin Chim Acta* **93**, 401.
4 DER KALOUSTIAN V.M., *et al* (1982) *Dermatologica* **164**, 293.
5 POWELL S, *et al* (1977) *J Pediatr* **91**, 242.
6 SHEFFIELD L.J., *et al* (1977) *Pediatrics* **91**, 578.

LABORATORY STUDIES IN THE PREMATURE AGEING SYNDROMES [6–14]

Fibroblasts from normal human skin have a limited life span in culture which is inversely proportional to the age of the donor [15] and it seems that the *in vitro* ageing of fibroblasts may serve as a model for the *in vivo* ageing of the whole body [8]. All the premature ageing syndromes studied to date have shown a marked reduction in fibroblast growth potential *in vitro*. These include pangeria [18, 19], progeria [19], poikiloderma congenitale [19], trisomy 2 [1, 22] and diabetes mellitus [14]. In addition, fibroblasts from progeria patients have shown a decrease in mitotic activity, rate of outgrowth from explants, DNA synthesis and cloning efficiency [2].

Another approach to the *in vitro* study of ageing is the assay of enzyme activity in cultured fibroblasts. Enzymes of the hexose monophosphate shunt have an increased heat-labile fraction in late passage cells, and this may be a manifestation of *in vitro* ageing [16, 17]. Other enzymes involved in purine metabolism alter during the ageing of human erythrocytes [4, 23]. Studies in fibroblasts from patients with progeria and pangeria have shown enzyme changes consistent with an accelerated ageing process [10–13].

In the normal ageing process, there is a threefold increase in the affinity of surface insulin receptors for native insulin between the first and seventh decades [21]. This accounts for the clinical finding of relative insulin resistance in the elderly. Patients with progeria also show increased insulin binding and relative insulin resistance [13, 21].

Other cellular abnormalities in pangeria and progeria include a decrease in surface-membrane HLA antigens [14] and a marked increase in the activity of a procoagulant which may predispose to atheroma [3].

Post-irradiation DNA repair appears to be normal in progeria and pangeria [14], although the cultured fibroblasts may have reduced karyotype stability [20]. A reduction in DNA stability might increase the rate of genomic deterioration, and this might accelerate cellular ageing.

The fact that the premature ageing syndromes have multiple features which are difficult to attribute to a single enzyme or protein defect suggests that they may result from a genetic defect in the regulation of various metabolic pathways [5].

REFERENCES

1 BOUÉ A., *et al* (1975) *In Vitro* **ii**, 409.
2 DANES B.S. (1971) *J Clin Invest* **50**, 2000.

3 EPSTEIN J., *et al* (1973) *Proc Natl Acad Sci USA* **70**, 977.

4 FORNAINI G., *et al* (1969) *Eur J Biochem* **7**, 214.

5 GILCHREST BARBARA A. (1981) *Birth Defects* **xvii** (2), 227.

6 GOLDSTEIN S. (1969) *Lancet* **i**, 424.

7 GOLDSTEIN S. (1978) In *The Genetics of Ageing*. Ed. Schneider E.L. New York, Plenum, p. 171.

8 GOLDSTEIN S. (1979) *J Invest Dermatol* **73**, 19.

9 GOLDSTEIN S., *et al* (1974) *Nature* **251**, 719.

10 GOLDSTEIN S., *et al* (1975) *Nature* **255**, 159.

11 GOLDSTEIN S., *et al* (1975) *N Engl J Med* **292**, 1305.

12 GOLDSTEIN S., *et al* (1976) *Interdiscip Top Gerontol* **10**, 24.

13 GOLDSTEIN S., *et al* (1976) *Nature* **260**, 711.

14 GOLDSTEIN S., *et al* (1978) *Science* **199**, 781.

15 HAYFLICK L. (1965) *Exp Cell Res* **317**, 614.

16 HOLLIDAY R., *et al* (1972) *Nature* **238**, 26.

17 HOLLIDAY R., *et al* (1974) *Nature* **248**, 762.

18 MARTIN G.M., *et al* (1965) *Fed Proc* **24**, 678.

19 MARTIN G.M., *et al* (1970) *Lab Invest* **23**, 86.

20 NORWOOD T.H., *et al* (1979) *J Invest Dermatol* **73**, 92.

21 ROSENBLOOM A.L., *et al* (1976) *Science* **193**, 412.

22 SCHNEIDER E.L., *et al* (1972) *Proc Soc Exp Biol Med* **141**, 1092.

23 YIP L.C., *et al* (1974) *Biochemistry* **13**, 2558.

FIBROMATOSIS, FIBROMA AND FIBROSARCOMA

Fibrous overgrowth of dermal and subcutaneous connective tissue occurs most readily in certain sites and at certain ages, and some of the resulting syndromes are clinically and histologically distinctive and well defined [1–3]. There are numerous cases, however, which defy precise classification and in which histological criteria may be a poor guide to prognosis [6]. Invasiveness and a high local recurrence rate may, or may not, be associated with a tendency to metastasize. The borderline between simple overgrowth and a benign tumour may be equally difficult to define.

The following classification may be useful:

Benign fibromatosis
  1. *Juvenile*
    (i) Congenital generalized fibromatosis
    (ii) Aponeurotic fibroma
    (iii) Infantile digital fibromatosis
    (iv) Fibrous hamartoma of infancy
    (v) Aggressive infantile fibromatosis
    (vi) Fibromatosis colli
  2. *Adult*
    (i) Dermatofibroma (p. 1706)
    (ii) Osteopoikilosis with connective tissue naevi
    (iii) Desmoid tumour (p. 2461)
    (iv) Palmar and plantar fibromatosis
    (v) Penile fibromatosis (Peyronie's disease)
    (vi) Knuckle pads
    (vii) Nodular fasciitis
    (viii) Elastofibroma
    (ix) Fibrous papule of the face

An attempt has been made [7] to group together, as hereditary polyfibromatosis, a number of these conditions which tend to occur in association and are perhaps determined by a dominant gene. There are certainly families in which many of the benign fibromatoses occur in increased incidence and in variable combination, but in general when they occur in isolation only palmar and plantar fibromatosis, cheloids and knuckle pads are unquestionably sometimes hereditary in origin.

Malignant fibroblastic tumours [5]
    (i) Dermatofibrosarcoma
    (ii) Subcutaneous fibrosarcoma
    (iii) Fibrosarcoma in radio-atrophic skin

The dermatofibroma, the desmoid tumour and the malignant fibroblastic tumours are described in other chapters.

REFERENCES

1 ALLEN P.W. (1977) *Am J Surg Pathol* **1**, 305.

2 FLEISCHMAJER R., *et al* (1973) *Arch Dermatol* **107**, 574.

3 FRETZIN D.F. & ESTERLY N.B. (1982) The Fibromatoses. In *Dermatology Update*. Ed. Moschella S.L. New York, Elsevier, p. 253.

4 GENTELE H. (1951) *Acta Derm Venereol (Stockh)* **31**, (Suppl. 27).

5 MACKENZIE D.H. (1970) *The Differential Diagnosis of Fibroblastic Disorders*. Oxford, Blackwell.

6 STOUT A.P. (1961) *Clin Orthop* **19**, 11.

7 TOURAINE A. & RUEL H. (1945) *Ann Dermatol Syphiligr* **5**, 1.

JUVENILE FIBROMATOSIS [1–4]

The term juvenile fibromatosis has been applied to a group of disorders occurring mainly in youngsters and characterized by proliferative activity of the fibroblasts. There is a tendency for local recurrence, but unlike fibrosarcomas they do not metastasize. Their classification is based predominantly on anatomical localization, as follows: generalized, palmoplantar and digital fibromatosis.

The group comprises a number of more or less well-defined clinical entities, but some cases still defy precise classification.

Juvenile hyaline fibromatosis is a separate entity

which is a disorder of glycosaminoglycan synthesis (p. 1852)

REFERENCES

1 FLEISCHMAJER R., *et al* (1973) *Arch Dermatol* **107**, 574.
2 FRETZIN D.F. & ESTERLEY N.B. (1982) The Fibromatoses. In *Dermatology Update*. Ed. Moschella S.L., New York, Elsevier, p. 253–4.
3 MACKENZIE D.H. (1970) *The Differential Diagnosis of Fibroblastic Disorders*. Oxford, Blackwell.
4 ROSENBERG H.S., *et al* (1978) *Perspect Pediatr Pathol* **5**, 269.

Congenital generalized fibromastosis [1–3]. In this very rare syndrome there is diffuse overgrowth of fibrous tissue with the formation of poorly circumscribed nodules in the subcutaneous tissue, bone, myocardium, lungs, liver and intestines. The nodules consist of loose bundles of elongated spindle-shaped fibroblasts.

Multiple small subcutaneous nodules are present at birth, but new ones may continue to appear for several months.

If the fibrous tumours spare the viscera the prognosis is good, even if muscle and bone are involved, but if the viscera are involved the prognosis is poor. The infant fails to thrive, and pulmonary or gastrointestinal symptoms develop [3]. The infant is likely to die within a few weeks or months.

Thirty-five cases had been described by 1978 [3], and virtually all were sporadic.

REFERENCES

1 BEATTY E.C. (1962) *Am J Dis Child* **103**, 620.
2 CONDON V.R. & ALLEN R.P. (1962) *Radiology* **76**, 444.
3 ROSENBERG H.S., *et al* (1978) *Perspect Pediatr Pathol* **5**, 269.

Aponeurotic fibroma (syn. Juvenile palmo-plantar fibromatosis; calcifying fibroma; cartilage anlage of fibromatosis). This is an invasive calcifying tumour of the palms and soles with a unique histological pattern [3, 4]. The proliferating fibroblasts, which have an abundant cytoplasm, are arranged in sheets, with plump dark nuclei all oriented in the same direction. Giant cells resembling osteoclasts, and amorphous linear or granular calcium deposits, are scattered throughout the tumour.

The condition generally occurs in young children, although it can occur in adolescence or even adults as late as the seventh decade [1]. The fibrous mass, which arises as a poorly marginated nodule, may be asymptomatic or painful. It is firm and fixed but not adherent to the overlying skin. Stippled cal-

cification seen on radiology provides a diagnostic clue.

The recurrence rate after excision is high, but metastasis does not occur.

REFERENCES

1 FRETZIN D.F. & ESTERLEY N.B. (1982) The Fibromatoses. In *Dermatology Update*. Ed. Moschella S.L., New York, Elsevier. p. 253.
2 GOLDMAN R.L. (1970) *Cancer* **26**, 1325.
3 KEASBEY L.K. & FANSELAU H.A. (1961) *Clin Orthop* **19**, 115.
4 ROSENBERG H.S., *et al* (1978) *Perspect Pediatr Pathol* **5**, 269.

Infantile digital fibromatosis (syn. Digital fibrous swellings [2, 5, 6])

Aetiology and pathology [1, 2, 4]. The histological appearances are distinctive. Collagen is abundant and apparently normal, but the sparse elastic fibres are abnormal. There are numerous spindle-shaped cells with indistinct outlines; the cytoplasm of some of these cells, which resemble fibroblasts, contains small dense round pyroninophilic bodies, the nature of which is uncertain, but no virus has been cultured [4]. They are probably by-products of the metabolically damaged cells. Electron microscopy suggests that the proliferating cell is a myofibroblast [1].

Clinical features [2, 3, 7]. Firm smooth pink or flesh-coloured nodules are found on one or more fingers or toes at birth or develop at any time up to the third year. The swellings, which are firmly attached to the skin, are on the extensor aspect of terminal phalanges.

Treatment. Spontaneous regression may occur in 2–3 yr and, if the diagnosis has been confirmed histologically, continued observation is justifiable. Recurrence after surgical excision has occurred in 75% of cases [6]. Some residual deformity may follow either spontaneous regression or surgical intervention.

REFERENCES

1 BHAWAN J., *et al* (1979) *Am J Pathol* **94**, 19.
2 COSKEY R.J., *et al* (1979) *Cutis* **23**, 359.
3 MCKENZIE A.W., *et al* (1970) *Br J Dermatol* **83**, 446.
4 MEHREGAN A.H., *et al* (1972) *Arch Dermatol* **106**, 375.
5 REYE R.D.K. (1965) *Arch Pathol* **80**, 288.
6 ROSENBERG H.S., *et al* (1978) *Perspect Pediatr Pathol* **5**, 269.
7 SHAPIRO L. (1969) *Arch Dermatol* **99**, 37.

Fibrous hamartoma of infancy [1, 3, 5, 7]. This affects boys more often than girls. It is present at birth or develops during the first 3 yr and in most cases involves the axillae, neck or trunk. The skin overlying the subcutaneous mass is normal. Histologically, there are bundles of fibrocollagenous material, cellular islands resembling primitive mesenchyme and mature adipose tissue. Recurrence after excision is infrequent and, if left untreated, spontaneous regression may recur. On electron microscopy, the cells have many of the features of myofibroblasts [1, 7].

Aggressive infantile fibromatosis [2, 3, 4, 5, 6]. It develops at any age up to about 16 yr as a firm subcutaneous swelling on any part of the body. The histological changes, with numerous mitoses, reflect the rapid growth of the lesion. Interlacing cords of spindle-shaped cells often form a whorled pattern, and reticulum fibres are prominent. On electron microscopy two cell types may be identified, an embryonic fibroblast with a relatively simple structure and a more complex cell with evidence of pinocytosis [3]. Recurrence may follow excision, but if metastases develop the case must be reclassified as fibrosarcoma [7].

Fibromatosis colli [3, 5]. This affects the lower third of the sternomastoid muscle. It develops in the first few months of life but often spontaneously regresses, although some patients are left with a wry neck deformity. It is thought that birth trauma may play a role in the pathogenesis, though the condition has occurred after Caesarean section. Early complete excision is the treatment of choice.

REFERENCES

1 BENJAMIN S.P., *et al* (1978) *Arch Dermatol* **114**, 1833.
2 ENZINGER F.M. (1965) *Cancer* (NY) **18**, 241.
3 FRETZIN D.F. & ESTERLEY N.B. (1982) The Fibromatoses. In *Dermatology Update*. Ed. Moschella S.L. New York, Elsevier, p. 253.
4 KING D.F., *et al* (1979) *J Dermatol Surg Oncol* **5**, 482.
5 MACKENZIE D.H. (1970) *The Differential Diagnosis of Fibroblastic Disorders*. Oxford, Blackwell.
6 REYE R.D.K. (1956) *J Pathol Bacteriol* **72**, 149.
7 ROSENBERG H.S., *et al* (1978) *Perspect Pediatr Pathol* **5**, 269.

ADULT FIBROMATOSIS

Osteopoikilosis and connective-tissue naevi (syn. Disseminated dermatofibrosis; Buschke–Ollendorf syndrome)

Definition and aetiology. This syndrome is characterized by the association of osteopoikilosis with various cutaneous lesions of connective-tissue origin [2], in particular juvenile elastoma [10] or extensive nodular fibrosis of the dermis [9]. It may be determined by an autosomal dominant gene of variable expressivity, for in some affected individuals the pathological changes appear to be confined to the skin [10] or to the skeleton [7].

Pathology. The histological changes are variable. They may be similar to those of the histiocytoma or solitary lenticular dermatofibroma (p. 1706). In some cases, dense fibrosis in the mid and lower dermis is associated with clumping of hypertrophic elastic fibres [5]. In one series of cases [10] all lesions submitted to biopsy showed broad interlacing bands of elastic fibres characteristic of juvenile elastoma. In others, the nodules consist of a disorderly arrangement of fibroblasts and collagen fibres in intertwining bands [14]. Others show phagocytic histiocytes containing lipid, and occasional giant cells [8]. These different histological changes represent, to some extent, stages in the maturation of the lesion, but it is clear that more than one form of cutaneous-tissue lesion may be associated with osteopoikilosis. The bone lesions consist of tightly meshed bony trabeculae.

Electron microscopy of the juvenile elastoma has shown marked abnormality of the microfibrillar component of the elastic fibres, with an increased desmosine content of the skin [3, 6, 12, 15]. It has been suggested that the same defect in synthesis of fibrillar components may produce osteopoikilosis in bone and juvenile elastoma in the dermis [12].

Clinical features [1, 4, 8, 9, 11, 13, 16]. The cutaneous features usually first occur in children but their later onset has been reported. The lesions are firm nodules up to 1 cm in diameter, but usually smaller. They are asymmetrically distributed and tend to be grouped in plaques, within which they are arranged in streaks or networks. They are skin-coloured or yellowish and may somewhat resemble the lesions of pseudoxanthoma elasticum. The distribution is variable, but the thighs, buttocks and abdominal wall are often involved, and the back, neck and arm in some cases. The pseudoxanthoma-like appearance on the thighs may contrast with the more irregular nodular pattern on the arms, where either the antecubital flexures or the extensor aspects may be involved.

Once the lesions have reached their full development they persist unchanged. The association with a tendency to cheloid scarring with other fibromatous disorders [9] and skin tags showing histologically epidermal cysts [16] have been reported.

Osteopoikilosis is detectable only radiologically. It consists of multiple circumscribed opacities each 1–10 mm. The mottling is more marked in the epiphyses and metaphyses of the long bones.

Diagnosis. The only important source of confusion is pseudoxanthoma elasticum, in which the papules are smaller, yellower and more uniform in size and more or less confined to the flexures. The diagnosis can be established by the associated features and by biopsy.

Treatment. None is available.

REFERENCES

1 ATHERTON D.J. & WELLS (1982) *Clin Exp Dermatol* 7, 109.
2 BUSCHKE A. & OLLENDORF H. (1928) *Dermatol Wochenschr* 86, 257.
3 COLE G.W. & BARR R.J. (1982) *Arch Dermatol* 118, 44.
4 CURTH H.O. (1934) *Arch Dermatol Syphil* 30, 552.
5 DANIELSON L., et al (1969) *Arch Dermatol* 100, 465.
6 DANIELSON L., et al (1977) *Acta Derm Venereol (Stockh)* 57, 93.
7 LANDBERG T. & AKESSON H.O. (1963) *Acta Genet Med Gemellol (Roma)* 12, 256.
8 LAUGIER P. & WORINGER F. (1964) *Hautarzt* 5, 214.
9 MARSHALL J. (1970) *S Afr Med J* 44, 775.
10 MORRISON J.G.L., et al (1977) *Br J Dermatol* 97, 417.
11 RAQUE C.J. & WOOD M.G. (1970) *Arch Dermatol* 102, 390.
12 REYMOND J.L., et al (1983) *Dermatologica* 166, 64.
13 SCHIMPF A., et al (1970) *Dermatologica* 141, 409.
14 SEROWY C. (1956) *Arch Klin Exp Dermatol* 203, 113.
15 UITTO J.U., et al (1981) *J Invest Dermatol* 76, 284.
16 VERBOV J. (1969) *Br J Dermatol* 81, 69.

Palmar fibromatosis (syn. Dupuytren's contracture)
Definition. This is a fibromatous hyperplasia of the palmar aponeurosis which is characterized by nodular thickening of the fascia with associated flexion contractures of one or more digits. The typical hand deformity was named after Baron G. Dupuytren [6].

Aetiology. The condition seems to be due to a reactive proliferation of fibroblasts with no inflammatory component and the basic cause is obscure. The contractures appear to follow the conversion of the fibroblasts to contractile myofibroblasts [4]. It is often familial and may be inherited as an autosomal dominant gene [11] with an incidence in the general population of around 2% [7, 12]. The condition occurs more commonly in patients with al-

coholic cirrhosis [19], epilepsy [5] and diabetes mellitus [11]. Plantar fibromatosis is also associated in about 5% of patients with other fibrosing conditions such as knuckle pads, plastic induration of the penis (Peyronie's disease) cheloid scarring or plantar fibromatosis [3, 18], and this has been termed the polyfibromatosis syndrome. Other conditions which have been less convincingly claimed to be associated with Dupuytren's contracture include periarthritis of the shoulder, chronic lung disease, gout, trauma and ulnar nerve damage [1, 17]. Phenytoin appears to stimulate fibrosis in the polyfibromatosis syndrome [16] and it may also cause gingival hypertrophy by stimulating fibroblasts and increasing collagen production [9].

Pathology [8]. In the early stages there are nodules in the subcutaneous tissue or within the fascia composed of proliferating fibroblasts with irregular hyperchromatic nuclei but with no excess of collagen. Later stages are characterized by the presence of myofibroblasts which have a fibrillary ultrastructure in the cytoplasm and seem to have some other properties of smooth muscle. The nuclei are deeply indented, and these constrictions may be related to the contractile properties of the cell. The cell also has surface membrane differentiations that provide attachment to neighbouring cells and stroma. Myofibroblasts have also been identified in the normal aorta and in granulation tissue, hypertrophic scars, cheloids, liver fibrosis, dermatofibroma etc. [10] in which their contractile properties may be important. The advanced stages of Dupuytren's contracture are characterized by dense fibrous connective tissue with a few elongated cells. An increased concentration of type III collagen is present in the nodules [2].

Clinical features. The age of onset is generally between 30 and 50 yr and the disease progresses more slowly in women [13, 14, 15]. The earliest sign is the development of a palmar nodule usually in the ulnar half of the hand. Insidious progression of the fibrosis causes flexion contractures of the affected fingers.

Diagnosis. There are few diagnostic difficulties. Juvenile aponeurotic fibroma may produce palmar or plantar nodules, but Dupuytren's contracture does not occur in young children.

Camptodactyly is a hereditary defect characterized by permanent flexion deformity at the interphalangeal joints of a finger, usually the fifth. It is not associated with fibromatosis.

Treatment. The advice of an orthopaedic or plastic surgeon should be sought. Surgical techniques available have been reviewed elsewhere [17].

REFERENCES

1 ALLEN P.W. (1977) *Am J Surg Pathol* 1, 255.
2 BAILEY A.J., *et al* (1977) *Clin Sci Mol Med* 53, 499.
3 BILLIG R., *et al* (1975) *Urology* 6, 409.
4 CHIN H.F. & MACFARLANE R.M. (1978) *J Hand Surg* 3, 1.
5 CRITCHLEY E.M., *et al* (1976) *J Neurol Neurosurg Psychiatry.* 39, 498.
6 DUPUYTREN G. (1834) *Lancet* ii, 222.
7 EARLY P.F. (1962) *J Bone Joint Surg* 44B, 62.
8 GABBIANI G. & MANJO G. (1972) *Am J Pathol* 66, 131.
9 HASSELL T.M., *et al* (1976) *Proc Natl Acad Sci USA* 73, 2909.
10 JAMES W.D. & ODOM R.B. (1980) *Arch Dermatol* 116, 807.
11 LING R.S.M. (1963) *J Bone Joint Surg* 458, 709.
12 MIKKELSEN O.A. (1972) *Acta Chir Scand* 138, 695.
13 MIKKELSEN O.A. (1976) *Hand* 8, 265.
14 MIKKELSON O.A. (1977) *Hand* 9, 11.
15 PIERARD G.E. & LAPIERE C.M. (1979) *Br J Dermatol* 100, 335.
16 VILJANTO J.A. (1973) *Semin Arthritis Rheum* 3, 155.
17 WILLIAMS J.L., *et al* (1970) *J Urol* 103, 75.
18 WOLFE S.J., *et al* (1956) *N Engl J Med* 255, 559.
19 YOST J., *et al* (1955) *Am J Surg* 90, 568.

Plantar fibromatosis [1, 3]. This is a much rarer condition than palmar fibromatosis. The lesions, which occur most often on the medial half of the midfoot, present as one or more nodules which may become painful and may even ulcerate. They rarely produce contractures but they tend to be locally invasive, with a tendency to recur. Total excision of the lesion and the entire plantar fascia seems to give the best results, with the lowest incidence of recurrence. The differential diagnosis includes keloid and fibrosarcoma, and in younger patients aggressive infantile fibromatosis and aponeurotic fibroma must also be considered [2].

REFERENCES

1 ALLEN R.A. (1955) *J Bone Joint Surg* 37, 14.
2 FLEISCHMAJER R. (1973) *Arch Dermatol* 107, 574.
3 WARTHAN T.L. (1973) *Arch Dermatol* 108, 823.

Hereditary camptodactyly [1, 3]. Hereditary camptodactyly has often been confused terminologically with Dupuytren's contracture, and on rare occasions the two conditions have occurred together. It has also been reported as forming part of the spectrum of developmental defects which constitutes the Marfan syndrome (p. 1844) and oculodentodigital dysplasia. Inheritance is determined by an autosomal dominant gene and the sexes are equally affected. It differs from Dupuytren's contracture in that it begins in childhood, that it involves the little finger and sometimes the ring and middle fingers, producing persistent flexion of the proximal interphalangeal joints, and that it spares the metacarpophalangeal joints and palmar fascia. It is only very slowly progressive. Defects frequently associated include pectus excavatum, scoliosis and ptosis. In one family taurinuria was associated [1].

Streblodactyly [2] is inherited as a sex-linked autosomal dominant character. The affected females show from birth a flexion deformity at the metacarpophalangeal joints of the thumbs and the proximal interphalangeal joints of the little fingers. Some fingers show swan-neck deformities and hyperextensible metacarpophalangeal joints. In one family there was an abnormal α-amino acid in the urine.

REFERENCES

1 NEVIN N.C., *et al* (1966) *J Med Genet* 3, 265.
2 PARISH J.G., *et al* (1963) *Br Med J* ii, 1247.
3 WELCH J.P. & TEMTAMY S.A. (1966) *J Med Genet* 3, 104.

Penile fibromatosis (syn. Peyronie's disease)
Aetiology. Penile fibromatosis may occur as an isolated abnormality or as one component of polyfibromatosis in association with palmoplantar fibromatosis, cheloids and knuckle pads [2]. A genetic factor is implicated, but reliable studies of the mode of inheritance are lacking, and some authorities [4] consider that the disease is essentially an inflammatory process. The condition is rare below the age of 20, and the highest incidence is between 40 and 60.

Pathology [5, 6]. The thickened plaque shows cellular fibroblastic proliferation surrounded by dense masses of collagen. Calcification and ossification may occur. The process appears to begin as a vasculitis in the areolar connective tissue beneath the tunica albuginea, whence it extends to adjacent structures.

Clinical features [1]. Painful erections and curvature of the erect penis often give the first indication of the disease, which is readily detectable as a thickened, subcutaneous plaque, rubbery or hard, 0·6–6·0 cm in diameter, usually on the dorsal aspect in its distal third. The condition is usually slowly progressive and the ultimate deformity may be considerable, but spontaneous regression may occur [4].

Treatment. Infiltration with steroids gives some improvement after repeated injections, especially in younger patients. The possibility of spontaneous cure makes it difficult to evaluate the claims [7] that radiotherapy is helpful. In persistently disabling cases plastic surgery may be advisable [3].

REFERENCES

1 CHESNEY J. (1963) *Br J Urol* **35**, 63.
2 GOSSRAU G. & SELLE W. (1965) *Dermatol Wochenschr* **151**, 1039.
3 HORTON C.E. & DEVINE C.J. (1973) *Plast Reconstr Surg* **52**, 503.
4 MACKENZIE D.H. (1970) *The Differential Diagnosis of Fibroblastic Diseases.* Oxford, Blackwell.
5 PUGH R.L.B. (1960) *Proc R Soc Med* **53**, 685.
6 SMITH B.H. (1966) *Am J Clin Pathol* **45**, 670.
7 VELTMAN G., *et al* (1968) *Hautarzt* **19**, 304.

Knuckle pads (syn. Tylositas articuli; coussinets des phalanges (Fr.))

Definition and aetiology. Knuckle pads are circumscribed fibromatous thickenings overlying the finger joints, often occurring as a sporadic, and apparently isolated, defect, but sometimes familial. Several pedigrees show autosomal dominant inheritance [3, 7]. The age of onset and the distribution of the lesions tend to be more or less constant in each family but show interfamily variation. Trauma is not a significant factor.

Pathology [2, 3]. The epidermis is grossly hyperkeratotic and acanthotic. The dermal connective tissue is hyperplastic and individual collagen fibres may be obviously thickened.

Clinical features [3, 4]. Flat or convex, smooth, circumscribed keratoses develop slowly and almost imperceptibly over the course of months or years. In some patients they become very much raised and obviously indurated, but in others the dermal component is not clinically apparent. They are most commonly seen over the dorsa of the proximal interphalageal joints, but occasionally develop over the knuckles or the distal interphalangeal joints. Any single site or combination of sites may be involved. Sites other than the hands are not often affected, but similar lesions on the knees were also present in one family [3] and we have seen them on the dorsa of the feet.

The age of onset is variable; it is usually between 15 and 30 but may be earlier. In some individuals the lesions may not be conspicuous until they have been present for some years.

An association with Dupuytren's contracture and other fibromatous lesions has been recorded in some families [6]. In one large family knuckle pads were associated with sensorineural deafness and with leukonychia [1]. Two affected individuals also had palmoplantar keratoderma.

In differential diagnosis occupational callosites must be carefully excluded [5].

Treatment. There is no satisfactory treatment. Excision may be followed by cheloidal scarring.

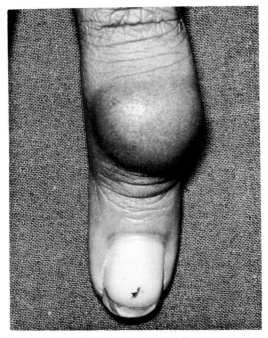

FIG. 49.19. Knuckle pads (Dr W. J. Cunliffe).

REFERENCES

1 BART R.S. & PUMPHREY R.E. (1967) *N Engl J Med* **276**, 202.
2 BELLAFIORE V. (1963) *Ann Ital Dermatol Sif* **17**, 105.
3 HERRMANN W.P. (1959) *Dermatol Wochenschr* **140**, 1165.
4 MORGINSON W.J. (1955) *Arch Dermatol* **71**, 349.
5 RONCHESE F. (1966) *G Ital Dermatol* **107**, 1227.
6 SCHWANDER R. (1953) *Arch Dermatol Syphil* **193**, 413.
7 VELTMAN G. (1954) *Dermatologica* **108**, 29.

Nodular fasciitis (syn. Subcutaneous pseudosarcomatous fibromatosis). This condition, of unknown origin, is probably not uncommon. It occurs mainly in adults aged 20–50 but has been reported in childhood and old age.

Histologically, poorly defined very vascular

nodules in the subcutaneous fat show fibroblastic proliferation with plump fibroblasts and poorly differentiated collagen fibres.

Clinically, there is a solitary, firm, mobile subcutaneous nodule, sometimes tender and painful, which reaches its maximum size of 1–2 cm in diameter in about 2 weeks and then persists unchanged. Multiple lesions may occur. The majority develop on the forearm or arm, but some occur on the legs or trunk or, less commonly, on the head and neck, even on the lips. Recurrence following surgery is infrequent.

REFERENCES

1 ABULAFIA J., *et al* (1968) *Arch Argent Dermatol* **18**, 139.
2 EMMERMANN H. (1968) *Der Chirurg* **39**, 360.
3 LUBRITZ R.R. & ICHINOSE H. (1975) *Cutis* **15**, 43.
4 MEHREGAN A.K. (1972) *Cutis* **10**, 305.
5 ROCKL H. & SCHUBERT E. (1971) *Hautarzt* **22**, 150.

Albopapuloid form of epidermolysis bullosa (syn. Pasini's syndrome). This rare form of epidermolysis bullosa is characterized by the development of ivory-white papules on the trunk which histologically show connective-tissue hyperplasia. Epidermolysis bullosa is discussed on p. 1620.

Elastofibroma [1–3]. Elastofibromas occur predominantly in elderly women and in most cases are situated beneath the lower angle of the scapula. The painless or slightly tender swelling, from 2 to 10 mm in diameter, is often discovered fortuitously. It may enlarge slowly, displacing neighbouring structures, and is prone to be clinically confused with a sarcoma. The histopathology, however, establishes the benignity of the lesion, despite its lack of circumscription. The growth is composed of mature fibrous tissue containing a number of fibres that behave tinctorially as elastic fibres.

Histologically the lesion contains abundant large elastic fibres, some broken into irregular masses, and large amounts of relatively acellular collagen. The condition is regarded as degenerative.

REFERENCES

1 BARR J.R. (1966) *Am J Clin Pathol* **45**, 679.
2 JARVI O.H., *et al* (1969) *Cancer NY* **23**, 42.
3 MacKENZIE D.H., *et al* (1968) *J Clin Pathol* **2**, 470.

Fibrous papule of the face (syn. Fibrous papule of the nose)
Definition and incidence. A small facial papule with a distinctive fibrovascular component on histological examination. The condition is uncommon, but not rare, and several large series have been reported [1, 2, 4].

Pathology [1, 2, 4]. The epidermis appears normal, although there may be an increased number of clear cells overlying the lesion. In the dermis there are broad bands of connective tissue oriented vertically to the surface. These are interspersed with multinucleate cells, often with a few cells resembling melanocytic naevus cells. There are prominent dilated capillaries but relatively few elastic fibres.

It has been suggested that the condition may be a variant of a melanocytic naevus [1, 4], but others disagree [2]. S-100 protein, which is an immunohistochemical marker of neuroepithelial elements, is present neither in the stellate cells in the papillary dermis nor in the mesenchymal 'naevus' cells [5]. It is possible that the fibrous papule represents a degenerate mole that can no longer synthesize S-100 protein, but the histogenesis of this lesion remains controversial [3].

Clinical features [1, 2, 4]. The lesions usually occur singly on the nose. Occasionally they may occur on the forehead, cheeks, chin or neck, and there may be several lesions. The lesion usually presents in middle life, and both sexes are equally affected.

The papule develops slowly as a dome-shaped skin-coloured or slightly red or pigmented lesion which is usually sessile. Most are asymptomatic, but about a third bleed on minor trauma.

Differential diagnosis. The lesions are not distinctive clinically, and they may simulate melanocytic naevus, angioma or pyogenic granuloma, but the histology is characteristic. The fibrovascular lesions of tuberous sclerosis have neither the cellular component nor the vertically arranged collagen bundles which typify fibrous papule of the face. The perifollicular fibroma is also easily distinguished histologically [6].

Treatment. The lesion is benign, but it may easily be excised or surgically 'pared' for cosmetic reasons.

REFERENCES

1 GRAHAM J.H., *et al* (1965) *J Invest Dermatol* **45**, 194.
2 MEIGEL W.N. & ACKERMAN A.B. (1979) *Am J Dermatopathol* **1**, 329.
3 OKUN M. (1984) *J Am Acad Dermatol* **10**, 680.
4 SAYLAN T., *et al* (1971) *Br J Dermatol* **85**, 111.
5 SPIEGEL J., *et al* (1983) *J Am Acad Dermatol* **9**, 360.
6 ZACKHEIM H.S. & PINKUS H. (1960) *Arch Dermatol* **82**, 913.

Reactive fibrous papule of the finger (syn. Irritation fibroma, giant cell fibroma). Saylan *et al* [1] have described small solitary papules of the fingers and palms which are very similar histologically to the fibrous papule of the face. These probably develop as a reaction to trauma.

Similar fibromatous papules of the oral mucosa have also been described [2].

REFERENCES

1 SAYLAN T., *et al* (1971) *Dermatologica* **143**, 368.
2 WEATHERS D.R. & CALLIHAN M.D. (1974) *Oral Surg* **37**, 374.

FASCIAL HERNIAS OF THE LEGS [1–2]

Small fascial hernias of the lower legs are not uncommon in athletes and heavy manual workers, and may present a problem in differential diagnosis. Herniation of muscle takes place through the hiatus in the deep fascia where it is perforated by communicating veins.

The hernias develop suddenly as nodules on the anterolateral aspect of the lower leg and are usually about 15 cm above the lateral malleolus. The nodules are soft, compressible and 1·5–2 cm in diameter. If bilateral they are strictly symmetrical. No treatment is required.

REFERENCES

1 KITCHIN I.D. & RICHMOND D.A. (1943) *Br Med J* i, 602.
2 OBERMAYER M.E. & WILSON J.W. (1951) *JAMA* **145**, 548.

CONSTRICTING BANDS OF THE EXTREMITIES
AINHUM AND PSEUDO-AINHUM

Definition. This is a constricting band around a digit or limb. The band may be shallow involving only the skin, or it may be deeper, involving fascia or bone, and in some cases amputation may result. The term *ainhum* is applied to a specific type in which a painful constriction of the fifth toe occurs in adults, with eventual spontaneous amputation. *Pseudo-ainhum* is the term applied to other constricting bands which are congenital or secondary to another disease [11, 17].

Ainhum (syn. dactylolysis spontanea)

Aetiology. The condition appears to be due to an abnormal blood supply to the foot, since arteri-ography has shown that in these patients the posterior tibial artery is attenuated at the ankle, and the plantar arch and its branches are absent [3]. Mechanical factors, including trauma from walking barefoot, may then precipitate the development of a groove in the ischaemic toe. There may be a genetic factor since a family history is common, and the disease is more common in certain races [2, 9]. Ainhum is most common in African Negroes, but many cases have been reported in American Negroes, and it can also occur in other races [7].

Various tropical infections, including leprosy, tuberculosis and yaws have been suggested as possible contributory factors [1], but these conditions are probably coexistent rather than causative [3, 4].

Pathology [1, 9, 10]. Fissuring and hyperkeratosis on the medial aspect of the digit is followed by fibrosis, distal degeneration and osteoporosis, ultimately leading to spontaneous amputation.

Clinical features. The condition is most common between the ages of 30 and 50, but the earliest stages may be seen in childhood. The presenting symptom is usually a painful fissure. The toe is held dorsiflexed at the metatarso-phalangeal joint, and gradually becomes clawed. Rest pain, coolness and cyanosis of the digit distal to the groove, suggest that ischaemia is present. Once the constricting band has encircled the toe, the condition tends to progress rapidly. The toe becomes globular, hangs by a thread of fibrous tissue and is eventually shed.

Diagnosis. The condition must be distinguished from pseudo-ainhum.

Treatment. Control of secondary infection and protection from trauma may prevent extension of the scarring process. If symptoms are severe, or the dangling digit is a disability, amputation is indicated.

Pseudo-ainhum. Congenital pseudo-ainhum may involve a digit, a limb or even the trunk, and it ranges in severity from a superficial groove to amputation *in utero* [6, 12, 14, 15]. The cause is unknown, but familial cases have been reported. Some cases of pseudo-ainhum may be due to amniotic bands or adhesions *in utero* which may arise as a result of tearing of the amnion in the first trimester [16]. Histology reveals broad finger-like projections of collagen, and coarse elastic bundles which penetrate deep into the subcutaneous fat [15]. Treatment with staged Z-plasty has been recommended [13]. Congenital pseudo-ainhum must be distinguished from aplasia of the limbs with rudimentary digits, from acromelia (in which part of the limb does not develop) and from hypoplasia (in which the parts, although formed, are poorly developed).

Pseudo-ainhum may also be acquired as a result of infection (particularly leprosy), trauma, cold injury, neuropathy, systemic sclerosis, etc. and it may occur in association with other hereditary diseases such as palmoplantar keratoderma (particularly Vohwinkel's disease), pachyonychia congenita, etc. Factitial pseudo-ainhum has also been reported [5].

REFERENCES

1 BROWNE S.G. (1976) *Int J Dermatol* **15**, 348.
2 COLE C.J. (1965) *J Bone Joint Surg* **47**, 43.
3 DENT D.M., *et al* (1981) *Lancet* ii, 396.
4 Editorial (1975) *Lancet* ii, 19.
5 FINDLAY G.H. (1951) *Trans R Soc Trop Med Hyg* **44**, 747.
6 GARCIA R.R. & HUBBELL C.G. (1979) *Cutis* **23**, 80.
7 GLESSNER J.R. (1963) *J Bone Joint Surg* **45**, 351.
8 HUCHERSON D.C. (1950) *Arch Surg (Chicago)* **132**, 312.
9 KEAN B.H. & TUCKER H.A. (1946) *Arch Pathol* **41**, 639.
10 KEAN B.M., *et al* (1946) *Arch Pathol* **41**, 637.
11 NEUMANN A. (1953) *Arch Dermatol Syphil* **58**, 421.
12 PETERKA E.S. & KARON I.M. (1964) *Arch Dermatol* **90**, 12.
13 PILLAY P.K. & HESKETH K.T. (1965) *J Bone Joint Surg* **47**, 514.
14 PRIESEL R. (1949) *Ost Z Kinderheilk* **3**, 107.
15 RAQUE C.J., *et al* (1972) *Arch Dermatol* **105**, 434.
16 RUSHTON D.I. (1983) *Br Med J* **286**, 919.
17 WELLS T.L. & ROBINSON R.C.V. (1952) *Arch Dermatol Syphil* **66**, 569.

HYPERTROPHIC SCARS AND CHELOIDS

Definition. A cheloid is an overgrowth of dense fibrous tissue which develops in the skin as a result of trauma, though in some cases the trauma may be trivial. A hypertrophic scar is a similar lesion and some workers use the terms synonymously, but others maintain that cheloids have a worse prognosis and are liable to spread laterally beyond the site of the initial trauma. The histology is similar and the two conditions probably differ only in degree.

Aetiology. The basic cause is unknown, but both local and constitutional factors appear to predispose to the excessive connective-tissue reaction.

Local factors. The presence of foreign material is liable to cause scar hypertrophy. This may be exogenous (e.g. suture material) or endogenous (e.g. embedded keratin from hair) and in some African tribes foreign bodies are deliberately introduced into tribal marks to induce a hypertrophic reaction.

Tension on a wound also favours hypertrophy, probably by disturbing the normal orientation of collagen bundles [8]. This is illustrated by the development of cheloids only at points of greatest tension in some scars [33] and by the fact that if cheloids are transplanted to the inner thigh, an area of relatively little tension, they may atrophy [4].

The type of trauma is significant. Cheloids commonly follow burns or scalds, and infection may also predispose to hypertrophy, though cheloids can follow an uncomplicated surgical incision.

Regional variations in skin structure are important. Scars on the eyelids, forehead, palms, soles, penis and scrotum are often inconspicuous, whereas hypertrophy readily occurs on the ear lobes, chin, neck, shoulders, upper trunk and lower legs.

Cheloids can result as a late consequence of the intramuscular injection of haematoporphyrin, which has been used to treat depression [29].

Systemic factors [24]. There is a familial tendency to cheloid formation, and both autosomal recessive [31] and autosomal dominant [2] inheritance have been reported. Among Europeans with cheloids a positive family history is obtained in 5–10% patients, more frequently in those with severe cheloids [7], but the incidence is higher in some Negro communities [14]. There is a genetic association between cheloids. Dupuytren's contracture and other manifestations of 'fibromatosis' (p. 1823).

Cheloids are rare in infancy and old age. Their incidence increases throughout childhood to reach a maximum between puberty and the age of 30. Women are more often affected than men, and cheloids may appear or enlarge during pregnancy [25]. They also occur after thyroidectomy, particularly in young patients, and they form readily in acromegalics, but the mode of action of endocrine factors remains speculative.

Pathology. The histology of normal wound healing and cheloid formation is similar in the early stages, but the orientation of the collagen fibres in the granulation tissue may indicate the type of scar that will eventually form [19]. Granulation tissue which forms a whorled or nodular arrangement of collagen is more likely to become hypertrophic than that which presents a parallel orientation of fibres. Hypertrophic scars and cheloids are characterized by increased cellularity and by a pattern of collagen which is not seen in normal skin or in non-hypertrophic scars [21]. They contain nodules of collagen which are highly compact, often with a capsule-like band around the periphery. There is vascular proliferation and the vessels are heavily cuffed by fibroblast clusters which enlarge and transform into a thickened nodular mass of collagen and proteoglycan. The number of mast cells is increased [17]. The epidermis is flattened by compression from collagen nodules but is otherwise normal [28].

By electron microscopy the nodule contains stellate fibroblasts, and in one study the cheloid was composed almost entirely of myofibroblasts [11]. The diameter of the collagen filaments is about half that seen in normal skin [1]. Scanning electron microscopy shows that in cheloids the organization of collagen bundles is more haphazard than in normal skin or mature scars [8].

The activity of several enzymes is increased in cheloids [13], but collagenase levels are not increased [24]. Abnormalities have been demonstrated in the types of collagen and the rate of collagen synthesis [1, 6]. A cross-linking amino acid, pyridinoline, is present in appreciable amounts in hypertrophic scars, but it is virtually absent in collagen from normal skin [26].

Possible mechanisms for the pathogenesis of cheloids have been reviewed elsewhere [27]. In summary, in hypertrophic scars and cheloids, more cells are making more collagen which may be protected from degradation by proteoglycan and specific protease inhibitors [20].

Clinical features. Scar hypertrophy may be evident within 3 or 4 weeks of the provocative stimulus. The scar becomes raised and thickened to form a well-defined, firm, pink or red plaque. Growth may continue steadily or intermittently for months or years, and huge irregular lesions of bizarre configuration may be formed. More commonly, growth ceases after a few months, the redness fades and no further change occurs. In the early stages it may be impossible to distinguish a hypertrophic scar from a potential cheloid. After 2 or 3 months, the cheloid becomes irritable and hypersensitive, its surface becomes smoother and rounder, and it extends beyond the area of the original lesion. In the absence of these signs, spontaneous regression remains a possibility.

Cheloids, particularly in the beard area, may occasionally undergo central suppurative necrosis [32] and they may rarely involute spontaneously. Malignant degeneration has also been reported [12]. Cheloids have been noted as a rare feature of Ehlers–Danlos syndrome, Rubinstein Taybi syndrome and pachydermoperiostosis [27].

Diagnosis. The diagnosis is usually simple if there is a history of trauma or an inflammatory skin lesion. The spontaneous cheloids with no such history usually develop in the pre-sternal region or upper chest. Basal cell carcinoma can mimic cheloid clinically and scar sarcoid can also cause confusion. Malignancy can also develop in scars.

Prophylaxis and treatment [27]. Non-essential surgery should be avoided in the sites of predilection in patients predisposed to cheloids. If surgery is necessary, simple excision, with careful planning to lessen skin tension and to control secondary infection is to be preferred to electrocoagulation or chemical caustics. If cheloid formation is anticipated, preoperative radiotherapy to the excision site may be useful.

Numerous treatments for the established cheloid

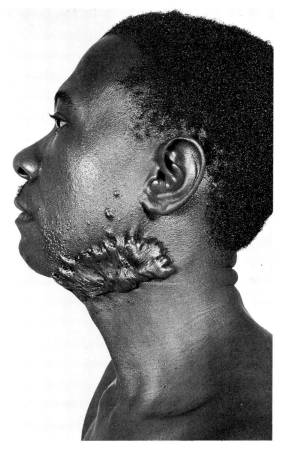

FIG. 49.20. Cheloids recurring after excision (Makere Medical School).

have been described, though few trials have been well controlled. Cheloids usually recur following simple surgical excision, but the results of surgery may be improved by combining excision with adjuvant therapy such as steroids, radiation or local compression, all of which may inhibit post-operative fibroplasia. Constant compression can also be used alone to treat cheloids [3, 16]. Ear lobe cheloids may respond well to surgical excision [34].

Superficial X-ray or electron beam therapy may be used to prevent cheloid recurrence [27], and radiotherapy with an iridium-192 wire has also been used successfully [22].

Intralesional triamcinolone injection is useful, particularly for early lesions, but the recurrence rate varies in different centres [10, 15]. This treatment can be combined with a liquid nitrogen spray prior to injection. This causes oedema which then allows the triamcinolone to be injected more readily [5].

Good results have also been obtained with repeated daily application of 0·05% retinoic acid [9], but systemic penicillamine is without effect [23]. Intralesional cytotoxic drugs have also been used but they may cause ulceration [30].

REFERENCES

1 BAILEY A.J., *et al* (1975) *Biochim Biophys Acta* **405**, 412.
2 BLOOM D. (1956) *NY State J Med* **56**, 511.
3 BRENT B. (1978) *Ann Plast Surg* **1**, 579.
4 CALNAN J.S., *et al* (1967) *Br J Surg* **54**, 330.
5 CEILLY R.I. & BABIN R.W. (1979) *J Dermatol Surg Oncol* **5**, 54.
6 CHAIG R.D.P., *et al* (1975) *Br J Surg* **62**, 741.
7 COSMAN B., *et al* (1961) *Plast Reconstr Surg* **27**, 335.
8 CRIKELAIR G.F. (1958) *Am J Surg* **96**, 631.
9 DE LIMPENS A.M. (1980) *Br J Dermatol* **103**, 319.
10 GRIFFITH B.H., *et al* (1970) *Plast Reconstr Surg* **46**, 145.
11 JAMES W.D., *et al* (1980) *J Am Acad Dermatol* **3**, 50.
12 KANAAR P. & OORT J. (1969) *Dermatologica* **138**, 312.
13 KEMBLE J.V. & BROWN R.F. (1976) *Br J Dermatol* **94**, 301.
14 KETCHUM L.D., *et al* (1974) *Plast Reconstr Surg* **53**, 140.
15 KIIL J. (1977) *Scand J Plast Reconstr Surg* **11**, 169.
16 KISCHER C.W., *et al* (1975) *Arch Dermatol* **111**, 60.
17 KISCHER C.W., *et al* (1978) *J Invest Dermatol* **70**, 355.
18 KNAPP T.R., *et al* (1977) *Am J Pathol* **56**, 47.
19 LINARES H.A. & LARSON D.L. (1974) *J Invest Dermatol* **62**, 514.
20 LINARES H.A. & LARSON D.L. (1978) *Plast Reconstr Surg* **62**, 589.
21 LINARES H.A., *et al* (1972) *J Invest Dermatol* **59**, 323.
22 MALAKER K., *et al* (1976) *Clin Radiol* **27**, 179.
23 MAYOU B.J. (1981) *Br J Dermatol* **105**, 87.
24 MILSOM J.P. & CRAIG R.D.P. (1973) *Br J Dermatol* **89**, 635.
25 MONSTAFA M.F.H., *et al* (1975) *Plast Reconstr Surg* **56**, 450.
26 MORIGUCHI T. & FUJIMOTO D. (1979) *J Invest Dermatol* **72**, 143.
27 MURRAY J.C., *et al* (1981) *J Am Acad Dermatol* **4**, 461.
28 NIKOLOWSKI W. (1961) *Arch Klin Exp Dermatol* **212**, 550.
29 NUNZI E., *et al* (1983) *Br J Dermatol* **108**, in press.
30 OLUWASANMI J.O. (1974) *Clin Plast Surg* **1**, 179.
31 OMA-DARE P. (1975) *J Natl Med Assoc* **67**, 428.
32 ONWUKWE M.F. (1978) *J Dermatol Surg Oncol* **4**, 333.
33 SHETLAR M.R., *et al* (1972) *Proc Soc Exp Biol Med* **139**, 544.
34 WEIMAR V.M. & CEILLEY R.I. (1979) *J Dermatol Surg Oncol* **5**, 522.

Cheloids, torticollis and renal dysplasia. Multiple large spontaneous Cheloids, appearing at puberty, are a feature of a syndrome apparently determined by an X-linked recessive gene. The other features are congenital torticollis, cryptorchidism and renal dysplasia.

REFERENCE

GOEMINNE L. (1968) *Acta Genet Med Gemell* **17**, 439.

MELORHEOSTOSIS

Melorheostosis is a rare disease of unknown aetiology characterized by dense cortical hyperostosis, usually affecting one limb but sometimes widespread. The distinctive radiological appearance has been compared with wax running down the side of a burning candle. The affected joints are deformed, and pain and stiffness are common. The disorder progresses rapidly in children and slowly in adults.

Skin changes occur in about 17% of cases [3] and these include proliferation or malformation of blood vessels or lymphatics, hypertrichosis and sclerodermatous changes. These usually precede the bone changes [1]. The histology suggests that linear melorheostotic scleroderma is a separate condition from morphoea [2, 5].

REFERENCES

1 CAMPBELL C.J. (1968) *J Bone Joint Surg Am* **50**, 1281.
2 MIYACHI Y., *et al* (1979) *Arch Dermatol* **115**, 1233.
3 MORRIS J.M. (1963) *J Bone Joint Surg Am* **45**, 1191.
4 SOFFA D.J., *et al* (1975) *Radiology* **114**, 577.
5 WAGERS L.T., *et al* (1972) *Br J Dermatol* **86**, 297.

HYPEREXTENSIBILITY, HYPERELASTICITY AND LAXITY OF THE SKIN

The capacity of the skin to adapt to local or general changes in body size and contour and to allow for movement of head and limbs and a wide range of facial expression, depends upon its tension, elasticity and tensile strength. One or all of these properties may be congenitally defective or modified by ageing or disease.

Tension [3]. The tension of the skin—its resistance to deforming forces—is provided by abundant elastic fibres and is reduced when they are defective or degenerate. Tension decreases with age.

Elasticity [1, 2, 3]. The elasticity of the skin is the measure of its ability to resume its original shape after deforming forces have ceased to act. There is wide individual variation but a tendency to decrease with age.

Tensile strength. The tensile strength of the skin is the degree to which it can be elongated before it tears. It is greatest in infancy and decreases with age but is also abnormally low in pregnancy and in Cushing's syndrome.

REFERENCES

1 GRAHAME R. (1970) *Clin Sci* **39**, 223.
2 JARRETT A. (1974) *The Physiology and Pathophysiology of the Skin.* Vol. 3. London, New York, Academic Press.
3 TREGEAR R.D. (1966) *Physical Functions of the Skin.* London, Academic Press.

Nomenclature. The complex interrelations, still incompletely understood, between tension, tensile strength and elasticity have contributed to the confused and inconsistent nomenclature and classification of those cutaneous disorders characterized by hyperextensibility, hyperelasticity or laxity of the skin. These abnormal properties may sometimes be associated but are not necessarily so. Lax skin can occur as a primary defect of the dermis or as a secondary feature following weight loss, in post-oedematous states, and inflammation. It may occur for example as a secondary manifestation in the later stages of various conditions affecting the dermis such as sarcoidosis and syphilis.

Primary increased laxity of the skin is uncommon and can be divided into three main groups:

Generalized cutis laxa
Localized {
  circumscribed cutis laxa
  blepharochalasis
  anetoderma (p. 1805)
}
Pseudoxanthoma elasticum (p. 1841)

CUTIS LAXA

SYN. GENERALIZED ELASTOLYSIS;
GENERALIZED ELASTORRHEXIS;
CHALAZODERMA; GENERALIZED
DERMATOCHALASIS

Definition. Cutis laxa is characterized clinically by lax pendulous skin and histologically by loss of elastic tissue in the dermis.

Aetiology. It may be inherited as an autosomal dominant [2], autosomal recessive [1, 11] or X-linked recessive [3]. It may also be acquired following inflammatory skin disease [13, 14] and it has occurred in babies born to women taking penicillamine [9]. It can also be a feature of an autosomal recessive form of pseudoxanthomas elasticum [15] or an autosomal dominant form of amyloidosis [12].

Pathology. The skin is of normal thickness but the elastic fibres are sparse, short, fragmented and clumped, particularly in the upper dermis, and they show granular degeneration [6, 11]. The elastic fibres are deficient in elastin but their microfibrils appear normal [10]. Similar changes in elastic fibres may occur in the lungs and aorta.

Abnormalities in collagen have been described in familial cutis laxa [10]. Two patients with X-linked recessive cutis laxa had deficiency of lysyl oxidase which is necessary for the cross-linking of both collagen and elastin [3].

Serum copper levels have been variously reported as increased, normal or decreased [10].

Clinical features [16]. This is a rare condition in which the skin becomes inelastic and hangs in redundant folds. The face and neck are often affected, which produces a 'bloodhound' appearance of premature senility (Fig. 49.21). The internal elastic tissues may also be affected and emphysema and cardiovascular abnormalities appear to be relatively common [20].

Congenital forms. In the autosomal dominant form the skin changes may begin at any age, involvement is usually limited to the skin, and life expectancy is unaltered [2]. The skin changes which may

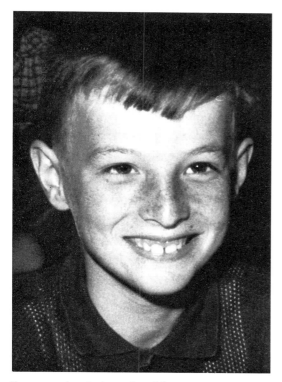 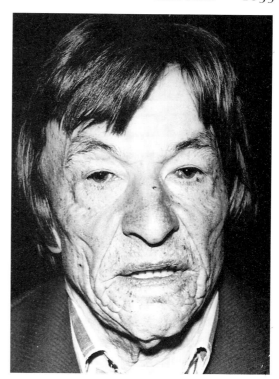

FIG. 49.21. Acquired cutis laxa following a reaction to penicillin: (a) the patient aged 11 yr before the penicillin reaction; (b) a few years later, showing the premature ageing due to elastolysis. (Courtesy of Dr H. Kerl, reproduced from *Am J Dermatopathol* (1983) **5**, 267.)

be preceded by episodes of oedema, usually develop within the first few months of life, and the child may look senile by the end of the second year. Affected males may be impotent with infantile genitalia and scanty body hair.

In the commoner autosomal recessive form, involvement begins in infancy and the disorder may be severe with progressive emphysema and cor pulmonale [5]. Hernias, diverticulae, aortic aneurysm and growth retardation may also occur [1].

In the rarer X-linked form there is joint hyperextensibility [3].

Acquired forms. Cutis laxa may rarely develop at any age following episodes of angio-oedema, extensive inflammatory skin disease [7] or febrile illness. It may also follow hypersensitivity reactions [8]. There may be widespread massive folds of lax skin, or the changes may be mild and confined to a limited area, in which case it cannot be distinguished from anetoderma. Purpura may follow slight trauma and fibrotic nodules may form over bony prominences. Organs other than the skin may also

be involved [5]. Emphysema, gastric fibromata and tracheobronchomegaly have been reported [19].

Post-inflammatory elastolysis also appears to develop as a distinctive syndrome in African children, with clinical features intermediate between anetoderma and cutis laxa [18]. This condition might represent an unusual reaction to an arthropod bite, since the lesions are preceded by urticaria or multiple red papules which slowly enlarge to form rings 2–10 cm in diameter.

Cutis laxa has also been reported in association with sarcoidosis, syphilis, multiple myeloma [4, 17] and the Klippel–Trenauny syndrome [10]. Focal elastolysis can also occur in association with lupus erythematosus.

Diagnosis. The diagnosis, which is suggested by finding loose skin which recoils only slowly after stretching, may be confirmed by histology. In the Ehlers–Danlos syndrome the skin is hyperextensible but not lax, and it recoils quickly. In pseudoxanthoma elasticum the skin may be lax, but it is yellowish and the face is usually spared. There may be circumscribed folds of lax skin in neurofibromatosis, and loose folded skin may also occur in leprechaunism (p. 1854), but these conditions are distinguished by their associated features.

Treatment. Plastic surgery ('face-lift') may reduce the cosmetic disability. Investigations for emphysema are indicated with referral to a pulmonary physician if necessary.

REFERENCES

1 AGHA A., *et al* (1978) *Acta Paediatr Scand* **67**, 775.
2 BEIGHTON P. (1972) *J Med Genet* **9**, 216.
3 BYERS P.H., *et al* (1976) *Birth Defects* **XII**, 293.
4 CHO S.Y., *et al* (1980) *Cutis* **26**, 209.
5 GOLTZ R.H., *et al* (1965) *Arch Dermatol* **92**, 373.
6 HASHIMOTO K. & KANZAKI T. (1975) *Arch Dermatol* **111**, 861.
7 JABLONSKA S. (1966) *Hautarzt* **17**, 341.
8 KERL H. & BURG G. (1975) *Hautarzt* **26**, 191.
9 LINARES A., *et al* (1974) *Lancet* **ii**, 43.
10 MARCHASE P., *et al* (1980) *J Invest Dermatol* **75**, 399.
11 MEHREGAN A.H., *et al* (1978) *J Cutan Pathol* **5**, 116.
12 MERETOJA J. (1969) *Ann Clin Res* **1**, 314.
13 NANKO H., *et al* (1979) *Acta Dermatol* **59**, 315.
14 O'BRIEN J.P. (1976) *Br J Dermatol* **95**, 105.
15 POPE F.M. (1974) *Arch Dermatol* **110**, 209.
16 REED W.B., *et al* (1971) *Arch Dermatol* **103**, 661.
17 SCOTT M.A., *et al* (1976) *Arch Dermatol* **112**, 853.
18 VERHAGEN A.R., *et al* (1975) *Br J Dermatol* **92**, 183.
19 WANDERER A.A., *et al* (1969) *Pediatrics* **44**, 709.
20 WEIR E.K., *et al* (1977) *Eur J Cardiol* **5**, 255.

Elastic tissue hypoplasia with dwarfism and oligophrenia (de Barsy's syndrome). In one patient, congenital cutis laxa with sparse dermal elastin was associated with degeneration of the anterior tunica elastica of the cornea, dwarfism and retarded psycho-motor development. The patient had a progeria-like facies but normal hair.

REFERENCE

DE BARSY A.M., *et al* (1968) *Helvetica Paediatr Acta* **23**, 305.

BLEPHAROCHALASIS [1, 2]

Definition. Laxity of the eyelid skin due to a defect in the elastic tissue.

Aetiology. The cause is unknown. Most cases are sporadic, but some pedigrees show autosomal dominant inheritance [4]. Some cases may be a localized form of post-inflammatory elastolysis (cutis laxa).

Pathology [5]. In the early stages there may be a mild dermal lymphocytic infiltrate, and in the later stages the elastic tissue in the lids becomes decreased and fragmented.

Clinical features [1, 4, 5]. Blepharochalasis is an uncommon condition that usually develops insidiously around the time of puberty. Repeated transient attacks of painless swelling of the eyelids lasting for 2 or 3 days are followed by laxity, atrophy, wrinkling and pigmentation, predominantly of the upper lids. There may be multiple telangiectasia.

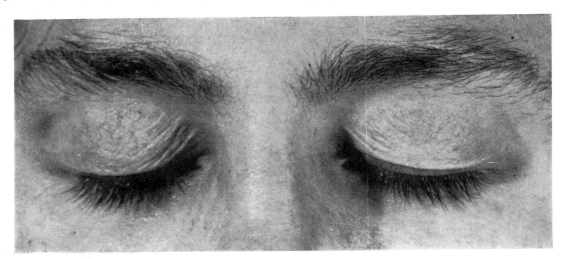

FIG. 49.22. Blepharochalasis in a boy aged 16. The skin of the lids is atrophic, finely wrinkled and telangiectatic (Addenbrooke's Hospital).

These changes produce an appearance of tiredness, debauchery or premature ageing.

Reduplication of the mucous membrane of the upper lid is associated with blepharochalasis in about 10% of cases, and this may make the eyelids appear thick.

Blepharochalasis is occasionally a manifestation of generalized cutis laxa, and it may form part of Ascher's syndrome (q.v.).

Diagnosis. The many other causes of eyelid swelling must be excluded (p. 2150). Ptosis is easily distinguished since the skin appears normal.

Treatment. Plastic surgery may be performed, but recurrence may occur [3].

REFERENCES

1 ALVIS B.Y. (1935) *Am J Ophthalmol* **18**, 238.
2 BRAZIN S.A., et al (1979) *Arch Dermatol* **115**, 479.
3 HARRIS W. (1975) *Ann Ophthalmol* **7**, 873.
4 LEVITT J.M. (1959) *Arch Ophthalmol* **62**, 506.
5 TAPASZTO I., et al (1963) *Acta Ophthalmol* **41**, 167.

ASCHER'S SYNDROME [1]

Ascher's syndrome is the association of blepharochalasis with progressive enlargement of the upper lip due to hypertrophy and inflammation of the labial salivary glands [2–4]. The lip feels soft and lobulated and there may be excessive salivation. In some cases the accessory lachrymal glands are also affected, with increased thickness of the eyelids. Enlargement of the thyroid has also been reported [1, 5].

REFERENCES

1 ASCHER K.W. (1920) *Klin Monatsbl Augenheilkd* **65**, 86.
2 BAZEX A. & DUPRÉ A. (1957) *Toulouse Méd* **58**, 89.
3 FINDLAY G.H. (1954) *Br J Dermatol* **66**, 129.
4 PAPANAYOTOU P.H. & HATZIOTIS J.C. (1973) *Oral Surg Med Oral Pathol* **35**, 467.
5 SCHIMPE A. (1955) *Dermatol Wochenschr* **132**, 1077.

CUTIS HYPERELASTICA
SYN. EHLERS–DANLOS SYNDROME

Definition. This is a group of inherited disorders of collagen metabolism showing clinical, genetic, biochemical and pathological heterogeneity which until recent years were thought to be a single disorder known as the Ehlers–Danlos syndrome (EDS). The characteristic clinical features include fragility of the skin and blood vessels, hyperelasticity of the skin and hyperextensibility of the joints, and these

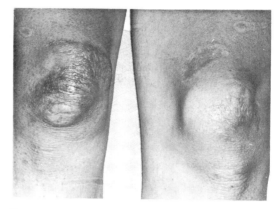

FIG. 49.23. Papyraceous atrophic scars of Ehlers–Danlos (Dr W. J. Cunliffe).

changes result from disorders of type I or type III collagen. At least 11 syndromes have now been identified [40], but many patients with the EDS do not meet the criteria for any of the 11 types.

Aetiology. Biochemical defects have been identified in some of the syndromes (see below), but the exact mechanisms involved are still obscure. In EDS VII there may be an analogy to dermatosparaxis in cattle [25, 28].

Pathology [49]. Histologically, the dermal collagen is scanty, whorled and disorderly, and elastic tissue is usually, but not invariably, increased. The ground substance stains only weakly for acid mucopolysaccharide. The pseudotumours consist of fat and mucoid material in fibrous capsules. They may be calcified. Collagen fibres in bone are irregular and mineralization is decreased [23].

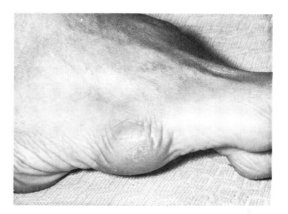

FIG. 49.24. Molluscoid pseudotumours of Ehlers–Danlos (Dr W. J. Cunliffe).

The essential defect is a quantitative deficiency of collagen [34, 38]. With the light microscope the fibres appear to be normal but form an inadequate weave of loose texture in the dermis, subcutis and joint capsules [22]. On electron microscopy an abnormal periodicity of the striations of the collagen fibres has been reported [21]. Elastic fibres may be increased in number but are quantitatively normal on histochemical and electron microscopy examination [20]. Study of the physical properties of the skin suggests that there may be defective binding of collagen fibrils [19].

Defects in the adventitia of small arteries and inadequate support from surrounding connective tissue probably account for the vascular vulnerability, which may be a conspicuous clinical feature.

The blood platelets in some patients show ultrastructural defects similar to those seen in thrombocytopathy A [24]. This defect may contribute to the abnormal bleeding tendency.

Mitral valve prolapse may occur [8].

Clinical features [5, 7, 11, 14, 26, 33, 40]. The distinctive features of the various types of EDS are summarized in Table 49.2.

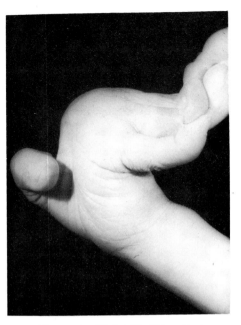

FIG. 49.25. Hyperextensible joint in Ehlers–Danlos syndrome (Dr W. J. Cunliffe).

TABLE 49.2. Cutis hyperelastica (Ehlers–Danlos syndrome)

Type	Inheritance	Ultrastructural findings	Biochemical disorder
I Gravis	Autosomal dominant	Large irregular collagen fibrils	Not known
II Mitis	Autosomal dominant	Large irregular collagen fibrils	Not known
III Benign hypermobile	Autosomal dominant	Not known	Not known
IV Ecchymotic	(i) Autosomal dominant (ii) Autosomal recessive	Small collagen fibres, fibrils of variable size	Decrease in type III collagen. Unstable triple helix
V X-linked	X-linked recessive	Not known	Not known
VI Ocular	Autosomal recessive	Small collagen bundles. Fibrils normal or similar to those in EDS I	Lysyl hydroxylase deficiency
VII Arthrochalasis multiplex congenita	(i) Autosomal dominant	Not known	Structural defect at the amino-terminal cleavage site of pro-α_2
	(ii) Autosomal recessive	Not known	Amino-terminal protease deficiency
VIII	Autosomal dominant	Not known	Reduced type III collagen
IX	? X-linked recessive	Not known	Increased copper incorporation and lysyl-oxidase deficiency

EDS I (gravis). This is inherited as an autosomal dominant. The skin is soft, velvety and hyperextensible, and if pulled out in a fold and then released it immediately springs back to its original position. The skin on the palms and soles may be redundant, like a loose glove. The skin is not otherwise lax until later in life, when redundant folds form at the elbows. Striae do not develop during pregnancy. Trivial lacerations form gaping wounds which heal very slowly to leave broad atrophic 'cigarette paper' scars. Sutures may tear out repeatedly. Blue–grey spongy tumours (molluscoid pseudotumours) due to accumulations of connective tissue may form in the skin, especially in scars or over pressure points. Smaller firm nodules may develop on the shins and forearms.

Easy bruising may be the presenting symptom, and pigmentation due to haemosiderin deposition is often found in areas of repeated trauma.

There is marked joint hypermobility, and in some cases this is so severe that walking is difficult. Subluxation of the large joints may occur, and genu recurvatum and kyphoscoliosis are frequent [47]. Muscle tone is often poor, and hernias readily develop. Varicose veins may develop in early life, and prematurity due to ruptured fetal membranes is common.

The facies may be distinctive, with widely spaced eyes, a wide nasal bridge and epicanthic folds. In older patients there may be redundant folds around the eyes. The sclerotics are sometimes blue.

Physical and mental development are normal and life expectancy is not reduced.

In EDS I, the dermal collagen fibres and bundles are small and disorganized [22], but at ultrastructural level the fibrils are larger than normal [48]. Many fibrils are irregularly shaped, with a 'flower-like' configuration on cross-section [43]. No biochemical defect has yet been identified, but it has been suggested that abnormal proteoglycan synthesis may affect collagen fibrillogenesis [44].

EDS II (mitis). In this type the clinical features are similar to EDS I but much milder. The ultrastructural findings are indistinguishable from EDS I, and the biochemical defect is unknown.

EDS III (benign, hypermobile). This type also resembles EDS I but the skin is only minimally affected whereas joint mobility is markedly increased and dislocation is common. The ultrastructural changes resemble those in EDS I [43].

EDS IV (ecchymotic, or arterial). This rare but severe type is clinically distinctive, but genetically heterogenous, and both autosomal dominant and autosomal recessive forms have been described [2, 9, 38, 39].

There is typically a hollow-cheeked, hollow-eyed appearance with a peaked nose and thin lips. In some cases the hands and feet appear prematurely aged (acrogeria). The skin is thin or translucent, or both, but it is not hyperextensible and the joints (except for the small joints in the hands) are usually of normal mobility. The surface veins are usually readily visible.

Marked bruising follows minor trauma, and the tissues are very friable so that rupture of the bowel (usually the colon), artery or uterus may occur. Dissecting aortic aneurysm or rupture of a large artery are common causes of death [4, 6, 32]. In one series the maternal mortality rate following pregnancy was 25% in EDS IV [42].

The condition is characterized by decreased production of type III collagen [9, 38].

In some patients the skin is reduced to 25% of normal thickness, with decreased size of collagen fibres and fibrils [10]. In others the fibril diameter is very variable. In many patients the rough endoplasmic reticulum in fibroblasts is increased, and cells in culture have abnormal and delayed secretion of type III collagen [9].

EDS V (X-linked). This rare variant is distinguished by its X-linked inheritance [5]. Clinically it resembles EDS II but bruising is more marked. The biochemical defect is unknown and skin collagen cross-links are normal [45]. Lysyl oxidase activity has been reported to be reduced in one family [13], but these patients appear to form a clinically distinct subgroup.

Genetic counselling is difficult in sporadic males with EDS II or V, since they are clinically similar but genetically different.

EDS VI (ocular). This type is distinguished clinically by its recessive inheritance, and the tendency to keratoconus and intra-ocular haemorrhage. The skin is soft and velvety and scoliosis is common.

These patients lack the enzyme lysyl hydroxylase, so that the lysyl residues in type I and type III collagens remain unhydroxylated, and the hydroxylysine-containing cross-links are not formed [17, 37]. Type II collagen (in cartilage) is hydroxylated normally, which suggests that there may be genetically distinct isoenzymes.

Some patients with EDS VI respond to treatment with ascorbic acid [16].

EDS VII (arthrochalasis multiplex congenita). This

rare type is characterized clinically by congenital hip dislocation and extreme hypermobility of both large and small joints [30]. The condition is genetically heterogenous. In one type, likely to be a recessive disorder, there is a defect in the enzyme which excises the amino-terminal propeptide from type I collagen [30]. This is analogous to dermatosparaxis in cattle [1, 3, 12]. In the other type there is a structural abnormality at or near the cleavage site in some of the pro-α chains, and this is presumably a dominant inheritance [46].

This disorder has shed light on the basic mechanism of collagen regulation. The observation that affected cells synthesized increased amounts of procollagen [30] suggested that the peptides normally cleaved from procollagen may act as a negative feedback control to regulate the rate of collagen synthesis. This idea has now been confirmed [35, 50], though the exact mechanism is still unclear.

EDS VIII. This type is characterized by hyperelastic fragile skin, moderate small joint hypermobility and severe periodontitis [31]. There is a reduced proportion of type III collagen [27].

EDS IX. The clinical manifestations include bladder diverticulae with spontaneous rupture, inguinal herniae, slight skin laxity and hyperelasticity, and various skeletal defects, the most characteristic being occipital horn-like exostoses [36]. This rare type appears to be inherited as an X-linked recessive.

Several disorders with defects of copper metabolism produce similar collagen defects. These disorders include Menke's syndrome, the mottled series of allelic mutant mice, EDS IX and some cases previously classified as X-linked cutis laxa. Because of the clinical and biochemical similarities it has been suggested that all these cases should be classified as EDS IX [36, 40].

In this group of disorders, the serum copper and caeruloplasmin concentrations are low, but most cells have increased copper levels. The connective tissue abnormalities are caused by a secondary reduction in the activity of lysyl oxidase [40].

Associated syndromes. The EDS has occurred with osteogenesis imperfecta, pseudoxanthoma elasticum, Marfan's syndrome [15, 18], renal tubular acidosis, medullary sponge kidney [24, 29] and osteolysis of the terminal phalanges [32], but it is not clear whether these abnormalities are associated with only one type of EDS.

Diagnosis. Cutis hyperelastica should not be confused with cutis laxa, in which the skin hangs in flaccid redundant folds. In cutis hyperelastica redundant folds may develop in late adult life, but they are usually limited to the elbows and the skin around the eyes.

The skin may be hyperelastic in Turner's syndrome (p. 116), but the dwarfism, unilateral valgus and webbing of the neck are distinctive.

Treatment. EDS VI may respond to oral ascorbic acid but no treatment is available for the other forms. The types with friable tissues may pose a problem to surgeons, and meticulous techniques and pressure dressings are needed. Re-excision of ugly scars can be cosmetically rewarding [41].

REFERENCES

1 ANSAY M., *et al* (1968 *Ann Med Vet* **122**, 449.
2 BARABAS A.P. (1967) *Br Med J* ii, 612.
3 BECKER U., *et al* (1976) *Biochemistry* **15**, 2853.
4 BEIGHTON P. (1968) *Br Med J* iii, 656.
5 *BEIGHTON P. (1970) *The Ehlers–Danlos Syndrome*. London, Heinemann.
6 BOPP P., *et al* (1965) *Circulation* **32**, 602.
7 BORNSTEIN P., *et al* (1980) In *Metabolic Control and Disease*. Eds Bowdy P.K. & Rosenberg L.E. 8th ed. Philadelphia, Saunders, p. 1089.
8 BRANDT K.D., *et al* (1975) *Am J Cardiol* **36**, 524.
9 BYERS P.H. (1981) *Birth Defects* xvii (2), 147.
10 BYERS P.H., *et al* (1979) *Hum Genet* **47**, 141.
11 CAPOTORTI L. & ANTONELLI M. (1966) *Acta Genet Med* **15**, 273.
12 COUNTS D.F., *et al* (1980) *J Invest Dermatol* **74**, 96.
13 DI FERRANTE N., *et al* (1975) *Connect Tissue Res* **3**, 49.
14 DUPERATT B., *et al* (1968) In *Maladies du Tissu Elastique Cutane*. Paris, Masson, p. 115.
15 EADY R.D. & CUNLIFFE W.J. (1977) *Clin Exp Dermatol* **2**, 117.
16 ELSAS L.J., *et al* (1978) *J Pediatr* **92**, 378.
17 EYRE D.R., *et al* (1972) *Proc Natl Acad Sci USA* **69**, 2594.
18 GOODMAN R.M., *et al* (1965) *N Engl J Med* **273**, 514.
19 GRAHAM E.R. & BEIGHTON P. (1969) *Ann Rheum Dis* **28**, 246.
20 HULT A.M., *et al* (1964) *Acta Dermatol Venereol (Stockh)* **44**, 415.
21 JACQUETI G., *et al* (1964) *Actas Dermosifilogr* **55**, 569.
22 JANSEN L.H. (1955) *Dermatologica* **110**, 108.
23 JULKONEN H., *et al* (1967) *Ann Med Intern Fenn* **56**, 55.
24 KASHIWAGI H., *et al* (1965) *Ann Intern Med* **63**, 249.
25 KERWAR S.S., *et al* (1973) *Proc Natl Acad Sci USA* **70**, 1378.
26 KRIEG T., *et al* (1981) *Int J Dermatol* **20**, 415.
27 LAPIERE C.M. & NUSGENS B.V. (1981) *J Invest Dermatol* **76**, 422.
28 LENAERS A., *et al* (1972) *Eur J Biochem* **23**, 533.
29 LEVINE A.S. & MICHEL A.F. (1967) *J Pediatr* **71**, 107.

30 LICHTENSTEIN J.R., *et al* (1973) *Science* **182**, 298.
31 LINCH D.C., *et al* (1979) *Br Dent J* **147**, 95.
32 MABILLE J.P., *et al* (1972) *J Ann Radiol* **15**, 781.
33 McKUSICK V.A. (1966) *Heritable Disorders of Connective Tisue*. 3rd ed. St Louis, Mosby, p. 179.
34 NORDSCHOW C.D. & MARSOLAIS E.G. (1969) *Arch Pathol* **88**, 65.
35 PAGLIA L., *et al* (1979) *Biochemistry* **18**, 5030.
36 PELTONEN L., *et al* (1983) *Biochemistry* **22**, 6156.
37 PINNELL S.R., *et al* (1972) *N Engl J Med* **286**, 1013.
38 POPE F.M., *et al* (1975) *Proc Natl Acad Sci USA* **72**, 1314.
39 POPE F.M., *et al* (1977) *J Med Genet* **14**, 200.
40 *PROCKOP D.J. & KIVIRIKKO K.I. (1984) *N Engl J Med* **311**, 376.
41 REIDY P.J. (1963) *Br J Plast Surg* **16**, 84.
42 RUDD P., *et al* (1983) *Lancet* **i**, 249.
43 SEVENICH M., *et al* (1980) *Arch Dermatol Res* **267**, 237.
44 SHINKAI H., *et al* (1976) *Arch Dermatol Res* **257**, 113.
45 SIEGEL R.C., *et al* (1979) *Biochem Res Comm* **88**, 281.
46 STEINMANN B., *et al* (1980) *J Biol Chem* **255**, 8887.
47 SVANE S. (1966) *Acta Orthop Scand* **37**, 49.
48 VOGEL A., *et al* (1979) *Lab Invest* **40**, 201.
49 WECHSLER H.L. & FISHER E.R. (1964) *Arch Pathol* **77**, 613.
50 WIESTNER M., *et al* (1979) *J Biol Chem* **254**, 7016.

PSEUDOXANTHOMA ELASTICUM

SYN. SYSTEMATIZED ELASTORRHEXIS; GRÖNBLAD—STRANDBERG SYNDROME

Definition. Pseudoxanthoma elasticum is an inherited disorder of connective tissue characterized by generalized elastorrhexis affecting the elastic tissue in the dermis, the blood vessels and Bruch's membrane of the eye.

Aetiology [3, 11, 27, 28]. Various modes of inheritance have been demonstrated including two autosomal dominant types and two autosomal recessive types [29]. The prevalence is estimated at one in 160,000 [8]. The disease is usually attributed to a basic defect in elastic tissue, although the collagen is also abnormal, and there may be increased degradation of connective-tissue components [12, 32].

Pathology [11]. One of the obvious changes in pseudoxanthoma is the deposition of calcium on elastic fibres which are otherwise normal in appearance. This, however, is probably not the primary change [23]. More likely some subtle changes in the fibres have provided suitable conditions for calcification to occur. In the fully developed lesion the elastic fibres in the mid-dermis are degenerate, fragmented and swollen, and mucopolysaccharide, mainly hyaluronic acid, is increased [17, 31]. The collagen fibres

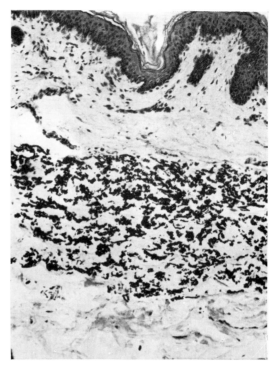

FIG. 49.26. Pseudoxanthoma elasticum. The mid-dermis contains a band of tangled elastotic fibres. These abnormal fibres stain positively for calcium (haematoxylin and eosin combined with von Kossa stain for calcium, ×65). (Professor E. Wilson Jones.)

are also abnormal, being split into small fibres. With the electron microscope most elastic fibres are grossly abnormal and often of irregular shape [25] and the early stage of elastogenesis is defective [15]. Similar changes in the elastic tissue occur in the media and intima of the blood vessels, Bruch's membrane of the eye and in the endocardium and pericardium. Mitral valve prolapse occurs in about 70% of cases [19].

The vascular involvement may be generalized but may involve predominantly the larger arteries, the mesenteric and visceral arteries or those of the extremities. Hypertension, cerebral vascular accidents and recurrent mucosal haemorrhages may result. The changes in Bruch's membrane give rise to angioid streaks, and rupture of the retinal vessels to haemorrhages and chorioditis.

Clinical features [1, 7, 9, 33]. The complete syndrome consists of distinctive skin lesions (pseudoxanthoma elasticum), retinal changes (angioid streaks) and vascular disturbances. Although pseudoxanthoma

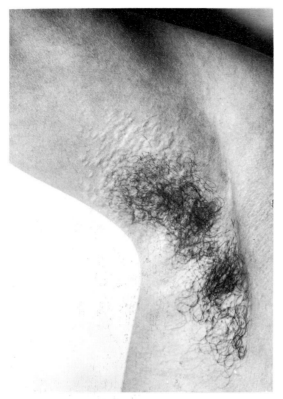

FIG. 49.27. Pseudoxanthoma elasticum (Dr I. B. Sneddon).

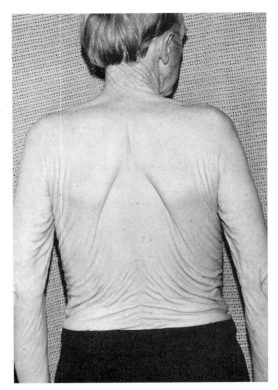

FIG. 49.28. Pseudoxanthoma elasticum showing lax folds of skin in an elderly patient (Dr J. Savin).

elasticum and angioid streaks have been reported as isolated findings, if the customary age of onset of the different manifestations is taken into account, it seems probable that the disorder is usually generalized. The relative severity of the cutaneous, ocular and vascular changes determines the wide variations in the clinical picture.

The skin lesions consist of small (1–3 mm) yellowish papules in linear or reticulate pattern in confluent plaques, often associated with telangiectasia. The skin is soft, lax and slightly wrinkled and may hang in folds, especially in the elderly. The sites of predilection are the sides of the neck, below the clavicles, the axillae, the abdomen, the groins, the perineum and the thighs. Although often limited, the eruption may involve most of the body. It may develop in early childhood, and usually does so before the age of 30, but may first appear in old age. It persists usually unchanged indefinitely. Similar changes may occur in the soft palate, inside the lips and in the mucous membranes of stomach, rectum and vagina. Rarely, chronic granulomatous nodules have developed in the skin lesions [14].

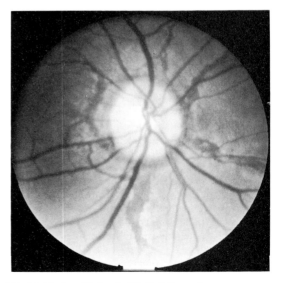

FIG. 49.29. Angoid streaks (Mr D. I. Bowen).

Angioid streaks [21] are seen as slate-grey, poorly defined streaks radiating from an incomplete greyish ring surrounding the nerve-head. They may be preceded by diffuse mottling of the fundus [10]. They are bilaterally symmetrical and usually first appear between age of 20 and 40. There may be no impairment of vision but progressive failure may occur, and haemorrhages and choroiditis occasionally result in total blindness. Loss of central vision is the most frequent disability and develops in over 70% of patients with angioid streaks [5].

A condition of abnormal visibility of the choroidal vessels has been present in some apparently unaffected members of affected families [3].

Arterial involvement may not be clinically manifest until adult life but intermittent claudication and angina has occurred in early childhood and recurrent gastrointestinal haemorrhages as early as 9. More usual are hypertension [24] or circulatory disturbances detectable by plethysmography or oscillometry [22]. Signs of arterial degenerations may be seen by the age of 30 and death may result from cerebral haemorrhage, coronary occlusion or massive haemorrhage into the gut. Some patients survive to old age. Hypercholesterolaemia with increased fatty esters has been reported in three patients [18].

The division of pseudoxanthoma into four genetic groups is of practical importance [29].

(a) *Dominant type I.* This type shows a flexurally distributed 'peau d'orange' pseudoxanthomatous rash, severe atheroma and a severe degenerative retinopathy, with early blindness.

(b) *Dominant type II.* This type, which is much less severe, typically has a canary-yellow macular rash or no rash at all, minimal vascular symptoms and mild retinal changes with prominent choroidal vessels. Increased cutaneous extensibility, blue sclerae, a high arched palate and myopia are also signs.

(c) *Recessive type I.* This resembles the dominant type I group, although vascular and retinal degeneration are milder. Haematemeses are common, especially amongst affected females.

(d) *Recessive type II.* This rare variant shows generalized cutaneous laxity and infiltration without systemic complications.

The physical properties of the apparently normal skin also differs in the groups but there is no difference in skin thickness [13].

Associated abnormalities. Angioid streaks may occur in Paget's disease of bone, in some cases of which pseudoxanthoma elasticum has been noted.

Angioid streaks may also occur in sickle cell disease, with which pseudoxanthoma may very rarely be associated [4]. Systemic, but not cutaneous, manifestations of pseudoxanthoma were present in a patient with Marfan's syndrome, and an association with perforating elastosis and systemic sclerosis has also been reported [22]. Multiple calcified cutaneous nodules had been present since childhood (onset 5–12) in three patients with angioid streaks and hyperphosphataemia but without pseudoxanthoma [20].

Skin changes of pseudoxanthoma elasticum are occasionally seen in adult patients with osteitis deformans (Paget's disease) [34]. It may also occur in association with *osteoectasia*, which is characterized by dwarfism, bizarre radiographic changes and elevated serum alkaline phosphatase levels [30].

Diagnosis. The clinical and histological changes of pseudoxanthoma elasticum are distinctive, and the diagnosis is usually readily made when skin lesions are present. If laxity of the involved skin is extreme other forms of dermatochalasis must be excluded (see p. 1834). In cases without skin lesions the diagnosis may be difficult. It should be suspected in obliterative arterial disease of early onset and unexplained gastrointestinal haemorrhage. The presence of angioid streaks or mucosal lessions should be sought. A skin biopsy from the side of the neck may be helpful even if no clinically evident changes are detectable. Soft tissue or vascular calcification may be detectable radiologically [16].

Treatment. The cosmetic appearance of the skin lesion may be improved by plastic surgery [6].

REFERENCES

1 ALTMAN L.K., *et al* (1974) *Arch Intern Med* **134**, 1048.
2 BARDSLEY J.L. & RUBEN-KOEHLER P. (1969) *Radiology* **93**, 559.
3 BERLYNE G.M., *et al* (1961) *Q Med* **30**, 201.
4 CAWLEY E.P. & WEARY P.E. (1962) *Arch Dermatol* **86**, 725.
5 CONNOR P.J., *et al* (1961) *Am J Med* **30**, 537.
6 CRIKELAIR G.F. (1953) *J Plast Reconstr Surg* **12**, 15.
7 EDDY D.D. & FARBER E.M. (1962) *Arch Dermatol* **86**, 729.
8 ENGELMANN M.W. & FLIEGELMAN M.T. (1978) *Cutis* **21**, 837.
9 GIBBS J.S.H. (1964) *Aust J Dermatol* **7**, 156.
10 GILLS J.P. & PATON D. (1963) *Arch Opthalmol* (NY) **73**, 792.
11 GOODMAN R.M., *et al* (1963) *Medicine* (Baltimore) **42**, 297.
12 GORDON S.G., *et al* (1975) *J Lab Clin Med* **86**, 638.
13 HARVEY W., *et al* (1975) *Br J Dermatol* **97**, 679.

14 HEYL T. (1967) *Arch Dermatol* **96**, 528.
15 HUANG S.N., *et al* (1967) *Arch Pathol* **83**, 108.
16 JAMES A.E., *et al* (1969) *Am J Roentgenol* **106**, 642.
17 KORTING G.W. & HOLZMANN H. (1968) *Arch Klin Exp Dermatol* **231**, 408.
18 KREYSEL H.W., *et al* (1967) *Hautarzt* **18**, 24.
19 LEBWAHL L.K., *et al* (1982) *N Engl J Med* **307**, 228.
20 McPHAULL J.J. & ENGEL F.L. (1961) *Am J Med* **31**, 488.
21 McWILLIAM R.J. (1955) *Br J Ophthalmol* **39**, 298.
22 NICHOLSON R. & BORK K. (1974) *Arch Dermatol Forsch* **249**, 301.
23 PAI S.H. & ZAK F.G. (1970) *Dermatologica* **140**, 54.
24 PALMER J.C., *et al* (1964) *N Engl J Med* **271**, 1204.
25 PIERARD J. & KINT A. (1970) *Ann Dermatol Syphiligr* **97**, 481.
26 POPE F.M. (1973) A study of pseudoxanthoma elastcum in England and Wales. *M.D. Thesis*, University of Wales.
27 POPE F.M. (1974a) *J Med Genet* **ii**, 152.
28 POPE F.M. (1974b) *Arch Dermatol* **110**, 209.
29 POPE F.M. (1975) *Br J Dermatol* **92**, 493.
30 SAXE N. & BEIGHTON P. (1982) *Clin Exp Dermatol* **7**, 605.
31 SMITH J.G., *et al* (1964) *J Invest Dermatol* **43**, 429.
32 UITTO J., *et al* (1971) *J Invest Dermatol* **57**, 44.
33 WHITCOMB F.F. & BROWN C.H. (1962) *Ann Intern Med* **56**, 834.
34 WOODCOCK C.W. (1952) *Arch Dermatol* **65**, 623.

Menke's disease (p. 2011). This rare metabolic disorder is usually recognized by the hair changes, but it also produces multiple connective-tissue defects including fragmentation and reduplication of the internal elastic lamina of the arteries [1]. The activity of lysyl oxidase in fibroblasts from patients with Menke's syndrome is reduced [3], suggesting that the basis of the connective-tissue abnormality could be defective cross-linking. This is secondary to the defective copper metabolism which characterizes the disease. It has been suggested that this condition may be related to Ehlers–Danlos syndrome type IX [2].

REFERENCES

1 OAKES B.W., *et al* (1976) *Exp Mol Pathol* **25**, 82.
2 *PROCKOP D.J. & KIVIRIKKO K.I. (1984) *N Engl J Med* **311**, 376.
3 ROYCE P.M., *et al* (1980) *Biochem J* **192**, 579.

Saltpetre-induced disease mimicking pseudoxanthoma elasticum. A condition which resembles pseudoxanthoma elasticum clinically, histologically and ultrastructurally has been described in a group of elderly farmers who years earlier had spread a fertilizer containing a mixture of various nitrates (Norwegian saltpetre). The patients developed cutaneous ulcers which quickly healed to leave yellowish-white papules and plaques. None of the patients had a positive family history or other signs of pseudoxanthoma elasticum.

REFERENCES

1 NEILSON A.O., *et al* (1978) *Acta Derm Venereol* **58**, 323.
2 CHRISTENSEN O.B. (1978) *Acta Derm Venereol* **58**, 319.

MARFAN'S SYNDROME

Definition. This is an inherited defect of connective-tissue metabolism determined by an autosomal dominant gene, but the expressivity of the gene varies widely [17, 18]. The full syndrome is characterized by abnormally long extremities, arachnodactyly, ocular and cardiovascular defects, but partial forms are not uncommon and there are no absolute diagnostic criteria [2, 21, 22].

Aetiology [23]. There is no doubt that collagen is defective in this condition but the exact defect is obscure [5]. Abnormalities in non-reducible cross-links have been described [3], and some patients (but not all) have increased levels of urinary hydroxyproline, an indication of accelerated collagen turnover [12]. Moreover animals fed lathyrogens or copper-deficient diets, both of which interfere with collagen cross-linking, have histological defects of the aortic media resembling those which occur in Marfan's syndrome. It has been suggested that the cross-link abnormalities are secondary to a primary gene-determined defect in the $\alpha_2(I)$peptide [3]. Other connective tissue components may also be abnormal including ground substance and elastin [1, 23]. Lysyl oxidase levels are normal [25].

Pathology. Fragmentation and sparsity of elastic fibres and the accumulation of mucinous material have been noted in the media of the aorta [19]. Histological abnormalities in other organs, including the skin, have not been thoroughly investigated.

Clinical features [13, 14, 20]. The full syndrome comprises skeletal, ocular and cardiovascular defects. The patient is often, but not invariably, exceptionally tall, but the skeletal proportions are abnormal. The extremities are long, the excess being greatest distally, giving rise to arachnodactyly, and the length of the hallux is often particularly conspicuous. The skull is dolichocephalic, the paranasal sinuses are large and the palate high and arched [28]. Lax capsules result in hyperextensible joints, kyphoscoliosis, pectus excavatus and flat foot.

Muscles may be underdeveloped and hypotonic, and subcutaneous fat is sparse.

The common ocular abnormalities [27] include ectopia lentis, myopia and retinal detachment; less frequent are blue sclerotics and heterochromia of the iris.

Aneurysmal dilatation of the ascending aorta is the most important abnormality of the cardiovascular system, and aortic and mitral incompetence are common. Aortic dilatation may begin in childhood. Mitral valve prolapse occurs in 80% of cases [2].

There are no constant or frequent cutaneous defects but perforating elastoma (p. 1851) may occur and the incidence and severity of striae atrophicae may be increased [16]. Several patients have been described with Ehlers–Danlos syndrome and Marfan's syndrome [89].

Other abnormalities are frequent—nerve deafness occurs in 6%; pulmonary malformations are often reported at autopsy; renal abnormalities [15] are manifest as proteinuria and raised blood urea.

The prognosis is related to the severity of the cardiac defects, the localization and progression of which are dependent on haemodynamic stresses [4]. Survival beyond the fifth decade is unusual, and some cases die in childhood. The average age at which dissection of the aorta develops is 30.

Diagnosis. The full syndrome is unmistakable, but diagnostic certainty is impossible in the partial forms. Dolichostenomelia is best estimated by the ratio of the lower segment (pubic ramus to floor) to the upper segment (height minus lower segment), but this ratio must be adjusted for the age and sex of the patient [20]. The metacarpal index as measured in the ring finger [28] is no longer considered worth while, but simple tests which may be helpful include the thumb sign (positive if the thumb when completely opposed in the clenched hand projects beyond the ulnar border) and the wrist sign (positive if the thumb and little finger overlap when wrapped around the opposite wrist) [21, 22]. The one-dimensional echocardiogram is more sensitive than a chest radiograph in detecting aortic dilatation [6].

Some tall people have high arched palates and some degree of arachnodactyly. This is probably of no consequence in many cases, though a Marfanoid habitus in women may be associated with mitral valve prolapse [2, 26].

Joint hypermobility may also be associated with mitral valve prolapse [11]. Other causes of joint hypermobility such as homocystinuria may be confused with the partial forms of the syndrome.

The Marfanoid habitus has been reported in association with distal pigmentation, neuroma of the eyelids and tongue, medullary carcinoma of the thyroid and phaeochromocytoma [7].

Management [21, 22]. Patients should be reviewed regularly by an ophthalmologist, a cardiologist and an orthopaedic surgeon. Hormonal therapy has been used to slow growth in the hope of preventing scoliosis, and propranolol may retard the development of aortic dilatation. Pregnancy is inadvisable, because of the 50% risk of inheritance in the fetus and because of the risk of acceleration of aortic degeneration and vascular rupture. Those with aortic or mitral valvular disease or dilatation of the aortic root are at high risk during pregnancy [24].

REFERENCES

1 ABRAHAM P.A., *et al* (1982) *J Clin Invest* **70**, 1245.
2 BEIGHTON P. (1982) *Br Med J* 284, 920.
3 BOUCEK R.J. (1981) *N Engl J Med* **305**, 988.
4 BOWDEN D.R., *et al* (1965) *Am Heart J* **69**, 69.
5 BYERS P.H., *et al* (1981) *Birth Defects* **xvii**, (2), 147.
6 COME P.C., *et al* (1977) *Chest* **72**, 789.
7 CUNLIFFE W.J., *et al* (1970) *Am Med J* **48**, 120.
8 DONALDSON L.B. & ALVAREZ R.R. (1965) *Am J Obstet Gynecol* **92**, 629.
9 EAD R. & CUNLIFFE W.J. (1977) *Clin Exp Dermatol* **2**, 117.
10 GOODMAN R.M., *et al* (1969) *Am J Cardiol* **24**, 734.
11 GRAHAME R, *et al* (1981) *Ann Rheum Dis* **40**, 451.
12 JONES C.R., *et al* (1964) *Proc Soc Exp Biol Med* **116**, 931.
13 KEECH M.K., *et al* (1966) *J Chronic Dis* **19**, 57.
14 LEHMANN O. (1960) *Acta Paediatr Scand* **49**, 540.
15 LOUGHRIDGE L.W. (1959) *Q Med* **28**, 531.
16 LOVEMAN A.B., *et al* (1963) *Arch Dermatol* **87**, 428.
17 LYNAS M.A. (1947) *Ann Hum Genet* **22**, 289.
18 MACEK M., *et al* (1966) *Humangenetik* **3**, 87.
19 MACLEOD M. & Wynn WILLIAMS A. (1956) *AMA Arch Pathol* **61**, 143.
20 McCUSISK V.A. (1972) *Heritable Disorders of Connective Tissue*. 4th ed. St Louis, Mosby, p. 61.
21 PYERITZ R.E., *et al* (1979) *N Engl J Med* **300**, 772.
22 PYERITZ R.E., *et al* (1979) *Brith Defects* **15** (5B), 155.
23 PYERITZ R.E., *et al* (1981) *N Engl J Med* **305**, 1011.
24 PYERITZ R.E. (1981) *Am J Med* **71**, 784.
25 ROYCE P.M. & DANKS D.M. (1982) *IRCS Med Sci* **10**, 41.
26 SCHUTTE J.E., *et al* (1981) *Am J Med* **71**, 533.
27 WACHTEL J.G. (1966) *Arch Opthalmol (NY)* **76**, 512.
28 WILNER H.J. & FINBY N. (1964) *JAMA* **187**, 490.
29 ZIMPRICH H. (1964) *Helv Paediat Acta* **19**, 483.

OSTEOGENESIS IMPERFECTA

Definition. This term is applied to a heterogeneous group of heritable disorders characterized by fragile bones due to a generalized disorder of connective tissue. Patients may also have blue sclerae, otosclerosis, skeletal deformity, imperfect dentine formation, mild joint hypermobility, hernias, mitral valve prolapse, arterial fragility and thin fragile skin [16]

Aetiology. The various forms of osteogenesis imperfecta are probably due to one or more of several basic biochemical defects in collagen metabolism [3, 13]. Details are given in a recent review [14]. Bone collagen is almost entirely type I, and nearly all the abnormalities in osteogenesis imperfecta affect either the α_1 or the α_2 chain of type I collagen. The biochemical abnormalities described include probable amino acid substitutions [7, 8, 9], short peptide deletions [1], abnormally migrating protein chains [7] and complete deletions of particular protein chains [6]. It is not clear why similar biochemical changes can apparently produce either mild or severe forms of the disease [13].

Pathology [2, 4, 17]. The bones are markedly collagen deficient, and often have a distorted architecture. The dermis is thin, with a relative increase of argyrophil and elastic fibres and a deficiency of adult collagen.

Clinical features [16]

Type 1: Mild form with blue sclerae. This is the commonest form. It is inherited as an autosomal dominant, though sporadic cases also occur [11]. Fractures are common in childhood. The sclerae are blue or grey and easy bruising and deafness are common, but skeletal deformity is absent or mild. Joint laxity is common. The incidence of mitral valve prolapse is increased [10, 15]. Most patients have decreased skin collagen, with an increased ratio of type I to type III collagen [5, 18]. Other patients have an abnormal α_2 chain which is unduly susceptible to proteolysis by pepsin [3, 7].

Type 2: Lethal perinatal form. This is the rarest form. There are multiple fractures *in utero* and infants rarely survive for more than a few days after birth. Avulsion of the limbs may occur during delivery due to a generalized connective-tissue fragility. Radiography shows beaded ribs, crumpled femora and little skull calcification. The inheritance is uncertain but may be autosomal recessive.

The defect in bone formation seems to be due to a decreased synthesis of type I collagen and secretion of an abnormal collagen which does not mineralize normally [19].

Type 3: Progressive deforming form. In this condition there are fractures *in utero* or at birth, and the long bones are thin and occasionally cystic. As the child grows older, progressive scoliosis and bowing of long bones cause crippling deformities. The sclerae are blue in childhood but become normal in the adult. The inheritance is uncertain, but the disease may be genetically heterogenous.

Some patients with this form seem unable to synthesize α_2 chains [6, 12].

Type 4: Mild form with normal sclerae. This condition is similar to type I in clinical features and inheritance, but the sclerae are not blue, dentinogenesis imperfecta is frequent and deafness is rare.

Diagnosis. Patients with short extremities and a large skull may be confused with achondroplasia, but bone fragility and thin skin do not occur in achondroplasia.

REFERENCES

1 BARSH G.S. & BYERS P.M. (1981) *Proc Natl Acad Sci USA* **78**, 5142.
2 BAUZE R.J., *et al* (1975) *J Bone Joint Surg* **57B**, 2.
3 BYERS P.H., *et al* (1981) *Birth Defects* **xvii** (2), 147.
4 FOLLIS R.H. (1953) *Bull Johns Hopkins Hosp* **93**, 225.
5 FRANCIS M.J.O., *et al* (1975). In *Disorders of Connective Tissue*. Ed. Bergsma D., Miami, The National Foundation March of Dimes, BD. OAS XI (6), pp. 15.
6 NICHOLLS A.C., *et al* (1979) *Lancet* **i**, 1193.
7 NICHOLLS A.C., *et al* (1983) *Br Med J* **288**, 112.
8 PELTONEN L., *et al* (1980) *Proc Natl Acad Sci USA* **77**, 162.
9 PELTONEN L., *et al* (1980) *Proc Natl Acad Sci USA* **77**, 6179.
10 PENTINNEN R.P., *et al* (1975) *Proc Natl Acad Sci USA* **72**, 586.
11 POPE F.M., *et al* (1975) *Proc Natl Acad Sci USA* **72**, 1314.
12 POPE F.M., *et al* (1980) *Lancet* **i**, 820.
13 POPE F.M., *et al* (1983) *J R Soc Med* **76**, 1050.
14 *PROCKOP D.J. & KIVIRIKKO K.I. (1984) *N Engl J Med* **311**, 376.
15 PYERITZ R.E. & LEVIN L.S. (1981) *Circulation* **64**, (Suppl 4), 311.
16 SILLENCE D.O., *et al* (1979) *J Med Genet* **16**, 101.
17 STEVENSON C.J., *et al* (1970) *Lancet* **i**, 860.
18 SYKES B., *et al* (1977) *N Eng J Med* **296**, 1200.
19 TRELSTAD R.L., *et al* (1977) *Lab Invest* **36**, 501.

WRINKLES

The facial skin responds to every movement of the facial muscles. This facility of response is achieved by the presence of a remarkably complex and dense intradermal elastic tissue mesh. This invisible sheath of elastic is unique to the face, not being found in such complexity elsewhere. With years of sunlight exposure the elastic tissue degenerates and with ageing there is an atrophy of the skin [2]. Not surprisingly, the effects of such a loss of elasticity and substance are most dramatically seen in the skin area most richly endowed with elastin. Thus, it is the face that mirrors the loss of the elastic recoil, and it is the face that wrinkles when both the normal elastic tissue and fat are reduced by the passage of years. Wrinkles are usually bilateral and symmetrical but one case of unilateral wrinkles has been described [3].

Widespread fine wrinkling with discrete perifollicular protrusions has been reported in association with elastolysis of the mid-dermal elastin [1].

REFERENCES

1 BRENNER W., *et al* (1978) *Br J Dermatol* **99**, 335.
2 FREEMAN R.G. (1971) *The Skin by 30 Authors*. Eds. Helwig E.B. & Mostofi F.K. Baltimore, Williams & Wilkins, p. 244.
3 SHELLEY W.B. (1974) *Arch Dermatol* **110**, 775.

The wrinkly skin syndrome. This rare familial condition is characterized by the appearance at birth of dry wrinkled skin of the hands, feet and ventral surfaces of the trunk. The veins are unduly prominent. There may also be mental retardation, ocular defects and poor muscle tone. The cause is unknown and the dermal collagen and elastin appear normal on light microscopy.

REFERENCE

GAZIT E., *et al* (1973) *Clin Genet* **4**, 186.

ACTINIC ELASTOSIS
SYN. SOLAR ELASTOSIS

Definition. This is a degenerative change caused by prolonged exposure to electromagnetic (usually solar) radiation. It is characterized clinically by yellowish discoloration and thickening of the skin and histologically by elastotic degeneration in the dermis.

Aetiology. Solar elastosis usually results from prolonged exposure to sunlight, though it can also result from infra-red radiation [5]. The biochemical mechanism which produces elastosis is poorly understood. The condition is related to the cumulative dose of irradiation. It becomes more common with increasing age and it is more common in outdoor workers and in sunny climates. There is considerable variation in susceptibility between individuals. Fair-skinned people are usually worst affected, though the condition can occur even in Negroes [7, 9]. Severe elastosis may occur in porphyria cutanea tarda.

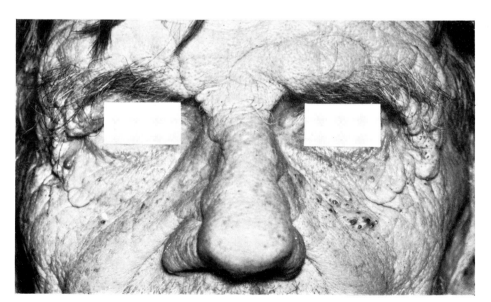

FIG. 49.30. Solar elastosis. The skin around the orbits is studded with comedones and follicular cysts—the Favre–Racouchot syndrome (Addenbrooke's Hospital).

Pathology. The essential abnormality is the so-called elastotic degeneration of collagen discussed on p. 76.

Clinical features. The condition is more common in later life. In temperate climates it is rare before the fourth decade, but it may occur earlier in sunnier climates. The light-exposed areas are affected, particularly the forehead and the back of the neck. Mild degrees of elastosis may not be apparent until the skin is pinched up, when it may assume a wrinkled appearance. Elastosis is usually more advanced in the tissue than the clinical appearance would suggest.

Several clinical patterns have been described, though the basic condition is probably similar in each.

In *cutis rhomboidalis* [11] the skin is thickened and yellow and divided by well-defined furrows into an irregular rhomboidal network. The back and sides of the neck are the usual sites.

Dubreuilh's elastoma consists of diffuse, but more or less sharply marginated, yellow thickened plaques on the face or neck. Plaques may be symmetrical, or there may be a single plaque on the dorsum of the nose [4].

Nodular elastoidosis [1, 3, 6] develops mainly around the orbits, especially in the malar regions and on and around the nose, but sometimes on the neck or behind the ears, and occasionally in other exposed areas. The skin is yellow and thickened and is studded with numerous comedones and follicular cysts (the Favre–Racouchot syndrome).

Elastotic nodules of the ear [2] commonly involve the antihelix.

All of these changes may be associated in variable degree. All may be complicated by solar keratoses and basal cell carcinoma. Actinic elastosis may also be complicated by actinic granuloma (see below).

Diagnosis. Plane xanthoma, pseudoxanthoma elasticum and colloid milium may sometimes cause confusion, but the combination of the clinical and histological features is distinctive.

Treatment. Sunscreens should be used by susceptible individuals [10].

REFERENCES

1 BORDA J.M., *et al* (1965) *Arch Argent Dermatol* **15**, 438.
2 CARTER V.H., *et al* (1969) *Arch Dermatol* **100**, 282.
3 CUCE L.C., *et al* (1964) *Arch Dermatol* **89**, 798.
4 DEGOS R., *et al* (1966) *Bull Soc Fr Dermatol Syphiligr* **73**, 123.
5 FINLAYSON G.R., *et al* (1966) *J Invest Dermatol* **46**, 104.
6 HELM F. (1961) *Hautarzt* **12**, 265.
7 KLIGMAN A. (1969) *JAMA* **210**, 2377.
8 MITCHELL R.E. (1967) *J Invest Dermatol* **48**, 208.
9 NURNBERGER F., *et al* (1978) *Arch Dermatol Res* **262**, 7.
10 PATHAK M.A. (1982) *J Am Acad Dermatol* **7**, 285.
11 TOSTI A. (1953) *Rass Dermatol Sifilogr* **6**, 175.

ACTINIC GRANULOMA
SYN. O'BRIEN'S GRANULOMA

Definitions. This is an annular inflammatory reaction with a giant cell dermal infiltrate, which develops in an area of actinic elastosis.

Aetiology [7]. It is thought that the inflammatory infiltrate develops in reaction to the elastotic changes in the sun-damaged dermis, and cells digest and absorb the elastotic fibres. The condition is more common in sunny countries, and fair-skinned or freckled subjects are particularly susceptible. A similar condition has been described in Negroes under the name of granuloma multiforme [2, 4, 5] (p. 1695). Contrary to popular belief, Negroes are not immune to actinic elastosis [3].

Pathology [1, 7]. A biopsy taken radially across the thickened edge of the lesion shows three distinct zones in the dermis. In the external 'normal' skin, there is actinic elastosis. In the thickened annulus there is a histiocytic and giant cell inflammatory reaction in relation to elastotic fibres, and in the centre, within the annulus, little or no elastic tissue remains. The cellular infiltrate slowly expands outwards, leaving behind a central area from which elastic fibres have been removed by 'elastoclasis'.

The epidermis may be normal or it may show signs of actinic damage.

Clinical features. Lesions develop in the exposed 'weather-beaten' skin of patients after the third decade, particularly in fair-skinned or freckled subjects. They start insidiously as small pink papules, which progress slowly to form an annulus of firm superficial dermal thickening. This is smooth, slightly raised and measures 0·2–0·5 cm in width. The ring may expand up to 6 cm in diameter. The centre may become slightly atrophic, and variable depigmentation may occur. The lesions are usually asymptomatic but a sunburn reaction may provoke severe erythema and irritation.

Diagnosis. The condition must be distinguished from granuloma multiforme, granuloma annulare, sarcoidosis and necrobiosis lipoidica [6, 8]. The lesions of actinic granuloma are confined to light-exposed skin, and the infiltrate lacks the tidy palisaded arrangement which is normally seen with granuloma annulare [8].

Treatment. Infiltration of the annular edge of the lesions with triamcinolone may be effective. Sunscreens should be used to prevent further damage.

REFERENCES

1 ALLEN T. (1966) *Aust J Dermatol* **8**, 252.
2 BROWNE S.G. (1966) *Int J Lepr* **34**, 27.
3 KLIGMAN A. (1969) *JAMA* **210**, 2377.
4 LEIKER D.L. (1964) *Int J Lepr* **32**, 368.
5 MARSHALL J., et al (1967) *Dermatologica* **134**, 193.
6 MEHREGAN A.H. & ALTMANN J. (1973) *Arch Dermatol* **107**, 62.
7 O'BRIEN J.P. (1975) *Arch Dermatol* **111**, 460.
8 PRENDIVILLE J., et al (1985) *Br J Dermatol* **113**, 353.

COLLOID MILIUM
SYN. COLLOID PSEUDOMILIUM; COLLOID DEGENERATION OF THE SKIN; ELASTOSIS COLLOIDALIS CONGLOMERATA

Definition. Colloid milium is a degenerative change characterized clinically by the development of yellowish, translucent papules or plaques on light-exposed skin and histologically by the presence of colloid in the dermal papillae.

Aetiology. The cause is uncertain, and the condition may not represent a single entity. The juvenile form, beginning before puberty and often familial, can be distinguished from a non-familial form occurring in later life [9]. Although light appears to play little part in provoking the lesions in the juvenile form, it is certainly implicated in older patients [8, 10] amongst whom the incidence is highest in fair-skinned outdoor workers in sunny climates [1, 5]. Cases among refinery workers in the tropics suggest that trauma and the photodynamic effects of phenols in oxide fuel (gas oil) may be contributory factors [4, 7]. Cases have also been reported after the long-term application of strong hydroxyquinone bleaching creams. These patients also had ochronosis [4].

Pathology [2, 6, 9, 11]. The earliest histological change is the appearance of colloid globules at the tips of the dermal papillae. Homogeneous fissured masses of colloid occupy the upper dermis, each surrounded by bands of collagen. The colloid is usually eosinophilic but may be basophilic. Within it small blood vessels and the nuclei of fibroblasts are well preserved. In the larger plaque-like lesions the colloid change occurs diffusely throughout the dermis.

In the juvenile form the colloid masses may also occur in the epidermis and elastosis is not present, whereas in the adult form the colloid is separated from the epidermis by a band of elastin and elastosis is present [2]. In the juvenile form 'immature' Civatte bodies occur in the epidermis [2].

The source of the colloid material is uncertain but *de novo* synthesis seems most likely. Histochemical and biochemical findings suggest that the colloid is a pathological protein differing from collagen and elastin and is probably a scleroprotein elaborated by dermal fibroblasts [5, 12].

The histological changes may require differentiation from those of amyloidosis and lipoid proteinosis.

Clinical features [1, 3, 10]. Small dermal papules 1–2 mm in diameter, yellowish and sometimes translucent, develop slowly and more or less symmetrically in irregular groups in areas exposed to sunlight. They feel soft and may release their gelatinous contents when punctured. The most frequently involved sites are the face, especially around the orbits, the backs of the hands, the back and sides of

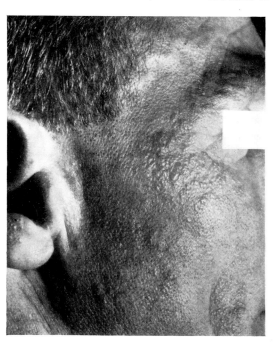

FIG. 49.31. Colloid milium. Extensive lesions on the face and ears of a young agricultural worker (Addenbrooke's Hospital).

the neck and the ears. There is some inconstant variation in the clinical features according to the age of onset. In young children [8, 10] the lesions are often confined to the face, with diffuse infiltration surmounted by innumerable small papules which may appear vesicular. In the older patients the papules are often fewer and larger and their potential distribution is much wider, although often only one or two sites are involved in each individual. The changes induced by prolonged light exposure are associated in varying degrees. Although colloid milium may become more severe and more extensive over the years, most cases reach their maximum development within 3 yr and then remain unchanged.

Diagnosis. The histological and clinical findings together are unmistakable though the former alone may be difficult to differentiate from amyloidosis. Trichoepithelioma, tuberous sclerosis and hydrocystoma are distinguished by biopsy.

Treatment. Destruction of the lesion with the diathermy or with cryotherapy has been advocated, but the cosmetic result is seldom satisfactory.

REFERENCES

1 BECK F. & WIFLING L. (1960) Z Haut GeschlKrankh **28**, 113.
·2 EBNER H. & GEBHART W. (1978) Arch Dermatol Res **261**, 231.
3 FERREIRA-MARQUES J. & VAN UDEN N. (1950) Arch Dermatol Syphil **192**, 2.
4 FINDLAY G.H., et al (1975) Br J Dermatol **93**, 613.
5 GRAHAM J.H. & MARQUES A.S. (1967) J Invest Dermatol **49**, 497.
6 HASHIMOTO K., et al (1972) Arch Dermatol **105**, 684.
7 HOLZBERGER P.C. (1960) Arch Dermatol **82**, 711.
8 MIEDZINSKI F., et al (1960) Dermatol Wochenschr **142**, 927.
9 PERCIVAL G.H. & DUTHIE D.A. (1948) Br J Dermatol **60**, 339.
10 WARIN R.P. (1961) Br J Dermatol **73**, 422.
11 ZAUN H. (1966) Arch Klin Exp Dermatol **224**, 408.
12 ZOON J.J., et al (1955) Br J Dermatol **67**, 212.

REACTIVE PERFORATING COLLAGENOSIS [2, 4, 6]

Definition. This is an unusual response to superficial trauma or cold in which abnormal collagen is extruded through the epidermis.

Aetiology. The cause is unknown, though the condition is often familial [3, 5]. The basic defect seems

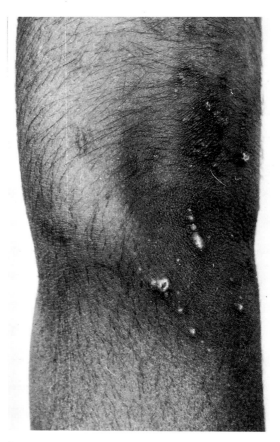

FIG. 49.32. Reactive perforating collagenosis (Dr Wojnarowska, High Wycombe).

to be a type of focal necrolysis of the epidermis and underlying dermis.

Clinical features. The condition usually starts in early childhood as small papules on the extensor surface of the hands, the elbows and the knees following superficial trauma. Each skin-coloured papule increases to a size of about 6 mm over 3–5 weeks and then becomes umbilicated with a keratinous plug. The lesions regress spontaneously in 6–8 weeks to leave a hypopigmented area or slight scar, but new lesions may appear. Lesions can be produced experimentally and Köbner's phenomenon may be present, with linear lesions. The papules can also be provoked by inflamed acne lesions, but deep incisions do not produce the lesions. The condition persists into adult life. In some cases the disease is associated with intolerance to cold and improves in warm weather.

Pathology. The lesion originates in the capillary dermis, where collagen which stains blue with haematoxylin is surrounded and engulfed by focal epidermal proliferation. The central crater which develops contains inflammatory cells and keratinous debris, and the abnormal collagen is eliminated by transepithelial migration [2]. The affected collagen fibres appear normal by electron microscopy [2].

Diagnosis. The condition may be mistaken for molluscum contagiosum, papular urticaria, elastosis perforans serpiginosa, perforating folliculitis, perforating granuloma annulare and Kyrle's disease, but the histology is characteristic [6]. Verrucous perforating collagenoma and acquired reactive perforating collagenosis must also be distinguished (see below).

Treatment. Topical retinoic acid may reduce the number of lesions [1]. Other treatments which may help include oral methotrexate, emollient creams and topical steroids under occlusion [6].

REFERENCES

1 CULLEN S.I. (1979) *Cutis* **23**, 187.
2 FRETZIN D.F., *et al* (1980) *Arch Dermatol* **116**, 1054.
3 KANAN M.W. (1974) *Br J Dermatol* **91**, 405.
4 MEHREGAN A.H. (1967) *Arch Dermatol* **96**, 277.
5 NAIR B.K.H., *et al* (1974) *Br J Dermatol* **91**, 399.
6 PATTERSON J.W. (1984) *J Am Acad Dermatol* **10**, 561.

Acquired reactive perforating collagenosis. There have been several recent reports [1, 2, 3, 5] of perforating disease of the epidermis in patients with chronic renal failure, most of whom were undergoing haemodialysis. The keratotic lesions developed on the trunk or extremities and were commonly associated with pruritus but were not necessarily related to superficial trauma. These cases have been variously reported as Kyrle's disease, reactive perforating collagenosis or perforating folliculitis. Patterson [4] has suggested that the presence or absence of the Köbner phenomenon, and the presence or absence of collagen fibres within the epidermis, do not reliably distinguish between these conditions in acquired cases with renal failure, and they may be variants of the same disease process.

REFERENCES

1 BRAND A. & BRODY N. (1981) *Cutis* **28**, 673.
2 COCHRAN R.J., *et al* (1983) *Cutis* **31**, 55.
3 HURWITZ R.M., *et al* (1982) *Am J Dermatopathol* **4**, 101.
4 PATTERSON J. (1984) *J Amer Acad Dermatol* **10**, 561.
5 POLIAK S.C., *et al* (1982) *N Engl J Med* **306**, 81.

Verrucous perforating collagenoma (syn. Collagenoma perforant verruciforme). In this rare condition, severe (as opposed to superficial) trauma to the skin produces verrucous papules which show transepithelial elimination of collagen. The eruption occurs as a single episode and is not familial.

REFERENCES

1 DELACRETAZ J. & GATTLEN J.M. (1976) *Dermatologica* **152**, 65.
2 LAUGIER P. & WORINGER F. (1963) *Ann Dermatol Syphiligr* **90**, 29.

PERFORATING ELASTOMA
SYN. ELASTOSIS PERFORANS SERPIGINOSA; ELASTOMA INTRAPAPILLARE PERFORANS

Definition. In this reactive perforating dermatosis the material extruded through the epidermis is derived from elastic fibres in the upper dermis.

Aetiology. The cause is unknown, but a genetically determined defect of elastic tissue may be involved. The altered elastin resembles that seen in experimental animals subjected to lathyrogens or copper deficiency [11]. Some 40% of reported cases have been associated with connective-tissue disorders, such as pseudoxanthoma elasticum, Ehlers–Danlos syndrome, Marfan's syndrome, osteogenesis imperfecta and acrogeria [9, 12, 13]. It has also been reported in otherwise healthy individuals and in mental deficiency, especially Down's syndrome [11]. Familial cases have occurred [1].

The disease is one of several conditions which exhibit the phenomenon of 'transepithelial elimination' [9]. It is probable that the primary abnormality is in the dermal elastin [4, 11, 13] which provokes a cellular response that ultimately leads to extrusion of the abnormal elastic tissue. It may be significant that the lesions are commonly seen in areas subjected to wear and tear. The lesions may follow an abrasion [2] and cases have been reported in which the lesions followed treatment of Wilson's disease with penicillamine [7].

Pathology [3, 9, 10, 14]. The earliest detectable change is the focal development of elastotic staining tissue and basophilic debris in the dermis. This is followed by a reaction of the overlying epidermis, which grows down to engulf the elastotic material. The epidermis surrounding the fully developed lesion is acanthotic and hyperkeratotic. The papule consists of a circumscribed area of epidermal hyperplasia traversed by a channel communicating directly with the dermis and containing a mass of tissue which projects above the surface. This plug consists of horny material in its upper third and of amorphous basophilic debris in its lower two-thirds. This material is derived from elastin [4, 6]. In the dermis beneath and around the lesion there is a foreign body giant cell reaction. The elastotic material is finally extruded to leave irregular scarring and warty thickening. Electron microscopy shows an increase in elastic fibres with fine filaments on the surface similar to those seen in normal embryos [10].

Clinical features [3, 5, 9, 14]. The age of onset ranges from 6 to 20 yr. Small horny or umbilicated papules are characteristically arranged in lines, circles or segments of circles in a serpiginous pattern. The individual papules may remain small or may enlarge slightly to assume a crateriform appearance with an elevated edge and a central plug, or further to leave an area of atrophic skin surrounded by smaller papules, each with a horny plug. The rings may reach a diameter of 15–20 cm but are usually smaller. The back and sides of the neck are most commonly affected, but the lesions may also occur on the cheeks or on the arms or thighs, and are sometimes bilaterally symmetrical. They may persist for several years but eventually involute spontaneously to leave reticulate atrophic scars. Biopsy scars readily become keloidal.

Diagnosis. The annular or linear arrangements of the papules and their distribution suggest the diagnosis, which is confirmed by the characteristic histology. Conditions which may cause confusion include porokeratosis of Mibelli, reactive perforating collagenosis and perforating granuloma annulare.

Treatment. Careful removal of the nodules with a curette under local anaesthesia may give a reasonable cosmetic result. Freezing has been recommended [9, 14]. Excision should be avoided, and dermabrasion may make the condition worse [11].

REFERENCES

1 AYALA F. & DONOFRIO P. (1983) *Dermatologica* **166**, 32.
2 BOVENMYER D.A. (1976) *Arch Dermatol* **102**, 313.
3 CATTERALL M.D. & PADLEY N.R. (1979) *Clin Exp Dermatol* **4**, 119.
4 COHEN A.S. & HASHIMOTO K. (1960) *J Invest Dermatol* **35**, 15.
5 GONCALVES A.P., et al (1963) *Dermatologica* **129**, 232.
6 HASHIMOTO K. (1960) *J Invest Dermatol* **35**, 7.
7 KIRSCH N. & HUKILL P.B. (1977) *Arch Dermatol* **113**, 630.
8 KORTING G.W. (1966) *Arch Klin Exp Dermatol* **224**, 437.
9 MEHREGAN A.H. (1968) *Arch Dermatol* **97**, 381.
10 MEVES C. & VOGEL A. (1972) *Dermatologica* **145**, 218.
11 PATTERSON J.W. (1984) *J Am Acad Dermatol* **10**, 561.
12 REED W.B. & PIDGEON J.W. (1964) *Arch Dermatol* **89**, 342.
13 RELIAS A., et al (1968) *Ann Dermatol Syphiligr* **95**, 491.
14 WHYTE H.J. & WINKELMANN R.K. (1960) *J Invest Dermatol* **35**, 113.

JUVENILE HYALINE FIBROMATOSIS
SYN. SYSTEMIC HYALINOSIS

Definition. This is a disorder of glycosaminoglycan synthesis which is characterized clinically by skin papules or tumours, gingival enlargement, osteolytic lesions and joint contractures, and histologically by deposition of amorphous hyaline material.

Aetiology. The cause is unknown, but increased chondroitin synthesis has been demonstrated in skin fibroblasts cultured from the tumour tissue [4]. The disease is very rare and occurs sporadically, but it has occurred in siblings [1, 5].

Pathology [3, 5]. The skin lesions contain 'chondroid' cells embedded in amorphous eosinophilic ground substance in the dermis. This hyaline material which probably consists of chondroitin is produced by the chondroid cells, which contain intracytoplasmic granules. The dermal collagen is decreased and the collagen fibrils are fewer and thinner than in normal skin. The hyaline material may also be present in the muscles and bones.

Clinical features [2, 5, 6]. Skin lesions are present at birth or develop in early childhood. There may be small pearly papules or nodules, particularly on the face or neck. Large subcutaneous tumours may also occur, particularly on the scalp. These may be hard or soft, fixed or mobile, and they may ulcerate. Gingival hypertrophy is commonly present, and flexion contractures of the fingers, elbows, hips and knees may develop. Osteolytic lesions can occur in the skull, long bones or phalanges. The musculature is poorly developed. The condition persists into adult life and the joint contractures are disabling.

Treatment. This is unsatisfactory. The tumours do not respond to radiotherapy, and they may recur after excision. Joint contractures may respond to intralesional steroid injections in the early stages

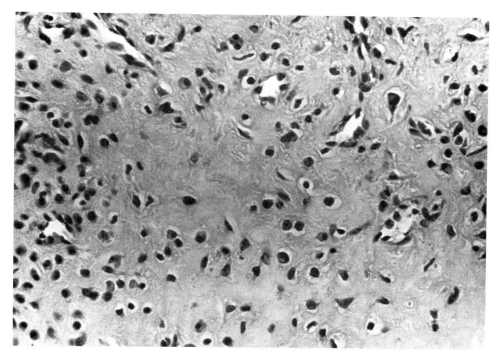

FIG. 49.33. Juvenile hyaline fibromatosis. Gingival biopsy, showing 'chondroid' cells embedded in hyaline material. (Dr P. Holt.)

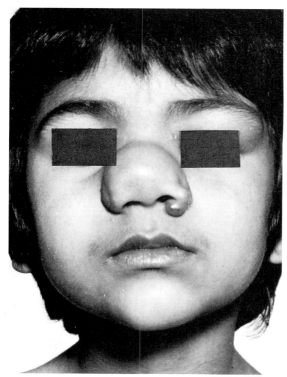

FIG. 49.34. Juvenile fibromatosis showing the bulbous deformity of the nose, a pearly papule arising from the rim of the nostril, and hyaline deposition in the left supra-orbital ridge (Dr P. Holt).

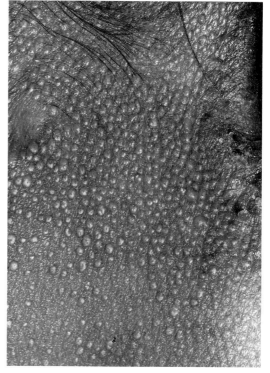

FIG. 49.35. Juvenile hyaline fibromatosis, showing multiple papules over the mastoid region (Dr P. Holt).

[6], and they may also respond to systemic steroids and physiotherapy.

REFERENCES

1 DRESCHER E., *et al* (1967) *J Pediatr Surg* **2**, 427.
2 FINLAY A.Y., *et al* (1983) *Br J Dermatol* **108**, 609.
3 ISHIKAWA, *et al* (1979) *Arch Dermatol Res* **265**, 195.
4 IWATA S., *et al* (1980) *Arch Dermatol Res* **267**, 115.
5 KITANO Y., *et al* (1972) *Arch Dermatol* **106**, 877.
6 KITANO Y. (1976) *Arch Dermatol* **112**, 86.

STIFF SKIN SYNDROME [1, 2]

This is a rare familial syndrome characterized by the development of localized areas of stony hard skin at birth or in early infancy accompanied by limited joint mobility and mild hypertrichosis. Skin biopsy shows an increased deposition of mucopolysaccharides in the dermis, but there is no increase in the urinary excretion of mucopolysaccharides and the patients do not show the other features of the congenital mucopolysaccharidoses (p. 2299).

The skin changes resemble those of scleroedema of Buschke but are distinguished by their early onset. The condition must also be distinguished from sclerema neonatorum, but this is a disorder of subcutaneous fat rather than the skin. The cases previously described as 'hereditary contractures with sclerodermatoid changes of the skin' were probably examples of the stiff skin syndrome [2].

REFERENCES

1 ESTERLY N.B. & McKUSICK V.A. (1971) *Pediatrics* **47**, 360.
2 PICHLER E. (1968) *Z Kinderheilk* **104**, 349.

LEPRECHAUNISM
SYN. DONOHUE'S SYNDROME

Definition. Leprechaunism is a rare and poorly defined syndrome characterized by severe intra-uterine and postnatal growth retardation, decreased subcutaneous tissue and muscle mass, and a characteristic facies [1, 4]. Tissue resistance to insulin appears to be an important feature, since hyperinsulinaemia and pancreatic β-cell hyperplasia are frequently present [4, 5].

Aetiology. The condition seems to be inherited, and familial cases have been reported [1]. There is some evidence that there is an intrinsic defect in the insulin receptor which results in a defective interaction between the insulin receptor and the affinity regulator [7]. The fibroblasts have a prolonged doubling time *in vitro*, and they respond poorly to the metabolic actions of insulin. They also respond poorly to the actions of several other growth factors, such as epidermal growth factor, and this suggests that there may be a defect at the post-receptor level which involves a pathway common to the action of several peptides [4].

Pathology [6]. In the skin, the elastic and collagen fibres are few and fragmented. On the extremities the horny layer is markedly thickened. The muscles show a proliferation of abnormal connective tissue. In some cases the ovaries are large and cystic, and there is β-cell hyperplasia of the pancreatic islets.

Clinical features [1, 2, 3, 6, 8]. The child is abnormal at birth with low birth weight. The nose is broad, the ears low set and large, the eyes widely spaced. There is hypertrichosis of the forehead and cheeks. The skin appears too large for the body and is loosely folded at the flexures and may be corrugated with gyrate folds on the hands and feet, which may be disproportionately large. Muscle wasting, often progressive, is usually present. The breasts and the penis or clitoris may be slightly hypertrophic. The bone age is retarded and there may be metaphyseal and epiphyseal dystrophy.

Growth is generally retarded, the nutritional status remains poor and susceptibility to infection is high. Early death is usual.

Diagnosis. The cutaneous changes could be confused with cutis laxa (p. 1834) but in leprechaunism the skin, although folded, is thickened and not lax. The diagnosis is confirmed by the associated features, and the finding of raised plasma insulin levels.

REFERENCES

1 DONOHUE W.L. & UCHIDA I. (1954) *J Pediatr* **45**, 505.
2 HARTDEGEN R.G., *et al* (1975) *Br J Dermatol* **93**, 587.
3 KALOUSTIAN V.M., *et al* (1971) *Am J Dis Child* **122**, 442.
4 KAPLOWITZ P.B. & D'ERCOLE (1982) *J Clin Endocrinol Metab* **55**, 741.
5 KOBAYISHI M., *et al* (1978) *Proc Natl Acad Sci USA* **75**, 3469.
6 PATTERSON J.H. & WATKINS W.L. (1962) *J Pediatr* **60**, 730.
7 TAYLOR S.I., *et al* (1982) *J Clin Endocrinol Metab* **55**, 1108.
8 TSUJINO G. & YOSHINAGA T. (1975) *Z Kinderheilk* **118**, 347.

MYXOID CYSTS

Definition and nomenclature. The myxoid cyst is a circumscribed mass of pathologically altered connective tissue, developing in the region of the finger joints. It has often been inappropriately described as a synovial cyst or a periungual ganglion.

Aetiology and pathogenesis [3]. The proliferation of fibroblasts in the corium is followed by increased production of hyaluronic acid and decreased or absent collagen formation. Hyaluronic acid accumulates and displaces the existing collagen fibres.

A convincing history of preceding trauma cannot always be elicited, but the sites involved are much exposed to friction and to minor injuries. There is nothing to suggest that the lesions are derived from the joints or tendon sheaths.

Women are affected more often than men. Most cases occur between the ages of 40 and 65, but onset in adolescence or old age is recorded.

Pathology. In the upper corium, and to a lesser extent in the mid-corium, is a localized or poorly

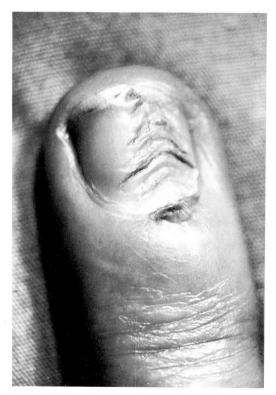

Fig. 49.36. Myxoid cyst producing nail dystrophy (Bristol Royal Infirmary).

marginated area in which spindle-shaped or stellate fibroblasts are scattered through an amorphous myxomatous matrix. There may be small or large cystic cavities. There are usually no inflammatory changes. The epidermis tends to be thin, though hyperkeratotic, occasionally with inspissated mucus in the keratinous lamellae.

Clinical features [1, 2, 4]. A myxoid cyst is a soft or rubbery nodule, skin-coloured or translucent, smooth or slightly warty, and from 3 to 15 mm in diameter. The nodule tends rapidly to reach its maximum size and then to fluctuate in size over short periods. It may burst to discharge thick mucoid material. The majority occur on the fingers and toes, especially on the terminal phalanges. When a cyst impinges on the nail matrix a deep longitudinal furrow may be formed in the nail. Most lesions are solitary, but two or more are sometimes present.

The treatment is largely cosmetic, but pain or tenderness are sometimes intermittently troublesome. Most lesions persist indefinitely, but spontaneous cure is possible.

Treatment. The recurrence rate after excision is high. Infiltration with triamcinolone should be tried [3]; it is often but not invariably effective. Flurandrenolone tape may be helpful [5]. Good results have also been obtained with liquid nitrogen spray cryosurgery [2].

REFERENCES

1 Bourns H.K. & Sanerkin N.G. (1963) *Br J Surg* **50**, 860.
2 Dawber R.P.R. (1983) *Clin Exp Dermatol* **8**, 153.
3 Johnson W.C., *et al* (1965) *JAMA* **191**, 15.
4 Newmayer W.L., *et al* (1974) *Plast Reconstr Surg* **53**, 313.
5 Ronchese F. (1974) *RI Med J* **57**, 154.

Focal mucinosis. This term has been introduced to describe a lesion essentially similar to a myxoid cyst in its pathogenesis and histology [1]. A flesh-coloured or white papule or nodule up to 2 cm in diameter, solitary and asymptomatic, develops on the face, neck, trunk or limbs and tends to persist.

If treatment is required excision is satisfactory, since recurrence is unusual.

A plaque-like form of cutaneous mucinosis may occur in reticular erythematous mucinosis (p. 2299) [2].

REFERENCES

1 JOHNSON W.C. & HELWIG E.B. (1966) *Arch Dermatol* 93, 13.
2 QUIMBY S.R. & PERRY M.O. (1982) *J Am Acad Dermatol* 6, 856.

RELAPSING POLYCHONDRITIS
SYN. ATROPHIC POLYCHONDRITIS;
SYSTEMIC CHONDROMALACIA;
VON MEYENBURG'S DISEASE

Definition. In this non-infective condition focal inflammatory destruction of cartilage is accompanied by fibroblastic regeneration. The condition characteristically affects the pinna and nose, but the eye may also be inflamed even though it normally contains no cartilage.

Aetiology. Relapsing polychondritis has been regarded as rare, but recent reports suggest that it is not so uncommon but is easily overlooked. The cause is unknown, but the association with rheumatoid arthritis, lupus erythematosus, vasculitis and Hashimoto's disease suggests that autoimmune mechanisms may be concerned [1, 14]. Antibodies to type II collagen have been detected in the serum in acute polychondritis [5, 7] and granular deposits of IgG, IgA, IgM and C_3 at fibrochondral junctions have indicated a possible role of immune complex deposits [20, 24]. The intravenous injection of papain into rabbits produces loss of cartilage rigidity, manifested by floppy ears [13], and it has been suggested that local protease activity may play some part in causing relapsing polychondritis [8].

Pathology [9, 11]. Areas of damaged cartilage, which have lost the normal basophilic staining, are separated by areas of predominantly lymphocytic infiltration. Later the fragments of cartilage are surrounded and replaced by abundant granulation tissue and even nascent cartilage.

Clinical features [1, 3, 4, 6, 12, 17, 18, 19, 22]. The condition affects both sexes equally and usually begins between the ages of 30 and 50. Chondritis ultimately involves three or more sites in most patients but may be limited to one or two for long periods. The following tissues may be involved in decreasing order of frequency: auricular, joint, nasal, ocular, respiratory tract, heart valves and skin [4]. During the acute stage the affected area is swollen, red and tender, and may be mistaken for cellulitis. Sparing of the ear lobe is a useful differentiating sign. Serous otitis media can occur, and there may be loss of hearing even in the absence of chondritis [1, 15]. Involvement of the nasal cartilage leads to obstruction and later to a saddle nose deformity. Cutaneous and systemic vasculitis, superficial thrombophlebitis and toxic erythema have been described [10, 12, 14, 21].

The joint changes, usually affecting the smaller peripheral joints, may simulate rheumatoid arthritis. Involvement of the larynx, trachea or bronchi produces respiratory embarrassment and recurrent infection. Permanent tracheostomy may be required [11, 15]. An association with granulomatous lung disease has also been described [16]. Ocular abnormalities are found in some cases—episcleritis, conjunctivititis and iritis or more rarely keratoconjunctivitis sicca or chorioretinitis. Proptosis occurs in 3% of cases [2, 12]. Involvement of the heart valves may cause serious complications [12].

The course of the disease is extremely variable. Relapses are the rule, but they vary in frequency and severity. Some cases continue to relapse for over 20 yr, but others become inactive within a short period. Deformity of the ears and nose is frequent, but in general the disease is a source of discomfort and disfigurement rather than a threat to life. The erythrocyte sedimentation rate is usually raised and anaemia is frequent. The rheumatoid factor is often positive. Leukocytosis is inconstant, but eosinophilia is found in 40% of cases. LE cells may be present. The characteristic biochemical finding is the increased urinary excretion of acid mucopolysaccharides during each relapse.

Radiological abnormalities are not pathognomonic, but evidence of extensive destruction of joint cartilage without changes in adjacent bone is suggestive. In some cases the changes are indistinguishable from rhematoid arthritis.

Diagnosis. Polychondritis may present to the dermatologist as 'chronic otitis externa with cellulitis of the pinna'. The diagnosis is established by biopsy, or by other associated changes, and by the examination of urine for acid mucopolysaccharides. Wegener's granulomatosis and lethal midline granuloma can produce a similar histology, but in these two conditions the involvement is more purely destructive.

Treatment. The progression of the acute relapse can be controlled with corticosteroids. An initial daily dose of 30 mg prednisone can be gradually reduced and finally discontinued as remission develops [23]. Remissions may also be induced with indomethocin [17] or dapsone [20].

REFERENCES

1 ARKIN C.R. & MASI A.T. (1975) *Semin Arthritis Rheum* 5, 41.
2 CROVATO F., *et al* (1980) *Arch Dermatol* 116, 383.
3 DAVIS R. & KELSALL A.R. (1960) *Ann Rheum Dis* 20, 189.
4 DOLAN D.L., *et al* (1966) *Am J Med* 41, 285.
5 EBRINGER R., *et al* (1981) *Am Rherum Dis* 40, 473.
6 FEINERMAN L.K., *et al* (1970) *Dermatologica* 140, 369.
7 FOIDART J.M., *et al* (1978) *N Engl J Med* 299, 1203.
8 GANGE R.W. (1976) *Clin Exp Dermatol* 1, 261.
9 HARWOOD T.R. (1958) *AMA Arch Pathol* 65, 81.
10 HUGHES R.A.C., *et al* (1972) *Q J Med* 41, 363.
11 KAYE R.L. & SONES D.A. (1964) *Ann Intern Med* 60, 653.
12 McADAM L.P., *et al* (1976) *Medicine* 55, 193.
13 McCLUSKEY R.T., *et al* (1958) *J Exp Med* 108, 371.
14 MEYRICK-THOMAS R.H., *et al* (1982) *Clin Exp Dermatol* 7, 519.
15 MOLONEY J.R. (1978) *J Laryngol Otol* 92, 9.
16 NIELD G.H., *et al* (1978) *Br Med J* i, 743.
17 NITZSCHNER H., *et al* (1970) *Dermatol Wochenschr* 157, 789.
18 OWEN D.S., *et al* (1970) *Arthritis Rheum* 13, 877.
19 PEARSON C.M. (1960) *N Engl J Med* 263, 1.
20 RIDGEWAY H.B., *et al* (1979) *Arch Dermatol* 114, 43.
21 ROWELL N.R. & COTTERILL J.A. (1973) *Br J Dermatol* 88, 387.
22 THURSTON C.S. & CURTIS A.C. (1966) *Arch Dermatol* 93, 664.
23 TRENTHAM D.E. & GOODMAN M.L. (1982) *N Engl J Med* 307, 1631.
24 VALENZUELA R. (1980) *Hum Pathol* 11, 19.

CHAPTER 50

The Subcutaneous Fat

J.L. BURTON & W.J. CUNLIFFE

The subcutaneous fat (syn. subcutis) occurs almost universally over the body surface between the skin and the deep fascia, but it is absent from the eyelids and the male genitalia. It acts as an insulating layer and a mechanical cushion, and it also acts as a store of readily available energy. The subcutaneous fat varies in thickness with the race, age, sex, endocrine and nutritional status of the individual.

Embryology. The first fat-containing cell, the lipoblast, appears in the mesenchyme around the 14th week of fetal life [12]. This cell matures to form the large unilocular lipocyte, the characteristic cell of adult fat. The primitive mesenchymal cell which forms the lipoblast is also capable of maturing to form a fibrocyte, a myocyte, a chondrocyte or an osteoblast. The distinction between adipocytes and fibroblasts is not always clear, and 'pre-adipocytes' which do not contain enough fat to be counted as fat cells by standard techniques have been described [2].

Brown fat is a special type of granular fat which differs from white fat in its distribution, histology and function. It is multilocular and is metabolically very active, with many mitochondria, so that it is capable of producing heat. It is most prominent in the neck and upper thorax of the fetus, and it may be homologous to the hibernating gland fat found in some animals [1]. Brown fat is now known to persist into adult life [5] and it may have a role in preventing obesity [7]. Warm patches develop in the skin 1 hour after taking ephedrine orally, and these warm patches may indicate the site of thermogenic brown fat.

Histology. The fat cells (lipocytes) form a specialized part of the reticulo-endothelial system [11] which is capable of fat synthesis as well as fat storage. The mature fat cell has a characteristic signet ring appearance due to the fact that the flat oval nucleus is displaced to the side by a single large intracellular vacuole which contains fat. Groups of lipocytes are arranged in lobules, which are separated by inter-lobular septa composed of collagen and reticulin fibres. Fat tissue has an abundant blood supply, each individual lobule being supplied by an arteriole which runs along the septa, before breaking up to form capillaries which come into close apposition with the individual fat cells. The subcutaneous fat also contains a rich lymphatic plexus which receives vessels from the dermis. These lymph vessels traverse the subcutaneous layer parallel to the skin surface for some distance before eventually penetrating the deep fascia and draining into the regional lymph nodes.

The fat tissue and the fat organ. The fat tissue is composed of lobules of fat cells with their supporting connective tissue, blood and lymph vessels and reticulo-endothelial cells. In addition to forming subcutaneous fat, fat tissue occurs in the mediastinal and retroperitoneal tissues, the mesentery and the bone marrow. This tissue, though it is widely scattered throughout the body, forms a true organ as regards both structure and function [8]. The thickest subcutaneous fat deposits are found over large muscles such as the gluteal muscles, and the blood supply in these areas comes mainly from the underlying muscle.

Physiology [6, 11]. Subcutaneous fat acts as an insulator to protect the body core from changes in environmental temperature, but in addition the fat tissue is the site of intense metabolic activity and it can produce heat. The synthesis and catabolism of fat in the subcutaneous depot depends on many factors, including nourishment, endocrine and nervous activity. Hormones which may affect the metabolism of fat cells include insulin, cortisol, noradrenaline, and several pituitary hormones, including somatotrophin, adrenocorticotrophin, thyrotrophin and lipotrophin [4, 9].

The fats contained within the lipocytes are predominantly triglycerides, especially those of palmitic and stearic acids and the unsaturated oleic acid. All the fatty acids have an even number of carbon

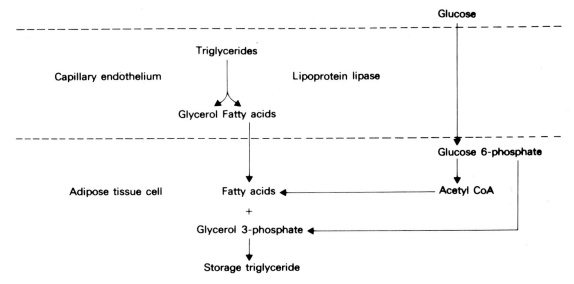

FIG. 50.1. The metabolic pathways related to adipose cells.

atoms, predominantly C_{16} and C_{18} with a few C_{14} and C_{12}. Adipose tissue contains 10–30% of water with a small proportion of lipochromes, and less than 2% cholesterol. Fat-soluble substances are also present in varying amounts. These include fat-soluble vitamins and traces of chlorinated hydrocarbons (aldrin, dieldrin, etc.) ingested with the diet. Adipose tissue *in vitro* has a metabolic rate similar to that of kidney tissue and about half that of liver. About half the triglyceride in the adipose tissue of rats and mice is catabolized and reconstituted in the course of a week or so. The turnover rate has not been measured in man, but it is likely to be very high because there is a high rate of turnover of non-esterified fatty acids (NEFA) in the plasma [3].

The fat for storage enters the lipocyte as fatty acids which combine with coenzyme A, using the energy of ATP, to form the corresponding acyl coenzyme A compounds. Some of these are then oxidized to provide energy for the regeneration of ATP, but most are converted to triglyceride by combination with glycerol 3-phosphate derived from glucose. Figure 50.1 shows the metabolic pathways related to adipose cells. When triglyceride is to be oxidized in the body for the provision of energy, it is converted to non-esterified fatty acids (NEFA) and conveyed in the blood to tissues such as liver and muscle, in which fatty acid oxidation readily takes place. In both tissues the essential part of the process consists of the oxidation in the mitochondria of the long chain fatty acids. The glycerol of the triglyceride molecule reacts with ATP to form glycerol phosphate which is oxidized to glyceraldehyde 3-

phosphate. This in turn may either be converted to glycogen by reversal of glycolysis or it may be converted to pyruvate. Skeletal muscle readily oxidizes fatty acids but glucose, if available, is preferentially used. In cardiac muscle fatty acids are a major source of energy.

REFERENCES

1 AHERNE W. & HULL D. (1964) *Proc R Soc Med* **57**, 1172.
2 ASHWELL (1978) *Int J Obesity* **2**, 69.
3 BELL G.H., *et al* (1976) *Textbook of Physiology and Biochemistry.* Edinburgh, Churchill Livingstone.
4 ENGEL F.L. (1960) *Vitamins Hormones* **19**, 189.
5 HEATON J.M. (1972) *J Anatomy* **112**, 35.
6 JEANRENAUD B. (1963) *Helv Med Acta* **30**, 1.
7 JUNG R.T., *et al* (1979) *Nature* **279**, 322.
8 KINSELL L.W. (1962) *Adipose Tissue as an Organ.* Springfield, Thomas.
9 LI C.H. (1964) *Nature* **201**, 924.
10 LI C.H., *et al* (1966) *Proc Sixth Pan Am Congr Endocrinol.* Ed. Gual C. Amsterdam, Excerpta Medica, p. 349.
11 RENOLD A.E. & CAHILL G.F. (1965) Adipose Tissue. In *Handbook of Physiology, Section 5.* Edinburgh, Livingstone.
12 WASSERMAN F. (1964) In *Fat as a Tissue.* Ed. Rodahl K. London, McGraw-Hill, p. 22.

OBESITY

Obesity is a condition in which there is excessive fat in the body. The most accurate method of measuring total body fat is to determine the average density of the body, using whole body plethysmography

[6, 7] but this method is not suitable for clinical practice. Measurement of skin fold thickness with calipers provides a more convenient method [23], but it must be remembered that the distribution of fat between subcutaneous and deep sites varies in different ethnic groups [12].

For epidemiological and clinical purposes obesity is usually defined in terms of excess weight. The ratio W/H^2, where W is body weight (in kg) and H is height (in m), gives a useful measure of weight-for-height. Actuarial data suggests that the range associated with greatest longevity is from about 19 to 24 for women and 20–25 for men [3]. A nomogram can be used to facilitate this calculation [3].

Aetiology. The cause of obesity remains uncertain but various possibilities have been suggested [6].

1. *Adipocytes.* Obese subjects may have an increased number of fat cells, or there may be metabolic differences between the fat cells of lean and obese subjects, even when fat cell size and diet are controlled [5]. Some authors maintain that hypercellular obesity, with an increased number of fat cells, has a worse prognosis than hypertrophic obesity, in which the fat content of each cell is increased [2].

2. *Genetic factors.* It is true that fat parents tend to have fat children, but the link is not necessarily genetic since fat dogs tend to have fat owners [18].

3. *Psychological factors.* The idea that food intake is solely determined by two centres in the hypothalamus is outmoded. It now seems that obese people are particularly susceptible to 'external' (i.e. non-nutritive) stimuli to eat, and the sensation of satiety is probably a learned response [6].

4. *Dietary fibre.* Refined carbohydrates have a high energy content relative to their bulk, and lack of dietary fibre might thus lead to obesity due to the increased energy intake [8].

It now remains uncertain how much a fibre-rich diet would contribute to the reduction of obesity [22].

5. *Exercise.* Obesity develops because the energy intake exceeds the energy expenditure. The level of physical activity is clearly relevant to a person's energy balance, but the resting metabolic rate is the main determinant of total energy expenditure, even in a very active man.

6. *Thermogenesis.* Contrary to what one would predict, obese subjects generally have a *higher* absolute resting metabolic rate than otherwise similar people of normal weight [10], but in human beings who are obese or prone to easy weight gain, the thermogenic responses to food and sympathetic drugs are subnormal [11, 13, 19].

7. *Virally-induced obesity.* After infection with canine distemper virus, mice may become greatly obese over the subsequent 5 months, and the catecholamine levels are depressed in the forebrain of the obese mice [16]. Catecholamine pathways are thought to regulate food intake and energy expenditure [17, 20].

Clinical features. Obesity predisposes to many systemic diseases, especially diabetes mellitus, ischaemic heart disease and hypertension, and fat people tend to die younger than their contemporaries of normal weight [10, 15]. In addition very obese patients pose difficult problems for surgeons and anaesthetists, and they appear to be more liable to wound infection and thromboembolism [21]. Obesity may also be a social and psychological handicap.

There are also dermatological complications. Increased friction and sweating between the skin folds encourage intertrigo and superadded secondary candidal or bacterial infection. Relative immobility and increased pressure in the veins may add to the risk of venous eczema and leg ulcers. Such pressure may also occasionally produce obstruction to the lymphatic system resulting in lymphoedema. These changes, along with the venous hypertension and the obesity itself, may also produce pachydermatous changes in the skin.

Treatment. The obesity must be treated. Recent advances in the management of obesity have been reviewed by Garrow [6]. For severe obesity the operation of jejuno-ileal bypass has been used, and though this causes satisfactory loss of weight, there is considerable long-term morbidity [1]. Some patients develop inflammatory skin lesions after the operation and these lesions may be associated with polyarthritis and fever (see p. 2356) [14].

REFERENCES

1 ALPERS D.H. (1983) *N Engl J Med* **308**, 1026.
2 BJORNTORP P. & SJOSTROM L. (1979) *Int J Obesity* **3**, 181.
3 BRAY G.A. (1978) *Int J Obesity* **2**, 99.
4 BRAY G.A. (1979) *Int J Obesity* **3**, 363.
5 BRAY G.A., *et al* (1977) *Metabolism* **26**, 739.
6 GARROW J.S. (1981) In *Recent Advances in Medicine*. Ed Dawson A.M. *et al*, vol. no. **18**. Edinburgh, Churchill Livingstone, p. 75.

7 GARROW J.S. *et al* (1979) *Br J Nutr* **42**, 173.
8 HEATON K.W. (1973) *Lancet* ii, 1418.
9 JAMES W.P.T. (1976) *Report on Obesity: A Report of the D.H.S.S.: M.R.C. Study Group.* London, HMSO.
10 JAMES W.P.T. *et al* (1978) *Lancet* i, 1122.
11 JEQUIER E., *et al* (1978) *Proc Nutr Soc* **37**, 45.
12 JONES P.R.M. *et al* (1976) In *Selected Topics in Environmental Biology.* Eds. Bhatia B., *et al.* New Delhi, Interprint Publications.
13 JUNG R.T., *et al* (1979) *Nature* **279**, 322.
14 KENNEDY C. (1981) *Br J Dermatol* **105**, 425.
15 LEVINSON M.I. (1977) *Preventive Med* **6**, 172.
16 LYONS M.J., *et al* (1982) *Science* **216**, 82.
17 MARSHALL J.F. (1977) *Adv Obesity Res* **2**, 6.
18 MASON E. (1970) *Vet Rec* **86**, 612.
19 MORGAN J. (1982) *Br J Nutr* **47**, 21.
20 ROTHWELL N.J. & STOCK M.J. (1981) *Ann Rev Nutr* **1**, 235.
21 STRAUSS R.J. & WISE I. (1978) *Surg Gynaecol Obstet* **146**, 286.
22 VAN ITALLIE T.B. (1978) *Am J Clin Nutr* **31** (Suppl. 10), S43.
23 WOMERSLEY J. & DURNIN J.V.G.A. (1977) *Br J Nutr* **38**, 271.

GENERAL PATHOLOGY OF ADIPOSE TISSUE

The pathological processes affecting the subcutaneous fat are in many respects similar to those involving the overlying dermis. The subcutis may be involved by simple spread from dermal disease, as part of a widespread disease affecting much of the fat organ, or as a strictly localized disease of the subcutaneous tissue.

In many instances of fat-cell damage, healing takes place quite uneventfully by fibrosis. In a proportion, however, once the fat cell is damaged, lipid is liberated which undergoes hydrolysis into glycerol and fatty acids. An inflammatory reaction may follow, even provoking a foreign body granuloma.

After the phase of reaction to the products of fat-cell disintegration there is a period of reconstitution, the ease of repair depending on the extent of the initial cell damage and the efficiency of the local circulation. Extensive fibrosis is inevitable if there is much loss of tissue. In certain cases a chain reaction is set up, fat-cell necrosis provoking a peripheral inflammatory reaction which leads to peripheral fat-cell necrosis and the spread of the lesion centrifugally. In other instances, fat-cell necrosis induces an excessive fibrosis which results in the formation of subcutaneous fibrotic nodules.

The diverse pathological changes which occur in the fat and are of importance to the dermatologist have been reviewed by several authors [1–5], but disorders of the subcutis remain a difficult problem for the histopathologist. A punch biopsy is inadequate, and a large, deep, scalpel biopsy is required.

REFERENCES

1 ELLIOTT R.I.K. (1964) In *Progress in the Biological Sciences in Relation to Dermatology.* Eds Rook A. & Champion R.H. Cambridge University Press, Vol. 2, p. 175.
2 FORSTROM L. & WINKELMANN R.K. (1977) *Arch Dermatol* **113**, 909.
3 LEVER W.F. & SCHAUMBERG-LEVER (1983) *Histopathology of the Skin.* 6th ed. Lippincott, Philadelphia, pp. 245–258.
4 MICHELSON H.E. (1957) *Arch Dermatol* **75**, 633.
5 REED R.J., *et al* (1973) *Human Pathol* **4**, 219.

INFLAMMATORY DISORDERS OF THE SUBCUTANEOUS FAT

Nodular panniculitis. This is a descriptive term which refers to inflammatory nodules in the subcutaneous fat (Figs 50.2 and 50.3). They may be single or multiple, localized or generalized, and they may vary in size from a few millimetres to several centimetres in diameter. They are generally firm, red and tender, but occasionally they become soft and may liquefy, or even ulcerate. They may resolve with or without scarring.

The definitive diagnosis is often difficult, since there are many causes and in many patients the cause cannot be found. The inflammatory process may begin in the fat lobule or in the interlobular septa and it has been traditional to separate 'septal' panniculitis, usually associated with erythema nodosum, from 'lobular' panniculitis, due to other causes. Even this simple classification is unsatisfactory, since lobular panniculitis can be a feature of erythema nodosum [3]. Panniculitis usually involves vessels of various sizes so that the distinction between the various forms of vasculitis and panniculitis is also sometimes blurred [3] (Fig 50.4). The classification of these disorders will probably remain unsatisfactory until our knowledge of their aetiology and pathogenesis improves. Not every case can be assigned to a definite entity, and some cases have to be called non-specific panniculitis [2]. The pathology of panniculitis has been reviewed recently by Eng and Aronson [1].

The following classification may be useful in the investigation of an individual case of nodular panniculitis:

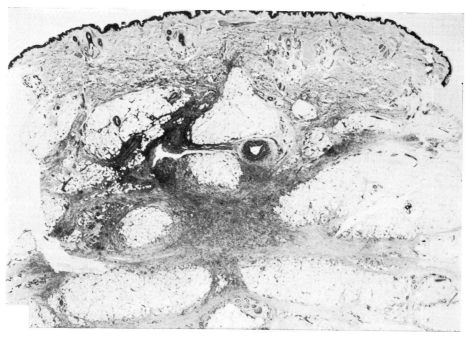

FIG. 50.2. Nodular panniculitis. H & E, × 8.

1. *Lipolytic enzyme release*
   (i) Enzyme panniculitis with or without pancreatic disease
   (ii) Alpha$_1$-antitrypsin deficiency

2. *'Immunological' panniculitis*
   (i)   Erythema nodosum and variants
   (ii) Lupus panniculitis
   (iii) Connective tissue panniculitis

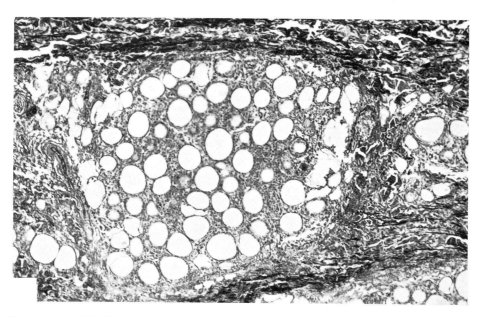

FIG. 50.3. Nodular panniculitis. Elastin stain, × 100.

3. *Cellular proliferative disease*
   (i) Lymphoma, malignant histiocytosis etc.
   (ii) Cytophagic histiocytic panniculitis
4. *Cold*
5. *Factitial*
6. *Jejuno-ileal bypass*
7. *Post-steroid panniculitis*
8. *Systemic nodular panniculitis*

REFERENCES

1 ENG A.M. & ARONSON I.K. (1984) *Semin Dermatol* **3**, 1.
2 NIEMI K.M., *et al* (1977) *Acta Derm Venereol* **57**, 145.
3 WINKELMANN R.K. & FORSTROM L. (1975) *J Invest Dermatol* **65**, 441.

1. NODULAR PANNICULITIS DUE TO LIPOLYTIC ENZYMES

(i) Pancreatic disease. Subcutaneous fat necrosis and painful nodular panniculitis may result from chronic pancreatitis or carcinoma of the pancreas, presumably due to the liberation of lipolytic enzymes into the circulation [7]. When lipase, trypsin and amylase are injected separately into fat, no lesion develops and all three enzymes are required to produce fat necrosis [6].

Panniculitis due to pancreatic disease may be associated with arthritis (especially of the ankles), pleural effusions, ascites and eosinophilia, and in patients with these systemic features the prognosis is poor [7].

The histology of the fat is pathognomonic. The necrotic fat characteristically contains 'ghost' cells with thick shadowy walls and no nuclei [4].

Cases have been recorded in which no pancreatic lesion was found even at autopsy, but increased levels of amylase and lipase activity were present in the skin and urine [3]. Subcutaneous fat necrosis of the abdominal wall secondary to leakage of pancreatic enzymes following paracentesis has also been described [5].

(ii) Deficiency of α_1-antitrypsin (AAT) inhibitor [1, 2, 8, 9]. This condition may also be associated with severe subcutaneous panniculitis, presumably secondary to the pancreatic disease which occurs in this disorder [8, 9]. Severe nodular panniculitis has been described in two brothers with marked AAT deficiency and phenotype PiZZ. In both brothers there was enhanced lymphocyte responsiveness to PHA stimulation with enhanced activation of neutrophils and monocytes [2]. Cases with moderate deficiency of AAT have been associated with the heterozygous phenotype PiMZ. It has been suggested that the deficiency of anti-proteolytic activity may enhance the panniculitis and also predispose to thrombosis. The panniculitis has a particular tendency to liquefaction of the nodules, with abscess formation and drainage [2, 9] and the lesions tend

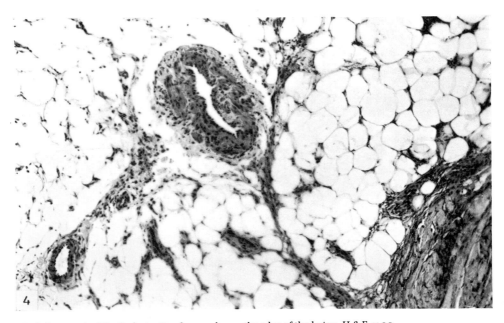

FIG. 50.4. Nodular panniculitis. Endarteritis of a vessel near the edge of the lesion. H & E, × 90.

to be induced by trauma [2, 9]. Another characteristic feature is the appearance of oedema, fragmentation and degeneration of collagen in the dermis.

REFERENCES

1 Balk E., *et al* (1982) *Neth J Med* **25**, 138.
2 Breit S.N., *et al* (1983) *Arch Dermatol* **119**, 198.
3 Forstrom L. & Winkelmann R.K. (1975) *Arch Dermatol* **111**, 497.
4 Hughes P.S.H., *et al* (1975) *Arch Dermatol* **111**, 506.
5 Levine N. & Lazarus G.S. (1976) *Arch Dermatol* **112**, 993.
6 Pannabokké R.G. (1958) *J Pathol Bacteriol* **75**, 319.
7 Potts D.E., *et al* (1975) *Am J Med* **58**, 417.
8 Rubinstein H.M., *et al* (1977) *Ann Intern Med* **86**, 742.
9 Warter J., *et al* (1972) *Ann Méd Interne* **123**, 877.

2. 'IMMUNOLOGICAL PANNICULITIS'

(i) **Erythema nodosum and variants.** This condition is described on p. 1156. Erythema nodosum may be associated with a variable degree of inflammation in the subcutaneous tissue, including phlebitis, acute panniculitis, lymphocytic infiltration and chronic granulomata of the fat lobules or septa [8]. It is now believed that *subacute nodular migratory panniculitis* (syn. erythema nodosum migrans) [1, 7] and *the chronic and granulomatous* forms of erythema nodosum are variants of the same pathological progress resulting from a hypersensitivity reaction to a variety of antigens [2, 3].

Some forms of nodular vasculitis, including erythema induratum, may also be associated with panniculitis.

The Rothman–Makai syndrome [4] (syn. subcutaneous lipogranulomatosis), characterized by multiple lipogranulomatous nodules with no systemic disturbance, probably does not exist as a separate nosological entity [5]. Some cases are probably minor variants of other conditions such as deep erythema nodosum, and those which cannot be classified are better referred to as non-specific panniculitis [6].

REFERENCES

1 Bafverstadt B. (1954) *Acta Derm Venereol* **34**, 181.
2 Forstrom L. & Winkelmann R.K. (1975) *Arch Dermatol* **111**, 335.
3 Hannuksela M. (1971) *Ann Clin Res* **3**, (Supp. 7), 1.
4 Laymon C.W. & Peterson W.C. (1964) *Arch Dermatol* **90**, 288.
5 Matukas T. & Reisner R.M. (1972) *Arch Dermatol* **105**, 287.
6 Niemi K.M., *et al* (1977) *Acta Derm Venereol* **57**, 145.
7 Vilanova X. & Piñol Aguadé (1959) *Br J Dermatol* **71**, 45.

8 Winkelmann R.K. & Forstrom L. (1975) *J Invest Dermatol* **65**, 441.

(ii) **Lupus panniculitis** (syn. LE profundus). About 2% of patients with systemic lupus erythematosus develop panniculitis, either as a presenting feature, or during the course of the disease [1, 4, 5]. The condition is described on p. 1316 and 1295.

The diagnosis may be suggested histologically by the presence of subcutaneous lymphoid follicles with germinal centres. These occur in about 25% of cases of lupus panniculitis, whereas they are infrequent in other forms of panniculitis [2]. Hyaline degeneration of the fat and blood vessels are also distinctive features [3]. Panniculitis can also occur in other connective-tissue disorders, such as systemic sclerosis and dermatomyositis [6].

REFERENCES

1 Diaz-Jouanen E., *et al* (1975) *Ann Intern Med* **82**, 376.
2 Harris R.B., *et al* (1979) *Arch Dermatol* **115**, 442.
3 Sanchez N.P., *et al* (1981) *J Am Acad Dermatol* **5**, 673.
4 Tuffanelli D.L. (1971) *Arch Dermatol* **103**, 231.
5 Winkelmann R.K. (1970) *JAMA* **211**, 472.
6 Winkelmann R.K. (1983) *Arch Dermatol* **119**, 336.

(iii) **'Connective tissue' panniculitis.** Winkelmann and Padhila-Goncalves [2, 3] have described two patients with lobular lymphohistiocytic panniculitis and caseation necrosis which progressed to subcutaneous atrophy. Both patients had antibody to extractable nuclear antigen, and the disease responded to antimalarial therapy. The authors felt this condition was related to, but differed from, lupus erythematosus and morphoea. Shelley's case of long-term nodular panniculitis responsive to antimalarials may also represent this disease [1].

REFERENCES

1 Shelley W.B. (1981) *J Am Acad Dermatol* **5**, 168.
2 Winkelmann R.K. (1983) *Arch Dermatol* **119**, 336.
3 Winkelmann R.K. & Padilha-Goncalves (1980) *Arch Dermatol* **116**, 291.

3. PANNICULITIS DUE TO CELLULAR PROLIFERATIVE DISEASE

Panniculitis associated with vasculitis has been associated with systemic lymphoma, leukaemia and multiple myeloma [1] Gastric carcinoma has also been reported in association with panniculitis [3].

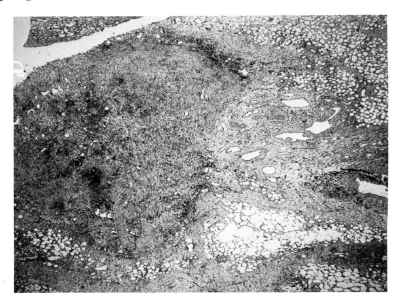

FIG. 50.5 Biopsy from a patient with a cytophagic panniculitis, showing lobular panniculitis with fat necrosis and haemorrhage (Dr Winkelmann, Mayo Clinic).

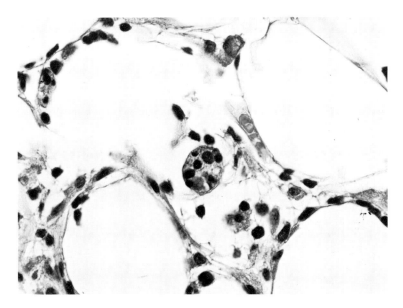

FIG. 50.6. A cytophagic histiocyte in the subcutaneous fat, showing erythrocytophagocytosis and lymphocytophagocytosis (Dr Winkelmann, Mayo Clinic).

Various histiocytic disorders may involve the subcutaneous fat, including malignant histiocytosis, histiocytosis X and a recently described disorder, cytophagic histiocytic panniculitis.

Cytophagic histiocytic panniculitis with fever and a haemorrhagic diathesis [2, 7].
Definition. Chronic visceral and cutaneous histiocytic cytophagic panniculitis which progresses to systemic histiocytosis with pancytopenia, abnormal liver function and a bleeding tendency.

Aetiology. Unknown.

Pathology. The condition involves the skin and sub-cutaneous tissues only for some years, but eventually spreads to invade the marrow, lymph nodes and reticulo-endothelial system. The affected tissues are gradually replaced by a syncytium of histiocytic cells, with associated lymphocytes and plasma cells (Fig. 50.5). The histiocytes are cytophagic, so that they become stuffed with white blood cells, red cells, nuclear fragments and platelets, and this gives them a characteristic 'bean-bag' appearance (Fig. 50.6) [2]. In the subcutis there may be lobular panniculitis and fat necrosis, together with massive hyaline necrosis, oedema and haemorrhage.

Clinical features. (Fig. 50.7). This is a rare condition which may in the past have been mistaken for systemic nodular panniculitis (Weber–Christian syndrome) [5, 6]. The condition begins with recurrent crops of red tender nodules associated with fever. After some years liver dysfunction develops,

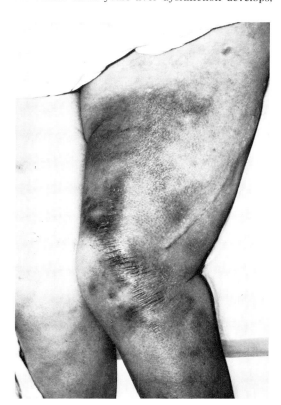

Fig. 50.7. Inflammatory plaques of cytophagic panniculitis with secondary ecchymosis (Dr Winkelmann, Mayo Clinic).

and this is associated with complex coagulation defects which are not fully understood. There may be thrombocytopenia or thrombocytosis, decreased factor VIII and fibrinogen levels and an increase in excretion of fibrin degradation products. It has been suggested that these abnormalities in coagulation may be due to a circulating proteolytic enzyme other than thrombin, which may originate from leukocytes [4].

Differential diagnosis. In its early stages the condition may be mistaken for systemic nodular panniculitis. Factitial panniculitis and erythema nodosum may be associated with bleeding into the tissues, but in these conditions coagulation is normal.

In its later stages the condition is distinguished from malignant histiocytosis by its chronic course and the benign appearance of the histiocytic infiltrate.

Treatment. The condition should be treated as a malignant histiocytosis [2] (p. 1704).

REFERENCES

1 CHRISTIANSON H.B. & FINE R.M. (1967) *South Med J* **60**, 567.
2 CROTTY C.O. & WINKELMANN R.K. (1981) *J Am Acad Dermatol* **4**, 181.
3 DOSTROVSKY A., et al (1957) *Dermatologica* **114**, 39.
4 HENRIKSSON P., et al (1975) *Scand J Haematol* **14**, 355.
5 MIYASAKI K., et al (1977) *Acta Pathol Jap* **27**, 213.
6 STEINBERG B. (1953) *Am J Pathol* **29**, 1059.
7 WINKELMANN R.K. & BOWIE E.J.W. (1980) *Arch Intern Med* **140**, 1460.

4. COLD PANNICULITIS

This is the result of cold injury to fat tissue. It is usually localized.

Clinical features. The affected areas become indurated with an ill-defined margin. The skin may be red or bluish, and the area is usually cold to the touch. The patient may complain of a cold sensation, or a dull ache. If the area is kept warm, the subcutaneous plaques slowly soften and resolve over several weeks without scarring.

Newborn infants are particularly susceptible to this condition (p. 254), as are adults with a chilblain type of circulation or paralysis.

Cold panniculitis of the thighs or buttocks may occur in skiers or horse-riders who wear inadequate clothing [1], although in this situation perniosis is more common than true panniculitis [4].

'Popsicle' panniculitis of the angle of the mouth

and the cheeks has been described in children who frequently suck ice-lollies [2, 3].

Differential diagnosis. The appearance may resemble other forms of panniculitis (including erythema induratum). It is distinguished from perniosis by the histology, since panniculitis is not a usual histological feature of perniosis [4].

Treatment. The condition resolves spontaneously if further exposure to cold is avoided. In horse-riders, tight jeans should be replaced by several layers of looser and thicker clothing. If the limb becomes thoroughly chilled, rapid rewarming should be avoided. Vasodilators are not helpful.

REFERENCES

1 BEACHAM B.E., *et al* (1980) *Arch Dermatol* **116**, 1025.
2 DUNCAN W.C., *et al* (1966) *Arch Dermatol* **94**, 722.
3 RAJKUMAR S.V., *et al* (1976) *Clin Pediatr* **15**, 619.
4 WALL J.M. & SMITH N.P. (1981) *Clin Exp Dermatol* **6**, 263.

5. FACTITIAL PANNICULITIS

This is a rare condition in which the panniculitis is self-inflicted or iatrogenic. It may be caused by injection of drugs such as morphine, pentazocine [3], meperidine [1] or by tetanus toxoid. Silicone injections (used by some patients to augment the size of the breasts or genitalia) may cause panniculitis, as may the accidental injection of various oily vehicles for therapeutic agents. Povidone, a synthetic polymer used as a dispersing or suspending agent for drugs, has also been reported to cause panniculitis associated with fever [2]. Mentally disturbed patients have been known to inject milk or faeces, which produce a severe cellulitis. Mechanical trauma, e.g. from an iron weight, can also cause fat necrosis and factitial panniculitis

The histology will depend on the substance injected, but in some cases there is a granulomatous reaction (p. 1870). The vessels are usually not involved, and in some cases birefringent crystals can be seen by polarized light [1].

Differential diagnosis. The diagnosis may be suggested by the personality of the patient, the chronic and recurrent nature of the panniculitis, and by its focal or bizarre site. In some cases there may be fever or systemic symptoms, and the condition may then be mistaken for systemic nodular panniculitis.

REFERENCES

1 FORSTROM L. & WINKELMANN R.I. (1974) *Arch Dermatol* **110**, 747.
2 KOSSARD S., *et al* (1980) *Arch Dermatol* **116**, 704.
3 PARKS D.L., *et al* (1971) *Arch Dermatol* **104**, 231.

6. JEJUNO-ILEAL BYPASS

Unusual forms of panniculitis can occur as a complication of jejuno-ileal bypass surgery (p. 2356).

REFERENCE

WILLIAMS H.J., *et al* (1979) *Arch Dermatol* **115**, 1091.

7. POST-STEROID PANNICULITIS

This type of panniculitis presents as subcutaneous nodules on the cheeks, arms and trunk from 1 to 13 days after the discontinuation of steroid therapy.

Clinical features [1, 2]. All reported cases have been in children who have received large doses of steroid over a short period, usually for rheumatic fever. The nodules vary in size from 0.5 to 4 cm. The overlying skin may be hyperaemic and there may be some pruritus [3]. Resolution is gradual, occurring over several weeks or months. There is a tendency for these nodules to localize in those areas in which there is the greatest accumulation of fat from steroid therapy. Although nodules appear after the discontinuation of steroids they are not associated with visceral manifestations of the steroid-withdrawal syndrome. A fatal case [2] showed, in addition to cutaneous lesions, damage to the intestinal fat tissue.

Differential diagnosis. See Table 31.8.

Treatment. There is no effective treatment.

REFERENCES

1 ROENIGK H.M., *et al* (1964) *Arch Dermatol* **90**, 387.
2 SMITH R.T. & GOOD R.A. (1956) *Clin Res Proc* **4**, 156.
3 SPAGNUOLO M. & TARANTA A. (1961) *Ann Intern Med* **54**, 1181.

8. SYSTEMIC NODULAR PANNICULITIS
SYN. WEBER CHRISTIAN DISEASE

Definition. The condition is characterized by recurrent crops of nodular non-suppurative panniculitis, accompanied by systemic features such as fever, malaise, abdominal pain and arthritis. The term 'Weber–Christian disease' has in the past often been applied to this idiopathic syndrome, but many of these cases would now be attributed to specific causes described above, and the term is probably best avoided [15, 17, 18].

Panniculitis due to pancreatic enzyme release is still included in the syndrome by some authorities, although it may have some distinguishing features (see above). Other conditions such as lupus panniculitis, cytophagic histiocytic panniculitis and factitial panniculitis are now considered to be separate entities.

Aetiology. Some cases are due to pancreatic disease, but more often no cause is found. In some cases there may be an immunologically mediated vasculitis affecting the vessels of the subcutis with secondary fat necrosis [15]. In many cases there is decreased fibrinolytic activity in skin and plasma, but this is thought to be secondary to the vasculitis rather than a primary event [13]. The immune responses may be abnormal in some cases [2, 4, 14].

Histopathology. The histological changes are non-specific [7]. In the early stages the fat lobules are infiltrated with inflammatory cells, mostly polymorphonuclear leukocytes, producing a pseudo-pyogenic reaction. Later, macrophages appear and ingest the fat released from damaged lipocytes; these lipophages have a characteristic foamy cytoplasm and produce a typical appearance of a lipophagic granuloma. There is no disorganization of the interlobular septa. Healing is by fibrosis, the fibrocytes invading the lobules from the connective tissue septa, depositing collagen and ultimately producing complete lobular fibrosis. In some instances careful examination of the interlobular septa will show vasculitis. Fat necrosis may also be present. In a review of 56 cases of systemic panniculitis who died, hepatic failure, haemorrhage and thrombosis were the predominant causes of death [7].

Clinical features. The disease is rare, whether or not it is associated with pancreatic disease. Cases have been reported at all ages, including infancy [10]. Most cases with pancreatic disease are middle-aged or elderly men, whereas the idiopathic disease is more common in middle-aged females. The usual presentation is with subcutaneous nodules, malaise, fever, arthralgia, tiredness, abdominal discomfort or loss of weight [16].

The subcutaneous nodules are usually about 1–2 cm in diameter, but they are sometimes much larger. They occur in crops at intervals of weeks or months, often with systemic symptoms. At first they are dull red, oedematous and tender, but over the course of a few weeks the oedema subsides, the nodule becomes firmer, and the erythema is suc-

ceeded by pigmentation. Sometimes the affected area becomes atrophic, leaving a central depression. The nodules are more or less symmetrically distributed, and they occur most commonly on the thighs and lower legs, although other areas may be involved. In a few cases the nodules may liquefy. The overlying skin then becomes necrotic and an oily yellow-brown liquid is discharged [11].

The visceral fat is also involved, but as a rule systemic localizing features do not appear until the visceral lesions are large. Systemic involvement may rarely develop before the subcutaneous nodules, and visceral involvement may be so extensive as to cause death [1, 7]. Myeloid involvement may cause anaemia of various types and this may rarely be associated with bone pain [19].

Osteolytic bone lesions may also occur [9]. Hepatomegaly can occur, possibly due to hyperlipaemia secondary to the breakdown of adipose tissue.

Necrotizing panniculitis has been reported as a result of pancreatic enzyme release [17]. Steatorrhoea [20], intestinal perforation [12] and severe granulomatous carditis [21] have also been described. There may be leukocytosis, leukopenia or increased circulating lipases.

Diagnosis. Systemic nodular panniculitis has to be distinguished from other forms of panniculitis (see below) and from other granulomatous diseases of the subcutis. (Table 50.1, p. 1871).

It is important to perform appropriate tests for pancreatic disease. Fever and other systemic symptoms are important features in systemic nodular panniculitis, but these may also occur in other forms of panniculitis such as lupus panniculitis, factitial panniculitis and cytophagic histiocytic panniculitis (see above). The finding of many subcutaneous 'foam' cells, some of which are multinucleated, is more helpful.

Disseminated lipogranulomatosis (Farber's disease) characteristically shows aphonia and joint manifestations, as well as cutaneous nodules.

Erythema induratum may simulate systemic nodular panniculitis, but the nodules are indolent and are usually confined to the lower leg. There are no constitutional symptoms, and the histology is characterized by a granulomatous tuberculoid infiltrate with vasculitis and caseation necrosis.

Liquefying panniculitis may simulate deep mycoses such as actinomycosis. A possible relationship between systemic nodular panniculitis and *systemic idiopathic fibrosis* has been suggested [16]. There is a striking correspondence in the anatomical distribution of these two disorders and adjoining organs are similarly affected. Systemic nodular panniculitis without skin involvement presents considerable diagnostic difficulties. *Massive visceral liposclerosis* is a similar and excessively rare disorder of unknown aetiology [3].

Prognosis. When only subcutaneous fat is involved the prognosis is good; it is also related to the underlying aetiology. Some cases recover after a few months and permanent remission within 2 to 5 years is usual. Rarely, recurrences may continue for 10 years or more but without serious deterioration of the general condition. Exceptionally, visceral involvement may be fatal.

Treatment. In cases where focal infection or drugs are possible antigens, antibiotic therapy or elimination of the offending drug is indicated. Once the possibility of systemic disease has been ruled out, the treatment is mainly symptomatic. Analgesics may be needed to alleviate pain and ulceration may need bland antiseptic dressings.

In severe cases corticosteroids may be effective, provided adequate dosage (up to 80 mg a day of prednisone) is employed for 7–10 days. The dose should then be slowly decreased over a period of 4–6 weeks. Steroids should be used only in acute attacks and for limited periods [5]. Fibrinolytic therapy (ethylestrenol 4 mg b.d. for 3 months) has been reported to help a third of patients [6]. Thalidomide [8] and chloroquine have also been recommended.

REFERENCES

1 Albrectson B. (1968) *Acta Derm Venereol* **40**, 474.
2 Allen-Mersh T.G. (1976) *J Clin Pathol* **29**, 144.
3 Blanc W.A. (1951) In *Syndromes Nouveaux de Pathologie Adipeuse*. Paris, Masson, p. 123.
4 Ciclitira P.J., *et al* (1980) *Br J Dermatol* **103**, 685.
5 Crosbie, S. (1955) *Ann Intern Med* **43**, 622.
6 Dodman B., *et al* (1973) *Br Med J* ii, 82.
7 Eng A.M. & Aronson I.K. (1983) *Semin Dermatol* **3**, 1.
8 Eravelly J. & Waters M.F.R. (1977) *Lancet* **i**, 251.
9 Gibson J., *et al* (1975) *J Rheumatol* **2**, 7.
10 Hendricks W.M., *et al* (1978) *Br J Dermatol* **98**, 175.
11 Hoyas N., *et al* (1965) *Arch Dermatol* **94**, 436.
12 Hutt M.S.R. & Pinniger J.L. (1956) *J Clin Pathol* **9**, 316.
13 Isacson S., *et al* (1970) *Acta Derm Venereol* **50**, 213.
14 Iwatsuki K., *et al* (1982) *Dermatologica* **164**, 181.
15 MacDonald A. & Feiwel M. (1968) *Br J Dermatol* **80**, 355.
16 Milner R.D.G. & Mitchinson M.K. (1965) *J Clin Pathol* **18**, 150.
17 Moore S. (1975) *J Rheumatol* **2**, 5.
18 Paraf A., *et al* (1965) *Rev Med Fr* **40**, 205.
19 Pinals R.S. (1970) *Arch Dermatol* **101**, 359.
20 Sandford H.N., *et al* (1952) *Am J Dis Child* **83**, 156.
21 Wilkinson P.J., *et al* (1974) *J Clin Pathol* **27**, 808.

OIL GRANULOMA
SYN. OLEOGRANULOMA; PARAFFINOMA;
OLEOMA; SCLEROSING LIPOGRANULOMA

Definition. A granulomatous reaction to the injection of a relatively bulky, oily liquid into the tissues. In some respects, such injections produce a tissue response comparable to that produced by the liberation of endogenous fatty substances.

Aetiology. Some years ago mineral oils, particularly liquid paraffin and soft paraffin, were in vogue for improving the contour of the body, being injected in the breasts of women and into the male scrotum for breast supplementation and testicular prostheses respectively. They have also been injected into the face and other areas for the correction of dimples and depressions. The inadvertent injection of grease gun oil also produces similar granulomatous reactions. Such granulomas are now uncommon since the development of less toxic silicones and bovine collagen for tissue replacement, and the reader is referred to older texts for further details [3].

Histopathology. A massive injection provokes an initial acute inflammation. Some mineral oils will remain in the tissue for a considerable time without any marked inflammatory reaction. Others form large oil droplets which become encysted and surrounded by many layers of collagen, producing conspicuous 'onion-skin cysts'. The classical 'paraffinoma' shows multiple small cysts which produce the characteristic 'Swiss-cheese appearance' with little inflammatory change, but massive fibrosis. Certain animal fats produce a tuberculoid granuloma, whereas vegetable oils, by virtue of irritant substances liberated by hydrolysis, often provoke inflammatory changes and a lipophagic granuloma. Differential diagnosis of an oil granuloma from the idiopathic sclerosing lipogranuloma may be impossible on histological grounds, although oil cysts are, as a rule, far more extensive in paraffinoma.

Clinical features. The nodules or plaques usually appear several months after injection, but their onset may be delayed for up to 20 years. The lesions may persist almost indefinitely. They form nodules and plaques which are firm and not tender; the overlying skin is usually normal; they may be fixed to both skin and deep fascia. Ulceration occasionally occurs. The common sites following cosmetic procedures are the face and breasts of women. Nodules on the thighs and buttocks are the result of injection of therapeutic agents in oily vehicles. In some patients the history of earlier injection for cosmetic or therapeutic purposes may be deliberately concealed.

The grease gun injury characteristically affects the dorsum of the left hand and appears as a nodule, plaque or sinus [6]. Perianal oil granulomas are reported [8] following injections for haemorrhoids. Dermatitis artefacta may also rarely be due to self injection with oils or silicones. An analysis of the lipid content in 23 cases of sclerosing lipogranuloma of the male genitalia demonstrated the presence of paraffin hydrocarbons in all specimens [4].

Differential diagnosis. The diagnosis may be difficult in the absence of a definite history. The causes of other granulomatous conditions of the subcutis are shown in Table 50.1. In the presence of fibrosis, morphoea must be excluded.

REFERENCES

1 BEST E.W., *et al* (1953) *Proc Staff Meet Mayo Clin* **28**, 623.
2 COLUMB D. (1962) *Ann Dermatol Syphiligr* **89**, 36.
3 CUNLIFFE W.J. & BLEEHEN S.S. (1979) In *Textbook of Dermatology*. Eds Rook A., Wilkinson D.S. & Ebling F.J.G. Oxford, Blackwell Scientific Publications, p. 1665.
4 OERTEL Y.C. & JOHNSON F.B. (1970) *Arch Pathol Lab Med* **101**, 321.
5 SCHUMACHERS R. (1965) *Hautdarzt* **10**, 458.
6 SMITH M.G.H. (1964) *Br Med J* **ii**, 918.
7 SWETANA H.F. & BERNHARD W.G. (1948) *Am J Pathol* **24**, 675.
8 SYMMERS W.ST.C. (1955) *Br Med J* **ii**, 1536.
9 WINER L., *et al* (1964) *Arch Dermatol* **90**, 588.

PRE-AGONAL INDURATION

Definition. A peculiar induration of the skin and subcutaneous tissues which may rarely occur in the terminal stages of any illness.

Aetiology. It has been suggested that hypothermia results in solidification of fat in the subcutis or that an alteration in the melting point of body fat pro-

TABLE 50.1. Granulomas of the subcutis

	Oil granuloma	Lipogranuloma	Foreign body	Sarcoidal	Tuberculoid	Rheumatoid-like
Aetiology	Liquid paraffin Soft paraffin Liquid silicones	Traumatic, toxic or vascular damage; fat-cell necrosis ensuing	Debris from injury (fabric, sutures)	Silica (talc, etc.) Beryllium sarcoidosis	Tuberculosis Gummata Deep mycosis	Nodules of rheumatoid arthritis, Deep granuloma annulare, Wegener's granulomatosis
	Grease gun oil	Idiopathic	Tatooed material	Tuberculoid leprosy		Granulomatous arteritis

Prognosis. The lesions remain essentially unchanged, almost indefinitely, although sarcomatous changes have been reported [2].

Treatment. If there is any doubt about the diagnosis biopsy should be performed. No effective treatment exists other than complete excision.

IDIOPATHIC SCLEROSING LIPOGRANULOMA [2, 4]

An idiopathic type of sclerosing lipogranuloma has also been reported, but the lack of recent reports may indicate that it really represents an oil granuloma in which, for some reason, the history is concealed [1, 4, 7].

duces semi-solidification. The condition is commoner in infants than in adults. Elliot [1] regards it as a special form of oedema affecting the septa rather than the fat lobules.

Histopathology. There is interlobular oedema with widening of the connective tissue septa. There is no lobular disorganization but slight lobular atrophy unaccompanied by any inflammatory cells.

Clinical features. The hardening of the skin is usually first perceptible in the legs and it then spreads upwards to involve the entire body. The affected skin is pale, cool and indurated.

Prognosis. Since the condition appears only in the

terminal stages of severe illness it is to be regarded as an ominous physical sign.

REFERENCE

1 Elliot R.I.K. (1959) *Proc R Soc Med* **52**, 1018.

FAT HYPERTROPHY

In this group are included obesity, Dercum's disease and fat hypertrophy due to insulin injections. Obesity has been discussed in the earlier parts of this chapter. Fat hypertrophy is an uncommon painless complication of diabetes treated with insulin. Although the mechanism is uncertain [1, 2] an immunological response to the insulin could be a factor. Although a change to a highly purified insulin may improve the appearance in half the patients, the change of therapy is less satisfactory than in insulin fat atrophy [1].

REFERENCES

1 Daggert P., *et al* (1977) *Br J Dermatol* **96**, 439.
2 Dixon K., *et al* (1975) *Q J Med* **176**, 543.

DERCUM'S DISEASE
SYN. ADIPOSIS DOLOROSA

Dercum's disease is a rare, progressive disease characterized by painful subcutaneous plaques and ecchymoses.

Aetiology. The mechanism of Dercum's disease is not known. It most commonly affects menopausal women; they are usually obese at the time of onset of the disorder and severe emotional disturbance is common. In some families there is a dominant inheritance [2].

Histopathology. The changes are non-specific; there is a combination of fat cell necrosis and interstitial tissue proliferation.

Clinical features [1, 3]. Although patients with Dercum's disease are usually obese at the time of onset, loss of weight and asthenia appear as the disease progresses. Painful subcutaneous plaques may be found on any site, except, perhaps, the face; they give a characteristic sensation on palpation, like a 'bag of worms'. Commonly associated symptoms in the patients include amenorrhoea, sparseness of the pubic and axillary hair and menopausal flushes. The majority of reported cases have psychoneurotic symptoms.

Juxta-articular lesions may cause joint pains [4].

Diagnosis. This is not difficult when the classical triad is present—painful plaques, ecchymoses and obesity, appearing in women with amenorrhoea and neurotic symptoms.

Cushing's disease with diffuse deposition of fat, plethora and hirsutes must be distinguished from Dercum's disease. Amenorrhoea and ecchymoses are common to both disorders.

Treatment. Weight reduction, surgical exision of individual tumours and intravenous lidocaine injection may be helpful [4].

REFERENCE

1 Atkinson R.L. (1982) *Int J Obes* **6**, 351.
2 Lynch H.T. (1963) *Am J Hum Genet* **15**, 184.
3 Palmer E.D. (1981) *Am Fam Phys* **24**, 155.
4 Nahir A.H. *et al* (1983) *Isr J Med Sci* **19**, 858.

FAT ATROPHY

The terms 'lipoatrophy' or 'lipodystrophy' have traditionally meant idiopathic atrophy of the subcutaneous tissue. The lipoatrophy may be part of a local panatrophy affecting all mesodermal layers [1] but in this chapter only true lipoatrophy will be considered. The atrophy may be *localized*, to the thighs, for example, or it can be widespread involving the upper part of the trunk (*partial lipodystrophy*) or it may affect the whole body (*total lipodystrophy*).

REFERENCE

1 Serup J., *et al* (1982) *Acta Derm Venereol (Stockh)* **55**, 135.

LOCALIZED ATROPHY

Localized atrophy may be seen in insulin-dependent diabetics, following certain inflammatory dermatoses, such as panniculitis and morphoea, or as primary idiopathic lipoatrophy. Failure to perform a biopsy in the early phases of the atrophy may explain why so many cases are labelled as idiopathic in origin. It has been suggested that many cases may be preceded by an inflammatory reaction in the fat [4].

1. **Insulin lipoatrophy** is a cosmetically distressing complication of insulin administration.

Aetiology. Insulin lipoatrophy is seen in women and children, rarely in men. The mechanism remains speculative but local changes induced by insulin or impurities are probably important [3]. Most cases are associated with high levels of insulin requirement and/or an increased insulin binding capacity.

Cross reaction of insulin antibodies with cells thus changed could result in further damage [2]. The subcutaneous damage is reduced if highly purified insulins are used, resulting in considerable clinical improvement and a reduction in insulin requirements and insulin binding capacity [1, 2, 4, 6, 7].

Histopathology. There is a loss of fat tissue and inflammatory changes are conspicuously absent.

Clinical features. Insulin atrophy is more frequently present than insulin fat hypertrophy although both features can occur in the same patient. Most cases present 6 months to 2 years after the start of insulin administration. The lesion may vary from only a dimple to an extensive disfiguring area; it is usually found only at the sites of injection but loss of fat may occur elsewhere. There is a definite tendency to spontaneous recovery at that site when the site of injection is changed.

Treatment. A change to a purified insulin, particularly the new human insulin, is often curative [4]. Prevention is either by the constant alteration in the site of injections so that no two injections are given in exactly the same area more frequently than once a month or by the use of the more purified insulins [2, 7].

REFERENCES

1 BLOOM S. (1976) *British Diabetic Association Spring Meeting.*
2 DAGGETT P., *et al* (1977) *Br J Dermatol* **96**, 439.
3 EISERT J. (1965) *Med Clinics North Am* **49**, 628.
4 KRISTENSEN J.S. & FALHOTT K. (1983) *Diabetes* **32**, (Suppl. 1), 66A.
5 PETERS M.S. & WINKELMANN R.K. (1980) *Arch Dermatol* **116**, 1363.
6 TANTILLO J.J., *et al* (1974) *Diabetes* **23**, 276.
7 TEUSCHER A. (1974) *Dermatologica* **211**, 15.

2. Localized 'idiopathic' lipoatrophy.

This group of disorders predominantly affects either the thighs, ankles or abdomen and all cases are possibly variants of the same process. To date two groups of localized lipoatrophy have been described. Both may represent the sequelae of a primary inflammatory process but more biopsies of very early cases are necessary to confirm this suggestion [11].

Lipoatrophia semicircularis [1, 3, 5, 9]. These patients show similar painless lesions on the antero-lateral aspects of the thighs, characterized by a bandlike circular depression 2–4 cm in width. The overlying skin is normal.

The loss of fat develops rapidly within several weeks, usually without associated symptoms, although rheumatic-like pains within the involved areas were reported by two women. Trauma is not responsible. Histological studies suggested that the primary cause was degeneration of fat cells which in turn induced a reactive inflammatory cellular infiltration and increased resorption of the fat.

Patients have also been described with lipoatrophy of the ankles [8]. These patients differ from other forms of annular lipoatrophy only in the site affected. Primary inflammatory vascular changes in the subcutaneous tissue have been demonstrated in these patients, and also during the early period of other lipoatrophies [11]. There is no treatment but considerable improvement may occur after the activity of the disease settles.

Lipodystrophia centrifugalis abdominalis infantalis (centrifugal lipodystrophy), is rare and has been seen predominantly in Japanese children [4, 5, 6, 7, 10] affecting the subcutaneous fat, usually of the abdomen and upper groin. A Chinese [2] and an English boy [13] have also been affected. The condition spreads in a centrifugal fashion with a central large bluish depressed area and slight erythema of the edge (Fig. 50.9). Histologically there is a decrease of the subcutaneous fat and an inflammatory cell infiltrate in the lower dermis and subcutis (Fig. 50.10). Further experience has shown that the original name is inappropriate, since the condition may affect other areas and may occur outside infancy. Regional lymphadenopathy may occur [6].

Treatment is disappointing although after the disease activity has ceased there seems to be regrowth of fat in 75% of cases. Some improvement has been reported in a majority of the cases treated with oral and topical corticosteroids [6].

3. Post-inflammatory lipoatrophy.

Several patients [10, 11] who have presented with lipoatrophy of the limbs have shown histologically clear-cut evidence of a lymphocytic panniculitis. One patient [12] had a lobular panniculitis, positive ANF and positive ENA and subsequently developed lipoatrophy. Lipoatrophy is also well recognized following lupus panniculitis and subcutaneous morphoea [11].

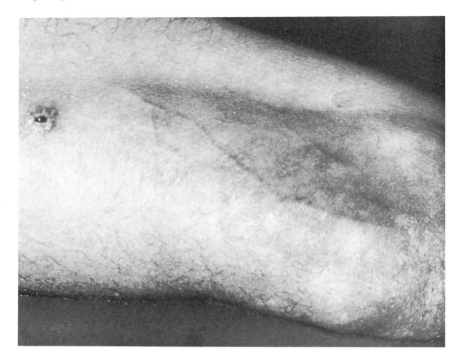

Fig. 50.8. Lipoatrophia semicircularis (General Infirmary, Leeds).

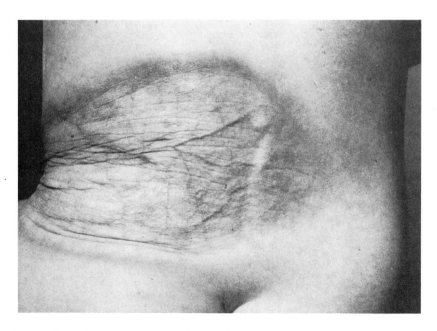

Fig. 50.9. Centrifugal lipodystrophy (Dr R.S. Wells, Guy's Hospital, London).

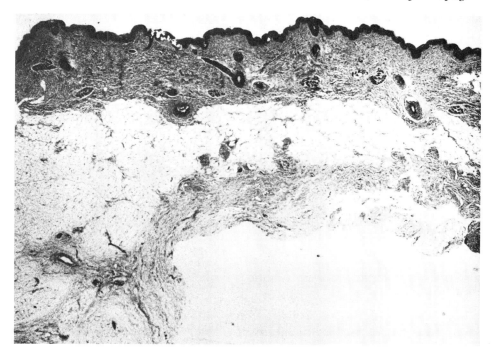

FIG. 50.10. Biopsy of centrifugal lipodystrophy shows the remarkable localized reduction in the subcutaneous fat (Dr R.S. Wells, Guy's Hospital).

REFERENCES

1 BLOCH P.H. & RUNNE U. (1978) *Hautarzt* **29**, 270.
2 GIAM Y.C., *et al* (1982) *Br J Dermatol* **106**, 461.
3 GSCHWANDTER W.R. & MUNZBERGER H. (1975) *Wien klin Wochenschr* **87**, 164.
4 IMAMURA S. & YAMADA M. (1977) *Br J Dermatol* **96**, 96.
5 IMAMURA S., *et al* (1971) *Arch Dermatol* **104**, 291.
6 IMAMURA S., *et al* (1979) *Der Hautzarzt* **30**, 360.
7 IMAMURA S., *et al* (1984) *J Am Acad Dermatol* **11**, 203.
8 JABLONSKA S., *et al* (1975) *Acta Derm Venereol (Stockh)* **55**, 135.
9 KARKARITAS C., *et al* (1981) *Br J Dermatol* **105**, 591.
10 MAKINO K., *et al* (1972) *Arch Dermatol* **106**, 899.
11 PETERS M.S. & WINKELMANN R.K. (1980) *Arch Dermatol* **116**, 1363.
12 WINKELMANN R.K. & PADILHA-GONCALVES A. (1980) *Arch Dermatol* **116**, 291.
13 ZACHARY C.B. & WELLS R.S. (1984) *Br J Dermatol* **110**, 107.

TOTAL LIPOATROPHY
SYN. LIPOATROPHIC DIABETES: LAWRENCE–SEIP SYNDROME [3, 5, 6]

A rare congenital or acquired lipoatrophy, sometimes familial, with loss of the subcutaneous and visceral fat, hepatomegaly, increased bone growth, hyperlipaemia and, later, diabetes mellitus [1, 3, 4, 5, 6].

Aetiology. The inheritance is probably autosomal recessive and it is suggested that patients with the full syndrome are homozygous; heterozygous subjects manifest hyperlipaemia only. The pathogenesis is unknown, but a defect in the diencephalon or hypothalamus has been suggested [2], since some patients have an increased level of hypothalamic releasing factors.

Histopathology. There is complete loss of subcutaneous and visceral fat.

Clinical features. There are two varieties: congenital and acquired lipoatrophy. In the congenital type there is complete loss of subcutaneous fat, noticeable at birth or before the age of 2 years. Hepatomegaly (occasionally with splenomegaly), hyperlipaemia and perhaps cutaneous xanthomas, hypermetabolism and excessive bone growth are characteristic. The younger patients show glycosuria only when given large amounts of glucose. Hyperglycaemia with excessive thirst and polyuria usually develop only after the age of 10. The diabetes is insulin resistant and ketosis is rare. Although there is complete loss of fat the skin retains its elasticity. There is often generalized hypertrichosis, even at birth, and the scalp hair becomes abundant and often curly with the onset of the disease. There is precocious enlargement of the genitalia, and in females marked enlargement of the clitoris.

As a result of increased bone growth the children are tall for their age; the somatic musculature is increased and the abdomen markedly protuberant, often with an umbilical hernia. All patients have a remarkably similar facial appearance; most have a dolichocephalic skull and luxuriant hair almost reaching the eyebrows and the loss of facial fat gives a very characteristic gaunt appearance. The joints, particularly of the hands and feet, are enlarged. Widespread pigmentation, particularly of the axillary and inguinal folds, may be associated with linear epidermal thickenings, giving the appearance of acanthosis nigricans [3].

A proportion of congenital cases have cardiomegaly, renal anomalies and neurological disorders (including mental deficiency and hemiplegia).

Some patients may have increased plasma levels of corticotrophin releasing factor, follicle stimulating hormone releasing factor and melanocyte stimulating hormone releasing factor, presumably due to neurological dysfunction [2].

Acquired total lipoatrophy. When the onset is in the adult, excessive height is not a feature, muscularity is less obvious and abdominal protuberance not so marked. However, acromegaloid features with enlargement of the skull, hands and feet may precede the diabetes. The acquired type is frequently heralded by a febrile illness. Death from hepatic failure or haematemesis is usual.

Differential diagnosis. In congenital cases differentiation from de Lange's disease may be difficult, especially if neurological features are present.

In adult cases the differential diagnosis is from acromegaly and thyrotoxicosis.

Insulin lipoatrophy in diabetics is focal and usually confined to the sites of insulin injection.

Treatment. Pimozide, a selective dopaminergic blocker, may be helpful in restoring the fat and decreasing the levels of hypothalamic releasing factors [2].

REFERENCES

1 Brunzell J.D., *et al* (1968) *Ann Intern Med* **69**, 501.
2 Corbin A., *et al* (1974) *Acta Endocrinol* **77**, 209.
3 Lawrence R.D. (1946) *Lancet* **i**, 724.
4 Reed W.B., *et al* (1965) *Arch Dermatol* **91**, 326.
5 Seip M. & Trygstad O. (1963) *Arch Dis Child* **38**, 447.
6 Senior B. & Gellis S.S. (1964) *Pediatrics* **51**, 593.

PARTIAL LIPOATROPHY
SYN. PARTIAL LIPODYSTROPHY;
BARRAQUER—SIMONS DISEASE;
PROGRESSIVE LIPODYSTROPHY [7, 8]

This rare affliction occurs either in childhood or in young adults as an incidental part of a widespread mesodermal atrophy.

Aetiology. Most patients are children or young adults when the disorder begins, but onset in the first year and in middle-age is reported. Females are affected four or five times more frequently than males [9] and the condition is sometimes familial. It may follow an acute specific fever such as measles but the common occurrence of specific fevers makes proof of this observation difficult. Partial lipodystrophy has followed damage to the region of the mid-brain or diencephalon [3]. The association of lipodystrophy with immunologically-related renal disease [4, 10], systemic sclerosis [2] and high titres of thyroid antibodies, supports the view of lipodystrophy being an immunological disorder [11]—but one which requires more investigation.

Histopathology. There is usually complete loss of adipose tissue over the affected areas.

Clinical features. The disease is characterized by the relatively slow symmetrical disappearance of the facial fat, producing a cadaverous appearance (Fig. 50.11) and complete loss of the subcutaneous fat in the upper half of the body (the Weir Mitchell type). In some cases there is a coincidental hypertrophy of the subcutaneous fat of the lower part of the body (Laignel–Lavastine and Viard type). Ten per cent may have 'hemi-lipodystrophy' involving half of the face or body. Up to 90% can develop progressive membranous mesangiocapillary glomerulonephritis [1, 5, 6, 9] and this can be precipitated by the contraceptive pill, pregnancy or the use of ergot derivatives [9]. Thus, such patients should be observed by a renal physician during pregnancy, and oral contraceptives are prohibited.

The association of hypocomplementaemia and mesangiocapillary glomerulonephritis is now well established [4, 10]. Approximately half of the

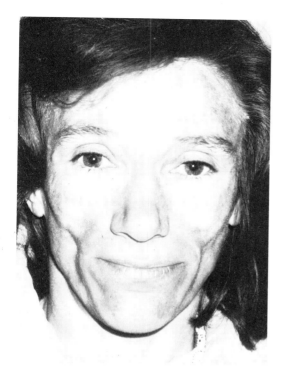

FIG. 50.11. The typical cadaveric facies of a patient with partial lipodystrophy. She also has melasma.

patients with this form of glomerulonephritis have a persistently low plasma concentration of the third component of complement (C3) while the concentration of the fourth component (C4) is normal. This is accompanied by the presence of a factor in serum which is capable of activating C3 without activation of the earlier components. This material has been termed 'nephritic factor' or C3NeF [4].

The relationship between C3NeF, persistently low C3 and mesangiocapillary glomerulonephritis is not clear. It has been suggested that the C3NeF predisposes the glomerulus to the development of mesangiocapillary glomerulonephritis in response to some other agent. Transplantation in one case resulted in normalization of C3 and the disappearance of C3NeF [5].

Diabetes mellitus develops in a third of the patients with partial lipodystrophy and retinitis pigmentosa is a rare complication.

Treatment. There is no effective treatment, other than the prevention of kidney disease and its appropriate treatment should these problems arise. In a series of 12 patients, 4 died from renal failure 10–25 years after the onset of the partial lipoatrophy [9].

REFERENCES

1 EISINGER A.J., et al (1972) *Q J Med* **41**, 343.
2 HALL W.S., et al (1978) *Arch Intern Med* **138**, 1303.
3 HAWES C.R., et al (1955) *J Pediatr* **45**, 393.
4 IPP M.M., et al (1976) *Immunol Immunopathol* 7, 281.
5 LJUNGHALL S., et al (1974) *Acta Med Scand* **195**, 493.
6 PETERS D.K., et al (1973) *Lancet* ii, 535.
7 POLEY J.R. & STICKLER G.B. (1963) *Am J Dis Child* **106**, 356.
8 SENIOR B. & GEDDIS S.S. (1964) *Pediatrics (Springfield)* 33, 593.
9 SIMPSON, N.B. et al (1979) *Br J Dermatol* **101**, (Suppl. 17), 11.
10 SISSONS J.G.P., et al (1976) *N Engl J Med* **294**, 461.
11 WILSON W.A. & SISSONS J.G.P. (1978) *Ann Intern Med* **89**, 72.

LIPOMA

Lipomas are benign tumours composed of mature fat cells found in the subcutaneous tissue and less commonly in internal organs.

Aetiology. The metabolic changes associated with benign tumours are varied but include fundamental defects responsible for the altered growth properties of the tumour. It has been demonstrated that loss of negative feedback control regulatory enzymes (by citrate or phosphofructokinase) may be an early feature in the development of lipoma [2].

Histopathology. Fat cells in groups slightly larger than the normal lobule are typically enclosed within a capsule of connective tissue but the capsule may be deficient and the tumour then appears locally invasive. Relatively large blood vessels are seen traversing the connective tissue septa. Primitive fat cells may be found in clinically benign lipomas in children [15]. Xanthomatous and mucinous changes appear in many lipomas.

Clinical features. A lipoma is a subcutaneous nodule, often lobulated, with a characteristic soft, putty-like consistency. The overlying skin is normal and moves freely over the tumour and feels cooler than the surrounding skin. The tumour grows very slowly to reach a diameter which is usually between 2 and 10 cm but may be considerably greater. The commonest sites are the neck, shoulders and upper arms, back and thighs. There are rarely any subjective symptoms, but pain from pressure on the nerves is sometimes experienced. Another rare event is infiltration of adjacent tissues, in particular muscle [7]. Fat necrosis may cause enlargement, pain and tenderness. A large lipoma on the exposed skin of the lower legs is susceptible to nodular perniosis.

There may be only one lipoma or large numbers [1] may develop at intervals over a period of years. Seven per cent of patients with lipoma have multiple lesions [10]. Such lipomas may be randomly distributed or more or less confined to one region of the body. In most patients the presence of multiple lipomas appears to have no special significance [3, 5]. They may, however, be associated with neurofibromatosis, or with visceral lipomas in the respiratory, alimentary or genito-urinary tract. They are an inconstant feature of Gardner's syndrome (p. 126) in which they are associated with multiple sebaceous cysts, osteomas and polyposis of the colon.

A diffuse multilobular lipomatosis involving the back of the neck and the shoulders in a cape-like distribution is sometimes seen in men. It classically afflicts wine porters in France and brewery workers elsewhere. It has been described as 'Madelung's neck'.

The prominent fat deposits over the buttocks which constitute the steatopygy of the Bushmen and Hottentots may be regarded as a racial form of physiological lipomatosis.

Malignant change in a lipoma is very rare. Liposarcoma usually arises *de novo* [14]. Some cases so diagnosed were probably embryonal adipose tissue which would have matured as the child grew.

Multiple symmetrical circumscribed lipomatosis [12, 13] is a well-defined and not uncommon syndrome beginning at any time between puberty and 40. The lipomas, which rarely exceed 5 cm in diameter, are limited to the arms, forearms, buttocks and thighs. Rarely multiple lipomatosis is familial and the inheritance is probably polygenic [11] or autosomal dominant [8].

Diagnosis. The diagnosis is usually easy but in cases of doubt a biopsy should be performed. Angiolipomas are morphologically similar to lipomas but are painful. Lipofascial herniae in the natal or perianal region simulate lipomas [9]. Excision and suture is required to prevent recurrence.

An epidermoid cyst can mimic a lipoma. However, the presence of the central punctum gives a clue to the correct diagnosis. The possibility of hibernoma (p. 1879) should be considered when fatty tumours appear in the neck and scapular region.

Treatment. This usually depends on the patient's desire for the lipoma to be surgically removed. Lipoma of the lumbar region may be associated with underlying spina bifida occulta and removal of the tumour is dangerous without simultaneous exploration of the cauda equina.

REFERENCES

1 ADAM B.A. & CHAN Y.S. (1974) *Br J Clin Pract* **28**, 101.
2 ATKINSON J.N.C., et al (1974) *Br Med J* i, 101.
3 GOLTZ R.W., et al (1962) *Arch Dermatol* **86**, 708.
4 JACOB M.I. (1962) *Fed Proc Fed Am Soc Exp Biol* **21**, 288.
5 KNOTH W. (1962) *Dermatologica* **125**, 161.
6 MARKS M.M. (1965) *South Med J* **58**, 442.
7 MATTEL S.F. & PERSKY M.S. (1983) *Laryngoscope* **93**, 205.
8 MOHAR N. (1980) *Acta Derm Venereol* **60**, 509.
9 MULLER R. (1951) *Dermatologica* **103**, 258.
10 OSMENT L.S. [1968) *Surg Gynecol Obstet* **127**, 129.
11 RABBIOSI G., et al (1977) *Acta Derm Venereol (Stockh)* **57**, 265.
12 SHAFAR J. & BEHR G. (1965) *Post Grad Med J* **41**, 15.
13 STOUT A.P. (1944) *Ann Surg* **119**, 86.
14 TEDESCHI C.G. (1946) *Arch Pathol* **42**, 320.
15 WAKELEY C. & SOMERVILLE P. (1952) *Lancet* **ii**, 995.

Congenital diffuse lipomatosis [1, 3, 4, 5]. Congenital diffuse lipomatosis has been infrequently recorded. Several syndromes, which may involve a neuroectodermal defect have been described in conjunction with various types of haemangioma or lymphangioma. In one case, congenital lipomatosis was associated with angiomatosis and macro-encephalia [2].

REFERENCES

1 BAKER A.B. & ADAMS J.M. (1938) *Am J Cancer* **34**, 214.
2 BANNAYAN G.A. (1971) *Arch Pathol* **92**, 1.
3 CAMERON A.H. & McMILLAN D.H. (1956) *J Bone Joint Surg* **38B**, 692.
4 SCHLICHT D. (1965) *Med J Aust* **2**, 959.
5 WISING P.J. (1954) *Nord Med* **51**, 279.

ANGIOLIPOMA

Angiolipoma is a benign encapsulated, lobulated tumour differing histologically from a lipoma in the excessive degree of vascular proliferation. The age of onset is relatively young, and in one series of 288 patients [2] averaged 17 years. Clinically, the lesions are from 0·5 to 5 cm in diameter and closely resemble lipomas but they are painful and tender and are sometimes bluish in colour [3]. They occur most frequently on the arms, legs and abdomen and are often multiple [1].

REFERENCES

1 DIXON A.Y., *et al* (1981) *Human Pathology* **12**, 739.
2 HOWARD W.R. & HELWIG E.B. (1960) *Arch Dermatol* **82**, 924.
3 KLEM K.K. (1949) *Acta Chir* **97**, 527.

HIBERNOMA

SYN. GRANULAR CELL LIPOMA [1]

A rare benign tumour which consists of primitive fetal brown fat. The histology is characteristic, showing masses of distinctive cells with fine granules and a solitary central nucleus [1, 2, 3]. The tumour is encapsulated and multilobular. It occurs in adults of either sex and presents as a firm, non-tender nodule, with vascular dilatation of the overlying skin. The sites of predilection are the cervical, axillary and interscapular regions. Surgical excision is the only treatment.

REFERENCES

1 ANGERVALL L., *et al* (1964) *Cancer* (NY) **17**, 685.
2 JENNINGS R.C. & BEHR G. (1955) *J Clin Pathol* **8**, 310.
3 NOVY F.G. & WILSON J.W. (1956) *Arch Dermatol* **73**, 149.

CHAPTER 51

Disorders of Sweat Glands

R.H. CHAMPION

COMPARATIVE ANATOMY AND PHYSIOLOGY

F.J. EBLING (pp. 1881–1884)

Sweat glands are described as merocrine because, unlike the holocrine sebaceous glands, their cells are not destroyed in the process of secretion. Merocrine glands have been further subdivided into two major types, usually known as apocrine and eccrine. The nomenclature is due to Schiefferdecker [58, 59] who believed apocrine glands to secrete by a decapitation of the apical cytoplasm in contrast to eccrine glands, in which no breakdown of any cellular material occurs. Such a distinction between modes of secretion has been denied for lack of evidence that necrobiotic secretory cycles occur in any mammal [12, 19, 20, 21, 24, 37, 42, 43]. However, in the rabbit chin gland [25] and in the lemur antibrachial organ [23] large portions of secretory epithelium do appear to be sloughed during secretion. In the axillary organ of man, on the other hand, although some authors have claimed that decapitation of apical cells can sometimes occur [18], most believe this to be abnormal. They favour the view that secretion occurs by small portions of apical cytoplasm becoming pinched off [2, 37].

Whatever the truth, it is convenient to divide tubular glands into those which—like the sebaceous gland—normally develop from the external root sheath of the hair follicle and remain attached to it, and those which develop from the superficial epidermis and remain independent of the follicle. If the functional connotation of 'apocrine' can be conveniently avoided by the description 'epitrichial' [5, 21], the logical substitution of 'atrichial' for 'eccrine' seems less justifiable. Gabe [13] has listed a number of other characteristic differences between the two types of gland.

Epitrichial (apocrine) glands occur in all the known orders of mammals except whales, elephants, sea cows and scaly ant-eaters [13]. Their density varies widely between species, ranging from 20–30 per cm² in the pig to over 2,000 per cm² in Zebu cattle [21].

Atrichial (eccrine) glands occur in the foot pads of most mammals; the exceptions again include whales, sea cows, elephants and scaly ant-eaters, with the addition of bats. Such glands probably serve to moisten the surface of the skin to improve the grip. In hairy skin, however, eccrine glands are found only in a few primates, including tree shrews,

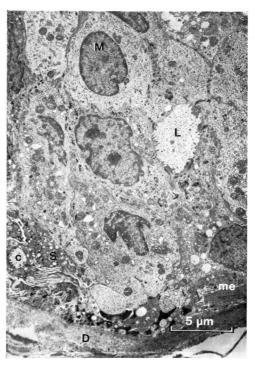

FIG. 51.1. Section of a secretory coil of an eccrine sweat gland, stained with osmium. The coil contains three types of cell, serous or clear cells (S) containing finger-like processes and bordering a canaliculus (c), mucous or dark cells (M) and myoepithelial cells (me). D = dermis; L = lumen of coil. Electron micrograph by Professor A. S. Breathnach.

Old World monkeys, apes and man [29, 38, 69]. There is insufficient evidence to conclude either that primate eccrine glands are homologues of foot-pad glands or that they are evolved from epitrichial glands, though the latter seems unlikely, since the human embryo possesses both rudiments. Within the primates, however, it is of interest that eccrine glands appear to replace epitrichial glands in the course of evolution; in the gibbon there are more epitrichial than eccrine glands [50], in the rhesus monkey [39] and the lutong [29] there are about equal numbers, and in the gorilla, chimpanzee [36] and the baboon [34] there are more eccrine than epitrichial. Only in man do eccrine glands completely replace epitrichial glands over the major areas of hairy skin. In the human embryo (Chapter 2, p. 35) such glands develop later than those on the palmar and plantar surfaces and thus they should probably be placed in a separate category from them and from mammalian foot-pad glands in general.

Specialized glands, i.e. aggregations of secreting units, are not only widespread amongst mammalian orders but, in different species, can be found in almost every area of the body from the head to the rump and the extremities [13, 51, 52, 65]. Some, as for example the chin and anal glands of the rabbit, contain only tubular units [14, 28, 44, 45, 46, 47, 48]; others, for example the supracaudal gland of the guinea pig, the flank organ of the golden hamster, the abdominal gland of the gerbil and the preputial glands of rodents are purely sebaceous (see Chapter 52). Both types of unit may be associated, as in the muzzle glands of certain bats [53], the side glands of shrews in which batteries of tubular glands underlie the sebaceous elements [9], and the inguinal glands of the rabbit which consist of a discrete pair of each type [28].

Similar glandular aggregations occur in primates. Lemurs have 'antibrachial' glands, composed of tubular units on the inner forearms, as well as paired 'brachial' glands, composed of sebaceous units, on the anterior chest [23, 33]. The male loris has units of both types concentrated in the scrotal region [35]. The New World owl monkey has both sternal glands which are tubular, and subcaudal organs with both tubular and sebaceous units [17], and the stump-tailed macaque has a high density of tubular glands on the scalp [40]. In man, rudiments of epitrichial tubular glands attached to each follicle appear during development but survive to become functional only in the axillae, the genital area and the areolae.

Epitrichial tubular glands perform two main functions: thermoregulation and odour-production.

The first function is confined to the glands of the general body surface; the second is a property of the specialized aggregates, though probably is not exclusive to them.

The extent to which the glands respond to environmental heat loads and the exact nature of the control mechanisms have been studied mainly in domestic animals. They vary widely. In horses, oxen and camels the glands secrete in response to a rise in ambient temperature, but in pigs, dogs and deer they do not [55]. Apart from the primates, Equidae and some Bovidae, sweat glands appear to play a minor role in the control of body temperature in warm conditions [21, 55, 56] though they may cool local areas, such as the scrotum in the sheep [66, 67]. By sympathetic denervation of the skin it has been shown that sweating is under adrenergic nervous control, even in species which lack a demonstrable nerve supply. In addition, in most species studied, the glands also respond to administration of adrenaline, though in contrast to human eccrine glands they are much less sensitive to acetylcholine [55, 56]. Though various interpretations have been made of the experimental results [69], it is now accepted that apocrine sweating is in general controlled by adrenergic nerves, and that in some species, e.g. the horse, adrenaline from the adrenal medulla supplements the sweating caused by exercise, though not that caused by heat exposure [55, 56].

Odour production is known to occur in fifteen out of nineteen mammalian orders, but has received detailed study in only a few species. Chemical signals serve a number of social purposes, of which the marking of territory, the maintenance of social hierarchy, alarm signals and individual group or species recognition are only a few [8, 10, 41, 49, 54, 65]. They are also concerned with sex attraction, either of the female by the male, as well established for example in the boar [62], or of the male by the female, as in the hamster [61] and the rhesus monkey [7, 22, 30, 31, 32]. For accounts of this rapidly expanding field the reader is referred to works by Albone [1], Doty [8], Müller-Schwarze and Mozell [41], Mykytowycz and Goodrich [49] and Thiessen and Yahr [65].

There seems little doubt that, notwithstanding social pressures to devalue its impact, odour is important in human communication [26, 57], as Havelock Ellis recognized in his comprehensive and entertaining, if almost entirely anecdotal, review [11]. The odorous steroids, 5α-androstenone and 5α-androstenol, known to act as pheromones in pigs, have been found in axillary sweat [3, 4, 15, 16] as well as in human urine, plasma and fatty tissue [6].

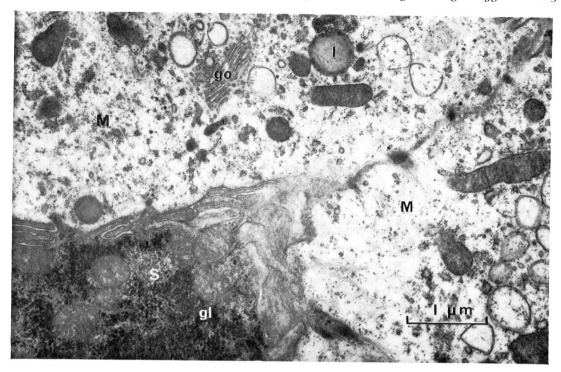

FIG. 51.2 Portions of two mucous ('dark') cells (M), one showing Golgi complex (go) and lipid globules (l), and a serous ('clear') cell (S) with glycogen granules (gl). Electron micrograph by Professor A. S. Breathnach.

Axillary odour appears to require the presence of diphtheroid bacteria, and apocrine sweat can be made odorous by inoculating it with diphtheroids [27].

The limited evidence available suggests that the epitrichial tubular glands are, like the sebaceous glands, controlled by hormones. In the rabbit all three sets of aprocrine glands are stimulated by androgens and inhibited by oestrogens [63, 68]. The glands are larger in males than in females, and start to become so at sexual maturity.

Phylogenetically, it is clear that the apocrine glands of the human axillary and pubic regions are more likely to be concerned with scent than with temperature control. Circumstantial evidence suggests that androgens play a part in controlling their secretion, since they do not become active until puberty, at the same time as the development of the sexual hair, which is part of the odour-disseminating apparatus. The report that implantation of androgens into the axillae of human males does not affect the activity of the apocrine glands [60] does not prove the contrary, since such glands, like the sebaceous glands in adult males [64], may already be under maximal stimulation by endogenous androgens.

REFERENCES

1 ALBONE E.S. (1984) *Mammalian Semiochemistry*. Chichester, John Wiley and Sons.
2 BELL M. (1974) *J Invest Dermatol* **63**, 147.
3 BIRD S. & GOWER D.B. (1981) *J Steroid Biochem* **14**, 213.
4 BIRD S. & GOWER D.B. (1982) *J Steroid Biochem* **17**, 517.
5 BLIGH J. (1967) *Environment Res* **1**, 28.
6 CLAUS R. & ALSING W. (1978) *J Endocr* **68**, 483.
7 CURTIS R.F., *et al* (1971) *Nature* **232**, 396.
8 DOTY R.L. (1976) *Mammalian Olfaction Reproductive Processes and Behaviour*, London & New York, Academic Press, p. 1.
9 DRYDEN G.L. & CONAWAY C.H. (1967) *J Mammal* **48**, 420.
10 EBLING F.J.G. (1981) In *The Biology of Aggression*. Eds. Brain P.F. & Benton D. Alphen aan den Rijn, Sijthoff & Noordhoff, p. 301.
11 ELLIS H. (1905) *Studies in the Psychology of Sex, IV Sexual Selection in Man*. Philadelphia, F.A. Davies, p. 44.

12 ELLIS R.A. (1967) In *Ultrastructure of Normal and Abnormal Skin.* Ed. Zelickson A.S. Philadelphia, Lea & Febiger, p. 132.

13 GABE M. (1967) in *Traité de Zoologie.* Vol. XVI. I: Mammifères. Ed. Grassé P. Paris, Masson et Cie, p. 1.

14 GOODRICH B.S. & MYKYTOWYCZ R. (1972) *J Mammal* **53**, 450.

15 GOWER D.B. (1972) *J Steroid Biochem* **3**, 45.

16 GOWER D.B. & COOKE G.M. (1983) *J Steroid Biochem* **19**, 1527.

17 HANSON G. & MONTAGNA W. (1962) *Am J Phys Anthropol* **20**, 421.

18 HASHIMOTO K., et al (1966) *J Invest Dermatol* **46**, 387.

19 HIBBS R.G. (1962) *J Invest Dermatol* **38**, 77.

20 JENKINSON D.M. (1967) *Br Vet J* **123**, 311.

21 JENKINSON D.M. (1973) *Br J Dermatol* **88**, 397.

22 KEVERNE E.B. & MICHAEL R.P. (1971) *J Endocrinol* **51**, 313.

23 KNEELAND J.E. (1966) *Z Zellforsch Microsk Anat* **73**, 521.

24 KUROSUMI K., et al (1959) *Arch Histol Jap* **16**, 523.

25 KUROSUMI K., et al (1961) *Z Zellforsch Microsk Anat* **55**, 297.

26 LE MAGNEN J. (1952) *Arch Sci Physiol* **6**, 125.

27 LEYDEN J.J., et al (1981) *J Invest Dermatol* **77**, 413.

28 LYNE A.G., et al (1964) *Aust J Zool* **12**, 341.

29 MACHIDA J. & MONTAGNA W. (1964) *Am J Phys Anthropol* **22**, 443.

30 MICHAEL R.P. & SAAYMAN G.S. (1968) *J Endocrinol* **41**, 231.

31 MICHAEL R.P. & WELEGALLA J. (1968) *J Endocrinol* **41**, 407.

32 MICHAEL R.P., et al (1971) *Science* **172**, 964.

33 MONTAGNA W. & YUN J.S. (1962) *Am J Phys Anthrop* **20**, 95.

34 MONTAGNA W. & YUN J.S. (1962) *Am J Phys Anthrop* **20**, 131.

35 MONTAGNA W. & YUN J.S. (1962) *Am J Phys Anthropol* **20**, 149.

36 MONTAGNA W. & YUN J.S. (1963) *Am J Phys Anthropol* **21**, 189.

37 MONTAGNA W., et al (1953) *Am J Anat* **92**, 451.

38 MONTAGNA W., et al (1962) *Am J Phys Anthropol* **20**, 431.

39 MONTAGNA W., et al (1964) *Am J Phys Anthropol* **22**, 307.

40 MONTAGNA W., et al (1966) *Am J Phys Anthropol* **24**, 71.

41 MÜLLER-SCHWARZE D. & MOZELL M.M. (1977) *Chemical Signals in Vertebrates.* New York, Plenum Press, p. 1.

42 MUNGER B.L. (1965) *Z Zellforsch* **67**, 373.

43 MUNGER B.L. (1965) *Z Zellforsch* **68**, 837.

44 MYKYTOWYCZ R. (1965) *Anim Behav* **13**, 400.

45 MYKYTOWYCZ R. (1966) *C.S.I.R.O. Wildl Res* **11**, 11.

46 MYKYTOWYCZ R. (1966) *C.S.I.R.O. Wildl Res* **11**, 49.

47 MYKYTOWYCZ R. (1966) *C.S.I.R.O. Wildl Res* **11**, 65.

48 MYKYTOWYCZ R. & DUDZINSKI M.L. (1966) *C.S.I.R.O. Wildl Res* **11**, 31.

49 MYKYTOWYCZ T. & GOODRICH B.S. (1974) *J Invest Dermatol* **62**, 124.

50 PARAKKAL P., et al (1962) *Anat Rec* **143**, 169.

51 QUAY W.B. (1962) *J Mammal* **43**, 303.

52 QUAY W.B. (1965) *J Mammal* **46**, 23.

53 QUAY W.B. (1970) In *Biology of Bats.* Ed. Wimsatt W.A. (1970) New York, Academic Press, Vol. 2, p. 1.

54 RALLS K. (1971) *Science* **171**, 443.

55 ROBERTSHAW D. (1974) *J Invest Dermatol* **63**, 160.

56 ROBERTSHAW D. (1983) In *Biochemistry and Physiology of the Skin.* Ed. Goldsmith L.A. New York, Oxford University Press, p. 642.

57 RUSSELL M.J. (1976) *Nature* **260**, 520.

58 SCHIEFFERDECKER P. (1917) *Biol Zbl* **37**, 534.

59 SCHIEFFERDECKER P. (1922) *Zoologica* **27**, 1.

60 SHELLEY W.B. & HURLEY H.J. (1957) *J Invest Dermatol* **28**, 155.

61 SINGER A.G., et al (1976) *Science* **191**, 948.

62 SINK J.D. (1967) *J Theoret Biol* **17**, 174.

63 STRAUSS J.S. & EBLING F.J. (1970) *Mem Soc Endocrinol* **18**, 341.

64 STRAUSS J.S., et al (1962) *J Invest Dermatol* **39**, 139.

65 THIESSEN D. & YAHR P. (1977) *The Gerbil in Behavioural Investigations.* Austin and London, University of Texas Press, p. 1.

66 WAITES G.M.H. & VOGLMAYR J.K. (1962) *Nature* **196**, 965.

67 WAITES G.M.H. & VOGLMAYR J.K. (1963) *Aust J Agricul Res* **14**, 839.

68 WALES N.A.M. & EBLING F.J. (1971) *J Endocrinol* **51**, 763.

69 WEINER J.S. & HELLMANN K. (1960) *Biol Rev* **35**, 141.

ANATOMY AND PHYSIOLOGY OF HUMAN ECCRINE GLANDS
[18, 20, 25, 33, 35]

Eccrine sweat glands are distributed over the whole skin surface, but not on mucous membranes. The numbers vary greatly with site from 620 per cm^2 on the soles to about 120 per cm^2 on the thighs [43]. The total numbers on the body surfaces are between 2 and 5 million and are the same in Negroids as in Caucasoids. Embryologically they are derived from a specialized down-growth of the epidermis at about the fourth month of intrauterine life. No new sweat glands develop after birth. Unlike the apocrine glands they have no developmental relationship with the pilosebaceous follicle, although some glands may eventually come to open into the follicle neck. The gland consists of a secretory coil in the lower dermis and subcutaneous tissue and a duct leading through the dermis to the intra-epidermal sweat duct unit.

The secretory coil contains two types of cell: large clear cells, which are the main secretory cells, and small dark cells, which resemble mucous-secreting cells of other organs [6, 13]. Their function is unknown. All the cells of the secretory coil, unlike those of the duct, are attached to the basement membrane, although individual sections may at times suggest a double layer. Outside the basement membrane are longitudinally arranged myoepithelial cells whose function is probably to support the gland, but they may also help propel the sweat towards the surface. The function of the coil is to produce from plasma a watery isotonic secretion which can subsequently be modified by the duct. The sodium pump in the gland can achieve a pressure up to 500 mmHg [11]. During active secretion, and in certain pathological conditions, well-marked histological changes occur in the gland [34].

The duct consists of two or more layers of relatively uniform cuboidal cells. About one-third of the coil has this histology, as well as the uncoiled part passing up to the epidermis. The duct is not an inert conducting channel; it has active enzyme systems e.g. sodium potassium ATPase, a liberal blood supply and performs an active part in modifying the secretion produced by the coil. On electron-microscopy the cells are found to resemble other cells concerned in sodium transport [13]. It has been suggested that sweat glands do not cool the skin only by evaporation of heat from the surface but also act as heat pipes. According to this theory evaporation of the fluid at the base of the duct allows water vapour to pass up the duct to condense nearer the surface and return to the deeper parts by capillary action. Such systems are a very effective way of transferring heat quickly [44]. The intra-epidermal sweat unit is lined by a layer of specialized cells which may be distinguished sometimes only with difficulty from the surrounding epidermis. On the palm and sole it has a well-developed coil structure which is not so apparent in other sites. Minor variations in the anatomy of sweat glands have been found in several genetically determined conditions [22].

The techniques [42,44,45] for studying the function of the eccrine sweat glands include the following:

1. Collection of sweat in bags or pads [10].
2. Direct measurement of water loss.
3. Microcannulae passed into the duct or coil [38].
4. Measurement of electrical potentials and electrical resistance of the skin, which depends on both the sweat present on the epidermis and the column present within the duct [7,26].
5. Visualization of the individual sweat droplets. This may be achieved by direct microscopy, by *in vivo* staining, by forming plastic impressions [19], or by indicators which become coloured

on contact with water, such as the starch/iodine technique [27], bromophenol blue [42] and quinizarin. The plastic or silicone impression techniques are probably the most reliable and can produce a permanent record.

A simple modification of the starch/iodine test is to dry the skin, paint it with 2% iodine in alcohol, allow it to dry and then to press the skin against a good quality paper. The starch in the paper reacts with iodine in the presence of water so that each sweat droplet shows up as a minute dark spot. Alternatively the starch may be suspended in castor oil (50 g in 100 ml) and painted onto the iodine-treated skin.

The functioning of the eccrine sweat gland is dependent on an intact sympathetic nerve supply. Glands deprived of their postganglionic nerve supply soon cease to respond to any stimuli although they remain histologically normal [40]. The sympathetic nerve supply to sweat glands is unusual in being cholinergic. Adrenergic agents also increase sweat gland activity [2,30,46,48], and a single isolated eccrine gland can respond to both cholinergic and adrenergic stimuli [35]. However, eccrine glands probably have no adrenergic nerve supply and this response seems to play little or no part in the normal control of eccrine sweating in man [35].

The activity of the sympathetic nerves to the sweat gland is controlled by stimuli of three types, thermal, mental and gustatory. Thermal sweating is controlled by the heat-regulating centre in the hypothalamus which is activated by changes in temperature of the blood perfusing it, and also by afferent stimuli from the skin. These afferent stimuli are not the same as those which produce the sensation of warmth. The efferent pathways from the hypothalamus involve nerve fibres relaying in the medulla, lateral horn of the spinal cord and sympathetic ganglia [33,37]. Thermoregulatory sweating occurs especially on the upper trunk and the face [21], but also occurs over the whole body surface, including the palms and soles.

The centres and pathways controlling mental sweating are not fully known. There are centres within the frontal region of the brain. Mental stimuli produce sweating, especially on the palms and soles, perhaps to improve the grip at times of activity. Mental activity also produces some general increase in sweating over the body surface. The activity may be emotional or intellectual, e.g. mental arithmetic. Gustatory sweating is considered on p. 1889.

Other factors may modify the quantity and quality of sweat in the presence of an intact sympathetic nerve supply [33], e.g. local temperature [4], hormones, circulatory changes, axon and spinal reflexes.

By these mechanisms the quantity and quality of sweat may be varied greatly. Under basal conditions there may be few or no impulses passing to the sweat gland. Some insensible perspiration always occurs, partly due to transepidermal water-loss and partly to sweat-gland activity. Only the latter can be suppressed by atropine. Under maximal stimulation the body can produce up to 12 litres in 24 h or for short periods 3 litres in 1 h, which rate exceeds the ability of man to drink [36].

The composition of sweat [16, 32, 33] varies greatly from person to person, time to time, and also from site to site. It has a basic similarity to the plasma from which it is derived. The sweat duct is largely responsible for the modification in concentration which occurs and this will therefore vary with how rapidly the sweat is passing through the duct. Sweat is hypotonic. The most important constituents are Na, Cl, K, urea and lactate. Lactate is found in a concentration of 4–40 meq/l, which greatly exceeds the concentration found in plasma. It is formed in the gland from glucose from the blood [17]. Glucose is present in small quantities only, usually 0–3 mg per 100 ml, although figures up to 11 mg per 100 ml may be found. The pH is 4–6·8.

The concentration of these substances varies greatly in health and disease. Such changes seldom give rise to any symptoms referable to the skin but may help in the understanding of the diseases.

Changes in electrolytes [23] may be found in Cushing's disease, Addison's disease, nephrosis, congestive cardiac failure, and after administration of various hormones, e.g. aldosterone [39] and antidiuretic hormone [14], although the mode of action of these hormones is quite different from that on the kidney. An increase in sweat NaCl has also been reported in patients with miliaria [24]. Of greater importance is the increase in sweat electrolytes which occurs in fibrocystic disease and is sufficiently constant to be a most useful diagnostic test [3, 9, 12, 31]. In the body fluids of these patients there may be CF (cystic fibrosis) factor(s) which disturb the transport capacity of the duct [9, 31]. Sweat may be collected after intradermal injection or iontophoresis of pilocarpine or mecholyl or after heating. In normal children it is most unusual to have sweat Na above 60 meq/l, but the majority of children with fibrocystic disease have levels above this, often above 90 meq/l. Sometimes a normal level is present but not the normal fall after Doca

or aldosterone. In adults the normal levels are higher and the tests of much less value. Initial suggestions that partial forms and carriers of fibrocystic disease could be diagnosed in this way have not been substantiated.

A variety of other substances may be excreted in sweat, e.g. drugs [8], various proteins, antibodies and antigens derived either from the sweat glands themselves or from external sources [5, 15, 28, 29, 41, 47] and substances attractive to insects of which lactate may be one [1].

REFERENCES

1 ACREE F., *et al* (1968) *Science* **161**, 1346.
2 ALLEN J.A. & RODDIE I.L. (1972) *J Physiol* **227**, 801.
3 ANDERSON C.M. & FREEMAN M. (1960) *Arch Dis Child* **35**, 581.
4 BEAUMONT W. VAN & BULLARD R.W. (1965) *Science* **147**, 1465.
5 BERRENS L. & YOUNG E. (1964) *Dermatologica* **128**, 3.
6 BREATHNACH A.S. (1971) *An Atlas of the Ultrastructure of Human Skin*. London, Churchill.
7 CHRISTIE M.J. (1981) *J R Soc Med* **74**, 616.
8 COMAISH J.S. & SHELLEY W.B. (1965) *J Invest Dermatol* **44**, 279.
9 DANN L.G. (1982) *Hosp Update* **8**, 131.
10 DOBSON R.L. & RATNER A.C. (1963) *J Appl Physiol* **18**, 1038.
11 DOBSON R.L. & SATO K. (1970) *Arch Dermatol* **105**, 366.
12 Editorial (1982) *Lancet* **ii**, 1196.
13 ELLIS R.A. (1967) In *Ultrastructure of Normal and Abnormal Skin*. Ed. Zelickson A.S. London, Kimpton.
14 FASCIOLO J.C., *et al* (1969) *J Appl Physiol* **27**, 303.
15 FORSTROM L., *et al* (1975) *J Invest Dermatol* **64**, 156.
16 GORDON R.S. & CAGE G.W. (1966) *Lancet* **i**, 1246.
17 GORDON R.S., *et al* (1971) *J Appl Physiol* **31**, 713.
18 GRICE K. & VERBOV J. (1977) In *Recent Advances in Dermatology*. Vol. 4. Ed. A. Rook. Edinburgh, Churchill Livingstone.
19 HARRIS D.R., *et al* (1972) *J Invest Dermatol* **58**, 78.
20 JARRETT A. (Ed) (1978) *The Physiology and Pathophysiology of the Skin*. Vol. 5. London, Academic Press.
21 KUNO Y. (1956) *Human Perspiration*. Springfield, Thomas.
22 LANDING B.H. & WELLS T.R. (1969) *J Chronic Dis* **21**, 703.
23 LOBITZ W.C. & DOBSON R.L. (1961) *Ann Rev Med* **12**, 209.
24 LOEWENTHAL L.J.A. (1963) *S Afr J Med* **38**, 315.
25 MONTAGNA W. & PARAKKAL P.F. (1974) *The Structure and Function of Skin*. 3rd ed. New York and London, Academic Press.
26 MONTAGNA W., *et al* (1962) *Advances in Biology of Skin*. Oxford, Pergamon.
27 MULLER S.A. & KIERLAND R.R. (1959) *J Invest Dermatol* **32**, 126.
28 PAGE C.O. & RIMINGTON J.S. (1967) *J Lab Clin Med* **69**, 634.

29 PENNEYS N.S., *et al* (1981) *J Am Acad Dermatol* **4**, 401.
30 RANDALL W.C. (1955) *Pharmacol Rev* **7**, 365.
31 Report of the Committee for a study for evaluation of testing for cystic fibrosis (1976) *J Pediatr* **88**, No. 4.
32 ROBINSON S. & ROBINSON A.H. (1954) *Physiol Rev* **34**, 202.
33 ROTHMAN S. (1954) *Physiology and Biochemistry of the Skin*. Chicago, University of Chicago Press.
34 SARGENT F. & DOBSON R.L. (1962) *J Invest Dermatol* **38**, 305.
35 SATO K. (1983) In Goldsmith L.A. *Biochemistry and Physiology of the Skin*. Oxford, Oxford University Press.
36 SCHMIDT-NIELSEN K. (1964) *Desert Animals. Physiological Problems of Heat and Water*. Oxford, Oxford University Press.
37 SCHLIACK H. & SCHIFFTER R. (1979) In *Jadassohn's Handbuch der Haut und Geschlechtskrankheiten*, Band 1 Teil 4A. Berlin, Springer.
38 SCHULZ I. (1969) *J Clin Invest* **48**, 1470.
39 SHUSTER S. (1962) *Proc R Soc Med* **55**, 719.
40 SILVER A., *et al* (1964) *J Invest Dermatol* **42**, 307.
41 SULZBERGER M.B. (1952) *Arch Dermatol Syphil* **66**, 172.
42 SULZBERGER M.B. & HERMANN F. (1954) *The Clinical Significance of Disturbances in the Delivery of Sweat*. Springfield, Thomas.
43 SZABO G. (1967) *Phil Trans R Soc B* **252**, 447.
44 THIELE F.A.J. *et al* (1981) In *Jadasshon's Handbuch der Haut und Geschlechtskrankheiten*. Band 1, Teil 4B. Berlin, Springer.
45 UTTLEY (1972) *J Soc Cos Chem* **23**, 23.
46 WARNDORFF J.A. & HAMER M. (1974) *Br J Dermatol* **90**, 263.
47 WILKINSON R.D., *et al* (1972) *J Invest Dermatol* **57**, 401.
48 WOLF J.E. & MAIBACH H.I. (1974) *Br J Dermatol* **91**, 439.

HYPERHIDROSIS [13, 33]

Hyperhidrosis is excessive production of sweat. In theory when there is over- or under-production of sweat it should be possible to determine whether the change is in the sweat glands, due to pharmacologically-active agents acting on the gland, to abnormal stimulation of the sympathetic pathway between the hypothalamus and the nerve ending, or to over-activity of one of the three different 'centres' responsible for thermoregulatory, mental and gustatory sweating. Any difficult case should be approached from first principles in this way. In practise most cases of hyperhidrosis fall into the following clinical groups:

Generalized or symmetrical hyperhidrosis, following one of the physiological patterns.

(a) Thermoreglutatory. There is marked physiological variation from person to person in the absence of disease. Increase in the temperature of blood bathing the hypothalamus increases heat loss by sweating and by vasodilatation. Some instability of the sweat regulating centre is caused by many febrile conditions, so that sweating may occur at times when there is no fever. This instability may persist for days, or even months, after the fever has subsided, and in some cases is such a prominent feature that the term 'sweating sickness' has been used [5]. Thermoregulatory sweating unlike emotional sweating is usually worse during sleep. Generalized sweating occurs during or after many infective processes, and may be the presenting manifestation of malaria, tuberculosis, brucellosis, etc. A similar mechanism may account for the hyperhidrosis associated with alcohol intoxication or gout and after vomiting. The mechanism of generalized hyperhidrosis which may be associated with diabetic autonomic neuropathy, hyperthyroidism, hyperpituitarism, obesity, the menopause and malignant disease is unknown. Two sisters have been reported who had generalized sweating in a thermal pattern but induced by cold [32].

(b) Mental sweating. Emotional or mental activity increases sweating, especially on the palms, soles, axillae and, to a lesser extent, groin and face. There may be some generalized increase in sweating [2]. Thermal stimuli increase this effect in many cases. Most cases of hyperhidrosis presenting to the dermatologist are of this type, affecting especially the palms, soles and axillae. Although mental or emotional factors are the usual trigger for this type of sweating and in some patients deep-seated emotional disturbances may be found, in many there seems to be no primary emotional disorder. Rather there seems to be some facilitation of the nervous pathway causing physiological mental sweating.

The sweating of the palms and soles may be either continuous or phasic [13]. When continuous it is worse in the summer and not so clearly precipitated by mental factors. When phasic it is usually precipitated by minor emotional or mental activity and is not markedly different in summer and winter. The hands may be cold and show a tendency to acrocyanosis.

Hyperhidrosis may be a real disability so that pools of water drip from the hands onto the floor, or clothing may be saturated. This disorder occurs in either sex and commonly begins in childhood or around puberty. Frequently there is a family history and it is one component of various syndromes in which palmoplantar keratoderma occurs (see Chapter 36). Hyperhidrosis may persist for some years but there is a tendency to spontaneous improvement after the age of 25. Apart from the embarrassing nature of the disorder, complications include pompholyx (see p. 394) and contact dermatitis. Sweating affects the hands, feet and axillae in any combination. Troublesome hyperhidrosis of the feet occurs especially in young adult men. When this is associated with vasomotor changes, so that the sodden skin is also cold and cyanotic, the name symmetrical lividity is sometimes applied. The condition of pitted keratolysis (p. 761) of the feet, due to a cornynebacterial or other infection, is associated with hyperhidrosis.

Axillary sweating is continuous, or more commonly phasic, and may be precipitated by heat or by mental activity. It is uncommon before puberty. Axillary sweating on undressing is very common. Axillary hyperhidrosis is due to over-activity of eccrine glands, unlike axillary odour which is mainly apocrine in origin.

Asymmetrical hyperhidrosis. Excessive sweating may be due to neurological lesions involving any part of the sympathetic pathway from the brain to the nerve ending. It may be the presenting symptom, but it is quite exceptional for this to occur as an isolated phenomenon in the absence of other neurological symptoms or signs. Such lesions may be within the central nervous system [11, 12, 22, 26, 27]—cortex, basal ganglia or spinal cord—or in the peripheral nerves [25]. It must be remembered that the distribution of the sympathetic nerves does not exactly correspond with sensory dermatomes. One sympathetic grey ramus may supply 10 or more sensory segments, and one white ramus extend over at least 5. Asymmetrical sweating may also occur reflexly from visceral disturbances [17], around an area of anhidrosis or due to axon reflex stimulation around, for example, a leg ulcer [26]. Compensatory hyperhidrosis occurs in normal sweat glands remaining when those elsewhere are not functioning because of neurological or skin disease, or after sympathectomy [29] and may then be the presenting symptom (see also Ross' syndrome p. 1891). Functioning sweat gland naevi have been reported [18].

Some bizarre cases of hyperhidrosis remain which cannot be explained in these ways. Areas of skin which may be localized [23] or even as extensive as one half of the body [4] may sweat continuously, or more commonly with mental activity. Sometimes some psychological disturbance accounts for the distribution [31] but more often such cases remain a mystery. They are not usually a manifestation of a progressive neurological lesion.

TREATMENT OF HYPERHIDROSIS

General management. Topical and systemic treatments are by no means satisfactory and at best only temporarily suppressive. In many patients all that is necessary is simple reassurance and explanation of the nature of the disorder, and that it is likely to improve spontaneously, perhaps in several years.

Topical treatment. Atropine-like drugs may be absorbed sufficiently to produce a beneficial local effect without producing systemic side-effects but none of those at present available can be relied upon [21]. Poldine methosulphate 1–4% in alcohol suppresses sweating experimentally, but unfortunately is less valuable on the palms, soles and axillae [10]. The use of dimethyl sulphoxide as a solvent for these drugs is still hardly beyond the experimental stage. Other drugs act by impeding the delivery of sweat to the surface. Formalin 1% soaks have long been used for hyperhidrosis of the feet, but are unsuitable for the hands and axillae. Glutaraldehyde 10% in a buffered solution pH 7·5 swabbed onto the feet thrice weekly has helped some patients [16], but may cause allergic sensitization and stains the skin, so that it is suitable only for the feet. For axillary hyperhidrosis (as opposed to bromhidrosis) the most commonly used topical applications are aluminium (or other metal) salts. Aluminium chloride, the first introduced, is in many ways the best but may be irritant to the skin and clothes. Many other salts, e.g. the chlorhydrate, are in use in cosmetic preparations [15]. Shelley and Hurley have achieved improved results by applying 20% aluminium chloride in absolute ethanol at night, when the axilla is dry, with or without polythene occlusion, at first nightly and later every 1 to 4 weeks [6, 28, 30]. Commercial preparations are available. The same treatment can also be tried on the hands and feet or other localized areas of hyperhidrosis but usually with rather less success. One of the more satisfactory methods of controlling hyperhidrosis of the hands and feet is by iontophoresis, either using tap water or using anticholinergic drugs such as glycopyrrhonium bromide [1, 20]. Once control has been achieved a single treatment may prove effective for some weeks. Minor systemic side-effects with dry mouth and eye symptoms are not uncommon.

Medical treatment. Atropine-like drugs [13] may be used to block the effect of acetylcholine on the sweat glands. They are helpful in some cases but their side-effects are often more troublesome than the hyperhidrosis itself. These include especially dryness of the mouth and disturbances of vision, due to paralysis of accommodation, but more serious side-effects, e.g. glaucoma, hyperthermia and convulsions, occur. Atropine itself is seldom employed. Propantheline (Probanthine) may be prescribed in doses of 15 mg three times daily, increasing if tolerated to as much as 150 mg daily. A variety of other similar drugs, e.g. poldine, have been employed. Ganglion-blocking drugs can inhibit sweating, but side-effects from hypotension are usually too troublesome. In cases with a pronounced emotional factor, sedative or tranquillizing drugs are often helpful, but psychiatric treatment may be necessary.

Surgical treatment. Sympathectomy, where complete, will cause anhidrosis [7, 9]. Unfortunately, sweating tends to return after a period of some years, due either to regeneration of sympathetic fibres or to fibres which do not pass through the sympathetic ganglia [8].

Other disadvantages, apart from the complications of the operation, are that the palms and soles become excessively dry and that all four limbs cannot be treated in this way because of the risk of severe compensatory hyperhidrosis on the body. This may follow an operation on only two limbs. In general only those cases where a severe disability is arising from the hands or feet, but not both, warrant operation, and in selected cases the results can be very gratifying. The bizarre and unexplained areas of localized hyperhidrosis are sometimes dramatically cured by surgical division of the sympathetic pathway.

Axillary hyperhidrosis may be greatly helped by local excision of the axillary vault [3, 14, 24]. The eccrine glands are mainly concentrated in a fairly small area, and excision of such an area, e.g. 4 × 1·5 cm, removes most of the sweat glands.

There is no place for radiotherapy in the treatment of hyperhidrosis.

REFERENCES

1 ABELL E. & MORGAN K. (1974) *Br J Dermatol* **91**, 87.
2 ALLEN J.A., et al (1973) *J Physiol* **235**, 749.
3 BRETTEVILL-JENSEN G., et al (1975) *Acta Derm Venereol (Stockh)* **55**, 73.
4 CHAMPION R.H. & HERXHEIMER A. (1960) *Acta Med (Scand)* **168**, 17.
5 DAVISON W.C. (1960) *Am J Dis Child* **100**, 934.
6 *Drugs and Therapeutics Bulletin* (1981) **19**, 101.
7 ELLIS H. (1979) *Am Surgeon* **45**, 546.
8 GILLESPIE J.A. (1961) *Br Med J* i, 79.
9 GJERRIS F. & OLESEN H.P. (1975) *Acta Neurol Scand* **51**, 167.
10 GRICE K.A. & BETTLEY F.R. (1966) *Br J Dermatol* **78**, 458.
11 GUTTMANN L. (1940) *J Anat* **74**, 537.
12 GUTTMANN L. & LIST C.F. (1928) *Z Ges Neurol Psychiat* **116**, 504.
13 HERXHEIMER A. (1958) *Trans St John's Hosp Dermatol Soc* **40**, 20.
14 HURLEY H.J. & SHELLEY W.B. (1966) *Br J Dermatol* **78**, 127.
15 JASS H.E. (1982) In *Principles of Cosmetics for the Dermatologist.* Eds. Frost P. & Horwitz S.N. St Louis, Mosby. Ch. 13.
16 JUHLIN L. & HANSON H. (1968) *Arch Dermatol* **97**, 327.
17 KORR I.M. (1949) *Fedn Proc Am Soc Exp Biol* **8**, 87.
18 LAPIERE S. (1957) *Dermatologica* **115**, 293.
19 LEIVY D.M., et al (1968) *J Neurosurg* **29**, 65.
20 LEVIT F. (1968) *Arch Dermatol* **98**, 505.
21 MACMILLAN F.S.K., et al (1964) *J Invest Dermatol* **43**, 363.
22 McCOY B.P. (1981) *Arch Dermatol* **117**, 659.
23 MELLINKOFF S.M. (1951) *Am J Med Sci* **221**, 86.
24 MUNRO D.D., et al (1974) *Br J Dermatol* **90**, 325.
25 POOL J.L.J. (1956) *J Neurosurg* **13**, 111.
26 ROTHMAN S. (1954) *Physiology and Biochemistry of the Skin.* Chicago, University of Chicago Press.
27 SCHLIACK H. & SCHIFFTER R. (1979) In *Jadassohn's Handbuch der Haut und Geschlectskrankheiten.* Band 1, Teil 4A. Berlin, Springer.
28 SCHOLES K.T., et al (1978) *Br Med J* ii, 84.
29 SHELLEY W.B. & FLORENCE R. (1960) *N Engl J Med* **263**, 1056.
30 SHELLEY W.B. & HURLEY H.J. (1975) *Acta Derm Venereol (Stockh)* **55**, 241.
31 SHORVON H.J. (1950) *Proc R Soc Med* **43**, 801.
32 SOHAR E., et al (1978) *Lancet* ii, 1073.
33 SULZBERGER M.B. & HERMANN F. (1954) *The Clinical Significance of Disturbances in the Delivery of Sweat.* Springfield, Thomas.

GUSTATORY HYPERHIDROSIS

Sweating on the lips, forehead and nose after eating certain foods occurs physiologically in many persons [5]. Hot, spicy foods are the most likely to cause it. The central connections of this reflex are not fully known.

Gustatory hyperhidrosis also occurs in pathological conditions involving the autonomic nervous system. Localized areas of intense hyperhidrosis may occur on the face [8], and even on the knee [7]. They are very rare, usually start in childhood, and are not progressive. Their nature is little understood. Also uncommon is gustatory hyperhidrosis due to a lesion within the central nervous system [12]. Much the commonest cause is damage to the sympathetic nerves around the head and neck. After damage to sympathetic nerves, regeneration occurs not only from the proximal ends of the dam-

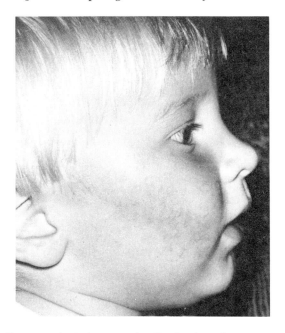

FIG. 51.3. Auriculo-temporal or Von Frey's syndrome, without detectable neurological disorder, presenting as flushing after eating (Dr P. Hudson).

aged sympathetic nerves, but also from damaged or undamaged parasympathetic nerves [2, 10]. In this way abnormal connections are made. Thus the reflex arcs which normally allow chewing or taste stimulation to cause parotid or gastric secretion, may cause sweating in a localized zone corresponding to the area of the skin in which the sympathetic innervation has been damaged. The commonest site is within the distribution of the auriculotemporal nerve following injury, abscess or operation in the parotid region (auriculotemporal or Von Frey's syndrome). Normally afferent impulses from taste stimuli pass via the 7th or 9th nerve and efferent fibres for the parotid gland via the tympanic branch of the 9th nerve, the lesser superficial petrosal nerve, and otic ganglion to the auriculotemporal nerve [1]. The sympathetic nerve supply to sweat glands from the superior cervical ganglion also passes with the auriculotemporal nerve from the external carotid plexus. Similarly, submental gustatory sweating [13, 14] follows injuries involving the chorda tympani, and sweating in the distribution of the greater auricular nerve commonly follows radical neck surgery [6]. On the upper arm, fibres from the vagus may cause gustatory sweating after cervical sympathectomy [3]. Gustatory sweating also occurs in diabetes as part of a widespread autonomic neuropathy [11].

Gustatory sweating is by no means uncommon and occurs in 50–80% of patients subjected to operations on the parotid gland [4, 9]. Usually the symptoms appear some 4–7 months after operation and either persist indefinitely or wane after 3–5 years. The stimuli required to initiate the reflex vary as does the severity. Sometimes chewing, without taste sensation, is the most important stimulus. In many cases it is merely a curiosity but in others a real disability. As well as sweating there is usually vasodilation which rarely occurs by itself in the absence of visible sweating.

Treatment of severe cases may require surgical interruption of the parasympathetic pathway, e.g. section of the glossopharyngeal nerve within the skull or tympanic neurectomy [2]. Excision of the auriculotemporal nerve is usually followed by recurrence. Topical therapy (see p. 1888) may be helpful.

REFERENCES

1 GLAISTER D.H., *et al* (1958) *Br Med J* ii, 942.
2 HARRISON K. & DONALDSON I. (1979) *J R Soc Med* **72**, 503.
3 HERXHEIMER A. (1958) *Br Med J* i, 688.
4 LAAGE-HELLMAN J.E. (1957) *Acta Otolaryngo* **48**, 234.
5 LIST C.F. & PEET M.M. (1938) *Arch Neurol Psychiat* **40**, 269, 443.
6 McGIBBON B.M. & PALLETA F.X. (1972) *Plast Reconstr Surg* **49**, 639.
7 MELLINKOFF S.M. & MELLINKOFF M.J. (1950) **143**, 901.
8 MONRO P.A.G. (1959) *Sympathectomy*. Oxford, Oxford University Press.
9 MOYSE P. (1955) *Mem Acad Chir* **81**, 999.
10 MURRAY J.G. & THOMPSON J.W. (1957) *J Physiol* **135**, 133.
11 WATKINS P.J. (1973) *Br Med J* i, 583.
12 WILSON W.C. (1956) *Clin Sci* **2**, 273.
13 YOUNG A.G. (1956) *Br Med J* ii, 976.
14 YOUNG A.G. (1960) *Br Med J* i, 620.

DYSHIDROSIS

The role of sweating in the production of pompholyx, or vesicular eczema of the palms or soles, is discussed on p. 394.

GRANULOSIS RUBRA NASI

The pathogenesis of this rare disease is obscure. Most cases are genetically determined, but the mode of inheritance is uncertain [3, 4].

The disease usually starts in early childhood from the sixth month to the tenth year [2]. Excessive sweating may precede other changes by several years [1]. Diffuse erythema first appears on the tip of the nose, gradually extends and may involve the cheeks, the upper lip and the chin. The erythema is covered by small beads of sweat which may also be evident over a wider area. Small red macules and papules, and sometimes vesicles, later form at the sweat duct orifices. The condition usually subsides spontaneously at puberty, but may persist indefinitely. In such cases telangiectasia becomes a conspicuous feature, and small cysts may be present. Many of those affected have poor peripheral circulation and hyperhidrosis of the palms and soles. Response to treatment is usually disappointing.

REFERENCES

1 GRIXONI F. (1955) *G Ital Derm Sif* **96**, 227.
2 MASCHKILLEISSON L.N. & NARADOW L.A. (1935) *Derm Z* **71**, 79.
3 TOURAINE A. (1955) *L'Hérédité en Médicine*. Paris, Masson et Cie, p. 551.
4 VELTMAN G. (1949) *Arch Klin Exp Dermatol* **188**, 188.

ANHIDROSIS [4, 10, 11]

Definition. Anhidrosis is the absence of sweat from the surface of the skin in the presence of an appropriate stimulus.

Aetiology. Anhidrosis may be due to an abnormality of the sweat gland itself or at any level in the nervous pathway. There are many causes [11]; some of the more important are as follows:

Brain
  Organic lesion at any level
  Hysteria
  Hyperthermia
Spinal cord and peripheral nerves
  Organic lesion, e.g. syringomyelia, leprosy, sympathectomy, diabetes mellitus and other causes of autonomic neuropathy [1, 7, 8]
  Ganglion-blocking and anticholinergic drugs
Sweat gland
  Aplasia
  Congenital ectodermal dysplasia, ichthyosis
    Any cause of atrophy, e.g. acrodermatitis atrophicans chronica, mepacrine eruption, scleroderma, myelomatosis, reticulosis, Sjögren's disease.
  Plugging
    Miliaria
    Eczema and atopic dermatitis
    Lichen planus
    Psoriasis
Uncertain
  Neonatal
  Sweat gland fatigue
  Idiopathic acquired anhidrosis [3]

Extensive anhidrosis may impair heat regulation to such a degree that hyperpyrexia occurs on exposure to heat. It characteristically occurs in anhidrotic ectodermal dysplasia and in otherwise normal premature or full-term infants under the age of 1 month [2]. It may be associated with compensatory hyperhidrosis of the remaining functionally active glands. It has been reported as an isolated finding [9]. Cessation of sweating is the cause of heat hyperpyrexia (see p. 1893). The anhidrosis associated with ichthyosis may be more apparent than real [13]. Localized areas of anhidrosis are of little clinical importance, except that they may help in the diagnosis of neurological lesions or of leprosy. Sweat retention is the cause of miliaria (see below), and plays an important part in producing crises of irritation in patients with atopic dermatitis, eczema and other dermatoses. It also occurs in psoriasis, where sweat-duct blockage and perhaps also impaired ductal absorption occur [6, 12].

Ross's syndrome [5]. This rare syndrome consists of widespread hypohidrosis combined with patchy sometimes very striking compensatory hyperhidrosis, together with a tonic pupil and loss of reflexes (Holmes–Adie syndrome). The changes are due to selective degeneration of the sympathetic pathways.

REFERENCES

1 EWING D.J. & CLARKE B.F. (1982) *Br Med J* **285**, 916.
2 FOSTER K.G., *et al* (1968) *J Physiol* **198**, 36 P.
3 GORDON B., *et al* (1964) *Arch Dermatol* **90**, 347.
4 GRICE K. & VERBOV J. (1977) In *Recent Advances in Dermatology*. Vol. 4. Ed. A Rook. Edinburgh, Churchill Livingstone.
5 HEATH P.D., *et al* (1982) *Neurology* **32**, 1041.
6 JOHNSON C. & SHUSTER S. (1969) *Br J Dermatol* **81**, 119.
7 JOHNSON R.H. & SPALDING J.M.K. (1974) *Disorders of the Autonomic Nervous System*. Oxford University Press.
8 JOHNSON R.H. & SPALDING J.M.K. (1976) *Br J Hosp Med* **15**, 266.
9 MAHLOUDJI M. & LIVINGSTON K.E. (1967) *Am J Dis Child* **113**, 477.
10 SHELLEY W.B. (1961) *Arch Dermatol* **83**, 903.
11 *SHELLEY W.B., *et al* (1950) *Medicine* **29**, 195.
12 SHUSTER S. & JOHNSON C. (1969) *Br J Dermatol* **81**, 846.
13 SULZBERGER M.F., *et al* (1959) *Int Arch Allergy Appl Immunol* **14**, 129.

MILIARIA

Aetiology and pathology [2, 4, 11]. The three forms of miliaria—miliaria crystallina (sudamina), miliaria rubra (prickly heat) and miliaria profunda (mamillaria)—represent different levels of obstruction of the sweat duct. In miliaria crystallina the obstruction is very superficial and the vesicle subcorneal. In miliaria rubra [2, 6, 9] the later changes include keratinization of the intra-epidermal part of the sweat duct, with leakage and then formation of a vesicle around the duct. In miliaria profunda there is rupture of the duct at the level of the dermo-epidermal junction.

Miliaria crystallina can easily be produced experimentally by minimal non-specific epidermal injury and profuse sweating [13]. It is often seen in febrile illnesses associated with profuse sweating.

The incidence of miliaria rubra is highest in hot, humid conditions but it may occur in desert regions. It affects up to 30% of people exposed to these climatic conditions [8, 10]. It may begin within a few days of arrival in a tropical climate but is maximal after 2–5 months [10]. There is a striking variation in individual susceptibility. Infants are especially prone. Lesions may be produced experimentally in susceptible subjects by epidermal injury. They can be reproduced regularly by occlusion of the skin under polythene for 3 to 4 days, following which anhidrosis lasts for about 3 weeks. Clinically prolonged exposure of the skin to sweat achieves the same effect. Hölzle and Kligman [2] have recently suggested that the first event is an increase in the skin flora, especially cocci, and that these may produce a toxin which damages the luminal cells and induces a PAS positive amorphous mass deep in the acrosyringium. The parakeratotic plugs which are a notable feature of the later stages of the disease are not the primary cause of the obstruction but arise in the repair process and may further aggravate the obstruction. Leakage of sweat into the epidermis is responsible for the final production of the lesions and for further aggravation of them.

Miliaria profunda is due to more severe damage to the sweat duct and usually follows repeated attacks of miliaria rubra. It may be reproduced by experimental injury [12].

Clinical features

Miliaria crystallina. Clear, thin-walled vesicles, 1–2 mm in diameter, without an inflammatory areola and symptomless, develop in crops, mainly on the trunk. In persistent febrile illnesses recurrent crops may occur. The vesicles soon rupture and are followed by superficial branny desquamation.

Miliaria rubra. The typical lesions develop on the body, especially in areas of friction with clothing and in flexures. They may also commonly be seen after occlusive therapy with polythene. The lesions are uniformly minute erythematous papules which may be present in very large numbers. Characteristically they lead to intense discomfort which is not so much itching demanding scratching as an unbearable pricking sensation. In infants lesions commonly appear on the neck, groins and axillae, but also occur on the face and elsewhere.

Miliaria profunda. This nearly always follows repeated attacks of miliaria rubra and is uncommon except in the tropics. The lesions are easily missed. The affected skin is covered with pale, firm papules 1–3 mm across, especially on the body, but sometimes also on the limbs. There is no itching or discomfort from the lesions.

Natural history. The course depends mainly on environmental factors. If continued sweating occurs, recurrent episodes lasting a few days are usual or discomfort may be continuous. However, after a few months some degree of acclimatization occurs and the disorder becomes less prevalent.

The most important complications of miliaria are secondary infection and disturbance of heat regulation. Secondary bacterial infection is common and sometimes serious. This may present as an ordinary impetigo. In other cases the pustules are more clearly related to sweat ducts, although in pustular miliaria factors other than bacterial infection are concerned [5]. Periporitis staphylogenes [7] is the name given to multiple staphyloccal abscesses superimposed on miliaria rubra in young infants. In most cases of miliaria rubra the changes are reversible if further sweating is avoided but permanent damage to the sweat duct may occur, especially after miliaria profunda.

Diagnosis. The diagnosis of typical miliaria seldom presents real difficulty. Sweat retention as a cause of itching in eczema and other dermatoses should be suspected when crises of irritation occur on heating, although it may be difficult to prove.

Treatment. The only really effective prevention or treatment for miliaria is avoidance of further sweating. Even if this is achieved only for a few hours a day, as in an air-conditioned office or bedroom, considerable relief is experienced. For the very susceptible person a move away from tropical climates may be essential. Avoidance of excessive clothing, friction with clothing, excessive soap and contact of the skin with irritants will reduce the incidence. Vitamin C 1 g daily has been reported to help many cases [1]. The large number of treatments advocated for prickly heat is the best indication of their relative ineffectiveness if sweating is not reduced. In the absence of gross secondary sepsis the effect of topical or systemic antibiotics or other antibacterial preparations on established miliaria is disappointing but they may have some role in prophylaxis [2]. Calamine lotion is probably as effective as anything for the relief of discomfort, but because of its drying effect a bland emollient, e.g. oily cream, may subsequently be required to prevent further epidermal damage.

REFERENCES

1 HINDSON T.C. & WORSLEY D.E. (1969) *Br J Dermatol* **81**, 226.
2 HÖLZLE E. & KLIGMAN A.M. (1978) *Br J Dermatol* **99**, 117.
3 LEITHEAD C.S. & LIND A.R. (1964) *Heat Stress and Heat Disorders*. London, Cassell.
4 LOBITZ W.C. (1962) In *Dermatoses due to Environmental and Physical Factors*. Ed. Rees R.B. Springfield, Thomas.
5 LOBITZ W.C. (1952) *JAMA* **148**, 1097.
6 LOEWENTHAL L.J.A. (1961) *Arch Dermatol* **84**, 2.
7 LUBOWE I.I. & PERLMAN H.H. (1954) *Arch Dermatol* **69**, 543.
8 LYONS R.E., *et al* (1962) *Arch Dermatol* **86**, 282.
9 O'BRIEN J.P. (1950) *J Invest Dermatol* **15**, 95.
10 SANDERSON P.H. & SLOPER J.C. (1953) *Br J Dermatol* **65**, 252.
11 SARGENT F. & SLUTZKY H.L. (1957) *N Engl J Med* **256**, 401, 451.
12 SHELLEY W.B. (1951) *J Invest Dermatol* **16**, 53.
13 SHELLEY W.B. & HORVATH P.N. (1950) *J Invest Dermatol* **14**, 193.

HEAT STRESS

A full consideration of the various problems of adaptation to hot climates [7] and syndromes caused by heat [6, 2] is beyond the scope of this book. Their terminology is confused. Although there is inevitably some overlap the classification in Table 51.1 is acceptable [5, 6]:

The mechanisms whereby acclimatization occurs are still largely unknown [2]. After a time in a hot climate the glands are able to secrete sweat containing much reduced quantities of sodium and chloride. This may be due partly to an effect of aldosterone. Experimentally after prolonged periods of secreting, sweat gland fatigue occurs. Again the mechanism is obscure but includes changes in the glands demonstrable histologically [1].

Table 51.1

1. Disorders secondary to thermoregulation which result from the processes of thermoregulation
    Heat syncope. Fainting due to loss of vasomotor tone in the absence of gross water or salt depletion; common and mild
    Heat oedema
    Water depletion heat exhaustion, i.e. dehydration
    Salt depletion heat exhaustion
    Heat cramps, similar to and usually part of salt depletion heat exhaustion, but clinically a distinct syndrome which may occur by itself
    Miliaria
    Anhidrotic heat exhaustion–the anhidrosis is usually considered secondary to severe miliaria
2. Failure of thermoregulation
    Heat stroke and heat hyperpyrexia
    Sudden failure of sweating due either to failure of the thermoregulatory centre, to sweat gland fatigue, or in some cases, to water depletion
3. Psychological effects
    Acute heat fatigue
    Chronic heat fatigue

REFERENCES

1 DOBSON R.L. (1960) *J Invest Dermatol* **35**, 195.
2 Editorial (1979) *Lancet* i, 910.
3 GOTTSCHALK P.G. & THOMAS J.E. (1966) *Mayo Clin Proc* **41**, 470.
4 JOHNSON B.B., *et al* (1969) *J Invest Dermatol* **53**, 116.
5 LEITHEAD C.S. (1964) *Lancet* ii, 637.
6 LEITHEAD C.S. & LIND A.R. (1964) *Heat Stress and Heat Disorders*. London, Cassell.
7 SCHMIDT-NIELSEN K. (1964) *Desert Animals. Physiological Problems of Heat and Water*. Oxford University Press.

APOCRINE SWEAT GLANDS

Anatomy and physiology [1, 4, 7]. Apocrine sweat glands derive their name from the way their secretion appears on light microscopy to be derived by pinching off parts of the cytoplasm. They are epidermal appendages and develop as part of the pilosebaceous follicle in the fourth to fifth month of intrauterine life [6]. In the embryo they are present throughout the skin surface but most of the glands subsequently disappear, so that in the adult the characteristic distribution in the axilla, perianal region and areola of the breasts is found. So-called ectopic glands may be found elsewhere. The mammary glands and glands in the external auditory meatus are modified apocrine glands. Apocrine glands are poorly developed in childhood and begin to enlarge with the approach of puberty. The activity of the glands is androgen dependent and the

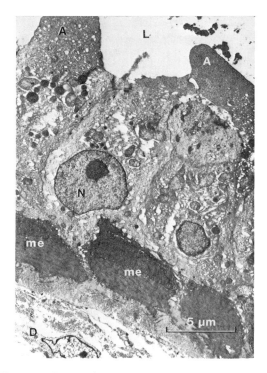

FIG. 51.4. Section of secretory coil of an apocrine gland from the human axilla. Lying next to the basement membrane are myo-epithelial cells (me), followed by cuboidal secretory cells, with prominent nuclei (N) and apical caps (A) projecting into the lumen (L). D = dermis. Electron micrograph by Professor A. S. Breathnach.

glands show marked testosterone 5α-reductase activity [10]. The glands are larger than eccrine glands and in the dissected specimen are visible to the naked eye. They are situated in the subcutaneous tissue. Each consists of a tubule and a duct which opens into the neck of the hair follicle above the sebaceous gland. Despite their embryological origin from the hair follicle, some apocrine glands eventually come to open on the surface of the skin. The secretory coil is a simple convoluted tube which may show some branching and anastomosis. It is lined by a single layer of columnar or cuboidal cells resting on a basement membrane. The free edge of the cells may show the appearance of apocrine secretion. Electron microscopy shows that this may be partly an artefact but evidence of eccrine, apocrine and even holocrine secretion may all be found in places [2, 7, 9]. The apocrine duct closely resembles the eccrine duct and consists of a double layer of cuboidal cells. Outside the basement membrane of the glands and duct is a longitudinal layer of myoepithelial cells. Their function is to support the

duct and to propel the secretion to the surface and waves of peristalsis have been seen in them [3]. Where the duct opens into the neck of the hair follicle there is the equivalent of the acrosyringium of the eccrine duct, although it is less obvious [11].

Apocrine glands secrete very small quantities of an oily fluid which may be coloured. This secretion is odourless on reaching the surface and bacterial decomposition is responsible for the characteristic odours. The glands have no apparent function in man, although they may play some part in human olfactory communication; they play no part in thermoregulation. The epithelium of the secretory coil produces its secretion continuously, with some variation depending on hormonal factors, e.g. menstruation and pregnancy. Nervous control of secretion is unimportant and it is even disputed whether the glands have any motor innervation [6, 8]. Expulsion of apocrine sweat may occur continuously or be provoked by emotional stimuli. The ducts have an adrenergic sympathetic nerve supply and are also stimulated by circulating adrenaline. It seems possible that histologically normal apocrine glands may fail to produce any secretion, and that only the axillary glands in man are important in producing body odour [5].

REFERENCES

1 BIEMPICA L. & MONTES L.F. (1965) *Am J Anat* **117**, 47.
2 HASHIMOTO K., *et al* (1966) *J Invest Dermatol* **46**, 378.
3 HURLEY H.J. & SHELLEY W.B. (1954) *J Invest Dermatol* **22**, 143.
4 *HURLEY H.J. & SHELLEY W.B. (1960) *The Human Apocrine Sweat Gland in Health and Disease*. Springfield, Thomas.
5 KLIGMAN A.M. & SHEHADEK N. (1964) *Arch Dermatol* **89**, 461.
6 MONTAGNA W. (1964) *J Invest Dermatol* **42**, 119.
7 MONTAGNA W. & PARAKKAL P.F. (1974) *The Structure and Function of Skin*. 3rd ed. New York and London, Academic Press.
8 ROBERTSHAW D. (1974) *J Invest Dermatol* **63**, 160.
9 SCHAUMBERG-LEVER G. & LEVER W.F. (1975) *J Invest Dermatol* **64**, 38.
10 TAKAYASU S., *et al* (1980) *J Invest Dermatol* **74**, 187.
11 TANI M., *et al* (1980) *J Invest Dermatol* **75**, 431.

Bromhidrosis. Osmidrosis [3, 5]. Odour of the skin in man is, to a large extent, determined by apocrine gland secretion, although there are other sources. Sebaceous secretion has some odour, and decomposition of products of keratinization, especially in the presence of hyperhidrosis, produces offensive smells. Eccrine secretion is usually odourless, but various substances may be excreted in it, e.g. garlic, drugs, arsenic. Characteristic odours may be associated with various uncommon amino-acidurias [1, 7]. Old textbooks of medicine report that sweat has a characteristic odour in gout, diabetes, scurvy, typhoid and other diseases [8]. An unusual case of generalized bromhidrosis due to a nasal foreign body has been recorded [2] and we have seen five such cases. Other patients complaining of body odour may be suffering from paranoia, phobias or from organic lesions of the central nervous system.

Apocrine secretion is often stated to be odourless as it reaches the surface, apart from excreted substances like garlic. Bacterial decomposition liberates fatty acids, etc., with characteristic smells. This process occurs only after some hours and frequent removal of apocrine sweat prevents its decomposition. A strong axillary odour tends to be associated with a richer bacterial flora and especially with more Corynebacteria [4, 6]. There is marked individual and racial variation in body odour and what is socially acceptable varies greatly with race and social upbringing. Treatment of axillary bromhidrosis includes omission of food-stuffs like garlic from the diet, frequent washing of the axillary regions, and local antibacterial substances [5]. There is little evidence that measures used to control axillary eccrine hyperhidrosis, e.g. aluminium salts and anticholinergic drugs, have much effect on the apocrine glands, although excessive eccrine excretion may favour spread of the apocrine secretion.

REFERENCES

1 CONE T.E. (1968) *Pediatrics* 41, 993.
2 GOLDING I.M. (1965) *Pediatrics* 36, 791.
3 HURLEY H.J. & SHELLEY W.B. (1960) *The Human Apocrine Sweat Gland in Health and Disease*. Springfield, Thomas.
4 JACKMAN P.J.H. (1982) *Semin Dermatol* 1, 143.
5 LABOWS J.N., et al (1982) In *Principles of cosmetics for the dermatologist*. Eds. Frost P. & Horwitz S.N. St Louis, Mosby, Ch. 12.
6 LEYDEN J.J., et al (1981) *J Invest Dermatol* 77, 413.
7 MARKS R., et al (1977) *Br J Dermatol* 96, 399.
8 SMITH M., et al (1982) *Lancet* ii, 1452.

Chromhidrosis [2, 3]. The more dramatic cases of coloured sweat are very rare and are due to coloured apocrine secretion. However, coloured sweat may have other origins. The term pseudo-chromhidrosis is applied when initially colourless sweat becomes coloured on the surface of the skin. The commonest origin is chromogenic bacteria, especially corynebacteria, which are not uncommonly present on the axillary skin and hair. Treatment is a matter of careful hygiene and, if neces-

sary, a topical antibacterial agent. Dyes may also be derived from clothing. Bacterial activity may liberate coloured material from uncoloured precursors excreted in eccrine sweat. True eccrine chromhidrosis is uncommon and when present is seldom of great intensity. The commonest causes are ingested drugs and dyes.

Apocrine sweat is coloured yellow, blue or green in 10% of normal persons, but this is not sufficient to give rise to any symptoms. Extremely rare are the cases where localized areas of skin become intensely discoloured. The sites are not usually those where apocrine glands normally occur. The face is the commonest. Ectopic apocrine glands can be found in these sites. The colour may be black, violet, blue, brown, yellow or green, but red is very rare. Different names have been applied according to the colours. The pigment is a lipofuscin. The patient complains of discoloration of the skin, continuously or intermittently. It is possible to see small beads of discoloration representing individual sweat droplets. This disorder starts at any age and usually persists. The only treatment is surgical. The phenomenon of coloured milk is essentially similar [1].

REFERENCES

1 GREIG D.M. (1930) *Edin Med J* 37, 524.
2 HURLEY H.J. & SHELLEY W.B. (1960) *The Human Apocrine Sweat Gland in Health and Disease*. Springfield, Thomas.
3 SHELLEY W.B. & HURLEY H.J. (1954) *Arch Dermatol* 69, 449.

Haematohidrosis. Bloody sweat is exceptionally uncommon. The red sweat of the hippopotamus is not due to blood. True haematohidrosis may occur in bleeding disorders [2]. The remarkable phenomenon of stigmatization [1], when blood wells from the skin of the palms and elsewhere, is not related to sweat gland activity.

REFERENCES

1 KLAUDER J.V. (1938) *Arch Dermatol* 37, 650.
2 RADCLIFFE-CROCKER H. (1903) *Diseases of the Skin*. 3rd ed. London, Lewis, p. 1031.

FOX-FORDYCE DISEASE

Aetiology and pathology [3]. Fox-Fordyce disease is a disorder of the apocrine glands comparable to prickly heat of the eccrine glands. The aetiology is unknown. Hormonal influences are important but there is little evidence of a primary hormonal abnormality. The earliest visible change histologically

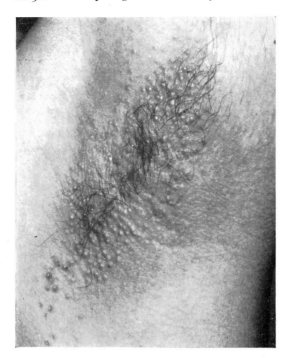

FIG. 51.5. Fox-Fordyce disease (Addenbrooke's Hospital).

is a small vesicle in the apocrine duct [7]. This progresses to an inflammatory lesion, followed by rupture and plugging of the duct. Apocrine sweat retention therefore follows.

Clinical features. The disease occurs mainly in women soon after puberty. It can occur in males or in children. It has been reported in identical twins [2]. Itching, which may be intense, occurs in the axillae and to a lesser extent in the anogenital region and around the breasts. Objectively there may be little to see at first but later there develop skin-coloured, or slightly pigmented dome-shaped follicular papules. The itching is often provoked by those emotional stimuli which normally cause apocrine secretion. The disease runs a very prolonged course and may persist until the menopause. Some remission may occur in pregnancy.

Treatment. Response to treatment is unsatisfactory. Topical corticosteroids help some cases. Treatment with 4–6 weekly doses of UVR, sufficient to cause exfoliation, helps some cases [6]. Topical retinoic acid may also be helpful [1], as may oral contraceptive agents [4, 5]. Other cases are sufficiently severe to require surgical excision of the affected skin or subcutaneous removal of the apocrine glands.

REFERENCES

1 GIACOBETTI R., *et al* (1979) *Arch Dermatol* **115**, 1365.
2 GRAHAM J.H., *et al* (1960) *Arch Dermatol* **82**, 212.
3 HURLEY H.J. & SHELLEY W.B. (1960) *The Human Apocrine Sweat Gland in Health and Disease*. Springfield, Thomas.
4 KRONTHAL H.L., *et al* (1965) *Arch Dermatol* **91**, 243.
5 LEYH F. (1973) *Hautarzt* **24**, 482.
6 PINKUS H. (1973) *JAMA* **223**, 924.
7 SHELLEY W.B. & LEVY E.J. (1956) *Arch Dermatol* **73**, 38.

HIDRADENITIS SUPPURATIVA

(see p. 785)

CHAPTER 52

The Sebaceous Glands

F. J. G. EBLING & W. J. CUNLIFFE

STRUCTURE, FUNCTION AND DISTRIBUTION

The sebaceous gland [25] is holocrine; its secretion is formed by complete disintegration of the glandular cells (Fig. 52.1). The cells are replaced by cell division at the periphery of the lobes or acini of the glands, with the consequence that differentiating cells are displaced towards the centres of the acinus. The average transit time of the cells, from formation to discharge, has been given as 7·4 days in the human gland [10], a figure similar to that estimated for the rat [3, 8]. However, the dynamics of the human gland are complicated. The gland consists of a series of lobes, each with a duct lined by a keratinizing squamous epithelium. The lobule ducts converge towards the main sebaceous duct, which normally opens into the pilary canal and whose epithelium is continuous with the surface epidermis. Within any one glandular unit the acini vary in differentiation and maturity; some are completely undifferentiated, showing little or no lipid accumu-

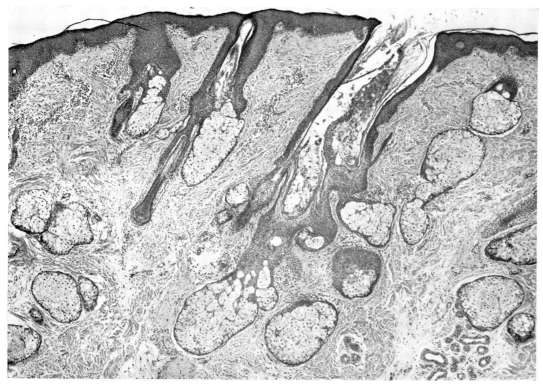

lation in any of their cells, and some are full of lipid-laden cells that extend to the outer periphery of the acinus [18]. New acini can apparently arise from the walls of the ducts, grow into sebaceous units, and fuse with adjacent ones. Three proliferative regions were recognized by Plewig *et al* [20, 21], using [³H] thymidine autoradiography. The duct displayed fast cellular migration with a renewal time of 2–4 days. An undifferentiated cell pool with a renewal time of 4–7 days could be distinguished from the differentiating lipid-producing cells in the glandular fundus with a replacement time of more than 14 and probably 21–25 days [22]. The synthesis and discharge of the lipid contained in the sebaceous cells require more than a week [7].

Sebaceous glands occur over much of the body, although not normally on the palms or soles and only sparsely on the dorsal surfaces of the hand and foot. Sebaceous glands are largest and most numerous in the midline of the back, on the forehead and face, in the external auditory meatus, and on the anogenital surfaces. On the scalp, forehead, cheeks and chin, for example, there are between 400 and 900 glands per square centimetre; elsewhere there are fewer than 100 glands per square centimetre [2, 17, 28].

In a number of sites sebaceous glands open directly to the surface of the skin and not by way of a hair follicle. Examples of such glands are the Meibomian glands of the eyelids and Tyson's glands of the prepuce [17]. Free sebaceous glands are also found on the mucocutaneous surfaces of the female genitalia, the areolae of the nipples and ectopic sites such as the tongue and the cervix uteri [13]. Free sebaceous glands in the margin of the upper lip are often visible to the naked eye as pale yellow bodies, which vary in size from minute specks to about 1·5 mm in diameter; they are known as Fordyce's spots [16] (p. 2079).

Many mammals have specialized aggregations of sebaceous units which function as scent glands [1, 6, 19, 23]. Some such glands also include tubular 'apocrine' units (see p. 32). Of special interest as possible models for the study of compounds which affect sebaceous activity [9] are the costovertebral organs of the golden hamster [9, 11, 12, 27], the supracaudal gland of the guinea-pig [14, 15], the abdominal gland of the gerbil [26], and the preputial glands of many species of rodents [5].

REFERENCES

1 ALBONE E.S. (1984) *Mammalian Sociochemistry.* Chichester, Wiley.

2 BENFENATI A. & BRILLANTI F. (1939) *Arch Ital Dermatol* **15**, 33.

3 BERTALANFFY R. D. (1957) *Anat Rec* **129**, 231.

4 BURDICK K.H. & HILL R. (1970) *Br J Dermatol* **82** (suppl. 6), 19.

5 CLEVEDON BROWN J. & WILLIAMS J.D. (1972) *Mamm Rev* **2**, 105.

6 DOTY R.L. (1976) *Mammalian Olfaction, Reproductive Processes and Behavior.* New York, Academic Press, p. 1.

7 DOWNING D.T., *et al* (1975) *J Invest Dermatol* **64**, 215.

8 EBLING F.J. (1963) In *Advances in Biology of Skin.* Vol. 4. *Sebaceous Glands.* Eds. Montagna W., *et al.* Oxford, Pergamon, p. 200.

9 EBLING F. J. (1977) In *Chemical Signals in Vertebrates.* Eds. Muller-Schwarze D. & Mozell M. M. New York, Plenum, p. 17.

10 EPSTEIN E. H. & EPSTEIN W. L. (1966) *J Invest Dermatol* **46**, 453.

11 FROST P. & GOMEZ E. C. (1972) In *Advances in Biology of Skin.* Vol. 12. *Pharmacology and the Skin.* Eds. Montagna W., *et al.* New York, Appleton–Century–Crofts, p. 403.

12 HSIA S. L. & VOIGT W. (1974) *J Invest Dermatol* **62**, 224.

13 HYMAN A. B. & GUIDUCCI A. A. (1963) In *Advances in Biology of Skin.* Vol. 4. *Sebaceous Glands.* Eds. Montagna, W., *et al.* Oxford, Pergamon, p. 78.

14 MARTAN J. (1962) *J Morph* **110**, 285.

15 MARTAN J. & PRICE D. (1967) *J Morph* **121**, 209.

16 MILES A. E. W. (1963) In *Advances in Biology of Skin.* Vol. 4. *Sebaceous Glands.* Eds. Montagna, W., *et al.* Oxford, Pergamon, p. 46.

17 MONTAGNA W. (1963) In *Advances in Biology of Skin.* Vol. 4. *Sebaceous Glands,* Eds. Montagna, W., *et al.* Oxford, Pergamon, p. 19.

18 MONTAGNA W. & PARAKKAL P. F. (1974) *The Structure and Function of Skin.* 3rd ed. New York, Academic Press.

19 MULLER-SCHWARZE D. & MOZELL M. M. (1977) *Chemical Signals in Vertebrates.* New York, Plenum.

20 PLEWIG G., *et al.* (1971) *Acta Derm Venereol (Stockh)* **51**, 413.

21 PLEWIG G., *et al.* (1971) *Acta Derm Venereol (Stockh)* **51**, 423.

22 PLEWIG G. & CHRISTOPHERS E. (1974) *Acta Derm Venereol (Stockh)* **54**, 177.

23 STRAUSS J. S. & EBLING F. J. (1970) *Mem Soc Endocrinol* **18**, 341.

24 STRAUSS J. S. & POCHI P. E. (1963) *Recent Prog Horm Res* **19**, 385.

25 STRAUSS J. S., *et al.* (1983) In *Biochemistry and Physiology of the Skin.* Ed. Goldsmith, L. A. New York, Oxford University Press, p. 569.

26 THIESSEN D. & YAHR P. (1977) *The Gerbil in Behavioral Investigations.* Austin, University of Texas Press.

27 VOIGT W. & HSIA S. L. (1973) *Endocrinology,* **92**, 1216.

28 YAMADA K. (1982) *Folia Anat Jpn* **10**, 721.

DEVELOPMENT OF SEBACEOUS GLANDS

The development of the sebaceous glands is closely related to the differentiation of hair follicles and epidermis [4, 8]. In about the third week of fetal life the epidermis consists of a single layer of undifferentiated cells, but by the fourth week an outer periderm and a basal stratum germinativum can be distinguished. At the 10th to 12th weeks a stratum intermedium becomes apparent, and at about the same time developing hair germs are quite distinct (see p. 32). In the following weeks the follicles extend downwards into the dermis and the rudiments of the sebaceous glands appear on the posterior surfaces of the hair pegs; by 13–15 weeks the glands are clearly distinguishable.

The cells at first contain glycogen. This lingers at the periphery of the gland, but is quickly lost at the centre, where large lipid drops are visible at 17 weeks [1, 3, 7]. At the point of its origin from the follicle, centrally positioned cells degenerate to form a lumen and surrounding cells keratinize to form the sebaceous duct [2]. The glands become multiacinar by the formation of buds on the peripheral wall.

The glands are functional from their formation; sebum is the first demonstrable glandular product of the human body. Their development and function before birth and in the neonatal period appear to be regulated by maternal androgens and by endogenous steroid synthesis by the fetus [11]. Hydroxysteroid dehydrogenases, which reduce testosterone to 5α-dihydrotestosterone, are present after 16 weeks [9, 10]. The glands reach a peak of activity in the third trimester and their secretion forms part of the vernix caseosa. The vernix lipids resemble sebum in their content of fatty acids, squalene and wax esters, but also contain sterols and sterol esters [5]. Sebaceous glands remain active in the neonatal period, but then involute and remain quiescent until puberty [6].

REFERENCES

1 BREATHNACH A. S. (1971) *J Invest Dermatol* **57**, 133.
2 BREATHNACH A. S. (1971) *An Atlas of the Ultrastructure of Human Skin*. London, Churchill.
3 FUJITA H., *et al.* (1972) *Acta Derm Venereol (Stockh)* **52**, 99.
4 HOLBROOK K. A. (1983) In *Biochemistry and Physiology of the Skin*. Ed. Goldsmith L. A. New York, Oxford University Press, p. 64.
5 NAZZARO-PORRO M., *et al* (1979) *J Invest Dermatol* **73**, 112.
6 RAMASATRY P., *et al* (1970) *J Invest Dermatol* **54**, 139.
7 SATO S., *et al* (1977) *Acta Derm Venereol (Stockh)* **57**, 279.
8 SERRI F. & HUBER W. M. (1963) In *Advances in Biology of Skin*. Vol. 4. *Sebaceous Glands*. Eds. Montagna W., *et al.* Oxford, Pergamon, p. 1.
9 SHARP F., *et al* (1970) *Br J Dermatol* **83**, 177.
10 SHARP F., *et al* (1976) *J Endocrinol* **70**, 491.
11 SOLOMON L. M. & ESTERLEY N. B. (1973) In *Major Problems in Clinical Pediatrics*. Philadelphia, W. B. Saunders, Vol. 9, p. 1.

HISTOCHEMISTRY AND ULTRASTRUCTURE

Undifferentiated sebaceous cells at the periphery of the gland are rich in ribonucleoproteins and stain with basic dyes [4]. As the cells move towards the centre of each lobe they come to contain more lipid and become progressively acidophilic. All the cells have numerous mitochondria, usually appearing as short or wavy rods. The undifferentiated cells contain coarse, osmium-staining particles around the nucleus; as differentiation proceeds these particles increase in number and size and develop lipid droplets in their centres, which gradually enlarge. This complex corresponds to the Golgi body; at completion of sebaceous synthesis it is no longer recognizable.

In studies with the electron microscope [1–3] the undifferentiated cells at the periphery of the gland can be seen to rest upon a basement membrane and to be connected with each other by desmosomes. The membranes of the granular endoplasmic reticulum are coated with ribosomes and there are in addition particles of ribonucleoprotein and glycogen scattered free in the cytoplasm. At this stage the Golgi zones are usually inconspicuous; the nucleus is relatively very large. Differentiation of the cell becomes evident with the appearance of one or more small sebum vacuoles within it. During the active phase of lipid synthesis the cytoplasm becomes packed with smooth-surfaced membranes of the endoplasmic reticulum. In some partially differentiated cells a large Golgi zone becomes apparent; typically it consists of parallel smooth-surfaced thick membranes, slightly dilated cisterns and small vesicles. The Golgi appears to be the centre where lipid aggregates to form sebum vacuoles. At an early stage of sebaceous transformation, one of the cisterns in the Golgi zone becomes more dilated than the others and forms the centre of the developing sebum vacuole. At a later stage the smooth membranes of the Golgi apparatus and the endoplasmic reticulum become oriented around the edge of the developing vacuole, forming a sort of 'husk'. The fully differentiated cells come to contain very large sebum vacuoles which each compare in size with the nucleus; the cell may have a complement of more than 60 (Fig. 52.2). In the final stages of differentiation the mitochondria become widely separated, indicating that their numbers have decreased, and the nucleus becomes irregularly shaped, with clumping of the nucleochromatin and dispersal of the nucleolar material. Lysosomes are prominent in peripheral and other cells in the early stages of differentiation, but are found at all stages [1]. They may be concerned with hydrolysing precursors of sebaceous lipids or the breakdown of mature cells.

The sebaceous cells of prepubertal and hypogonadal males are qualitatively similar to those of normal adults, even though the glands are smaller [4].

REFERENCES

1 BELL M. (1974) *J Invest Dermatol* **62**, 132.
2 BREATHNACH A.S. (1971) In *Atlas of the Ultrastructure of Human Skin*. London, Churchill, p. 340.
3 ELLIS R.A. & HENRIKSON R.C. (1963) In *Advances in Biology of Skin*. Vol. 4. *Sebaceous Glands*. Eds. Montagna W., *et al.* Oxford, Pergamon, p. 94.
4 MONTAGNA W. (1963) In *Advances in Biology of Skin*. Vol. 4. *Sebaceous Glands*. Eds. Montagna W., *et al.* Oxford, Pergamon, p. 19.

COMPOSITION OF SEBUM

Sebum is a complex mixture of lipids which varies widely from species to species [1, 11, 17]. The

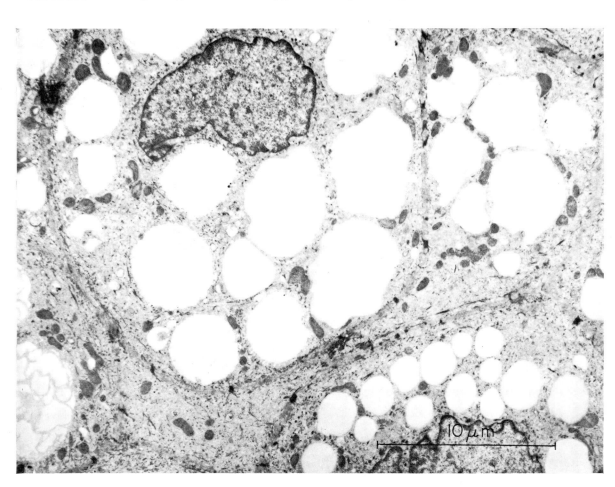

FIG. 52.2. Transverse section of the sebaceous gland of a 24-week-old human fetus. The cytoplasm of the cells is honeycombed with spaces occupied by lipid droplets which have been leached away during processing. (Electron micrograph by Professor A. S. Breathnach.)

analysis of human sebum is complicated by several factors. The principal difficulty is that the surface film contains not only sebum but also lipid from the keratinizing epidermis and possibly from apocrine and eccrine glands. In addition, the pure sebaceous secretion may undergo degradation as it passes through the ducts or on the skin surface, and some material, e.g. hydrocarbons, may also accrue from environmental sources.

Human skin surface lipid consists of glycerides, free fatty acids, wax esters, squalene, cholesterol esters and cholesterol. Lipid production varies according to site: e.g. 5–10 $\mu g/cm^2$ were recovered from the trunk and limbs of subjects who washed 3 h prior to extraction, compared with 150–300 $\mu g/cm^2$ from the forehead [3]. When amounts were in the range 5–10 $\mu g/cm^2$, the skin surface lipid contained virtually no wax esters or squalene. However, as the quantity of surface lipid increased, so did the proportion of wax esters and squalene, while at the same time the proportions of cholesterol esters decreased. The proportion of each of the constituents became nearly constant when the amount of lipid reached 50–100 $\mu g/cm^2$.

These results are consistent with the view that wax esters and squalene are produced by the sebaceous glands only, and not by the epidermis. When the surface lipid is as low as 4–10 $\mu g/cm^2$ no sebum is present, and this level of lipid represents that contributed by the epidermis. However, when the surface lipid is greater than 100 $\mu g/cm^2$, its composition approximates to that of sebum. The percentage proportions of constituents are thus as follows.

Constituents	Sebum	Epidermal lipid
Glycerides (plus free fatty acids)	57·5	65
Wax esters	26·0	—
Squalene	12·0	—
Cholesterol esters	3·0	15
Cholesterol	1·5	20

It may be concluded from these figures that the sebaceous glands do not to any great extent convert squalene to sterols, whereas in the epidermis squalene synthesized in the lower layers is rapidly and totally converted to sterols, either to precursors of vitamin D or to cholesterol.

Between birth and sexual maturity, surface lipid undergoes two distinct changes [15, 16]. Shortly after birth it resembles adult sebum, presumably because the sebaceous glands have been activated by maternal hormones. Between 2 and 8 yr of age, the wax esters and squalene decline, and cholesterol and its esters become prominent. In this age range, then, sebum apparently constitutes less than half the total surface lipid of the forehead, compared with 95% or more in the adult. Between 8 and to 10 yr of age the wax esters and squalene rise to about two-thirds of the adult level and between 10 and 15 yr the composition comes to resemble that of the adult.

Free fatty acids make up as much as 30% of the human skin surface fat [6, 7, 19] but occur in only small amounts in the hair lipids of rabbits, sheep and rodents [18] and are not demonstrable in the chimpanzee, baboon, hamster, guinea-pig, dog, cat, goat or cow [8]. Analysis of pure sebum from isolated human sebaceous glands showed the presence of triglycerides, but not free fatty acids, monoglycerides or diglycerides [4, 5]. It thus seems that prior to secretion all the fatty acids are combined as triglycerides which are subsequently subjected to lipolytic activity by enzymes present in the sebaceous ducts and on the skin surface. This conclusion is reinforced by the demonstration that the skin surface can hydrolyse triglycerides of exogenous origin; when ^{14}C-labelled tripalmitin was spread on the back, labelled free fatty acids were isolated from the surface fat 3 h later [6].

The fatty acid components [1, 9, 11, 17] have both odd and even numbered carbon chains up to C_{25} in length although more than half are C_{16} and C_{18} compounds. They are both saturated and unsaturated, and of particular interest is the presence in both classes of unusual branched chains. These are of two kinds, one having an even number of carbons with the methyl group attached to the penultimate (iso series), the other having an odd number of carbons with the methyl group attached to the antepenultimate (antieso series). Such branches are present in the chains of the wax esters, which are virtually limited to 18 carbons and produced only by the sebaceous glands and, in higher proportion, in the longer chains of the sterol esters which probably arise from both sebaceous glands and epidermis.

Though various effects have been ascribed to diet, there is no evidence from either man or experimental animals that any components of sebum are directly derived from ingested fats. In man, most of the unsaturated fatty acids in the surface film are Δ^6 compounds, whereas dietary lipids are Δ^9 compounds [17]. Prolonged starvation of human subjects [2, 14] decreased the rate of sebum synthesis by about 40% without any decrease in the actual amount of squalene, which thus rose as a proportion of the total surface lipid. When a fat-free diet was given to rats, they showed a significantly *higher* rate of sebaceous secretion than animals given diets containing 20% of stearic acid, oleic acid, linoleic acid, linolenic acid or cholesterol, respectively. No appreciable amounts of any fed lipids were found to be incorporated as such into the skin surface fats. The only effects exerted on composition were related to the amount of linoleic acid in the diet: a number of significant changes, of which the clearest was the reduction of the longer-chain alcohols and of octadecadienoic acid, occurred as a result of linoleic acid deficiency [10].

The composition of the skin surface fat can also be influenced, in rats, by administered hormones. Thus testosterone, at the same time as increasing the amount of sebaceous secretion (see below), increases the ratio of palmitate to stearate and the ratio of oleate to stearate; oestrogens and antiandrogens antagonize these effects [12, 13, 20]. However, in man, the maximum changes in sebum production which could be produced by oral administration of oestrogens or androgens had no noticeable effect on sebum composition [1].

REFERENCES

1 DOWNING D. T. & STRAUSS J.S. (1974) *J Invest Dermatol* **62**, 228.
2 DOWNING D.T., *et al* (1972) *Am J Clin Nutr* **25**, 365.
3 GREEN R.S., *et al* (1970) *J Invest Dermatol* **54**, 240.
4 KELLUM R. E. (1966) *Arch Dermatol* **93**, 610.
5 KELLUM R.E. (1967) *Arch Dermatol* **95**, 218.
6 NICOLAIDES N. (1963) In *Advances in Biology of Skin.* Vol. 4. *Sebaceous Glands.* Eds. Montagna W., *et al.* Oxford, Pergamon, p. 167.
7 NICOLAIDES N. (1974) *Science* **186**, 19.
8 NICOLAIDES N., *et al* (1968) *J Invest Dermatol* **51**, 83.
9 NICOLAIDES N., *et al* (1972) *Lipids* **7**, 506.
10 NIKKARI T. (1965) *Scand J Clin Lab Invest* **17** (Suppl. 85).
11 NIKKARI T. (1974) *J Invest Dermatol* **62**, 257.
12 NIKKARI T. & VALAVAARA M. (1970) *J Endocrinol* **48**, 373.
13 NIKKARI T. & VALAVAARA M. (1970) *Br J Dermatol* **83**, 459.
14 POCHI P. E., *et al* (1970) *J Invest Dermatol* **55**, 303.
15 RAMASASTRY P., *et al* (1970) *J Invest Dermatol* **54**, 138.
16 SANSONE-BASSANO G., *et al* (1980) *Br J Dermatol* **103**, 131.
17 STRAUSS J. S., *et al* (1983) In *Biochemistry and Physiology of the Skin.* Ed. Goldsmith L. A. New York, Oxford University Press, p. 569.
18 WHEATLEY V. R. (1956) *Am Perfumer* **68**, 37.
19 WHEATLEY V.R. (1963) In *Advances in Biology of Skin.* Vol. 4. *Sebaceous Glands.* Eds. Montagna W., *et al.* Oxford, Pergamon, p. 135.
20 WILDE P.F. & EBLING F.J. (1969) *J Invest Dermatol* **52**, 362.

FUNCTIONS OF SEBUM

Several functions have been ascribed to sebum but they are by no means undisputed. In hairy mammals the sebum may be important in waterproofing the hair and perhaps, as in cattle, it may seasonally reduce thermal insulation by the coat [10]. In man it has been stated that the lipid film both controls moisture loss from the epidermis and protects the skin from fungal and bacterial infection. Aggregations of holocrine gland units play an important part in scent production in many mammals (see Chapter 51) and components of sebum may possibly contribute to body odour.

Cornified epithelium, such as a cutting from a plantar callus, becomes hard and brittle if it is allowed to dry out, but remains pliable as long as it contains 10% by weight of water [1]. The stratum corneum receives moisture from below and loses it by evaporation at the skin surface, but the major barrier against water loss through the skin is not at the surface but is either near the base of the stratum corneum or throughout the entire cornified layer. At relative humidities of about 60% and higher the moisture content remains high enough to maintain the pliability of the keratin. Under the lower relative humidity of winter weather, or in rapidly flowing air, the stratum corneum can, however, dry out, with consequent chapping of the skin surface.

If the cornified epithelium is treated with organic solvents and then extracted with water, the water-holding capacity of the epithelium is greatly decreased [2]. This suggests that the water-holding power of the cornified epithelium depends on the presence of lipids, but an alternative explanation might be that lipid solvents damage natural barriers. There may be little reason to doubt that under adverse environmental conditions the application of lipid materials helps to keep the stratum corneum pliable and to prevent chapping of the skin, but it is debatable how far naturally occurring lipids play such a role and, if they do, whether sebum contributes to any protective surface film.

Kligman [5] has calculated that the thickness of the natural sebum film is of the order of only 0·45 μm on the forehead and considerably less on the abdomen, and has questioned whether this is of any protective value. He pointed out that in the prepubertal child the sebaceous glands remain undeveloped, yet the epidermis is smooth and flexible; sufficient lipid is derived from the epidermis itself. Others disagree, providing the evidence that, if the skin of women is defatted with alcohol–ether, the anhidrosis produced by aluminium salts is intensified [8]. To complicate the issue still further it may be pointed out that the hydrolysis of triglycerides on the skin surface must produce a small quantity of glycerol which, by reason of its hygroscopic properties, would retain moisture [6].

It is widely believed that free fatty acids on the skin surface hinder the growth of pathogenic organisms [7]. Circumstantial evidence supports the view that sebum, or at least the product of its hydrolysis, is fungistatic. Fungi causing tinea pedis preferentially colonize areas which are not supplied with sebaceous glands; ringworm of the scalp becomes rare after puberty, when sebum production increases. It is also evident that free fatty acids have a limited action against certain bacteria, e.g. *Streptococcus pyogenes* [7]. Both these properties of sebum have been challenged by Kligman [5]. Admitting that fatty acids by themselves are antifungal *in vitro*, he claims that this potential is inactivated in the presence of horny material. He also states that the addition of sebum has no effect on streptococci or staphylococci growing on discs of isolated stratum corneum in agar culture. He therefore suggests that the sterilizing power of the skin is due largely to desiccation, a process supported equally by a wide range of inanimate surfaces. A criticism of these studies is that they may only demonstrate the self-evident proposition that sebum does not prevent the growth of organisms which normally occur on the skin surface, and that they tell us nothing about the possible role of sebum in prevention of infection by other organisms which might prove pathogenic [4]. A finding that the bacterial population was correlated with the production rate of free fatty acids but not with the sebum excretion rate was interpreted to indicate that free fatty acids are the product rather than the cause of the bacterial presence [3].

Shuster [9] has made the interesting suggestion that the capacity to develop delayed immune hypersensitivity may be augmented and maintained by the corynebacteria which colonise active sebaceous glands in acne.

REFERENCES

1 BLANK I.H. (1952) *J Invest Dermatol* **18**, 433.
2 BLANK I.H. (1953) *J Invest Dermatol* **21**, 259.
3 CAVE J.H., *et al* (1980) *Br J Dermatol* **103**, 383.
4 JARRETT A. (1964) *Br J Dermatol* **76**, 295.
5 KLIGMAN A. (1963) In *Advances in Biology of Skin*. Vol. 4 *Sebaceous Glands*. Eds. Montagna W., *et al.* Oxford, Pergamon, p. 110.
6 NICOLAIDES N. (1963) In *Advances in Biology of Skin*. Vol. 4. *Sebaceous Glands*. Eds. Montagna W., *et al.* Oxford, Pergamon, p. 167.
7 ROTHMAN S. (1954) *Physiology and Biochemistry of the Skin*. Chicago, Chicago University Press, Chapter 13.
8 SCHMID N., *et al* (1964) *Br J Dermatol* **76**, 395.
9 SHUSTER, S. (1978) *Lancet* **i**, 1328
10 YEATES N.T.M. (1955) *Aust J Agric Res* **6**, 891.

MEASUREMENT OF SEBACEOUS ACTIVITY AND SEBUM PRODUCTION

Various methods have been used for collecting lipids from human skin and for measuring their production [14]. They include swabbing by pads soaked in solvent [23], washing lipid solvents over areas of skin circumscribed by rings, caps or apertures of bottles [9, 19, 21, 22], absorption on paper [28, 29] and removal by pressing a ground-glass plate on the skin followed by photometric assessment [7, 12, 25–27]. The rate of sebum production has also been calculated from the squalene content of skin biopsies [10] and by measuring sebaceous lipogenesis

A simple and practical method for measuring human sebaceous secretion is to place a pad of cigarette papers for 3 h on a delimited area of the forehead and then to extract the sebum with diethyl ether. In view of circadian changes in secretion [4], the measurement should be carried out between standard times. It does not give the absolute sebum production rate which is indefinitely sustainable [11], but it is valuable for comparative purposes and appears to give more reproducible results than the glass plate methods at high levels of sebum [5]. The method that follows was originally devised by Strauss and Pochi [8, 28, 29].

(a) The forehead is wiped several times with dry gauze sponge squares.

(b) A square area is delimited by non-perforated cloth adhesive tape or micropore tape. The mask may conveniently be assembled on a glass plate.

(c) A pad of four or five cigarette papers is previously prepared for use by cutting off the gummed edges. The papers are covered with gauze sponges 7·5 cm square, and these in turn are held in place by a 7·5 cm rubber or stocking weave bandage encircling the head (Fig. 52.3).

(d) Packs of papers are discarded after each of two preliminary successive periods of 15 min.

(e) A pad of papers, which is prepared by washing in ether and being allowed to dry, is then applied. At the end of a 3-hour collection period, the central lipid-containing portion of the papers is cut out and repeatedly extracted with anhydrous ethyl ether. The combined

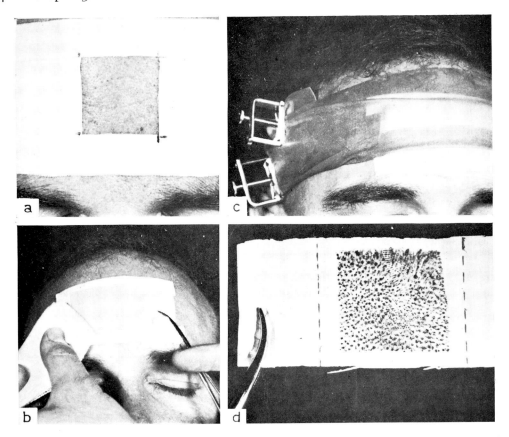

FIG. 52.3. Technique for the collection of sebum: for an explanation of (a), (b) and (c), see the text; (d) the central lipid-containing area of the cigarette papers, which has been stained with osmic acid vapour for photographic purposes (from Strauss J. S. & Pochi P. E. [28, 29]).

washings are evaporated to dryness in weighed aluminium cups of the type sold as baking cases. The cups and sebum are finally weighed at room temperature. Control papers must also be subjected to the extraction and subsequent procedures.

Sebum production in the rat has been measured by total immersion of animals in lipid solvents [1], by changes in hair fat [15, 16], or by absorption of lipid on paper from areas denuded of hair [17].

To study responses to hormones, the size of the sebaceous glands has also been estimated from histological sections either by planimetry [13, 20] or by superimposing a grid with sampling points [24]. Mitotic activity, estimated after injecting the rats with colchicine which arrests mitoses in the metaphase, has also been used as a measure of glandular activity [13]. Other experimental models, such as the preputial glands of rodents [6] which can be

dissected out and weighed, or the visible costovertebral glands of the hamster [3, 18] to which hormones can be topically applied, have been reviewed by Ebling [14].

In interpreting the results of animal experiments it is important to realize that the reactions of supposed homologues of the sebaceous glands may vary not only from species to species but also within species. Thus the responses to hormones of the preputial and sebaceous glands of the rat may not be identical. Moreover, because of the miscellaneous parameters involved it is also important to understand the relationships between the different facets of sebaceous activity. The rate of secretion of sebum depends on two factors: the synthetic capacity of each sebaceous cell and the rate of production of the cells. The size of the glands depends partly on both these things, but also of critical importance is the time taken for each cell to mature and pass through the gland; i.e. the turnover time or cell life. If, for example, the rate of production of cells were doubled, with a consequent increase in sebum production, no alteration in gland size need occur if at the same time cell life were halved. As a general principle, it seems to be true that, the greater the mitotic rate, the lower is the turnover time [2]; but in practice the changes do not keep pace with each other, and glands under stimulation do increase in size as well as in secretory rate.

REFERENCES

1 ARCHIBALD A. & SHUSTER S. (1970) *Br J Dermatol* **82**, 146.

2 BULLOUGH W. S. (1965) *Cancer Res* **25**, 1683.

3 BURDICK K. H. & HILL R. (1970) *Br J Dermatol* **82**, 19.

4 BURTON J. L., *et al* (1970) *Br J Dermatol* **82**, 497.

5 CHIVOT M., *et al* (1981) *Br J Dermatol* **105**, 701.

6 CLEVEDON BROWN J. & WILLIAMS J. D. (1962) *Mamm Rev* **2**, 105.

7 CUNLIFFE W. J. & SHUSTER S. (1969) *Br J Dermatol* **81**, 697.

8 CUNLIFFE W. J., *et al* (1980) *J Invest Dermatol* **75**, 394.

9 DOWNING D. T., *et al* (1969) *J Invest Dermatol* **53**, 322.

10 DOWNING D. T., *et al* (1981) *J Invest Dermatol* **77**, 358.

11 DOWNING D. T., *et al* (1982) *J Invest Dermatol* **79**, 226.

12 EBERHARDT H. (1974) *Arch Dermatol Forsch* **251**, 155.

13 EBLING F. J. (1963) In *Advances in Biology of Skin.* Vol. 4. *Sebaceous Glands.* Eds. Montagna W., *et al.* Oxford, Pergamon, p. 200.

14 EBLING F. J. (1977) In *Dermatotoxicology and Pharmacology.* Eds. Marzulli F. N. & Maibach H. I. Washington, Hemisphere Publishing, p. 55.

15 EBLING F. J. & SKINNER J. (1967) *Br J Dermatol* **79**, 386.

16 EBLING F. J. & SKINNER J. (1975) *Br J Dermatol* **92**, 321.

17 EBLING F. J., *et al* (1981) *J Invest Dermatol* **77**, 458.

18 FROST P., *et al* (1973) *J Invest Dermatol* **61**, 159.

19 GREENE R. S., *et al* (1970) *J Invest Dermatol* **54**, 240.

20 HASKIN D., *et al* (1953) *J Invest Dermatol* **20**, 207.

21 JARRETT A. (1955) *Br J Dermatol* **67**, 165.

22 JARRETT A. (1959) *Br J Dermatol* **71**, 102.

23 RAMASASTRY P., *et al* (1970) *J Invest Dermatol* **54**, 138.

24 SAUTER L. S. & LOUD A. V. (1975) *J Invest Dermatol* **64**, 9.

25 SCHAEFER H. (1973) *J Soc Cosmet Chem* **24**, 331.

26 SCHAEFER H. & KUHN-BUSSIUS H. (1970) *Arch Klin Exp Dermatol* **238**, 429.

27 SIMPSON N. B. & MARTIN A. R. (1983) *Br J Dermatol* **109**, 647.

28 STRAUSS J. S. & POCHI P. E. (1961) *J Invest Dermatol* **36**, 293.

29 STRAUSS J. S. & POCHI P. E. (1963) *Recent Prog Horm Res* **19**, 385.

ENDOCRINE CONTROL OF SEBACEOUS ACTIVITY [26, 28, 30, 31, 79, 91, 95, 96]

Androgens. The fact that sebaceous activity is stimulated by androgens has been established by many studies in animals and man. Androgens have been shown to enlarge the sebaceous glands of the rat [17, 20, 21, 50], the mouse [61] and the rabbit [68], as well as homologues such as the supracaudal gland of the guinea-pig [66, 67], the abdominal gland of the gerbil [47], the costovertebral glands of the hamster [45, 54, 57], and the preputial glands of rodents [6, 15, 58]. Studies of the action of testosterone in the rat show that it increases the incidence of cell division and the size of the cells [20, 21], as well as the production of sebum [2, 4, 25, 33].

In man, the level of sebum excretion at birth is similar to that in adults [1]. The sebaceous glands regress to become minute during the prepubertal period, but undergo vast enlargement at puberty when the sebum output of males increases more than fivefold [84]. The levels remain essentially unchanged until around the age of 80, when they decline [84]; paradoxically the sebaceous glands become larger, but cell turnover is decreased [73, 84].

Administration of testosterone increases the size of the glands and the sebum output of prepubertal boys (Fig. 52.4a) but not of adult males, where the glands appear to be under maximal stimulation by endogenous androgen [53, 85, 94, 97].

Eunuchs secrete about half as much sebum as normal males, but substantially more than prepubertal boys. Sebum production by eunuchs is correlated with the urinary excretion of 17-hydroxycorticoids and 17-oxosteroids [81]; thus the activity of the sebaceous glands of eunuchs appears to be dependent on adrenal androgens.

The secretion of sebum by adult women is only a little less than that by normal men. Up to the age of 50 it is greater than in castrated men, but after that age it falls [82]. This pattern, and the fact that women do not normally produce more adrenal androgens than men, suggest that the sebaceous glands are affected by extra-adrenal sources of androgen. Circumstantial evidence implicates the ovary, although significant changes in sebum secretion have not been demonstrated after bilateral ovariectomy [74, 96].

Androgens other than testosterone also stimulate sebaceous activity. 5α-Dihydrotestosterone was shown to be at least as effective as testosterone in stimulating sebaceous secretion in castrated rats; androstenedione was much less potent, though not without significant effect [3, 39, 71]. In hypophysectomized castrated rats 5α-dihydrotestosterone, 5α-androstane-3β,17β-diol and androstenedione were each more potent than testosterone [39, 40]. These researchers failed to detect any significant effect of dehydroepiandrosterone, 5α-androstanedione or androsterone on sebaceous secretion, though each stimulated sebaceous mitosis and increased preputial gland weight. In man, both dehydroepiandrosterone and androstenedione have been shown to stimulate sebum production, although androsterone had no such effect [77, 83].

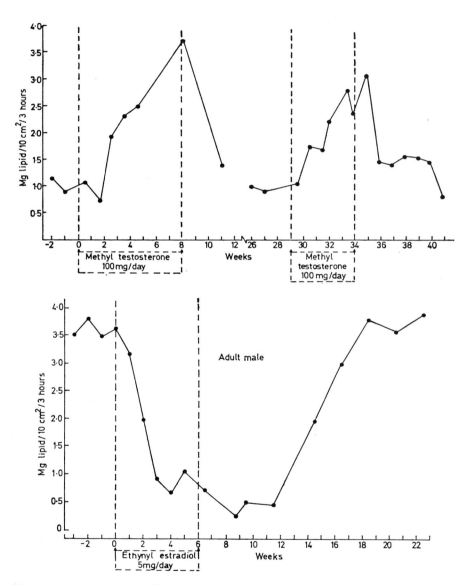

FIG. 52.4. (a) Sebum output of an 11-year-old boy given two courses of methyltestosterone orally (100 mg per day). Sebaceous secretion promptly rose with androgenic stimulation and quickly declined to the original level when the drug was stopped. (b) Suppression of sebum production in an adult male given 5 mg of ethinyloestradiol orally daily for 6 weeks. In this subject the decrease was readily detectable in 2 weeks and was nearly maximal after 3 weeks. Sebum production returned to pre-oestrogen levels approximately 11–12 weeks following discontinuation of oestrogen. (From Strauss J. S. & Pochi P. E. [94].)

Progesterone. Whether progesterone affects the sebaceous glands has been a matter of dispute. The statement of some researchers that sebum production in women fluctuates during the menstrual cycle [56] has not been confirmed by others. It has been claimed that the administration of progesterone can produce acne [115], and that given to senile women it increases sebum production [90], but no such effect could be demonstrated by other investigators [60, 93]. In the rat, large doses of the order of 10 mg per day have been shown to increase gland volume [23, 55], though without significant changes in sebum secretion [36]; 1 mg per day or less was ineffective [22, 52]. The lack of response to this dose was shared by immature and mature, intact and spayed rats, and was unaffected by previous treatment with oestrogen [22]. Other researchers have claimed that even a low dose of progesterone has some stimulating effect provided that gonadectomy is carried out at 3 weeks of age [87]. Even so, it seems reasonable to conclude that progesterone cannot, except possibly in very large doses, stimulate sebaceous excretion. Moreover, the evidence that progesterone can inhibit testosterone metabolism and lipogenesis in animal sebaceous glands [46], and may actually suppress human sebum when applied topically [16, 89], cannot be ignored.

Adrenocortical hormones. As stated above, androgens of adrenocortical origin, such as dehydroepiandrosterone or androstenedione, have been shown to stimulate sebaceous secretion in both the rat and man. These facts explain the finding that sebum production was decreased after adrenalectomy in three women with Cushing's syndrome [83]. They are also compatible with the findings that administration of ACTH causes hypertrophy of sebaceous glands in prepubertal human males and postpubertal human females [92], and increases the size of sebaceous glands [51, 55] and sebum production [37] in hypophysectomized and gonadectomized rats.

The role of glucocorticoids, however, is less easy to assess. Whereas some researchers [5, 14, 55] reported that in the rat sebaceous gland size was decreased by cortisone, others found sebum secretion to be unchanged by corticosterone [87]. Administration of 20 mg per day of prednisone suppressed sebum secretion in castrated—though not in normal—men and to a lesser extent in women [76], although since excretion of 17-oxosteroids was lowered the researchers attributed this effect to suppression of adrenal androgens. Combined glucocorticoid–oestrogen treatment has been shown to suppress sebum excretion in female acne patients [8, 80].

The evidence thus supports the view that adrenal androgenic steroids, or their precursors, stimulate sebaceous activity, and suggests that exogenous glucocorticoids may inhibit it either by suppressing adrenal androgen production or by a direct effect. There is some contrary evidence, however. In an adult male with Addison's disease, replacement therapy with cortisone or hydrocortisone was followed by a marked increase in sebum production; thus it remains possible that glucocorticoids could act in a permissive capacity for the response of the sebaceous glands to endogenous androgens [83].

Pituitary hormones. That pituitary hormones affect sebaceous activity is incontestible. What is less certain is how the variety of evidence from animal experiments should be interpreted and the extent to which any conclusions are relevant to man, for whom the evidence is usually sparse or indirect.

It is important to recognize that there are several different routes or modes of action of pituitary hormones. First, if gonadal, adrenal or thyroid hormones influence sebaceous activity, then the demonstrable effects of gonadotrophic [79, 88, 96], adrenocorticotrophic [42, 51, 55, 92, 102, 103] or thyrotrophic [38, 106, 107] hormones are likely to be *indirect* by way of the endocrine organs which they respectively control (Fig. 52.5). Second, as distinct from such actions, pituitary hormones may also exert *direct* effects at the site of the sebaceous glands. Lastly, irrespective of whether the effect is indirect or direct, it may be either *independent* of the presence of another hormone, or *dependent* on it, in which case its action may be described as *permissive* or *synergistic*.

The concept of permissive or synergistic factors for sebaceous activity was first established by the discovery that the response to testosterone of the rat sebaceous glands, as measured by changes in size, was absent or impaired after hypophysectomy [21, 62, 63]. Notwithstanding some debate about the extent of this effect [70, 101, 104, 105], the finding appears to be amply confirmed by experiments (Fig. 52.6) in which sebum production was measured [28, 35]. Lorinez and his associates [64, 65] proposed the name of *sebotropic factor* for the pituitary factor necessary to facilitate this response and, using pig pituitary, claimed to have prepared such a material which was free from somatotrophic, thyrotrophic and gonadotrophic activity [112, 113]. However, one such preparation made by other workers using similar methods had neither synergistic nor independent actions [35] and others had only slight independent effects

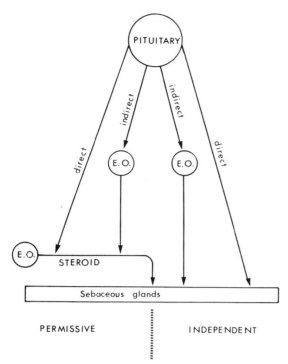

FIG. 52.5. Possible ways in which pituitary hormones may affect the sebaceous glands: E.O., endocrine organ. The effect may be direct or indirect, and in addition may be either independent or permissive, in the sense that the pituitary hormone facilitates the response of another hormone, e.g. a steroid. (From Ebling *et al* [41] by permission of the *British Journal of Dermatology*.)

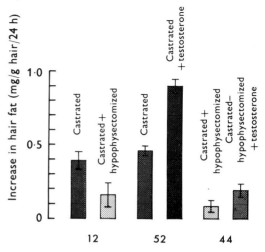

FIG. 52.6. Effects on sebum secretion of hypophysectomy in castrated rats (left-hand group), of testosterone in castrated rats (centre group) and of testosterone in hypophysectomized castrated rats (right-hand group). The numbers of compared litter-mate pairs are shown below each pair of histograms. (From Ebling [28] by permission of the *Journal of Investigative Dermatology*.)

which, in their makers' opinion, could be accounted for by their gonadotrophic, adrenocorticotrophic and somatotrophic activity [87].

There is thus little reason to support the existence of a sebotrophic factor free from other hormonal activity. At the same time there is ample experimental evidence that several pituitary peptides directly influence the sebaceous glands, both independently and synergistically. For example, in hypophysectomized castrated rats a pure bovine growth hormone (Fig. 52.7) completely restored the responses of both the sebaceous and preputial glands to testosterone [41,42]. The action was mainly synergistic, though for the sebaceous glands a small but significant component could be attributed to growth hormone acting independently. A porcine growth hormone had a similar synergistic effect [35] but was without detectable independent action. According to one report [35], but not confirmed by another [72], so did ovine prolactin.

Evidence that growth hormone affects human sebaceous secretion is limited, but positive. In four men and seven women with untreated acromegaly, the mean rates of sebaceous secretion within each group were above normal [11]. Five patients had their pituitaries irradiated with yttrium implants and in all of them sebum secretion diminished. Data for 20 treated and untreated acromegalics revealed that sebum production was significantly correlated with the logarithm of the serum growth hormone concentration. Sebum secretion has been measured in only a few subjects with isolated growth hormone deficiency: in one study [48] two of three had extremely low rates; in another of three males and four females [79] the rates were a little, but not significantly, below normal.

The clinical evidence from man backed by the experimental evidence from animals raises the possibility that growth hormone as well as androgen might play some role in the genesis of adolescent acne [29]. Such a view receives support from the finding that, while growth of boys before puberty is dependent on growth hormone only, the adolescent spurt requires the synergistic action of both growth hormone and testosterone [100]. Even more relevant is the finding that GH-deficient boys and girls are less than normally responsive to androgens and that growth hormone is necessary as a synergistic factor to permit a full response to tes-

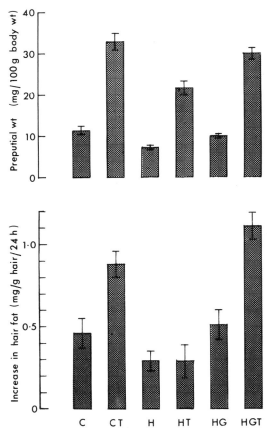

FIG. 52.7. Sebum production as measured by the increase in hair fat and relative preputial gland weight. Values are means ± standard errors for groups of 11 rats: C, castrated; CT, castrated + testosterone; H, hypophysectomized castrated; HT, hypophysectomized castrated + testosterone; HG, hypophysectomized castrated + growth hormone; HGT, hypophysectomized castrated + growth hormone + testosterone. (Data from Ebling *et al* [41, 42].)

pophysectomized castrated but not in thyroidectomized animals [107], the possibility of a synergistic effect with testosterone cannot be ruled out. TSH increases sebum production of hypophysectomized castrated or castrated rats treated with testosterone [38]. The results may simply reflect the additive effects of testosterone and thyroid hormone. However, they do not explain why treatment of castrated rats with propylthiouracil, which inhibits thyroid activity but might be expected to increase secretion of TSH, appeared to enhance rather than reduce the response to testosterone as measured by sebum secretion [38].

The situation is further complicated by the undoubted evidence that melanocyte-stimulating hormones, which are relatively short peptides, also have marked effects in experiments on rats. Sebum secretion in the rat is reduced by posterior as well as total hypophysectomy [108]. In hypophysectomized castrated rats synthetic α-MSH has both a significant independent effect on sebaceous secretion and a marked synergistic effect with testosterone [40, 109–111]. The knowledge that human sebum secretion is increased in pregnancy [10] and suckling [13], both states when MSH secretion is believed to be increased [86, 99], and a presumed association between seborrhoea and an increase in plasma MSH in Parkinson's disease [9, 12, 81], led Shuster and his associates [88] to postulate that MSH was sebotrophic in man. However, the finding that in patients with Addison's disease or bilaterally adrenalectomized for Cushing's disorder [49] sebum production was normal or even, in females, much below normal, notwithstanding increases in α-MSH levels, lends no support to this view. The finding that β-lipotropin [105] increased sebum production in hypophysectomized rats without causing significant changes in adrenal weight suggests that this peptide, also, may have a direct effect on sebaceous activity.

Oestrogens. Oestrogens undoubtedly depress sebaceous activity. They decrease the size of the sebaceous glands when injected into rats [17–19, 24] or mice [7] or when given orally to adult human males [95] and have also been shown to reduce sebum production in both animals [25, 33, 69] and man [59, 75, 78, 94, 97]. On the grounds that it was not possible to demonstrate a local, as distinct from a systemic, effect by topical application of oestrogen ointment to the human forehead [97], it has been suggested that oestrogens may act by reducing endogenous androgen production [95]. This view that they suppress gonadotrophin secretion by the pituitary receives support from the finding that

tosterone with respect to protein in anabolism and androgenicity as well as growth promotion [114].

Growth hormone and prolactin are not the only pituitary hormones which may act directly and synergistically with testosterone. While reported effects of gonadotrophins on sebum secretion in the rat [88] were undoubtedly mediated through the testis, there is some evidence that sebum production may be related to rising gonadotrophin titres in orchiectomized men [74]. Similarly, while there is clear evidence that thyrotrophic hormone acts indirectly by way of the thyroid gland to stimulate sebum production in rats, since it is effective in hy-

sebum-suppressing doses of oestrogen reduced the levels of testosterone in the plasma and urine of normal men [44], though not from the evidence that they suppressed sebum secretion in eunuchs [82].

The evidence from animal experiments favours the hypothesis that oestrogens act peripherally and directly upon the sebaceous glands. First, their suppressive action is no less in hypophysectomized [19] or adrenalectomized castrated rats [26] than in intact ones. Second, notwithstanding a claim that they reduce uptake of radioactive thymidine by human sebaceous cells [98] they do not appear to reduce sebaceous cell division in the rat [20]. Third, their suppressive action can be clearly demonstrated against the stimulating effects of exogenous androgen in castrated animals [25, 27]. Last, the local effect of topically applied oestrogen has been demonstrated in the rat [32, 34]. In summary, oestrogens appear to act independently of androgens at the peripheral site and independently of the existence of androgen-secreting glands. However, the possibility that in man they also influence hormonal levels by some systemic mechanism cannot be excluded.

REFERENCES

1 AGACHE P., *et al* (1980) *Br J Dermatol* **103**, 643.
2 ARCHIBALD A. & SHUSTER S. (1967) *J Endocrinol* **37**, 22p.
3 ARCHIBALD A. & SHUSTER S. (1969) *Proc R Soc Med* **62**, 887.
4 ARCHIBALD A. & SHUSTER S. (1970) *Br J Dermatol* **82**, 146.
5 BAKER B.L. & WHITAKER W.L. (1948) *Anat Rec* **102**, 333.
6 BEAVER D.L. (1960) *J Exp Zool* **143**, 153.
7 BULLOUGH W.S. & LAURENCE E.B. (1960) *J Invest Dermatol* **35**, 37.
8 BURTON J.L. & SAIHAN E. (1980) *Br J Dermatol* **103**, 139
9 BURTON J.L. & SHUSTER S. (1970) *Lancet* ii, 19.
10 BURTON J.L., *et al* (1970) *Br Med J* ii, 769.
11 BURTON J.L., *et al* (1972) *Br Med J* ii, 406.
12 BURTON J.L., *et al* (1973) *Br J Dermatol* **88**, 475.
13 BURTON J.L., *et al* (1973) *Nature* **243**, 349.
14 CASTOR C.W. & BAKER B.L. (1950) *Endocrinology* **47**, 234.
15 CLEVEDON BROWN J. & WILLIAMS J.D. (1972) *Mamm Rev* **2**, 105.
16 CUNLIFFE W.J. & SIMPSON N.B. (1980) In *Percutaneous Absorption of Steroids*. Eds. Mauvais-Jarvis P., *et al*. London, Academic Press, p. 149.
17 EBLING F.J. (1949) *J Endocrinol* **5**, 297.
18 EBLING F.J. (1951) *J Endocrinol* **7**, 288.
19 EBLING F.J. (1955) *J Endocrinol* **12**, 38.
20 EBLING F.J. (1957) *J Embryol Exp Morph* **5**, 74.
21 EBLING F.J. (1957) *J Endocrinol* **15**, 297.
22 EBLING F.J. (1961) *Br J Dermatol* **73**, 65.
23 EBLING F.J. (1963) In *Advances in Biology of Skin*. Vol. 4. *Sebaceous Glands*. Eds. Montagna W., *et al*. Oxford, Pergamon, p. 200.
24 EBLING F.J. (1964) In *Hormonal Steroids, Biochemistry, Pharmacology and Therapeutics, Proceedings of the First International Congress on Hormonal Steroids*. New York, Academic Press, Vol. 1, p. 537.
25 EBLING F.J. (1967) *J Endocrinol* **38**, 181.
26 EBLING F.J. (1970) In *Advances in Steroids*. Ed. Briggs M.H. London, Academic Press, Vol. 2, p. 1.
27 EBLING F.J. (1973) *Acta Endocrinol* **72**, 361.
28 EBLING F.J. (1974) *J Invest Dermatol* **62**, 161.
29 EBLING F.J. (1976) *Cutis* **17**, 469.
30 EBLING F.J. (1977) In *Chemical Signals in Vertebrates*. Eds. Muller-Schwarze D. & Mozell M.M. New York, Plenum, p. 17.
31 EBLING F.J. (1977) In *Dermatotoxicology and Pharmacology*. Eds. Marzulli F.N. & Maibach H.I. Washington, Hemisphere Publishing, p. 55.
32 EBLING F.J. & RANDALL V.A. (1983) *J Steroid Biochem* **19**, 587.
33 EBLING F.J. & SKINNER J. (1967) *Br J Dermatol* **9**, 386.
34 EBLING F.J. & SKINNER J. (1983) *J Invest Dermatol* **81**, 448.
35 EBLING F.J., *et al* (1969) *J Endocrinol* **45**, 245.
36 EBLING F.J., *et al* (1969) *J Endocrinol* **45**, 257.
37 EBLING F.J., *et al* (1970) *J Endocrinol* **48**, 73.
38 EBLING F.J., *et al* (1970) *J Endocrinol* **48**, 83.
39 EBLING F.J., *et al* (1971) *J Endocrinol* **51**, 181.
40 EBLING F.J., *et al* (1973) *J Invest Dermatol* **60**, 183.
41 EBLING F.J., *et al* (1975) *Br J Dermatol* **92**, 325.
42 EBLING F.J., *et al* (1975) *J Endocrinol* **66**, 401.
43 EBLING F.J., *et al* (1975) *J Endocrinol* **66**, 407.
44 FORCHIELLI E., *et al* (1965) *Acta Endocrinol* **50**, 51.
45 FROST P. & GOMEZ E.C. (1972) In *Advances in Biology of Skin*. Vol. 12. *Pharmacology and the Skin*. Eds. Montagna W., *et al*. New York, Appleton–Century–Crofts, p. 403.
46 GIRARD J., *et al* (1980) *Arch Derm Res* **269**, 281.
47 GLENN E.M. & GRAY J. (1965) *Endocrinology* **76**, 115.
48 GOOLAMALI S.K., *et al* (1973) *Br J Dermatol* **89**, 21.
49 GOOLAMALI S.K., *et al* (1974) *J Invest Dermatol* **63**, 253.
50 DE GRAAF H.J. (1943) *Ned Tijdschr Geneeskd* **87**, 1450.
51 DE GRAAF H.J. & KOOIJ R. (1955) *Acta Physiol Pharmacol Néerl* **4**, 201.
52 DE GROOT C.A., *et al* (1965) *Br J Dermatol* **77**, 617.
53 HAMILTON J.B. (1941) *J Clin Endocrinol Metab* **1**, 570.
54 HAMILTON J.B. & MONTAGNA W. (1950) *Am J Anat* **86**, 191.
55 HASKIN D., *et al* (1953) *J Invest Dermatol* **20**, 207.
56 HODGSON-JONES I.S., *et al* (1952) *Acta Derm Venereol* [*Suppl. 29*] (*Stockh*) **32**, 151.
57 HSIA S.L. & VOIGT W. (1974) *J Invest Dermatol* **62**, 224.
58 HUGGINS C., *et al* (1955) *Endocrinology* **57**, 25.

59 JARRETT A. (1955) *Br J Dermatol* **62**, 165.

60 JARRETT A. (1959) *Br J Dermatol* **71**, 102.

61 LAPIÈRE C. (1953) *C R Séances Soc Biol Paris* **147**, 1302.

62 LASHER N., *et al* (1954) *J Invest Dermatol* **22**, 25.

63 LASHER N., *et al* (1955) *J Invest Dermatol* **24**, 499.

64 LORINCZ A.L. (1963) In *Advances in Biology of Skin*. Vol. 4. *Sebaceous Glands*. Eds. Montagna W., *et al*. Oxford, Pergamon, p. 188.

65 LORINCZ A.L. & LANCASTER G. (1957) *Science* **126**, 124.

66 MARTIN J. (1962) *J Morph* **110**, 285.

67 MARTIN J. & PRICE D. (1967) *J Morph* **121**, 209.

68 MONTAGNA W. & KENYON P. (1949) *Anat Rec* **103**, 365.

69 NIKKARI T. (1965) *Scand J Clin Lab Invest* **17** (Suppl. **85**).

70 NIKKARI T. & VALAVAARA M. (1969) *J Endocrinol* **43**, 113.

71 NIKKARI T. & VALAVAARA M. (1970) *Br J Dermatol* **83**, 459.

72 NIKKARI T. & VALAVAARA M. (1970) *J Endocrinol* **48**, 373.

73 PLEWIG G. & KLIGMAN A.M. (1978) *J Invest Dermatol* **70**, 314.

74 POCHI P.E. & STRAUSS J.S. (1963) *Arch Dermatol* **88**, 729.

75 POCHI P.E. & STRAUSS J.S. (1966) *J Invest Dermatol* **47**, 582.

76 POCHI P.E. & STRAUSS J.S. (1967) *J Invest Dermatol* **49**, 456.

77 POCHI P.E. & STRAUSS J.S. (1969) *J Invest Dermatol* **52**, 32.

78 POCHI P.E. & STRAUSS J.S. (1973) *Arch Dermatol* **108**, 210.

79 POCHI P.E. & STRAUSS J.S. (1974) *J Invest Dermatol* **62**, 191.

80 POCHI P.E. & STRAUSS J.S. (1976) *Arch Dermatol* **112**, 1108.

81 POCHI P.E., *et al* (1962) *J Invest Dermatol* **38**, 45.

82 POCHI P.E., *et al* (1962) *J Invest Dermatol* **39**, 475.

83 POCHI P.E., *et al* (1963) *J Invest Dermatol* **41**, 391.

84 POCHI P.E., *et al* (1979) *J Invest Dermatol* **73**, 108.

85 RONY H.R. & ZAKON S.J. (1943) *Arch Dermatol* **48**, 601.

86 SHIZUME K. & LERNER A.B. (1954) *J Clin Endocrinol Metab* **14**, 1491.

87 SHUSTER S. & THODY A.J. (1974) *J Invest Dermatol* **62**, 172.

88 SHUSTER S., *et al* (1973) *Lancet* i, 463.

89 SIMPSON N.B., *et al* (1979) *Br J Dermatol* **100**, 687.

90 SMITH J.G. (1959) *Arch Dermatol Syphil* **80**, 663.

91 STRAUSS J.S. & EBLING F.J. (1970) *Mem Soc Endocrinol* **18**, 341.

92 STRAUSS J.S. & KLIGMAN A.M. (1959) *J Invest Dermatol* **33**, 9.

93 STRAUSS J.S. & KLIGMAN A.M. (1961) *J Invest Dermatol* **36**, 309.

94 STRAUSS J.S. & POCHI P.E. (1961) *J Invest Dermatol* **36**, 293.

95 STRAUSS J.S. & POCHI P.E. (1963) In *Advances in Biology of Skin*. Vol. 4. *Sebaceous Glands*. Eds. Montagna W., *et al*. Oxford, Pergamon, p. 220.

96 STRAUSS J.S. & POCHI P.E. (1963) *Recent Prog Horm Res* **19**, 385.

97 STRAUSS J.S., *et al* (1962) *J Invest Dermatol* **39**, 139.

98 SWEENEY T.M., *et al* (1969) *J Invest Dermatol* **53**, 8.

99 TALEISNIK S. & ORFAS R. (1966) *Endocrinology* **78**, 522.

100 TANNER J.M. & WHITEHOUSE R.H. (1972) In *Growth and Growth Hormone*. Eds. Pecile A. & Muller E.E. Amsterdam, Excerpta Medica, p. 429.

101 THODY A.J. & SHUSTER S. (1970) *J Endocrinol* **47**, 219.

102 THODY A.J. & SHUSTER S. (1970) *J Endocrinol* **48**, 139.

103 THODY A.J. & SHUSTER S. (1971) *J Endocrinol* **49**, 325.

104 THODY A.J. & SHUSTER S. (1971) *J Endocrinol* **49**, 329.

105 THODY A.J. & SHUSTER S. (1971) *J Endocrinol* **50**, 533.

106 THODY A.J. & SHUSTER S. (1971) *J Endocrinol* **51**, 6p.

107 THODY A.J. & SHUSTER S. (1972) *J Endocrinol* **54**, 239.

108 THODY A.J. & SHUSTER S. (1972) *Nature* **237**, 346.

109 THODY A.J. & SHUSTER S. (1973) *J Endocrinol* **58**, 35.

110 THODY A.J. & SHUSTER S. (1973) *Nature* **245**, 207.

111 THODY A.J. & SHUSTER S. (1975) *J Endocrinol* **64**, 503.

112 WOODBURY L.P., *et al* (1965) *J Invest Dermatol* **45**, 362.

113 WOODBURY L.P., *et al* (1965) *J Invest Dermatol* **45**, 364.

114 ZACHMANN M., *et al* (1976) In *Growth Hormone and Related Peptides*. Eds. Pecile A. & Muller E.E. Amsterdam, Excerpta Medica, p. 286.

115 ZELIGMAN I. & HUBENER L.F. (1957) *AMA Arch Derm* **76**, 652.

INHIBITORS OF SEBACEOUS ACTIVITY

Sebaceous activity can be inhibited not only by oestrogens but also by certain synthetic non-oestrogenic steroids which antagonize the action of androgens at the target site [12, 42], as well as by some other compounds, notably derivatives of Vitamin A such as 13-cis-retinoic acid (isotretinoin).

Anti-androgens include A-norprogesterone [28, 29], 17α-methyl-B-nortestosterone [8] and its 6α,6-ethylene substituent [40], cyproterone acetate [10, 11, 35, 36] and Δ_1-chlormadinone acetate [3, 9], all of which have been shown to reduce sebaceous activity in animal experiments. Their action differs from that of oestrogens in that it involves a clear reduction in sebaceous mitosis, and requires a much larger dose. Thus in castrated rats treated with 0·2 mg/24 h of testosterone, 5·0 mg/24 h of cyproterone acetate suppressed sebum production to a lesser extent than 2 μg of oestradiol did (Fig. 52.8). The demonstration that when such doses of cyproterone acetate and oestradiol are given concomitantly their effects are additive [11] reinforces the conclusion that their points of action

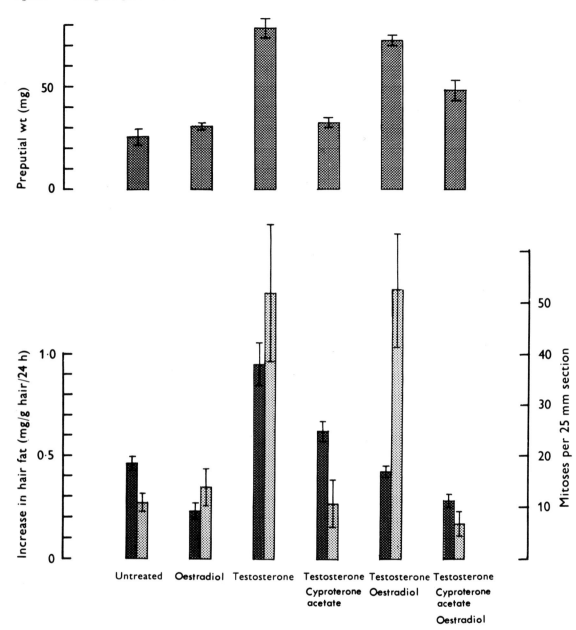

FIG. 52.8. Effects of oestradiol (2–4 μg/24 h), testosterone (0·2 mg/24 h) and cyproterone acetate (50 mg/24 h) on (a) the weight of the preputial glands and (b) the secretion of sebum (left-hand columns) and mitosis in the sebaceous glands (right-hand columns). Means ± standard errors for groups of six rats. (Data from Ebling [11].)

are distinct. That cyproterone acetate acts locally has been unequivocally demonstrated after topical administration in ethanol to rats [16].

In man, sebum production has been significantly reduced by oral administration of 17α-methyl-B-nortestosterone [38, 43, 44, 48], chlormadinone acetate [43] and cyproterone acetate [4, 7, 14, 15, 46, 47]. The anti-androgenic action may not be solely peripheral, since plasma testosterone is also lowered [1, 14, 15, 44].

The effectiveness of the topical application of anti-androgens is debatable. 17α-Methyl-B-nortestosterone was shown to act topically in man [44] and the degree of sebum suppression was not always correlated with the lowering of plasma testosterone, implying a peripheral effect. Cyproterone acetate appeared to be ineffective when applied in 50% DMSO [6] or in cetomacrogel [39] but to have some effect in oil-in-water emulsion [46,47] or ethanol [2].

Various other agents have been proposed. 17α-Propyltestosterone has been shown to cause regression of the hamster flank organ [17] and to reduce sebum secretion by 20% when applied to the human forehead for 4 weeks [33]. Flutamide, a non-steroidal anti-androgen, is similarly effective in the hamster [31], but produced equivocal results when tested in human subjects [34]. Novel 17α-chloro and 17β-sulphinyl steroids have recently been suggested as inhibitors of sebaceous activity [24]. Spironolactone, given systemically, has been shown to inhibit the hamster flank organ [30], and the H_2 receptor antagonists ranitidine and cimetidine to inhibit sebum secretion in man [19, 32]. The possibility must also be considered that 5α-reductase inhibitors, which inhibit the conversion of testosterone to 5α-dihydrotestosterone without blocking attachment of the steroid to the intracellular receptor (see Chapter 2), similarly reduce sebum production [13, 25]. The reduction in the rate of sebum excretion by topically applied progesterone [5, 18, 41] may involve such a mechanism.

Certain derivatives of vitamin A, in particular 13-cis-retinoic acid, have marked affects on the sebaceous glands when given systemically. They have been shown to reduce the size of the hamster flank organ [21–23, 37] and the human sebaceous glands [27] and to cause a profound inhibition of sebaceous excretion [20, 26, 45].

REFERENCES

1 Barnes E.W., *et al* (1975) *Clin Endocrinol (Oxf)* **4**, 65.
2 Bingham K.D., *et al* (1979) *Lancet* ii, 304.
3 Burdick K.H. & Hill R. (1970) *Br J Dermatol* **82**, 19.
4 Burton J.L., *et al* (1973) *Br J Dermatol* **89**, 487.
5 Cunliffe W.J. & Simpson N.B. (1980) In *Percutaneous Absorption of Steroids*. Eds. Mauvais-Jarvis P., *et al*. London, Academic Press, p. 149.
6 Cunliffe W.J., *et al* (1969) *Br J Dermatol* **81**, 200.
7 Dowd P.M., *et al* (1983) *Br J Dermatol* **109**, 709.
8 Ebling F.J. (1967) *J Endocrinol* **38**, 181.
9 Ebling F.J. (1970) *Br J Dermatol* **82** (Suppl. 6), 10.
10 Ebling F.J. (1970) In *Advances in Steroids*. Ed. Briggs M.H. London, Academic Press, Vol. 2, p. 1.
11 Ebling F.J. (1973) *Acta Endocrinol* **72**, 361.
12 Ebling F.J. (1977) In *Androgens and Antiandrogens*. Eds. Martini L. & Motta M. New York, Raven Press, p. 341.
13 Ebling F.J. (1980) In *Percutaneous Absorption of Steroids*. Eds. Mauvais-Jarvis, P., *et al*. London, Academic Press, p. 139.
14 Ebling F.J., *et al* (1977) *Br J Dermatol* **97**, 371.
15 Ebling F.J., *et al* (1979) In *Androgenisierungserscheinungen bei der Frau*. Eds. Hammerstein J., *et al*. Amsterdam, Excerpta Medica, p. 243.
16 Ebling F.J., *et al* (1981) *J Invest Dermatol* **77**, 458.
17 Ferrari R.A., *et al* (1978) *J Invest Dermatol* **71**, 320.
18 Girard J., *et al* (1980) *Arch Derm Res* **269**, 281.
19 Gloor M., *et al* (1981) *Acta Derm Venereol (Stockh)* **61**, 262.
20 Goldstein J.A., *et al* (1982) *J Am Acad Dermatol* **6**, 760.
21 Gomez E.C. (1980) *J Invest Dermatol* **76**, 68.
22 Gomez E.C. (1982) *J Am Acad Dermatol* **6**, 746.
23 Gomez E.C. & Moskowitz R.J. (1980) *J Invest Dermatol* **74**, 392.
24 Green M.J., *et al* (1983) *J Med Chem* **26**, 78.
25 Hsia S.L. & Voigt W. (1974) *J Invest Dermatol* **62**, 224.
26 King K., *et al* (1982) *Br J Dermatol* **107**, 583.
27 Landthaler M., *et al* (1980) *Arch Derm Res* **269**, 281.
28 Lerner L.J. (1964) *Recent Progr Horm Res* **20**, 435.
29 Lerner L.J., *et al* (1960) *Proc Soc Exp Biol Med* **103**, 172.
30 Luderschmidt C., *et al* (1982) *J Invest Dermatol* **78**, 253.
31 Lutsky B.N., *et al* (1975) *J Invest Dermatol* **64**, 412.
32 Lyons F. & Shuster S. (1980) *Br J Dermatol* **102**, 730.
33 Lyons F. & Shuster S. (1981) *Br J Dermatol* **104**, 685.
34 Lyons F. & Shuster S. (1982) *Br J Dermatol* **107**, 697.
35 Neumann F. (1977) *Horm Metab Res* **9**, 1.
36 Neumann F. & Elger W. (1966) *J Invest Dermatol* **46**, 561.
37 Plewig G. (1980) *Arch Derm Res* **268**, 239.
38 Pria S.D., *et al* (1969) *J Invest Dermatol* **52**, 348.
39 Pye R.J., *et al* (1976) *Br J Dermatol* **95**, 427.
40 Saunders H.L. & Ebling F.J. (1969) *J Invest Dermatol* **52**, 163.
41 Simpson N.B., *et al* (1979) *Br J Dermatol* **100**, 687.
42 Stewart M.E. & Pochi P.E. (1978) *Int J Dermatol* **17**, 167.
43 Strauss J.S. & Pochi P.E. (1970) *Br J Dermatol* **82** (Suppl. 6), 33.
44 Strauss J.S., *et al* (1969) *J Invest Dermatol* **52**, 95.
45 Strauss J.S., *et al* (1980) *J Invest Dermatol* **74**, 66.
46 Winkler K. (1968) *Ann Dermatol Syphiligr* **95**, 147.
47 Winkler K. (1968) *Arch Klin Exp Dermatol* **233**, 296.
48 Zarate A., *et al* (1966) *J Clin Endocrinol Metab* **26**, 1394.

ACNE VULGARIS

Definition. Acne is a chronic inflammatory disease of the pilosebaceous units, which is characterized by the formation of comedones, erythematous papules and pustules.

The condition usually starts in adolescence and resolves by the mid-twenties [4]. Four major aetiological factors are involved: increased sebum production, an abnormality of the microbial flora, hyperkeratinization of the pilosebaceous duct and the production of inflammation. Treatments are related logically to its cause [5] and should be gratifying for the patient and physician; only a few patients are likely to prove difficult to treat with present therapies.

Natural history. Acne develops earlier in females than in males [1, 13]. This may reflect the earlier onset of puberty in females. However, some subjects may show small non-inflamed lesions by the age of 8–9 yr [15]. The age of greatest incidence and severity is 16–18 yr for women and 18–19 yr for men [1, 9]. The incidence of clinical acne in females at 17 yr is 40% and in males at 18 yr is 35%. Thereafter the acne resolves only slowly but some patients still have problems worthy of treating up to the age of 25–35 yr [5]. At the age of 40 yr, lesions are present in 1% of males and 5% of females [5, 6]. It is not known why acne resolves or why it is more persistent in females. These problems are worth investigation, as this could yield a new pharmacological approach to treatment [3].

Genetic factors. The preponderant importance of genetic factors in determining susceptibility to acne is suggested by racial studies [2, 11] and is confirmed by the very high degree of concordance between identical twins [14]. A survey in Essen, Germany [8], showed that acne had been present in one or both parents of 45% of schoolboys with acne, but in parents of only 8% of boys without acne. Similar findings were recorded in a later survey of both girls and boys [10]. The mode of inheritance is unknown but is assumed to be multifactorial. The decreased incidence of atopic dermatitis in acne sufferers [12] may be genetically determined but could be otherwise explained. The association of very severe acne with the XYY syndrome [7, 16] has been recorded.

Epidemiology. Acne occurs in all races of man, but not in other primates. The incidence and severity are very significantly lower in the Japanese than in Caucasoids [11]. In a study in the United States of prisoners aged 15–21 yr, severe or very severe acne was found in 5% of Caucasoids but in only 0·5% of Negroes.

REFERENCES

1 BURTON J.L., *et al* (1971) *Br J Dermatol* **85**, 119.
2 CRANDALL B.F., *et al* (1974) *J Med Genet* **11**, 393.
3 CUNLIFFE W.J. (1981) *Acne. Update Postgraduate Series*. London, Update Publications.
4 CUNLIFFE W.J. & COTTERILL J.A. (1975) *The Acnes*. London, W.B. Saunders.
5 CUNLIFFE W.J. & GOULD D.J. (1979) *Br Med J* **166**, 1.
6 EPSTEIN E. (1968) *Dermatol Digest* **7**, 49.
7 FUNDERBURK S.J. (1976) *Arch Dermatol* **112**, 859.
8 GLOOR M., *et al* (1974) *Hautarzt* **25**, 391.
9 GÖTZ H., *et al* (1971) *Minerva Dermatol* **2**, 35.
10 GÖTZ H., *et al* (1974) *Hautarzt* **25**, 288.
11 HAMILTON J.B. (1964) *J Clin Endocrinol Metab* **23**, 267.
12 LIDDELL K. (1976) *Br J Dermatol* **94**, 633.
13 MUNRO-ASHMAN D. (1963) *Trans St. John's Hosp Dermatol Soc* **49**, 144.
14 NIERMANN H. (1958) *Z. Mensch. Vererb.-U, Konstit. Lehre* **34**, 483.
15 POCHI P.E. & STRAUSS J.S. (1974) *J Invest Dermatol* **62**, 191.
16 VOORHEES J.J., *et al* (1972) *Arch Dermatol* **105**, 913.

Aetiology

Increased sebum production. Whatever the relative importance of the various aetiological factors that may be involved in acne vulgaris, one fact is indisputable: active sebaceous glands are a prerequisite. Acne patients, male and female, excrete on average more sebum than normal subjects [51] and the level of secretion correlates well with the severity of the acne (Fig. 52.9) [3, 8]. The question of why this

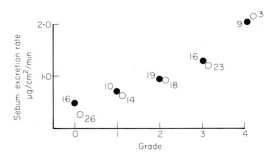

FIG. 52.9. The correlation between sebum excretion and acne in males (●) and females (○) between 15 and 25 years of age.

should be so is less easy to resolve. Sebaceous activity is dependent on male hormones of gonadal or adrenal origin [12, 13, 52, 61]. Abnormally high levels of sebum secretion could thus result from high overall androgen production or increased availability of free androgen because of deficiency in sex-hormone-binding globulin (SHBG). Equally, they could involve an amplified target response mediated either through 5α-reduction of testosterone or the capacity of the intracellular receptor to bind the hormone.

There is general agreement that plasma testosterone levels are not abnormally high in males with acne [14, 39, 53]. In females with acne the situation is more complicated. Some investigators have found testosterone levels to be normal [43, 49] whilst others have found the means to be significantly above normal [14, 34, 39, 40, 58], albeit only a fraction of the concentration in the male. There is more general agreement that mean SHBG levels are significantly below normal, with free testosterone consequently above normal [34, 40, 49]. However, for each endocrine assay, there is a considerable overlap between the acne and normal ranges. Thus Lawrence et al. [34] found that only 41% of their acne patients had free testosterone levels above normal. Lucky et al. [40] measured a number of androgens and their precursors, as well as SHBG, and found that 52% of non-hirsute women with acne had at least one abnormal hormone level. Darley et al. [10] found high testosterone in 26%, low SHBG in 45% and high prolactin in 45% of 38 women with acne. However, 24% of the total had no abnormality.

It may reasonably be concluded that abnormally high sebum excretion could be accounted for by systemic hormonal disbalance in between 50% and 75% of all cases of female acne. At least for the substantial residue, as well as for males, the probability of an enhanced peripheral response must be considered. The possible role of increased 5α-reduction of testosterone to its more active metabolite is indicated both by the demonstration that sebaceous glands in acne-prone regions show abnormally high 5α-reductase activity *in vitro* [57] and by the finding of abnormally high amounts of 5α-androstanediols in the urine of female acne patients [43].

Finally, the possibility that other hormones affect the sebaceous glands either directly or by enhancing their response to androgens should not be neglected [12, 13, 41, 62]. Most of the evidence for this view comes from animal experimentation and has already been discussed (p. 1905). A role for pituitary hormones is supported by the findings that in acromegalics the rate of sebum excretion correlates well with the logarithm of the serum growth hormone concentration [4] and that sebum excretion appears to be low in individuals with isolated growth hormone deficiency [17].

Irrespective of the rate of sebum excretion, could acne be related to changes in lipid composition? Sebum consists of a mixture of squalene, wax and sterol esters, cholesterol, polar lipids and triglycerides [11]. As the sebum moves up the duct, bacteria, especially *Propionibacterium acnes* (*P. acnes*), hydrolyse the triglycerides to free fatty acids. The precise roles of the individual lipid components are not clear. They may be involved in ductal hypercornification or may be essential to the growth of bacteria. No consistent differences are reported between acne subjects and controls, but patients with acne tend to have higher levels of squalene and wax esters, lower levels of fatty acids [1, 5, 28, 63] and a more frequent occurrence of particular free fatty acids [29, 47].

Ductal hypercornification. Acne patients show hypercornification, evident clinically by the presence of blackheads and whiteheads and from the finding that there is a significant correlation between the severity of acne and the number and size of follicular casts [24].

The reason for this ductal hypercornification is unclear. Electron microscopy of early non-inflamed lesions taken from prepubertal and early pubertal individuals has demonstated few or no bacteria [33]. Quantification of comedonal bacteria suggests that colonization is an extension of the follicular flora and may be unrelated to the event of comedogenesis [56]. Biopsy and culture of early non-inflamed lesions has shown that 30% of these are also without bacteria [36], suggesting that initiation of cornification is not related, in most instances, to the presence of ductal bacteria. The stimulus to hypercornification could possibly be androgen mediated [60], or result from an irritant effect of sebaceous lipids as they move through the duct [27, 31], as demonstrated in the rabbit ear model [44]. The development of a human model for comedogenecity [45] has suggested that the rabbit model is over-reactive. Animals do not develop whiteheads or inflamed lesions, whereas the rabbit's ear readily produces comedones [15]. Nevertheless, as hypercornification increases, so does ductal colonization with *P. acnes* and *Staphylococcus epidermidis* (*S. epidermidis*), whose lipases hydrolyse the sebaceous triglycerides to free fatty acids which may contribute to the cornification.

Hypercornification appears to involve persistence of desmosomes, desmosomal bodies and a decrease in the number of membrane-coated granules [32, 48, 68], but it is not clear whether such changes are primary or secondary. What converts a normal follicle into either a whitehead (closed comedone) or a blackhead (open comedone) is equally obscure. Possibly hydration of the ductal exit may precipitate the development of a non-inflamed into an inflamed lesion [66, 67].

Acne and bacteria. Acne is not infectious. The three major organisms isolated from the surface of the skin and the duct of patients with acne are *P. acnes*, *S. epidermidis* and *Pityrosporum ovale* [42]. There are three major subgroups of the propionibacteria (*P. acnes*, *P. granulosum* and *P. avidum*). Almost certainly *P. acnes* and, to a lesser extent, *P. granulosum*, are the most important. Nevertheless, as they live in association with the staphylococci and *Pityrosporum* it is likely that these organisms have some control over the growth of *P. acnes* [22].

Adolescence and its attendant seborrhoea are associated with a significant increase in *P. acnes* [38] but, in contrast with sebum excretion rate and ductal cornification, there is little or no relationship between the number of bacteria on the skin surface or in the ducts and the severity of acne [6, 7, 37].

The environment of the bacteria is probably more important than their absolute numbers for the development of lesions. Oxygen tension, pH and nutrient supply markedly affect the growth of *P. acnes in vitro* and its production of substances with potential biological activity such as lipases, proteases, hyaluronate lyase and phosphatase [7, 23, 25]. *In vivo* the pH of blackheads markedly varies between 3·6 and 6·7 [20], and this is likely to affect the functioning of the bacteria. Such physiological variability could determine whether or not a follicle develops into a non-inflamed comedo and subsequently into an inflamed lesion [22].

The 'lipase' theory for acne was fashionable [16] but no longer has many supporters, since injection of fatty acids into the skin produces only mild inflammatory reactions [54]. Lipids are not seen in the infiltrate associated with inflammation and a specific lipase inhibitor does not help acne [65].

Mediation of inflammation. From the viewpoint of the patient, the inflamed lesions are usually the more important. The inflammation is not caused by bacteria in the dermis, since these are rarely demonstrable by routine and immunofluorescent methods [59]. It probably results from biologically active mediators which diffuse from the follicle where they are produced by *P. acnes*. Alternatively, *P. acnes* proteases [26] may degrade the ductal keratin to produce eukaryotic mediators.

Most inflamed lesions probably arise from non-inflamed lesions [61], but the precise factors which induce inflammation and the detailed morphogenesis of acne lesions are unknown [50]. *P. acnes* produces many enzymes, including three proteases, lipase, phosphatases and hyaluronate lyase, all of which might in theory be implicated [22]. *P. acnes*, especially its cell wall fraction, is a potent chemoattractant for polymorphonuclear and mononuclear cells [35, 55, 64]. It also produces a prostaglandin-like substance [18, 63.]; that this could be involved is suggested by the evidence that non-steroidal anti-inflammatory drugs have an anti-acne effect [19, 46].

Whatever the initiating factor(s), direct immunofluorescent studies have shown that in early non-inflamed and inflamed lesions there is activation of the classical and alternative complement pathways [9, 59, 64]. As the lesions progress type 3 and 4 reactions become more evident at the expense of the complement pathways [59]. Circulating immune complexes are not evident in acne sera [2]. Skin testing with a heat-killed suspension of *P. acnes* demonstrated that subjects with severe acne produced a greater inflammatory response at 48 h than other subjects, suggesting that the host response may also be important [30]. It is uncommon to see females with very severe acne and this may be due to the observation that females muster a better defence mechanism against *P. acnes* than males do [21].

Resolution of acne. While the evolution of acne has received considerable attention, there has been virtually no work on why it resolves. Limited studies suggest that the resolution is not related to reduction of sebum production [62] or surface bacteria [42]. There is no published work relating resolution to ductal hypercornification, inflammatory mediators or to changes in the host response.

REFERENCES

1 BEVERIDGE G.W. & POWELL, E. (1969) *Br J Dermatol* **81**, 525.
2 BURKHART C.G. & LEHMANN P.F. (1982) *Br J Dermatol* **106**, 120.
3 BURTON J.L. & SHUSTER S. (1971) *Br J Dermatol* **84**, 600.
4 BURTON J.L., *et al* (1972) *Br Med J* i, 406.
5 COTTERILL J.A., *et al* (1972) *Br Med J* ii, 444.
6 COVE J.H., *et al* (1980) *Br J Dermatol* **103**, 383.
7 COVE J.H., *et al* (1980) *J App Bacteriol* **49**, 29.
8 CUNLIFFE W.J. & SHUSTER S. (1969) *Lancet* i, 685.
9 DAHL M.G.C. & McGIBBON D.H. (1979) *Br J Dermatol* **101**, 633.
10 DARLEY C.R., *et al* (1982) *Br J Dermatol* **106**, 517.
11 DOWLING D.T., *et al* (1969) *J Invest Dermatol* **53**, 322.
12 EBLING F.J. (1974) *J Invest Dermatol* **62**, 161.
13 EBLING F.J.G. (1979) In *Acne: Update for the Practitioner*. Ed. Frank S.B. New York, Yorke Medical Books, p. 53.
14 FÖRSTROM L., *et al* (1974) *Acta Derm Venereol (Stockh)* **54**, 369.
15 FRANK S.B. (1982) *J Am Acad Dermatol* **6**, 373.

16 FREINKEL R.K. & SHEN Y. (1969) *J Invest Dermatol* **53**, 422.

17 GOOLAMALI S.K., *et al* (1973) *Br J Dermatol* **89**, 21.

18 HELLGREN L., *et al* (1979) *Experimentia* **35**, 196.

19 HINDSON C., *et al* (1982) *Lancet* i, 1415.

20 HOLLAND D.B. & CUNLIFFE W.J. (1983) *Acta Derm Venereol (Stockh)* **63**, 155.

21 HOLLAND D.B., *et al* (1983) *Br J Dermatol* **109**, 199.

22 HOLLAND K.T., *et al* (1978) *Clin Exp Dermatol* **65**, 382.

23 HOLLAND K.T., *et al* (1979) *J Appl Bacteriol* **47**, 383.

24 HOLMES R.L., *et al* (1972) *Br J Dermatol* **87**, 327.

25 INGHAM E., *et al* (1979) *J Gen Microbiol* **115**, 411.

26 INGHAM E., *et al* (1983) *J Appl Bacteriol* **54**, 263.

27 KANAAR P. (1971) *Dermatologica* **142**, 14.

28 KANAAR P. (1971) *Dermatologica* **143**, 121.

29 KELLUM R.L. & STRANGFELD K.E. (1972) *J Invest Dermatol* **58**, 315.

30 KERSEY P., *et al* (1980) *Br J Dermatol* **103**, 651.

31 KLIGMAN A.M. & KATZ A.G. (1968) *Arch Dermatol* **98**, 53.

32 KNUTSON D.D. (1974) *J Invest Dermatol* **62**, 288.

33 LAVKER R.M. *et al* (1981) *J Invest Dermatol* **77**, 325.

34 LAWRENCE D.M., *et al* (1981) *J Clin Endocrinol* **15**, 87.

35 LEE W., *et al* (1982) *Infect Immun* **71**, 78.

36 LEEMING J., *et al* (1982) Data presented at SID/ESDR, Washington, May 1982.

37 LEYDEN J.L., *et al* (1975) *J Invest Dermatol* **65**, 379.

38 LEYDEN J.L., *et al* (1975) *J Invest Dermatol* **65**, 382.

39 LIM L.S. & JAMES V.H.T. (1974) *Br J Dermatol* **91**, 135.

40 LUCKY A.W., *et al* (1983) *J Invest Dermatol* **81**, 70.

41 LUDERSCHMIDT C., *et al* (1983) *Arch Derm Res* **275**, 175.

42 MARPLES R. (1974) *J Invest Dermatol* **62**, 326.

43 MAUVAIS-JARVIS P., *et al* (1973) *J Clin Endocrinol Metab* **36**, 452.

44 MILLS O.H. & KLIGMAN A.M. (1975) In *Animal Models in Dermatology*. Ed. Maibach H.I. New York, Churchill Livingstone, p. 176.

45 MILLS O.H. & KLIGMAN A.M. (1982) *Br J Dermatol* **107**, 543.

46 MILLS O.H. & KLIGMAN A.M. (1983) *Br J Dermatol* **108**, 371.

47 MORELLO A.M., *et al* (1976) *J Invest Dermatol* **66**, 319.

48 MOTOYOSHI K. (1983) *Br J Dermatol* **109**, 191.

49 ODLIND V., *et al* (1982) *J Clin Endocrinol* **16**, 243.

50 ORRENTREICH N. & DURR N.P. (1974) *J Invest Dermatol* **62**, 316.

51 POCHI P.E. & STRAUSS J.S. (1964) *J Invest Dermatol* **43**, 383.

52 POCHI P.E. & STRAUSS J.S. (1974) *J Invest Dermatol* **62**, 191.

53 POCHI P.E., *et al* (1965) *J Clin Endocrinol Metab* **25**, 1660.

54 PUHVEL S.M. & SAKAMOTO M. (1977) *J Invest Dermatol* **69**, 401.

55 PUHVEL S.M. & SAKAMOTO M. (1978) *J Invest Dermatol* **71**, 324.

56 PUHVEL S.M., *et al* (1979) *J Invest Dermatol* **65**, 525.

57 SANSONE G. & REISNER R.M. (1971) *J Invest Dermatol* **56**, 366.

58 SCHIARONE F.E., *et al* (1983) *Arch Dermatol* **119**, 799.

59 SCOTT G.C., *et al* (1979) *Br J Dermatol* **101**, 315.

60 SHUSTER S., *et al* (1980) *Br J Dermatol* **103**, 127.

61 STRAUSS J.S. & POCHI P.E. (1970) *Arch Dermatol* **82**, 779.

62 STRAUSS J.S., *et al* (1983) In *Biochemistry and Physiology of the Skin*. Ed. Goldsmith L. New York, Oxford University Press, p. 569.

63 TRONNIER H. & BRUNN G. (1972) *Berufsdermatosen* **20**, 79.

64 WEBSTER G. & LEYDEN J.J. (1980) *Inflammation* **4**, 261.

65 WEEKS J.G., *et al* (1979) *J Invest Dermatol* **69**, 236.

66 WILLIAMS M. & CUNLIFFE W.J. (1973) *Lancet* iv, 1055.

67 WILLIAMS M., *et al* (1974) *Br J Dermatol* **90**, 1.

68 WOO-SAM P.C. (1977) *Br J Dermatol* **97**, 609.

Clinical picture. There are many myths about factors which might help or aggravate acne.

Diet. Considerable folklore has blamed acne on certain foods, in particular, chocolate and pork fat. Scientific proof is generally lacking. Chocolate appears to have no significant influence [4, 6]. Excessive dietary restriction resulting in weight loss reduces seborrhoea but cannot be considered of physiological or pharmacological benefit [10]. A link between diet and acne has recently been suggested again [12], and it is true that acne occurs less frequently in Zambia, Nigeria and Japan [11], where dietary habits differ markedly from those in Western Europe. However, such studies cannot distinguish between the effect of diet and genetic factors. The possible effect of diet on the age of puberty may be relevant. Acne is more likely after the start of sexual development, which occurs when the body weight attains about 48 kg [5].

Premenstrual flare. About 70% of women complain of a flare 2–7 days premenstrually and this subjective observation has been confirmed objectively [3]. It is unlikely that variations in sebum excretion during the menstrual cycle [2,13], even if substantial, could explain the flare. Possibly it is related to the effect of well-recognized premenstrual fluid changes on the epidermal hydration of the pilosebaceous duct [17]. Progesterone and oestrogen also have both pro- and anti-inflammatory effects.

Sweating. Up to 15% of acne patients notice that sweating causes a deterioration in their acne, especially if they live or work in hot humid environments (e.g. as cooks) [1, 3, 15]. Ductal hydration may be the responsible factor [16].

UV radiation. Patients and doctors alike accept that natural UV radiation often improves acne but objective evidence is relatively lacking. The cosmetic effect may be the entire explanation. Artificial UV radiation appears to be less satisfactory than natural radiation and PUVA has been reported actually to induce acne lesions [8]. Furthermore, UV radiation may enhance the comedogenicity of sebum [9].

Mental stress. Although primary induction has occasionally been observed, it is unlikely that stress in general induces the formation of *de novo* acne lesions [7]. However, acne itself induces stress, and 'picking' of the spots will aggravate the appearance. This is particularly obvious in young females who present with acne excoriée [14].

Occupation. Hydration of the ductal stratum corneum may induce acne in such occupations as catering. Patients dealing with oil undoubtedly develop an oil folliculitis [18], particularly on their trunks and limbs. The induction of chloracne by accidental release of halogenated hydrocarbons or other chemicals (see p. 573) is discussed elsewhere.

REFERENCES

1 BELISARIO J.C. (1951) *Aust J Dermatol* **1** (2), 86.
2 BURTON J.L., *et al* (1972) *Acta Derm Venereol (Stockh)* **52**, 81.
3 CUNLIFFE W.J. & COTTERILL J.A. (1975) *The Acnes*. London, W.B. Saunders.
4 FRIES J.H. (1978) *Ann Allergy* **41**, 120.
5 FRISCH R.E. (1972) *Pediatrics* **50**, 445.
6 FULTON J.E., *et al* (1969) *JAMA* **210**, 11.
7 KENYON F.E. (1966) *Br J Dermatol* **76**, 344.
8 MILLS O.H. & KLIGMAN A.M. (1978) *Arch Dermatol* **114**, 221.
9 MILLS O.H., *et al* (1978) *Br J Dermatol* **98**, 145.
10 POCHI P.E., *et al* (1970) *J Invest Dermatol* **55**, 303.
11 RATNAM A.V. & JAYARAJU K. (1979) *Br J Dermatol* **101**, 449.
12 ROSENBERG W.E. & KIRK B.S. (1981) *Arch Dermatol* **117**, 193.
13 SCHAEFFER H. (1973) *J Soc Cosmet Chem* **24**, 331.
14 SNEDDON J. & SNEDDON I. (1983) *Clin Exp Dermatol* **8**, 65.
15 SULZBERGER M.B., *et al* (1946) *US Naval Med Bull* **46**, 1178.
16 WILLIAMS M., *et al* (1974) *Br J Dermatol* **90**, 1.
17 WILLIAMSON D. & CUNLIFFE W.J. (1973) *Br J Dermatol* **88**, 253.
18 WULF K. & FEGELER F. (1953) *Hautarzt* **4**, 371.

Clinical appearance. Acne is a polymorphic disease occurring predominantly on the face (99%) and less so on the back (60%) and chest (15%) [4, 11]. In

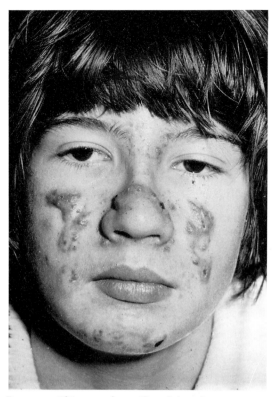

FIG. 52.10. This young boy with nodulocystic acne should be initially given isotretinoin or, if this is not available, tetracycline (1 g per day) plus benzoyl peroxide topically.

young males it predominantly affects the face, and in older males the back [11]. Seborrhoea is an almost universal feature [3]. Non-inflamed lesions are more frequent in the younger patients and consist of blackheads (the black colour is due to melanin, not dirt [6]), whiteheads and the so-called intermediate non-inflamed lesions which show features of both blackheads and whiteheads [1]. Inflammatory lesions may be superficial or deep and some arise from non-inflamed lesions [10]. The superficial lesions are usually papules and pustules, and the deep lesions are deep pustules, nodules and cysts (Figs. 52.10 and 52.11). Often forgotten is the macule, a lesion well on the way to regression, but one which can last for many weeks and contribute markedly to the general inflammatory appearance. Classification of lesions is arbitrary and the types may merge. Nodules and cysts are particularly disfiguring (Fig. 52.12). They may extend over areas of a few to many centimetres and the nodules may be remarkably deep with very little surface involvement. The deeper inflammatory lesions are often

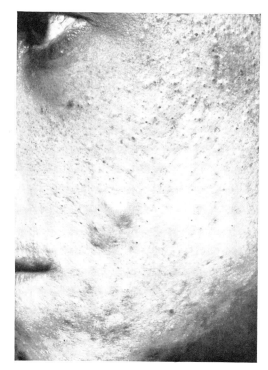

FIG. 52.11. Acne vulgaris in a boy aged 17. Comedones predominate but there are a few deep nodular lesions (Addenbrooke's Hospital).

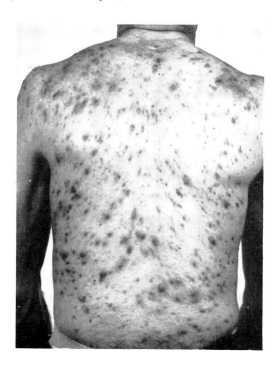

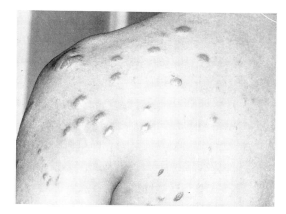

FIG. 52.13. Extensive keloids in a person who had extensive acne which is now under control.

associated with scarring. Rarely they develop into pyogenic granulomata [5].

Scars may be atrophic macules, ice-pick scars (especially on the face) or keloids. Keloids (Fig. 52.13) are the least common and are most prevalent on the trunk. Atrophic macules normally retain a purple colour for many months before becoming white and less conspicuous. Ice-pick scars probably change very little, but—except for keloids—scarring tends to improve even in the absence of treatment. A further common type of scarring on the back and chest is the small perifollicular atrophic lesion—the so-called perifollicular elastolysis [12].

A rare complication of scarring is calcification [7, 8, 9]. A common feature of darkly pigmented skin is the relatively persistent post-inflammatory pigmentation. Hidradenitis suppurativa may be associated [2]

REFERENCES

1 BURKE B.M. & CUNLIFFE W.J. (1984) *Br J Dermatol* 111, 83.
2 CHALMERS R.J.G., *et al* (1983) *Br Med J* ii, 1347.
3 CUNLIFFE W.J. & SHUSTER S. (1969) *Lancet* i, 685.
4 GOTZ H. (1971) *Minerva Dermatol* 2, 35.
5 HAGEDOM M. & KIRCHNER S. (1979) *Dermatologica* 158, 93.
6 KAIDBEY K.H. & KLIGMAN A.M. (1974) *J Invest Dermatol* 62, 31.
7 LEIDER M. (1950b) *Arch Dermatol Syphil* 62, 406.
8 MACGREGOR A.J. (1971) *Oral Surg Oral Med Pathol* 32, 829.

FIG. 52.12. Nodular acne with severe scarring in a man aged 35 who had suffered from acne of the trunk for 17 yr but whose face had never been affected (Addenbrooke's Hospital).

9 MOBAYEN M.M. & COPEMAN P.W.M. (1983) *Clin Exp Dermatol* **8**, 107.
10 ORRENTREICH N. & DURR N.P. (1974) *J Invest Dermatol* **62**, 316.
11 TAAFFE A., *et al* (1983) *Br J Dermatol.* **109**, (Suppl. 24) 43.
12 VARADI D.P. & SQUETON A.C. (1970) *Br J Dermatol* **83**, 143.

Differential diagnosis. Acne is rarely misdiagnosed. The commonest mistaken diagnosis is rosacea, which occurs in an older group. There are no comedones, nodules or cysts, and scarring does not occur. Occasionally patients may have both rosacea and acne. Rosacea patients may also have ocular involvement, but rarely truncal lesions. In females, confusion with perioral eczema is possible, but in these patients the lesions itch, the skin is dry, and non-inflamed lesions are lacking. Whiteheads may be confused with milia. The milia predominantly occur infra-orbitally, are whiter and can occur in association with, although they are unrelated to, acne. Acneiform drug eruptions (p. 1245) can easily be misdiagnosed. Folliculitis due to Gram-negative organisms can complicate acne therapy [3, 4] and the rare folliculitis due to *Candida* may also present as multiple pustular eruptions. Localized pustular eruptions may be due to animal ringworm infection resulting in a kerion. Occurring particularly on the back, a folliculitis due to *Pityrosporum* has been described [2] which may respond well to ketoconazole. Plane warts, particularly on the face, can also cause confusion, as can pseudo-folliculitis barbae [1]. Rare diseases producing difficulties include acne agminata, adenoma sebaceum and a micropapular sarcoidal facial eruption, which has been reported to be due to the selective perifollicular absorption of oils present in certain bubble gums [5]. The severe papulopustular eruption associated with zinc deficiency can be mistaken for severe acne [6]. Several cases have been reported after prolonged intravenous feeding.

REFERENCES

1 CONTE M.S. & LAWRENCE J.E. (1979) *JAMA* **241**, 53.
2 FORD, G.P., *et al* (1982) *Br J Dermatol* **107**, 691.
3 FRIES J.H. (1978) *Ann Allergy* **41**, 120.
4 FULTON J.E., *et al* (1968) *Arch Dermatol* **98**, 349.
5 GEORGOUSAS K. & KOCSARD E. (1978) *Acta Derm Venereol (Stockh)* **58**, 433.
6 SCHLAPPER O.L.A. (1972) *JAMA* **219**, 877.

Treatment [9]. Acne is a most treatable disease. Mild acne requires only topical therapy. Patients with moderate or severe acne need both oral and topical therapy; oral antibiotics must be given for 6 months but topical therapy will be required throughout the duration of the disorder. Further courses of oral antibiotics can and must be given if needed.

Topical treatment. The most widely used topical therapies are benzoyl peroxide, vitamin A acid and antibiotics. Topical antibiotics include tetracycline, chloramphenicol, erythromycin and clindamycin [12, 15, 18, 23, 31]. They are used in concentrations of 1–4% in a cream or lotion base. Benzoyl peroxide is available in concentrations of 2.5, 5 and 10%, either alone or with a combination of sulphur, imidazole or hydroxyquinolone [3, 6, 10, 16]. Adequate dose response studies with benzoyl peroxide are lacking, and the clinical value of combined therapy remains insufficiently investigated. Retinoic acid is available in a 0·025 and 0·05% concentration as either a gel or a cream.

In general, topical therapy appears less effective than adequate oral treatment. However, one study has shown topical clindamycin to be as effective as 500 mg per day of tetracycline [20]. Vitamin A acid acts by removing non-inflamed lesions, and thereby Non-inflamed lesions can thereby make the microenvironment less favourable for the development of inflammation [8, 21, 22, 28]. Benzoyl peroxide is primarily antimicrobial [7, 16] and also reduces the number of non-inflamed lesions [20], but it is unlikely that it affects sebum production [7, 14, 19]. Topical antibiotics appear to have comparatively less effect on the non-inflamed lesions [2, 4]. In the U.K. and many European countries, benzoyl peroxide seems to be the favourite treatment; in the USA benzoyl peroxide is also widely used, but so are retinoic acid and topical antibiotics. Currently topical antibiotics (with the exception of one chloramphenicol, one tetracycline and one neomycin preparation) are not yet commercially available in the U.K., perhaps because of the possible risk of producing resistant organisms [11, 13]. Comparative studies between benzoyl peroxide, vitamin A acid and topical antibiotics are not yet comprehensive [1]. Benzoyl peroxide appears to be therapeutically superior to topical erythromycin [20], but only equivalent to vitamin A acid [24, 25]. Of the topical antibiotics, clindamycin appears to be the most and tetracycline the least effective, with erythromycin in second place [18, 31]. Chloramphenicol proved less effective than benzoyl peroxide in a single study [8].

The efficacy of other topical treatments has not been established by controlled studies. Sulphur continues to be used, although it may be both comedogenic [25] and comedolytic [32]. Salicylic acid in propylene glycol (5%) [26] is probably useful but the many formulations of resorcin appear to be totally ineffective [27]. A few topical preparations contain weak corticosteroids but proof of their efficacy is lacking.

Recently, ethyl lactate, in combination with zinc sulphate as a stabilizer, has been reported to help acne. The drug appears to be metabolized by *P. acnes* into lactic acid, which is unfavourable for survival of the bacterium [17]. Azelaic acid cream (1,7-heptanedicarboxylic acid) seems to help some patients but has not yet undergone controlled studies [29].

The conclusion of the authors is that the topical therapies, benzoyl peroxide, vitamin A acid and antibiotics (erythromycin and clindamycin), should be used alone in patients with mild acne, in conjunction with oral antibiotics in patients with more severe acne and as a maintenance treatment after stopping oral therapy [30].

REFERENCES

1 BELKNAP B.S. (1981) *Cutis* 82, 856.
2 BERNSTEIN J.E. & SHALITA A.R. (1980) *Acta Derm Venereol (Stockh)* 60, 537.
3 BOSSCHE H.V. *et al* (1982) *Br J Dermatol* 107, 342.
4 BURKE B.M. *et al* (1983) *Br J Dermatol* 108, 199.
5 CHRISTIANSEN J.V., *et al* (1974) *Dermatologica* 149, 121.
6 CUNLIFFE W.J. (1981) *Acne. Update Postgraduate Series.* London, Update Publications.
7 CUNLIFFE W.J. & HOLLAND K.T. (1981) *Acta Derm Venereol (Stockh)* 61, 267.
8 CUNLIFFE W.J., *et al* (1980) *Practitioner* 224, 952.
9 CUNLIFFE W.J., *et al* (1981) *Clin Exp Dermatol* 6, 461.
10 DEGREEF H. & BUSSCHE G.V. (1982) *Dermatologica* 164, 201.
11 DOBSON R.L. (1981) *J Am Acad Dermatol* 5, 458.
12 DOBSON R.L. & BELKNAP B.S. (1980) *J Am Acad Dermatol* 3, 478.
13 EADY E.A., *et al* (1982) *J Antimicrob Chemother* 10, 89.
14 FANTA D. & JURECKA W. (1978) *Acta Derm Venereol (Stockh)* 58, 361.
15 FEUCHT C.L., *et al* (1980) *J Am Acad Dermatol* 3, 483.
16 FULTON J.E. & PABLO G. (1974) *Arch Dermatol* 110, 83.
17 GEORGE D., *et al* (1984) *Br J Dermatol* 110, 475.
18 GLOOR M., *et al* (1978) *Dermatologica* 157, 96.
19 GOLDSTEIN J.A. & POCHI P.E. (1981) *Dermatologica* 162, 287.
20 GRATTON D., *et al* (1982) *J Am Acad Dermatol* 1, 50.
21 KLIGMAN A.M., *et al* (1969) *Arch Dermatol* 99, 469.
22 LEYDEN J.L., *et al* (1982) Data presented at the American Academy of Dermatology, New Orleans, December.
23 LLORCA M.A., *et al* (1982) *Curr Therap Res* 32, 14.
24 LYONS R.E. (1978) *Int J Dermatol* 17, 246.
25 MILLS O.H. & KLIGMAN A.M. (1972) *Br J Dermatol* 86, 620.
26 MILLS O.H. & KLIGMAN A.M. (1983) *Acta Derm Venereol (Stockh)* 63, 68.
27 MILLS O.H. & KLIGMAN A.M. (1983) *Br J Dermatol* 108, 371.
28 MILLS O.H., *et al* (1972) *Arch Exp Pathol Pharmakol* 141, 501.
29 NAZZARO-PORRO M., *et al* (1983) *Br J Dermatol* 109, 45.
30 OLSEN T.G. (1982) *Med Clin North Am* 66, 851.
31 STOUGHTON R.B. (1979) *Arch Dermatol* 115, 486.
32 STRAUSS J.S., *et al* (1978) *Br J Dermatol* 114, 1340.

Oral therapy. The main oral treatments for acne are antibiotics but other compounds, including dapsone [10, 20], zinc sulphate, clofazimine and vitamin A acid in doses of 10–20 mg per day [13, 19, 22] have been used. These less conventional drugs are discussed later. Isotretinoin and hormonal preparations are discussed on pp. 1924 and 1923.

Treatment with oral antibiotics has evolved more by chance than by good scientific studies. Tetracyclines remain the antibiotics of choice [14, 18, 24], erythromycin is satisfactory [2, 7, 12] and cotrimoxazole, although successful, is now used less often because of its value in urinary tract infections. Trimethoprim is as beneficial as tetracycline [7]. Clindamycin, most helpful because of its lipid solubility [1], should not be used routinely because of the possible risk of pseudomembranous colitis [15, 21].

Not all patients respond equally; e.g. young males with a marked seborrhoea and truncal acne respond less well [5]. Patients who require antibiotics should be given 1 g per day of tetracycline or erythromycin [8]. The major disadvantage of tetracycline (and less so of erythromycin) is the need to take the tablet with water, not milk, half an hour before food; otherwise there is reduced absorption [11].

Oral therapy should be given for a minimum of 6 months [8]. In combination with topical benzoyl peroxide, improvement should be 40% by 2 months, 60% by 4 months and 80–90% by 6 months. With 1 g per day relapse is significantly less than with smaller doses [8]. In general, brand name antibiotics offer few or no advantages [3, 6]. However, some such as minocycline are better absorbed since chelation with calcium-containing food is much less of a problem. A dose of 200 mg of minocycline appears to be marginally more beneficial than 1 g of tetracycline [16]. If the acne recurs, repeated courses of antibiotics can be given as resistance of *P. acnes* is rare.

Mechanism of action. Tetracycline and erythromycin are bacteriostatic, especially in larger doses [17]. In smaller doses (500 mg per day or less) they do not reduce the number of organisms but they affect their function [4]. The antibiotics can also inhibit various enzyme activities [23] and affect chemotaxis and lymphocyte function [15, 23].

REFERENCES

1 ASHTON H., *et al* (1970) *Br J Dermatol* **85**, 585.
2 COTTERILL J.A., *et al* (1971) *Br J Dermatol* **85**, 130.
3 CULLEN S.I. (1978) *Cutis* **21**, 101.
4 CUNLIFFE W.J., *et al* (1973) *Br Med J* iv, 332.
5 CUNLIFFE W.J., *et al* (1981) *Clin Exp Dermatol* **6**, 461.
6 DEGREEF H. (1983) *Curr Therap Res* **33**, 8.
7 GIBSON J.R., *et al* (1982) *Br J Dermatol* **107**, 221.
8 GREENWOOD R., *et al* (1983) In press.
9 HASSING G.S. (1971) *J Invest Dermatol* **56**, 189.
10 KAMINSKY C.A., *et al* (1974) *Cutis* **13**, 869.
11 KIRBY W.M., *et al* (1961) *Antimicrob Agents Chemother* **286**, 292.
12 KLIGMAN A.M., *et al* (1974) *Postgrad Med* **55**, 99.
13 KLIGMAN A.M., *et al* (1974) *Postgrad Med* **55**, 104.
14 LANE P. & WILLIAMSON D. (1969) *Br Med J* ii, 76.
15 LASSON H.E. & PRICE A.B. (1977) *Lancet* ii, 1312.
16 LEYDEN J.L., *et al* (1971) *J Invest Dermatol* **56**, 127.
17 MARPLES R., *et al* (1971) *J Invest Dermatol* **56**, 127.
18 OLSEN T.G. (1982) *Med Clin North Am* **66**, 851.
19 PLEWIG G., *et al* (1979) *Arch Dermatol* **265**, 37.
20 ROSS C.M. (1961) *Br J Dermatol* **73**, 367.
21 SACO L.S., *et al* (1981) *J Am Acad Dermatol* **4**, 619.
22 SCHUMACHER A. & STUTTGEN D.M. (1971) *Dtsch Med Wochenschr* **96**, 1547.
23 WEBSTER G.F., *et al* (1982) *Antimicrob Agents Chemother* **21**, 770.
24 WITOWSKI J.A. & SIMONS H.M. (1966) *JAMA* **196**, 397.

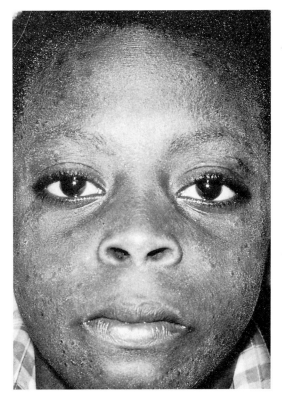

FIG. 52.14. The scaling which often occurs on treatment with benzoyl peroxide or retinoic acid. It usually settles on reducing the frequency of application.

Side effects of conventional therapy. Many topical preparations produce a primary irritant dermatitis (Fig. 52.14) [1, 12, 14, 15] and the patient must be warned so that treatment will not be prematurely ended. An allergic contact dermatitis is rare; e.g. with benzoyl peroxide the incidence is 1:450 cases [4]. The suggestion that both benzoyl peroxide and vitamin A acid induce skin carcinomas has been refuted by more adequately controlled studies and continued use of these two drugs is recommended [11].

Oral therapy with tetracycline or erythromycin has gastrointestinal effects, especially colic and diarrhoea in 5% (easily controlled with a diphenoxylate HCl, atropine sulphate combination (Lomotil®)) and vaginal candidiasis in 6% [5]. Pseudomembranous colitis is a very rare consequence of long-term treatment.

Uncommon complications of oral therapy include onycholysis, widespread or fixed drug eruptions [6, 8, 9] and photosensitivity, including porphyria-like cutaneous changes [7] especially with the longer acting tetracyclines. Tetracyclines, especially minocycline, may produce benign intracranial hypertension [10]; this normally presents with headache, loss of concentration and sometimes papilloedema, and quickly disappears on stopping therapy. Other rare iatrogenic problems are oesophageal ulceration with tetracycline [2] and a blue–black pigmentation in resolving acne lesions and on the legs with minocycline [14].

Tetracycline produces a bowel flora resistant to antibiotics [16], but this does not appear to be of clinical significance.

The possible clinical interactions between oral antibiotics and the contraceptive pill have not been adequately studied [3], but they are probably insignificant [13]. Patients should be advised about the risk of contraceptive failure if they develop diarrhoea, and the need for additional contraceptive measures.

REFERENCES

1 BOSSCHE H.V., *et al* (1982) *Br J Dermatol* **107**, 343.
2 CHANNER K.S. & HOLLANDER D. (1981) *Br Med J* **282**, 1359.
3 COSKEY R.J. (1982) *J Am Acad Dermatol* **7**, 23.
4 CUNLIFFE W.J., *et al* (1980) *Practitioner* **224**, 952.
5 CUNLIFFE W.J., *et al* (1981) *Clin Exp Dermatol* **6**, 461.
6 DELANEY T.J. (1970) *Br J Dermatol* **83**, 357.
7 EPSTEIN H.H., *et al* (1976) *Arch Dermatol* **112**, 661.
8 FRANK S.B., *et al* (1971) *Arch Dermatol* **103**, 520.
9 JOLLY H.W., *et al* (1978) *Arch Dermatol* **114**, 1484.
10 MEACOCK D.J. (1981) *Br Med J* **282**, 271.
11 NELSON K.R. & SLAGA T.J. (1982) *Carcinogenesis* **3**, 1315.
12 OLSEN T.G. (1981) *Med Clin North Am* **66**, 851.
13 ORME M.E. & CUNLIFFE W.J. (1983) Unpublished observations.
14 RIDGEWAY H.A., *et al* (1982) *Br J Dermatol* **107**, 95.
15 RIETSCHEL R.L. & DUNCAN S.H. (1982) *Contact Dermatitis* **8**, 323.
16 SCHMIDT H., *et al* (1973) *Acta Derm Venereol (Stockh)* **53**, 153.

The difficult acne patient. The most common causes of failure are poor education of the doctor on how to treat acne and lack of compliance by the patient. Otherwise, only 5–10% of people will respond unsatisfactorily [11] and in these patients various possibilities should be considered. Resistance of *P. acnes* is rare [3]. The patient may develop a Gram-negative folliculitis (Fig 52.15) [8a] (see p. 1935) due to either a *Klebsiella*, *Escherichia coli* or *Proteus* organism. Treatment is often difficult and requires stopping the current antibiotic and giving ampicillin (up to 1 g per day) or cotrimoxazole. Relapse is common, but 13-cis-retinoic acid (isoretinoin) then often proves successful [19].

Doubling the dose of antibiotic to 2 g per day [1] or the use of alternatives such as minocycline [14] can be tried. Alternatively, for females, hormonal therapy and, for either sex, 13-cis-retinoic acid can be considered.

Various hormonal regimes exist for reducing sebaceous production [7, 21]. Only contraceptive pills with 50 μg or more of ethinyl oestradiol will significantly reduce sebum production [20]; the switch to such a pill might ameliorate acne in females unresponsive to conventional therapy. Continuous low dose glucocorticosteroids (i.e. 2·5 mg prednisolone

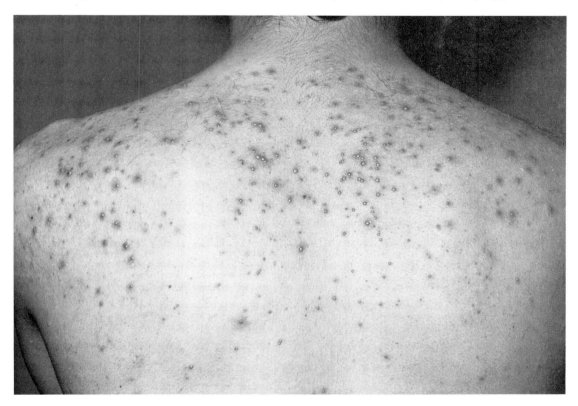

FIG. 52.15. Florid Gram-negative folliculitis.

on waking and 5 mg on retiring) to suppress adrenal androgens with or without a combined pill will reduce sebum production by up to 50% with a concomitant improvement in the acne [22]. Cyclical oestrogens (30 μg) with medroxyprogesterone acetate (5 mg for 7 days) significantly increases SHBG, thereby reducing available testosterone, and this regime also is of considerable help in the female with difficult acne [7].

Anti-androgens are a logical approach to the treatment of acne [4, 12]. In most European countries, but not in the U.S.A., the anti-androgen cyproterone acetate is available. Clinically effective topical anti-androgens are not available [6], although it appears possible to reduce sebum production slightly by topical applications [2, 23]. Cyproterone acetate (2 mg) combined with 50 μg ethinyl oestradiol (Diane®) is an oral contraceptive [15] which ameliorates acne [17, 24], although this opinion is not universally shared [16]. It is probably as clinically effective as 1 g per day of oral tetracycline over a 6-month period, although slower in action [9]. Diane® appears to be of value in women with acne resistant to other therapies [13] and in males 25 mg cyproterone acetate has been used with success [5]. In women, the side effects of cyproterone acetate with oestrogen appear to be small [5, 17] and no different from those of conventional contraceptive pills. However, should a patient taking Diane® become pregnant, then an abortion may be indicated because of the risk of feminizing a male fetus with the anti-androgen. In the male, gynaecomastias, loss of libido and azoospermia are obviously potential hazards.

Diane® should be given for 24 months and a conventional contraceptive pill thereafter. Since Diane® only reduces sebum production by about 30% it is possible that its action is via additional mechanisms [9]. In female patients over the age of 30 yrs oral spironolactone 100 mg bd, for 6 months, is of considerable benefit [8b]. Its prime effect is by reducing sebum excretion.

For the patient with intractable moderate or severe acne, or if anti-androgens are unavailable, 13-cis-retinoic acid is the treatment of choice [10]. Comparison of Diane® and 13-cis-retinoic acid has shown that the retinoid is the preferred treatment for such patients [10].

REFERENCES

1 BAER R.L., et al (1974) Arch Dermatol **110**, 85.
2 BINGHAM K.D., et al (1979) Lancet **ii**, 304.
3 BROWN J.M. & POSTON S.M. (1983) J Med Microb. **16**, 271

4 BURTON J.L. (1979) Clin Exp Dermatol **4**, 501.
5 CORMANE R.H. & VAN DER MEEREN L.M. (1981) Arch Derm Res **271**, 83.
6 CUNLIFFE W.J., et al (1981) Clin Exp Dermatol **6**, 461.
7 DARLEY C.R., et al (1983) Br J Dermatol **108**, 345.
8a FULTON J.E., et al (1968) Arch Dermatol **98**, 349.
8b GOODFELLOW A. et al (1984) Br J Derm **111**, 209
9 GREENWOOD R., et al (1983) Lancet **ii**, 796.
10 GREENWOOD R., et al (1984) In Retinoid Therapy. Ed. Cunliffe W.J. & Miller A.J. Lancaster, MTP Press. In press.
11 GREENWOOD R., et al (1985) In press.
12 HAMMERSTEIN J. & CUPCEANCU B. (1969) Dtsch Med Wochenschr **94**, 829.
13 HANSTEAD B. & REYMANN F. (1982) Dermatologica **164**, 117.
14 LEYDEN J.J., et al (198?) Arch Dermatol **118**, 19.
15 LUDERSCHMIDT C., et al (1982) J Invest Dermatol **78**, 253.
16 MARSDEN J.R., et al (1983) Lancet **ii**, 215.
17 MUGGLESTONE C.J. & RHODES E.L. (1982) Clin Exp Dermatol **7**, 593.
18 ORME M.E. & CUNLIFFE W.J. (1986) Unpublished observations.
19 PLEWIG G., et al (1982) Am Acad Dermatol **6**, 766.
20 POCHI P.E. & STRAUSS J.S. (1973) Arch Dermatol **108**, 210.
21 PYE R.J., et al (1977) Br Med J **ii**, 1581.
22 SAIHAN E.M. & BURTON J.L. (1980) Br J Dermatol **103**, 139.
23 TAMM J., et al (1982) Br J Dermatol **107**, 63.
24 WOJNAROWSKA F.T., et al (1983) Lancet **ii**, 458.

The retinoids. The retinoids have revolutionized the management of severe and intractable acne. The aromatic retinoid, etretinate, has only a minimal effect on acne [1] whereas isotretinoin (13-cis-retinoic acid) produces a striking benefit and appears superior both to conventional treatment [15] and to Diane® [9]. Recommended doses and duration of treatment vary [5, 6, 14, 18, 23, 24, 26, 27]: 0·1 mg/kg is too low whereas 2·0 mg/kg has a dramatic effect but considerable side effects. 1·0 mg/kg is now the dose of choice. Detailed studies are recorded in three symposia [2, 20, 32]. Adequate responses are seen with a dose of 1·0 mg/kg for 4–5 months (Fig. 52.16) Residual acne continues to improve after cessation of treatment. Up to 75% of patients will show a remission for up to 2–4 yr [12, 31]. The relapse rate is much less than that seen with conventional treatment [3]. The drug is recommended only for patients with (a) the most severe acne, (b) moderate to severe acne which has not responded to 3–4 months of conventional therapy, (c) moderate to severe acne which has quickly relapsed after several successful courses of conventional therapy, (d) dysmorphophobic acne and (e) intractable Gram-negative folliculitis [19, 29].

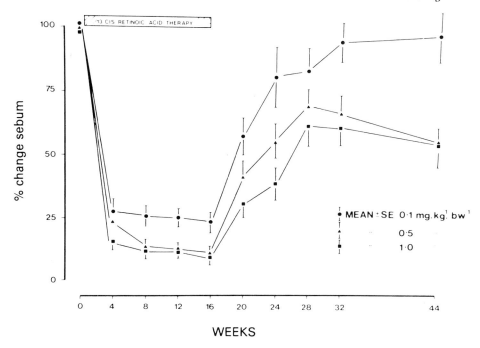

FIG. 52.16. The dramatic effect of three different doses of isotretinoin on sebum excretion whilst on and off therapy: ●, 0·1 mg/kg; ▲, 0·5 mg/kg; ■, 1·0 mg/kg. The mean values and the standard deviations are shown.

As yet, clinical effects have not been achieved with topical isotretinoin and the third generation of retinoids (e.g. arotenoid) seems unlikely to be better than isotretinoin [17].

Mechanisms of action. Isotretinoin influences all the major aetiological factors involved in acne. In doses of 0·5–2·0 mg/kg it reduces sebum excretion by 90% within 1 month [14, 30, 32]. The populations of surface and ductal bacteria, especially of *P. acne* [13, 16], fall gradually and ductal cornification also gradually decreases [4a, 29]. In addition, isotretinoin has anti-inflammatory actions [1, 23, 28]. It stimulates the T helper cells with a consequent increase in immunoglobulins [11] and reduces chemotaxis [25]. Its effects on bacteria, ductal keratin and inflammation may all be secondary; the chief

function is probably its sebo-suppressive effect. It reduces the sebaceous glands to epithelial buds. The drug is not an anti-androgen [8]; it somehow affects cellular differentiation. On stopping treatment sebum production slowly returns to pretreatment levels in a dose-dependent manner. In patients who have received 0·5 mg/kg or more, the sebum excretion often returns to only 50% of the original level and this correlates with a low relapse rate [12].

Side effects. The many side effects are summarized in Table 52.1. Most are mucocutaneous (Fig. 52.17) and the patients must be told to apply emollients to the skin and the lips. In extreme cases a moderate strength steroid ointment combined with an antibiotic and/or antiseptic helps considerably. Petroleum jelly (Vaseline[R]) reduces the nose bleeds, which

TABLE 52.1. Clinical side effects (and their incidence) in patients treated with isotretinoin (0·5–1·0 mg/kg)

Cheilitis	100%	Dermatitis elsewhere	20%
Facial dermatitis	95%	Anorexia	10%
Arthralgia and myalgia	60%	Cutaneous staphylococcal infections	6%
Epistaxes	50%	Weight loss	1%
Conjunctivitis	40%	Pyogenic granuloma	1%
Headaches	40%		

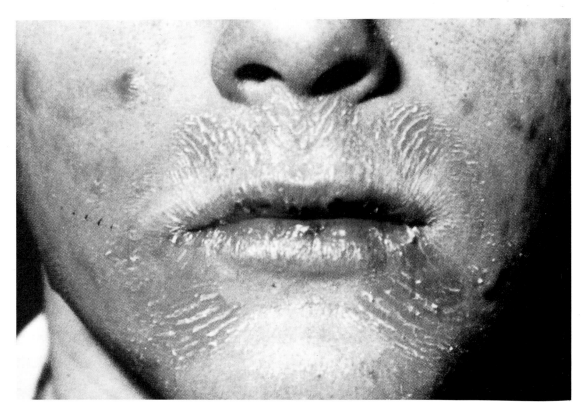

FIG. 52.17. Cheilitis and facial dermatitis, the most common mucocutaneous side effects of isotretinoin.

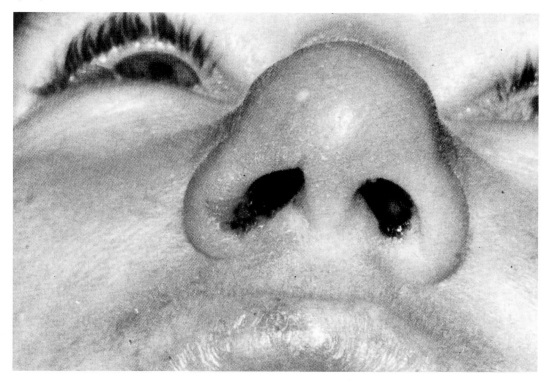

FIG. 52.18. Typical nasal crusting in a patient receiving isotretinoin.

are due to epithelial crusts (Fig 52.18). Colonization of the skin with *S. aureus* is not uncommon and may explain the scalp folliculitis. The uncommon pyogenic granulomas [33]. The uncommon pyogenic granulomas occur usually on the face and can be treated with cautery, 1% silver nitrate or potent steroid ointments. Rarely do any of these side effects necessitate a reduction in the dose. The polyarthropathy and headaches often respond to aspirin or non-steroidal anti-inflammatory drugs. A rare side effect is depression [10].

Most patients develop a small increase in liver enzymes, alkaline phosphatase, fasting cholesterol and triglycerides [7, 14, 23]. The side effects are dose dependent but the abnormalities rarely rise much beyond the upper limit of normal. The significance of an elevated lipid for 4 months has been highlighted [17, 18], but probably has little practical significance. Nevertheless, fasting lipids and liver function must be monitored before treatment and at monthly intervals thereafter. Patients who are overweight, or have a pre-existing hyperlipidaemia, a strong family history of diabetes or coronary artery disease should be given the drug only with circumspection; elevated levels of triglycerides ($\times$ 5–6) may induce pancreatitis. Diffuse interstitial skeletal hyperostosis (DISH) has been reported but the risk is small. [4b]

13-Cis-retinoic acid is teratogenic in rats at 10 times the human dose; females must take adequate contraception when on the drug and for 1 month afterwards. Fortunately, there is no evidence of drug interaction between 13-cis-retinoic acid and the contraceptive pill [21]. Many cases of malformed fetuses have been recorded. The drug is neither mutagenic nor carcinogenic.

REFERENCES

1 Camissa C., et al (1982) *J Am Acad Dermatol* **6**, 620.
2 Cunliffe W.J. & Miller A. (1984) *The Retinoids.* Lancaster, MTP Press.
3 Cunliffe W.J., et al (1983) *Lancet* (In press).
4a Cunliffe W.J., et al (1984) In *The Retinoids.* Eds. Cunliffe W.J. & Miller A. Lancaster, MTP Press.
4b Ellis C.N. et al (1985) In *Retinoids: New Trends in Research and Therapy.* Karger Basle.
5 Farrell L.N., et al (1980) *J Am Acad of Dermatol* **3**, 602.
6 Goldstein J.A., et al (1982) *J Am Acad Dermatol* **6**, 760.
7 Gollnick H., et al (1981) *Arch Derm Res* **271**, 189.
8 Gomez E.C. & Moschowitz R.J. (1980) *J Invest Dermatol* **74**, 397.
9 Greenwood R., et al (1984) In *The Retinoids.* Eds. Cunliffe W.J. & Miller A. Lancaster, MTP Press.
10 Hazen P.G., et al (1983) *J Am Acad Dermatol* **9**, 278.
11 Holland D.B., et al (1984) *Br J Dermatol* **110**, 343.
12 Jones D.H. & Cunliffe W.J. (1984) In *The Retinoids.* Eds. Cunliffe W.J. & Miller A. Lancaster, MTP Press.
13 Jones D.H., et al (1981) In *Retinoids.* Berlin, Springer-Verlag, p. 255.
14 Jones D.H., et al (1983) *Br J Dermatol* **108**, 333.
15 Jones D.H., et al (1984) In *The Retinoids.* Eds. Cunliffe W.J. & Miller A. Lancaster, MTP Press.
16 King K., et al (1982) *Br J Dermatol* **107**, 583.
17 Kingston T., et al (1983) *Lancet* i, 472.
18 Marsden J.R., et al (1983) *Lancet* i, 134.
19 Neubert U. & Plewig G. (1980) *Z Haut Geschlechtskr* **38**, 144.
20 Orfanos C.E., et al (1981) In *Retinoids.* Berlin, Springer-Verlag.
21 Orme M.E., et al (1984) In *The Retinoids.* Eds. Cunliffe W.J. & Miller A. Lancaster, MTP Press.
22 Ott F. & Geiger J.M. (1982) *Ann Dermatol Vénéréol* **109**, 849.
23 Peck G.L., et al (1979) *New Engl J Med* **300**, 329.
24 Peck G.L., et al (1982) *J Am Acad Dermatol* **6**, 735.
25 Pigatto P.D., et al (1983) *Dermatologica* **167**, 16.
26 Plewig G. & Wagner A. (1981) *Arch Derm Res* **270**, 179.
27 Plewig G., et al (1980) *Munchen Med Wochenschr* **122**, 1287.
28 Plewig G., et al (1981) In *Retinoids: Advances in Basic Research and Therapy.* New York, Springer-Verlag, p. 279.
29 Plewig G., et al (1982) *J Am Acad Dermatol* **6**, 766.
30 Puhvel S.M. (1983) Data presented at SID/ESDR, Washington, May 1983.
31 Shalita A.R., et al (1983) *J Am Acad Dermatol* **9**, 629.
32 Strauss J.S., et al (1982) *J Am Acad Dermatol* (Suppl), **6**.
33 Valentine J.P., et al (1983) *Arch Dermatol* **119**, 871.

Other oral treatments. Until the advent of the retinoids and anti-androgens, a number of therapies were proposed which now merit little consideration. They will occasionally be tried in difficult cases of acne if the newer drugs are either contra-indicated or unobtainable.

Oral zinc was of supposed benefit, but on balance probably has little value [3, 4, 9, 15, 16].

Certain non-steroidal anti-inflammatory drugs, such as ibuprofen and benoxaprofen, have been shown to reduce inflamed lesions [5]. Ibuprofen reduces inflamed lesions in a dose-dependent way but less so than 5% benzoyl peroxide [2]. Clofazimine (200 mg three times a week) has been shown to improve acne fulminans [12] but should not be given as a first option. Dapsone (100–300 mg per day for 6 months) has also been tried with varied success but, as with clofazimine, controlled studies are limited [6, 10, 13].

Oral vitamin A has been advocated [7, 8, 14] but failed in other controlled studies [1, 11]. Certainly doses of less than 40 mg per day are not effective. In our experience oral vitamin A proved considerably less effective than 1 g per day of either tetracycline or erythromycin in controlled studies. Its side effects are similar to but less than those of the retinoids and the period of therapy should not exceed 6 months.

Oral corticosteroids have been used successfully in acne fulminans and as an immediate measure to reduce an acute flare of the acne quickly [10]. Doses of 40–60 mg are required and treatment should not be prolonged beyond 3 weeks because of side effects, which paradoxically include steroid acne.

REFERENCES

1 ANDERSON J.A.D. & STOKOE I.M. (1963) *Br Med J* ii, 294.
2 BURKE B.M. & CUNLIFFE W.J. (1983) Personal observations.
3 CUNLIFFE W.J., *et al* (1979) *Br J Dermatol* 101, 321.
4 HILLSTROM L., *et al* (1977) *Br J Dermatol* 97, 679.
5 HINDSON C., *et al* (1982) *Lancet* i, 1415.
6 KAMINSKY C.A., *et al* (1974) *Cutis* 13, 869.
7 KLIGMAN A.M., *et al* (1974) *Postgrad Med* 55, 99.
8 KLIGMAN A.M., *et al* (1981) *Int J Dermatol* 20, 278.
9 MICHAELSSON G., *et al* (1977) *Br J Dermatol* 97, 561.
10 OLSEN T.G. (1982) *Med Clin North Am* 66, 851.
11 PLEWIG G., *et al* (1979) *Arch Dermatol* 265, 37.
12 PRENDIVILLE J. & CREAM J.J. (1983) *Br J Dermatol* 109 (Suppl. 24) 90.
13 ROSS C.M. (1961) *Br J Dermatol* 73, 367.
14 SCHUMACHER A. & STUTTGEN G. (1971) *Dtsch Med Wochenschr* 96, 1547.
15 VAHLQUIST A., *et al* (1978) *Acta Derm Venereol (Stockh)* 58, 437.
16 WEIMAR V.M., *et al* (1978) *Arch Dermatol* 114, 1776.

Physical modalities. Some of the physical modalities often require considerable skill and must be used only as an adjunct to treatment. The many abrasive materials, usually based on polyethelene and aluminium oxide, are of little or no value. Facial saunas, heat and massage probably worsen the condition by precipitating the development of inflamed lesions.

Visible comedones are a cosmetic nuisance but do not usually give rise to inflammatory lesions. Some patients wish them to be removed, which may, where practical, be aided by hot compresses. Comedo removal can be surprisingly uncomfortable and a variety of specially shaped tools are available. Some patients have very visible closed comedones, which are the more likely to become inflamed; under a good light the eccentrically placed pore may be widened with a small blade to allow enucleation of the keratin plug with a comedo remover.

Objective assessment of treatment by UV radiation does not support the common opinion that it is highly beneficial. A combination of UVA and UVB is probably the best but not as good as natural sunlight. Deep X-ray treatment must not be prescribed because of its carcinogenic risk. Superficial X-ray therapy (no more than 1,000 R to any given area of skin in a lifetime) is of questionable benefit.

Superficial freezing with carbon dioxide–acetone slush, or with liquid nitrogen on a cotton wool pledget or using specially designed equipment will hasten the resolution of nodular cystic lesions and is comparatively painless [1]. Two freeze cycles of 15 s each are recommended. It is uncertain how the treatment works, but it may invoke an inflammatory reaction to break down the indolent tissue surrounding the nodulocystic lesion.

The authors consider cryotherapy to be superior to intralesional injections in the treatment of nodulocystic lesions, although others prefer steroids [5]. Triamcinolone, 2·5 mg/ml, may be administered from a syringe with a 30 gauge needle. Placement too superficially or too deeply may cause atrophy; 0·025–0·1 ml should be injected into the middle of the lesion, causing slight distension [5]. Drainage often follows the injection and this is desirable.

Treatment of scars. Many scars, over a period of many months, become much less conspicuous; keloids are one exception. Nevertheless, some scars need surgery.

Dermabrasion. Dermabrasion [7] may be of value for scars of even depth. Multiple ice-pick or keloid scars respond badly, hypertrophic scars variably. The procedure involves the use of a high-speed wire brush or diamond fraise to plane the skin to different levels. Surgery is probably best performed when the disease is under good control, although some advocate it even for active lesions [6]. It is best avoided in summer because of the risk of post-inflammatory pigmentation, and, if sunlight could pose a problem, a topical sunscreen should be applied post-operatively. Hypopigmentation and therapeutic failures may also be problems. Improvement ranges from 30 to 75%; the patient's estimate of improvement often surpasses that of the surgeon.

Excision of scars. Small, well-defined scars can be satisfactorily excised.

Collagen injection. Injections of purified bovine dermal collagen to augment tissues defects have recently been introduced. Thirty days after an intradermal test for possible hypersensitivity, 0·5–2·0 ml of collagen are injected. Deep ice-pick scars do badly. Repeated treatments are needed, as is technical expertise. The precise value of the procedure remains to be objectively assessed.

Cosmetic camouflage. Although certain cosmetics may induce acne, it is not unreasonable, and often psychologically necessary, for the female patient to be told that she can wear light, non-greasy make-up.

Cosmetic camouflage is also essential, especially for women, when scarring is a physical and psychological problem. In certain countries professional advice is available, and in the U.K. the cosmetics are available on prescription. Make-up is often needed for the post-inflammatory pigmentation which may occur in the skin of coloured people. Indeed, where this risk occurs, even mild acne should be treated aggressively with long-term antibiotics to reduce it. Much of this post-inflammatory pigmentation will mostly remit over a period of many months.

REFERENCES

1 DETLER K. & GOETTE K. (1973) *South Med J* 66, 1131.
2 KLEIN A. (1983) *J Am Acad Dermatol* 9, 224.
3 KLIGMAN A.M. & MILLS O.H. (1979) *Dermatology Insight* 1, 21.
4 Leading article (1983) *Lancet* ii, 555.
5 OLSEN T.G. (1982) *Med Clin North Am* 66, 851.
6 ORENTREICH N. & DURR N.P. (1979) In *Acne*. Ed. Frank S.B. New York, Yorke Medical Books.
7 ORENTREICH N. & DURR N.P. (1983) *Dermatol Clin* 1(3), 405.

ACNE VARIANTS

Acne excoriée. This variant (Fig. 52.19) occurs predominantly in females. Two subgroups exist: those with a few primary acne lesions and those with almost none at all. Both groups consist of neurotic females who fiddle with the skin to exacerbate even the smallest lesions. There is often some considerable underlying personality or other psychiatric problem [72]. Treatment with 1 g per day of tetracycline for six months and advice not to pick the spots is of considerable benefit to those females with mild acne. Topical treatment tends to irritate the skin. By markedly reducing the number of lesions the regimen leaves the patient fewer to 'play' with. In the second group with few or no spots, trifluoperazine hydrochloride (5–30 mg daily) or pimozide (2 mg b.d.) and appropriate psychotherapeutic procedures may help.

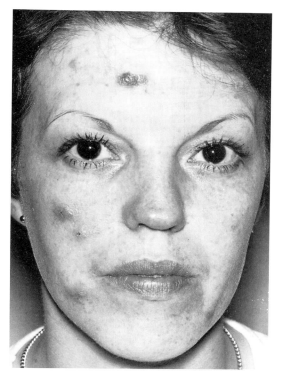

FIG. 52.19. Acne excoriée.

Drug-induced acne. The many drugs which have been incriminated as possible aggravators of acne are listed in Table 52.2 [8, 28]. The evidence is often based upon isolated case reports [12, 67]. Since many other patients on the same drugs develop no acne whatever, many of the reported reactions are idiosyncratic and have little general relevance. Only those substances which definitely

TABLE 52.2. Drugs reported to cause acne or acne-like eruptions

Hormones and steroids	*Antituberculous drugs*
Gonadotrophins	Isoniazid
Androgens	Rifampicin
Anabolic steroids	
Oral and topical steroids	*Miscellaneous*
	Chloral hydrate
Halogens	Cyanocobalamin
Bromides	Disulfiram
Iodides	Lithium
Halothane	Psoralens (with UVA)
	Quinine
Epileptic drugs	Sulphur
Diphenylhyldantoin	Thiouracil
Phenobarbitone	Thiourea
Troxidone	

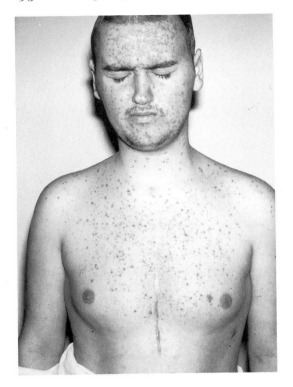

FIG. 52.20. Acne induced by oral steroids.

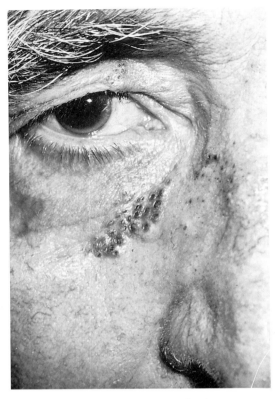

FIG. 52.21. A sarcoid granuloma treated with a potent fluorinated corticosteroid which induced comedonal acne.

induce acne will be discussed. Corticosteroids, both orally and topically, may do so (Figs. 52.20 and 52.21) [62], although the precise mechanism is uncertain. They do not affect the number of surface bacteria [23] but do induce keratinization in the upper part of the pilosebaceous duct [62]. Steroid acne is usually more monomorphic than acne vulgaris.

Androgens, gonadotrophins and ACTH, given early in puberty, may precipitate acne, especially in females. Contraceptive pills which reduce SHBG may also result in a deterioration of pre-existing acne.

Anti-epileptic drugs, especially phenytoin, have often been incriminated but recent data indicate that severe epileptics on several anticonvulsants are no more at risk of acne than the normal population [32]. Patients on isoniazid, especially those who slowly inactivate the drug, appear prone to acne [15, 68] and 5% of patients receiving PUVA treatment appear to develop a perioral dermatitis and/or an acneform eruption on the face [38, 56]. The administration of iodides and bromides used to be a common cause of follicular pustules; such lesions may evolve quickly and affect any age group [59].

The ideal therapy is to reduce the dose of the drug, but this may not be possible; conventional therapy, according to the severity of the acne, with oral antibiotics and topical benzoyl peroxide or vitamin A acid often proves quite successful.

Ectopic sebaceous glands. These are commonly seen in the mouth—the so-called Fordyce's disease—as multiple, symmetrical, barely elevated, discrete yellow papules. They are present in 25% of the population over the age of 35 yr and are asymptomatic.

Similar lesions are common on the penile shaft, especially on the ventral surface and at this site an inflamed acne lesion, usually requiring no more than reassurance, may be seen.

Endocrine acne. The role of the endocrine system in the aetiology of acne has already been discussed [2, 24, 47, 58]. While there is no doubt that acne is sometimes associated with menstrual abnormalities and hirsutism, the majority of female patients must be regarded as endocrinologically normal and requiring no further investigation. The term 'endocrine acne' should be reserved for cases of clinically manifested endocrine abnormality and include the Stein–Leventhal syndrome, Cushing's disease and adrenogenital syndrome.

Externally-induced acne

Acne cosmetica. This variant is more recognized as a problem in the U.S.A. [14, 40, 42] than in Europe and elsewhere. This may be due to the greater usage of potentially comedogenic cosmetics in the U.S.A. The lesions occur characteristically in the perioral area of mature females (Fig. 52.22), especially those who had acne as adolescents and have

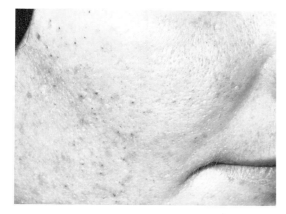

FIG. 52.22. Cosmetic acne: multiple blackheads in a middle-aged lady, who had had no previous acne, following the application of a comedogenic moisturizer.

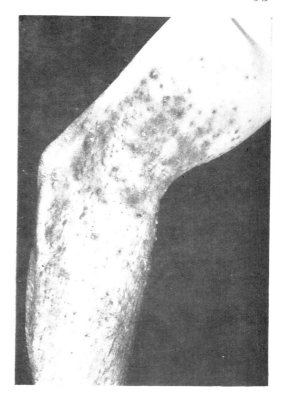

FIG. 52.23. Oil acne. The trousers were constantly saturated in machine oil. Note the sparsity of lesions where the skin was protected by the underpants (Radcliffe Infirmary).

used cosmetics for a long time. The rabbit ear model has shown that many make-ups, especially those containing lanolin, petrolatum, certain vegetable oils, butylstearate, lauryl alcohol and oleic acid, are comedogenic. Many cosmetics are now screened by the rabbit ear test [40] and, if appropriate, are labelled as being non-comedogenic [14].

Switching to a non-comedogenic cosmetic will not bring rapid clinical results. Treatment, especially with topical vitamin A or benzoyl peroxide, is required.

Pomade acne. This is similar to cosmetic acne but consists of non-inflamed lesions around the forehead and other areas where greasy pomades may extend onto the non-hairy skin [63]. The rabbit ear model has shown that certain pomades are comedogenic. Pomade acne often presents as part of acne vulgaris and advice on the restrictive use of pomades is essential, as well as acne therapy.

Occupational acne due to oils and tars. Areas in con-

tact with oils and crude tars may show conspicuous comedones (Fig. 52.23) [10]. Only occasionally do frank inflammatory lesions arise and these are usually superficial; not suprisingly men are more often affected than women. Lesions can occur within 6 weeks of exposure on almost any site, but especially on the thighs and lower arms. It is also suggested, but not proven, that individuals prone to acne vulgaris are more prone to oil acne.

The commonest oils involved are the impure paraffin mixtures used in the engineering industry [83]. Crude petroleum can affect oil field and refinery workers, and heavy coal tar distillates, especially pitch and creosote, are also acnegenic. Other occupational acnegenes include DDT, asbestos and heavy water distillate [33].

Chloracne. This variant is part of a syndrome in which there are characteristically acne-like lesions, usually comedones, inflammatory lesions being infrequent [18, 19]. They are often localized on both sides of the face, especially the temporal regions, but in more severe cases may occur on other parts of the body. In addition to chloracne other skin lesions may be seen and these include porphyric changes, melanin pigmentation, hypertrichosis, phrynoderma, ophthalmic chloracne (due to the Meibomian gland involvement) and palmar and plantar hyperhydrosis. Systemic abnormalities are less frequent and include fatigue, anorexia, neuropathy, impotence, disturbed liver function and hyperlipidaemia. In many cases the chloracne and systemic disturbances may last for many years.

Chloracne has been reported following exposure to chlornaphthalenes, polychlorbiphenyls, polychlorinated dibenzofurans, chlorophenol contaminants and chlorobenzenes [14, 18, 19, 25, 77] and the contamination is often the result of an explosion resulting in the uncontrolled liberation of the chemical [37]. Recent studies have failed to identify the chloracnegen in the pilosebaceous apparatus but in one instance the agent, dioxin, produced a hyperproliferative reaction of the cutaneous epithelium with squamous metaplasia of the pilosebaceous duct [21, 60] and subsequent atrophy of the sebaceous gland.

The skin lesions are relatively persistent. Topical therapy with vitamin A acid is probably the best treatment but occasionally oral antibiotic therapy is needed. Litigation is frequent.

Acne mechanica. This term covers a mixed group of disorders in which the acne occurs at the site of physical trauma, as indicated by the pattern of the lesions [54]. Examples are so-called fiddler's neck [61] on the neck of violin players, which is also characterized by lichenification and pigmentation. Head bands, as worn by sportsmen and 'hippies', and tight brassière straps are other causes [28, 80]. Continuous friction from turtle neck sweaters may localize acne to the neck [31]. The mechanism of acne mechanica is unclear. Most patients have a tendency to acne and its localization may be caused by an irritant dermatitis of the upper part of the pilosebaceous duct or excessive hydration at that site. Adolescent patients lying in bed for a long time, such as in the orthopaedic ward, frequently develop a flare of acne, probably due to a change in the environment of the skin, which may enhance bacterial colonization of the duct—the so-called immobility acne [49]. Treatment of these conditions in no way differs from that of other forms of acne; in addition, advice on reducing or modifying the additional stimulus is essential.

Acne detergicans. This acne develops in patients who -wash many times daily, hoping to moderate their existing acne. Certain bacteriostatic soaps contain weak acnegenic compounds, such as hexachlorophene. Pustular and papular lesions are most noticeable [53].

Hydration acne or tropical acne. Certain occupations may aggravate pre-existing acne; workers in a hot humid environment, such as cooks, are at risk. Troops in the Second World War were at risk when posted to the Far East, but not U.S. Marines in Vietnam, possibly because non-prone individuals had been preselected [43, 57, 76]. A common aetiological event linking these clinical observations is hydration of the pilosebaceous duct pores, which in turn may accentuate blockage of the duct and so precipitate inflamed lesions [81]. A similar explanation may apply to Mallorca acne, in which small follicular papules appear, especially on the upper trunk, in summer. Potentially comedogenic sunscreens may be an additional factor in these patients [36].

Infantile and juvenile acne. This condition, in which males are mainly affected, presents as facial acne at around 3 months and may last up to 5 yr of age (Fig. 52.24) [7, 8]. The lesions are more localized than in adults, but may demonstrate the entire acne spectrum, even occasionally with scarring. It is suggested that juvenile acne initially

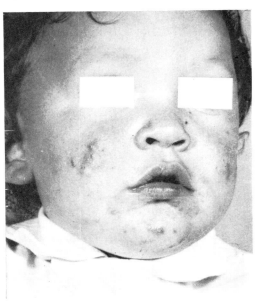

FIG. 52.24. Acne present for 6 months in a girl aged 10 months. No hormonal abnormality was detected (Addenbrooke's Hospital).

results from transplacental stimulation of the adrenal, and most sufferers have elevated plasma adrenal androgens [7, 8]; it is uncertain why the acne lasts for up to 5 yr. Occasionally, a drug such as phenytoin has been incriminated [73]. Infantile acne can rarely be a feature of a virilizing tumour or congenital adrenal hyperplasia. Treatment may have to consist of oral erythromycin (125 mg t.d.s.) for 6 months, and topical therapy, preferably with benzoyl peroxide or vitamin A acid, is essential until lesions have totally disappeared. Such patients may develop severe acne as teenagers [34].

Pilosebaceous naevoid disorders. Some of these disorders are only tenuously linked with the pilosebaceous system and so are only briefly mentioned here, but they are described elsewhere (Chapter 6).

Non-acne naevus. Two patients have been described [16, 22]: one had symmetrical areas of normal looking skin set in the midst of severe acne on the back; the other had extensive acne on one side of the back but not on the other. A reduced rate of sebum excretion in the affected areas associated with a smaller number of surface bacteria was demonstrated.

Acne naevus. We have also seen one patient who has had for many years an an area of slightly undulating skin on the anterior chest. This naevoid area developed extensive acne at puberty, even though the condition was elsewhere mild.

Naevus comedonicus. This uncommon naevus has had several descriptive names, including comedone naevus, naevus follicularis and naevus unilateralis comedonicus [9, 79]. It has been suggested that the comedo naevus is a developmental defect of the hair follicle and that the sebaceous glands may be normal, hypoplastic or hyperplastic. In one case the sweat duct was the origin of the lesions [6, 50]. They are usually present on the scalp, face and trunk but occasionally at unusual sites, such as the penis [1]. The individual lesions are large comedones, usually linear in arrangement. Occasionally inflammatory lesions develop. Although usually present at birth they can present much later in life. Symptoms are of a cosmetic nature and treatment with keratolytics produces only limited success. In a patient with an extensive naevus the lesions improved considerably with an oral contraceptive [5]. An association with epidermolytic hyperkeratosis is documented [4].

Familial comedones. These are an uncommon disorder, usually with an autosomal inheritance [69]. The earliest lesions are monoporous but later the face may be extensively involved with polyporous comedones and cysts, and scarring may follow. New lesions may continue into middle age.

Naevus sebaceus of Jadassohn. This is an organoid naevus, consisting of a mixture of relatively normal looking epidermis, dermis, sweat and sebaceous glands. It presents on the scalp as a small area of alopecia associated with a pinkish flat fleshy swelling (Fig. 52.25) [52]. At puberty the sebaceous

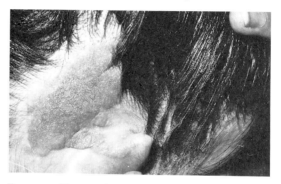

FIG. 52.25. Naevus sebaceus of Jadassohn.

glands enlarge and the epidermis becomes verrucous. Although debated, excision is recommended because of the risk of malignant change into a squamous or basal cell carcinoma [27]. Trichoepithelioma may also arise in the naevus.

Lesions occurring in the mid-line are often associated with mental subnormality and epilepsy [46].

'Sebaceous' cysts and steatocystoma multiplex. The classical 'sebaceous' cyst is an epidermoid structure and is discussed in Chapter 64. However, true sebaceous cysts do occur as the so-called steatocystoma multiplex, a naevoid condition which histologically shows a mixture of a keratinizing epithelium and sebaceous lobules attached to the epidermis by a thin epidermal strand [2, 26, 65]. The condition is uncommon and may be inherited as an autosomal trait, although most cases seen by the authors had no family history.

The lesions are multiple, smooth, elastic, yellow dermal swellings varying from a few to 20 mm in size. They appear or enlarge at puberty and mainly occur on the trunk or limbs. They last indefinitely, and whether they resolve with old age is uncertain. Inflamed lesions due to rupture of the cysts are common and, when extensive, can produce the so-called steatocystoma multiplex suppurativa, which may mimic acne conglobata. Treatment is not easy [26]; excision of the larger cysts is possible, but total removal of all cysts is impractical because of their multiplicity. Tetracycline (1 g per day) for 6 months is required if the lesions suppurate excessively. Topical antibiotics or benzoyl peroxide are of benefit in less severe cases, but for the really difficult patient 13-cis-retinoic acid (1 mg/kg) can be most helpful.

Sebaceous gland tumours. These are uncommon and may be associated with some systemic tumours.

Sebaceous gland hyperplasia. Small papules are occasionally found on the face, especially on the forehead of persons at or beyond middle age [69]. These lesions, which are mature sebaceous glands, are 1–3 mm in size, red–yellow in appearance and of little clinical significance. Usually no treatment is requested.

Sebaceous adenoma. This is a benign tumour, composed of incompletely differentiated sebaceous cells, which affects both sexes and is seen mainly in elderly patients on the face or scalp [78]. The tumours are round, raised, sessile or pedunculated; they are usually 10 mm or less in size but may form plaques and ulcerate. Their colour is fleshy or waxy yellowish. Excision is the best treatment but they are radiosensitive.

Sebaceous carcinoma. This is an uncommon malignant tumour usually involving men over the age of 40 yr. It presents as a solitary, firm tumour, yellow–orange in colour, especially on the face and scalp. The tumour grows slowly but those arising near the eye (from the Meibomian glands) have a greater predilection for metastasizing [11]. Treatment is by excision but there is a definite, if ill-understood, link between sebaceous and visceral carcinoma, especially that of the colon [3, 11, 35, 78].

Seborrhoea. Excessive grease production is an uncommon reason for referral but many patients with severe acne complain bitterly of seborrhoea. It can persist after the acne has regressed [20] and patients with post-encephalitic Parkinsonism also often have a seborrhoea [66]. The conventional treatment of acne does not really influence the seborrhoea and detergent washes are of limited (30 min) benefit. 13–Cis-retinoic acid, and to a lesser extent, anti-androgens, do significantly reduce the seborrhoea (see p. 1924).

SEVERE ACNE VARIANTS

Pyoderma faciale. Explosive post-adolescent facial acne (Fig. 52.26) is an uncommon clinical situation in which mild acne suddenly erupts producing many purulent nodulocystic lesions, especially on the face [51]. It mainly affects post-adolescent women (aged 20–40 yr) and, in contrast with acne fulminans, involves no systemic symptoms. The reason for the sudden flare is unknown, but the prognosis is good; 1 g per day of tetracycline or erythromycin plus intralesional steroids or liquid nitrogen to the cysts and topical benzoyl peroxide are of considerable benefit. However, if available, 13-cis-retinoic acid (1 mg/kg) for 4–6 months will bring the disease under quick control and so minimize the inevitable scarring.

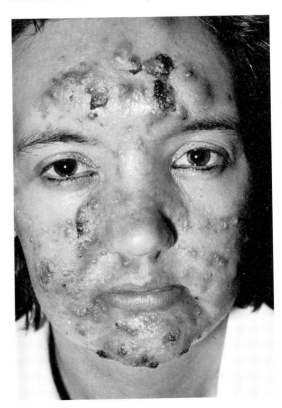

FIG. 52.26. A young woman with aggressive pyoderma faciale.

Acne conglobata. This is a most severe form of acne, found particularly in males; the lesions usually occur on most of the trunk, face and limbs. Nodules and cysts are characteristic and may fuse to form multiple draining sinuses. Grouped multiple fused blackheads and scarring are also features. Some patients have hidradenitis suppurativa and familial cases have been reported, but there are no HLA associations [30, 70]. Therapy with 2 g per day of oral tetracycline or erythromycin is indicated, but 13-cis-retinoic acid (1 mg/kg for 4–6 months) is the drug of choice, if it is available.

Acne fulminans. Acute febrile ulcerative acne conglobata is an uncommon systemic disease in which the offending antigen is *P. acnes*. The patients are predominantly males who have extensive inflammatory lesions, especially on the trunk [13, 39, 75]. Associated features are fever, polyarthropathy, marked leukocytosis (even a leukemoid reaction), weight loss, anorexia and general malaise [44, 74]. Bone pain due to aseptic osteolysis and erythema nodosum [82] have also been reported. Blood cultures are universally sterile. Skin tests with *P. acnes* demonstrate a very extensive, immediate and delayed reaction, immunohistology of which reveals a type III or type IV reaction [82]. The acute myalgia and arthralgia usually respond well to supportive treatment with salicylates and graduated physical exercise; the underlying skin condition requires a minimum of 1 g per day of tetracycline or erythromycin and topical retinoic acid or benzoyl peroxide. Many cases have responded well to oral steroids, up to 40 mg per day, and, while experience with 13-cis-retinoic acid is limited, it is probably not the initial treatment of choice. Dapsone may also be useful [71].

Gram-negative folliculitis. This is a complication of the long-term treatment of conventional acne [29]. It presents either as a sudden eruption of multiple small follicular pustules or as a development of many nodular cystic lesions. Occasionally it appears as a worsening of acne which may have been under good control. Microbiological sampling from the nose and lesions will reveal one or more Gram-negative organisms, including *Klebsiella*, *E. coli*, *Proteus* or *Pseudomonas* [29, 45]. Therapy usually involves stopping the current antibiotics and replacing them with either ampicillin (250 mg q.i.d.) or cotrimoxazole (4 tablets a day). However, the response may be slow, relapse is common, and 13-cis-retinoic acid now appears to be the treatment of choice [64].

(Solar) senile comedones. These are not uncommon in elderly people (Fig. 52.27), especially in the periorbital areas. Most patients have had high exposure to UV radiation and the solar damage to the supporting damage to the supporting dermis allows the pilosebaceous duct to become more easily distended

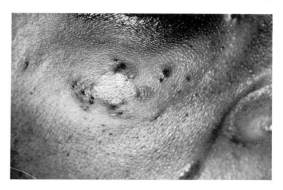

FIG. 52.27. This patient has many senile comedones.

with impacted corneocytes. Similar lesions may be seen in pseudoxanthoma elasticum. In the unwary, the edge of the adjacent comedonal skin may be mistaken for the pearly edge of a basal cell carcinoma. Treatment, if requested, is reasonably easy with a comedo expressor, and by using topical retinoic acid to suppress the formation of future comedones.

Uncommon associations with acne. A small number of patients with dysmorphophobia have acne as their prime symptom [17]. However, the acne is very mild and the patient's complaint is out of all proportion to the physical signs. Such patients require sympathy, especially since they have a significant risk of suicide; they are often depressed or schizophrenic. However, they usually tolerate psychiatric treatment badly, and the dermatologist must treat their acne firmly with 1 g per day of tetracycline for 6 months, or even with 13-cis-retinoic acid (1 mg/kg per day) for 4 months. The results can be quite rewarding.

A rare complication of healing severe nodulocystic lesions is pyogenic granuloma [85]. The lesions either need no treatment or respond well to 1% silver nitrate. Calcification, i.e. osteoma cutis, is also a rare event and usually needs no treatment [48].

A somewhat more common association is hidradenitis suppurativa (see p. 785), particularly in association with acne conglobata. Unfortunately, hidradenitis suppurativa is a much more difficult condition to treat and even the newer retinoids have little effect on the disease process. There is also a possible increased association between acne and Apert's syndrome [84]. These subjects develop early epiphyseal closure which, like acne, is an androgen-mediated event. Consequently, the patient has an unusual appearance with a flat face and fused digits as well as extensive acne. The acne requires 1 g per day of tetracycline and topical treatment, and in one case 13-cis-retinoic acid produced a dramatic improvement of the skin.

REFERENCES

1 ABDEL-AAL H. & ABDEL-AZIZ A.H.M. (1975) *Acta Derm Venereol (Stockh)* **55**, 78.
2 AMERLINCK F. (1949) *Arch Belg Dermatol Syphilog* **5**, 187.
3 BAKKER P.M., et al (1971) *Dermatologica* **142**, 50.
4 BARSKY S., et al (1981) *Arch Dermatol* **117**, 86.
5 BECK M.H. & DAVE V.K. (1980) *Arch Dermatol* **116**, 1048.
6 BEERMAN H. & HOMAN J.B. (1959) *Arch Clin Exp Dermatol* **208**, 325.
7 BESSONE L. (1974) *Chron Dermatol* **1**, 77.
8 BESSONE L & ANSELM L. (1970) *Chron Dermatol* **3**, 3.
9 BETTMAN C. (1906) *Arch Dermatol Syphil* **80**, 63.
10 BHUTANI L.K., et al (1970) *Indian J Dermatol* **36**, 119.
11 BRAUNINGER G.E., et al (1973) *Arch Ophthalmol* **77**, 326.
12 BURKEHART C.C. (1981) *Arch Dermatol* **117**, 603.
13 BURNS R.E. & COLVILLE J.M. (1959) *Arch Dermatol* **79**, 361.
14 CARAMASCHI F., et al (1982) *Int J Epidemiol* **10**, 135.
15 COHEN L.K., et al (1974) *Arch Dermatol* **109**, 377.
16 COOPER M.F., et al (1976) *J Invest Dermatol* **66**, 261.
17 COTTERILL J.A. (1981) *Br J Dermatol* **104**, 611.
18 CROW K.D. (1970) *Trans St John's Hosp Dermatol Soc* **56**, 79.
19 CROW K.D. (1981) *Clin Exp Dermatol* **6**, 243.
20 CUNLIFFE W.J. & SHUSTER S. (1969) *Lancet* **i**, 685.
21 CUNLIFFE W.J., et al (1975) *Acta Derm Venereol (Stockh)* **55**, 211.
22 CUNLIFFE W.J., et al (1977) *Br J Dermatol* **96**, 287.
23 DALTREY D.C. & CUNLIFFE W.J. (1981) *Acta Derm Venereol (Stockh)* **61**, 575.
24 DARLEY C.R., et al (1982) *Br J Dermatol* **106**, 517.
25 DEEKEN J.H. (1974) *Arch Dermatol* **109**, 245.
26 EGBERT D.M. & PRICE N.M. (1979) *Arch Dermatol* **115**, 334.
27 FERGIN P.E., et al (1981) *Clin Exp Dermatol* **6**, 111.
28 FRANK S.B. (1974) *Cutis* **14**, 817.
29 FULTON J.E., et al (1968) *Arch Dermatol* **98**, 349.
30 GOLD S. & DELANEY J. (1974) *Br J Dermat*, **91**, (Suppl. 10) 54.
31 GOLDMAN L. (1977) *Arch Dermatol* **113**, 109.
32 GREENWOOD R., et al (1983) *Br Med J* **287**, 1669.
33 HEGZI E. & FARKAS J. (1965) *Berufsdermatosen* **13**, 46.
34 HELLIER F.F. (1954) *Br J Dermatol* **66**, 25.
35 HERNÁNDEZ-PÉREZ E. & BÀNOS E. (1978) *Dermatologica* **156**, 184.
36 HJORTH N., et al (1972) *Acta Derm Venereol (Stockh)* **52**, 61.
37 JENSEN N.E., et al (1972) *Trans St John's Hosp Dermatol Soc* **58**, 172.
38 JONES C. & BLEEHEN S.S. (1977) *Br Med J* **ii**, 866.
39 KELLY A.P. & BURNS R.E. (1971) *Arch Dermatol* **104**, 182.
40 KLIGMAN A.M. & KATZ A.G. (1968) *Arch Dermatol* **98**, 53.
41 KLIGMAN A.M. & MILLS O.H. (1972) *Arch Dermatol* **106**, 843.
42 KLIGMAN A.M. & MILLS O.H. (1978) *Dermatology* **7**, 43.
43 LAMBERG S.I. (1971) *Cutis* **7**, 655.
44 LANE J.M., et al (1976) *J Bone Joint Surg* **58**, 673.
45 LEYDEN J.J., et al (1979) *Arch Dermatol* **115**, 1203.
46 LOVEJOY F.H. & BOYLE W.E. (1974) *Pediatrics* **52**, 382.
47 LUCKY A.W., et al (1983) *J Invest Dermatol* **81**, 70.
48 MACGREGOR A.J. (1971) *Oral Surg Oral Med Path* **32**, 829.
49 MACGREGOR A.J., et al (1976) *Br Med J* **i**, 130.
50 MARSDEN R.A., et al (1979) *Br J Dermatol* **77**, 722.
51 MASSA M.C. & SU D.W.P. (1982) *J Am Acad Dermatol* **6**, 84.
52 MEHREGAN A.H. & PINKUS H. (1965) *Arch Dermatol* **91**, 574.
53 MILLS O.H. & KLIGMAN A.M. (1975) *Arch Dermatol* **111**, 65.
54 MILLS O.H. & KLIGMAN A.M. (1975) *Arch Dermatol* **111**, 481.
55 MOBAYEN M.M. & COPEMAN P.W.M. (1983) *Clin Exp Dermatol* **8**, 107.
56 NIELSON E.B. & THORMANN J. (1978) *Acta Derm Venereol (Stockh)* **58**, 374.
57 NOVY F.G. (1946) *Calif Med J* **115**, 274.
58 ODLIND V., et al (1982) *Clin Endocrinol* **16**, 243.
59 PAPA C.M. (1976) *Arch Dermatol* **112**, 555.
60 PASSI S., et al (1981) *Br J Dermatol* **105**, 137.
61 PEACHEY R.D.G. & MATTHEWS C.N.A. (1978) *Br J Dermatol* **98**, 669.
62 PLEWIG G. & KLIGMAN A.M. (1973) *Arch Dermatol Forsch* **247**, 29.
63 PLEWIG G., et al (1970) *Arch Dermatol* **101**, 580.
64 PLEWIG G., et al (1982) *J Am Acad Dermatol* **6**, 766.
65 PLEWIG G., et al (1982) *Arch Derm Res* **272**, 363.
66 POCHI P.E., et al (1962) *J Invest Dermatol* **39**, 475.
67 PONTE C.D. (1982) *Am J Psychiat* **139**, 141.
68 RIEBEL A.F. (1963) *Med Welt* **35**, 1749.
69 ROOK A.J. (1972) *Textbook of Dermatology*. Eds. Rook A., Wilkinson D.S. & Ebling F.J.F. Oxford, Blackwell Scientific.
70 SCHACKERT K., et al (1974) *Arch Dermatol* **110**, 458.
71 SIEGEL D., et al (1982) *J Rheumatol* **92**, 344.
72 SNEDDON J. & SNEDDON I. (1983) *Clin Exp Dermatol* **8**, 65.
73 STANKLER L. & CAMPBELL A.G.M. (1980) *Br J Dermatol* **103**, 453.
74 STATHAM B.N., et al (1983) *Clin Exp Dermatol* **8**, 401.
75 STRÖM S., et al (1973) *Acta Derm Venereol (Stockh)* **53**, 306.
76 SULZBERGER M.B., et al (1946) *US Naval Med Bull* **46**, 1178.
77 TAYLOR J.S. (1974) *Cutis* **13**, 585.
78 TORRE D. (1968) *Arch Dermatol* **98**, 549.
79 WHITE C.J. (1914) *J Cutan Dis* **32**, 187.
80 WILENTZ J.M. & BERGER R.A. (1971) *Cutis* **8**, 42.
81 WILLIAMS M., et al (1974) *Br J Dermatol* **90**, 1.
82 WILLIAMSON D.M., et al (1977) *Clin Exp Dermatol* **2**, 351.
83 WULF K. & FEGELER F. (1953) *Hautarzt* **4**, 371.

CHAPTER 53

The Hair

F. J. G. EBLING, R. DAWBER & A. ROOK

INTRODUCTION [1–9]

Hair has no vestige of vital function in man, yet its psychological functions seem immeasurable. If the inevitability of scalp baldness makes it reluctantly tolerable to genetically disposed men, in women loss of hair from the scalp is no less distressing than growth of body or facial hair in excess of the culturally acceptable amount.

The evolutionary history of hair is no less enigmatic. Whatever its origin, it is clear that the warm-blooded mammals owe much of their evolutionary success to the properties of the hairy pelage as a heat insulator. Paradoxically, man's radiation from his ancestral forest home to populate the globe is linked with a reversion to relative nudity and an ability to keep cool. Moreover, hair serves other purposes. In particular, it is concerned with sexual and social communication by constructing adornments such as the mane of the lion or the beard of the human male, or assisting in the dispersal of scents secreted by complexes of sebaceous or apocrine glands.

For these evolutionary reasons, hair follicles are not all under identical control mechanisms. To match the animal pelage to seasonal changes in ambient temperature or environmental background requires moulting and replacement of the hairs. The process appears to involve an inherent follicular rhythm, modified by circulating hormones such as steroids or thyroxine, whose secretion is, in turn, geared to environmental cues through the hypothalamus and hypophysis.

The control of sexual hair growth must be clearly differentiated from that of the moult cycle. The development of pubic, axillary and other body hair is delayed until puberty because it is dependent upon androgens in both sexes: that 'male' hormones are, in contrast, also a prerequisite for the manifestation of pattern baldness still defies adequate explanation.

Hair grows from follicles which are stocking-like inpushings of the superficial epithelium, each of which encloses at its base a small stud of dermis known as the dermal papilla. The cylinder of hair may be regarded as a holocrine secretion arising by division of cells surrounding the papilla, in a region known as the bulb. The follicles are slanted in the dermis, and the longer ones extend into the adipose layer. An oblique muscle, the arrector pili, runs from a point in the mid-region of the follicle wall to the dermo-epidermal junction. Above the muscle one or more sebaceous glands, and in some regions of the body an apocrine gland also, open into the follicle.

In all mammals, including man, but with the possible exception of the merino sheep, hair follicles show intermittent activity. Thus each hair grows to a maximum length, is retained for a time without further growth, and is eventually shed and replaced.

REFERENCES

1 EBLING F.J. (1976) *J Invest Dermatol* **67**, 98.
2 HAMILTON J.B. (1950) *Ann NY Acad Sci* **53**, 461.
3 LUBOWE I.I. (1959) *Ann NY Acad Sci* **83**, 539.
4 LYNE A.G. & SHORT B.F. (Eds.) (1965) *Biology of the Skin and Hair Growth*. Sydney, Angus & Robertson.
5 MONTAGNA W. & ELLIS R.A. (Eds.) (1958) *The Biology of Hair Growth*. New York, Academic Press.
6 MONTAGNA W. & DOBSON R.L. (Eds.) (1969) *Advances in Biology of Skin*. Vol IX. *Hair Growth*. Oxford, Pergamon.
7 ORFANOS C.E. (Ed.) (1979) *Haar und Haarkrankheiten*. Stuttgart, Gustav Fischer.
8 ORFANOS C.E., *et al* (Eds.) (1981) *Hair Research: Status and Future Aspects*. Berlin, Springer.
9 ROOK A. & DAWBER R. (1982) *Diseases of the Hair and Scalp*. Oxford, Blackwell Scientific.

DEVELOPMENT AND DISTRIBUTION OF HAIR FOLLICLES

Rudiments of hair follicles appear first in the regions of the eyebrows, upper lip and chin at about 9 weeks of embryonic development, and in other regions in the fourth month [4]; by 22 weeks the full complement of follicles is established. A fuller account of embryonic development is given in Chapter 2. As the body surface increases, there is a decrease in the actual density of follicles [5,6]. It is generally accepted that new follicles cannot develop in adult skin; the evidence for and against neogenesis of follicles has been reviewed [3]. The total number of follicles in an adult man has been estimated at about 5 million, of which about 1 million are in the head and perhaps 100,000 in the scalp. There appear to be no significant sexual or racial differences in follicle number [5, 6].

A significant loss of hair follicles occurs with advancing age [1]; in adults aged 20–30 an average of 615 per square centimetre has been noted, but between 30 and 50 the mean density falls to 485, and by 80–90 it is only 435 [2]. There are undoubtedly fewer follicles in baldness; a comparison of bald with hairy scalps for the whole range of 30–90 yr gave means of 306 per square centimetre and 459 per square centimetre respectively [2].

REFERENCES

1 BARMAN J.M., *et al* (1969) In *Advances in Biology of Skin*. Vol. IX: *Hair Growth*. Eds. Montagna W. & Dobson R.L. Oxford, Pergamon, p. 211.
2 GIACOMETTI L. (1965) In *Advances in Biology of Skin*. Vol. VI. *Ageing*. Ed. Montagna W. Oxford, Pergamon, p. 97.
3 MULLER S.A. (1971) *J Invest Dermatol* **56**, 1.
4 PINKUS H. (1958) In *The Biology of Hair Growth*. Eds. Montagna W. & Ellis R.A. New York, Academic Press, p. 1.
5 SZABO G. (1958) In *Advances in Biology of Skin*. Vol. IX. *Ageing*. Ed. Montagna W. Oxford, Pergamon, p. 33.
6 SZABO G. (1967) *Philos Trans R Soc Lond Ser B* **252**, 447.

THE ACTIVE FOLLICLE [4, 5]

The bulk of any hair is formed by a thick cortex made up of elongated keratinized cells cemented together, which in pigmented hairs contain granules of melanin. The cortex is surrounded by a cuticle, and may also have a continuous or discontinuous core or medulla (Fig. 53.1). Although the cuticle is formed as a single layer, the cells become progressively imbricated as they move peripherally. The outer cells overlap with their free edges directed towards the tip, and they interlock with the cuticle of the surrounding inner root sheath. The inner root sheath consists, in addition to its cuticle, of Henle's and Huxley's layers; it is formed in pace with the hair and its keratinized cells are ultimately desquamated (Figs. 53.1 and 53.2). Investing it is the outer root sheath, which is continuous with the superficial epithelium, and this is itself enclosed in a non-cellular partition known as the vitreous or glassy membrane. The entire follicle is surrounded by a connective-tissue sheath formed of collagenous fibres, a few elastic fibres and fibroblasts.

Cell formation in hair follicles has been studied by intracutaneous injection of 10 µCi of tritiated thymidine into sites on the human scalp [2]. In biopsy samples taken 40 min later, labelling of cells was observed in the lower half of the hair bulb but not elsewhere. However, labelled cells were distributed diffusely within the area and not in a well-defined basal layer along the papilla, and no labelled mitotic figures were observed. Six hours after injection, the number of labelled cells had increased, labelled mitotic figures were seen and some movement was detected in cells of the outer bulb destined to become inner root sheath. Subsequently, a stream of cells moving into the cortex could also be perceived, but it moved much more slowly. In general, these results confirm earlier suggestions that new cells are formed by division in the region of the bulb surrounding the lower two-thirds of the dermal papilla, but they do not settle the question of whether only cells adjacent to the dermal papilla are capable of division [1]. The fact that the number of grains per cell is reduced as labelled cells move peripherally suggests that further divisions take place, and the assumption that at each division one daughter cell remains capable of further division and attached to the dermal papilla is also questionable in the light of studies of the behaviour of cells in the basal layer of the superficial epidermis [3].

REFERENCES

1 BULLOUGH W.S. & LAURENCE E.B. (1958) In *The Biology of Hair Growth*. Eds. Montagna W. & Ellis R.A. New York, Academic Press, p. 171.
2 EPSTEIN W.L. & MAIBACH H.T. (1969) in *Advances in Biology of Skin*. Vol IX. *Hair Growth*. Eds. Montagna W. & Dobson R.L. Oxford. Pergamon p. 83.
3 GREULICH R.C. (1964) In *The Epidermis*. Eds. Montagna W. & Lobitz W.C. New York, Academic Press, p. 117.
4 MONTAGNA W. & VAN SCOTT E.J. (1958) In *The Biology of Hair Growth'* Eds. Montagna W. & Ellis R.A. New York, Academic Press, Chapter 3.
5 ODLAND G.F. (1983) In *Biochemistry and Physiology of the Skin*. Ed. Goldsmith L.A. Oxford, Clarendon Press, p. 3.

COMPOSITION AND MOLECULAR STRUCTURE OF HAIR KERATIN [1–5]

Keratins are a group of insoluble cystine-containing proteins produced in the epidermal tissues of verte-

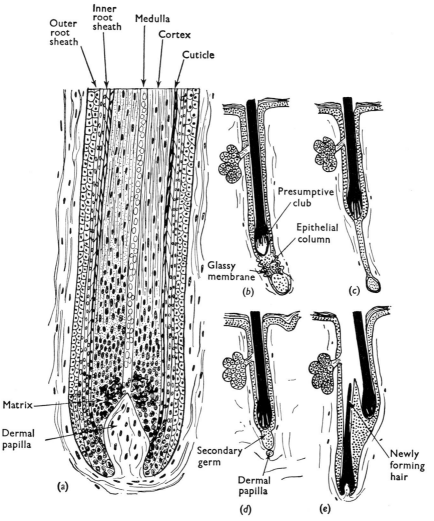

FIG. 53.1. The human hair cycle: (a) an active follicle; (b) early catagen; (c) late catagen, showing ascent of the presumptive club; (d) telogen; (e) early anagen. (From Ebling F.J. (1964) *Progress in the Biological Sciences in Relation to Dermatology.* Vol. 2. Eds. Rook A & Champion R.H. Cambridge, University Press, p. 303.)

brates. Hair contains *hard* keratin, which differs from the *soft* keratin of desquamating tissues (see p. 1393) by its higher sulphur content.

X-ray crystallography of hair gives a so-called *α-diffraction pattern* indicating an axial repeat of 0·51 nm units. If the hair is stretched or heated in water it gives the *β-pattern* with an axial repeat of 0·33 nm. This bears some similarity to the 'feather pattern' characteristic of keratin in avian and reptilian tissues, which has a repeat of 0·31 nm. A fourth pattern, described as *amorphous* because it lacks discrete reflections, occurs in the keratin of the hair cuticle.

It can be concluded from the X-ray diffraction pattern that the polypeptide chains of α-keratin have a geometrically regular secondary structure. The hypothesis is that they are arranged in an α-helix, with 3·6 amino acid residues in each turn of 0·54 nm. The 0·51 nm repeat could be explained if the helices were tilted, which led to the suggestion that they were intertwined to form a two-stranded or, more probably, a three-stranded rope [1]. Some researchers have even favoured seven or more strands [6]. The change to the β-pattern when hair is stretched can be explained by assuming that the helix is pulled into a straight-chain configuration.

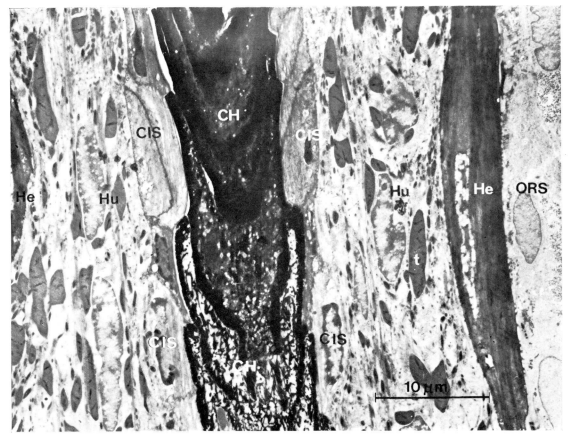

FIG. 53.2. Longitudinal section of the suprabulbar portion of a hair follicle in the scalp of a human fetus at $16\frac{1}{2}$ weeks: ORS, outer root sheath; He, Henle's layer of inner root sheath, keratinized; Hu, Huxley's layer of inner root sheath, unkeratinized at this level; t, trichohyalin granule; CIS, cuticle of inner root sheath, unkeratinized below and keratinized above; CH, cuticle of the, hair, partially keratinized below and fully keratinized above. (Electron micrograph by Mrs E.J. Robbins.)

Chemical analysis of keratin is complicated by the fact that the procedures to render it soluble by breaking disulphide links of an interchain, intramolecular or intermolecular nature may also cleave the peptides. Three soluble fractions, respectively designated low sulphur, high sulphur and high glycine tyrosine have been obtained from wool. Molecular weights are of the order of 10,000–28,000 for high sulphur fractions and 45,000–50,000 for low sulphur fractions. There appear to be more than 50 different proteins in hard keratin, most of the variety being due to the high sulphur group. While the complete amino acid sequences are known for at least 21 wool proteins, the components of human or other hair have not yet been fully purified or sequenced [2].

The keratinizing cells contain small filaments about 7 nm in diameter, which are usually known as *microfibrils*. A bundle of such microfibrils is known as a *fibril* or *macrofibril*. The filaments or microfibrils appear to be set in a matrix which is osmiophilic and sulphur rich; it is well known that such fibre–matrix composites confer great strength. Hence it is concluded that low sulphur proteins containing the α-helices are associated with the filaments and high sulphur proteins with the matrix. Further evidence indicated that within each microfibril a central core about 2 nm in diameter can be discerned and that this is surrounded by a tubular framework about 2 nm thick with an outer diameter of 7·3 nm. It is suggested that the microfibril might contain *protofibrils* about 2 nm in diameter arranged in the form of a core and an annular ring, and that the helical sections of the low sulphur proteins are confined to these units. The dimensions of the ring are such that it could accommodate about nine sections of the coiled core rope, consonant with the proposal that the protofibrils are dispersed in the 9 + 2 pattern of those found in cilia, though this is far from established.

REFERENCES

1 FRASER R.D.B., *et al* (1972) *Keratins: their Composition, Structure and Biosynthesis.* Springfield, Thomas.
2 GILLESPIE J.M. (1983) In *Biochemistry and Physiology of the Skin.* Ed. Goldsmith L.A. Oxford, Clarendon Press, p. 475.
3 MERCER, E.H. (1958) In *The Biology of Hair Growth.* Eds. Montagna W. & Ellis R.A. New York, Academic Press, p. 113.
4 MERCER E.H. (1961) *Keratin and Keratinization.* Oxford, Pergamon.
5 RUDALL K.M. (1964) In *Progress in the Biological Sciences in Relation to Dermatology.* Vol 2, Eds. Rook A. & Champion R.H. Cambridge, Cambridge University Press, p. 355.
6 SWANBECK G. (1964) In *The Epidermis.* Eds. Montagna W & Lobitz W.C. Jr. New York, Academic Press, p. 339.

ULTRASTRUCTURE [1–20]

The medulla. The cells of the medulla begin to show vesicles within their cytoplasm in the suprabulbar region. Such cells contain glycogen and may include melanosomes (Fig. 53.3). Ultimately, above the level of the epidermis, the cells appear to dehydrate and the vacuoles become air filled.

The cortex. In the zone just below the tip of the dermal papilla the microfibrils can already be seen in the cells which give rise to the cortex. They rapidly aggregate to form clusters; in the upper bulb region aggregates a few tenths of a micron wide can be seen as fibrils in the light microscope. At this level the fibrils are birefringent and give the oriented α-type X-ray diffusion pattern; thus the synthesis of the basic structure is virtually complete. Subsequently the denser sulphur-rich matrix develops, coincident with the intense sulphydryl reaction which indicates the presence of cysteine

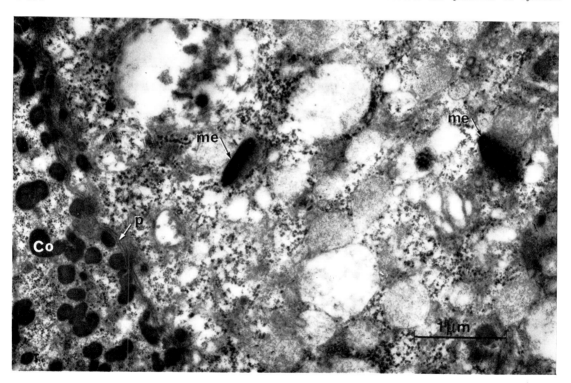

FIG. 53.3. Transverse section of adult hair, just above the bulb. Part of a cortical cell (Co) is separated by a plasma membrane from a cell of the medulla containing vesicles and melanosomes (me). (Electron micrograph by Professor A.S. Breathnach.)

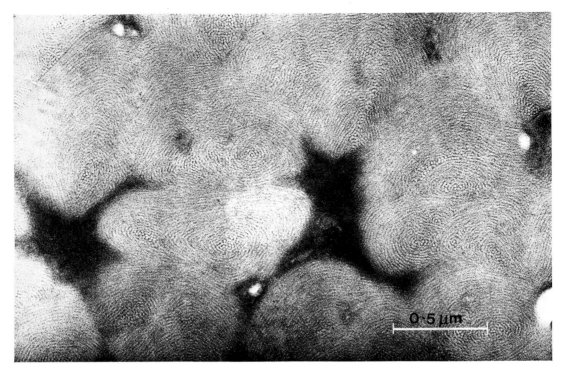

FIG. 53.4. Transverse section of transformed cortical cells of human hair. The relatively translucent filaments, set in a more dense amorphous matrix, appear as concentric lamellae, giving a characteristic 'thumb print' pattern. (Electron micrograph by Professor A.S. Breathnach.)

links. In contrast with the superficial epidermis (see p. 1393) and the inner root sheath, keratohyalin granules do not appear at any stage. On examination in the electron microscope the fully mature cortex can be seen to consist of closely packed spindle-shaped cells with their boundaries separated by a narrow gap (20–25 nm) containing a dense central plasma membrane or intercellular lamella (10–15 nm), generally believed to be proteinaceous and to cement the cells together. Within the cells most of the microfibrils are closely packed and oriented longitudinally in lamellae, though some remain in loose bundles. In transverse section these concentric lamellae have a characteristic 'thumb print' appearance (Fig. 53.4).

The cuticle of the hair. The cuticle consists of five to ten overlapping cell layers, each 350–450 nm thick. The mature cells are thin scales consisting of compact cuticular keratin which shows outer and inner zones of different densities (Fig. 53.5). Between the cell boundaries is a narrow gap (30 nm) containing a dense central intercellular lamella. From the outside the scales can be seen to be im-

bricated like the tiles on a roof. Over the newly formed part of the hair the scale margins are intact, but as the hair emerges from the skin they become jagged (Fig. 53.6) and progressively break off ('weathering').

The 'environmental' outer surface of each cuticular cell has a very clear A layer which is rich in high sulphur protein; this protects the cuticular cells from premature breakdown due to chemical and physical 'insults'.

Inner root sheath. Each of the three layers of the inner root sheath keratinizes, and though the rates of maturation are different the patterns of change are identical. Filaments about 7 nm thick and, in contrast with the hair cortex, amorphous trichohyalin granules appear in the cytoplasm. As the cells move up the follicle, the filaments become more abundant and the number and size of the granules increase. In the hardened cytoplasm, however, only filaments can be seen. The changes occur first in the outermost Henle layer, then in the innermost cuticle and lastly in Huxley's layer, which is situated between them (Fig. 53.7).

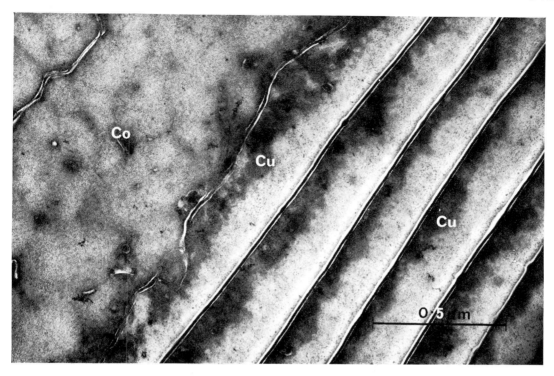

FIG. 53.5. Transverse section of the cuticle and cortex of adult hair from the eyebrow. Both the cortical cells (Co) and the cuticular cell (Cu) are separated by plasma membranes and dense intracellular material. The keratinized cuticular cells show outer and inner zones of different densities. (Electron micrograph by Professor A.S. Breathnach.)

The inner root sheath hardens before the presumptive hair within it, and it is consequently thought to control the definitive shape of the hair shaft in health and in many genetic diseases with abnormal hair morphology.

REFERENCES

1 BIRBECK M.S.C. & MERCER E.H. (1957) *J Biophys Biochem Cytol* **3**, 203.
2 BIRBECK M.S.C. & MERCER E.H. (1957) *J Biophys Biochem Cytol* **3**, 215.
3 BIRBECK M.S.C. & MERCER E.H. (1957) *J Biophys Biochem Cytol* **3**, 223.
4 BREATHNACH A.S. (1971) *An Atlas of the Ultrastructure of Human Skin*. London, Churchill.
5 FORSLIND B. & SWANBECK G. (1966) *Expl Cell Res* **43**, 191.
6 FRASER R.D.B., *et al* (1972) *Keratins: their Composition, Structure and Biosynthesis*. Springfield, Thomas, p. 1.
7 MAHRLE G., *et al* (1969) *Arch Klin Exp Dermatol* **235**, 295.
8 MERCER E.H. (1958) In *The Biology of Hair Growth*. Ed. Montagna W. & Ellis R.A. New York, Academic Press, p. 91.
9 MERCER E.H. (1961) *Keratin and Keratinization*. Oxford, Pergamon.
10 ODLAND G.F. (1983) In *Biochemistry and Physiology of the Skin*. Ed. Goldsmith L.A. Oxford, Clarendon Press, p. 3.
11 ORFANOS C. & RUSKE H. (1968) *Arch Klin Exp Dermatol* **231**, 97.
12 ORFANOS C. & RUSKE H. (1968) *Arch Klin Exp Dermatol* **231**, 264.
13 ORFANOS C. & RUSKE H. (1968) *Arch Klin Exp Dermatol* **231**, 279.
14 PARAKKAL P.F. & MATOLTSY A.G. (1964) *J Invest Dermatol* **43**, 23.
15 PUCCINELLI V.A., *et al* (1967) *G ital Dermatol Sifilol* **108**, 453.
16 ROGERS G.E. (1964) In *The Epidermis*. Eds. Montagna W. & Lobitz W.C. Jr. New York, Academic Press, p. 179.
17 ROTH S.I. & CLARK W.H. Jr. (1964) In *The Epidermis*. Eds. Montagna W. & Lobitz W.C. Jr. New York, Academic Press, p. 303.
18 SWIFT J.A. (1967) *J R Microsc Soc* **88**, 449.
19 VAN SCOTT E.J. (1968) *Annu Rev Med* **19**, 337.
20 ZELICKSON A.S. (1967) *Ultrastructure of Normal and Abnormal Skin*. Philadelphia, Lea & Febiger.

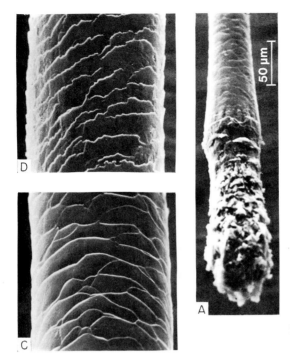

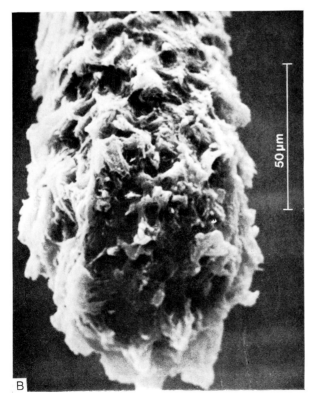

Fig. 53.6. A, Surface view of the proximal part of a club hair from the human scalp. B, Surface view of the basal part of the club. C, Surface view of cuticular scales in the region adjacent to the club (on the same scale as B). D, Surface view of jagged cuticular scales in the distal portion of the hair (on the same scale as B). (Electron-scan micrographs by Dr D. Jackson.)

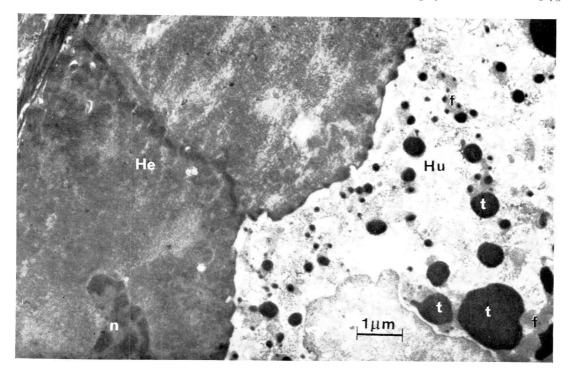

FIG. 53.7. Transverse section of adult human eyebrow to show transformed Henle layer (He) with nuclear remnant (n), and Huxley layer (Hu) with trichohyalin (t) and filaments (f) in cytoplasm. (Electron micrograph by Professor A.S. Breathnach.)

CYCLIC ACTIVITY OF THE FOLLICLE

The duration of the activity of follicles, or anagen, varies greatly from species to species, and in any species from region to region, and with age [3, 4, 6, 9, 18]. For example, in the rat the dorsal hair is fully formed in 3 weeks and the shorter ventral hair in only 12 days [8], whereas in the guinea-pig anagen lasts from 20 to 40 days [7]. In the human scalp anagen may occupy 3 yrs or more [10, 11]. However, the transition from terminal hair to vellus in ageing must clearly involve a change in the periodicity of the follicle as well as in follicular architecture; thus on the vertex of a 60-yr-old man the growing period of coarse hairs ranged between 17 and 94 weeks, and that of finer hairs between 7 and 22 weeks [18]. Elsewhere on the body the periods of anagen are considerably less. In a young male they ranged from 19 to 26 weeks on the leg, 6 to 12 weeks on the arm, 4 to 13 weeks on the finger, 4 to 14 weeks in the moustache and 8 to 24 weeks in the region under the temple [18]. Seago and Ebling [19] estimated averages of 54 and 28 days, respectively, for the thighs and arms of nine males, and 22 days for each of these sites in eleven females.

Activity is followed by a relatively short transitional phase, catagen, occupying a few days in rodents and only about 2 weeks in the human scalp, and a resting phase or telogen (Figs. 53.1 and 53.8). Towards the end of anagen, scalp follicles show a gradual thinning and lightening of pigment at the base of the hair shaft [10, 14]. The melanocytes in the region of the tip of the dermal papilla cease producing melanin, resorb their dendrites and become indistinguishable from the matrix cells. The middle region of the bulb now starts to become constricted; distal to the constriction the expanded base of the hair becomes keratinized as a 'club', and below the epithelial column can be seen the dermal papilla which becomes released from its epidermal investment. From the onset of catagen [20] the connective-tissue sheath of the follicle, in particular the vitreous membrane, thickens enormously and causes a characteristic corrugation in the epithelial strand. Subsequently the club hair moves towards

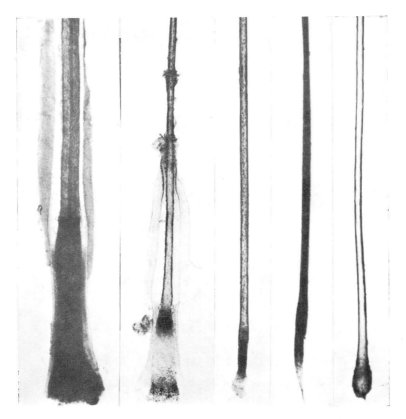

FIG. 53.8. Appearance of the hair root in plucked hairs: (a) normal anagen hair; (b) dysplastic anagen hair with the root sheath still attached to it, from a female scalp showing chronic diffuse alopecia; (c) dysplastic anagen hair without root sheath; (d) dystrophic hair without root sheath and lacking matrix, but with pointed proximal end; (e) club hair. (From Braun Falco O. & Zaun H. (1962) *Arch Klin Exp Dermatol* **215**, 165.)

the skin surface so that the epithelial column lengthens. After the ascent of the presumptive club, the epithelial strand shortens progressively from below and finally is reduced to a little nipple, the secondary germ. This resting stage, or telogen, lasts only a few weeks in the human scalp. When the next hair cycle starts the secondary germ elongates by cell division, grows downwards, becomes invaginated by the papilla and gives rise to a new bulb. The keratinized dome of newly forming hair subsequently emerges by the side of the old club, which is lost.

In the adult human scalp the activity of each follicle is independent of its neighbours [1, 10, 15]; such a pattern is known as a mosaic. At any one time, on average about 13% of the follicles are in telogen, though the range is large; it has been recorded as 4–24% [1, 10, 15, 17]. Only 1% or less are in catagen. If there are about 100,000 follicles in the scalp and their period is about 1,000 days,

about 100 hairs ought to be lost each day; in practice, the average recovery of shed hairs is usually rather less and over 100 can be regarded as high [10, 11]. Follicles throughout the body, as well as those on the scalp, are out of synchrony and, indeed, have different periodicities. It is of particular interest, however, that the cycles of the hair comprising each 'Meijéres trio group' are in phase [18] (Figs. 53.9 and 53.10).

The guinea-pig has been said to resemble man, in that moulting of the adult appears to take place in a mosaic. However, in the newborn animal all follicles are simultaneously active [7], and it seems that, for at least 50 days after birth and probably for much longer, follicles producing a single fibre type show a measure of synchrony with each other but are out of phase with those producing different fibre types (Fig. 53.11). The finding is of interest, for in man there is frequently a more or less synchronous moult of scalp hairs during the early

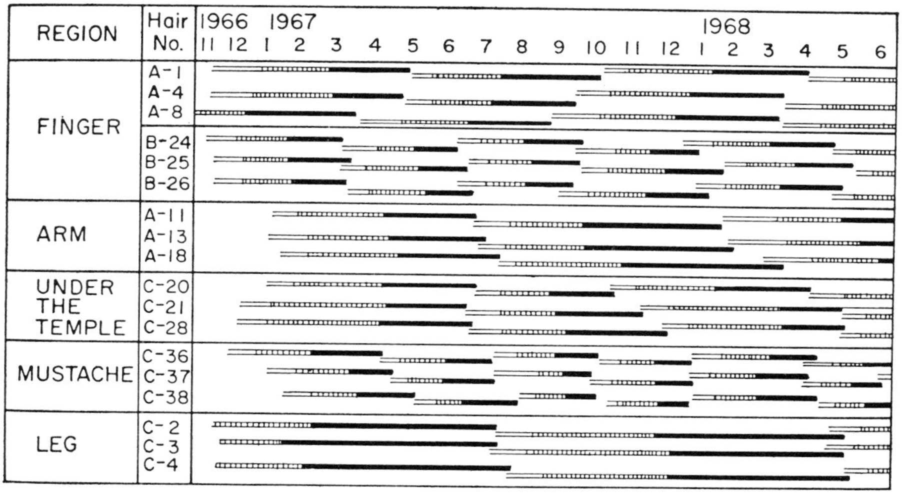

REGION	Hair No.	1966		1967											1968					
		11	12	1	2	3	4	5	6	7	8	9	10	11	12	1	2	3	4	5 6
FINGER	A-1 A-4 A-8 B-24 B-25 B-26																			
ARM	A-11 A-13 A-18																			
UNDER THE TEMPLE	C-20 C-21 C-28																			
MUSTACHE	C-36 C-37 C-38																			
LEG	C-2 C-3 C-4																			

FIG. 53.9. Cycles of three hairs in a Meijéres trio group. The white bar indicates the time for the emergence of a new hair from the shedding of the club. The shaded bar indicates the period of activity of the follicle subsequent to emergence and the black bar indicates the resting period. (From Saitoh M., *et al* (1970) *J Invest Dermatol* (**54**, 65.)

months of life as well as the shed of lanugo in development [11], and there is evidence of the passage of a growth wave from front to back in the scalp of newborn infants [2, 11, 16]. Thus it may be that in both the guinea-pig and man asynchrony gradually develops from synchrony.

Many animals moult in a characteristic wave pattern; in the rat, for example, replacement of hairs starts in the venter and bands of activity and shedding move over the flanks to the dorsum, subsequently spreading to the head and tail regions (Fig. 53.12). Initially, whilst the animal is growing

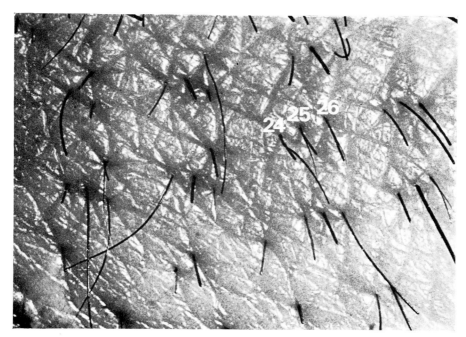

FIG. 53.10. Meijéres trio group from the finger of a man of 30. (From Saitoh M. *et al* (1970) *J Invest Dermatol* **54**, 65.)

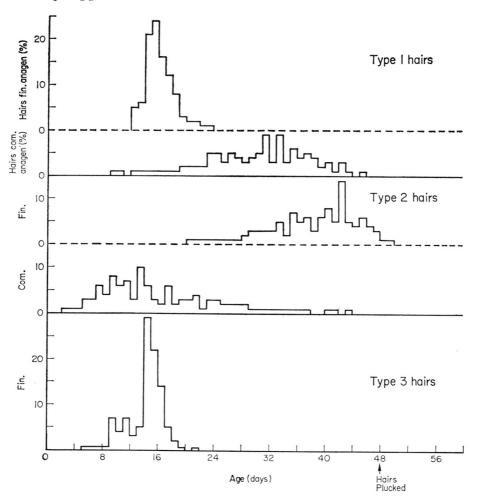

FIG. 53.11. Cycles in hair follicles of the dorsal skin of the guinea-pig. The graphs show the number of follicles of each of three types finishing activity (Fin.) and commencing activity (Com.) on each day. For details of the experiment see legend to Fig. 53.15. (From Jackson D. & Ebling F.J. (1971) *J Soc Cosmet Chem* **22**, 701.)

the moults are correlated with age and such spontaneous cycles continue throughout life in laboratory rodents [4, 5, 12]. However, in wild mammals of temperate zones the adult moult becomes seasonal, so that by changing the physical nature and colour of pelage the animal becomes adapted to changes in temperature and background. The skin cycle seems to resemble the sexual cycle, in that it is influenced through the hypothalamus and probably the pineal, the anterior hypophysis and the endocrine system; the important and overriding environmental influence is the photoperiod, though ambient temperature may exert a slight modifying effect [4, 5]. Of particular interest is the demonstration that hair fall in man can show significant seasonal fluctuations [13, 18], suggesting that follicular activity in the scalp is not entirely free of environmental influences.

Undoubtedly changes in the hair cycle may be involved in transient hair loss in man. Some of the conditions formerly grouped under the description 'alopecia symptomatica', which can result from a variety of mental and physical stresses, involve the simultaneous precipitation of many follicles into catagen, Kligman [11] has described several cases of postfebrile alopecia in which shedding of club hairs began about 3–4 months after the fever and continued for 3–4 weeks. At the height of shedding the

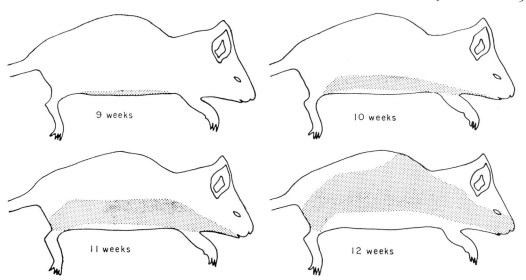

FIG. 53.12. Passage of the second replacement wave of hair growth in the albino rat. The area of active follicles is shown stippled. The age of the animal is given in each case.

telogen counts made from scalp biopsies ranged from 34 to 53%; regeneration was well under way 6 weeks later. Similarly, a prisoner who underwent a series of trials for murder began to lose hairs at the rate of over 1,000 per day about 10 weeks after conviction; there were no histological abnormalities except for an increased proportion of follicles in telogen. The phenomenon has been given the name 'telogen effluvium' (p. 1978). The nature of the neuroendocrine or other mechanisms by which it is brought about remains to be elucidated. The condition bears some similarity to postpartum alopecia, which is presumed to follow hormonal changes and is considered further below (p. 1951).

REFERENCES

1 BARMAN J.M., *et al* (1965) *J Invest Dermatol* **44**, 233.
2 BARMAN J.M., *et al* (1967) *J Invest Dermatol* **48**, 138.
3 EBLING F.J. (1964) In *Progress in the Biological Sciences in Relation to Dermatology* Vol. 21, Eds. Rook A. & Champion R.H. Cambridge, Cambridge University Press, p. 303.
4 EBLING F.J. (1965) In *The Comparative Physiology and Pathology of the Skin*. Eds. Rook A.J. & Walton G.S. Oxford, Blackwell, p. 87.
5 EBLING F.J. & HALE P.A. (1970) *Mem Soc Endocrine* **18**, 215.
6 EBLING F.J. & JOHNSON E. (1964) *Symp Zool Soc Lond* **12**, 97.
7 JACKSON D. & EBLING F.J. (1971) *J Soc Cosmet Chem* **22**, 701.
8 JOHNSON E. (1958) *J Endocrinol* **16**, 337.
9 JOHNSON E. (1981) In *Hair Research: Status and Future Aspects*. Eds. Orfanos C.E., *et al.* Berlin, Springer, p. 183.
10 KLIGMAN A.M. (1959) *J Invest Dermatol* **33**, 307.
11 KLIGMAN A.M. (1961) *Arch Dermatol* **83**, 175.
12 LING J.K. (1970) *Q Rev Biol* **45**, 16.
13 ORENTREICH N. (1969) In *Advances in Biology of Skin*. Vol. IX. *Hair Growth*. Eds. Montagna W. & Dobson R.L. Oxford, Pergamon, p. 99.
14 PARAKKAL P.F. (1970) *Z Zellforsch Mikrosk Anat* **107**, 174.
15 PECORARO V., *et al* (1964) *J Invest Dermatol* **42**, 427.
16 PECORARO V., *et al* (1964) *J Invest Dermatol* **43**, 145.
17 PECORARO V., *et al* (1969) In *Advances in Biology of Skin*. Vol. IX. *Hair Growth*. Eds. Montagna W. & Dobson R.L. Oxford, Pergamon, p. 203.
18 SAITOH M., *et al* (1970) *J Invest Dermatol* **54**, 65.
19 SEAGO S.V. & EBLING F.J.G. (1985) *Br J Dermatol* **113**, 9.
20 SUGIYAMA S., *et al* (1976) *J Ultrastruct Res* **54**, 359.

HORMONAL INFLUENCES

It is important to make a clear distinction between the effects of a range of hormones on the follicular cycle, in evolutionary terms related to the adaptive function of moulting, and the particular role of androgens in the induction of sexual and other adult hair which is an adaptation for delaying until puberty the associated socio-sexual signals [5]. Most dermatological problems centre around androgen-dependent hair, which will be considered separately below. Knowledge of other hormonal mechanisms is, however, relevant not only to understanding the control of the moult cycle but also to the problems of human hair loss in thyroid disorder and following pregnancy.

Each hair follicle appears to have an intrinsic rhythm. In rats, this has been shown to continue when the site is changed [7] or even, under some circumstances, when the follicle is transplanted to another animal in a different phase of the moult [8]. Plucking of hairs from resting follicles brings forward the next period of activity, and such follicles continue out of phase with their neighbours, at

least for a time [19]. The nature of this intrinsic control, and the mechanism by which epilation or wounding affect it, are unknown. One hypothesis is that a mitotic inhibitor accumulates during anagen and is gradually used up or dispersed during telogen [2, 3]; another is that growth-promoting wound hormones are released by epilation [1]. The finding that removal of residual club hairs after follicular activity has commenced does not affect the anagen in progress but does advance the next eruption of hairs [13, 14] appears to be irreconcilable with the inhibitor hypothesis.

Plucking of rat hairs during telogen has been

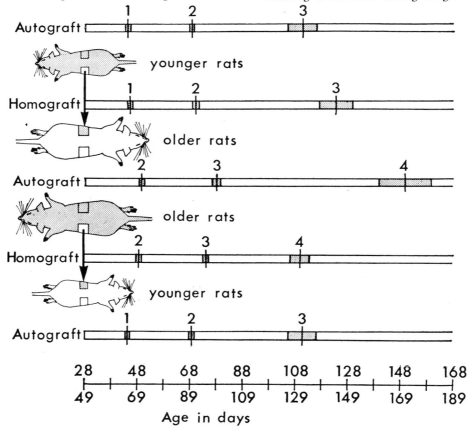

FIG. 53.13. Successive eruptions of hair on homografts exchanged between rats aged 28 and 49 days respectively, and on autografts made at the same time. The top channel, for example, shows the mean time of eruption on autografts made on the right flank of the younger rats, and below it is shown the eruption on homografts taken from the left flank and put into older hosts. The shaded limits represent $\pm 1 \cdot 5$ times the standard errors. In comparing homografts with autografts, when the limits do not overlap, the differences are significant with $P < 0 \cdot 05$. The minimum number of observations was nine.

The experiments show that the follicles in homografts retain the rhythm of the donor for a substantial period after grafting, but that their activity is gradually brought into phase with that of symmetrically situated follicles in the host. (From Ebling F.J. (1965). In *Biology of the Skin and Hair Growth*. Eds. Lyne A.G. & Short B.F. Sydney, Angus & Robertson, p. 507.)

shown to induce high levels of ornithine decarboxylase within 4 h [23], although during the first 60 min the enzyme actually decreases in activity [21]. This decrease is at first very rapid and about 30% of the activity is lost within 5 min. There is no great change in other enzymes or in the protein synthetic capacity of the skin. It appears that an inhibitor of ornithine decarboxylase is produced, and the extraction of such an enzyme from epilated skin [20] raises the possibility that it is involved in the intrinsic mechanism.

Irrespective of intrinsic control, the overall timing of the cyclic events also appears to be influenced by systemic factors, for follicles on homografts gradually come into phase with their hosts [8] (Fig. 53.13), and parabiotic rats gradually come to moult in phase with each other [6]. This systemic control mechanism may embody components as yet unknown, but it could be accounted for by facts that can be demonstrated. In rats, oestradiol, testosterone and adrenal steroids delay the initiation of follicular activity [17, 18] and oestradiol also delays the shedding of club hairs [18], so that the moult is accelerated by gonadectomy or adrenalectomy; conversely, thyroid hormone advances onset of follicular activity and thyroidectomy or inhibition of the thyroid delays passage of the moult [10]. Oestradiol has similarly been shown to delay the onset of follicular activity in the guinea-pig [15]. In the rat, hypophysectomy advances it, so the influence of the gonadal system appears to override that of the thyroid [10]. The hypothalamus and the hypophysis may thus exert their influence by way of the thyroid, with the adrenal cortex and the gonads forging a link between environmental, reproductive and moulting cycles [4, 9].

Hormones also influence follicles in anagen. Studies in which rat hairs were pulse labelled with ³⁵S cysteine [13] showed that oestradiol or thyroxine each similarly reduced the duration of the active phase, their effects being additive when they were administered simultaneously. In contrast, whereas oestradiol decreased the rate of hair growth, thyroxine had the opposite effect. The findings suggest that the two hormones do not have the same point of action.

Human hair is profoundly affected by thyroid hormones. In a study carried out in Sheffield [11], 16 out of 150 women who complained of hair loss were diagnosed as hypothyroid on the basis of serum protein bound iodine levels confirmed by radio-iodine tracer studies. Mean hair diameter was reduced [16]. Whereas diameters in normal subjects had a symmetrical distribution with a marked peak at 0·08 mm, in all subjects with hair loss, and especially in those with hypothyroidism, their spread was much wider, with separate peaks at 0·04 and 0·06 mm. The proportion of roots in telogen has been shown to be abnormally high in hairs plucked from the occipital and parietal areas of hypothyroid subjects; treatment with thyroid hormone restored it to normal after 8 weeks [12]; this fact contradicts the idea that decreased scalp hair in hypothyroidism is due to increased 'free' androgen levels resulting from decreased sex hormone binding globulin (SHBG).

The phenomenon of post-partum hair loss also appears to result from a hormonally mediated change in the cycles of scalp follicles. A loss of hairs at about two to three times the normal rate gives rise to a transient alopecia about 4–6 months after parturition. At this time the proportion of hairs in telogen can be as much as 35% [22], whereas in late pregnancy it may be less than 5% which is only about a third of normal (Fig. 53.14). This suggests that the passage of follicles into catagen, followed by shedding of club hairs, is slowed down by pregnancy, but occurs precipitously after parturition when hormonal conditions are altered, particularly by a rapid fall in oestrogen levels. The pattern of fluctuation in the anagen-to-telogen ratio has been observed over three consecutive pregnancies in one subject over a period of 9 yr; the change became less marked in each successive pregnancy [24].

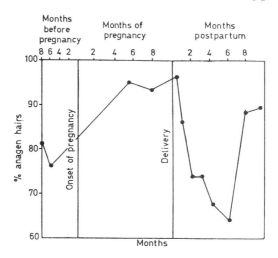

FIG. 53.14. Percentage of anagen hairs in a 25-yr-old woman before, during and after pregnacy. (From Lynfield Y.L. (1960) *J Invest Dermatol* **35**, 323.

REFERENCES

1 ARGYRIS T.S. (1969) In *Advances in Biology of Skin.* Vol. IX. *Hair Growth.* Eds. Montagna W. & Dobson R.L. Oxford, Pergamon, p. 339.

2 CHASE H.B. (1954) *Physiol Rev* **34**, 113.

3 CHASE H.B. & EATON G.J. (1959) *Ann NY Acad Sci* **85**, 365.

4 EBLING F.J. & HALE P.A. (1970) *Mem Soc Endocrinol* **18**, 215.

5 *EBLING F.J. & HALE P.A. (1983) In *Biochemistry and Physiology of the Skin.* Ed. Goldsmith L.A. Oxford, Clarendon, p. 522.

6 EBLING F.J. & HERVEY G.R. (1964) *J Embryol Exp Morphol* **12**, 425.

7 EBLING F.J. & JOHNSON E. (1959) *J Embryol Exp Morphol* **7**, 417.

8 EBLING F.J. & JOHNSON E. (1961) *J Embryol Exp Morphol* **9**, 285.

9 EBLING F.J. & JOHNSON E. (1964) *Symp Zool Soc Lond* **12**, 97.

10 EBLING F.J. & JOHNSON E. (1964) *J Endocrinol* **29**, 193.

11 ECKERT J., *et al* (1967) *Br J Dermatol* **79**, 543.

12 FREINKEL R.K. & FREINKEL N. (1972) *Arch Dermatol Syphilol.* **106**, 349.

13 HALE P.A. & EBLING F.J. (1975) *J Exp Zool* **191**, 49.

14 HALE P.A. & EBLING F.J. (1979) *J Exp Zool* **207**, 49.

15 JACKSON D. & EBLING F.J. (1972) *J Anat* **111**, 303.

16 JACKSON D., *et al* (1972) *Br J Dermatol* **87**, 361.

17 JOHNSON E. (1958) *J Endocrinol* **16**, 351.

18 JOHNSON E. (1958) *J Endocrinol* **16**, 360.

19 JOHNSON E. & EBLING F.J. (1964) *J Embryol Exp Morphol* **12**, 465.

20 LESIEWICZ J. & GOLDSMITH L.A. (1983) *J Invest Dermatol* **80**, 97.

21 LESIEWICZ J., *et al* (1980) *J Invest Dermatol* **75**, 411.

22 LYNFIELD Y.L. (1960) *J Invest Dermatol* **35**, 323.

23 MORRISON D.M. & GOLDSMITH L.A. (1978) *J Invest Dermatol* **70**, 309.

24 PECORARO V., *et al* (1969) In *Advances in Biology of Skin.* Vol. IX. *Hair Growth.* Eds. Montagna W. & Dobson R.L. Oxford, Pergamon, p. 203.

ANDROGEN-DEPENDENT HAIR

The growth of facial, trunk and extremity hair in the male, and of pubic and axillary hair in both sexes, is clearly dependent on androgens. The development of such hair at puberty is, in broad terms, and at least initially, in parallel with the rise in levels of androgen from testicular, adrenocortical and ovarian sources which occurs in both sexes and is somewhat steeper in boys than girls [41].

That testosterone from the interstitial cells of the testis is responsible for growth of beard and body hair in male adolescence and that testicular activity is itself initiated by gonadotrophic hormones of the pituitary is unquestioned. However, the findings that growth-hormone deficient boys and girls are less than normally responsive to androgens and that growth hormone is necessary as a synergistic factor to allow testosterone to be fully effective with respect to protein anabolism, growth promotion and androgenicity [42] suggest that hypophysial hormones might also play a more direct role. In support of such a view is the evidence that the pubertal spurt in human body growth requires both growth hormone and androgen [39], and that the change from infantile to adult pelage can be prevented by hypophysectomy in both the dog [20] and the rat in which it can be restored by prolactin [32]. Moreover, the response of the rat sebaceous glands to testosterone is also reduced by hypophysectomy and can be restored by hypophysial hormones (see p. 1945).

Direct evidence of the role of testicular androgen is that castration reduces growth of the human beard [15], whereas testosterone stimulates it in eunuchs and old men [5]. Since facial and body hair is normally absent from women, it appears to require high levels of the hormone and, since it is usually deficient in cases of 5α-reductase deficiency [12], it seems that metabolism of the testosterone to 5α-dihydrotestosterone is mandatory (see p. 22). This view is further supported by the finding that in patients with coeliac disease the rate of beard growth was correlated with the level of 5α-dihydrotestosterone in the plasma but not with that of testosterone [11]. The role of androgen is further demonstrated in the treatment of hirsute women with the antiandrogen cyproterone acetate [18, 19] which reduces the definitive length, rate of growth, diameter and extent of medullation of the thigh hairs [9, 10]. While the plasma androgen levels are lowered, the major part of the action appears to be by competition for the androgen receptors in the hair follicle [2, 7, 15, 36].

Pubic and axillary hair is also undoubtedly androgen dependent. It is deficient in testicular feminization, a condition in which genetic males develop as females because of a lack of intracellular androgen receptor, and in women suffering from adrenal insufficiency [25]. However, it appears to be present in the condition Type 11 incomplete hermaphroditism in which genetic males lack 5α-reductase even though their plasma testosterone is normal [12]. Therefore it seems probable that growth of the pubic hair requires only low levels of androgen and is not dependent on 5α-reductase.

Scalp hair differs in that its growth does not require any androgenic stimulus. However, in genetically ordained subjects androgen is, paradoxically, responsible for post-pubertal hair deficiency on the vertex of the scalp [13, 14, 17]. The existence of testosterone receptors in scalp hair follicles is implied by the fact that female diffuse alopecia can be alleviated by oral antiandrogens [8, 43]. The additional necessity for 5α-reductase is suggested by the evidence that male bald scalp has a greater capacity than non-bald scalp to convert testosterone to 5α-dihydrotestosterone [3], that isolated hair roots have a similar capacity [38] and that recession of the frontal hairline does not occur in cases of familial male pseudohermaphroditism involving 5α-reductase deficiency [25]. However, the oxidative pathway may also be important, since the major metabolite produced by isolated hair roots *in vitro* is androstenedione [35, 37].

If growth of hair on the face and body and deficiency of hair on the scalp are both androgen dependent, the question arises whether hirsutism and baldness are provoked by excess androgen or by an enhanced peripheral response. When hirsutism is associated with other gross signs of virility or with menstrual disorder, it clearly has an endocrine pathology. Much more frequently the hirsutism is described as idiopathic because there is no obvious 'central' hormonal disturbance. In idiopathic hirsutism the concentration of plasma testosterone is usually within or only slightly above the normal range; androstenedione is more often found to be elevated [1, 22, 33]. The possibility that free androgen may be higher is suggested by the finding that SHBG is, on average, lower [36]. However, although such minor abnormalities are frequently associated with hirsutism, they cannot account for every case since about 40% of all patients appear to show all hormonal parameters within the normal range [26]. The finding that hirsute women with no evidence of ovarian or adrenal dysfunction excreted about four times as much 5α-androstanediol as non-hirsute women [28] suggested that increased 5α-reductase activity in the hair follicle might be involved; this was borne out by the demonstration that suprapubic skin from such patients, when incubated with tritiated testosterone, produced 5α-reduced metabolites at about four times the rate of skin from normal women [23, 24, 27].

The question of whether male pattern baldness is associated with other signs of virility or abnormal androgen levels has been similarly debated. Evidence that it is correlated with hairiness of the chest [34] appears to be contradicted by a failure to find any association with density of body hair, skin and muscle thickness or rate of sebum excretion [4]. However, the finding that, despite normal plasma testosterone, bald men tend to have lower SHBG

and higher salivary testosterone does suggest that they might enjoy more available androgen [6].

Most female diffuse alopecia is androgenetic. While it may be associated with virilism and high androgen levels resulting from disorders of the adrenal cortex or ovaries, plasma androgens are more usually normal. However, as in males, there is a tendency for SHBG to be lower, though with a considerable overlap of the normal range [29].

Since human hair itself so clearly differs between regions in its response to androgens, it is obvious that any possible animal models must be viewed with caution. The vibrissae of rats [21], the hairs of the gerbil ventral gland [30] and, presumably, the mane of the lion are all androgen dependent. Even if male baldness is truly mimicked by the stumptailed macaque, the model is not particularly accessible [31, 40], and the wattled starling, which loses feathers from its head, can hardly be considered as a greatly superior alternative [16].

REFERENCES

1 BARDIN C.W. & LIPSETT M.B. (1967) *J Clin Invest* **46**, 891.
2 BARNES E.W., *et al* (1975) *Clin Endocrinol* **4**, 65.
3 BINGHAM K.D. & SHAW D.A. (1973) *J Endocrinol* **57**, 111.
4 BURTON J.L., *et al* (1979) *Br J Dermatol* **100**, 567.
5 CHIEFFI M. (1949) *J Gerontol* **4**, 200.
6 CIPRIANI R., *et al* (1983) *Br J Dermatol* **109**, 249.
7 CITTADINI E. & BARRECA P. (1977) In *Androgens and Antiandrogens.* Eds. Martini L. & Motta M. New York, Raven Press, p. 309.
8 DAWBER R.P.R., *et al* (1982) *Br J Dermatol* **107** (Suppl. 22), 20.
9 EBLING F.J., *et al* (1977) *Br J. Dermatol* **97**, 371.
10 EBLING F.J., *et al* (1979) In *Androgenisierungserscheinungen bei der Frau.* Eds. Hammerstein J., *et al.* Amsterdam, Excerpta Medica, p. 243.
11 FARTHING M.J.G., *et al* (1982) *Br J Dermatol* **107**, 559.
12 GRIFFIN J.E. & WILSON J.D. (1977) *J Clin Endocrinol Metab* **45**, 1137.
13 HAMILTON J.B. (1942) *Am J Anat* **71**, 451.
14 HAMILTON J.B. (1951) *Ann NY Acad Sci* **53**, 708.
15 HAMILTON J.B. (1958) In *The Biology of Hair Growth.* Eds. Montagna W. & Ellis R.A. New York, Academic Press, p. 399.
16 HAMILTON J.B. (1959) *Ann NY Acad Sci* **83**, 429.
17 HAMILTON J.B. (1960) *J. Clin Endocrinol Metab* **20**, 1309.
18 HAMMERSTEIN J. & CUPCEANCU B. (1969) *Dtsch Med Wochenschr* **94**, 829.
19 HAMMERSTEIN J., *et al* (1975) *J Steroid Biochem* **6**, 827.
20 HOUSSAY B.A. (1918) *Endocrinology* **2**, 497.
21 IBRAHIM L. & WRIGHT E.A. (1983) *Br J Dermatol* **108**, 321.
22 JAMES V.H.T. & ANDRE C.M. (1974) In *Biochemistry in*

Women: Clinical Concepts. Eds. Curry A.S. & Hewlett J.V. Boca Raton, FL, CRC Press, p. 23.

23 KUTTENN F., *et al* (1977) *J Endocrinol* **75**, 83.

24 KUTTENN F., *et al* (1980) In *Percutaneous Absorption of Steroids.* Eds. Mauvais-Jarvis P., *et al.* London, Academic Press, p. 99.

25 LESHIN M. & WILSON J.D. (1981) In *Hair Research.* Eds. Orfanos C.E., *et al.* Berlin, Springer, p. 205.

26 LUCKY A.W., *et al* (1983) *J Invest Dermatol* **81**, 70.

27 MAUVAIS-JARVIS P. (1977) In *Androgens and Antiandrogens.* Eds. Martini L. & Motta M. New York, Raven Press, p. 229.

28 MAUVAIS-JARVIS P., *et al* (1973) *J Clin Endocrinol Metab* **36**, 452.

29 MILLER J.A., *et al* (1982) *Br J Dermatol* **106**, 331.

30 MITCHELL O.G. & BUTCHER E.O. (1966) *Anat Rec* **156**, 11.

31 MONTAGNA W., *et al* (1966) *Am J Phys Anthropol* **24**, 71.

32 RENNELS E.G. & CALLAHAN W.P. (1959) *Anat Rec* **135**, 21.

33 ROSENFELD R.L. (1971) *J Clin Endocrinol Metab* **32**, 717.

34 ŠALAMON T. (1968) In *Biopathology of Pattern Alopecia.* Eds. Baccaredda-Boy A., *et al.* Basel, Karger, p. 39.

35 SANSONE-BAZZANO G., *et al* (1972) *J Clin Metab* **34**, 512.

36 SAWERS R.S., *et al* (1982) In *Androgens and Anti-androgen Therapy.* Ed. Jeffcoate S.L. New York, Wiley, p. 145.

37 SCHWEIKERT H.U. & WILSON J.D. (1974) *J Clin Endocrinol Metab* **38**, 811.

38 SCHWEIKERT H.U. & WILSON J.D. (1981) In *Hair Research.* Eds. Orfanos C.E. *et al.* Berlin, Springer, p. 210.

39 TANNER J.M. & WHITEHOUSE R.H. (1972) In *Growth and Growth Hormone.* Eds. Pecile A & Muller E.E. Amsterdam, Excerpta Medica, p. 429.

40 UNO H., *et al* (1969) In *Advances in Biology of Skin.* Vol. IX. *Hair Growth.* Eds. Montagna W. & Dobson R.L. Oxford, Pergamon, p. 221.

41 WINTER J.S.D. & FAIMAN C. (1973) *Pediatr Res* **7**, 948.

42 ZACHMANN M., *et al* (1976) In *Growth Hormone and Related Peptides.* Eds. Pecile A. & Muller E.E. Amsterdam, Excerpta Medica, p. 286.

43 ZAUN H. (1983) In *Proc. 16th Int. Congr of Dermatology.* Eds. Kukita A. & Seiji M. Tokyo, University of Tokyo Press, p. 113.

ENERGY METABOLISM IN HAIR FOLLICLES [1-3]

Studies in which freshly plucked hair follicles from the human scalp were incubated with ^{14}C-labelled glucose or other substrates indicate that, in common with many other tissues and organs, hair follicles utilize glucose via the Emden–Meyerhoff pathway, the pentose cycle and the tricarboxylic acid cycle. However, hair follicles differ from muscle in several respects. They have a faster glycolytic rate, a slower respiration rate and considerable pentose cycle activity, although this is insignificant in muscle.

Active and resting follicles differ remarkably. In active follicles, compared with resting follicles, glucose utilization is increased by 200%, glycolysis by 200%, activity of the pentose cycle by 800%, metabolism by other pathways 150% and ATP production via the respiratory chains by 270% [2].

REFERENCES

1 ADACHI K. & UNO H. (1969) In *Advances in Biology of Skin.* Vol. IX. *Hair Growth.* Eds. Montagna W. & Dobson R.L. Oxford, Pergamon, p. 511.

2 ADACHI K., *et al* (1970) *J Soc Cosmet Chem* **21**, 901.

3 UNO H., *et al* (1969) In *Advances in Biology of Skin.* Vol. IX. *Hair Growth.* Eds. Montagna W. & Dobson R.L. Oxford, Pergamon, p. 221.

TYPES OF HAIR

Different types of hair may be produced by different kinds of follicle, and the type of hair produced in any particular follicle can change with age or under the influence of hormones. Animals characteristically have both an overcoat of stiff guard hairs and an undercoat of fine hairs [1], but many kinds of follicle and fibre have been described. Many species also have large vibrissae or sinus hairs, which are sensory and are produced from special follicles containing erectile tissue. There are no strictly comparable follicles in man, but there are occasional large so-called tylotrich follicles [6] with a structure suggesting a sensory function; they are most numerous in abdominal skin [7].

The infantile pelage of animals is usually fine, and such 'puppy' fur is retained in the adult if the young animal is hypophysectomized [2]. In the absence of precise knowledge about species differences in pituitary hormones the question of whether growth hormone or prolactin induces the change to adult pelage may be unrealistic [4]; moreover, steroid hormones also influence the type of hair produced [3].

In man, a prenatal coat of fine, soft, unmedullated and usually unpigmented hair, known as *lanugo*, is normally shed *in utero* in the eighth to ninth month of gestation; however, lanugo may be retained throughout life in the rare hereditary syndrome hypertrichosis lanuginosa (p. 1959). Postnatal hair may be divided at the extreme into two kinds: vellus, which is soft, unmedullated, occasionally pigmented and seldom more than 2 cm long, and terminal hair, which is longer, coarser, and often medullated and pigmented. However, there is a range of intermediate kinds [5]. Before puberty terminal hair is normally that limited to the scalp, eyebrows and eyelashes. After puberty secondary sexual 'terminal' hair is developed from vellus hair in response to androgens.

REFERENCES

1 DRY F.W. (1926) *J Gener* **16**, 287.
2 HOUSSAY B.A. (1918) *Endocrinology* **2**, 497.
3 MOHN M.P. (1958) In *The Biology of Hair Growth*. Eds. Montagna W. & Ellis R.A. New York, Academic Press.
4 RENNELLS E.G. & CALLAHAN W.P. (1959) *Anat Rec* **135**, 21.
5 ROOK A. (1965) *Br Med. J* **i**, 609.
6 STRAILE W.E. (1960) *Am J Anat.* **106**, 133.
7 WINKELMANN R.K. (1959) *Ann NY Acad Sci* **83**, 400.

RACIAL AND INDIVIDUAL VARIATION

Wide genetically determined variations in the patterns and amount of hair growth can be observed both between races and between individuals. The most striking differences are seen in scalp hair. It is a common observation that Mongoloids tend to have coarse straight hair, Negroids curly hair (at the extreme the intertwined shafts give rise to the 'peppercorn' pattern) and Caucasoids a range of textures and curl. The macroscopic appearance of hair is related to its cross section. Mongoloid hair is the most massive and circular, Negroid hair is oval, and Caucasoid hair is moderately elliptical and finer than Mongoloid hair [12, 13, 15]. Significant variations between populations can be shown for a number of other measurements such as medullation, cuticular scale count, kinking and average curvature [7].

A hypothesis [5] that hair form is controlled by only three or four genes (straight, wavy, spiral and peppercorn) is not currently accepted. On the one hand, Dyer [3], while accepting that the genes have major as opposed to biometric or polygenic effects, concludes that a number of genes are involved. On the other hand, Hardy [7] states that hair form is undoubtedly polygenic, but suggests that relatively few genes are involved.

Mongoloids, both male and female, have less pubic, axillary, beard and body hair than Caucasoids. The surface area covered by coarse beard hairs and the weight of hairs grown per day are less in Japanese than Caucasians, as are the mean number of axillary hairs and their daily growth [6]. Not only amounts of hair but also the patterns of distribution may vary between populations. Thus Setty [9, 10] has shown that absence of hair on the foot combined with presence of hair on the thighs and lower leg is three times more frequent in blacks than in whites.

The growth of coarse hairs on the rim of the helix (*hypertrichosis of the pinna*) occurs between the ages of 17 and 45 in many males among the Bengali and Sinhalese [2, 8, 14]. The character is well known to geneticists as a possible example of Y-linked inheritance. In other races, few or many coarse hairs may grow on the helix or on other regions of the pinna, usually after the third decade. The patterns have been classified [11] but their modes of inheritance are unknown. An unexplained phenomenon is the presence of pronounced hypertrichosis of the pinna in most infants born of diabetic mothers and showing the features of macrosomia [4].

A syndrome of 'hairy elbows' (hypertrichosis cubiti) has been described in two of five siblings [1]. The mode of inheritance is uncertain. Hypertrichosis of the elbow region was noticed soon after birth. It reached its greatest extent and severity at the age of 5 yr and then slowly regressed.

Such individual variations in the patterns of hair growth can now be accurately recorded and correlated with other hereditary traits. They will be of undoubted genetic interest and may, like certain variations in the pattern of the eyebrows, prove to have clinical implications.

REFERENCES

1 BEIGHTON P. (1970) *J Med Genet* **7**, 158.
2 DRONAMRAJA K.R. (1963) *J Genet* **53**, 324.
3 DYER K.F. (1974) *The Biology of Racial Integration*. Bristol, Scientechnica.
4 EKLUND J., *et al* (1960) *Ann Paediat Fenn* **6**, 233.
5 FISCHER E. (1939) *Z Induct Abstamm Vererb* **76**, 47.
6 HAMILTON J.B. (1958) In *The Biology of Hair Growth*. Eds. Montagna W. & Ellis R.A. New York, Academic Press, p. 399.
7 HARDY D. (1973) *Am J Phys Anthropol* **39**, 7.
8 SARKAR S.S., *et al* (1961) *Am J Hum Genet* **13**, 214.
9 SETTY L.R. (1966) *Am J Phys Anthropol* **25**, 131.
10 SETTY L.R. (1968) *Am J Phys Anthropol* **29**, 51.
11 SETTY L.R. (1969) *Am J Phys Anthropol* **31**, 153.
12 STEGGERDA M. (1940) *J Hered* **31**, 474.
13 STEGGERDA M. & SEIBERT H.C. (1941) *J Hered* **32**, 315.
14 STERN C., *et al* (1964) *Am J Hum Genet* **16**, 455.
15 VERNALL D.G. (1961) *Am J Phys Anthropol* **19**, 345.

CHANGES WITH AGE

At puberty, terminal hair gradually replaces vellus, starting in the pubic region. In both boys and girls [17] the first pubic hair is sparse, long, downy, slightly pigmented and almost straight. It later becomes darker, coarser, more curled and extends in area to form an inverse triangle. A British study [7, 8] showed that boys had the first recognizable pubic hair at an average age of 13·4 yr and the full adult 'female' pattern at 15·2 yr about 3½ years after the start of development of the genitalia. The corresponding mean ages for girls were considerably earlier, namely 11·7 yr and 13·5 yr. In about 80% of men and 10% of women the pubic hair continues spreading until the mid-twenties or later; there is no absolute distinction between male and female patterns, only one of degree [18]. Of 3,858 normal young men, 4·7% were found to have a horizontal upper border to the pubic hair, and a further 10·3% had a convex border [9]. In another study, 3% of women aged 25–34 were found to have an acuminate upper border [1].

Axillary hair first appears about 2 yr after the start of pubic hair growth. The amount, as measured by the weight of the fully grown mass, continues to increase until the late twenties in males as well as in females, in whom, however, it is less at any age [4]. The mean amounts grown per day increase from late puberty until the mid-twenties and thereafter decrease steadily.

Facial hair in boys first appears at about the same time as the axillary hair, starting at the corners of the upper lip, and spreading medially to complete the moustache and then the cheeks and beard.

Terminal hair development is continued in regular sequence on the legs, thighs, forearms, abdomen, buttocks, back, arms and shoulders [10]. The patterns of distribution of terminal hair on the neck, chest, back and limbs have been effectively differentiated and classified by Setty [12–16]. The extent of terminal hair tends to increase throughout the years of sexual maturity, but most patterns occur over a wide age range. The adult pattern is not achieved until the fourth decade, when the androgen levels are already somewhat lower than in early adult life. Moreover, aural hairs do not appear until late middle age, and a detailed study [6] of coarse sternal hair in men showed that the hairs continue to increase in length and number from puberty to the fifth or sixth decade.

Certain follicles of the scalp may regress with age to produce only fine short vellus hair [3]. This condition of patterned baldness is inherited and requires male hormone [2]; it is prevented by castration before puberty [2], though not substantially reversed by castration in maturity [5]. Some 35% of men of Caucasoid stock [11] develop, during the third and fourth decades, sharply defined patches of alopecia in the peroneal area of the lower leg, and often smaller patches on the calves.

REFERENCES

1 BEEK C.H. (1950) *Dermatologica* 93, 213.
2 HAMILTON J.B. (1942) *Am J Anat* 71, 451.
3 HAMILTON J.B. (1951) *Ann NY Acad Sci* 53, 708.
4 HAMILTON J.B. (1958) In *The Biology of Hair Growth.* Eds. Montagna W. & Ellis R.A. New York, Academic Press, p. 399.
5 HAMILTON J.B. (1960) *J. Clin Endocrinol Metab* 20, 1309.
6 HAMILTON J.B., *et al* (1969) In *Advances in Biology of Skin.* Vol IX. *Hair Growth.* Eds. Montagna W. & Dobson R.L. Oxford, Pergamon, p. 129.
7 MARSHALL W.A. & TANNER J.M. (1969) *Arch Dis Child* 44, 291.
8 MARSHALL W.A. & TANNER J.M. (1970) *Archs Dis Child* 45, 13.
9 MCGREGOR D. (1961) *Br J Dermatol* 73, 61.
10 REYNOLDS E.L. (1951) *Ann NY Acad Sci* 53, 576.
11 RONCHESE F. & CHACE R.R. (1937) *Arch Dermatol Syphilol* 40, 416.
12 SETTY L.R. (1961) *Am J Phys Anthropol* 19, 285.
13 SETTY L.R. (1962) *Am J Phys Anthropol* 20, 365.
14 SETTY L.R. (1964) *Am J Phys Anthropol* 22, 143.
15 SETTY L.R. (1966) *Am J Phys Anthropol* 24, 321.
16 SETTY L.R. (1968) *Am J Phys Anthropol* 29, 51.
17 TANNER J.M. (1962) *Growth at Adolescence* 2nd edn. Oxford, Blackwell.
18 THOMAS P.K. & FERRIMAN D.G. (1957) *Am J Phys Anthropol* 15, 271.

THE TRICHOGRAM

The proportion of active to resting follicles in the scalp can be determined from plucked hairs and is a useful clinical parameter [6]. Barman *et al* [1] first described such an analysis as a 'trichogram' but included within the term data on the density of hair follicles, thickness of hair and rate of growth. In fact, the systematized use of epilation to study hair roots stems from Van Scott [16, 17] and has been exploited by several other workers [4–15], each of whom has developed individual techniques.

For the prospective investigator the literature is confusing, because in addition to the normal phrases of the hair follicle cycle, so-called *dysplastic* and *dystrophic* hair roots have been described not only in pathological conditions but also in some healthy persons; if the hair is pulled out slowly more (artefactual) dystrophic roots will be seen. The existence of such 'abnormal' hair roots may be of considerable interest in some conditions of the scalp and in systemic diseases of which hair changes are a symptom. However, for monitoring the status and progress of so-called 'androgenetic alopecia', whether the hair thinning is patterned or diffuse, only the simple determination of anagen-to-telogen ratios in the vertex and occipital regions is necessary, i.e. the proportion of telogen hairs in the sample (the so-called telogen count) which is easy to use in clinical practice [12].

Examinations should be carried out at a standard time (at least 4 days) after the last washing of the hair [5, 14]. The areas should be carefully selected and specified. The hair should be cut to about 0·5 cm above the scalp surface and about 4–7 hairs extracted with a rapid tug with tightly closing spade-ended epilating forceps placed as close to the skin as possible. The procedure must be repeated in contiguous areas to obtain a sample of not less than 50 hairs [2, 3]. The hairs can be immediately examined in water, but are better mounted on glass slides under a cover slip using a medium such as Depex; for telogen count analysis alone, the hairs can be mounted dry.

For diagnosis of the hair root status the overall shape is of primary importance, but the presence or absence of root sheaths and the external contours are also useful evidence [10, 14]. The principal features are as follows.

Anagen (Fig. 53.8(a)). The root is usually largest at its base, though it may have an equal diameter throughout. The inner root sheath is usually present and firm. The plucked roots may show an angle of 20° or more with the shaft [14].
Telogen (Fig. 53.8(e)). The root is clearly characterized by its club shape, with smooth contours, lack of angulation and loose sheath.
Dysplastic (Figs. 53.8(b) and 53.8(c)). The matrix is diminished in diameter and often deformed; the root sheath is loose or absent.
Dystrophic (Fig. 53.8(d)). The changes are so severe that the root has broken off at the narrowest level and tapers to a point; root sheaths are never present.

The highest ratio of anagen to telogen hairs, over 90%, occurs in children. In adult men, even those not clinically bald, the ratio is lowest in the frontovertical region, but non-bald women—as distinct from those with alopecia androgenetica—show no regional differences [4]. A study of scalp hairs from 146 clinically normal subjects [18] revealed that the overall proportion of hairs in anagen was 83% in men and 85% in women; the corresponding figures for telogen were 15% and 11%. Catagen hairs accounted for only 2·9% of the total in men and 2·1% in women, and were only demonstrable in 31% of males and 19% of females. Dystrophic anagen hairs were found in 46% of men, where they accounted for 3·2% of the total, and in 48% of women, where they accounted for 2·5%.

REFERENCES

1 BARMAN J.M., *et al* (1964) *J Invest Dermatol* **42**, 421.
2 BOSSE K. (1967) *Hautarzt* **18**, 35.
3 BOSSE K. (1967) *Hautarzt* **18**, 218.
4 BRAUN-FALCO O. (1966) *Arch Klin Exp Dermatol* **227**, 419.
5 BRAUN-FALCO. O & FISCHER C. (1966) *Arch Klin Exp. Dermatol* **226**, 136.
6 BRAUN-FALCO O. & HEILGEMEIR G.P. (1985) In *Seminars in Dermatology*. Vol. 4. Eds. Dawber R. & Rook A. New York, Thieme–Stratten, p. 19.
7 BRAUN-FALCO O. & RASSNER B. (1965) *Arch Klin Exp Dermatol* **223**, 50.
8 BRAUN-FALCO O. & ZAUN H. (1962) *Hautarzt* **13**, 342.
9 BRAUN-FALCO O. & ZAUN H. (1962) *Arch Klin Exp Dermatol* **215**, 165.
10 EBLING F.J.G. & RANDALL V.A. (1984) In *Methods in Skin Research*. Eds. Skerrow D. & Skerrow C.J. New York, Wiley, p. 297.
11 MEIERS H.G. (1967) *Arzt Kosmetol* **6**, 22.
12 MORTIMER C.H., *et al* (1984) *Clin Exp Dermatol* **9**, 342.
13 ORFANOS C.E. (1979) In *Haar und Haarkrankheiten*. Ed. Orfanos C.E. Stuttgart, Gustav Fischer, p. 586.
14 PEEROBOOM-WYNIA J.D.R. (1982) Hair root characteristics of the human scalp hair in health and disease. M.D. Thesis. University of Rotterdam.
15 ROOK A & DAWBER R. (1982) *Diseases of the Hair and Scalp*. Oxford, Blackwell Scientific.
16 VAN SCOTT E.J. (1958) In *The Biology of Hair Growth*. Eds. Montagna W. & Ellis R.A. New York, Academic Press, p. 441.
17 VAN SCOTT E.J., *et al* (1957) *J Invest Dermatol* **29**, 187.
18 WITZEL M. & BRAUN-FALCO O. (1963) *Arch Klin Exp Dermatol* **26**, 221.

RATE OF GROWTH OF HAIR

The rate of growth of hair varies from species to species, and within one species from region to region, as well as with sex and age. For example, in the rat it can be more than 1 mm [6, 9, 17] and in the guinea-pig up to 0·6 mm [8] in 24 h, whereas in man it is much less. The rate has been determined by direct measurement of marked hairs *in situ* [18, 20], by shaving and clipping at selected intervals [1, 3, 5, 9] or by pulse labelling with ^{35}S cystine [2, 6, 8, 11, 13, 17]. In experimental mammals parenteral doses of 0·1 μCi of ^{35}S DL-cystine per kilogram body weight at daily intervals have given satisfactory autoradiographs of hairs exposed for 3 or 4 weeks, but up to 20 times this amount with exposures of only 3 days has been used [6, 11, 17]. In the human scalp, results have been obtained by giving eight intradermal injections, each containing 0·05 μCi of ^{35}S L-cystine in 0·05 ml isotonic saline, over an area of about 2 cm^2, and repeating the process after 3 or 4 weeks [13].

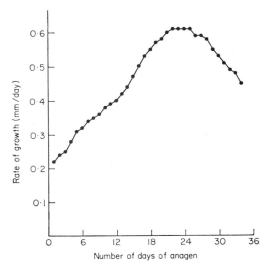

FIG. 53.15. Mean daily rates of type 2 hairs from the dorsal region of the guinea-pig, based on 20 complete hairs from each of six animals. Hairs were pulse labelled by daily injections of ^{35}S cysteine, starting 2–7 days after birth, and samples were plucked at 48 days and autoradiographed. (From Jackson D. & Ebling F.J. (1971) *J Soc Cosmet Chem* **22**, 701.)

Comparable measurements are obtained by all methods. The average rate of hair growth has been stated to range from about 0·21 mm per 24 h on the female thigh to 0·38 mm per 24 h on the chin of a young male [1]. On the crown of the scalp it averaged about 0·5 mm per 24 h, being slightly less on the margins [1]. In another study [18] in which graduated capillary tubes were fitted around the growing hairs the average growth per 24 h in males was as follows: vertex, 0·44 mm; temple, 0·39 mm; chest, 0·44 mm; beard, 0·27 mm. The average rate on the vertex of women was 0·45 mm per 24 h, and there were no variations diurnally or during the menstrual cycle [18]. Though scalp hair grows faster in women than in men [14, 18], the rate before puberty is greater in boys than in girls [15]. The average rate over the whole body is greater in men than in women [16]. Irrespective of sex, growth appears to be highest in the two decades between 50 and 69 yr of age [16]. Some workers believe that the growth rate remains constant in any individual follicle [18], whereas others have found that most hairs either increase or decrease their growth rates [2]. From studies on the guinea-pig [8] it seems clear that the growth rate depends upon the time for which the activity of the follicle has been in progress (Fig. 53.15).

There is agreement that shaving has no effect on the rate of growth [12, 18]. Various endocrine factors have been shown to influence the rate of hair growth in animals; for example, oestrogens reduce it [6,7, 10] and thyroxine increases it [3] (see p. 1961).

Hair diameter, as well as the rate of growth, has proved a useful measure of follicular output [4, 19].

REFERENCES

1 BARMAN J.M., *et al* (1964) *J Invest Dermatol* **43**, 421.
2 COMAISH S. (1969) *Br J Dermatol* **81**, 283.
3 EBLING F.J. & JOHNSON E. (1964) *J Endocrinol* **29**, 193.
4 EBLING F.J.G. & RANDALL V.A. (1984) In *Methods in Skin Research*. Eds. Skerrow D. & Skerrow C.J. New York, Wiley, p. 297.
5 EBLING F.J., *et al* (1977) *Br J Dermatol* **97**, 371.
6 HALE P.A. & EBLING F.J. (1975) *J Exp Zool* **191**, 49.
7 JACKSON D. & EBLING F.J. (1970) *J Endocrinol* **48**, iv.
8 JACKSON D. & EBLING F.J. (1971) *J Soc Cosmet Chem* **22**, 701.
9 JOHNSON E. (1958) *J Endocrinol* **16**, 337.
10 JOHNSON E. (1958) *J Endocrinol* **16**, 351.
11 JOHNSON E. (1965) In *Biology of the Skin and Hair Growth*. Eds. Lyne A.G. & Short B.F. Sydney, Angus & Robertson, p. 491.
12 LYNFIELD Y.L. (1970) *J Invest Dermatol* **55**, 170.
13 MUNRO D. (1966) *Arch Dermatol* **93**, 119.
14 MYERS R.J. & HAMILTON J.B. (1951) *Ann NY Acad Sci* **53**, 562.
15 PECORARO V., *et al* (1964) *J Invest Dermatol* **42**, 427.
16 PELFINI C., *et al* (1969) In *Advances in Biology of Skin*. Vol. IX. *Hair Growth*. Eds. Montagna W. & Dobson R.L. Oxford, Pergamon, p. 153.
17 PRIESTLEY G.C. (1966) *J Anat* **100**, 147.
18 SAITOH M., *et al* (1969) In *Advances in Biology of Skin*. Vol. IX. *Hair Growth*. Eds. Montagna W. & Dobson R.L. Oxford, Pergamon, p. 183.
19 SIMS R.T. (1968) *Br J Nutr* **22**, 229.
20 TROTTER M. (1924) *Am J. Phys. Anthropol* **7**, 427.

EXCESSIVE GROWTH OF HAIR, HYPERTRICHOSIS AND HIRSUTISM
[1–3]

Growth of hair which in any given site is coarser, longer or more profuse than is normal for the age, sex and race of the individual is regarded as excessive. The terms hirsutism and hypertrichosis are often applied interchangeably and indiscriminately to excessive hair growth of any type in any distribution. On phylogenetic grounds, and on the basis of its specific androgenic induction, the growth in the female of coarse terminal hair in the male adult sexual pattern should be differentiated clearly from the numerous other forms of excessive hair growth of widely varying aetiology. The term hirsutism will be restricted to androgen-dependent hair patterns, and the term hypertrichosis will be applied to other patterns of excessive hair growth.

REFERENCES

1 *BROOKSBANK B.W.L. (1961) *Physiol Rev* **41**, 623.
2 FENTON D.A. (1985) In *Seminars in Dermatology*. Vol. 4. Eds. Dawber R. & Rook A. New York, Thieme–Stratton, p. 43.
3 *PHILBERT M. (1965) *Ann Biol Clin (Paris)* **23**, 429.

HYPERTRICHOSIS LANUGINOSA

In congenital hypertrichosis the fetal pelage is not replaced by vellus and terminal hair but persists, grows excessively and is constantly renewed throughout life. In the acquired form the previously normal follicles of all types revert at any age to the production of lanugo.

CONGENITAL HYPERTRICHOSIS LANUGINOSA
SYN. HYPERTRICHOSIS UNIVERSALIS CONGENITA

Aetiology. Only about 50 cases of this rare syndrome have been reported. Traditionally, the cases have been classified into two groups—'dog faced' and 'simian'—but a survey [3] suggests that there may be only a single genotype, with considerable interfamily variation in the phenotype. With one exception [4] all published pedigrees suggest autosomal dominant inheritance.

Clinical features [1, 3, 5]. The child is usually noticed to be excessively hairy at birth. The hair gradually lengthens until by early childhood the entire skin, apart from the palms and soles, is covered by silky hair which may be 10 cm or more long. Long eyelashes and thick eyebrows are conspicuous features. Some affected individuals are normal at birth, and sometimes for the first few years of life, before the universal replacement of other hair types by lanugo. Once established the hypertrichosis is permanent, but some diminution of hairiness of trunk and limbs may be noted in later childhood. At puberty axillary, pubic and beard hairs retain their downy character. Hypodontia or anodontia and deformities of the external ear are apparently associated in some families, but the physical and mental development of most patients has been normal. In a Mexican family hypertrichosis was associated with an osteochondral dysplasia [2].

The status of the apparently recessive form is still more uncertain. Three children of a normal mother were densely hairy at birth and died within a week.

REFERENCES

1 BEIGHTON P. (1970) *Arch Dermatol* **101**, 669.
2 CANTU J.M., et al (1982) *Hum Genet* **60**, 36.
3 *FELGENHAUER W.-R. (1969) *J Genet* **17**, 1.
4 JANSSEN T.A.E. & DE LANGE C. (1945) *Acta Paediatr Scand* **33**, 69.
5 TOURAINE A. (1955) *L'Hérédité en Médecine*. Paris, Masson, p. 525.

ACQUIRED HYPERTRICHOSIS LANUGINOSA

Aetiology. In its dramatic severe forms this syndrome is rare. It has usually accompanied a serious and often fatal illness. Fine downy hair grows over a large area of the body, replacing normal hair and primary and secondary vellus. About 50 cases have been reported and all except two, of which there has been no follow-up, were suffering from malignant disease of the gastrointestinal tract [1, 5, 7, 9], bronchus [6, 8], breast, gall-bladder [7], uterus [12], bladder [10] or other organs. One patient with lymphatic leukaemia had acquired ichthyosis [11] as well as hypertrichosis, and one had a lymphoma [12]. The hypertrichosis may precede the diagnosis of a neoplasm by up to 2 yr.

Pathology. In one case [2] the lanugo follicles lay almost parallel to the surface, and were apparently derived from mantle follicles.

Clinical features [3, 4, 13]. In the milder forms ('malignant down' [2]) the growth of long fine silky hair is confined to the face, where it attracts attention by its appearance on the nose and eyelids and other sites which normally are clinically hairless. As the growth of hair continues it may ultimately involve the entire body, apart from the palms and soles. Existing terminal hair of scalp, beard and pubes may not be replaced and may contrast in colour and texture with the very fine white or blonde lanugo. Such hair may grow abundantly even on the previously bald scalp. The hair may grow exceedingly rapidly, up to 2·5 cm weekly [10], and may be more than 10 cm long.

REFERENCES

1 CHADFIELD H.W. & KHAN A.V. (1970) *Trans Rep St John's Hosp Dermatol Soc Lond* **56**, 30.
2 DAVIS R.A., et al (1978) *Can Med Assoc J* **118**, 1090.
3 GONZALES J.J., et al (1980) *Arch Intern Med* **140**, 969.
4 GOODFELLOW A., et al (1980) *Br J Dermatol* **103**, 431.
5 HEGEDUS S.I. & SCHORR W.F. (1970) *Arch Dermatol* **106**, 84.

6 HENSLEY G.T. & GLYNN K.P. (1969) *Cancer NY* **24**, 1051.
7 HERTZBERG J.J., *et al* (1968) *Arch Klin Exp Dermatol* **232**, 176.
8 KNOWLING M.A., *et al* (1980) *Can Med Assoc J* **126**, 1308.
9 LUGT H. VAN DER & DUDOK DER WIT C. (1973) *Dermatologica* **146**, 46.
10 LYELL A. & WHITTLE C.H. (1951) *Proc R Soc Med* **44**, 576.
11 RICKEN K.H. (1979) *Z Hautkr* **54**, 819.
12 SAMSON M.K., *et al* (1975) *Cancer NY* **36**, 1519.
13 SINDHUPAK W. & VIBHAGOOL A. (1983) *Int J Dermatol* **21**, 599.

UNIVERSAL HYPERTRICHOSIS

This term describes a condition in which the hair pattern is normal but in any site the hairs are larger and coarser than usual. The eyebrows may be double. Inheritance is determined by an autosomal dominant gene. The condition is not very rare, and modern fashions in clothing are bringing to hospital patients who would previously have been content to keep their bodies covered.

The condition is most often seen in dark-skinned Caucasians in the Mediterranean and Middle East.

NAEVOID HYPERTRICHOSIS

The growth of hair abnormal for the site and the age of the patient in its length, shaft diameter and colour may occur as a circumscribed developmental defect, either isolated or associated with other naevoid abnormalities (Figs. 53.16 and 53.17).

Melanocytic naevi (p. 181) may be accompanied by a vigorous growth of coarse hair. The hair may be present from infancy or may develop at puberty or later.

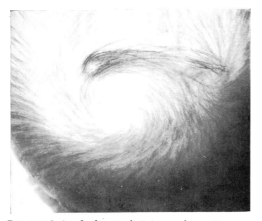

FIG. 53.16. A tuft of coarse hair in a melanocytic naevus of the scalp (Stoke Mandeville Hospital).

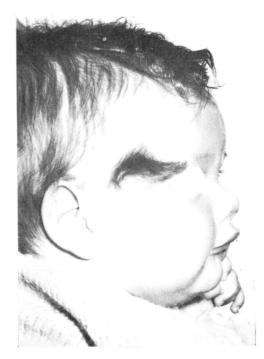

FIG. 53.17. Naevoid circumscribed hypertrichosis (Stoke Mandeville Hospital).

Less often, circumscribed hypertrichosis may occur as the only clinical abnormality. Histologically the epidermis is acanthotic and the follicles are large but there is no excess of melanocytes.

Hypertrichosis is a characteristic feature of Becker's naevus (p. 186). The coarse hairs develop in the same body regions as the pigmentation, usually the thoracic or pelvic girdle, but pigmentation and hypertrichosis are not coextensive.

A tuft of hair in the lumbosacral region, the so-called faun-tail naevus, is often associated with diastematomyelia (Fig. 53.18).

SYMPTOMATIC HYPERTRICHOSIS

Hypertrichosis, symmetrical and usually widespread, occurs as a sequel to or manifestation of a wide variety of pathological states. In none is the mechanism by which the growth of hair is induced fully understood. In some an endocrine mechanism can be assumed. In others an abnormality of dermal connective tissue, including the hair papilla, provoked by some biochemical agency can be postulated with some degree of probability. In the remaining conditions the pathogenesis of the hypertrichosis is even more obscure.

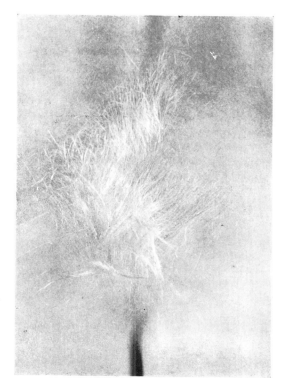

FIG. 53.18. Lumbosacral hypertrichosis in a girl with diastematomyelia. The circumscribed overgrowth of lanugo is as significant as the more conspicuous coarse long hair of the classical 'faun tail' (Addenbrooke's Hospital).

Hereditary disorders

Porphyria (p. 2271). Hypertrichosis of exposed skin is a common feature of the very rare erythropoietic porphyria; appearing first on the forehead it later extends to the cheeks and chin, and, to a lesser degree, to other exposed areas. It is also present in many cases of the much more common erythropoietic protoporphyria [7].

In porphyria cutanea tarda, hypertrichosis is an inconstant finding, but may accompany the pigmentation, blistering and scleroderma-like changes on exposed skin and is well marked in some children with the disease [14]. In Negroes hypertrichosis and pigmentation may be present without blistering [23]. The most extreme degree of hypertrichosis is seen in children with hepatic porphyria induced by hexachlorobenzene or other chemicals. Hypertrichosis is frequent in porphyria variegata. The temples, forehead and cheeks are covered with downy hair. There is also increased pigmentation.

Epidermolysis bullosa [5]. Gross hypertrichosis of the face and limbs has occurred in association with epidermolysis bullosa of the dystrophic type.

Hurler's syndrome and other mucopolysaccharidoses [11] (p. 2299). Hypertrichosis is usually present from early infancy or early childhood on the face, trunk and limbs, and may be a conspicuous feature. The eyebrows are often bushy and confluent. In abortive forms the hair growth may first appear after puberty and be more limited in extent.

Congenital macrogingivae [3] (p. 2080). Exuberant overgrowth of the gingivae as an isolated congenital defect is not uncommon. The association with profuse hypertrichosis of trunk, limbs and lower face has been reported on several occasions. Some patients have markedly acromegaloid features [22].

Cornelia de Lange syndrome (p. 160). These mildly microcephalic mentally defective children show a low hair-line and profuse overgrowth of the eyebrows. The forehead is covered with long fine hair. Hypertrichosis is usually also conspicuous on the lower back and may be generalized.

Winchester syndrome. This rare hereditary disorder is characterized by dwarfism, joint destruction and corneal opacities. The skin in many parts of the body becomes thickened, hyperpigmented and hypertrichotic [6].

Trisomy 18 [20] (p. 115). Generalized hypertrichosis of variable degree is present in these patients.

Endocrine disturbances

Hypothyroidism [13] A profuse growth of hair on the back and the extensor aspects of the limbs develops in some children with hypothyroidism.

Hyperthyroidism. Coarse hair often grows over the plaques of pretibial myxoedema.

Berardinelli's syndrome [2]. From early life growth and maturation are accelerated, and there is lipodystrophy with muscular hypertrophy. An enlarged liver and hyperlipidaemia are other constant features. The skin is coarse and often hypertrichotic.

Possible diencephalic or pituitary mechanisms. Severe generalized hypertrichosis has been reported in young children after encephalitis [18] and after mumps followed by the sudden onset of obesity [12]. A diencephalic disturbance is postulated. Generalized hypertrichosis occurred in a girl after traumatic shock [16] and remitted in 6 months. There are many reports of hypertrichosis after head injuries, especially in children [1, 20]. The hair growth is first noticed 4–12 weeks after the injury, which seems to be of no consistent type, and appears as fine silky hair on the forehead, cheeks, back, arms and legs and may be asymmetrical [21]. It is sometimes shed after a few months but may persist.

Hypertrichosis has been reported in the rare hereditary globoid leucodystrophy (Krabbe's disease). Most patients die in infancy [19].

Teratogenic syndromes

Fetal alcohol syndrome [8, 10]. Mental and physical retardation affects the infants of many mothers with chronic alcoholism. The cutaneous changes include hypertrichosis and capillary haemangiomatosis.

Other conditions

Malnutrition [4, 9]. Gross malnutrition, which may be primary or occur in coeliac disease or other malabsorption states or in severe infections, may cause profuse generalized hypertrichosis in children.

Anorexia nervosa [17]. An increased growth of fine downy hair on face, trunk and arms, sometimes of severe degree, has been reported in about 20% of cases, but is now rarely seen.

Acrodynia [9]. Some increased growth of hair on the limbs is common. In severe cases the hypertrichosis

may be very conspicuous on face, trunk and limbs. One child was described as monkey-like.

Dermatomyositis [15]. Excessive hair growth has been noted mainly in children and principally on the forearms, legs and temples, but it may be more extensive.

REFERENCES

1 BARTUSKA D.G. (1953) *J Am Med Wom Assoc* **18**, 711.
2 BERARDINELLI W. (1954) *J Clin Endocrinol Metab* **14**, 193.
3 BYARS L.T. & JURKIEWICZ M. (1962) *Plast Reconstr Surg* **27**, 608.
4 CASTELLANI A. (1938) *J Trop Med Hyg* **41**, 400.
5 COFANO A.R. (1955) *Ann Ital Dermatol Sifilol* **10**, 195.
6 COHEN A.H., et al (1975) *Archs Dermatol* **111**, 230.
7 DEAN G. (1963) *The Porphyrias*. London, Pitman.
8 HANSON J.W., et al (1976) JAMA **235**, 1458.
9 HOLZEL A. (1951) *Acta Paediatr Scand* **40**, 59.
10 JONES K.L. & SMITH D.W. (1975) *Trichology* **12**, 1.
11 KORTING G.W. & KORRINTHENBERG I. (1964) *Z Haut GeschlKrankh* **37**, 65.
12 LESNÉ E., et al (1930) *Bull Soc Pediatr Paris* **28**, 94.
13 PERLOFF W.H. (1955) *JAMA* **157**, 651.
14 PINOL AGUADE J., et al (1973) *Med Cutan Iber Lat Am* **7**, 37.
15 REICH M.G. & REINHART J.B. (1948) *Arch Dermatol Syphilol* **57**, 725.
16 ROBINSON R.C.V. (1955) *Arch Dermatol* **71**, 401.
17 RYLE J.A. (1938) *Lancet* **ii**, 893.
18 STEGANO G. & VIGNETTI P. (1955) *Arch Ital Pediatr Pueric* **17**, 421.

TABLE 53.1. Hypertrichosis in infancy—hereditary syndromes

	Age of onset of hypertrichosis	Distribution	Associated features
Hypertrichosis lanuginosa	Birth or infancy	Generalized; long, silky hair	Dental defects or none (p. 1959)
Leprechaunism	Birth	Forehead	Low-set ears
		Limbs	Grotesque facies
			Cutis gyrata on large hands and feet (p. 1854)
Berardinelli's syndrome	Early infancy	Forehead	Lipodystrophy
		Limbs	Diabetes
			Gigantism (p. 1961)
Cornelia de Lange syndrome	Early infancy	Low hair-line, neck and forehead	Mentally and physically retarded
		Long, fine hair; back, shoulders and limbs	Characteristic facies (p. 160)
		Bushy, confluent eyebrows	
Hurler's syndrome	Infancy	Low hair-line; forehead and limbs	Coarse facies
			Mentally retarded

19 TAORI G.M., *et al* (1970) *Ind J Med Res* **58**, 993.
20 TARNOW G. (1957) *Nervenarzt* **28**, 327.
21 TARNOW G. (1971) *J Neurovisc Relat Suppl* **10**, 549.
22 VONTOBEL F. (1973) *Helv Paediatr Acta* **28**, 401.
23 ZELIGMAN I. (1963) *Arch Dermatol* **88**, 616.

IATROGENIC HYPERTRICHOSIS

Certain therapeutic agents may induce the growth of hair in extensive areas of the trunk and limbs, or occasionally on the face. The hair, which is of intermediate status, coarser than the vellus but less coarse than terminal hair, may reach a length of 3 cm. The hair usually reverts to the normal for the sex, age and site 6 months to 1 yr after the drug is discontinued. Such hypertrichosis must be differentiated from drug-induced hirsutism, which occurs in part or all of the male secondary sexual hair pattern and is usually not reversible.

Diphenylhydantoin [8]. Hypertrichosis is frequently observed in epileptic children, usually beginning after treatment for 2 or 3 months. It appears first on the extensor aspects of the limbs and later on the trunk and face. The pattern is the same as that sometimes induced by head injury.

Diazoxide. This hypoglycaemic agent induces generalized hypertrichosis in over 50% of children but rarely does so in adults [7].

Streptomycin [1, 4]. Hypertrichosis has been reported in many children treated with streptomycin for tuberculous meningitis. It is probable that the streptomycin is responsible because the pattern and the time of onset and reversal of the hypertrichosis in relation to the antibiotic are essentially similar to those observed with diphenylhydantoin.

Cortisone. Patients receiving intensive and prolonged cortisone therapy may develop hypertrichosis, which is most marked on the forehead, the temples amd the sides of the cheeks, but may also involve in slight degree the back and the extensor aspects of the arms. It is usually reversible within a few months of the end of treatment.

Penicillamine. This may cause lengthening and coarsening of the hair on trunk and limbs.

PUVA [9, 11]. Clinically obvious increased growth may be seen with prolonged PUVA therapy.

Minoxidil [2, 6, 10]. This antihypertensive drug may cause well-marked hypertrichosis affecting even the bald scalp.

Benoxaprofen [3]. This drug caused hypertrichosis and also accelerated growth of the nails.

Cyclosporin-A [5]. Hypertrichosis occurs in the majority of renal transplant patients receiving this immunosuppressive agent; it has also been described after the use of the drug in graft *versus* host disease.

Universal hirsutism. This is a severe degree of hirsutism, the inheritance of which is determined by an autosomal dominant gene. The sites affected are the normal ones; the hair is longer and coarser, and young men of Mediterranean or Middle Eastern Caucasoid race sometimes seek treatment.

REFERENCES

1 BUFFONI L. (1951) *Minerva Pediatr* **3**, 710.
2 BURTON J.L. & MARSHALL A. (1979) *Br J Dermatol* **101**, 593.
3 FENTON D.A., *et al* (1982) *Br Med J* **284**, 1128.
4 FONO R. (1950) *Ann Pediatr (Pans)* **174**, 389.
5 HARPER J.I., *et al* (1984) *Br J Dermatol* **110**, 469.
6 INGLES R.M. & KAHN T. (1983) *Int J Dermatol* **22**, 120.
7 KOBLENZER P.J. & BAKER L. (1968) *Ann NY Acad Med* **150**, 373.
8 LIVINGSTONE S., *et al* (1955) *J Pediatr* **47**, 351.
9 RAMPEN F.H.J. (1983) *Br J Dermatol* **109**, 657.
10 SEIDMAN M., *et al* (1981) *Cutis* **28**, 551.
11 SINGH G. & LAL S. (1967) *Br J Dermatol* **79**, 501.

ACQUIRED CIRCUMSCRIBED HYPERTRICHOSIS

Cutting or shaving hair influences neither the rate of growth nor the calibre of the hair shaft [6]. However, repeated or long-continued inflammatory changes involving the dermis, whether or not clinically evident scarring is produced, may result in the growth of long and coarse hair at this site. Although rarely reported, the phenomenon is of common occurrence. The cause of the hair growth is usually obvious but may be overlooked when the trauma is occupational, e.g. circumscribed patches of hypertrichosis on the left shoulder in men carrying heavy sacks [1]. A patch of hypertrichosis on one forearm or hand is sometimes seen in mental defectives who have acquired the habit of chewing the site [8]. Sometimes the hypertrichosis, which may involve too few follicles to have attracted the patient's attention, develops at the site of an accidental wound or a vaccination scar [5]. We have seen it surrounding a meniscectomy scar. Hypertrichosis of this type is often persistent but may disappear after a few months [3].

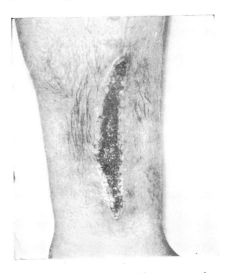

FIG. 53.19. Hypertrichosis surrounding a surgical wound of the leg (Addenbrooke's Hospital).

Long-continued cutaneous hyperaemia without permanent dermal change can also induce increased hair growth which is usually reversible. Hypertrichosis of this type may occur in the neighbourhood of inflamed joints and has been reported particularly in association with gonococcal arthritis [4]. It is also seen on the lower legs in some patients with chronic venous insufficiency [9]. Very exceptionally, inflammatory dermatoses, especially in children, may induce a temporary overgrowth of hair. It has been observed after eczema [2] and after varicella [7]. It may also occur in patients with acne treated by procedures which induce hyperaemia.

REFERENCES

1 CSILLAG J. (1921) *Arch Dermatol Syphilol* **134**, 147.
2 EDEL K. (1939) *Ned Tijdscher Geneeske* **82**, 2466.
3 FRIEDERICH H.C. & GLOOR M. (1970) *Z Haut Geschl-Krankh* **45**, 10.
4 HEIDEMANN H. (1934) *Ugeskr Laeg* **96**, 556.
5 LINSER A.G. (1926) *Klin Woschr* **5**, 1490.
6 LYNFIELD Y.L. & MACWILLIAMS P. (1970) *J Invest Dermatol* **55**, 170.
7 NAVEH Y. & FRIEDMAN A. (1972) *Pediatrics* **50**, 487.
8 RESSMAN A.C. & BUTTERWORTH T. (1952) *Arch Dermatol Syphilol* **65**, 458.
9 SCHRAIBMAN I.G. (1967) *Postgrad Med J* **43**, 545.

HIRSUTISM

Hirsutism is defined as the growth in the female of coarse terminal hair in part of or the whole adult male sexual pattern. This patterned transition of vellus to terminal hair is induced by androgen, and its degree and extent depend in part on the level of androgenic stimulation and in part on the capacity of the follicles to respond. This capacity is genetically determined and is influenced by ageing and perhaps by pituitary or diencephalic factors. It was formerly believed that in the great majority of women with hirsutism without genital virilization or other clinical evidence of abnormal endocrine function the essential abnormality was an increased susceptibility of certain follicles to androgen. There is little doubt that there is indeed wide genetic variation in follicular response, but more refined methods of investigation of endocrine function have established that in a proportion of women with hirsutism circulating androgen is increased; in many of them other manifestations of masculinization can be discovered if carefully sought. It follows that so-called idiopathic hirsutism, though still a diagnostic label of some practical value, is not an aetiological entity. Patients with hirsutism form a continuous spectrum: at one end are the few in whom even the most sophisticated investigations can detect no systemic androgen excess; the largest proportion are women with slight or moderate excess of androgen production and with minimal clinical evidence of masculinization; at the other end of the spectrum are those women in whom marked excess of androgen production is associated with obvious or even gross clinical evidence of androgenic stimulation.

Genetics of hirsutism [2]. When patients after investigation were classified in three groups—adrenal dysfunction, ovarian dysfunction and 'idiopathic'—familial aggregation of hirsutism was evident in all three groups. This finding suggests that the inheritance of most forms of hirsutism is multifactorial, and makes it clear that a family history of hirsutism cannot in itself be accepted as evidence that hirsutism is racial or 'idiopathic'.

Sources of androgen in the female [1]. Testosterone is the most potent of the C-19 (androgenic) steroids. However, the estimation of testosterone secretion by adrenal cortex and ovary does not give a true picture of the effective level of androgenic activity. Both adrenal and ovary secrete testosterone. The main source of androgen in the female is dehydroepiandrosterone, which is converted in the skin into androstenedione and other steroids. The skin is also capable of converting testosterone to dihydrotestosterone, and a hereditary or acquired regional increase in this capacity may be an important factor in the development of hirsutism.

TABLE 53.2. The normal figures for androgens for men and women.

	Women	Men
Plasma testosterone (μg/10 ml)	0·02–0·2	0·4–1·0
Testosterone glucuronide excretion (μg/24 h)	4–10	40–200
Testosterone production rate (mg/24 h)	1–3	4–12

The interpretation of published reports on the endocrine basis of hirsutism is further complicated by the variable relationship between plasma testosterone and urinary testosterone glucuronide levels. Whilst most testosterone is excreted as the glucuronide, some is converted to etiocholanolone and some androstenedione is converted to testosterone glucuronide without first circulating as free testosterone.

REFERENCES

1 *Ferriman D. (1969) *Anovulatory Infertility*. London, Heinemann.

2 Lorenzo E.M. (1970) *J Clin Endocrinol Metals* 31, 556.

THE CAUSES OF HIRSUTISM

1. Idiopathic
2. Adrenal
   Congenital adrenal hyperplasia of early or delayed onset
   Virilizing adrenal tumours
   Cushing's syndrome
   Borderline adrenal dysfunction
3. Ovarian
   Virilizing ovarian tumours
   Polycystic ovary syndrome
   Pure gonadal dysgenesis
4. Pituitary
   Acromegaly
5. Achard–Thiers syndrome
6. Male pseudohermaphroditism
7. Turner's syndrome with androgenic manifestations
8. Iatrogenic

IDIOPATHIC HIRSUTISM

Definition [16]. This term is reluctantly retained to describe the growth in the female of coarse terminal hair in part of the male sexual pattern in the absence of gross clinical evidence of disturbed endocrine function. In fact, some hormonal abnor-mality can be found in about 60% of cases [12]. The critical factor probably concerns androgen metabolism at the target site, and the terms primary hirsutism or primary cutaneous virilism have been proposed [21].

Incidence. The incidence of hirsutism in any population cannot be assessed from hospital statistics, for the criterion of excessive growth is largely social—what is accepted as normal in one community is a source of distress in another. A survey of women students in Wales, using objective criteria [13], showed that 26% had some terminal hair on the face; in 4% it was considered disfiguring. Other sites in which terminal hair was present were as follows: the chest, usually on the breasts, 17%; the abdomen, 35%; the upper back, 3%. Terminal hairs were found on forearms and lower legs in 84%. There are few precisely comparable figures but there is certainly considerable variation in incidence within the Caucasoid race. The incidence is highest in the peoples of the Mediterranean region. In other races the incidence is lower; hirsutism is rare in the Japanese.

The extent and severity of hirsutism of trunk and limbs increases into middle age and then decreases. Facial hirsutism, however, continues to increase in old age and was present in over 40% of elderly Caucasoid women in the United States.

Endocrine biochemistry [9, 19]. The biochemical findings reflect the fact that idiopathic hirsutism is not a single entity, and that authorities differ in their application of this diagnosis.

The mean resting levels of 17-oxosteroids and 17-hydroxycorticosteroids tend to be higher than in controls [8], but are not necessarily so, and the adrenal response to ACTH stimulation tends to be increased [10].

Testosterone production is increased in the majority of hirsute women [3, 6, 7]. Stimulation and suppression tests show that either ovary or adrenal or both may be the source of the testosterone [1, 2, 17]. In the presence of normal adrenal function the failure of dexamethasone suppression after 7 days strongly suggests that the testosterone is ovarian in origin [11].

Quantitative assessment of hirsutism. The growth of coarse hair in each region of the body involves a fairly constant sequence of changes in pattern, and it is therefore possible to grade the degree of hirsutism in any one region semiquantitatively [4]. For example, hirsutism of the chest can be classified as follows: grade 1, circumareolar hairs; grade 2, with midline in addition; grade 3, fusion of these areas with three-quarters cover; grade 4, complete cover. Ferriman and Gallwey [4] have also proposed appropriate grades for other regions. The sequence in which different regions become hirsute shows some consistency, but wide individual variation occurs. It is possible, for example, for hirsutism to be confined to a single site, such as the breast, or less commonly the upper and inner thighs. Further quantitative studies are required before such differences can be confidently attributed to either genetic or hormonal factors.

Clinical features. The onset of idiopathic hirsutism is usually at or soon after the menarche, and it may become slowly more extensive over the next three decades. In some women hirsutism first develops in pregnancy, regresses only partially after parturition and extends after each successive pregnancy. Hirsutism confined to the face is common at or after the menopause.

The rapid onset of hirsutism has followed severe emotional stress, and Segré [20] claims that 'lack of peace of mind is ... both a cause and a result of hirsutism'.

Although by definition patients with genital virilization or other gross clinical evidence of endocrine dysfunction are not diagnosed as exhibiting idiopathic hirsutism, the incidence of other less dramatic androgen-influenced defects is significantly increased in hirsute women. Androgenetic alopecia was present in 27·9% of hirsute women [14]. Anovulatory cycles [10] and reduced fertility [3, 18] are more common than in normal controls. The bisacromial diameter of the pelvis also correlates with hirsutism [5]. Muscle mass tends to be increased; hirsutism was present in 67·8% of 143 women athletes examined in Poland [15].

REFERENCES

1 COOKE C.W., *et al* (1972) *Am J Obstet Gynecol* **114**, 65.
2 ETTINGER B., *et al* (1973) *Am J Med* **54**, 195.
3 *FERRIMAN D. (1969) *Anovulatory Infertility*. London, Heinemann.
4 FERRIMAN D. & GALLWEY J.D. (1961) *J Clin Endocrinol Metab* **21**, 1440.
5 FERRIMAN D., *et al* (1962) *J Endocrinol* **25**, 351.
6 FLEETWOOD J.A., *et al* (1974) *Clin Endocrinol* **3**, 457.
7 ISMAIL A.A.A., *et al* (1969) *Acta Endocrinol (Copenh)* **61**, 283.
8 JAMES V.H.T., *et al* (1962) *J Endocrinol* **24**, 463.
9 *LIPSETT M.B., *et al* (1968) *Ann Intern Med* **68**, 1327.
10 LLOYD C.W., *et al* (1963) *J Clin Endocrinol Metab* **23**, 413.
11 LOPEZ J.M., *et al* (1967) *Am J Obstet Gynecol* **98**, 749.
12 LUCKY A.W. *et al* (1983) *J Invest Dermatol* **81**, 70.
13 McKNIGHT E. (1964) *Lancet* i, 410.
14 MICHALOWSKI R. & HENDZEL G. (1966) *Minerva dermatol* **41**, 196.
15 MICHALOWSKI R. & HENDZEL G. (1966) *Gaz Méd France* **73**, 1531.
16 MULLER S.A. (1973) *J Invest Dermatol* **60**, 457.
17 NICHOLS T., *et al* (1966) *J Clin Endocrinol Metab* **26**, 79.
18 ROSENFIELD R.L. (1973) *J Reprod Med* **11**, 87.
19 RUBENS R. (1984) *Clin Endocrinol* **20**, 313.
20 *SEGRÉ E.J. (1967) *Androgens, Virilization and the Hirsute Female*. Springfield, Thomas.
21 SHUSTER S. (1972) *Br Med J* i, 285.

ADRENAL SYNDROMES

In the *congenital forms of the adrenogenital syndrome* varying degrees of female pseudohermaphroditism of the genitalia are associated with general masculinism and hirsutism, which is usually not severe [5]. The ability of the adrenal to synthesize cortisol is impaired [1, 2]. The urinary excretion of testosterone glucuronide and of 17-oxosteroids is increased and pregnanetriol and pregnanetriolone are also excreted. The defect of biosynthesis is probably determined by an autosomal recessive gene [1, 6].

In the *postnatal adrenogenital syndrome* menstruation is established normally but subsequently becomes irregular. Hirsutism of variable degree is usual and some genital virilization may occur. Moderate elevation of 17-oxosteroid excretion is accompanied by excess of pregnanetriol, accentuated by ACTH [1].

The changes induced by *adrenal tumours* also depend on the age of onset [4]. With early onset there is some genital virilization, but hirsutism is often limited to the genitals; physical growth is advanced. In older girls menstruation often fails to start at puberty, and breast development fails; hirsutism is more extensive. During the years of sexual maturity the extent and severity of the hirsuties and of male-pattern alopecia are determined by genetic predisposition, and if the tumour develops after the menopause there may be little or no hirsutism, apart from the face. Large quantities of 17-oxosteroids are excreted, and suppression by corticosteroids cannot be obtained. Pregnanetriol is excreted, but not pregnanetriolone.

In *Cushing's syndrome* significant hirsutism is present in only 25% of cases [7]. In these cases the characteristic features of the syndrome, which are caused by excessive secretion of cortisol, are added to the features of the adrenogenital syndrome. The cortisol excess can usually be demonstrated chemically and the overactivity of the adrenal cortex is abnormally resistant to cortisone suppression. Further investigation is required to determine whether the primary defect is adrenal or pituitary.

In the so-called *borderline adrenogenital syndrome* [3] hirsutism and virilization are slight. Menstrual disorders are common and fertility is low. The ovaries may be polycystic. The urinary excretion of 17-oxosteroids is in the high normal range and urinary pregnanetriol excretion is definitely elevated. Therapy with corticosteroids restores ovulatory cycles but does not reduce the hirsutism.

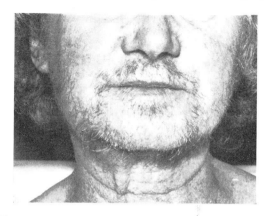

FIG. 53.20. Hirsutism of ovarian origin in a woman aged 60 (Addenbrooke's Hospital).

REFERENCES

1 BROOKS R.V., *et al* (1960) *Br Med J* i, 1294.
2 CHRISTAENS L., *et al* (1963) *Arch Fr Pédiatr* 20, 169.
3 GOLD J.J. (1963) In *The Hirsute Female*. Ed. Greenblatt R.B. Springfield, Thomas, p. 101.
4 GREENBLATT R.B. & ROY S. (1963) In *The Hirsute Female*. Ed. Greenblatt, R.B. Springfield, Thomas, p. 109.
5 JAILER J.W. & HOLUB D.A. (1963) In *The Hirsute Female*. Ed. Greenblatt R.B. Springfield, Thomas, p. 77.
6 KLEVIT H.D. (1960) *Am J Dis Child* 100, 415.
7 LIDDLE G.W. (1963) In *The Hirsute Female*. Ed. Greenblatt R.B. Springfield, Thomas, p. 62.

OVARIAN SYNDROMES

Virilizing ovarian tumours. The normal ovary [4] secretes Δ^4-androstenedione and after ovariectomy urinary androsterone and etiocholanolone levels are lowered. Three main types of virilizing ovarian tumour occur [3]; all are uncommon but early diagnosis is of great importance and hirsutism is often the presenting symptom.

The *arrhenoblastoma* is derived from remnants of male-directed cells which have persisted at the hilum. The majority occur between the ages of 20 and 30. Defeminization is followed by masculinization and hirsutism may be moderate or severe. Plasma testosterone is elevated; 17–oxosteroid excretion is variable and often but little raised. The ovarian tumour may be palpable. Surgical treatment is essential. The recurrence rate exceeds 20%. Menstruation returns to normal but the hirsutism is usually not lost.

The *adrenal-rest tumour* (including masculinovoblastoma [2]), gives rise to a similar but more variable clinical picture. The tumour is small, unilateral and benign. It secretes cortisol and testosterone, and sometimes oestrogens as well. Features of Cushing's syndrome may therefore be present. Urinary excretion of 17-oxosteroids is higher than with arrhenoblastomas, and as in those tumours testosterone output is increased. The prognosis after surgery is good, but loss of hirsutism cannot be prom-

ised although complete recovery from male-pattern alopecia has occurred [1].

Hilus cell tumours are found mainly in patients over 40. The clinical picture is that of uncomplicated virilization. The excretion of 17-oxosteroids may be normal. Testosterone output is elevated. Malignancy is exceptional and the prognosis after surgery is usually excellent.

REFERENCES

1 DOUGLAS M. (1947) *Am J Obstet Gynecol* 53, 190.
2 NOVAK E.R. (1963) In *The Hirsute Female*. Ed. Greenblatt R.B. Springfield, Thomas, p. 195.
3 SANDBERG E.C. & JACKSON J.R. (1963) *Am J Surg* 105, 784.
4 TOURNIARE J. & PUGEAT M. (1983) *Horm Res* 18, 125.

Polycystic ovary syndrome [3, 8]. The term Stein–Leventhal syndrome is widely used to describe the association of hirsutism with amenorrhoea or oligomenorrhoea, infertility, obesity and enlarged polycystic ovaries. However, as these manifestations are extremely variable, and as hirsutism and infertility can occur in the absence of polycystic ovaries, the term is probably best abandoned. The polycystic ovary syndrome comprises those cases of polycystic ovarian disease which are apparently primary.

Aetiologically, the polycystic ovary syndrome is not a single entity. In some cases the primary defect appears to be ovarian [7, 9]. Usually the ovaries contain much androstenedione, the conversion of which to oestradiol has failed to occur [10]. In other cases a block appears to have affected only the earlier stage of conversion of dehydroepiandrosterone to androstenedione. These two substances may thus be metabolized to testosterone. However, in some patients showing such changes increased production of androgen by the adrenal is also demonstrable. The possibility that in many cases the primary defect is hypothalamic has been discussed and the onset of the syndrome after a head injury has been reported [1]. In some cases the onset has followed an acute depressive illness.

Luteinizing hormone (LH) levels may be low, normal or elevated [4]. High levels of LH could be a result of increased production of testosterone by ovary or adrenal. However, a hypothalamic mechanism could disturb the pattern of gonadotrophin release, giving rise to the ovarian changes, and the secretion of androstenedione by the ovary could further disturb hypothalamic function.

Plasma testosterone levels are elevated more consistently than the urinary oxosteroids. Levels of testosterone are usually higher in ovarian veins than in peripheral blood [6, 9] but in some cases the testosterone is largely derived from the adrenals. A single estimation of plasma testosterone may be misleading because of irregular diurnal variation [5].

The clinical features are variable [2, 3]. Hirsutism, ranging from slight to severe, is present in most patients and begins at or within 10 years of puberty. In the genetically predisposed acne may be the presenting feature and the hirsutism be slight. In some patients androgenetic alopecia is also present and the severity of the acne, the alopecia and the hirsutism is not necessarily proportionate. Amenorrhoea, oligomenorrhoea or menorrhagia are common; by no means all patients are obese. Many patients seek medical advice on account of infertility.

REFERENCES

1 BARTUSKA D.G., *et al* (1967) *Am J Obstet Gynecol* **99**, 387.
2 CHAMBERLAIN G. & WOOD C. (1964) *Br Med J* i, 96.
3 *FERRIMAN D.G. (1969) *Anovulatory Infertility.* London, Heinemann.
4 GAMBRELL R.D., *et al* (1973) *Obstet Gynecol* **42**, 429.
5 ISMAIL A.A.A., *et al* (1974) *J Clin Endocrinol Metab* **39**, 81.
6 LLOYD W., *et al* (1966) *J Clin Endocrinol Metab* **26**, 314.
7 MAHESH V.B. (1963) In *The Hirsute Female.* Ed. Greenblatt R.B. Springfield, Thomas, p. 179.
8 RENTOUL J.R., *et al* (1983) *Br J Dermatol* **108**, 224.
9 RIVAROLA M.A., *et al* (1967) *Johns Hopkins Med J* **121**, 82.
10 SHORT E.V. & LONDON D.R. (1961) *Br Med J* i, 1724.

Pure gonadal dysgenesis [1]. In this form of defective gonadogenesis in phenotypic females develop-

ment is normal until puberty, after which the body becomes eunuchoid and there is amenorrhoea. Hirsutism develops in 5–10% of cases in which the oestrogen deficiency leads to increased gonadotrophin secretion, which stimulates excess androgen production by gonadal streak issue.

REFERENCE

1 JUDD H.L., *et al* (1970) *N Engl J Med* **282**, 881.

Achard–Thiers syndrome [2]. The status and pathogenesis of this syndrome are uncertain, but it differs significantly both from the adrenogenital syndrome and from Cushing's syndrome. The essential manifestations are obesity of more or less uniform distribution, hirsutism involving principally the face, hypertension and diabetes. The obesity and hirsutism become evident between the ages of 15 and 30; the diabetes may not be manifest until some years later. Menstrual disorders are inconstant. Osteoporosis, muscle wasting and purple striae are absent. The urinary excretion of 17-oxosteroids and of 17-oxogenic steroids is normal; prednisone suppression and the response to ACTH are good.

The probable authenticity of the syndrome is endorsed by the reports [1] on the diabetic syndrome of the Natal Indians, which is characterized by obesity and a high incidence of hirsutism.

REFERENCES

1 CAMPBELL G.D. & McKECHNIE J. (1961) *S Afr Med J* **35**, 1008.
2 GREENBLATT R.B., *et al* (1963) In *The Hirsute Female.* Ed. Greenblatt R.B. Springfield, Thomas, p. 251.

Morgagni's syndrome [1]. The association of hyperostosis frontalis with hirsutism and obesity has been elevated to syndromal dignity and the term is still occasionally employed. The association of the three components of the syndrome is now regarded as fortuitous.

REFERENCE

1 HENSCHEN F. (1949) *Morgagni's Syndrome.* Edinburgh, Oliver & Boyd.

IATROGENIC HIRSUTISM

The administration of known androgens in adequate dosage will inevitably result in the development of that degree of hirsutism to which the patient's age and genetic constitution predispose her. Some proprietary 'tonics' contain significant quantities of androgen [2], the presence of which may be unsuspected; these are now rarely used.

Many of the anabolic steroids have androgenic activity [1], notably dihydrotestosterone, methylandrostenediol, 19-nortestosterone and 17-α-ethyl-17-hydroxy-19-nor-4-androsten-3-one. Any claims that an anabolic steroid is free from androgenic activity should be accepted with reserve [2].

Progestogens derived from progesterone are seldom androgenic but may be abnormally metabolized by some women. Those derived from nortestosterone are more likely to show androgenic activity, and although the majority show no tendency to produce hirsutism, even when taken for prolonged periods, some may occasionally do so.

REFERENCES

1 HAMBLEN E.C. (1963) In *The Hirsute Female*. Ed. Greenblatt R.B. Springfield, Thomas, p. 269.
2 WILKINS L. (1962) *Am J Dis Child* **104**, 449.

DIAGNOSIS [2, 5, 7]

The differential diagnosis of hirsutism is often difficult, and the degree of diagnostic precision which can be achieved is, to some extent, dependent on the available laboratory facilities. However, the correct interpretation of a detailed history and physical examination should at least allow a decision to be made as to whether the patient is one of the minority in whom full investigation is essential or one of the majority in whom such investigations cannot be justified, except for research purposes, since they increase apprehension and serve no practical purpose.

Family history and racial origins. These may indicate a genetic predisposition to idiopathic hirsutism, but a positive family history may also be given by patients with hirsutism of ovarian or adrenal origin [3]. Congenital adrenal hyperplasia may occur in siblings.

Age of onset
Childhood
    Congenital adrenal hyperplasia
    Virilizing adrenal tumours
    Iatrogenic
Puberty to 20
    Congenital adrenal hyperplasia of delayed type
    Polycystic ovary syndrome
    Idiopathic hirsutism
    Achard–Thiers syndrome

    Male pseudohermaphroditism
    Turner's syndrome
    Pure gonadal dysgenesis
Reproductive period
    Adrenal tumours
    Cushing's syndrome
    Polycystic ovary syndrome
    Ovarian tumours (peak 20–30)
    Iatrogenic

Mode of onset. A very rapid onset suggests a tumour, adrenal or ovarian, but in patients with borderline adrenal hyperplasia hirsutism of sudden onset may develop with severe stress or in pregnancy.

Menstrual history. Menstrual abnormalities are frequent, except in idiopathic hirsutism.

Primary amenorrhoea
    Congenital adrenal hyperplasia (untreated)
    Prepubertal adrenal tumour
    Polycystic ovary syndrome of early onset
    Turner's syndrome
    Pure gonadal dysgenesis
    Male pseudohermaphroditism

Secondary amenorrhoea
    Virilizing ovarian or adrenal tumours
    Polycystic ovary syndrome
    Cushing's syndrome

Menstrual disorders of many types are frequent in the polycystic ovary syndrome.

Physical examination. The degree and extent of the hirsutism should be carefully noted; although not of specific diagnostic value they may provide useful indications. Moderate to severe hirsutism is usual in ovarian and adrenal tumours and in many cases of adrenal hyperplasia. Mild to moderate hirsutism is found in most cases of adrenal hyperplasia, in borderline adrenal dysfunction and in the polycystic ovary syndrome. Idiopathic hirsutism is often mild, as is the hirsutism which may occur in Turner's syndrome. In congenital adrenal hyperplasia the full pattern of hirsutism is reached only slowly by the third decade. In Cushing's syndrome moderate to severe hirsutism may be associated with hypertrichosis of the temples and forehead—cortisol induced.

The genitalia should be examined carefully. In congenital adrenal hyperplasia there is ambiguity. In congenital adrenal hyperplasia of delayed onset, and in adrenal and ovarian tumour, some degree of virilization is usual. In Turner's syndrome the external and internal genitalia are often infantile, and in male pseudohermaphroditism normal female external genitalia are present but the vagina usually ends in a blind pouch.

The ovaries may be palpably enlarged in the polycystic ovary syndrome and in ovarian tumours.

Short stature, a broad shield-shaped chest with small widely separated nipples, a low hair-line, webbing of the neck and other stigmata of Turner's syndrome should be sought but are not invariably present.

Biochemical investigations

17-oxosteroid excretion is moderately elevated in
Congenital adrenal hyperplasia
Cushing's syndrome

Greatly increased in
Malignant adrenal tumours, and in some adrenal rest tumours

Slightly elevated or normal in
Polycystic ovary syndrome
Idiopathic hirsutism
Borderline adrenal dysfunction
Arrhenoblastoma and hilus cell tumour

Pregnanetriol excretion is elevated in
Cushing's syndrome
Congenital and postpubertal adrenal hyperplasia

Plasma testosterone (total and free) is increased in
Idiopathic hirsutism (many cases)
Polycystic ovary syndrome
Adrenal and ovarian tumours
Adrenal hyperplasia

ACTH stimulation test
Exaggerated response in Cushing's syndrome owing to adrenal hyperplasia
Congenital adrenal hyperplasia
Usually no response in adrenal tumours
The test may also uncover latent borderline adrenal hyperplasia

Adrenal suppression test
Suppression of urinary excretion of steroids of adrenal origin by small doses of corticosteroids—normal subjects
Suppression by large doses in adrenal hyperplasia, not in adrenal tumours
Failure to suppress, if adrenal tumour has been excluded, suggests ovarian source

Urinary gonadotrophins are elevated in
Turner's syndrome
Pure gonadal dysgenesis

Prolactin levels are raised in
Prolactinoma

Chromosome studies. In the presence of stigmata of Turner's syndrome, or of sexual ambiguity, the nuclear sex should be determined and chromosome studies undertaken.

Other investigations. Many other investigative techniques are often required—more intensive biochemical investigation, radiological studies, and, sometimes, laparotomy.

TREATMENT

When hirsutism is attributable to a well-defined endocrine disorder in which practicable surgical treatment will eliminate the source of excess androgen, further extension of the hirsutism will be prevented. Carefully planned investigation to identify such cases is therefore of the utmost importance. Removal of the androgen-secreting lesion is occasionally followed by partial or, more rarely, complete regression of the hirsutism. However, this fortunate outcome should never be promised, since in many cases the hirsutism persists unchanged.

In such cases, and in the far more numerous cases of idiopathic hirsutism, treatment is disappointing. In the many young women self-conscious about mild degrees of hirsutism repeated reassurance is the kindest expedient. In the more severe forms various physical procedures are available [6]. Where the coarse hairs are relatively few, electrolysis or diathermy in the hands of a fully trained and experienced technician is useful. Both methods are effective, but the shaft diameter of any hairs that regrow is smaller after diathermy than after electrolysis [4]. Regular courses of treatment at intervals of 6–9 months are usually necessary.

Under no circumstances should radiotherapy be employed in the treatment of hirsutism. Permanent depilation can be achieved only at the expense of eventual radiodermatitis, which is both disfiguring and dangerous.

Where many coarse hairs are present depilation with waxes or lotions containing barium sulphide is often advised (p. 2569). Troublesome folliculitis is a frequent complication unless the procedure is carried out under skilled supervision. Some women find abrasion with sandpaper pads convenient and moderately effective.

In general, if the hair is profuse and the disfigurement severe, shaving provides the best available, though admittedly inadequate, solution. It is a fallacy that shaving hair causes it to grow faster or more coarsely.

The oral administration of the antiandrogen cyproterone acetate in combination with ethinyl oestradiol (reversed sequential method) significantly reduced hirsutism in some women but did not influence androgenetic alopecia where this was also present [1]. Many studies have since confirmed this initial success with such combined therapy; the antiandrogen status of spironolactone is not yet proven in practical therapeutic terms [5].

REFERENCES

1 HAMMERSTEIN J. & CUPCEANCU B. (1969) *Dtsch Med Wochenschr* **94**, 829.
2 LIPSETT M.B., *et al* (1968) *Ann Intern Med* **68**, 1327.
3 LORENZO E.M. (1970) *J Clin Endocrin Metab* **31**, 556.
4 PEEREBOOM-WYNIA J.D.R. (1975) *Arch Dematol Res* **254**, 15.
5 RENTOUL J.R. (1983) *Int J Dermatol* **22**, 265
6 RIDLEY C.M. (1969) *Br J Dermatol* **81**, 146.
7 TOURNIAIRE J. & PUGEAT M (1983) *Horm Res* **18**, 125.

ANDROGENETIC ALOPECIA
SYN. COMMON BALDNESS
MALE-PATTERN ALOPECIA

Nomenclature. Androgenetic alopecia is widely referred to as male-pattern alopecia, but this term is too restrictive and leads to missed diagnoses, especially in females. Androgenetic alopecia more accurately describes common baldness.

Aetiology. Androgenetic alopecia occurs in chimpanzees, orangs and other primates as well as in man [24]. The display of bare skin is a secondary sexual character.

Androgenetic alopecia is induced as its name implies by androgenic stimulation of hair follicles predisposed to this response by the interdependent influences of genetic factors and of ageing.

The essential role of androgen is established [12] by the complete absence of baldness in males castrated before puberty, by its development in some such individuals when testosterone is administered and by the higher incidence in women with increased androgen secretion. The presence of more 'free' circulating androgens in men with common baldness—has been outlined in one report [8]. The influence of ageing is demonstrated by the progressive extension of the area of baldness with increasing age under physiological conditions, and the limitation of the baldness in the testosterone-treated castrate to the area appropriate to the normal male of the same age.

The initial stage in the condemned follicles [25] is probably the accumulation of 5α-dihydrotestosterone, the tissue-active androgen which inhibits the metabolism of such follicles. What determines this accumulation is not clear; 5α-reductase which catalyses the conversion of testosterone to dihydrotestosterone is not the controlling factor [1].

The genetic background of androgenetic alopecia has not been fully elucidated [31, 33]. According to Osbourne's hypothesis, which incriminates a single pair of sex-influenced factors [33] in genotype Bb, baldness develops only with male levels of androgen [3]; in genotype BB with female levels and in

MALE PATTERN ALOPECIA

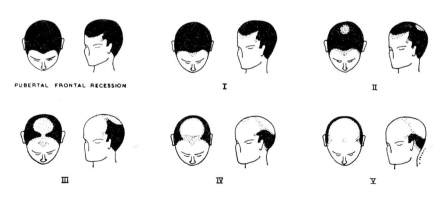

PUBERTAL FRONTAL RECESSION   I   II

III   IV   V

modified from Hamilton, 1951.

FIG. 53.21. A diagrammatic representation of the patterns of hair loss in androgenetic alopecia in males. (After Hamilton [13].)

genotype bb it never occurs. Genetic factors also influence the age of onset of baldness [16] and the pattern of its extension. The tendency to uniform recession of the frontal hair-line at puberty is independently inherited. It is probable that the Osbourne hypothesis oversimplifies a complex situation and that either inheritance is multifactorial [31] or there are several distinct genotypes.

There is marked racial variation in the incidence of androgenetic alopecia, which is most frequent and severe in Caucasoids [14]. Baldness is rare in Mongoloid females and extensive baldness is uncommon in males. Frontal recession is also unusual. Negroids show less baldness than Caucasoids but more than Mongoloids [32].

Local factors play no essential role in determining the onset or progression of baldness. Seborrhoea may be associated but is not causally related. Hats and hairdressing styles are irrelevant.

Pathology [10, 11]. The earliest detectable change in the potentially bald areas is a reduction in the duration of anagen, manifest as an increase in the percentage of telogen follicles [7, 30]. These club hairs are loosely held and are easily shed. Over successive cycles the size of the follicles is progressively reduced and terminal hairs are replaced by vellus. Ultimately many of the vellus follicles disappear. The earliest histological change [19, 22] is the appearance of foci of degeneration in the lower part of the connective-tissue sheath of the follicles, with perivascular basophilic change. The follicle gradually shrinks, leaving beneath it a strand of sclerosed and hyaline connective tissue. However, even in areas of scalp in which almost all follicles are short and small, producing at best only tiny vellus hairs, there remain a few quiescent terminal follicles which can be stimulated into growth to give false hopes of a cure [25]. Eventually only sebaceous glands and sweat glands appear normal. The total number of sebaceous glands decreases significantly, but the proportion of small glands [29] and the level of sebum production appears to be unchanged [23]. The epidermis becomes thin, the dermo-epidermal junction flattens and the subepidermal capillary plexus almost disappears [9]. There is increased deposition of sulphated mucopolysaccharides in the

dermis [16]. In general the enzymatic activity of the vellus follicles is normal [2].

Incidence and clinical features. Uniform recession of the frontal hair-line occurs during adolescence in 96% of males and about 80% of females. It does not represent the first stage of androgenetic alopecia.

Males. In some 5% pf Caucasoid males alopecia is first observed before the age of 20, usually as symmetrical frontotemporal recession. There may also be some loss along the frontal margin (type I). During the third decade the incidence of this pattern of loss increases rapidly and it is frequently associated with some loss on the crown (type II). With increasing age hair loss in both regions tends to become more extensive and the two areas become confluent (types III–V). By the seventh decade 80% of males show at least type I alopecia, but the rate of extension shows wide genetically determined individual variation. Some who develop type I or II alopecia by the age of 30 may show only very slow extension thereafter. Some 12–15% of males ultimately develop types IV and V, and in 1% or 2% this degree of alopecia has been achieved by the age of 30.

Total androgen production is no higher in men with alopecia than in those with full hair [13]; 'free' testosterone may, however, be higher than for those with no overt hair loss [8]. The administration of testosterone to the normal adult male produces no extension of alopecia. Castration after the onset of alopecia prevents further extension but there is no recovery of terminal hair in the frontoparietal regions and only rarely some partial regrowth on the crown [15].

Females. In Caucasoid females alopecia is of later onset and less rapid progression than in males. The picture is usually that of diffuse thinning, most marked on the vertex. Gross bitemporal recession is unusual but there are fewer hairs at the temples, and those that remain are small and poorly pigmented. Reduction in shaft diameter regularly occurs [17] and many patients spontaneously complain that their hair is becoming finer. Many complain also that the scalp is becoming increasingly greasy. Type I alopecia has developed in about 25% of women by the age of 40 [5, 13], and may occasionally begin soon after puberty. The incidence increases to 50% by the age of 50 and only slowly thereafter. Alopecia of type II reaches a peak in the fifth decade. The more severe degrees of alopecia are rare.

The incidence of hirsutism is increased in women

TABLE 53.3. Inheritance of androgenetic alopecia

	Male	Female
Baldness	BB Bb	BB
No baldness	bb	Bb bb

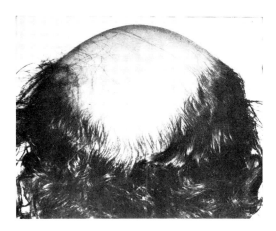

FIG. 53.22. Severe androgenetic alopecia in a woman aged 45. This degree of alopecia rarely, possibly never, occurs in women whose androgen production is within the normal female range (Addenbrooke's Hospital).

with androgenetic alopecia. Alopecia of grades IV or V is always associated with hirsutism, but although these two androgen-influenced changes in hair pattern tend to be of proportionate severity, alopecia of grade II or even grade III may occur without hirsutism. We have seen alopecia as the presenting manifestation of the polycyctic ovary syndrome; some of the women were hirsute whereas others were not.

Testosterone production is increased in some women with androgenetic alopecia [3, 6, 28]. Of women with diffuse frontovertical alopecia some 50% excrete about twice as much testosterone as normal controls [21]. Women with complete frontovertical baldness tend to have urinary testosterone levels approaching those of normal males.

Diagnosis. The differential diagnosis of alopecia is discussed on p. 2018. The commonest errors arise from the failure to appreciate that the so-called 'diffuse' alopecia in women is in the great majority of cases androgenetic [18]. Increased shedding of club hairs is a feature of androgenetic alopecia in both sexes. It should not be confused with a fortuitously associated moult induced by fever or drugs (p. 1978). Vertical alopecia in post-menopausal women is androgen dependent [21]: at this stage decreased oestrogen levels with lower SHBG give more 'free' androgens as in some younger women [24].

In all cases in women careful clinical assessment is required to determine whether full endocrinological investigation is advisable.

Treatment. There is no very effective treatment for this form of alopecia in the male or the endocrinologically normal female, and surgical treatment of a virilizing syndrome in a female is followed at the best by only partial regrowth; oral cyproterone acetate and ethinyl oestradiol may help early cases [27]. Topical minoxidil can induce some regrowth [36].

In a young man the onset of alopecia causes severe distress and may precipitate an anxiety state in the predisposed. Careful examination and repeated reassurance are valuable in discouraging recourse to futile and expensive proprietary treatments. Associated seborrhoea or pityriasis capitis should be treated on cosmetic grounds, although the course of the alopecia will not be influenced.

In exceptional circumstances it may be justifiable to advise a young man, if his baldness genuinely handicaps his professional advancement, to submit to grafting from the occipital and parietal regions to the bald areas [4, 10]. The results of such transplant procedures may be satisfactory if the patients are selected with care and the operation is carried out by a qualified and experienced practitioner. Reported complications include bleeding, infection, fistula formation and scarring [20]; in recent years scalp reduction procedures have become widely used in countries in which 'cosmetic' surgery is freely practised.

REFERENCES

1 ADACHI K. (1973) *Curr Prob Dermatol* **5**, 37.
2 ALLEGRA F. (1968) In *Biopathology of Pattern Alopecia*. Eds. Baccaredda-Boy A., *et al*. Basel, Karger, p. 107.
3 APOSTOLAKIS M., *et al* (1965) *Klin Wochenschr* **43**, 9.
4 AYRES S. (1964) *Arch Dermatol* **90**, 492.
5 BEEK C.H. (1946) *Dermatologica* **93**, 213.
6 BINAZZI M. & CALANDRA P. (1968) *Ital G Rev Dermatol* **8**, 15.
7 BRAUN-FALCO O. & CHRISTOPHERS E. (1968) In *Biopathology of Pattern Alopecia*. Eds. Baccaredda A., *et al*. Basel, Karger, p. 141.
8 CIPRIANI R., *et al* (1983) *Br J Dermatol* **109**, 249.
9 ELLIS R.A. (1958) In *The Biology of Hair Growth*. Eds. Montagna W. & Ellis R.A. New York, Academic Press, p. 469.
10 FRIEDRICH H.C. (1970) *Hautarzt* **21**, 197.
11 *GOERTTLER K. (1965) *Der menschliche Glatze im Altersformwandel der behaarten Kopfhaut*. Stuttgart, Thieme.
12 HAMILTON J.B. (1942) *Am J Anat* **71**, 451.
13 HAMILTON J.B. (1951) *Ann NY Acad Sci* **53**, 708.
14 HAMILTON J.B. (1958) In *The Biology of Hair Growth*. Eds. Montagna W. & Ellis R.A. New York, Academic Press, p. 399.
15 HAMILTON J.B. (1960) *J Clin Endocrinol Metab* **20**, 1309.

16 HARRIS H. (1946) *Ann Eugen* **13**, 172.
17 JACKSON D., *et al* (1972) *Br J Dermatol* **37**, 361.
18 KUHN B. (1972) *J Am Med Wom Assoc*, **27**, 357.
19 LATTANAND A. & JOHNSON W.C. (1975) *J Cutan Pathol* **2**, 58.
20 LEPAW M.I. (1973) *Cutis* **11**, 88.
21 LUDWIG E. (1968) In *The Biology of Hair Growth*. Eds. Montagna W. & Ellis R.A. New York, Academic Press, p. 50.
22 MAGUIRE H.C. & KLIGMAN A.M. (1963) *Geriatrics* **18**, 329.
23 MAIBACH H., *et al* (1968) In *The Biology of Hair Growth*. Eds. Montagna W. & Ellis R.A. New York, Academic Press.
24 MILLER J.A., *et al* (1982) *Br J Dermatol* **106**, 331.
25 MONTAGNA W. & PARAKKAL P.F. (1974) *The Structure and Function of Skin* 3rd edn. New York, Academic Press, p. 307.
26 MONTAGNA W. & UNO H. (1968) *J Soc Cosmet Chem* **19**, 173.
27 MORTIMER C.H., *et al* (1984) *Clin Exp Dermatol* **9**, 342.
28 PIERARD J., *et al* (1968) *Arch Belg Dermatol Syphiligr* **24**, 409.
29 RAMPINI E., *et al* (1968) In The *Biology of Hair Growth*. Eds. Montagna W. & Ellis R.A. New York, Academic Press, p. 155.
30 RASSNER B., *et al* (1963) *Arch Clin Exp Dermatol* **216**, 307.
31 SALOMON T. (1968) In *The Biology of Hair Growth*. Eds. Montagna W. & Ellis R.A. New York, Academic Press, p. 39.
32 SETTY L.R. (1970) *Am J Phys Anthropol* **33**, 49.
33 SMITH M.A. & WELLS R.S. (1964) *Arch Dermatol* **89**, 95.
34 SNYDER L.H. & YINGLING H.C. (1935) *Hum Biol* **7**, 608.
35 UNO H., *et al* (1969) In *Hair Growth*. Eds. Montagna W. & Dobson R.L. Oxford, Pergamon, p. 221.
36 VANDERVEEN E.E. (1984) *J Acad Dermatol* **11**, 416.

CONGENITAL ALOPECIA AND HYPOTRICHOSIS

Total or partial absence of hair of developmental origin occurs in a bewildering variety of clinical forms, either as an apparently isolated defect or in association with a wide range of other anomalies. A logical classification must be based on detailed histological and genetic investigations and these, unfortunately, have seldom been carried out. Provisionally, a purely clinical classification is useful to enable the clinician at least to understand the clearly defined types.

Diffuse alopecia
Total alopecia—complete absence of hair
    A. As an isolated abnormality
    B. With associated defects
Hypotrichosis—hair sparse

Circumscribed alopecia. Circumscribed alopecia of congenital origin is usually the result of a local aplasia of all layers of the skin of an epidermal naevus, but aplasia or hypoplasia of the hair follicles in an otherwise grossly normal epidermis can also occur.

TOTAL ALOPECIA
SYN. ATRICHIA CONGENITA

As an isolated abnormality

Aetiology. Total alopecia as an apparently isolated defect is usually determined by an autosomal recessive gene [8]. Some pedigrees have been traced back to the early 19th century [3]. Dominant or irregular dominant inheritance has occurred in some families [2, 10, 11]. The two genotypes seem to be phenotypically indistinguishable, but detailed investigation would probably reveal differences. The term 'total' is relative, but if any hairs are present they are extremely few. Many isolated cases and families reported under the diagnosis of congenital alopecia are found on review of the original reports to be unquestionably examples of other syndromes; many were hidrotic ectodermal dysplasia.

Pathology [8]. The hair follicles are absent in adult life, even when the fetal hair-coat has been normal. Sebaceous glands are smaller than normal. When a few stray hairs have survived the structure of the shaft appears to be normal.

Clinical features [8, 10]. The scalp hair is often normal at birth but is shed between the first and sixth months, after which no further growth occurs. In some cases the scalp has been totally hairless at birth and has remained so [6]. Eyebrows, eyelashes and bodyhair may also be absent [5], but more often there are a few straggling pubic and axillary hairs and scanty eyebrows and eyelashes. Teeth and nails are normal, and general health, intelligence and expectation of life are unimpaired.

With associated defects. Total or almost total alopecia is unusual in hereditary syndromes.

Progeria (pp. 135 and 1817). Scalp and body hair is totally deficient.

Hidrotic ectodermal dysplasia (p. 135). Total or almost total alopecia is associated with palmoplantar keratoderma and thickened discoloured nails. Any hairs that are present are structurally normal but are often finer in diameter than the average.

REFERENCES

1 BARAITSER M., *et al* (1983) *J Med Genet* **20**, 64.
2 BIRKE G. (1954) *Archs Dermatol Syphilol* **197**, 322.
3 CALVO MELENDRO J. (1955) *Med Clin (Barc)* **24**, 253.
4 DAMSTÉ T.J. & PRAKKEN J.R. (1954) *Dermatologica* **108**, 114.
5 FRIEDERICH H.C. (1950) *Dermatol Wochenschr* **121**, 408.
6 LINN H.W. (1964) *Aust J Dermatol* **7**, 223.
7 LOEWENTHAL L.J.A. & PRAKKEN J.R. (1961) *Dermatologica* **122**, 85.
8 LUNDBÄCH H. (1944) *Acta Derm Venereol (Stockh)* **25**, 189.
9 MOYNAHAN E.J. (1962) *Proc R Soc Med* **55**, 411.
10 PAJTAS J. (1950) *Dermatologica* **101**, 90.
11 TILLMAN W.G. (1952) *Br Med J* ii, 428.

HYPOTRICHOSIS

Aetiology and pathology. Congenital hypotrichosis of sufficient degree to cause social embarrassment but not to reach clinical meetings is not uncommon, and is probably determined by an autosomal dominant gene. Severe degrees of congenital hypotrichosis without associated defects are rare. Dominant inheritance has been recorded [2, 14], but many cases have occurred sporadically [4, 8, 11]. There are a number of distinct syndromes.

Hypotrichosis is a relatively common feature of many hereditary syndromes, usually in association with other ectodermal defects. In the majority the hair is not only sparse but is structurally abnormal. Where hypotrichosis is the most prominent manifestation and the structural defect is distinctive and well characterized it has given its name to the syndrome, as in monilethrix and pili torti. In other syndromes the scanty scalp hair is a minor and sometimes inconstant manifestation, and the shaft defect is usually less specific, although often gross. The follicles are sparse and are reduced in size, and the hair shafts are brittle and deficient in pigment. The nature of the disturbance in keratinization is not known.

Clinical features. When hypotrichosis occurs as an isolated abnormality the scalp hair at birth is normal in quantity and quality, but is shed during the first 6 months and never adequately replaced. It is sparse, fine, dry and brittle and seldom exceeds 10 cm in length. The eyebrows, eyelashes and vellus may be absent, sparse or normal. In exceptional cases improvement or recovery has taken place at puberty, but the condition is usually permanent.

In some families the hair is normal until the age of 5 or later, when growth becomes retarded and

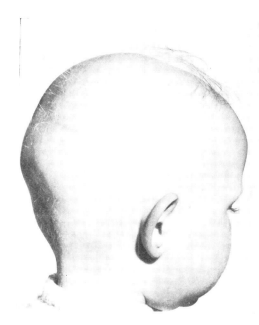

FIG. 53.23. Almost total alopecia in a girl aged 20 months with hidrotic ectodermal dysplasia. The mother was similarly affected (Addenbrooke's Hospital).

Moynahan's syndrome [10]. This autosomal recessive syndrome, reported in male siblings, is associated with mental retardation, epilepsy and total baldness of the scalp; the hair may regrow in childhood between 2 and 4 years of age.

Atrichia with keratin cysts [5, 8]. This rare syndrome, comparable with the condition found in certain hairless mice, has been reported only in girls, but the mode of inheritance is unknown. Total and permanent alopecia develops after the first hair-coat is shed. At any age between 5 and 18 numerous small horny papules appear, first on the face, neck and scalp, and then gradually over the great part of the limbs and trunk. Histologically the papules are thick-walled keratin cysts.

Baraitser's syndrome [1]. This autosomal recessive syndrome presents as almost total alopecia following the loss of some downy scalp hair present at birth.

Three cases are reported in an inbred family [1]; all had almost total alopecia of all sites including eyebrows and lashes. There were occasional isolated hairs. Mental and physical retardation were associated.

TABLE 53.4. Alopecia or hypotrichosis in hereditary syndromes*

	Main features of syndrome	Characteristics of hair
Hidrotic ectodermal dysplasia	Nail thickened, striated, discoloured. Palmoplantar keratoderma	Scalp hair sparse and fine; may be completely absent
Progeria	Normal first year, then gross retardation of physical growth. Senile appearance, thin, dry, wrinkled skin, bird-like features	Total alopecia
Monilethrix	Keratosis pilaris—especially on occiput and nape	Normal at birth, later brittle, beaded hair 1–2 cm in length. Microscopy diagnostic
Pili torti	Hair defect main manifestation	Onset usually in second or third year. Hair sparse and brittle. Spangled in reflected light. Microscopy diagnostic
Anhidrotic ectodermal dysplasia	Usually male. Reduced sweating. Sunken nose, conical teeth. Smooth, finely wrinkled skin	Sparse, dry, fine, short, scalp and eyelashes; hair may sometimes be normal
Rothmund–Thomson syndrome	Erythema cheeks, hands, feet from 3 to 6 months, followed by poikiloderma. Light sensitivity	Scalp hair sparse; eyebrows, eyelashes and body hair very sparse
Werner's syndrome	Sclerodermiform changes face and extremities. Cataracts	Premature greying 14–18. Progressive alopecia from adolescence
Hallermann–Streiff syndrome	Dyscephaly. Aplasia of mandible. Proportionate dwarfism	Normal at birth; later sparse with patchy alopecia, often sutural
Marinesco–Sjögren syndrome	Cerebellar ataxia. Mental retardation. Cataract. Small stature	Scalp hair fine, sparse, short, deficient in pigment
Netherton's syndrome	Females, Eczema	Sparse, brittle; often bamboo-hairs; trichorrhexis invaginata or nodosa
Cartilage–hair hypoplasia	Dwarfism, skeletal abnormalities	Sparse, brittle, fine and light in colour, but hair may be normal
Trichorhinophalangeal syndrome	Pear-shaped nose	Hair sparse, fine, brittle (may be normal)
AEC syndrome	Ankyloblepharon, cleft lip and palate	Hair sparse, coarse, wiry
EEC syndrome	Ectrodactyly, cleft lip and/or palate	Hair sparse
Follicular atrophoderma	Depressions at follicular orifices. Basal cell naevi	Sparse and fine
Menkes' syndrome	Retarded growth. Symptoms of cerebral and cerebellar degeneration	Sparse, brittle, poorly pigmented

*Hypotrichosis is sometimes present in the following syndromes: focal dermal hypoplasia (p. 154); oral facial digital syndrome (p. 140); chondroectodermal dysplasia (p. 138); oculodentodigital dysplasia (p. 141); pachyonychia congenita (p. 155); popliteal-web syndrome (p. 164); polydysplastic epidermolysis bullosa (p. 1625); disorders of amino acid metabolism (p. 2315); Cockayne's syndrome (p. 148); dyskeratosis congenita (p. 149).

the scalp is progressively denuded so that baldness is almost total by the age of 25 [14].

Many of the hereditary syndromes of which hypotrichosis is a constant or frequent feature are listed in Table 53.4. In the majority the hair is not only sparse but fine and brittle, and is often hypopigmented. The hair shafts are often defective but may show no consistent well-characterized structural abnormality. Since the hypotrichosis is not the most prominent feature of these syndromes they are described more fully in other chapters.

There are also other syndromes, as yet incompletely investigated, in which hypotrichosis is associated with other defects.

Hypotrichosis with keratosis pilaris [6, 9]. The hair is apparently normal at birth but after the birth-coat has been shed, between the second and sixth months, it fails to grow satisfactorily and remains sparse, short, brittle and poorly pigmented. Eyebrows and eyelashes may be normal or sparse. Keratosis pilaris is present in the occipital region and neck, and sometimes in the trunk and limbs. Nails, teeth and general physical development are normal. The hairs show no beading or other distinctive abnormality.

Hypotrichosis with keratosis pilaris and lentiginosis [5]. Seven females in three generations in a family of three males and 13 females developed hypotrichosis at or just after puberty, which progressed until the menopause. Axillary and pubic hair was completely lost. There was keratosis pilaris of the scalp and axillae, brittleness and longitudinal striation of the nails and centrofacial lentiginosis.

Eyelid cysts, hypodontia and hypotrichosis [3]

Hypomelia, hypotrichosis, facial haemangioma syndrome [7]. This 'pseudothalidomide' syndrome, which is probably determined by an autosomal recessive gene, associates gross reduction defects of the limbs, a midfacial capillary naevus and sparse silver-blonde hair.

Hypotrichosis, Marie–Unna type [1, 10, 12, 13]. This rare but very distinctive syndrome is determined by an autosomal dominant gene. Affected individuals may be normal at birth or be completely or almost completely hairless. Hair becomes or remains sparse or absent until about the third year when coarse flattened irregularly twisted hair appears on the scalp. This coarse hair is gradually lost with the approach of puberty as follicles are progressively destroyed by a scarring process. The hair loss is greatest around the scalp margins and on the vertex, but may be patchy. Lashes, eyebrows and body hair are sparse, and often virtually absent from birth. General physical and mental development are normal. Scanning electron microscopy shows that the hair shafts are coarse, irregularly twisted and fluted [10].

Hypotrichosis in disorders of amino acid metabolism (see p. 2315). In many disorders with aminoaciduria the hair is hypopigmented and is often also fine, friable and sometimes sparse. Fine sparse hair has been reported in phenylketonuria, arginosuccinic aciduria and hyperlysinaemia.

A number of case reports associate hypotrichosis with a variety of ectodermal defects. Some such cases may represent partial forms of recognized syndromes but it is probable that many additional distinct syndromes remain to be identified and characterized.

Differential diagnosis of hypotrichosis. Microscopy of plucked hairs will exclude the more distinctive structural defects (pili torti, monilethrix and pili annulati). Other ectodermal defects should be carefully sought and relatives should be examined. Many of the syndromes of which hypotrichosis is a constant or frequent feature are listed in Table 53.4.

REFERENCES

1 BORELLI S. (1954) *Hautarzt* **5**, 18.
2 BRAIN R.T. (1938) *Proc R Soc Med* **32**, 87.
3 BURKET J.M. (1984) *J Am Acad Dermatol* **10**, 922.
4 DOCHAO L.A. & MONUX R.M. (1956) *Actas Dermosifilogr* **47**, 396.
5 GREITHER A. (1960) *Arch Klin Exp Dermatol* **210**, 123.
6 HADIDA E. (1948) *Alger Med* **51**, 115.
7 HALL B.D. & GREENBERG M.H. (1972) *Am J Dis Child* **123**, 602.
8 LANDES E. & LANGER I. (1956) *Hautarzt* **7**, 413.
9 OLIVER E.A. & GILBERT N.C. (1926) *Arch Dermatol Syphilol* **13**, 359.
10 PEACHEY R.D.G. & WELLS R.S. (1971) *Trans Rep St John's Hosp Dermatol Soc Lond* **57**, 157.
11 SAINT-PAUL J. (1962) *Bull Soc Fr Dermatol Syphiligr* **69**, 149.
12 SOLOMON L.M., *et al* (1971) *J Invest Dermatol* **57**, 387.
13 STEVANOVIC D.V. (1970) *Br J Dermatol* **83**, 331.
14 TORIBO J. & QUINONES P.A. (1974) *Br J Dermatol* **91**, 687.

CIRCUMSCRIBED ALOPECIA OF CONGENITAL ORIGIN

The differential diagnosis of circumscribed alopecia of developmental origin presents little difficulty if a reliable history is available. Without it alopecia areata and the acquired cicatrical alopecias must be considered.

1. The commonest forms are *naevoid*. Epidermal naevi are usually devoid of hair and present as warty or smooth but slightly indurated plaques (p. 169). A zone of non-cicatricial alopecia sometimes develops around melanocytic naevi [6].

2. Aplasia (p. 225) of all layers of the skin gives rise to a congenital defect, usually a circular or rectilinear area of scarring somewhat depressed below the scalp surface and commonly on the vertex.

3. Irregular areas of cicatrical alopecia not preceded by clinically apparent inflammatory changes produce the syndrome known as pseudopelade (p. 2001). Pseudopelade may develop during early infancy in association with certain hereditary syndromes, e.g. incontinentia pigmenti (p. 1559) and Conradi's syndrome (p. 163).

4. Circumscribed non-cicatricial alopecia is uncommon. It is the result of hypoplasia or aplasia of a group of follicles. The scalp is clinically normal and histologically shows no change other than a reduced number of follicles. Any follicles present are usually small and of vellus rather than terminal type. The first hair-coat is normal and the patches develop between the third and sixth months, although if they are small and not completely bald

they may not be noticed by the parents until considerably later.

Several clinical forms occur [2].

In *vertical alopecia* a small and often irregular patch of alopecia is present on the vertex at birth. It has been confused with aplasia cutis, but the skin is normal apart from the absence of appendages.

In *sutural alopecia*, which is one component of the Hallermann–Streiff syndrome (p. 217), multiple patches overlie the cranial sutures.

Triangular alopecia [1, 3, 5] was first recognized by Sabouraud. In the usual form a triangular area overlying the frontotemporal suture just inside the anterior hair-line, and with its base directed forwards, is completely bald or covered by sparse vellus hairs. Rarely, similar triangular patches have occurred on the nape of the neck.

Single or multiple [4] small patches of total alopecia or hypotrichosis may occasionally occur in other sites but are often inconspicuous.

REFERENCES

1 CANIZARES O. (1941) *Arch Dermatol Syph* **44**, 1106.
2 FRIEDERICH H.C. (1949) *Dermatol Wochenschr* **120**, 712.
3 FUERMAN E.J. (1981) *Cutis* **28**, 196.
4 GEDDA L., *et al* (1954) *Acta Genet Mea Gemell* **3**, 117.
5 KUBBA R. & ROOK A. (1976) *Br J Dermatol* **95**, 657.
6 QUIROGA M. & PECORARO V. (1958) *Hartarzt* **9**, 377.

DISTURBANCES OF THE HAIR CYCLE: TELOGEN EFFLUVIUM

Aetiology. In the normal young adult scalp 80–90% of follicles are in the anagen phase of hair cycle, although there is some variation with site and age. Kligman [3] introduced the term telogen effluvium to describe the shedding of normal club hairs which follows the premature precipitation of anagen follicles into telogen, a process which may be regarded as the common response of the follicle to many different types of stress. Fever, prolonged and difficult childbirth [4], surgical shock, haemorrhage (including blood donation), sudden severe reduction of food intake ('crash' dieting) and emotional stress, including perhaps that of prolonged jet flights, may all induce this response; the proportion of follicles affected, and hence the severity of the subsequent alopecia, depends partly on the duration and severity of the stress and partly on unexplained individual variation in susceptibility. The club hairs may be retained for about 3 months until the affected follicles are well advanced in a new anagen or may be shed prematurely.

The most frequent form of postpartum effluvium is probably due to the withdrawal of factors which have prevented normal entry to catagen during later pregnancy. It is universal in some degree, but is often subclinical. A similar state of affairs prevails when the contraceptive pill is discontinued after it has been taken continuously for some time [1, 2].

Pathology. Histological examination shows no abnormality other than an increase in the proportion of follicles in telogen. The shed hairs are normal clubs.

Clinical features [5, 6]. Diffuse shedding of hairs is the only symptom. The patient may be aware of increased loss on the brush or comb or during a shampoo. The daily loss ranges from under 100 to over 1,000. If the lower rates of shedding are continued for only a short period there may be no obvious baldness in the previously normal scalp, since loss of over 25% of the total complement of hairs is never attained. In the patient of either sex with androgenetic alopecia, previously inapparent, the added diffuse loss may deceptively unveil it, or a previously recognized slight baldness may become more conspicuous. If shedding occurs at higher rates, or is long continued, obvious diffuse baldness is produced. It may be severe but is seldom, if ever, total. Unless the stress is repeated spontaneous complete regrowth takes place almost invariably in about 6 months. Exceptionally, prolonged or high fevers, such as typhoid, may destroy some follicles completely so that only partial recovery is possible. If postpartum effluvium is severe and recurs after successive pregnancies regrowth may ultimately be incomplete [1].

Diagnosis. The diagnosis is usually simple. Increased shedding of hair is clearly related to the stressful episode which preceded it by 6–16 weeks. Plucked hairs show a large proportion of normal clubs until the shedding is complete. The alopecia induced by heparin is very similar but the time interval is often shorter. Other chemical alopecias are discussed on p. 1980. They can sometimes be excluded by the examination of plucked hairs. Alopecia areata of very rapid onset is usually patchy at first but may become total within a week. Telogen effluvium is always diffuse and never total [6]. Acute syphilitic alopecia is patchy. Increased shedding of club hairs is of course a variable but often very obvious symptom of early androgenetic alopecia.

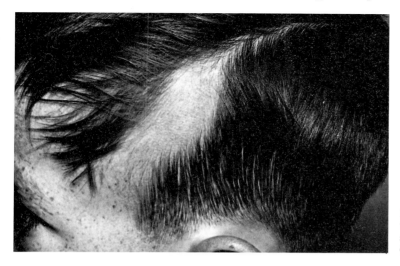

FIG. 53.24. Triangular alopecia. In this patient it was bilaterally symmetrical (Addenbrooke's Hospital, Cambridge).

Treatment. Spontaneous regrowth takes place and recovery is not accelerated by any available treatment.

REFERENCES

1 DAWBER R.P.R. & CONNOR B.L. (1971) *Br Med J* iv, 234.
2 GRIFFITHS W.A.D. (1973) *Br J Dermatol* 88, 31.
3 KLIGMAN A.M. (1961) *Arch Dermatol* 83, 175.
4 SCHIFF B.L. & KERN A.B. (1963) *Arch Dermatol* 87, 609.
5 STECK W.D. (1978) *Cutis* 21, 543.
6 STEIGLEDER G.K. & MAHRLE G. (1973) *Fortschr Prakt Dermatol Venereol* 7, 237.

DIFFUSE ALOPECIA OF ENDOCRINE ORIGIN

Diffuse alopecia occurs in many endocrine syndromes, but the mechanisms have not been fully investigated in man [8]. In many case reports the criteria for the diagnosis of the endocrine disorder have been inadequate.

Hypopituitary states. The hypopituitary dwarf is usually totally hairless. In pituitary deficiency beginning after puberty, as in Sheehan's syndrome, the scalp hair becomes very thin, and pubic and axillary hair is totally lost. The skin is yellowish and dry, and lacks turgidity.

Hypothyroidism [2, 7, 10, 11] Diffuse loss of scalp hair and later of body hair is frequent in hypothyroidism. Sparsity of the eyebrows may be conspicuous and a decrease in axillary hair is evident in about 50% of cases [11]. The trichogram shows the proportion of roots in telogen to be abnormally high, suggesting either prolonged telogen or premature catagen or both [5]. Regrowth is usual when the hypothyroidism is controlled, but may be incomplete. Reports to the contrary probably apply to the association of androgenetic alopecia, possibly owing to more 'free' androgen due to decreased

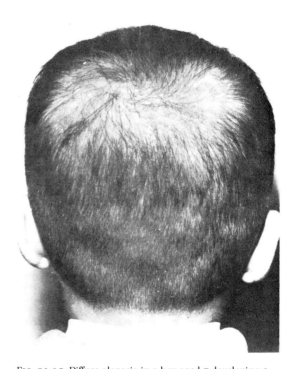

FIG. 53.25. Diffuse alopecia in a boy aged 7 developing 3 months after a severe febrile illness (Addenbrooke's Hospital).

SHBG. Diffuse alopecia may be the only clinical manifestation of hypothyroidism. The diagnosis of hypothyroidism must be based on critical clinical assessment, together with estimation of the thyroxin level and thyroid-stimulating hormone (TSH). Alopecia has occurred in iodine-induced hypothyroidism [1] in which the serum protein-bound iodine level was high.

Hyperthyroidism [2, 9]. In hyperthyroidism, diffuse alopecia develops in 40–50% of cases, but is rarely severe. It is reversible. Alopecia areata (see p. 1985) and vitiligo occur with increased frequency.

Hypoparathyroidism. The scalp hair is coarse, sparse and dry. It is easily shed with slight trauma and the alopecia may appear irregularly patchy. Similar changes have been reported in pseudo-hypoparathyroidism [3].

Diabetes mellitus. In poorly controlled diabetes diffuse alopecia may occur.

Pregnancy. The hair changes in pregnancy are described on p. 1951.

Oral contraceptives. Diffuse alopecia has been attributed to oral contraceptives [4] but the evidence is conflicting. Studies of anagen–telogen counts [12, 13] showed a variable response; some women showed a temporary and some a more prolonged increase in telogen ratio, and in others no change was observed. In general no clinically significant changes are induced, but in some women diffuse hair shedding follows 3–4 weeks after the contraceptive is discontinued as after pregnancy [6]; recovery occurs spontaneously.

REFERENCES

1 CHAPMAN R.S. & MAIN R.A. (1967) *Br J Dermatol* **79**, 103.
2 COMAISH J.S. (1985) In *Seminars in Dermatology*, Vol. 4. Ed. Dawber R. New York, Thieme–Stratton, p. 32.
3 COREA L. & LUPATTELLI L. (1972) *Folia Endocrinol* **25**, 347.
4 CORMIA F.A. (1967) *JAMA* **201**, 635.
5 FREINKEL R.K. & FREINKEL N. (1972) *Arch Dermatol* **106**, 349.
6 GRIFFITHS W.A.D. (1973) *Br J Dermatol*, **88**, 31.
7 HOLT P.J.A. & MARKS R. (1977) *J Invest Dermatol* **68**, 299.
8 *ROOK A. (1965) *Br med J* i, 609.
9 SAINTON P. & SIMONNET H. (1931) *Ann Metab* **7**, 52.
10 SAITO R., *et al* (1976) In *Biology and Diseases of Hair*. Eds. Kobori T. & Montagna W. Baltimore, MD, University Park Press, p. 279.
11 WILLIAMS R.H. (1947) *J Clin Endocrinol Metab* **7**, 52.
12 ZAUN H. & GERBER T. (1969) *Arch Klin Exp Dermatol* **234**, 353.
13 ZAUN H. & RUFFING H. (1970) *Arch Klin Exp Dermatol* **238**, 197.

ALOPECIA OF CHEMICAL ORIGIN

Many chemicals which are capable of inducing alopecia are in frequent use in therapeutics [36]. Man is only rarely and accidentally exposed to others. Together they account for a small but increasing proportion of cases of diffuse alopecia [11, 31]. In many instances their mode of action is uncertain and a logical classification is therefore impracticable.

Thallium. Thallium salts are no longer prescribed in Britain for the depilation of the scalp infected with ringworm, and are not contained in any preparation on sale to the public. In many other countries they are still used as pesticides, and serious outbreaks of poisoning have followed the contamination of grain stores and other food [4, 15]. Thallium salts are tasteless and have been used in homicide and suicide [13]. Thallium is rapidly taken up by anagen follicles and disturbs keratinization [30, 38]. Many hairs break within the follicle; irregularity of the dark keratogenous zone and air bubbles within the shaft near the tapered tip give a distinctive appearance. Many other follicles enter catagen prematurely. Surface keratinization is also disturbed [33]. Alopecia is the most constant symptom. The loss of hair begins after 10 days as diffuse shedding of abnormal anagen hairs. It may rapidly become complete or, with lower doses, may be followed by the gradual shedding of club hairs over a period of 3 or 4 months. In severe poisoning death may result from acute cerebral and renal damage before hair loss can occur. In less severe cases the associated symptoms are very variable [4, 30]; ataxia, weakness, somnolence, tremor, headache, and nausea and vomiting are among the most constant. In mild poisoning alopecia may be the only symptom [17]. In all cases the hair regrows completely within 6 months, but there may be persistent signs of residual cerebral damage. The diagnosis may be suspected on clinical grounds but can be confirmed only by the detection of the thallium in the urine and faeces, in which it may continue to be excreted for 4 or 5 months [1]. There is no specific treatment.

Thyroid antagonists [22]. Some patients with thyrotoxicosis treated with thirouracil or carbimazole

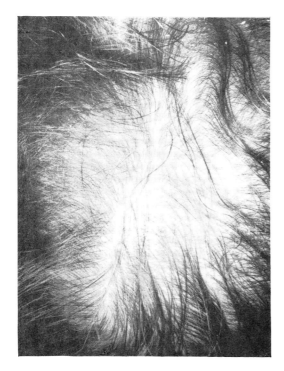

FIG. 53.26. Severe diffuse alopecia in a woman receiving anticoagulants for femoral thrombophlebitis (Addenbrooke's Hospital).

develop a diffuse alopecia. Long continued administration of iodides has induced hypothyroid alopecia [5].

Anticoagulants. All the anticoagulant drugs (heparin, heparinoids, and coumarins) will induce alopecia [10, 11, 39]. Coumarins such as warfarin are widely used as rodent poisons and are sometimes accidentally ingested by children [31]. The highest dose, and not the duration of the exposure, determines the degree of hair loss. Apparently normal club hairs are shed some 2–3 months after the effective blood level is achieved. There is often moderately increased shedding without obvious alopecia, but with high dosage moderate or severe alopecia may occur. Full recovery follows omission of the drug.

Cytostatic agents [6]. Many cytostatic agents employed therapeutically [8] or given with criminal intent can cause hair loss. Experimental and clinical studies with cyclophosphamide [3, 20] show that some anagen follicles enter catagen prematurely; in others the inhibition of mitosis in the matrix results in a constriction in the shaft or a complete break.

A similar constriction is produced by aminopterin [16, 40]. Clinically, alopecia is frequently observed after cyclophosphamide therapy. It has also been reported after therapeutic doses of colchicine [24, 27], after an abortifacient dose of aminopterin [23] and after cantharidin [28]. Hairs with broken constricted shafts may be shed diffusely as early as 4–6 days after the first effective dose, and shedding of apparently normal telogen hairs may continue for some months.

When cytostatic drugs are indicated the expected loss of hair will be minimized by scalp hypothermia, e.g. applying ice packs to the scalp for 30 min before the drug is injected [7].

Triparanol. Triparanol [42], and the chemically unrelated antipsychotic drug fluorobutyrophenone [34], disturb keratinization by inhibiting cholesterol synthesis. Scalp and body hair becomes dry and sparse, and light in colour. The skin is generally dry and ichthyotic. Cataracts develop later in some cases.

Hypervitaminosis A. Excessive consumption of vitamin A gives rise to a variable syndrome [35] in which the principal features are dryness, irritability and, sometimes, pigmentation of the skin, and slowly progressive thinning of scalp and body hairs, eyebrows and eyelashes. Loss of weight, fatigue, anaemia and bone pain are frequent, and the liver and spleen are sometimes enlarged. The symptoms develop insidiously after doses in excess of 50,000 units daily—usually very much higher—have been ingested for many months. The mode of action of vitamin A on hair growth is unknown [11]. Diagnosis is established by estimation of the fasting blood level of the vitamin. Slow recovery takes place when the vitamin A is discontinued.

Boric acid. Occupational exposure to sodium borate has caused diffuse alopecia [37]. Boric acid mouthwashes have caused a similar pattern of hair loss. Serum boric acid levels were elevated. Boric acid taken with suicidal intent caused total alopecia after 10 days [32].

Other chemicals. Reversible alopecia is occasionally induced by other chemicals [36]: potassium thiocyanate, formerly prescribed for hypertension [2]; trimethadione employed in the control of epilepsy [16]; bismuth after prolonged overdosage [12]; industrial exposure to the cyclic condensation products of monomeric chloroprene in the manufacture of rubber [21]. The possible effects of oral contraceptives are discussed on p. 1980. Other drugs described as inducing hair loss include lithium carbonate, pyridostigmine [9], dixyrazine [29] and etretinate.

Propranolol [14] and metoprolol [12], levadopa [25] and cimetidine [41], have all been suspected of causing diffuse alopecia after several months of administration, as has ibuprofen [26].

The amino acid mimosine in *Leucaena glauca* and some other leguminous plants and the toxic substance in the nut *Lecythis* [16], which appears to be selenocystathionine [2], have also caused alopecia. Seleniferous plants are a well-known cause of hair loss in cattle, and there are occasional reports of a similar effect in man.

REFERENCES

1 ARNOLD W., *et al* (1964) *Arch Klin Exp Dermatol* **218**, 396.
2 ARONOW L. & KERDEL-VEGAS F. (1965) *Nature* **205**, 1185.
3 BRAUN-FALCO O. (1961) *Arch Klin Exp Dermatol* **212**, 194.
4 CHAMBERLAIN P.H., *et al* (1958) *Paediatrics, Springfield* **22**, 1170.
5 CHAPMAN R.S. & MAIN R.A. (1967) *Br J Dermatol* **79**, 103.
6 CROUNSE R.G. & VAN SCOTT E.J. (1960) *J Invest Dermatol* **35**, 83.
7 DEAN J.C., *et al* (1983) *J Clin Oncol* **1**, 33–37.
8 FALKSON G. & SCHULZ E.J. (1964) *Br J Dermatol* **76**, 309.
9 FIELD L.M. (1980) *Arch Dermatol* **116**, 1103.
10 FISCHER R., *et al* (1953) *Schweiz Med Wochenschr* **83**, 509.
11 FLESCH P. (1963) *Pharmacol Rev* **15**, 653.
12 GÖLTNER E. (1961) *Z Haut GeschlKrankh* **31**, 164.
13 HEYROTH E.F. (1947) *Rep US Publ Hlth Serv* (Suppl **197**).
14 HILDER M.J. (1979) *Cutis* **24**, 63.
15 HOLLANDER L., *et al* (1949) *Arch Dermatol Syphulol* **59**, 112.
16 HOLOWACH J. & SANDEN H.V. (1960) *N Engl J Med* **263**, 1187.
17 HUBLER W.R. (1966) *South Med J* **59**, 436.
18 KERDEL -VEGAS F. (1964) *J Invest Dermatol* **42**, 91.
19 KHALSE J.H., *et al* (1973) *Int J Dermatol* **22**, 203.
20 KOSTANECKI W., *et al* (1967) *Arch Klin Exp Dermatol* **230**, 896.
21 LIJHANCOVA G. (1967) *Berufsdermatosen* **15**, 280.
22 LUNDBACK K. (1946) *Acta Med Scand* **124**, 266.
23 MAIBACH H.I. & MAGUIRE H.C. (1964) *N Eng J Med* **220**, 1112.
24 MALKINSON E.D. & LYNFIELD Y.L. (1959) *J Invest Dermatol* **33**, 371.
25 MARSHALL A. & WILLIAMS M.J. (1971) *Br Med J* ii, 47.
26 MEYER H.C. (1979) *JAMA* **242**, 142.
27 MIKKLESON W.M., *et al* (1956) *N Engl J Med* **255**, 766.
28 PINETTI P. & BIGGIO P. (1967) *Rass Med Sarda* **70**, 433.
29 POULSEN J. (1981) *Acta Derm Venereol (Stockh)* **61**, 85.
30 REED D., *et al* (1963) *JAMA* **183**, 516.
31 *ROOK A. (1965) *Br J Dermatol* **77**, 115.
32 SCHILLINGER B.M., *et al* (1982) *J Am Acad Dermatol* **7**, 667.
33 SCHWARTZMAN R.M. & KIRSCHBAUM J.O. (1962) *J Invest Dermatol* **39**, 169.
34 SIMPSON G.M., *et al* (1964) *Clin Pharmacol Ther* **5**, 310.
35 SOLER-BECHARA J. & SOSCIA J.L. (1963) *Arch Intern Med* **112**, 462.
36 STROUD J.D. (1985) In *Seminars in Dermatology* Vol. 4. Eds. Maibach H. & Rook A.J. New York, Thieme–Stratton, p. 37.
37 TAN T.G. (1970) *Acta Derm Venereol (Stockh)* **50**, 55.
38 THYRESSON N. (1952) *Acta Derm Venereol (Suppl) (Stockh)*, **29**, 370.
39 TUDHOPE G.R., *et al* (1958) *Br Med J* i, 1034.
40 VAN SCOTT E.J., *et al* (1957) *J Invest Dermatol* **29**, 197.
41 VIRCBURGER C., *et al* (1981) *Lancet* i, 1160.
42 WINKELMANN R.K., *et al* (1963) *Arch Dermatol* **87**, 372.

ALOPECIA OF NUTRITIONAL AND METABOLIC ORIGIN [12]

Hair is affected early in protein deficiency, since protein is conserved for more essential purposes. Malnutrition influences the hair cycles, the structure of the hair shaft and, sometimes, the colour of the hair. Short-term experimental protein deprivation causes atrophy of the bulb and loss of internal and external root sheaths but no changes in the anagen-to-telogen ratio, although these would probably develop if the protein deprivation were continued [4].

Marasmus is the result of protein calorie deficiency, usually in the first year of life. The hair is fine and dry; the diameter of the hair bulbs is reduced to a third of normal and almost all follicles are in telogen [2]. Kwashiorkor occurs during the second year of life in children suddenly weaned to a diet very low in protein and high in carbohydrate. The hair changes are grossly similar to those in marasmus, but there are more anagen follicles although most are atrophic [4]. The differences between the findings in these two states of malnutrition may be related to the degree and rapidity of protein deprivation. In both states the hair is brittle and easily shed, and partial or complete alopecia may occur; the hair is lustreless and, if normally black, may assume a reddish tinge [11, 17]. Many hair shafts may show constrictions which increase their vulnerability to trauma. Hair cuticle changes that are observed in the electron microscope appear not to contribute usefully to nutritional assessment [6].

Surveys of hair-root morphology may provide a

simple and inexpensive way of assessing the nutritional status of a community [3, 5], but root changes reflect only relatively gross differences [14].

Iron deficiency is occasionally associated with diffuse alopecia, even in the absence of anaemia [13]. The association is often difficult to prove because it is not always easy to evaluate other possible factors, but in some cases the apparent response to the administration of iron is convincing [9].

Zinc deficiency resulting from a failure in absorption gives rise to alopecia and cutaneous changes in acrodermatitis enteropathia. Zinc deficiency may result from prolonged parenteral alimentation with erythema, scaling, bullae and hair loss [18]. Parenteral alimentation may also cause deficiency of essential fatty acids. This results in erythema, scaling of the scalp and eyebrows, and diffuse alopecia. The remaining hair is dry and unruly, but this may be reversed by the topical application of safflower oil.

Defects of hair growth occur in certain metabolic disorders but the alleged finding of arginosuccinic acid in the urine of patients with monilethrix has been proved to be due to technical error [8, 10], and a similar finding claimed in other defects of the hair shaft requires confirmation [19]. Changes resembling trichorrhexis nodosa (p. 2016) have been more reliably related to arginosuccinic aciduria.

In homocysteinuria [7], which is an inborn error in the metabolic pathway of methionine, the hair is sparse, fine and fair. It appears normal on microscopy but shows an orange–red fluorescence when stained with acridine orange and examined under ultraviolet light. Affected children are mentally retarded, have a shuffling duck-like gait, a malar flush and a wide variety of skeletal defects.

In hereditary orotic aciduria [1], which is a rare inborn error of pyrimidine metabolism characterized by retarded physical and mental development and macrocytic anaemia, the hair is fine, short and sparse.

A genetically determined defect in the incorporation of histidine, tyrosine and arginine into hair keratin has been found in a syndrome in which dry lustreless tightly curled hair is associated with flat, fragile dystrophic nails and enamel hypoplasia of the teeth [15, 16].

REFERENCES

1 BECROFT D.N.O. & PHILLIPS L.I. (1965) *Br Med J* i, 547.
2 BRADFIELD R.B., *et al* (1969) *Lancet* ii, 1395.
3 BRADFIELD R.B. (1974) *J Pediatr* 89, 294.
4 *BRADFIELD R.B. & BAILEY M.A. (1969) In *Hair Growth*. Eds. Montagna W. & Dobson R.L. Oxford, Pergamon. p. 109.
5 BRADFIELD R.B. & GRAY S.O. (1975) *Lancet* i, 406.
6 BRADFIELD R.B. & MONTAGNA W. (1974) *Lancet* ii, 1026.
7 CARSON N.A.J., *et al* (1965) *J Pediatr* 66, 565.
8 COMAISH J.S. (1966) *Lancet* i, 97.
9 COMAISH J.S. (1971) *Br J Dermatol* 84, 83.
10 EFRON M.L. & HOEFNAGEL D. (1966) *Lancet* i, 321.
11 EL-HEFNAWI H., *et al* (1965) *Br J Dermatol* 77, 137.
12 GUMMER C.L. (1985) In *Seminars in Dermatology*, Vol. 4. Eds. Maibach H. & Rook A.J. New York, Thieme–Stratton, p. 53.
13 HARD S. (1963) *Acta Derm Venereol (Stockh)* 43, 562.
14 JOHNSON A.A., *et al* (1975) *J Invest Dermatol* 65, 311.
15 ROBINSON G.C., *et al* (1966) *Pediatrics* 37, 478.
16 SALAMON T., *et al* (1967) *Arch Klin Exp Dermatol* 230, 60.
17 SIMS R.T. (1967) *Arch Dis Child* 42, 397.
18 WEISMANN K. (1980) *Recent Advances in Dermatology*, Vol. 5. Eds. Rook A. & Savin J. Edinburgh, Churchill Livingstone, p. 109.
19 WINTHER A. & BUNDGAARD L. (1968) *Acta Derm Venereol (Stockh)* 48, 567.

CHRONIC DIFFUSE ALOPECIA

More or less evenly distributed loss of hair occurring continuously, but sometimes fluctuating in severity [7], is common in both sexes. It is seen more frequently in women over the age of 25, either because certain forms occur more often in women or because women are more eager to seek advice [4, 10].

'Chronic diffuse alopecia' is not an acceptable diagnosis. This clinical state may be brought about by a number of different factors, singly or in combination; in many cases no fully convincing cause can be established.

A factor which is usually ignored, but which probably makes a significant though small contribution in many cases, is the diffuse reduction in follicle density which occurs from the third decade onwards (p. 1971).

Other factors which must be carefully assessed in each case are as follows.

1. *Androgenetic alopecia.* Endocrine investigations, notably the estimation of plasma testosterone levels (free and total) have shown [1–3, 9] that androgenetic alopecia is common in women. The diagnosis has tended to be overlooked when, as is usually the case, the pattern of loss is a diffuse frontovertical thinning differing from the typical more sharply bitemporal and vertical alopecia seen in men. The latter occurs in women only when androgen output approaches the male levels. In our experience the great majority of women presenting with chronic

diffuse alopecia have androgenetic alopecia as the principal or only defect.

2. *Other endocrine factors* (p. 1979). Hypothyroidism is a relatively frequent factor in some series of cases [6] but there are regional variations in its prevalence and it is often diagnosed on inadequate evidence. Hyperthyroidism, hypopituitarism and perhaps, diabetes mellitus are occasionally incriminated. Diffuse hair loss has appeared to be related to oophorectomy, though there is no evidence that it follows a normal menopause.

3. *Telogen effluvium* (p. 1978). Acute telogen effluvium following 3 or 4 months after a clearly defined episode such as childbirth or severe stress is not a diagnostic problem, but it is uncertain whether prolonged emotional stress can maintain an increased rate of hair loss by the regular precipitation of small numbers of follicles prematurely into telogen. A high telogen count alone does not establish this diagnosis, for high counts may be found in hypothyroidism, protein deficiency and in other conditions, including androgenetic alopecia.

4. *Chemical agents.* The chemicals known to produce hair loss are mentioned on p. 1980. It is probable that others may have a similar effect; amphetamines have been suspected [6].

5. *Nutritional deficiency* (p. 1982).

6. *Impaired liver function* [13]. In many patients with impaired liver function from hepatitis or cirrhosis the telogen ratio is increased, and in some there is clinically evident alopecia. Disturbed amino acid metabolism has been postulated as its cause.

7. *Severe chronic illness* may be associated with alopecia. Neoplastic disease may result in mild or moderate alopecia [12], the severity of which cannot as yet be related to such factors as the degree of anaemia or of cachexia [11] and which may prove to be determined by secondary endocrine effects. Occasionally alopecia may be a presenting symptom of neoplasia, e.g. Hodgkin's disease [8], either owing to increased telogen shedding, or from specific tumour infiltration, i.e. alopecia neoplastica.

8. *Chronic diffuse alopecia of unknown origin.* When all these factors have been excluded many cases remain unexplained, the majority of them in woman aged 30–50. The age group concerned, the occasional association with seborrhoea and the reduction in hair shaft diameter of which the patient herself is sometimes aware, suggest that further studies of androgen metabolism may be informative, but in some such cases testosterone excretion has already been shown to be within normal limits; however, the intermediary metabolism of androgen may prove to be abnormal.

This group of unexplained cases certainly does not represent a single uniform entity. In some the alopecia fluctuates in severity over months or years but eventually recovers more or less completely. In others, notably those in whom the hair is becoming finer, the alopecia tends to be progressive, though often occurring extremely slowly.

This group of cases includes what may be a distinct clinical entity and which has been so regarded in some countries for many years under the name of 'widow's cap alopecia'. The patients are post-menopausal women, and the alopecia, which has been shown not to be androgen dependent [4, 13], is markedly accentuated on the vertex, rather than in the whole frontovertical region as in androgenetic alopecia.

Some women who are deeply distressed about 'loss of hair' show no evidence of alopecia or at least no greater sparsity than their uncomplaining contemporaries; this is known as the dysmorphophobic state. Some such women are often depressed and others are in need of help with marital problems [5].

REFERENCES

1 APOSTOLAKIS M., *et al* (1965) *Klin Wochenschr* **43**, 9.
2 BINAZZI M. & CALANDRA P. (1968) *Ital G Rev Dermatol* **8**, 1.
3 BINAZZI M. & WIERDIS T. (1960) *G Ital Dermatol Sifol* **101**, 244.
4 BRAUN-FALCO O. & ZAUN H. (1962) *Arch Klin Exp Dermatol* **215**, 165.
5 ECKERT J. (1976) *Acta Psychiatr Scand* **83**, 321.
6 ECKERT J., *et al* (1967) *Br J Dermatol* **79**, 543.
7 GUY W.B. & EDMUNDSON W.F. (1960) *Arch Dermatol* **81**, 205.
8 KLEIN A.W., *et al* (1973) *Arch Dermatol* **108**, 702.
9 MILLER J.A., *et al* (1981) *Br J Dermatol* **106**, 331.
10 ROOK A. (1965) *Br J Dermatol* **77**, 115.
11 SULZBERGER M.B., *et al* (1960) *Arch Dermatol* **81**, 556.
12 VAN SCOTT E.J. (1958) In *The Biology of Hair Growth.* Eds. Montagna W. & Ellis R.A. New York, Academic Press, p. 441.
13 ZAUN H., *et al* (1969) *Arch Klin Dermatol* **235**, 386.

ALOPECIA IN DISORDERS OF THE CENTRAL NERVOUS SYSTEM

Alopecia has been described in association with a number of diseases of the central nervous system but in many instances the association was probably fortuitous. There are four forms of hair loss in which the association appears to be valid, although the mechanism is unknown.

Total and permanent alopecia has accompanied lesions of the midbrain and brain stem [2]—a glioma in the region of the hypothalamus or post-encephalitic damage to the midbrain.

Temporary diffuse alopecia may follow head injuries, particularly in children [4], and may be associated with reversible hirsutism.

Total loss of hair occurred at about annual intervals for 20 years in a patient with syringomyelia and syringobulbia [3].

Androgenetic baldness occurs early in myotonic dystrophy [5]. A genetic linkage rather than a direct effect of the neurological changes is probably concerned.

Piloerection [1]. Episodes of piloerection may occur in patients with lesions close to the hypothalamus or involving some portion of the limbic system, but the symptom has no precise localizing value.

REFERENCES

1 Brody L.A., *et al* (1960) *Neurology* **10**, 993.
2 Hoff H. & Riehl G. (1937) *Arch Dermatol Syph* **176**, 196.
3 Mikula F. & Steidl L. (1961) *Dermatol Wochenschr* **143**, 543.
4 Tarnow G. (1971) *J Neurovis Relat* (Suppl X), 549.
5 Waring J.J., *et al* (1940) *Ann Intern Med* **65**, 763.

ALOPECIA AREATA

Aetiology. Alopecia areata (AA) accounts for about 2% of new dermatological outpatient attendances in Britain and the United States. Figures from Portuguese and Spanish hospitals show an incidence of 2·5% [3] to 3·5% [48], but the differences may not be significant.

Cockayne [9] stated that 'all authorities are agreed that AA almost always occurs in dark-haired people', but a controlled study in Britain [1] failed to confirm this assertion.

In some 70–80% of cases the first attack is between the ages of 5 and 40 but it may occur from infancy to old age. From the age of 5 the incidence remains uniform for about three decades and then declines [1, 19, 38, 42, 48, 61]. In Britain and the United States the sexes are equally affected at all ages but figures from France [12], Italy and Spain [38, 48] show a considerably higher incidence (approximately 2:1) in males.

Heterogeneity. In an elaborate long-term investigation Ikeda [27] of Japan found that, on the basis of associated abnormalities, her cases could be classified into four types, which proved to differ in their age incidence, clinical features and prognosis. This work has been repeated in Nijmegen, the Netherlands [45], and in Cambridge, England, and the findings have lent some support to Ikeda's claims. If Ikeda is correct, it is probable that the relative incidence of the four types differs from country to country, and this would account for incompatible discrepancies between published reports, particularly in relation to prognosis and apparent response to treatment.

The main features of Ikeda's four types, which are rearranged here, can be summarized as follows (the percentages indicate their relative incidence in Japan).

Type I—Atopic (10%). The onset was usually early and the course was prolonged. Alopecia totalis developed in 75% of cases.

Type II—Combined (5%). The onset was usually after 40 and the course was prolonged, but alopecia totalis developed in only 10% of cases. This type would now be called 'autoimmune'.

Type III—Prehypertensive (4%). The patients were young adults with one or both parents hypertensive. The course was rapid, and the incidence of alopecia totalis was 39%.

Type IV—Common (83%). This type was characterized negatively by the absence of the systemic associations of Types I–III. The onset was in later childhood or young adult life, and the total course was usually under 3 years. Individual patches regrew in less than 6 months. Alopecia totalis occurred in 6% of cases.

Genetic factors. Although many workers report a positive family history in 10–20% of cases [43, 47], others obtained such a history in only 6.3% [3] or in none [48]. Identical twins have been affected simultaneously and in the same site [25]. HLA studies tend to confirm the heterogeneity of the disorder; in Finland HLA B12 was associated with AA, but not with alopecia universalis [30]. In Jews in Israel, AA was significantly associated with particular HLA types [22].

Immunological factors [18]
(i) *The atopic state.* The significant association of the atopic state with AA in some populations has been stressed only relatively recently. The criteria for the diagnosis of the atopic state have varied and the published figures are not comparable. Eczema or

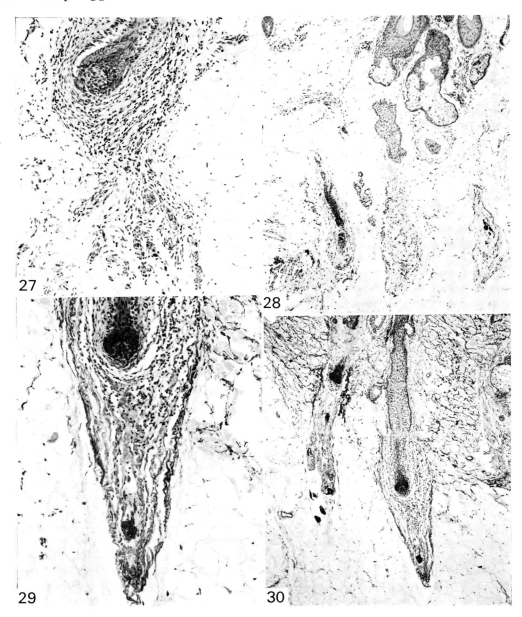

ALOPECIA AREATA

FIG. 53.27. The hairs, smaller than normal, move upwards, leaving empty papillary connective-tissue sheaths in the upper fat. Shed melanin has been picked up by macrophages. This is particularly noticeable in the papillary connective tissues near the right-hand margin of the picture. (H & E; × 100) (Professor E. Wilson Jones).

FIG. 53.28. AA, showing complete retraction of the hair bulb with surrounding inflammatory infiltrate. In the lower half of the picture dilatation of the capillaries is noticeable at the original site of the hair bulb. (H & E. × 40) (Professor E. Wilson Jones).

FIGS. 53.29 & 53.30. A hair in the process of moving upwards. The elastica shows clumping and retraction. A loose perivascular lymphocytic infiltrate is seen around the hair bulb. (H & E, orcein, saffron; × 100 and × 40) (Professor E. Wilson Jones).

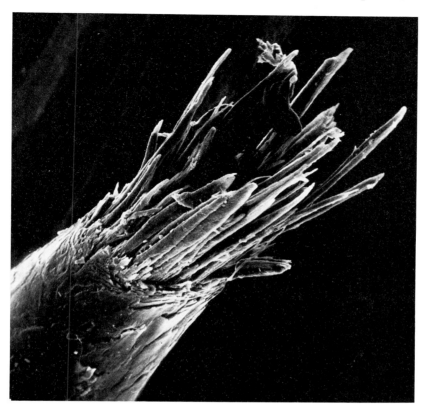

FIG. 53.31. AA. Fractured (!) hair as seen with an electron microscope (David Jackson, Sheffield).

asthma or both were present in 18% of children with AA and in 9% of adults, but in 23% of children with alopecia totalis in the U.S.A. [43]: 10% of Japanese with AA were atopics [27], but in the Netherlands [45], where positive skin tests together with a family history of atopy were accepted as evidence of presence of the atopic constitution, 52.4% were atopic.

(ii) *Autoimmunity* [18, 49]. The association of AA with certain endocrine disorders, some cases of which are of autoimmune origin, has long been recognized. The reported association of thyroid disease with AA has ranged from 2.8% [10] to 8% [43] to 0% [40]. An increased incidence of diabetes has been noted in relatives of patients themselves. Vitiligo, which is associated with AA in about 4% of cases as compared with 1% of control subjects [1, 43], is also significantly associated with pernicious anaemia, diabetes mellitus and Addison's disease.

The search for autoantibodies in patients with AA has provided similarly inconsistent findings. Although a significant association between AA and the presence of autoantibodies has been reported [27], most workers [4, 10, 40] have failed to confirm these findings.

The claim that an antibody is formed against matrix cells [54, 55] awaits confirmation [35].

A reduction in T-cell number has been demonstrated [35], and it has been suggested that AA results from a defect in immune response.

(iii) *Down's syndrome.* The increased incidence of AA in Down's syndrome established in 1965 [64] has been confirmed [60]. The high incidence of AA often total or universal, and the significantly increased occurrence of autoantibodies in such patients remain unexplained.

Endocrine factors [6]. Endocrine influences on the course of alopecia areata have been little studied by modern methods, but valid clinical observations have established that, although pregnancy usually does not influence the course of alopecia, there are

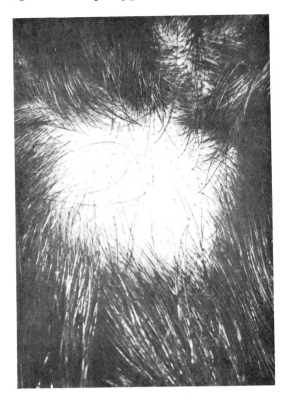

FIG. 53.32. A typical early patch in AA. Some club hairs have not yet fallen. A few exclamation-mark hairs can be seen (Addenbrooke's Hospital).

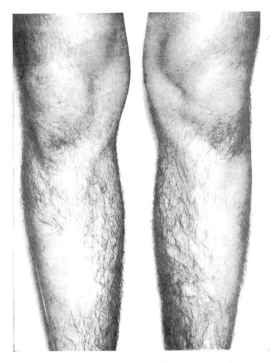

FIG 53.34. AA affecting the legs. This Iranian student, aged 16, was unusually hirsute and multiple patches of alopecia on trunk and limbs were conspicuous. They are often present but easily overlooked when the hair is less profuse and dark (Addenbrooke's Hospital).

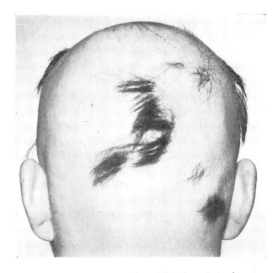

FIG. 53.32. AA in a boy aged 15. The alopecia is almost total (Addenbrooke's Hospital).

patients in whom regrowth occurs only during pregnancy, the hair being shed after parturition.

AA is significantly associated with testicular abnormalities leading to impaired fertility.

Psychological factors [17]. Some investigators consider that emotional factors play no significant role in alopecia areata [39], whereas others [15] claim that most patients are psychologically abnormal. A very detailed psychosomatic study of eight patients [26] does not convincingly resolve the problem. We believe that stress may precipitate attacks.

Other factors. Reflex irritation of ocular or dental origin and focal sepsis have been incriminated in uncontrolled investigations and without convincing evidence. The possibility that physical trauma, notably head injuries, may precipitate attacks [43, 50] requires further investigation.

Pathology (Figs 53.27–53.30). The lesion of AA starts at a focal point. When hairs are plucked at intervals from a developing patch, a high proportion of club hairs is at first found at the centre, and this zone moves centrifugally [14]. The effect could result from either a premature entry of follicles into telogen [13] or a breakage of growing hairs leaving only clubs susceptible of removal. Breakage of the shaft of hairs entering catagen gives rise to *exclamation-mark hairs* [7]. In an established lesion, clinically bald, the affected hair follicles lie higher in the dermis and are smaller than normal, the reduction in size of the matrix being relatively greater than that of the papilla [59]. The follicles are in anagen, but the majority fail to advance beyond a stage roughly equivalent to anagen IV [56, 59]. The internal root sheath is formed, but only keratinous debris or a small imperfectly keratinized hair. These changes may be found in a proportion of follicles in apparently normal scalp in some affected individuals [5, 34] and an intense cellular infiltrate has also been observed around follicles in the clinically normal skin of the upper arm [37]. In many cases, however, the disease is localized and clinically unaffected follicles even in the scalp are histologically normal.

Melanin and melanocytes are lost from the hair bulb [41] and migrate to the dermal papilla [58]. The connective tissue around the vessels leading to the papilla shows degenerative changes, and some of the vessels appear to be occluded [54, 57]. Alkaline phosphatase in the papillae is diminished or absent during the early stages but later returns to normal levels [33]. Also, during the early stages the bulb is heavily infiltrated with lymphocytes [57, 61], as is the spongiotic epidermis around the opening of the follicle [20], and there may be a lymphocytosis of the peripheral blood. In long-standing cases the number of follicles may be reduced, but the majority of follicles permanently retain the ability to form normal hair. In persistent patches the activity of the sebaceous gland progressively declines [51].

Shed hairs may include a proportion of normal clubs, but most show abnormal proximal ends, some of which are brushlike and some tapering.

The upper part of the exclamation mark is a broken shaft of normal diameter; below this the poorly pigmented shaft tapers to end in an atrophic or shrunken bulb, or a more or less normal club. Scanning electron microscopy of such hairs [5, 28] shows that up to the point of fracture the cuticular scale pattern is more or less normal, but thereafter strands of cortical and medullary tissue are evident, giving a frayed rope appearance (Fig. 53.31).

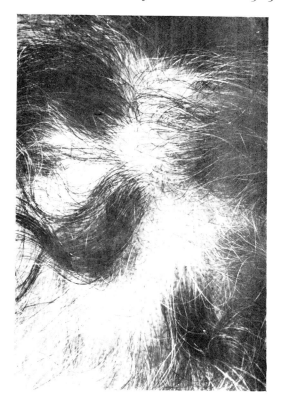

FIG. 53.35. AA in a reticular pattern in a woman aged 60. The white hairs in the bald patches have been retained (Addenbrooke's Hospital).

Clinical features. The alopecia commonly develops without subjective symptoms and is often first noticed by a relative or a hairdresser. Occasionally there may be paraesthesiae. The primary patch, which may appear anywhere but is usually on the scalp, is circumscribed and clearly defined, and is often rounded or oval in shape. Characteristically, the skin is smooth, soft and ivory white, and is totally devoid of hair. Rarely, slight erythema or oedema may be found at an early stage. Around the margins of the patch exclamation-mark hairs may be present, where the patch is actively extending, together with many easily extracted normal club hairs. Extension may continue for a few weeks. The patch may regrow after 4–10 months. More often, after 2–6 weeks a succession of further patches appears more or less simultaneously in any part of the scalp. The course is infinitely variable. Further patches may develop whilst the earlier ones are regrowing, or gradual extension may lead to total alopecia. Particularly in children the initial patches are sometimes atypical, lacking a regular outline, and with scattered long hairs retained within the bald areas. Sometimes, indeed, the initial loss is diffuse and patches become apparent only after 1 or 2 weeks or not at all.

If regrowth and extension occur simultaneously in one region of the scalp, they may result in a reticular pattern of alopecia (Fig. 53.35), which like ophiasis has unfavourable prognostic implications.

The clinical form known as *ophiasis* occurs mainly in children. The primary patch usually develops in the occipital region and the alopecia extends in a band along the scalp margins. Like other forms it may be followed by total alopecia.

The growth of very fine vellus hair implies that the unknown pathogenic stimulus is still active and that the follicles have not reverted to their normal size and function.

Alopecia totalis, the loss of all scalp hair, ultimately develops in 5–10% of all cases of partial alopecia. The onset may be acute, all the scalp hair falling within a few days, or it may develop after months of partial alopecia, and usually within 2 yr. Progression to the total form occurs more slowly, but more frequently, in children than adults [40].

In 10% of cases only sites other than the scalp are affected—eyelashes, eyebrows, beard or pubic or general body hair. Such sites may be involved singly or in any combination, and alopecia of the beard or bilateral or unilateral loss of eyelashes or eyebrows may be the only manifestation of the disease. Far more commonly, alopecia of one or more other sites occurs in association with partial or total scalp alopecia. *Alopecia universalis*, the loss of all scalp and body hair, may result from slow extension of the partial form or may develop within a few days [50].

In patients with vitiligo or canities the white hairs may be retained for some time after the pigmented hairs are shed or may be completely spared. If the alopecia is of acute onset the patient may appear 'to go white overnight' [31] In a patient over 40 all the hairs in a regrown patch may remain white indefinitely.

Perinaevoid alopecia, the shedding of hair immediately surrounding a melanocytic naevus, has rarely been reported but is not very uncommon [42].

Nails (p. 2072). Nail changes occur in a high proportion of cases of acute alopecia totalis, but are not uncommon in partial forms [32] and may even precede the alopecia [42]. Pits, larger and less deep than in psoriasis, longitudinal ridging and irregular thickening are most frequent, but the changes may be gross with opacity and friability [10]. Occasionally the nails are shed or thicken to give a pseudo-mycotic appearance.

Eyes. Posterior subcapsular cataracts occur as a rare complication of alopecia universalis [36] in atopic subjects. Other changes have been described, but the association is probably fortuitous. Asymptomatic punctate lens opacities are no more common in patients with alopecia areata than in controls [52].

Pigmentary changes. Vitiligo is present in about 4% of cases, which is certainly significant [44]. Both conditions occur in association with uveitis in the Vogt–Koyanagi syndrome (p. 1590). An apparent total vitiligo may occur with alopecia universalis and severe nail dystrophy [11]. It is possible that the pallor is due to downward migration of pigment.

Prognosis [2]. The prognosis is always uncertain and no reliable opinion can be given at any early stage. Atopic AA tends to have a poor prognosis. This form of AA may be identified by the presence in the patient of classical atopic disorders. In such cases a prolonged course may be anticipated. Most of the cases in which alopecia becomes total before puberty belong to this form of AA, and such cases have long been recognized as rarely regrowing fully and permanently.

The simple form of AA in which hair loss usually remains confined to one region of the scalp is far more common, and the short- and long-term prognosis is good.

Taking all cases together the duration of the initial attack is less than 6 months in a third and less than a year in a half, and within 5 yr in 70–80%; 20–30% fail to recover completely from the original attack. The immediate prognosis is significantly better for females than for males. Relapses occur within a few months to 5 yr in 40–50% of cases. Apparently complete recovery, with freedom from attacks for 10–15 yr, occurs in about a third of cases [16]. Rapid progression, the loss of eyebrows and eyelashes or severe nail changes usually indicate a poor prognosis. Cases, usually in women, have been seen where trichotillomania developed in the 'regrowth' phase of AA. The early appearance of fine vellus hair is a feature of these cases.

Diagnosis. The circumscribed patches of complete alopecia, without scarring, are easily recognized. In ringworm the patches are seldom totally bald, and scaling and broken and lustreless hairs are usually

exclude this diagnosis [7]. Traumatic alopecias are usually identified by the twisted and broken hairs, but the irregular type of AA may not be easy to differentiate and a period of observation may be necessary. Congenital triangular alopecia (p. 1978) may first be noticed in early childhood. The site and shape of the bald area are distinctive. The persistence of traces of the central inflammatory lesion identifies the temporary patchy hair loss, which may develop around furuncles, insect bites or varicella vesicles. The marginal patches of alopecia in some severe cases of sickle-cell anaemia must be distinguished from the ophiasic forms of AA. In the former the hair loss in the denuded area is seldom total and the shaft defects of AA are lacking. Lupus erythematosus of the scalp may sometimes, in its early stages, mimic AA very closely [4].

The most difficult problems are presented by certain cases of acute onset in which the hair fall is at first diffuse. Unless exclamation-mark hairs are detected a confident diagnosis may be impossible without a short period of observation.

If the hair loss is diffuse, but with some patchy accentuation, the possibility of secondary syphilis must be considered (p. 852). There are usually other signs, including mucosal lesions.

The scarring alopecias are excluded by careful examination. Exceptionally a biopsy may be advisable.

Treatment. The treatment of AA is disappointing and the widely conflicting claims for the success of many different measures merely reflect the very great variations in the spontaneous course of the disease [29].

Systemic corticosteroids will induce regrowth in a large proportion of cases but the regrowth is maintained after the corticosteroid is discontinued only in those cases which have, on the basis of their clinical features and associated disorders, a good prognosis. Alopecia totalis is an atopic subject may show no response even to high doses of systemic corticosteroids. Similar observations have been made with intralesional triamcinolone acetonide and hexacetonide [46]; a total or zero response was noted and, if the hair regrew, growth was maintained for at least 6 months. Intralesional steroids can be regarded as a means of accelerating spontaneous regrowth, and can be used for this purpose when one or more conspicuous patches cause a patient embarrassment. They are not helpful in alopecia totalis, except perhaps to restore the growth of the eyebrows which may be of great cosmetic benefit. In most cases the injections will need to be repeated at intervals of a few months.

The treatment of AA by first inducing allergic sensitivity to a chemical agent and then applying the same substance to the bald patches to induce dermatitis has been used with variable success. Promising results have been claimed. Dinitrochlorbenzene (DNCB) was used in this way by several investigators [21, 23] but the possible teratogenicity of DNCB led others to substitute squaric acid, dibutyl ester [24] or primin, the potent sensitizing agent in *Primula obconica*. The leaves of this plant are applied directly to the skin. A wide variety of irritants have been used for many years, and many of them such as dithranol (buthralin), may stimulate regrowth, but it has yet to be shown that such measures modify the long-term cure of alopecia. An allergic contact dematititis gives a better response than a primary irritant dermatitis [53]. UV radiation has long been used and is of some value, but only in those cases in which the prognosis is in any way favourable. PUVA treatment also has its advocates but the beginning growth of hair makes future treatment less effective. If PUVA is to be used the whole body should be exposed [8]. Empirically, zinc sulphate (220 mg daily) is claimed to be helpful in some cases, but this observation has not been reliably confirmed [63]; after only 6 months of treatment these patients were no better than matched controls. Minoxidil is a drug which causes hypertrichosis in a proportion of patients when administered for hypertension. The local application of 1% solution is followed by some regrowth and appears to be harmless. Further evaluation is required [62].

The patient with AA should be carefully assessed and if necessary examined at intervals for several weeks before a prognosis is given. If history and observation suggest, as they usually do, that a patient has the simple form, then an optimistic prognosis may be given with some confidence. Patches which are slow to recover may be injected with a corticosteroid if the patient wishes. If the history and the course suggest that AA is of the atopic type or has other unfavourable associations, the prognosis should be guarded but not despairing. The patient or his parents should be warned against desperate and useless measures which will put the child's development at risk to no purpose. We have seen patients with severely scarred scalps resulting from repeated misguided corticosteroid injections. Regular supervision is desirable if only to maintain morale. The advice of a child psychiatrist may be needed to assist adjustment to the cosmetic disability, or, less frequently, to resolve problems which appear to be playing a part in inducing relapses.

REFERENCES

1 ANDERSON I. (1950) *Br Med J* ii, 1250.
2 ARNOLD H.L. (1952) *AMA Arch Dermatol* 66, 191.
3 BASTOS ARAUJO A. & POIARES BAPTISTA A. (1967) *Trab Soc Port Venereol* 15, 135.
4 BETTERLE C., *et al* (1975) *Arch Dermatol* 111, 927.
5 BRAUN-FALCO O. & ZAUN H. (1962) *Hautarzt*, 13, 342.
6 BROWN A.C. (1985) In *Seminars in Dermatology*, Vol. 4. Eds. Rook A.J. & Maibach H.I., New York, Thieme–Stratton, p. 1.
7 CARTEAUD J.P. (1969) *Bull Soc Fr Dermatol Syphiligr* 76, 660.
8 CLAUDY A.L. & GAGNAIRE D. (1983) *Arch Dermatol* 119, 975.
9 COCKAYNE E.A. (1933) *Inherited Abnormalities of the Skin and Appendages*. London, Oxford University Press.
10 CUNLIFFE W.J., *et al* (1969) *Br J Dermatol* 81, 879.
11 DEMIS D.J. & WEINER M.A. (1963) *Arch Dermatol* 88, 195.
12 DESAUX A. (1953) In *Affections de la Chevelure et du Cuir-Chevelu*. Ed. Desaux A. Paris, Masson.
13 EBLING F.J. (1976) *J Invest Dermatol* 67, 98.
14 ECKERT J., *et al* (1968) *Br J Dermatol* 80, 203.
15 FELDMAN M. & RONDON LUGO A.J. (1975) *Med Cutan Iber Lat Am* 7, 95.
16 FENTON D.A. & WILKINSON J.D. (1983) *Br Med J* 287, 1015.
17 FORNASA C.V. & CIPRIANI R. (1982) *G Ital Dermatol* 117, 211.
18 FRIEDMANN P.S. (1985) In *Seminars in Dermatology*, Vol 4. Eds Rook A.J. & Maibach, H.I. New York, Thieme–Stratton, p. 58.
19 GIP L., *et al* (1969) *Acta Derm Venereol (Stockh)* 49, 180.
20 GOOS M. (1971) *Arch Dermatol Forsch* 24, 160.
21 GU S.B., *et al* (1981) *Int Arch Allergy Appl Immunol* 66, 448.
22 HACHAM ZADEK S. (1980) *Tissue Antigens* 18, 21.
23 HAPPLE R., *et al* (1978) *Arch Dermatol* 110, 629.
24 HAPPLE R., *et al* (1980) *Dermatologica* 261, 289.
25 HENDREN O.S. (1949) *Arch Dermatol Syphilol* 60, 793.
26 *HOMMES O.P. & PRICK J.J.G. (1968) Alopecia Maligna *Verhand K Ned Akad Wet* 57, no 2.
27 IKEDA T. (1965) *Dermatologica* 131, 421.
28 JACKSON D., *et al* (1971) *Br J Dermatol* 85, 242.
29 KERN F. (1973) *Archs Dermatol* 107, 407.
30 KIANTU U., *et al* (1977) *Arch Dermatol* 113, 1716.
31 KLINGMÜLLER G. (1958) *Dermatologica* 117, 84.
32 KLINGMÜLLER G. & RECHE E. (1955) *Arch Klin Exp Dermatol* 201, 574.
33 KOPE A.W. & ORENTREICH N. (1957) *Arch Dermatol* 76, 288.
34 KOSTANECKI W. & KWIATKOWSKA E. (1966) *Arch Klin Exp Dermatol* 226, 21.
35 *Lancet* (1984) 1, 1335.
36 LASSUS A., *et al* (1980) *Dermatologica* 161, 298.
37 LAZOVIC-TEPAVOC O. SALOMON T. (1970) *Dermatol Wochenschr* 156, 665.
38 LOPEZ B. (1951) *Actas Dermosifilogr* 42, 589.
39 MACALPINE I. (1958) *Br J Dermatol* 70, 117.
40 MAIN R.A., *et al* (1975) *Br J Dermatol* 92, 389.
41 MESSENGER A.G. & BLEEHEN S.S. (1984) *Br J Dermatol* 110, 155.
42 MULLER S.A. & BRUNSTING L.A. (1963) *Arch Dermatol* 88, 202.
43 MULLER S.A. & WINKLEMANN R.K. (1963) *Arch Dermatol* 88, 290.
44 PECORARO V. (1963) *Arch Argent Dermatol* 13, 297.
45 PENDERS A.J.M. (1968) *Dermatologica* 136, 395.
46 PORTER D. & BURTON J.L. (1971) *Br. J Dermatol* 85, 272.
47 SABOURAUD R. (1929) *Pelades et Alpécies en Aires*. Paris, Masson.
48 SAENZ H. (1963) *Actas Dermosifilogr* 54, 357.
49 SANDER D.N., *et al* (1980) In *Hair Trace Elements and Human Elements*. Eds. Brown A.S.U. & Crowns R.G. New York, Praeger, p. 334.
50 SCHMIDT C.L. (1953) *Penn Med J* 56, 975.
51 SCHWEIKERT H.U. (1967) *Arch Klin Exp Dermatol* 230, 96.
52 SUMMERLY R., *et al* (1966) *Arch Dermatol* 93, 411.
53 SWANSON N.A., *et al* (1981) *Acta Dermatol* 117, 384.
54 THIES W. (1966) *Arch Klin Exp Dermatol* 227, 541.
55 THIES W. & KLASCHKA F. (1970) *Arch Klin Exp Dermatol* 237, 51.
56 UCHIYAMA M. (1967) *Jpn J Dermatol* 72, 281.
57 VAN SCOTT E.J. (1958) *J Invest Dermatol* 31, 35.
58 VAN SCOTT E.J. (1959) *Ann NY Acad Sci* 83, 480.
59 VAN SCOTT E.J. & EKEL T.M. (1958) *J Invest Dermatol* 31, 281.
60 DU VIVIER A. & MUNRO D.D. (1975) *Br Med J* i, 191.
61 WALKER S.A. & ROTHMAN S. (1950) *J Invest Dermatol* 14, 403.
62 WEISS V.C., *et al* (1984) *Arch Dermatol* 120, 457.
63 WOLOWA F. & STACKOWA A. (1984) *Z Hautkr* 55, 1125.
64 WUNDERLICH C. & BRAUN-FALCO O. (1965) *Med Welt* 10, 477.

TRAUMATIC ALOPECIA

Definition and nomenclature [5]. Traumatic alopecia results from the forcible extraction of hairs or the breaking of hair shafts by traction, friction or other physical or chemical trauma [8, 17].

Physical trauma is a common and often unrecognized cause of alopecia, and is often the sole significant factor. However, the identification of a traumatic factor excludes neither an underlying defect of the hair of developmental or chemical origin which increases its vulnerability nor a primary disorder of the scalp which induces the patient to rub. A careful history is essential and must include details of recent hairdressing and cosmetic procedures. Routine microscopy of the broken hairs is advisable.

The number of patterns of traumatic alopecia increases with the ingenuity of the cosmeticians. A purely clinical classification is convenient.

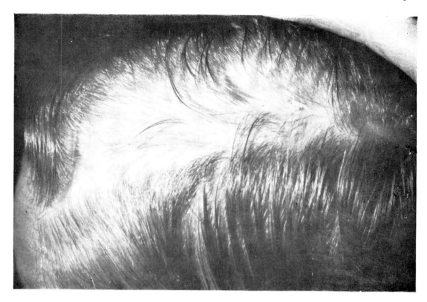

FIG. 53.36. Traumatic alopecia in a boy aged 9, with a hair-pulling tic. The site is characteristic in a right-handed child (Addenbrooke's Hospital).

Neonatal occipital alopecia. Thinning of the hair in the occipital region by friction on the pillow is common during the early months of life. The friction merely accelerates normal postnatal shedding but the bald patches may alarm the inexperienced mother.

Hair-pulling tics (syn. trichotillomania)

In children [14, 16]. Some children develop a nervous tic of pulling the hair and twisting it round the fingers, and eventually produce a patch of partial alopecia (Fig. 53.36). It occurs in children of both sexes, usually between the ages of 4 and 10 but sometimes as early as the second year. The habit is usually practised when the child is reading or writing, or in bed before falling asleep, and it may escape the observation of the parents. It is perhaps most common in retarded children, but is often seen in those of normal intelligence. Most are under emotional stress and a few are seriously disturbed. One affected child also plucked hair from other children her own age [21]; another patient inflicted damage similar to that on her own scalp on her doll [28]. Extensive alopecia and other self-mutilations are seen in children with familial sensory neuropathy [20]. Trichotillomania may develop following alopecia areata [29]. The patches, which are usually single, are often frontoparietal or frontotemporal. Exceptionally they are in other

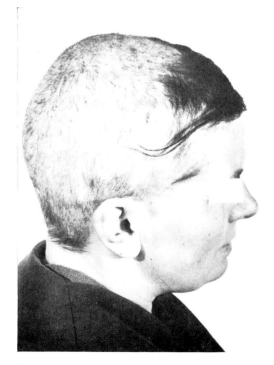

FIG. 53.37. Extensive traumatic alopecia in a severely disturbed woman aged 43 (Addenbrooke's Hospital).

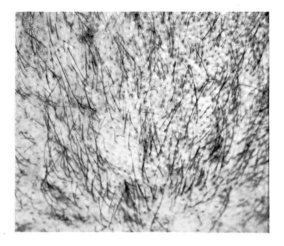

FIG. 53.38. Close-up of the scalp in the same patient as Fig. 53.37. Note the broken and twisted hairs (Addenbrooke's Hospital).

parts of the scalp. Some patients complain of tenderness of the scalp. The hairs on the patch show great variation in length; some are normal and others are broken at varying lengths above the scalp. Characteristically the direction of growth of many hairs does not conform to the normal hair streams and they point irregularly in all directions. The scalp is normal or slightly scaly. Very rarely the eyebrows [22] or eyelashes may be plucked [27].

The tic is often rapidly amenable to reassurance

and explanation, but occasionally the advice of a psychiatrist may be required.

In adults [24]. In older children and adults hair pulling is rare in the absence of severe emotional disturbance. The patients are usually women. Characteristically hair is plucked from the central region of the scalp, perhaps because the pain threshold is higher there than at the scalp margins. The hairs are uniformly about 3 cm long, partly because this is the shortest the patient can grasp in her fingers and because of synchronization of most follicles in the affected areas. This so-called 'tonsure' alopecia may continue for many years. Exceptionally other regions of the body are plucked—the pubes or perianal skin [7]. Expert psychiatric advice is always essential.

The diagnosis of trichotillomania is usually readily established, but if there is any doubt biopsy may be helpful [15]. In the earlier stages the follicles show evidence of severe traumatic damage, but the hair shafts are normal and show some trichorrhexis. Many follicles are in catagen and dilated follicular infundibula contain horny plugs [19]. Later, there is atrophy of many follicles which provide only soft hairs (trichomalacia).

Alopecia and lichen simplex [3]. A circumscribed patch of broken and twisted hairs is often associated with lichen simplex (p. 412) of the scalp. The pruritus, the frequent hyperpigmentation and often profuse scaling should suggest the diagnosis, which is

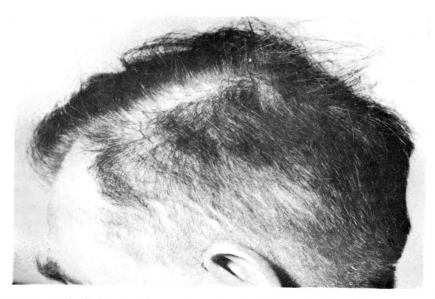

FIG. 53.39. Alopecia in a patch of lichen simplex in the temporal region (Addenbrooke's Hospital).

readily made when the patch occurs on the nape of the neck in a woman, but is often overlooked when other sites are affected (Fig. 53.39).

Massage alopecia [2]. Repeated vigorous massage may produce patchy baldness with short broken lustreless hairs. The condition is usually seen in adolescents but occasionally at any age in those who have made over-enthusiastic applications of proprietary hair restorers in the treatment of real or imagined baldness. Excessive use of heavy brushes with sharp-angled bristles may produce similar but more diffuse changes [25].

Traction alopecia [13]. Experimental studies of the effects of prolonged traction on wool fibres in sheep show an increase in growth rate but a decrease in diameter and overall volume [12].

Hairdressing styles or traditional [26] or sophisticated procedures which involve prolonged traction on the hair may give rise to a characteristic succession of changes—perifollicular erythema and occasional pustules, scaling and many broken hairs during the earlier stages, and follicular scarring and permanent alopecia if the practice is continued. In some cases *peripilar casts* are formed. These are fine yellowish-white keratin cylinders 3–7 mm in diameter surrounding the hair shaft [4] (p. 0000).

The part of the scalp affected depends on the hair style [13].

Marginal alopecia (syn. alopecia liminaris frontalis). This is produced by tight curlers or rollers, or, in

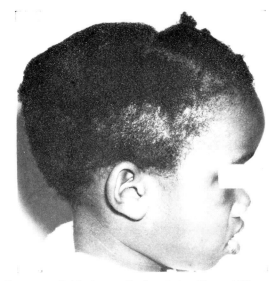

FIG. 53.41. Patchy traumatic alopecia in a Negro child produced by the regular application of 'straighteners' (Addenbrooke's Hospital).

Negro girls, by 'straighteners'. Symmetrical areas just within the hair margin, immediately in front of the ears, gradually extend forward in a band 1–3 cm wide. There may be irritation and crusting. The short peripheral hairs are often spared. In the 'pony-tail' hair style, which resembles the traditional style of the women of Greenland, alopecia with folliculitis and scarring develops at both temples [9, 23]. Small patches of alopecia, scattered

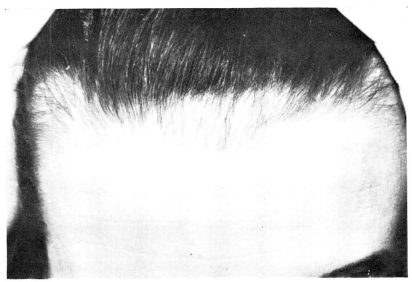

FIG. 53.40. Marginal traction alopecia (Stoke Mandeville Hospital).

through the scalp, are sometimes produced by brush rollers [10]. They are often irregular in outline and may be linear. The *chignon alopecia* of the crown has become as uncommon as the fashion which produced it.

The traditional hair styles of many races cause unusual patterns of alopecia. Morgan [18] has described the consequences of tight braiding in the Sudan.

Hot-comb alopecia. This is seen in women who use hot combs to straighten their hair [11]. Patches of scarring on the crown of the head slowly extend centrifugally.

Pressure alopecia. Continued pressure on a circumscribed area may cause oedema, exudation, crusting and temporary alopecia. Pressure alopecia has been reported in infants as a consequence of birth trauma [6] and in women who have undergone prolonged pelvic operations in the Trendelenburg position [1]. Oedema and crusting develop at or near the vertex a few days after the operation and the hair is shed 1–4 weeks later. Regrowth occurs spontaneously.

REFERENCES

1 Abel R.R. (1964) *Anesthesiology* **25**, 869.
2 Bowers R.E. (1950) *Br J Dermatol* **62**, 262.
3 Braun-Falco O. & Hasenpflug K. (1960) *Dermatol Wochenschr* **141**, 201.
4 Costa O.G. (1946) *Br J Dermatol* **58**, 280.
5 Dawber R.P.R. (1985) In *Seminars in Dermatology*. Vol 4. Eds. Rook A.J. & Maibach H. New York, Theime–Stratton, p. 80.
6 Friederich H.C. (1950) *Dermatol Wochenschr* **121**, 344.
7 Galewsky W. (1928) *Dermatol Wochenschr* **53**, 208.
8 Garcia M.L., et al (1978) *J Soc Cosmet Chem* **29**, 155.
9 Hjorth N. (1957) *Br J Dermatol* **69**, 319.
10 Lipnik M.J. (1961) *Arch Dermatol* **84**, 493.
11 Lo Presti P., et al (1968) *Arch Dermatol* **98**, 234.
12 Lyne A.G. & Jolly M. (1969) In *Hair Growth*. Eds. Montagna W. and Dobson R.L. Oxford, Pergamon, p. 247.
13 Malhotra Y.K. & Karwas A.J. (1980) *Arch Dermatol* **116**, 987.
14 Mannino F.V. & Delgardo R.A. (1969) *Am J Psychiatr* **126**, 505
15 Mehregan A.H. (1970) *Arch Dermatol* **102**, 129.
16 Meiers H.G., et al (1973) *Hautarzt* **24**, 248.
17 Menkart J. (1979) *Cutis* **23**, 276.
18 Morgan H.V. (1960) *Br Med J* ii, 115.
19 Muller S.A. & Winkelmann R.K. (1972) *Arch Dermatol* **105**, 535.
20 Pinsky L. & Di George A.M. (1966) *J Pediatr* **68**, 1.
21 Reuter K. (1951) *Z Hautkr Geschlkrankh* **10**, 287.
22 Rohebach D. (1963) *Hautarzt* **14**, 122.
23 Rollins T.G. (1961) *Am J Dis Child* **101**, 639.
24 Sanderson K.V. & Hall-Smith P. (1970) *Br J Dermatol* **82**, 343.
25 Savill A. (1958) *Br J Dermatol* **70**, 296.
26 Singh G. (1975) *Br J Dermatol* **92**, 232.
27 Sonck C.E. (1958) *Hautarzt* **9**, 183.
28 Tabatabai S.E. & Salari-Lak M. (1981) *Cutis* **28**, 206.
29 Wilkins J.K. (1983) *Cutis* **31**, 65.

CICATRICIAL ALOPECIA

Cicatricial alopecia is the end result of a wide variety of pathological processes which cause destruction of the hair follicles. The destruction may be the result of a developmental defect or of physical trauma, or of acute or chronic inflammatory changes of proved infective origin, or of a benign or malignant neoplasm. It may have followed a well-defined and identifiable but more mysterious process, lupus erythematosus, lichen planus or necrobiosis lipoidica. It may, in contrast, conform to one of several easily recognizable clinical syndromes such as pseudopelade and folliculitis decalvans, the cause and even the nature of which are often unknown.

The essential clinical features of all cicatricial alopecias are obviously the presence of scarring and the absence of follicles. The detection of small areas of scarring may require some experience and the use of a hand lens; in alopecia areata the scalp may appear deceptively atrophic. The scarring may be the only abnormal physical sign, as in many cases of pseudopelade, but other changes should be carefully sought both in and around the bald areas—telangiectasia or pigmentation, follicular inflammatory changes, plugging or broken hairs. When scarring is the only abnormality, the history, or the presence of lesions elsewhere on the skin or of other abnormal physical signs, may allow the cause of the scarring to be established with a high degree of probability. Examination of the whole skin surface and a general physical examination are therefore essential in all cases of doubt.

In some patients, despite every possible effort, all evidence is lacking, and a morphological diagnosis of pseudopelade or of cicatricial alopecia of unknown origin must be accepted.

If the diagnosis is in doubt ringworm must be excluded by the microscopy and culture of hairs plucked from the margins of scarred areas. More than one dermatologist has blushed when favus has been demonstrated in his 'familial cicatricial alopecia'.

Biopsy may sometimes be helpful [1–3], but the

site should be carefully selected. The older lesions, whatever their origin, may show non-specific changes.

REFERENCES

1 IOANNIDES G. (1982) *Int J Dermatol* **21**, 316.
2 PINKUS H. (1978) *J Cutan Pathol* **5**, 93.
3 POMPOSIELLO I.M. (1949) *Rev Argent Dermatosifilol* **33**, 1.

THE CAUSES OF CICATRICIAL ALOPECIA

Developmental defects and hereditary disorders

Aplasia cutis (p. 225)
Lumpy scalp syndrome (p. 2032)
Conradi's disease (p. 163)
Incontinentia pigmenti (p. 1559)
Epidermal naevi (p. 169)
Porokeratosis of Mibelli (p. 1465)
Keratosis pilaris atrophicans (p. 1437)
Ichthyosis (p. 1416)
Icthyosiform erythroderma (p. 1420)

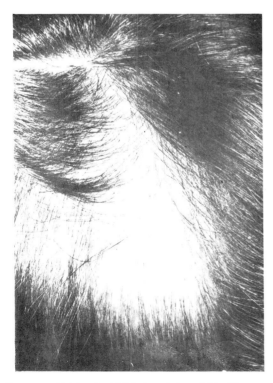

FIG. 53.42. Patchy cicatricial alopecia in a child with ichthyosis of sex-linked recessive type (Dr G.B. Mitchell-Heggs, S. John's Hospital).

Darier's disease (p. 1438)
Hair follicle hamartomas

In aplasia cutis the deficiencies, often rectilinear, are present at birth and heal slowly to leave scars. In Conradi's disease and in incontinentia pigmenti, cicatricial alopecia of the vertex is present from early infancy. Crusting of the scalp is present from birth and after separation of the crusts the alopecia remains unchanged throughout life. It is found in about 25% of cases of Conradi's disease [2]. Epidermal naevi are present at birth or develop during childhood; the nature of the naevus is often obvious, but some flat but extensive sebaceous naevi are referred to the dermatologist as alopecia. Porokeratosis of Mibelli may fortuitously involve the scalp [4] but is otherwise typical.

In keratosis pilaris atrophicans, facial keratosis pilaris, often with numerous milia, develops in infancy or childhood in association with cicatricial alopecia of the scalp and brows.

Some scarring with heavy scaling of the scalp may accompany ichthyosis of the sex-linked recessive type. In ichthyosiform erythroderma extensive alopecia of pseudopelade type may occur as a rare complication [3, 5].

The greasy-brown papules of Darier's disease often involve the scalp. Rarely, they give rise to extensive alopecia [6].

Generalized hair follicle hamartomas have caused extensive alopecia [1].

REFERENCES

1 BROWN A.L., *et al* (1969) *Arch Dermatol* **99**, 478.
2 CURTH H. (1949) *J Invest Dermatol* **13**, 233.
3 LONGHIN S., *et al* (1962) *Arch Belg Dermatol Syphiligr* **24**, 1.
4 ROSEN I. (1942) *Arch Dermatol Syphilol* **45**, 782.
5 STEVANOVIC D. & KONSTANTINOVIC S. (1959) *Arch Dermatol* **80**, 56.
6 WALTON D.G. (1943) *Arch Dermatol Syphilol* **47**, 398.

Physical injuries

Mechanical trauma
Burns
Radiodermatitis

The diagnosis is usually readily established by the history, but may be overlooked when unusual injuries are involved. The use of a vacuum extractor in obstetrics has resulted in cicatricial alopecia of the vertex [2], as has the use of fetal scalp electrodes [1]. Marginal or vertical alopecia in women may be produced by certain hairdressing procedures (p. 1995).

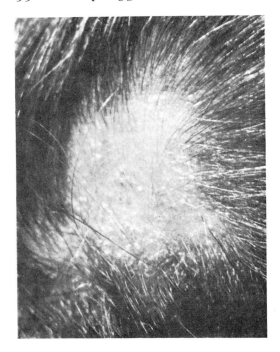

FIG. 53.43. One of many patches of alopecia around mosquito bites in a child's scalp. The hair regrew, except on the small central scar (Addenbrooke's Hospital).

Radiodermatitis as a sequel of X-ray epilation carried out before the days of accurate dosimetry is still encountered. The diagnosis is unlikely to be overlooked except in those few cases in which the X-ray damage to the follicles was marginal and atrophy developed only after an interval of some years as a result of added age changes. The distribution of the alopecia should suggest the cause.

REFERENCES

1 BROWN Z.A., *et al* (1977) *Am J Obstet Gynecol* **129**, 351.
2 HALL-SMITH P. & FOULKES J.F. (1964) *Arch Dermatol* **89**, 473.

Infections

Fungus infections (p. 911)	Kerion—many species of dermatophyte
	Trichophyton violaceum
	Trichophyton sulphureum
	Favus
Bacterial infections	Lupus vulgaris (p. 809)
	Leprosy (p. 823)
	Tertiary syphilis (p. 854)
	Yaws (p. 871)
	Pyogenic infections
	Carbuncle (p. 740)
	Furuncle (p. 739)
	Folliculitis (p. 742)
	Acne necrotica (p. 743)
	Gonococcus (p. 753)
Protozoal infections	Leishmaniasis (p. 1020)
Virus infections	Herpes zoster (p. 680)
	Variola (p. 693)
	Varicella (p. 680)

The infective causes of cicatricial alopecia are numerous, and their retrospective identification is often difficult. A distinction must be drawn between the scarred footsteps of a past infection—a kerion, a carbuncle or herpes zoster—and the scarring which may be associated with continuing active infection with the ectothrix trichophytons, lupus vulgaris or syphilis. The lesions of varicella, furuncles or secondarily infected excoriated insect bites may give rise to multiple patches of alopecia up to 5 cm in diameter. The hair shed from the zone of hyperaemia is soon regained and only the

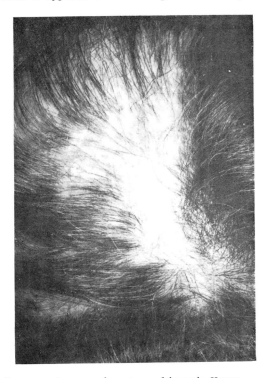

FIG. 53.44. Lupus erythematosus of the scalp. Horny plugs fill many follicles in patches of erythema and scaling (Addenbrooke's Hospital).

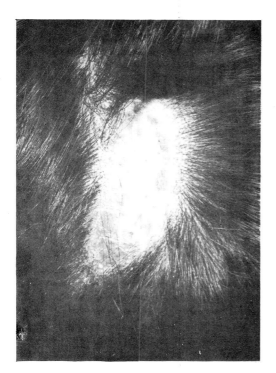

Loss of hair without scarring may occur over a variety of benign and malignant tumours of the scalp, but cicatricial alopecia is unusual. The development of a single sclerotic plaque in an elderly patient should suggest the possibility of primary or secondary neoplasm [1, 2, 5], which should be confirmed by biopsy. Rarely, metastatic carcinoma can cause very extensive cicatricial alopecia [4]. In the younger patient also biopsy may be necessary to differentiate morphoea from morphoeic basal cell carcinoma, which may occur in early childhood [3]. Squamous carcinoma has developed in chronic scarring caused by lupus erythematosus [6].

REFERENCES

1 Baran R. (1969) *Dermatologica* **138**, 169.
2 Baum E.M., *et al* (1981) *J Am Acad Dermatol* **4**, 688.
3 Botvinik I., *et al* (1967) *Arch Dermatol* **95**, 67.
4 Martin J. & Ross J.B. (1983) *Int J Dermatol* **22**, 687.
5 Nelson C.T. (1963) *Arch Dermatol* **90**, 249.
6 Vidal Lliteras J. & Carre J. (1971) *Actas Dermosifilogr* **62**, 63.

Fig. 53.45. A plaque of scleroderma (morphoea) histologically confirmed (Addenbrooke's Hospital).

small central scar remains, often less than 2 mm in diameter and of little or no cosmetic significance. The loss of hair around furuncles is first noted after 7–10 days. It has been suggested [1] that staphylococcal toxins have a direct effect on the hair follicles.

Alopecia surrounding tick bites [2, 3] differs in its more rapid and wider extension. The hair is shed a few days after the bite over an area up to 5 cm in diameter. Regrowth occurs rapidly except in the small central scar at the site of the bite itself. It is possible that anticoagulants are responsible for the hair loss (p. 1981).

REFERENCES

1 Butterworth T. & Fowler J.C. (1959) *AMA Arch Dermatol* **80**, 570.
2 Heyl T. (1982) *Clin Exp Dermatol* **7**, 537.
3 Marshall J. (1966) *S Afr Med J* **40**, 555.

Neoplasms

Cicatrizing basal cell carcinoma
Morphoeic basal cell carcinoma
Metastatic carcinoma

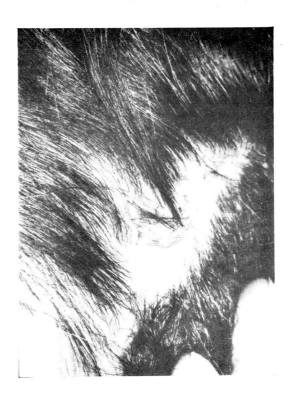

Fig. 53.46. Cicatricial alopecia caused by sarcoidosis (Addenbrooke's Hospital).

Dermatoses of unknown origin
  Lichen planus (and lichenoid drug eruptions)
  Lupus erythematosus (p. 1289)
  Scleroderma (p. 1336)
  Necrobiosis lipoidica (p. 1692)
  Sarcoidosis (p. 1755)
  Benign mucosal pemphigoid (p. 1644)
  Follicular mucinosis (pp. 2004, 2297)
  Erosive pustular dermatosis
  Eosinophilic cellulitic
  Syringoma [2, 4] (p. 2407)

Lichen planus and lupus erythematosus involve the scalp relatively frequently (see below). Both may give rise to distinctive changes or to pseudopelade. Scleroderma is usually seen as a single paramedian plaque (p. 1338), but the diagnosis has also been applied to multiple small lesions on histological criteria [6] and on the subsequent development of systemic sclerosis [7].

In lichenoid drug eruptions irregular cicatricial alopecia occurs only in the more severe and prolonged reactions. It has been reported after mepacrine, after gold and after PAS [5].

Necrobiosis lipoidica and sarcoidosis very rarely involve the scalp, and in the absence of typical lesions elsewhere the diagnosis is unlikely to be made on clinical grounds alone. The cicatricial alopecia in sarcoidosis may show no distinctive features clinically, although the characteristic infiltrate is present histologically [1]. It occurs predominately in Negro women with intrathoracic and other cutaneous sarcoidosis [3].

In benign mucosal pemphigoid recurrent bullae are ultimately followed by scarring. The eyes and mouth are frequently involved.

Rarely, follicular mucinosis results in the permanent destruction of follicles with the formation of bald areas which may be studded with horny plugs.

REFERENCES

1 BLUEFARB S.M., *et al* (1955) *Arch Dermatol* **71**, 602.
2 DUPRE, *et al* (1981) *Arch Dermatol* **117**, 315.
3 GOLITZ L.E., *et al* (1973) *Arch Dermatol* **107**, 758.
4 NOBLE J.P. & LEIBOWITCH M.L. (1979) *Ann Dermatol Vénéréol* **106**, 275.
5 PINOL AGUADE J. (1968) *Med Cutan Iber Lat Am* **3**, 275.
6 RINALDI V.G. (1955) *Dermatologica* **116**, 448.
7 TSVETANOV T. (1967) *Dermatol Venereol (Sofia)* **6**, 134.

LICHEN PLANUS OF THE SCALP

Incidence and nomenclature [9, 10]. Cicatricial alopecia of the scalp may be associated with lesions of the ordinary form of lichen planus elsewhere on the skin or mucous membrane, but is found in only a small proportion of such cases. It occurs more frequently in association with lichen planopilaris (syn. lichen planus et acuminatus atrophicans) in which the scalp is involved in about 40% of cases.

The present evidence, which is necessarily circumstantial since the nature of lichen planus is unknown, suggests that ordinary lichen planus, lichen planopilaris and some cases of the Lassueur–Graham–Little syndrome (p. 2004) are variants of the same process showing an increasing degree of follicular involvement.

Lichen planus of the scalp is usually seen between the ages of 30 and 60 and is diagnosed considerably more often in women than in men. It may occasionally begin in childhood but some of the cases so reported are examples of keratosis pilaris atrophicans (p. 1437).

Pathology [8]. The histological changes are essentially the same as those of lichen planus in other sites (p. 1666) but the lymphocytic infiltrate, which may not be present beneath the surface epidermis, extends deeply around the follicles and involves the papillae. Lacunae may appear outside the oedematous external sheath but a saw-toothed outline is never well defined. Connective tissue of the dermis and around the follicle becomes hyaline and later sclerotic. In the later stages the appearance is not diagnostic of lichen planus and in many cases some apparently recent lesions may show only sclerosis and destruction of the follicles with or without horny plugging of the follicular orifices. In the scanning electron microscope hairs from areas of the scalp are affected by lichen planus and show longitudinal furrows and gross disturbance of the cuticular scale pattern [5].

Clinical features [1, 4, 6, 7]. The chance discovery of a small bald patch is the usual presenting manifestation, for subjective symptoms are uncommon.

The morphology of the lesions shows wide variations which cannot be consistently related to the stage of the lesion, and lesions of more than one type may be found in the same patient. Most frequently, multiple small areas of white scarring are associated with conspicuous plugging of the follicles around their margins and sometimes elsewhere on the scalp. In other cases the plugging is absent and the appearance is that of pseudopelade. Other cases show some erythema and oedema with adherent scale and dilated follicular orifices. When atrophic scarring is added later the appearance may be indistinguishable from lupus erythematosus.

Cicatricial alopecia without clinically certain [3] or evident follicular keratosis is often a feature of that uncommon variant of lichen planus in which atrophic lesions of the feet are also accompanied by loss of the nails [2].

Although in most cases the lesions extend only very slowly and have produced no socially embarrassing baldness even after many years, in some the scalp may be largely denuded within a year or two. Some cases eventually become totally quiescent. Rapid extension during the first year often implies an unfavourable prognosis, but there are no certain criteria.

Diagnosis. It is rarely possible to make a confident clinical diagnosis of the scalp lesions alone, and although histological appearances may provide confirmation they may be non-specific. The diagnosis must often be based on the presence of typical lesions of skin or mucous membranes, and these should always be sought.

Treatment. The intralesional injection of corticosteroids may be of benefit in those in whom lichen planus is still active.

REFERENCES

1 BORDA J.M., *et al* (1961) *Arch Argent Dermatol* 11, 251.
2 CRAM D.L., *et al* (1966) *Arch Dermatol* 93, 692.
3 EBNER H. (1973) *Dermatologica* 147, 219.
4 ELLIS F.A. & KIRBY-SMITH H. (1941) *Arch Dermatol Syphilol* 43, 628.
5 FIMIANI M., *et al* (1982) *Ann Ital Dermatol* 36, 219.
6 SACHS W. & DE OREO W. (1942) *Arch Dermatol Syphilol* 45, 1081.
7 SANNICANDRO G. (1954) *Ann Dermatol Syphilol* 41, 380.
8 SANNICANDRO G. (1955) *Hautarzt* 6, 401.
9 SILVER H., *et al* (1953) *AMA Arch Dermatol Syphilol* 67, 346.
10 *SPIER H.W. & KEILIG W. (1953) *Hautarzt* 4, 457.

Clinical syndromes

Pseudopelade
Folliculitis decalvans
Lassueur–Graham-Little syndrome
Alopecia parvimaculata
Perifolliculitis capitis abscendens et suffodiens
   (syn. dissecting cellulitis of the scalp)

PSEUDOPELADE

Aetiology. Pseudopelade is a morphological syndrome and not an aetiology entity. With the help of a detailed history and careful examination

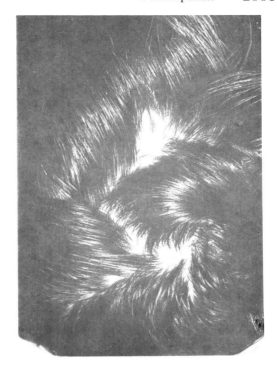

FIG. 53.47. Pseudopelade. Small patches of cicatrical alopecia of unknown origin (Addenbrooke's Hospital).

of the whole surface of the skin it is possible to attribute pseudopelade more or less confidently to a known pathological process in some 70% of cases [2]. However, it is not proven that pseudopelade is necessarily always the end result of such processes. We have examined cases of less than 3 months' duration in which there was neither clinical nor histological evidence of any other disorder. Pseudopelade is best regarded as a pattern of follicular response to a wide variety of insults, known and unknown. It is convenient to reserve the unqualified term for cases of unknown origin and to classify the remainder according to their presumed cause. The age and sex incidence of the syndrome as a whole varies with the incidence of the initiating processes. Cases of unknown origin are seen mainly between the ages of 30 and 55, and rather more frequently in women than in men.

The conditions which can give rise to, or occur in association with, pseudopelade include [2, 3] lupus erythematosus, lichen planus (which some authorities [4] consider accounts for the majority of cases), scleroderma and keratosis pilaris, clinically and histologically typical lesions of which in the scalp or elsewhere may be associated with typical pseudopelade. Other cases follow suppurative folliculitis or the less well-defined folliculitis decalvans. We have observed several cases in which alopecia areata and pseudopelade coexisted. This association has been previously reported [2].

Pathology [2, 6]. The earliest change is an infiltrate of lymphocytes around the upper two-thirds pf the hair follicle, sparing the bulb. Later, the epidermis is atrophic and flattened and the dermis is densely sclerotic. The sebaceous glands and the hair follicles are destroyed but the arrectors and sweat glands persist. Dense foci of lymphocytes may be seen around the follicular remnants. Later these also disappear.

Clinical features [2, 5]. Pseudopelade begins insidiously and there are usually no subjective symptoms; occasionally, pruritus may accompany periods of extension. Small, round or oval bald areas, which are smooth, white, soft and slightly depressed and up to 1 cm in diameter, appear singly or in small groups. The absence of inflammatory signs is characteristic but there may be some erythema. Neighbouring patches coalesce to form irregular plaques several centimetres in diameter. Scattered follicles in these plaques are often spared. The vertex is most frequently affected but the patches may develop anywhere in the scalp and in several areas simultaneously. In most cases the alopecia extends extremely slowly, with long remissions and irregular periods of activity, and in some patients is not severe enough to be a serious cosmetic disability even after 20 yr. However, the course is unpredictable and rapid extension can occur. Rarely, the greater part of the scalp may be denuded within 2 or 3 yr.

Diagnosis. The small size of the initial bald patches and the usual absence of inflammatory signs make the diagnosis an obvious one in many cases. In others the many other causes of cicatricial alopecia must be considered. Favus is the diagnosis most commonly overlooked. Since pseudopelade may accompany or follow many other disorders, the presence in some areas of scaling, follicular plugging or even folliculitis does not exclude the diagnosis. In the present state of our knowledge the diagnosis to be applied should be either pseudopelade, without qualification, or pseudopelade with lupus erythematosus or lichen planus.

Biopsy may be useful at an early stage but in later stages the points of distinction between pseudopelade, lichen planus and scleroderma tend to be lost.

Treatment. Pseudopelade itself is irreversible and there is at present no evidence that any treatment will prevent the extension of the process. The cosmetic disfigurement may be reduced by autografts from unaffected areas of the scalp [1].

Precision in diagnosis is important, since it may be possible to control any associated disorder and thus limit further extension of the alopecia.

REFERENCES

1 CURBAN G.V. & GOLLMAN B. (1973) *Med Cutan Iber Lat Am* **7**, 65.
2 *DEGOS R., *et al* (1954) *AMA Arch Dermatol Syphilol* **81**, 5.
3 GAY PRIETO J. (1955) *J Invest Dermatol* **24**, 323.
4 KAMINSKY A., *et al* (1967) *Med Cutan Iber Lat Am* **2**, 135.
5 LAYMON C.W. & MURPHY R.J. (1947) *J Invest Dermatol* **8**, 99.
6 MIESCHER G. & LENGGENHAGER R. (1947) *Dermatologica* **94**, 122.

FOLLICULITIS DECALVANS

Definition and nomenclature [2–5, 9]. Folliculitis decalvans is characterized by clinically evident follicular inflammation which leads to destruction of the follicle and consequent permanent alopecia. The *folliculite épilante* originally described by Quinquaud involved the scalp predominantly. Brocq described a similar process involving the beard as *lupoid sycosis*, which has generally been accepted as identical with Unna's *ulerythema sycosiforme*. *Folliculitis depilans* of the glabrous skin as described by Arnozan occurs mainly on the legs. Although some authorities claim that these conditions represent separate entities we believe that they are variants of a single clinical syndrome. They may indeed all occur in the same patient.

Aetiology. The cause is unknown. Many of those affected have seborrhoea and a long history of seborrhoeic dermatitis. *Staphylococcus aureus* may often be isolated from the pustules, and hypersensitivity to this organism has been postulated but not proven [1]. It is more likely that the predisposing factor is a defect in the immune response; the cell-mediated response was impaired in two severely affected brothers who also had oral candidiasis [8]. All forms of the syndrome are rare. In women it occurs between the ages of 30 and 60 and in men it usually begins in adult life, but may first appear at adolescence or even in infancy [6]. The marginal folliculitis decalvans of the female scalp is a traction alopecia (see p. 1995). In one report hypocomplementaemia was associated [4].

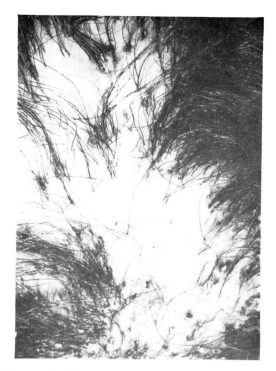

Fig. 53.48. Folliculitis decalvans in a woman aged 42. Extensive cicatricial alopecia with follicular pustules (Addenbrooke's Hospital).

Pathology. Follicular abscesses with numerous polymorphonuclear leucocytes are rapidly succeeded by a granulomatous infiltrate around and involving the follicles and sweat glands, and consisting largely of lymphocytes, but often with a large proportion of plasma cells and occasional giant cells. Later only follicular remnants can be found within the scarred areas and the changes may be indistinguishable from pseudopelade.

Clinical features. Folliculitis decalvans can involve any hairy region and may indeed involve them all in the same patient [3]. More often it is confined to one region. In any form seborrhoeic dermatitis may be associated or may accompany recrudescences, but not all patients are obviously seborrhoeic.

In the scalp, small, rounded or oval patches of scarring are surrounded by perifollicular pustules. As the hairs are shed the pustules are followed by red macules which fade to leave scars. The pustules may develop in crops with pruritus, but there are usually no symptoms. Slow intermittent extension over many years may result in extensive baldness but the disease sometimes remains limited to a few small patches.

In the beard the process usually begins in front of one ear and may be restricted to the temple, but may extend downwards to the chin and up to the back and sides of the scalp. Occasionally it is bilateral. In the advancing edge are brown or red lupoid papules or pustules. The scarring may be cheloidal.

The axillary and pubic hair may be involved in association with the scalp alone or in generalized forms.

The lower legs, thighs and arms may rarely be the only sites affected [7] but may be involved together with the beard or with the scalp, axillae and pubes. Rarely, other parts of the body are also involved.

In all forms the condition tends to persist indefinitely. In women extension is often limited and the cosmetic disability is minimal, but the severe forms in men, particularly those of early onset, may be grossly disfiguring.

Diagnosis. Other causes of cicatricial alopecia are discussed on p. 1997. Favus and other related ringworm infections must always be excluded. Marginal folliculitis in women throws suspicion on hairdressing procedures (p. 1995).

In the beard lupus vulgaris may need exclusion.

Follicular mucinosis (pp. 2004 and 2297) does not give rise to scarring but the patchy hair loss could cause confusion.

Treatment. There is no procedure which can produce a permanent cure. In cases of limited extent the application of ointment containing the antibiotic Fucidin in combination with a steroid has provided effective control. For extensive lesions the oral administration of antibiotics alone may be effective but a maintenance dose is usually required. The most severe forms will respond only to the combination of an antibiotic and a steroid, and their continued administration is sometimes hazardous.

REFERENCES

1 Bizzorero E. & Leone R. (1947) *Dermatologica* **92**, 269.
2 Binazzi M. (1954) *Ann Ital Dermatol Sifilol* **9**, 325.
3 *Bogg A. (1963) *Acta Derm Venereol (Stockh)* **43**, 14.
4 Frazer N.G. & Grant P.W. (1982). *Brit J Dermatol (Suppl 22)* **107**, 88.
5 Hoffman E. (1931) *Arch Dermatol Syphilol* **164**, 317.
6 Loewenthal L.J.A. (1957) *Br J Dermatol* **69**, 443.
7 Miller R.F. (1961) *Arch Dermatol* **83**, 777.
8 Shitara A., et al (1974) *Jpn J Dermatol* **28**, 133.
9 Suter L. (1981) *Hautarzt* **32**, 429.

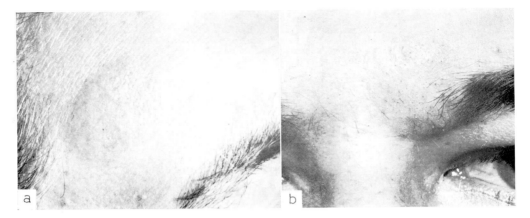

FIG. 55.49. Follicular mucinosis: (a) a single plaque of the right temple; (b) a plaque involving the eyebrow with loss of hair from many of the affected follicles (Addenbrooke's Hospital).

PICCARDI–LASSUEUR–GRAHAM-LITTLE SYNDROME

This rare syndrome, which is usually associated eponymously with Graham-Little [2], was previously described by Piccardi [6]. Some reports suggested that the condition might be a variant of lichen planopilaris, and this suggestion has received some support from immunofluorescence studies [3]. However, there are cases in which no evidence of lichen planus is discovered [1, 4, 5, 7, 8] and the syndrome is clinically distinctive.

Most patients have been women aged 30–70, but a boy aged 10 has also been affected [5]. Cicatricial alopecia is commonly the presenting symptom and may or may not be associated with follicular plugging or scaling of the scalp. After months or years keratosis pilaris develops on the trunk and limbs; the horny papules, prolonged upwards into spines, are usually grouped in well-defined plaques but may be more irregularly distributed. They may involve the face and eyebrows [5, 7].

Loss of pubic and axillary hair is often noted. There is no clinically evident scarring, although histologically the follicles are found to be destroyed [9].

In differential diagnosis other causes of cicatricial alopecia must be excluded (p. 1997).

In younger patients the various forms of keratosis pilaris atrophicans should be considered (p. 1437).

REFERENCES

1 ALESSI E. & DAL POZZO V. (1968) *G Ital Dermatol* **109**, 493.
2 GRAHAM-LITTLE E. (1915) *Br J Dermatol* **27**, 181.
3 HORN R.T., et al (1982) *J Am Acad Dermatol* **7**, 203.
4 JUOCADO L., et al (1971) *Arch Argent Dermatol* **31**, 155.
5 PAGES F., et al (1961) *Ann Dermatol Syphilol* **88**, 271.
6 PICCARDI G. (1914) *G Ital Dermatol* **35**, 416.
7 REISS F., et al (1958) *AMA Archs Dermatol* **78**, 616.
8 VALENTINO A., et al (1974) *G Minerva Dermatol* **109**, 588.
9 WALDORF D.S. (1966) *Arch Dermatol* **93**, 684.

ALOPECIA PARVIMACULATA

This uncommon and rather mysterious disorder is usually associated with the name of Dreuw, who described two epidemics in boys' schools. Other school and family outbreaks have been reported [1, 2]. No pathogenic agent has been isolated. The histology is that of pseudopelade (p. 2001).

Multiple small irregular angular or linear patches of alopecia develop rapidly. Some regrow but others persist as permanent scars.

REFERENCES

1 HÖFER W. (1964) *Dermatol Wochenschr* **149**, 381.
2 LOEWENTHAL L.J.A. & LURIE H.I. (1956) *Br J Dermatol* **68**, 88.

ALOPECIA MUCINOSA

This condition is fully described as follicular mucinosis on p. 2297. Alopecia is a conspicuous clinical feature only when the scalp, eyebrows or adult male beard are involved. In the acute benign forms diagnosis is relatively simple if there are multiple plaques on the face, neck and shoulders, but a solitary plaque in the scalp invites confusion with ringworm; erythema and scaling are associated with partial or complete loss of hair. Difficulties may also arise when the skin lesions are atypical, e.g. disseminated ungrouped keratotic follicular papules of the trunk and limbs with scaling of the scalp and patchy alopecia of the eyebrows [1] or scattered erythematous papules of the face and scalp with patchy alopecia [2].

Although in the acute forms and in many cases of the chronic forms there is usually complete recovery, in some chronic lesions the follicles are largely destroyed to leave cicatrical alopecia in which there may be follicular plugs.

REFERENCES

1 BAZEX A., *et al* (1962) *Bull Soc Fr Dermatol Syphiligr* **69**, 484.
2 GOLDSCHLAG F. & JABLONSKA S. (1960) *Aust J Dermatol* **5**, 173.

PERIFOLLICULITIS CAPITIS ABSCEDENS ET SUFFODIENS

SYN. DISSECTING CELLULITIS OF THE SCALP

This aggressively scarring condition is possibly an abnormal host response to bacterial infection seen in Negroid individuals [1]. It is four times more common in men than in women.

Progressive spread of deep 'cellulitis' occurs on the scalp and more rarely the axillae and groin.

Oral oxytetracycline may be of benefit.

REFERENCE

1 JOLLIFFE D. & SARKANY I. (1977) *Clin Exp Dermatol* **2**, 291.

THE HAIR SHAFT [7]

Hairs emerge from the skin either singly or in groups of two or more; on the scalp several individual pilosebaceous units may converge and share a common follicular opening. Hairs show extreme variations in diameter and bore, some being flattened or oval and others rather round. In general, hair is straight in Mongoloids, curly in Negroids and wavy in Caucasoid individuals [7]—asymmetrical keratinization is the most likely basis of such contour variation.

The main part of the fully keratinized hair fibre is the cortex which is made up of closely packed interdigitating spindle-shaped cells whose axis is parallel to the hair axis [5]. The main structures within cortical cells are the closely packed macrofibrils—longitudinal microfibrils in a matrix of high sulphur protein. Melanin granules are positioned between macrofibrils. The cortex is the part of the shaft which contributes most to the mechanical properties of hair [6].

The outer layer of each fibre is the cuticle [4] consisting of imbricated overlapping flattened cells; the free margin of each cell points towards the tip of the hair. Because of the length of each cell and the degree of overlap, in cross section the cuticle appears as six to ten layers. The exocuticle of each cell, particularly the A layer, is rich in high sulphur protein enabling the fibre to withstand frictional forces [6]. The surface epicuticle (2·5 nm thick), which was thought to cover the entire surface of the hair, has been shown to be part of the cuticular cell membrane complex [6].

The core of each hair fibre is the medulla; in many lower animals, e.g. porcupine quill, the medulla is continuous along the whole fibre. In human terminal hair, the medulla may be continuous, discontinuous or even absent. Appleyard [1], using Wildman's system, has subdivided medullary types into a 'latticed' and 'simple' pattern for continuous medulla, and a 'fragmented' and 'ladder' pattern for discontinuous medulla. Vellus and lanugo hair generally have no central medulla. Evidently, the androgen-mediated conversion of vellus to terminal hair at puberty is associated with the acquisition of a central medulla in the secondary sexual hair; the reverse is true on the vertex of the scalp if androgenic alopecia occurs to a significant degree.

The technical advances of the last 20 yr have enabled the fine structure of hair—physical [7] and chemical [2, 3]—to be defined in great detail. Much of the pioneer work has been done by cosmetic and wool scientists, and many of the techniques are now being applied in disease as will be seen in the following sections.

REFERENCES

1 APPLEYARD H.M. (1976) *Guide to the Identification of Animal Fibres*. Leeds WIRA.
2 FRAZER R.D.B., *et al* (1972) In *Keratins, Their Composition, Structure and Biosynthesis*. Springfield, Thomas.
3 GILLESPIE J.M. & MARSHALL R.C. (1979) In *Hair Research*. Eds. Orfanos C.E., *et al*. Berlin, Springer.
4 MUTO H., *et al* (1981) *Acta Anat* **109**, 13.
5 ORFANOS C. & RUSKA H. (1968) *Arch Klin Exp Dermatol* **231**, 234.
6 ROBBINS C.R. (1979) *The Chemical and Physical Behaviour of Human Hair*. New York, Van Nostrand–Reinhold.
7 SWIFT J.A. (1977) In *Chemistry of Natural Protein Fibres*. Ed. Asquith R.A. New York, Wiley, Chapter 3.

ABNORMALITIES OF THE HAIR SHAFT

Variations in the structure of the hair shaft are of common occurrence and are often of little clinical significance. The diameter of the shaft, the degree of curl and the character of the medulla are genetically determined traits of this kind. Structural variations become clinically significant when they are unsightly or when they reduce the resistance of the shaft to the minor traumas to which it is daily exposed.

Certain rare genetically determined defects easily recognizable with the light microscope have long been known to dematologists—monilethrix and pili torti are perhaps the most striking examples.

The defects of the shaft in some other hereditary syndromes such as anhidrotic ectodermal dysplasia are not detectable by light microscopy, but it has been shown that the hair is of low tensile strength with low elastic modulus [5].

Scanning electron microscopy [6] has revealed that even in normal healthy hair there is progressive disruption of the cuticular scale pattern from normal weathering and from the trauma of simple cosmetic procedures. In hair which is congenitally abnormal such trauma may produce greater abnormalities [1, 2].

Defects in the physicochemical properties of the shaft have been reported in a number of metabolic and endocrine disorders and in nutritional deficiencies. The wide variety of investigative techniques employed and the limited number of conditions to which any of them has been applied make it impossible as yet to draw any general conclusions of practical value to the clinician.

Many years ago Pinkus [3] reported detailed investigations of the effects of systemic illness on the diameter of the hair shaft. His neglected work has been confirmed by Sims [4] who has demonstrated the frequency with which a systemic illness or a surgical operation produces an immediate constriction in the hair shaft, presumably by disturbing protein synthesis.

These structural weaknesses of the hair shaft must be clearly distinguished from the patterns of response to trauma to which they may predispose but to which even the normal shaft is susceptible if the trauma be severe or frequently repeated. The traditional nomenclature of the injured hair is complex, but in fact the number of ways in which the hair shaft can respond to injury is very limited. The shaft may be frayed and split longitudinally (*trichoptilosis*) or transversely (*trichoclasis*), or the cortex may be swollen and dissociated at circumscribed points along the shaft (*trichorrhexis nodosa*). The term *trichoschisis* has been used for a clean transverse fracture. Finally, individual hairs may be knotted (*trichonodosis*). In dystrophies with congenitally fragile hair, a mixture of the above may be seen.

REFERENCES

1 GARCIA M.L., *et al* (1978) *J Soc Cosmet Chem* **29**, 155.
2 MENKART J. (1979) *Cutis* **23**, 276.
3 PINKUS F. (1917) *Die Einwirkung von Krankheiten auf das Kopfhaar des Menschen.* Berlin, Karger.
4 SIMS R.T. (1967) *Br J Dermatol* **79**, 43.
5 SWANBECK G., *et al* (1970) *J Invest Dermatol* **54**, 248.
6 SWIFT J.A. & BROWN A.C. (1972) *J Soc Cosmet Chem* **23**, 695.

MONILETHRIX

Definition. Monilethrix (Latin *monile* (necklace) + Greek-*thrix* (hair)) is a developmental defect of the hair shaft, which is beaded and breaks prematurely where the shaft is narrowed.

Aetiology [6, 19]. Monilethrix is usually determined by an autosomal dominant gene of high penetrance but variable expressivity. Apparent monohybrid recessive inheritance has been reported [10] and it is possible that the phenotype of this rarer recessive gene differs in some respects from classical monilethrix. Several reports have appeared of arginosuccinicaciduria [17] in patients with monilethrix; in one such report a technical error was responsible [7]. No metabolic abnormality is known to be consistently associated with monilethrix [22].

Pathology. The affected hair shafts are uniformly beaded; elliptical nodes 0·7–1 mm apart are separated by very narrow internodes (Fig. 7.1 of Rook & Dawber [18]). Even within families there are differences in internode distance and width at nodes [12]. Scanning electron microscopy has shown that the wider nodes have a normal surface structure whilst the narrow nodes show increasing fluting, longitudinal ridging and, terminally, transverse fissures and fracture [4, 5, 15]. The distance between two internodes appears to equate in some cases with 48 h growth [14] and in others with 24 h [2], but Comaish [3] was unable to establish a simple time cycle of any length for the beading. He also noted that beaded fibres grew faster than normal scalp hair.

Histologically [19] the follicles, which frequently show horny plugging, present correspondingly wide and narrow zones; many studies have demonstrated essentially normal follicular architecture. Electron histochemical studies [8] have shown that struc-

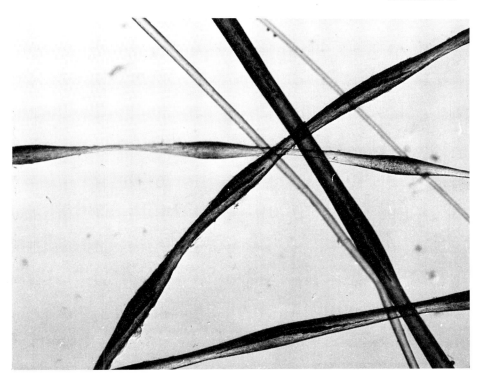

FIG. 53.50. Monilethrix; an electron micrograph of the hair (Dr A. Messenger, Royal Hallamshire Hospital, Sheffield).

tural abnormalities manifest in the cortex and cuticle of the hair shaft can be traced to the 'zone of keratinization' of the follicle; abnormal orientation of the cortical cell proteins, folding of the cuticle cell membrane and varying amounts of endocuticular material were all observed in this region.

Clinical features [13, 21]. The hair is usually normal at birth but when this is shed it is replaced within months by short, sparse, deformed and brittle hair. In a minority of cases onset may be delayed until later in childhood or early adult life. In typical cases small reddish horny follicular papules gradually develop and brittle beaded hair fibres which usually break before attaining a length of 1–2 cm emerge from a proportion of these. The nape and occipital region are commonly affected most severely (Fig. 7.2 of Rook & Dawber [18]). Terminal hair on any body site may be affected; rarely, the scalp is spared and one or more areas on the trunk or limbs are the only manifestation. The extent and severity may vary widely even within a single family; some affected individuals may be virtually bald whilst others show only a minority of follicles affected. In one family only body hair was affected [9].

Follicular keratosis is an associated sign in most cases though its severity does not usually equate with the severity of the beading or brittleness; it may precede the shaft defect.

Most affected individuals show a slow increase in severity and extent throughout childhood. Some cases persist throughout life with little change [1] apart from slight improvement during summer [21]. Pregnancy may give considerable temporary improvement [22]. Complete recovery has been reported in late childhood or early adult life [11].

Many associated defects have been recorded; nail and tooth abnormalities and cataract are probably more common than in controls [19]. Concurrent mental retardation has been described [20]. Studies of the reported pedigrees suggest, but do not prove, that oligophrenia may be significantly associated with the recessive type.

Diagnosis. Microscope examination of the hairs confirms the diagnosis which is suggested by short broken hair with follicular keratosis. Pili torti must be excluded microscopically. Other types of hereditary alopecia are listed on p. 1976.

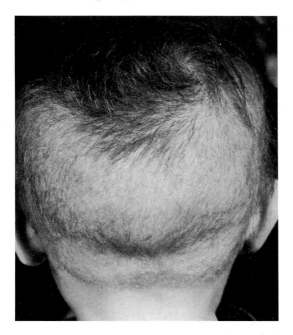

FIG. 53.51. Monilethrix: the nape of the neck showing horny follicular papules and sparse short beaded hairs (Dr S. Bleehen, Royal Hallamshire Hospital, Sheffield).

Treatment. There is no effective treatment, but minimizing cosmetic physical and chemical damage may improve the length of the hair. Pregnancy can be accompanied by considerable improvement, and therefore oral contraceptives of the combined type—oestrogen and progestogen together—may enhance hair growth in affected adult women [16]. Aromatic retinoids (etretinate) certainly improve the follicular keratosis but cannot correct the beading and hair fragility.

REFERENCES

1 ALEXANDER L. O'D. & GRANT P.W. (1958) *Scott Med J* **3**, 356.
2 BAKER H. (1962) *Br J Dermatol* **74**, 24.
3 COMAISH S. (1969) *Br J Dermatol* **81**, 443.
4 DAWBER R.P.R. (1979) In *Hair Research*. Eds. Orfanos C, *et al*. Berlin, Springer.
5 DAWBER R.P.R. & COMAISH S. (1970) *Arch Dermatol* **101**, 316.
6 DERAEMARKER R. (1957) *Am J Hum Genet* **9**, 195.
7 EFRON M.L. & HOEFNAGEL D. (1966) *Lancet* **i**, 321.
8 GUMMER C. (1981) *Br J Dermatol* **105**, 529.
9 HAMM H., *et al* (1984) *Z Hautkr* **59**, 1177.
10 HANHART E. (1955) *Arch Julius Klaus–Stift Vererbungsforsch* **30**, 1.
11 HEYDT G.E. (1964) *Arch Klin Exp Dermatol* **319**, 415.
12 HORN-HEYDT G.E., *et al* (1967) *Arch Klin Exp Dermatol* **229**, 256.
13 INGRAM J.T. (1934) *Br J Dermatol* **46**, 272.
14 KLINGMÜLLER G. (1954) *Hautarzt* **5**, 23.
15 LUBACH D. & GLOWIENKA F. (1982) *Dermatologica* **164**, 1.
16 PRICE V.H. (1978) *Pediatr Clin North Am* **25**, 305.
17 RONDON LUGO A.J., *et al* (1977) *Dermatol Venezol* **15**, 23.
18 ROOK A. & DAWBER R. (1982) *Diseases of the Hair and Scalp*. Oxford, Blackwell Scientific, pp. 181, 182.
19 SALAMON T. & SCHNYDER U.W. (1962) *Arch Klin Exp Dermatol* **215**, 105.
20 SFAELLO Z. & HARIGA J. (1967) *Arch Belg Dermatol Syphiligr* **23**, 363.
21 SOLOMON I.L. & GREEN O.C. (1963) *N Engl J Med* **269**, 1279.
22 SUMMERLY R. & DONALDSON E.M. (1962) *Br J Dermatol* **74**, 387.

PSEUDOMONILETHRIX

This term has been applied to a complex defect of hair shaft formation observed in several large families of European or Indian descent in South Africa [1, 2]. The defect, inheritance of which is determined by an autosomal dominant gene of high penetrance, is manifest by the development of three abnormalities.

(i) *Pseudomonilethrix*: irregularly distributed nodal 'swellings' each 0·75–1 mm in length are present. On electron microscopy the 'nodes' are seen to be depressions with sides protruding beyond the normal diameter of the shaft. Similar changes may be seen in an artefact when hair fibres overlapping each other are mounted and pressed against each other for light microscopy.

(ii) *Twisted hairs*: the hairs are twisted irregularly through 25–200° with no flattening of the shafts.

(iii) *Broken hairs*: the breaks, which leave brush-like ends, occur in microscopically normal shafts.

Clinical features. Most patients present with a degree of alopecia, dependent on the vigour and frequency of hair brushing which breaks the excessively fragile shafts. It is usual for each affected individual to show only one of the three abnormalities, but broken hairs as well as either pseudomonilethrix or twisted hairs are seen in some. Clinically evident alopecia first develops most often between the ages of 8 and 14.

Microscopy differentiates the twisted hairs from classical pili torti in which the twists are regular and with flattening. Keratosis pilaris is absent.

If physical and chemical trauma to the hair can be reduced to a minimum, a considerable improvement in the alopecia may result.

REFERENCES

1 BENTLEY-PHILLIPS B. & BAYLES M.A.H. (1973) *Br J Dermatol* **89**, 159.
2 BENTLEY-PHILLIPS B. & BAYLES M.A.H. (1975) *Br J Dermatol* **92**, 113.

PILI ANNULATI
SYN. RINGED HAIR; BANDED HAIR; LEUCOTRICHIA ANNULARIS

Aetiology and pathology. The first accurate description of pili annulati was given by Wilson [7]. It is a rare developmental anomaly of the hair shaft, in most cases inherited as an autosomal dominant trait; in one report autosomal recessive inheritance was suggested [1]. Sporadic examples have occurred but mostly without adequate family studies.

Routine transmitted light microscopy reveals alternate light (normal) and dark (abnormal) bands of varying length, most being approximately 1 mm long [1, 5]; in reflected light—naked eye or microscopy—this band colour is reversed, the abnormal bands being light. Immersing the hairs in liquid of similar refractive index to hair keratin abolishes the optical banding [1]—in this way early workers proved that the 'colour' abnormality was due to air spaces and this was confirmed by scanning electron microscopy of transverse sections [1]. Electron microscopy and histochemistry have revealed normal keratinization but intermacrofibrillar spaces [2, 5]. The surface of some abnormal bands has a 'cobble-stoned' appearance with irregular cuticular cells [2].

Clinical features. Pili annulati may be present from birth or only noted as hair grows during the first 2 yr of life. Typically the majority of scalp hairs are affected; axillary hair involvement has been described. The hair grows to a normal length in most cases; if fragility is present even the shortest hairs tend to be at least 5 cm long. The alternate light and dark bands give the hair a distinctive sheen, described by one affected family as 'sandy'.

The condition is usually only diagnosed incidentally unless the hair is unduly fragile. Most affected individuals are otherwise normal; in one family inherited scalp blue naevi were associated [1]. Ringed hair was detected in some hair shafts in patients with woolly hair [4].

Diagnosis. Examination of hairs using low power microscopy establishes the diagnosis and differentiates ringed hair from pseudo pili annulati [6].

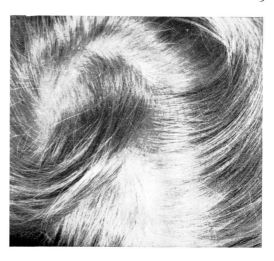

FIG. 53.52. Ringed hair in a girl aged 8 (Addenbrooke's Hospital).

Treatment. None is required in most cases. In those with fragile hair, cosmetic, chemical and physical trauma must be minimized.

REFERENCES

1 DAWBER R.P.R. (1972) *Trans St John's Hosp Dermatol Soc (Lond)* **58**, 51.
2 DAWBER R.P.R. & COMAISH S. (1970) *Arch Dermatol* **101**, 316.
3 GUMMER C.L. & DAWBER R.P.R. (1981) *Br J Dermatol* **105**, 401.
4 HUTCHINSON P.E., *et al* (1974) *Trans St John's Hosp Dermatol Soc (Lond)* **60**, 160.
5 PRICE V.H., *et al* (1968) *Arch Dermatol* **98**, 640.
6 PRICE V.H., *et al* (1970) *Arch Dermatol* **102**, 354.
7 WILSON E. (1867) *Proc R Soc Lond* 12th March.

PILI TORTI

Definition. Pili torti describes a structural defect in which the hair shaft is twisted on its own axis. It occurs in many variants, the morphological differences between which may prove to be of diagnostic significance.

Aetiology. Most commonly twisted hairs are a developmental defect which may be only one manifestation of a complex syndrome, e.g. Menkes' syndrome (p. 2011), Bjornstad's syndrome (p. 2012), Crandall's syndrome (p. 2012), pseudomonilethrix (p. 2008) or hypodrotic ectodermal dysplasia (p. 130).

When such cases have been excluded, there remain many in which pili torti appears to be the

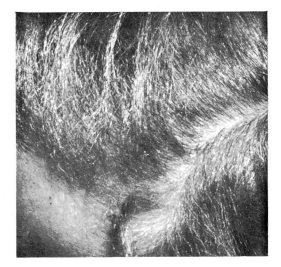

FIG. 53.53. Pili torti; the spangled appearance of the twisted hairs is well shown (Stoke Mandeville Hospital).

only abnormality. Most such cases appear to be determined by an autosomal dominant gene [1]. There are some reports of apparently sporadic cases [7], but relatives have not been carefully screened for subclinical involvement. Some cases have affected siblings of related parents. It seems probable that there are two distinct genotypes but the pub-lished evidence does not yet allow them to be differentiated phenotypically. Certain cases [9, 12] have unusually associated features and are, perhaps, distinct.

Irregularly twisted hairs may be formed as the result of deformation of the follicles in scarring inflammatory processes, as at the edge of patches of cicatricial alopecia [6].

Pathology [2, 5]. The affected hairs are flattened or ridged and the shaft is twisted on its axis at a few or many points along its length. The only histological abnormality is some curvature of the follicle. X-ray diffraction studies have shown only normal α-keratin patterns, but the polypeptide chains must show frequent deviation from parallelism, as in merino wool, which would explain the brittleness of the affected hair. With the scanning electron microscope, the cuticle appears normal [2, 3]. Arginosuccinicaciduria [9] and citrullaemia may be found. In those cases with fragile hair the fractures tend to occur within the twist.

Clinical features [5]. The hair is usually normal at birth but is progressively replaced by abnormal hair which becomes clinically evident by the second or third year. Onset, or perhaps recognition, has sometimes been delayed until adolescence or adult life. In some cases the child has been hairless at birth

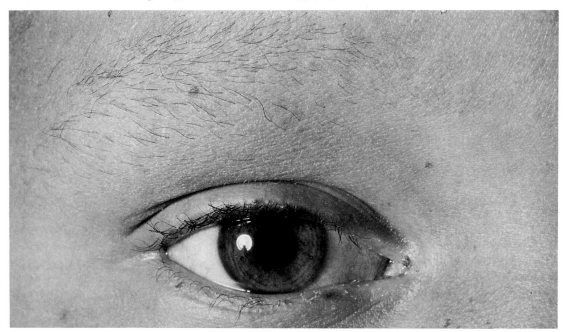

FIG. 53.54. Pili torti; involvement of eyebrows and eyelids (Dr Darrell Wilkinson).

and for the first few years of life. The affected hairs have a spangled appearance in reflected light. They are usually brittle and may break off at a length of 4 or 5 cm, or in some cases much less. The gross clinical appearance is very variable. There may be extensive stubble-like baldness, an occipital traumatic alopecia from friction on the pillow [8], an irregular and patchy baldness [11] or a more or less normal scalp in which the affected hairs must be carefully sought [10]. Some cases improve after puberty but others remain grossly abnormal throughout life. The eyebrows, eyelashes, and axillary and pubic hair are sometimes involved; rarely, vellus hairs are also affected [13].

Diagnosis. The diagnosis is established by microscope examination of several hairs. Ringed hair may give a similar appearance in reflected light.

Other hereditary causes of alopecia are listed in Table 53.4.

Treatment. None is available. Patients should be advised to avoid physically or chemically traumatic hairdressing procedures; careful use of conditioners can give quite long hair and minimize brittleness.

REFERENCES

1 APPEL B. & MESSINA S.J. (1942) *N Engl J Med* **226**, 912.
2 BJORNSTAD R.T. (1941) *Acta Derm Venereol (Stockh)* **22**, 242.
3 DAWBER R.P.R. (1977) *Clin Exp Dermatol* **2**, 271.
4 DAWBER R.P.R. & COMAISH S. (1970) *Arch Dermatol* **101**, 316.
5 HELLIER F.F., *et al* (1940) *Br J Dermatol* **52**, 173.
6 KURWA A.R. & ABDEL-AZIZ A.H.M. (1973) *Acta Derm Venereol (Stockh)* **53**, 585.
7 LYONS J.B. & DAWBER R.P.R. (1977) *Br J Dermatol* **96**, 197.
8 NICHAMIN S.J. (1958) *Am J Dis Child* **95**, 612.
9 PHILLIPS M.E., *et al* (1981) *J Roy Soc Med* **74**, 221.
10 SCOTT M.J., *et al* (1983) *Pediatr Dermatol* **1**, 45.
11 SISKIND W.M. (1947) *Arch Dermatol Syphilol* **56**, 540.
12 WHITING D.A. *et al* (1980) In *Hair, Trace Elements and Human Illness.* Eds. Brown A.C. & Crounse R. New York, Praeder, p. 238.
13 ZAUN H. & BURG G. (1969) *Aesthetic Med* **18**, 95.

MENKES' SYNDROME

Nomenclature and incidence. This distinctive syndrome was first described by Menkes and his colleagues in 1962 [6]. It is variously known as the 'kinky hair', 'stubbly hair' or 'steely hair' disease. It is probably not excessively rare, since seven cases in 5 families were seen at a children's hospital in Melbourne, Australia, over a period of 3 yr [3]. The frequency of the disease was established to be 1 in 35,000 live births.

Aetiology and pathology [1, 3, 7]. The basic defect, inheritance of which is determined by a sex-linked recessive gene, appears to be an abnormality of copper storage, with the observed defects resulting from inappropriate systemic copper distribution. It is probable that the presence of pili torti in a female relation is evidence of heterozygosity [2]. Metachromasia was seen in fibroblasts cultured from patients and from heterozygotes [3]. The primary abnormality may be in the metabolism of metallothionein, a metalloprotein involved in cellular copper transport [4]. Serum levels of copper and caeruloplasmin are low [5]. One patient [4] was able to absorb copper when given a daily dose 10 times larger than the normal requirement, but could synthesize caeruloplasmin only after copper was given intravenously. The copper deficiency is believed to be responsible for the extensive pathological changes present in many organs, including the diffuse neuronal damage, gliosis and cystic degeneration of the brain, and fragmentation of the elastin lamina in arterial walls. The abnormal hair, which is deficient in copper, shows an excess of sulphydryl groups [3].

Clinical features [3, 4, 6, 7]. Progressive psychomotor retardation, convulsions, instability of temperature and a general failure to thrive may for the first few weeks of life be accompanied by no clearly definable clue to the diagnosis. However, the facies may be recognizable—pale podgy cheeks lacking expressive movements and rather horizontal and twisted eyebrows [3]. The hair present at birth is normal. As this is in due course shed and replaced the new hair is found to be short, brittle, stubby and light in colour; under the light microscope the presence of pili torti (p. 2009) is readily demonstrable. Other associated structural defects such as monilethrix and trichorrhexis nodosa were mentioned in some early reports. One child, whose parents were black, had a very light coloured skin [7]. The disease is usually fatal before the age of 5 yr.

Treatment. It was suggested that intravenous copper may be of therapeutic value [2]. This has unfortunately not proved successful [4, 7].

REFERENCES

1 AGUILAR M.J., *et al* (1966) *J Neuropathol Exp Neurol* **25**, 507.

2 BUCKNALL W.E., *et al* (1973) *Pediatrics* **52**, 653.
3 DANKS D.M., *et al* (1972) *Pediatrics* **50**, 188.
4 HART D.B. (1983) *J Am Acad Dermatol* **9**, 145.
5 LOTT I.T., *et al* (1975) *N Engl J Med* **292**, 197.
6 MENKES J.H., *et al* (1962) *Pediatrics* **29**, 764.
7 WHEELER E.M. & ROBERTS P.F. (1976) *Arch Dis Child* **51**, 269.

BJORNSTAD'S SYNDROME AND CRANDALL'S SYNDROME

Pili torti occurs in association with sensorineural deafness. The syndrome is determined by an autosomal recessive gene. The hair shafts are ridged and twisted and their brittleness results in alopecia, the severity of which correlates with the degree of deafness [1, 4].

Similar defects of hair and of hearing [3] are associated with hypogonadism in a syndrome described by Crandall [2], which probably has a sex-linked recessive inheritance. There is a deficiency of luteinizing and growth hormones.

REFERENCES

1 BJORNSTAD R.T. (1965) *Proc Fennoscand Assoc Dermatol (Copenh)*, p. 3.
2 CRANDALL B.F., *et al* (1973) *J Pediatr* **82**, 461.
3 REED W.B., *et al* (1967) *Arch Dermatol* **95**, 456.
4 SCOTT M.J., *et al* (1983) *Pediatr Dermatol* **1**, 45.

WOOLLY HAIR

Woolly hair lacks any precise quantified definition; the term is used to describe tightly curled hair with some features of negroid hair rather than the 'crimped' contour of sheep wool [1]. Three syndromes in which such hair occurs have been more or less clinically characterized [3], but many case reports lack essential details and it is therefore possible that more than four distinct entities will ultimately be recognized. The nomenclature proposed by Hutchinson *et al* [3] has been adopted.

Hereditary woolly hair. This inherited condition is determined by an autosomal dominant gene; there is no consistent association with any hair colour. From birth to early infancy the hair is tightly curled, but tends to become less so in adult life. It is fine and brittle and may break as a result of associated trichorrhexis nodosa.

Pili annulati and pili torti have been reported in association with woolly hair but in different pedigrees [7]. Cataracts have been reported in some cases [4]. Recently, woolly hair has been reported in association with keratosis pilaris atrophicans and Noonan's syndrome [6].

Familial woolly hair. The lack of adequate case reports precludes dogmatism, but autosomal recessive inheritance is probable. The hair, which is fine, brittle and poorly pigmented, is tightly curled from birth; it may break at a length of 2 or 3 cm [3, 7].

Woolly hair naevus. This is not known to be inherited [2, 4, 5]. From birth or early infancy the hair in a circumscribed area of the scalp is tightly curled, and is lighter in colour than that of the remainder of the scalp. Over the next few years the size of the affected area, which may be scaly and irritable [5], may increase, but it usually does so only in proportion to general growth.

In over half the pigmented cases a pigmented or epidermal naevus has been present, not in the affected area of the scalp, but usually on the same side of the body [5]. Ocular defects may be present [4].

REFERENCES

1 FURANDO J., *et al* (1979) *Actas dermosifilogr* **70**, 203.
2 HASPER M.G. & KLOKKE A.H. (1983) *Br J Dermatol* **108**, 111–3.
3 HUTCHINSON P.E., *et al* (1974) *Trans St John's Hosp Dermatol Soc (Lond)* **60**, 160.
4 JACOBSEN L. & LOWES S. (1975) *Dermatologica* **151**, 249–52.
5 LANTIS S.D.H. & PEPPER M.G. (1978) *Arch Dermatol* **114**, 233.
6 NIELD V.S., *et al* (1984) *Br J Dermatol* **110**, 357.
7 VERBOV J. (1978) *Dermatologica* **157**, 42.

STRAIGHT HAIR NAEVUS

Straight hairs with a short anagen have been found within an epidermal naevus of the scalp in a negro child [2]; in another case only the focal straight hair was present [1].

REFERENCES

1 DOWNHAM T.F., *et al* (1976) *Int J Dermatol* **5**, 438.
2 GIBBS R.L. & BERGER R.A. (1970) *Int J Dermatol* **9**, 47.

ACQUIRED PROGRESSIVE KINKING OF HAIR

Definition. This is a progressive postpubertal transformation of terminal hair of the scalp from its normal contour into a 'kinked' or pubic hair type of morphology.

Aetiology and pathology. The name was first coined by Wise & Sultzberger [3]. The entity described as whisker hair [2] appears to be synonymous. The aetiology of acquired progressive kinking is unknown. The hairs in the affected region show both structural and functional abnormalities [1]; affected fibres are irregularly kinked with half twists visible in the microscope. The reported cases have all been in men.

Clinical features. Onset is typically in the second or third decade of life. The patient gradually becomes aware of the change in hair character; usually it is first noticed on the vertex and hair margins. The boundaries between affected and unaffected areas remain ill defined.

In most cases this morphological change predates the development of androgenetic alopecia.

Treatment. None is known.

REFERENCES

1 COUPE R.L. & JOHNSTON M.N. (1969) *Arch Dermatol* **100**, 191.
2 NORWOOD O.T. (1981) *Cutis* **27**, 651.
3 WISE F. & SULZBERGER M.B. (1932) *Arch. Dermatol. Syphilol* **25**, 99.

'CHAND' SYNDROME

This syndrome has been reported to be inherited as an autosomal dominant trait. It has associated curly hair (not woolly hair), ankyloblepharon and nail dysplasia [1].

REFERENCE

1 BAUGHMAN F.A. (1971) *Birth Defects* **7**, 160.

CURLY HAIR IN OTHER HEREDITARY SYNDROMES

Tricho-dento-osseous (TDO) syndrome [1–3]. The characteristic features of this syndrome, determined by an autosomal dominant gene, are strikingly curly hair, small widely spaced teeth with defective enamel, dolichocephaly, frontal bossing, a square jaw and increased bone density. Children are born with a full head of hair described as 'kinky' but showing no abnormality under the microscope; it tends to straighten during childhood.

Curly hair has been recorded as a presenting sign in giant axonal neuropathy.

REFERENCES

1 GEBHART W., *et al* (1979) In *Hair Research*. Eds. Orfanos C., *et al*. Berlin, Springer, p. 420.
2 LICHSTENSTEIN J., *et al* (1972) *Am J Hum Genet* **14**, 569.
3 ROBINSON G.C., *et al* (1966) *Pediatrics* **37**, 498.

TRICHONODOSIS

Trichonodosis (knotting) is a relatively common condition well known to hairdressers which is more common in Negroid or curly hair [1, 2]. It is probably induced by frictional forces between adjacent fibres. Scanning electron microscopy shows degenerative changes within each knot—longitudinal fissures, fractures and loss of cuticular scales.

The condition is not conspicuous and must be deliberately sought. Usually, only a minority of scalp hairs are affected. Pubic and other body hair may also be affected, particularly when pediculosis induces rubbing and scratching [3].

Brushing and combing may pull out the knotted fibres or cause enhanced weathering and ultimate shaft breakage.

(See also Matting, p. 2031.)

REFERENCES

1 DAWBER R.P.R. (1974) *Br J Dermatol* **91**, 169.
2 ENGLISH D.T. & JONES H.E. (1973) *Arch Dermatol* **107**, 77.
3 SCOTT M.J. (1951) *Arch Dermatol* **63**, 769.

TRICHOSTASIS SPINULOSA

Aetiology and pathology. Trichostasis spinulosa is inconspicuous and therefore rarely diagnosed, but it is not uncommon [2] in young and middle-aged adults; recent experience [5] does not support the contention that it is most frequent over the age of 50 [1]. The term was coined in the belief that the disorder resulted from the retention within a single follicle of successive vellus hairs. It is more probable that the condition represents a physiological involutionary stage in a variant form of follicle; histological studies show multiple matrices with a common follicular orifice.

Clinical features. Numerous comedo-like black dots develop in the 'seborrhoeic regions'—the vertex, the forehead, temples, nose and cheeks, the neck, the upper chest and back, and the shoulders and upper arms [3]. With a hand lens the dots are seen to be small projecting tufts of fine hairs. The tufts are easily extracted and are found to contain up to 50 short hairs embedded in a horny plug [2]. In one report seborrhoeic keratoses were associated [3].

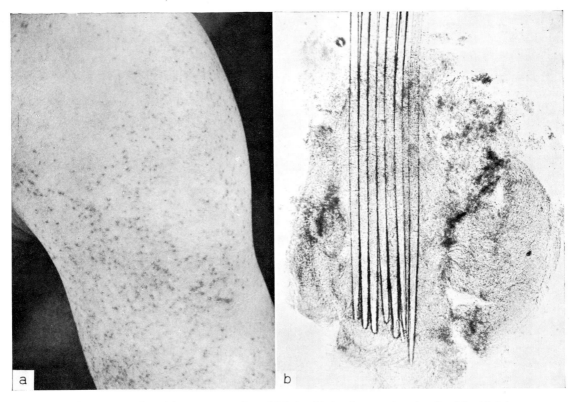

FIG. 53.55. Trichostasis spinulosa: (a) conspicuous plugged follicles: (b) the plug contains a bundle of short hairs.

Treatment [4, 5] Keratolytics are of little value, but depilatory wax has been used successfully, and topical retinoic acid is also effective [4].

REFERENCES

1 GOLDSCHMIDT H., *et al* (1974) In *First Human Hair Symposium.* Ed. Brown A.C. New York, Medcom, p. 50.
2 KAILASAM, *et al* (1979) *Int J Dermatol* **18**, 297.
3 KOSSARD S., *et al* (1979) *J Cutan Pathol* **6**, 492.
4 MILLS O.H. & KLIGMAN A.M. (1973) *Arch Dermatol* **108**, 378.
5 SARKANY I. & GAYLARDE P.M. (1971) *Br J Dermatol* **84**, 311.

BAYONET HAIRS

Bayonet hairs appear to represent a developmental defect of the hair shaft, possibly associated with some degree of excessive keratinization of the upper third of the follicle [1]. A few may be detected in normal scalps, especially near the vertex; their frequency is said to be increased in both seborrhoea and ichthyosis.

Just below the hair tip is a spindle-shaped thickening of the shaft, and above this the shaft tapers off to a fine point. The spindle is 2 or 3 mm long and can be seen under the microscope to result from thickening of the cortex, which is also hyperpigmented.

REFERENCE

1 PINKUS F. (1910) *Dermatol Z* **18**, 253.

TRICHOTHIODYSTROPHY

Definition. Trichothiodystrophy (sulphur-deficient brittle hair) is a clinical marker of a severe congenital syndrome with complex and variable neuro-ectodermal changes.

The BIDS, IBIDS [4] and PIBIDS [1, 7] syndromes and the Marinesco–Sjögren syndrome [5] are specific subtypes.

Aetiology. Most cases described show no family history; where family cases have occurred, the pattern suggests autosomal recessive inheritance.

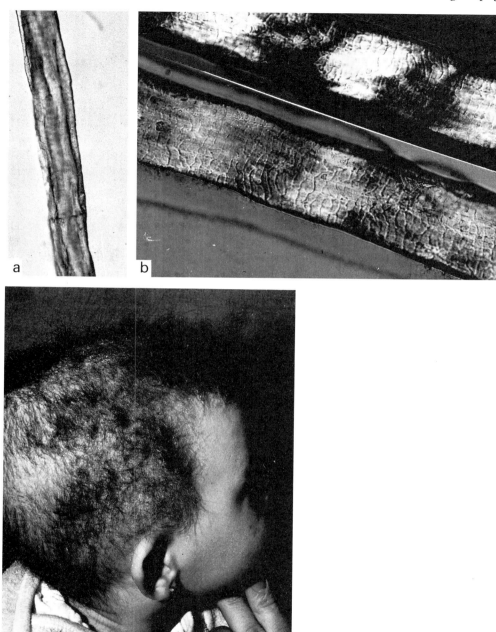

FIG. 53.56. Trichothiodystrophy.
(a) In the scanning electron microscope the hairs are seen to be flattened and irregularly ridged and fluted (Dr Van Neste, Lille).
(b) Alternating bright and dark zones in the polarizing microscope (Dr Van Neste, Lille).
(c) Moderately severe alopecia in trichothiodystrophy (Dr Van Neste, Lille).

Pathology and biochemistry [2, 6]. The hair is typically short, brittle and flattened ('ribbon like') with both trichorrhexis nodosa and trichoschisis fractures, together with advanced cuticular weathering. When viewed with plane-polarized light the hair usually shows alternating light and dark ('zigzag') bands. Light and scanning electron microscopy may show twists; this is not pili torti in which the twists are 'fixed' in the follicle but is due to the floppiness of the ribbon-like hairs.

The total sulphur content of the hair is reduced to about half normal levels. Two-dimensional electrophoresis has shown a reduction in the high sulphur protein fraction [2]. Electron histochemical studies have demonstrated that this reduction is specifically located in the cuticular A layer and the cortex matrix protein [3].

It is not known whether sulphur deficiency is the basis of the defects in the nervous system.

Clinical features. The affected individuals show neuro-ectodermal abnormalities from birth. As well as the characteristic short brittle hair, the clinical signs may include atrophic nails, koilonychia, lamellar ichthyosis, photosensitivity [1], dental caries, dwarfism, mental retardation, congenital cataracts, spasticity, ataxia and decreased fertility.

REFERENCES

1 CROVATO F., *et al* (1983) *Br J Dermatol* **108**, 247.
2 GILLESPIE J.M. & MARSHALL R.C. (1983) *J Invest Dermatol* **80**, 195.
3 GUMMER C.L., *et al* (1984) *Br J Dermatol* **110**, 439.
4 JORIZZO J.L., *et al* (1982) *Br J Dermatol* **106**, 705.
5 PRICE V.H., *et al* (1980) *Arch Dermatol* **116**, 1375.
6 VAN NESTE D. (1983) *Ann Dermatol Vénéréol* **110**, 409.
7 VAN NESTE D. *et al* (1985) *J Amer Acad Derm* **12**, 372.

TRICHORRHEXIS NODOSA

Definition. Trichorrhexis nodosa is a distinctive response of the hair shaft to physical or chemical trauma, and is characterized by the development of cuticular fissuring and fractures, and of nodes consisting of cortical cells protruding through the cuticular defect [4].

Aetiology [1, 3, 6, 10]. The essential provocative factor is trauma. Previously normal hair is damaged only by trauma of some severity, such as the repeated application of heat, bleaches or thioglycollates, or by frequent rubbing, as in a patch of lichen simplex. In one patient seasonal recurrences were related to the cumulative effect of sunlight, seabathing and brushing [11].

In the presence of an abnormal brittle shaft, the minor trauma of normal friction, brushing and combing may induce node formation and fracture. Such is the situation in development defects such as monilethrix, pseudomonilethrix and trichothiodystrophy. Occasionally, congenital susceptibility to node formation may be inherited as a dominant character [5] in the absence of any other gross defect of the shaft. It occurs in otherwise normal individuals, but has been reported in Apert's syndrome [1]. Nutritional deficiencies or systemic illnesses [8] may temporarily increase susceptibility.

Trichorrhexis nodosa induced by trivial trauma occurs very readily in some patients with a hereditary metabolic disorder manifest as arginosuccinic aciduria [13]; mental retardation is associated. Most children with this disease do not have abnormal hair [2].

Pathology. At the nodes the cuticle is damaged and cortical cells protrude through. Fracture of the hair occurs at a node to leave an end like a paint brush. The remainder of the hair shaft shows a disorderly scale pattern and other evidence of wear and tear—excessive 'weathering' [4].

Clinical features [1, 3, 10, 12, 14]. Nodes, usually one but sometimes more, on each affected shaft appear as white or yellow points. The total clinical picture depends on the degree of inherent fragility of the hair, its length and natural form, and the amount and type of trauma to which it has been subjected. Several clinical syndromes may be differentiated.

In Negroid hair the 'proximal type' occurs [12] and there may be patches of irregular alopecia in which hairs with nodes 1–5 cm above the scalp are associated with broken stumps. There is always a history of physical and chemical trauma, often over a long period. Hair straightening has frequently been attempted [7].

In adults of most other races the nodes tend to be nearer the tips of the hairs—the 'distal type'. If they are few they are subclinical and an incidental finding. Often they are associated with hairs that are fractured or split longitudinally (trichoptilosis). The patient may complain that her hair is dry and brittle.

Where trichorrhexis complicates a hereditary defect of the hair shaft, dry, brittle and broken hair—patchy or throughout the scalp—may be present from early childhood.

In circumscribed traumatic alopecia, such as may complicate lichen simplex, many hairs show trichorrhexis nodosa and fracture. Node formation may occur in any hairy region as the result of rubbing or scratching [3]. In the literature there are many reports, usually under the diagnosis of idiopathic trichoclasis, in which patchy alopecia with trichorrhexis in children is said not to be attributed to trauma. Dominant inheritance of this condition is reported [5, 6]. The evidence excluding trauma is not conclusive.

Finally, there is an acquired syndrome [14] in which the hairs in a circumscribed patch of scalp, beard and moustache show multiple nodes and readily fracture; generalized nodes have been described [9]. Spontaneous recovery ultimately occurs.

Diagnosis and treatment. Microscopy readily excludes nits and hair casts, monilethrix and other developmental defects.

The only practicable treatment in most cases is the avoidance of physical and chemical trauma. Abnormalities of amino acid metabolism should be excluded by urine examination.

REFERENCES

1 AOYASI T. & PORTER P.S. (1976) In *Biology and Diseases of the Hair.* Eds. Toda K., *et al.* Baltimore, University Park Press, p. 473.
2 CEDERBAUM S.D., *et al* (1973) *Am J Ment Defic* **77**, 395.
3 CHERNOSKY M.E. & OWENS D.W. (1966) *Arch Dermatol* **94**, 577.
4 DAWBER R.P.R. & COMAISH S. (1970) *Arch Dermatol* **101**, 316.
5 DORN H. (1956) *Z Haut GeschlKrankh* **20**, 129.
6 FRIEDRICH H.C. (1950) *Z Haut GeschlKrankh* **8**, 163.
7 JOLLY H.W. & CARPENTER C.L. (1967) *Cutis*, **3**, 359.
8 LEIDER M. (1950) *Arch Dermatol Syphilol* **62**, 510.
9 LEONARD J., *et al* (1980) *Br J Dermatol* **103**, 85.
10 OWENS D.W. & CHERNOSKY M.E. (1966) *Arch Dermatol* **94**, 586.
11 PAPA C.M., *et al* (1972) *Arch Dermatol* **105**, 888.
12 PRICE V. (1975) *Cutis* **15**, 231.
13 RAUSCHKOLB E.W., *et al* (1967) *J Invest Dermatol* **48**, 260.
14 SABOURAUD R. (1921) *Ann Dermatol Syphilol* **2**, 445.

TRICHORRHEXIS INVAGINATA
SYN. BAMBOO HAIRS

The bamboo hairs of Netherton's syndrome may appear similar to trichorrhexis nodosa. The hair is sparse and brittle, and in addition to other defects shows bamboo-like nodes with 'telescoping' preceding fracture. The other features of the syndrome (p. 1428) establish the diagnosis.

TRICHOPTILOSIS

Trichoptilosis is longitudinal splitting of the distal end of the hair shaft. In some cases the split extends a considerable distance along the shaft. It is extremely common in those with long hair, for its incidence and severity are related to the cumulative physical and chemical trauma to which the hair has been subjected during its lifetime [1]. It is often associated with trichorrhexis nodosa, trichoclasis and other evidence of hair damage.

The split ends may be cut off. Only reduction in the degree of further chemical and physical trauma will prevent recurrence.

REFERENCE

1 FREIDERICH H.C. & FRÖB G. (1949) *Dermatol Wochenschr* **120**, 674.

TRICHOSCHISIS

This term has been coined to describe a clean transverse fracture of the hair shaft in contrast with trichoclasis which is an irregular transverse, sometimes 'greenstick', fracture [1].

Trichoschisis has been reported [2] in a girl aged 4 with extreme fragility of the scalp hair. This was the result of deficient synthesis of high sulphur matrix type hair protein—probably an example of the syndrome of trichothiodystrophy (p. 2014). It also occurs in the IBIDS syndrome [3].

REFERENCES

1 BROWN A.C. (1971) *Birth Defects* **7**, 52.
2 BROWN A.C., *et al* (1970) *J Invest Dermatol* **54**, 496.
3 JORIZZO J.L., *et al* (1982) *Br J Dermatol* **106**, 705.

TRICHOMALACIA

The status of this condition, which was described by Miescher [2] in 1942, is still uncertain. It was associated with a hair-pulling tic in an elderly woman. Although this has not been an obvious factor in other cases, which have occurred in young children [1, 3], histological studies in trichotillomania (p. 1993) support the assumption that trichomalacia is usually the result of traumatic injury to hair follicles. A similar localized and temporary alopecia reported in a strain of mice [4] is unexplained.

Histologically, some follicles are plugged and contain coiled deformed swollen hairs and there may be some perivascular lymphocytic infiltration.

Irregular and poorly defined patches of total or partial alopecia develop in the occipital or parietal region. The scanty remaining hairs are soft, fragile and considerably larger than normal. The condition eventually remits spontaneously.

REFERENCES

1 HAENSCH R. & BLAICH W. (1960) *Arch Klin Exp Dermatol* **210**, 447.
2 MIESCHER G. (1942) *Arch Dermatol Syphilol* **183**, 117.
3 MULLER R. & GIRARDET P. (1957) *Dermatologica* **115**, 717.
4 PINKUS H. (1965) In *Biology of the Skin and Hair Growth.* Eds. Lyne A.G. & Short B.F. Sydney, Angus & Robertson.

UNCOMBABLE HAIR SYNDROME
SYN. CHEVEUX INCOIFFABLES

This unusual hair defect was simultaneously described in the U.S.A. as spun-glass hair [4] and in France as cheveux incoiffables [3]. Based on microcope findings it is sometimes also termed pili trianguli et canaliculi [1, 5].

Scanning electron microscopy shows two essential abnormalities: a triangular section with rounded angles and a longitudinal groove along one or several sides of the hair. These changes affect the majority of scalp hairs [3].

Clinically, the condition is characterized by short, sparse, unruly and frizzy hair [2, 4]. It is usually an isolated defect but has been reported in association with Wilson's disease [3] and atopic eczema with hamartomas [2].

Differential diagnosis is from pili torti which is easily diagnosed using low power light microscopy.

REFERENCES

1 BRAUN-FALCO O., et al (1982) *Hautarzt* **33**, 336.
2 CRONIN J. (1982) *Ann Dermatol Vénéréol* **109**, 373.
3 DUPRE A. & BONAFE J.L. (1978) *Arch Dermatol Res* **261**, 217.
4 STROUD J.D. & MEHREGAN A.H. (1973) In *The First Human Hair Symposium.* Eds. Brown A.C. & Crounse R. New York, Medcom, p. 103.
5 VAN NESTE D., et al (1981) *Arch Dermatol Res* **271**, 225.

UNCHARACTERIZED DEFECTS

Many defects of the hair shaft remain uncharacterized. It is indeed often difficult to distinguish with certainty between primary defects in hair formation and changes induced by trauma in abnormally vulnerable hairs which are structurally normal at least on light microscopy. To try to define intrinsic defects, it is therefore important always to examine plucked or close-cut hair to view proximal changes.

Two abnormalities which have been described [1] are the fragile banded hairs of citrullinaemia and the abruptly narrowed hairs sometimes seen in association with other hereditary defects.

REFERENCE

1 PORTER P.S. & LOBITZ W.C. (1970) *Br J Dermatol* **83**, 225.

Rolled hairs (syn. 'Poils en spirale'). Rolled or spiral hairs [3] are commonly associated with ichthyosis of autosomal dominant type or with keratosis pilaris of other origins. The tightly coiled hairs lie beneath the horny plug obstructing the mouth of the follicle [2], especially on the back or the extensor aspects of the limbs. They are frequently to be found on the thighs and abdomen of men aged 50 and over [1] without other evident abnormality of the follicles.

REFERENCES

1 ADATTO R. (1963) *Dermatologica* **127**, 145.
2 FERGUSON A.G. & DERBLAY P.R. (1963) *Arch Dermatol* **87**, 311.
3 LEVIT F. & SCOTT M.J. (1983) *J Am Acad Dermatol* **8**, 423.

Hair casts (syn. Peripilar keratin casts). These are firm yellowish-white accretions [2] ensheathing but not attached to scalp hairs and freely movable up and down the hair shaft [1]. They are very common in 'parakeratotic' hair disorders, e.g. psoriasis and seborrhoeic dermatitis, and with traction hair styles and following the use of hair 'lacquers'. They may be misdiagnosed as *Pediculosis capitis* ova capsules [3] which are easily differentiated microscopically—also 'nits' are firmly attached to the hair.

The classification of hair casts has recently been revised, differentiating keratin and non-keratin types [4].

REFERENCES

1 DAWBER R.P.R. (1979 *Br J Dermatol* **100**, 417.
2 KLIGMAN A.M. (1957) *Arch Dermatol* **75**, 509.
3 KOHN S.R. (1977) *JAMA* **238**, 2058–9.
4 SCOTT M.J. & ROENIGK H.H. (1983) *J Am Acad Dermatol* **8**, 27.

DIFFERENTIAL DIAGNOSIS OF ALOPECIA

The term alopecia is derived from the Greek word for fox, allegedly because foxes may suffer from patchy loss of hair. It was originally applied only to the disorder now known as alopecia areata, but current usage applies the unqualified term alopecia to loss of hair of any type and any origin.

Patients with alopecia account for from 3% to 8% of new outpatient attendances at most dermatological clinics in Europe, but so many social factors influence hospital attendance that no valid conclusions can be drawn as to possible geographical variations in incidence.

In the differential diagnosis of alopecia, the dermatologists should first determine the pattern of hair loss, then the state of the scalp and finally the presence of any abnormality of the hair itself.

The pattern of alopecia. The patterns of hair loss can be broadly classified in four groups.

(1) *Bitemporal and frontovertical.* This is the classical pattern of male baldness. The onset is invariably slow, and the apparent rapid development of androgenetic alopecia over the course of a few weeks should always suggest the possibility that diffuse loss of hair is unveiling a previously subclinical alopecia, i.e. the patient has in fact two types of alopecia. If this possibility can be excluded see p. 1971.

(2) *Diffuse.* The loss of hair is distributed evenly over the entire scalp. Pre-existing androgenetic alopecia is a source of diagnostic error. A careful history must be taken with special reference to recent illness, pregnancy or stress and the ingestion of drugs or other chemicals (p. 1980). Exceptionally the hair loss is initially diffuse in alopecia areata

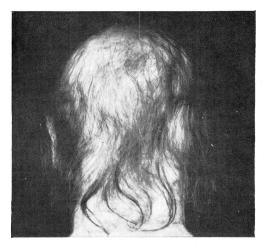

FIG. 53.57 Secondary syphilis: severe diffuse alopecia (Dr G. Lomholt).

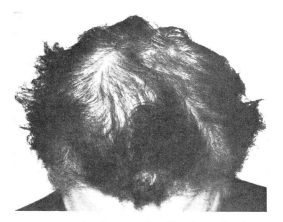

FIG. 53.58. Patchy alopecia induced by chemical and physical trauma—too frequent dyeing and waving. Many hairs show trichorrhexis nodosa and almost all show extensive fraying of the cuticle of the cortex (Addenbrooke's Hospital).

(p. 1985), secondary syphilis (p. 852), lichen planus (p. 2000) and lupus erythematosus (p. 1289).

Diffuse alopecia present from infancy is often associated with defects of the hair shaft in the various forms of congenital alopecia (p. 1976).

Diffuse alopecia with abnormalities of the hair shafts beginning in adult life should suggest external physical or chemical injury (p. 1992).

(3) *Marginal.* The loss of hair is confined to a strip along the margin of the scalp. Alopecia areata may assume this form. Irregular marginal alopecia with twisted hairs, folliculitis and some scarring may be produced by some hairdressing procedures (p. 1995).

(4) *Patchy.* The loss of hair occurs in patches which are single or multiple, rounded, oval or irregular. This pattern of loss can be produced by so many disorders that careful examination of the scalp and microscopy of hair are usually required before a diagnosis can be made.

The state of the scalp. Whatever the pattern of alopecia, the whole scalp should be carefully examined, and particular attention must be given to its state in the bald areas, which should be inspected with a magnifying lens. The scalp is usually normal in androgenetic and diffuse alopecias, and in alopecia areata of classical or marginal distribution. Scaling in the form of pityriasis is an extremely common finding and is not causally related to any form of alopecia. The scaly plaques of psoriasis are also an incidental finding and are not the cause of any alopecia which may be present, although hair shedding may be increased in plaques of psoriasis as shown by a raised telogen ratio, and scarring may develop following inflammatory changes after the sudden withdrawal of strong corticosteroids. Scaling more or less confined to the areas of alopecia is a characteristic feature of some forms of ringworm (p. 911) and is often seen in traumatic alopecia, particularly in association with lichen simplex of the scalp). In both ringworm and traumatic alopecia the hairs may be twisted and broken, but in ringworm they may be of abnormal texture and colour, whereas in traumatic alopecias the hair shafts are essentially normal.

The scalp may be scarred and the hair follicles destroyed. The recognition of scarring is of the greatest diagnostic and prognostic importance (see cicatricial alopecias (p. 1996)). The scarring may be gross and unmistakable, but if only small areas are involved it may be difficult to identify with confidence. Repeated observation and sometimes histological examination may be required.

Other scalp changes must be carefully noted. Follicular plugging, telangiectasia or pigmentary anomalies may assist the diagnosis.

The hair. Microscope examination of the hair is essential in the reliable diagnosis of most forms of alopecia. A minimum of five to ten hairs should be plucked; if obviously abnormal hairs are present these will be selected, but if the hair appears grossly normal hairs should be plucked from the edge of the patch of alopecia or, if the hair loss is diffuse, from the parietal region. The hairs should be mounted dry and examined first under low power and then under high power of the microscope in a suitable microscopy mounting medium. In patchy alopecia, whether the scalp surface be normal, scaly or scarred, some of the hairs should be mounted in 20% potassium hydroxide and examined for the presence of fungus (p. 888).

By simple direct microscopy of the hair shaft it is possible to identify a variety of developmental and acquired defects (p. 2006). Physical or chemical injury to the hair shafts can be recognized; ringworm can be excluded or direct support for a diagnosis of alopecia areata can be obtained.

Polarized light microscopy may unmask a shaft biochemical defect (see trichothiodystrophy (p. 2014)).

Examination of the bulbs of plucked hairs may be of diagnostic value in some forms of diffuse alopecia. Distinctive changes produced by antimitotic agents may be indentifiable by anagen root analysis (p. 1981) and androgenetic alopecia treatment monitored by standardized telogen counting.

Other diagnostic procedures
Wood's light. The use of Wood's light is fully described in Chapter 24 (p. 892). In the presence of patchy hair loss, particularly in the presence of scaling, this procedure can be of the greatest value in the diagnosis of ringworm.

Biopsy. This is helpful in the differential diagnosis of cicatricial alopecias and occasionally in other forms. If biopsy is considered advisable the specimen taken should not be too small and sections should be cut in the direction of slope of the hair follicles. Serial sections will often be necessary if accurate pathogenic and diagnostic information is to be obtained.

HAIR PIGMENTS

The colour of hair depends on the number, size and distribution of pigment granules in the cortex and the nature of the pigment present and various optical effects [1, 3]. The granules in black and blonde hair also differ in their internal structure [6, 7]. The pigment may be masked by defects in the structure of the shaft, by keratinophilic artificial dyes or by exogenous substances which coat the hair shaft.

The wide range of shades in human hair is produced largely by two pigments—the brown-black eumelanin, and pheomelanin which gives the light shades and reds; the latter pigment is produced initially by a similar pathway to eumelanin but later by a condensation reaction with cysteine [8, 9], i.e. via the condensation of dopa quinone with cysteine to produce cysteine dopa and the oxidation and polymerization of cysteine dopa [5].

Each follicle's complement of melanocytes is said to be diffusely distributed throughout the dermal papilla during the telogen phase of the hair cycle. During the early stages of anagen they become aligned along the margin and apex of the matrix, and by anagen III tyrosinase activity can normally be demonstrated. However, at least in the rabbit [9] the melanocytes remain at the surface of the papilla throughout telogen, but in a shrunken inconspicuous form without dendrites. In anagen these cells enlarge and develop dendrites. There may be species differences in the behaviour of melanocytes during the hair cycle but in all species investigated the melanocytes transfer melanin granules to the migrating columns of epithelial cells of the hair during the later stages of anagen, i.e. to prospective cortical cells. The dendritic processses of the melanocytes play an important part in effecting the transfer of melanin, but the mechanism is not fully elucidated. Melanocytes without dendrites may also transfer pigment [9]. The follicular melanocytes respond like the epidermal melanocytes to α-MSH, which darkens light-coloured hair [2]. For a fuller account of these processes the papers by Fitzpatrick and his colleagues [4] and Straile [9] may be consulted.

It is evident that even our present limited knowledge allows us to envisage on theoretical grounds a wide variety of possible disturbances of hair pigmentation. Not all have yet been shown actually to occur.

(1) Absence of melanocytes
(2) Structural abnormalities of the melanocyte
    (a) Genetically determined—piebaldism
    (b) Acquired $\begin{cases} \text{vitiligo} \\ \text{ageing} \\ \text{after ionizing radiation} \end{cases}$
(3) Tyrosine deficiency
    (a) Genetically determined—albinism
    (b) In nutritional deficiency of copper. Copper is the prosthetic group of tyrosinase. Achromotrichia occurs in some animals on diets low in copper.
(4) Tyrosine inhibition
    Phenylketonuria. The tyrosine–tyrosinase reaction is inhibited by phenylalanine. Phenylthiourea inhibits melanin formation.
(5) Inhibition of phaeomelanin formation
    Chloroquine inhibits the formation of phaeomelanin but not of eumelanin.
(6) Abnormal keratinization of the hair shaft
    The epithelial cells may be unable to accept melanin granules from normal melanocytes. This could account for the loss of hair pigment induced by cholesterol-lowering agents and by the relative lack of pigment in some hereditary defects of the hair shaft. Keratinization defects may give optical colour changes with abnormal melanogenesis, e.g. in pili annulati (p. 2009).

REFERENCES

1 BIRBECK M.S.C. & BARNICOT N.A. (1959) In *Pigment Cell Biology: Proceedings of the Fourth Conference on Normal and Atypical Pigment Cell Growth*. Ed. Gordon M. New York, Academic Press, p. 54.
2 CLIVE D. & SNELL R. (1967) *J Invest Dermatol* **49**, 314.
3 FINDLAY G.H. (1982) *Br J Dermatol* **107**, 517.
4 FITZPATRICK T.B., *et al* (1958) In *The Biology of Hair Growth*. Eds. Montagna W. & Ellis R.A. New York, Academic Press.
5 MENON I.A., *et al* (1983) *J Invest Dermatol* **80**, 202.
6 MOTTAZ, J.H. & ZELICKSON A.S. (1969) In *Hair Growth*. Eds. Montagna W. & Dobson R.L. Oxford, Pergamon, p. 471.
7 ORFANOS C. & RUSKA H. (1968) *Arch Klin Exp Dermatol* **232**, 279.
8 PROTA G. (1980) *J Invest Derm* **75**, 122.
9 STRAILE W.E. (1964) *Dev Biol* **10**, 45.

VARIATIONS IN HAIR COLOUR

The importance of hair colour to the happiness of a steadily increasing proportion of women and men is reflected in the vast expenditure of time and money on efforts to change it. If such deliberate interference with the designs of nature be excluded, gross variation in hair colour is very largely genetically determined. Metabolic and nutritional disorders and certain drugs are occasionally implicated, and accidental discoloration can also occur.

Hereditary variation. Little is known about the inheritance of hair colour in man, but detailed investigations in many laboratory and domestic animals have shown a general conformity in the complement of genes affecting hair colour [2, 11], and it is reasonable to assume that a somewhat similar complex of genes may be involved in man. The anatomical and biochemical basis of hair colour has been described above; the colour depends on the chemical nature and quantity of pigment and its distribution in the hair shaft. Each of these factors must be influenced by several genes, some of which are pleiotropic and also affect other parts of the body.

The association between hair colour and hair form and other racial characteristics primarily of interest to the anthropologist is discussed on p. 1955. There are also obvious associations between hair colour and the colour of the iris [7]. Of greater significance to the dermatologist is the association between hair colour and the degree of pigmentation and other properties of the skin.

Red hair (syn. rutilism). This is easily recognized, and its associations have therefore attracted more attention than have other hair colours. Red hair appears to be recessive to non-red [9, 12], but the masking of red pigment by melanin could explain apparently contradictory findings [10]. There is some evidence that the gene for red hair gives rise to freckling with brown hair in the homozygote [8]. The incidence of red hair ranges from about 0·3% in Northern Germany, 1·6% in Paris and 3·7% in England to up to 11% in parts of Scotland. The skin of the redhead tends to be fair and sensitive, with a poor tanning response to sunlight, often forming freckles on exposed skin, and a poor resistance to chemical irritants. Traditionally, the redhead is ab-

normally susceptible to rheumatic fever and tuberculosis, but recent statistically controlled studies are
lacking.

**Planning investigations on the inheritance and
associations of hair colour.** Large-scale cutaneous
and systemic investigations of hair colour could
make an important contribution to our knowledge
of racial factors in disease, but most of the reports
in the clinical literature are anecdotal. Future surveys should be planned with the cooperation of an
anthropologist and a statistician. Hair colour may
be classified by subjective visual matching with an
internationally accepted scale, such as the Fischer–
Saller scale, or more reliably by spectrophotometry
of solutions of hair pigment [4–6]. Allowance must
be made for the darkening of hair by approximately
1 Fischer–Saller unit with each year of age from 6
to 18 [13] and the effects of sun bleaching and
chemical contaminants.

Physiological and pathological greying (canities)
and circumscribed loss of hair pigment (poliosis) are
largely genetic in origin, and are considered fully
below.

Heterochromia. This term describes the growth of
hair of two distinct colours. A colour difference between the hairs of scalp and moustache is not uncommon. Rarely, the hair in a circumscribed patch
or patches in the scalp differs distinctively in colour
from the surrounding hair. These cases fall into five
groups:

(a) dark, often black, hair, frequently of coarse
texture, grows in a tuft from a melanocytic naevus;
(b) patches of heterochromic hair arising in normal scalp may be an hereditary trait, usually determined by an autosomal dominant gene (e.g. tufts of
red hair at the temples in an otherwise black head
or a single black patch in a blonde [3];
(c) partial bilateral asymmetry of hair and eye
colour may occur sporadically, perhaps as a result
of somatic mosaicism [1];
(d) the white forelock in piebaldism (p. 1587);
(e) the 'flag sign' in kwashiorkor (p. 2328).

REFERENCES

1 AHUJA Y.R. (1960) *Acta Genet Stat Med* 9, 427.
2 FITZPATRICK T.B. (1958) In *The Biology of Hair Growth.*
Eds. Montagna W. & Ellis R.A. New York, Academic
Press.
3 FROHN W. (1938) *Dermatol Z* 77, 4.
4 HANNA B.L. (1956) *Am J Phys Anthropol* 14, 153.
5 HANNA B.L. (1961) *Am J Phys Anthropol* 19, 351.
6 LEA A.J. (1954) *Ann Hum Genet* 19, 97.
7 MANNY H. (1942) *Ann Eugen* 11, 189.
8 NICHOLLS E.M. (1969) *Hum Hered* 19, 36.
9 REED T.E. (1952) *Ann Eugen* 17, 115.
10 RIFE D.C. (1967) *Acta Genet Med Gemmellol (Roma)* 16,
342.
11 SEARLE A.G. (1968) *Comparative Genetics of Coat Colour
in Mammals.* London, Logos Press.
12 SINGLETON W.R. & ELLIS B. (1964) *J Hered* 55, 261.
13 STEGGERDA M. (1941) *J Hered* 32, 402.

CANITIES
SYN. GREYING OF THE HAIR

Aetiology [4–6]. Canities is a physiological manifestation of the ageing process. There is a gradual dilution of pigment in the greying hairs so that in
different hairs the full range of colours from normal
to white can be found. The loss of pigment in the
hair shafts is associated with a progressive loss of
tyrosinase activity by the melanocytes of the hair
bulbs. On electron microscopy grey hairs contain
numerous melanocytes in their normal position, but
some contain large vacuoles in their cytoplasm and
others many apparently normal melanosomes, few
of which are fully melanized. In white hairs melanocytes are scarce or absent, and there are no melanocytes or melanophores in their papillae.

The association of premature greying with certain organ-specific autoimmune processes [3]
prompted a statistical investigation which suggested
that normal greying may also be induced by an
autoimmune mechanism [2].

The process of greying is sometimes reversed in
Addison's disease or, very rarely, spontaneously.
Some patients receiving massive doses of para-aminobenzoic acid may also recover normal hair pigmentation [11]; non-steroidal anti-inflammatory
agents may also induce repigmentation.

The age of onset of canities is largely determined
by inheritance, but other factors are probably implicated. Some of them are discussed below. Lerner
[8] observed fewer grey hairs on the sympathectom-
ized side of a scalp than on the normal; Ortonne
and colleagues [9] also noted this finding.

Clinical features. The first white hairs commonly
appear at the temples and slowly involve the remainder of the scalp over a period of years. Greying
of the beard and of the body hair usually follows
after an interval of some years, but chest, pubic and
axillary hairs may retain their pigment even in old
age.

Among the Caucasoid races, white hairs first
appear at the age of 34.2 ± 9.6 [1]. By the age of 50,
50% of the population have at least 50% grey hairs

[7]. The rate at which the pigment content of hair diminishes is independent of its initial concentration; visual impressions to the contrary are influenced by contrast. Among the Negroids the age of onset is 43.9 ± 10.3. In the Japanese the onset of canities occurs between the ages of 30 and 34 in males and 35 and 39 in females [10]. In all races there is wide variation in the rate of progression.

Treatment. There is no treatment other than dyeing the hair.

REFERENCES

1 BOAS F. & MICHELSON N. (1932) *Am J Phys Anthropol* **17**, 213.
2 BURCH P.R.J. & JACKSON D. (1966) *J Gerontol* **21**, 522.
3 DAWBER R.P.R. (1970) *Br J Dermatol* **82**, 221.
4 FITZPATRICK T.B., *et al* (1958) In *The Biology of Hair Growth*. Eds. Montagna W. & Ellis R.A. New York, Academic Press, p. 255.
5 FITZPATRICK T.B., *et al* (1965) In *Advances in Biology of Skin*. Vol. V. *Ageing*. Ed. Montagna W. Oxford, Pergamon.
6 HERZBERG J. & GUSEK W. (1970) *Arch Klin Exp Dermatol* **236**, 368.
7 KEOGH E.U. & WALSH R.J. (1965) *Nature* **207**, 877.
8 LERNER A.B. (1966) *Arch Dermatol* **93**, 235.
9 ORTONNE J.P., *et al* (1982) *Arch Dermatol* **118**, 876.
10 TERADA H. (1956) *Folia Anat Jpn* **28**, 435.
11 ZARAFONETIS C. (1950) *J Invest Dermatol* **15**, 399.

POLIOSIS

Poliosis results from absence or deficiency of melanin in a group of neighbouring hair follicles. Clinically, it presents as a strand or mesh of white hairs. The underlying disturbance in melanogenesis is essentially the same as in hypomelanosis of surface epidermis.

Hereditary defects
Piebaldism (p. 1587). A white forelock—a paramedian frontal mesh of white hair—is associated with white skin patches. The white forelock is usually present from birth, but may develop rapidly in later childhood [2]. Similar changes in Waardenburg's syndrome (p. 1588) are combined with widely spaced medial canthi and deafness. Rarely, a white forelock is an isolated defect of dominant inheritance [1].

Vitiligo (p. 1591). Patchy loss of skin pigment develops in childhood or adult life. The hairs on the affected patches are usually, but not necessarily, white. A halo naevus of the scalp may present clinically as poliosis [6]. Vitiligo and poliosis are increased in incidence in patients presenting with uveitis [5].

Vogt–Koyanagi syndrome (p. 1590). The poliosis may be limited to eyebrows and eyelashes or may involve scalp and body hair. Onset in young adults

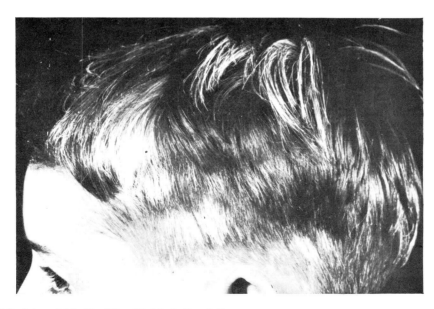

FIG. 53.59. Poliosis in a child with vitiligo (St. John's Hospital).

follows a febrile illnesss with uveitis. Vitiligo usually develops.

Alezzandrini's syndrome (p. 1595). Poliosis of brows and lashes accompanies unilateral facial vitiligo and retinitis.

Poliosis with multiple malformations. This new syndrome has been described in siblings, and consists of a white forelock associated with congenital malformations of the eye, hair, lungs and skeletal system [3].

Alopecia areata (p. 1985). The first hair to regrow is often pigment free and may remain so.

Tuberous sclerosis (p. 122). Poliosis is relatively frequent; absence of hair pigment may be the earliest sign [4, 5].

Neurofibromatosis (p. 119). Poliosis may overlie a neurofibroma of the scalp [3].

Acquired abnormalities. Permanent loss of hair pigment may follow the destruction of melanocytes by inflammatory processes or X-rays. The site of herpes zoster involving the scalp is not uncommonly marked by a tuft of white hair.

Reversible patchy loss of pigment in the beard or moustache has been associated with acute dental conditions.

REFERENCES

1 CROMWELL A.M. (1940) *J Hered* **31**, 94.
2 GILMAN R.S. & PERLMAN H.H. (1952) *J Pediatr* **40**, 101.
3 GOODMAN R.M., *et al* (1980) **17**, 437.
4 KOPLON B.S. & SHAPIRO L. (1968) *Arch Dermatol* **98**, 631.
5 McWILLIAM T.S. & STEPHENSON J.B.P. (1978) *Arch Dis Child* **53**, 961.
6 NATHANSON R. & JOHNSON W.C. (1973) *Cutis* **11**, 317.

NUTRITIONAL, METABOLIC AND CHEMICAL INFLUENCES ON HAIR COLOUR

Nutritional deficiencies. The effects of nutritional deficiency on hair colour have not been effectively studied in man, because specific lack of a single nutrient rarely occurs and experimental investigations are usually impracticable [5]. The tentative interpretation of scattered clinical observations must be based on work on laboratory and domestic animals.

An inadequate diet may disturb hair pigment formation by depleting the follicle of tyrosine and/or tryptophan or by inhibiting the action of tyrosinase. In gross protein malnutrition the hair is sparse, fine and dry and appears hypopigmented, but the effects of impaired keratinization probably overshadow any consequences of reduced melanin synthesis. Deficiency of copper, the prosthetic group of tyrosinase, produces achromotrichia in many laboratory species and in cattle [15]. Deficiency of pantothenic acid rapidly produces achromotrichia in rats [9].

Essential fatty acid deficiency in a patient receiving long-term fat-free hyperalimentation resulted in dermatitis of the scalp with some alopecia and lightening of the colour of the hair [16].

In man discoloration of the hair is a characteristic though inconstant feature of kwashiorkor [10]. In this variable syndrome of protein malnutrition the hair tends to be sparse, dry, brittle and easily plucked and lacks lustre and curl. Discoloration, usually reddish but sometimes blonde or grey depending on the intensity and shade of the normal colour, may affect most scalp hair or only a marginal fringe. Fluctuations in food supply may produce bands of different colour—the so-called flag sign [13]. The biochemical basis of the colour changes is not understood. The cysteine content of the hair may be reduced, but there is no correlation with the degree of dyschromia and the amino acid content of the hair usually appears to be normal [10]. Gummer *et al* [6], using sensitive electron histochemical methods, could not find any abnormality of incorporation of amino acids into the hair of severely affected children.

Protein depletion in ulcerative colitis [8] or after extensive surgical resection of the bowel [14] is sometimes followed by similar hair changes.

Extreme anaemia from iron deficiency alone is said to have produced a reversible change of hair colour from black to brown [19].

The evidence that isolated deficiences of components of the vitamin B complex will produce hair dyschromias in man is questionable.

Metabolic disorders. In phenylketonuria (p. 2315) excess phenylalanine inhibits the tyrosine–tyrosinase reaction. The hair is usually appreciably lighter than in normal siblings and may be pale blonde.

In homocystinuria, an inborn error on the pathway of the metabolism of methionine, the hair is fine and fair and may be sparse. The hair appears normal under the microscope but gives an orange–red fluorescence when stained with acridine orange and examined under ultraviolet radiation [3].

The hair is light, almost white, in the rare amino-aciduria called oasthouse disease.

In many genetically determined syndromes characterized by hypotrichosis the hair is hypopigmented and in some may be white or almost white. Structural defects of the hair shaft are also present and disturbed keratinization rather than primary hypomelanization may be responsible.

Drugs and other chemical agents [11, 18]. Several drugs have been found which produce changes in hair colour by interference with the synthesis of phaeomelanin or of eumelanin. The mode of action of others is quite unknown.

Chloroquine diphosphate [7, 12] may produce silvery or white bleaching, often irregular and first noticed at the temples or in the eyebrows, in blonde hair after 3 or 4 months' administration. No colour change is produced in black or dark brown hair and specific inhibition of phaeomelanin synthesis is therefore postulated. The change is fully reversible.

Mephenesin [17], an aromatic glycerol ether used in the treatment of multiple sclerosis, produces loss of pigment in patients with dark hair. Since the drug has no known effect on melanin synthesis the mechanism is unknown.

The anticholesterolaemic agent triparanol, which is no longer available commercially, and the antipsychotic compound fluorobutyrophenone are chemically unrelated drugs which block cholesterol synthesis and disturb keratinization. Scalp and body hair become sparse, but also hypopigmented. The study of these effects may throw light on the cause of the hypopigmentation in some hereditary hypotrichotic syndromes.

Minoxidil and diazoxide, two potent antihypertensive drugs, cause hypertrichosis and darkening of hair [2].

Postinflammatory pigmentation. Local inflammatory changes in the scalp, induced by infection or trauma, may be followed by darkening of the hair, which regains its previous colour gradually over a period of months or years [1, 4].

REFERENCES

1 BEAN W.B. (1959) *AMA Archs Dermatol* **79**, 681.
2 BURTON J.L. & MARSHALL A. (1979) *Br J Dermatol* **101**, 543.
3 CARSON N.A.J., et al (1965) *J Pediatr* **66**, 565.
4 FROHN W. (1938) *Dermatol Z* **77**, 4.
5 GUMMER C.L. (1985) In *Seminars in Dermatology*. Vol. 4. Eds. Rook A.J. & Maibach H. New York, Thieme–Stratton, p. 104.
6 GUMMER C.L., et al (1982) *Br J Dermatol* **106**, 407.
7 JAHRIG K. (1963) *Kinderarztl Prax* **31**, 495.
8 MELKNIKOFF S.M. (1957) *Am J Dig Dis* **2**, 738.
9 MUSKETT L.W. & UNNA K. (1941) *J Nutr* **22**, 565.
10 RAO B.S.N. & GOPALAN C. (1957) *Indian J Med Res* **45**, 85.
11 ROOK A. (1965) *Br J Dermatol* **77**, 115.
12 SANDERS T.S., et al (1959) *J Invest Dermatol* **33**, 87.
13 SCRIMSHAW N.S. & BEMAR M. (1961) *Science* **133**, 2039.
14 SILVERBLATT C.W. & BROWN H.E. (1960) *Am J Med* **28**, 847.
15 SJOLLERNA B. (1937) *Biochem Z* **295**, 372.
16 SKOLNIK P., et al (1977) *Arch Dermatol* **113**, 939.
17 SPILLANE J.D. (1963) *Br Med J* i, 997.
18 STROUD J.D. (1985) In *Seminars in Dermatology*. Vol. 4. Eds. Rook A.J. & Maibach H. New York, Thieme–Stratton, p. 88.
19 TASKER P. & POLUNIN I. (1954) *Br Med J* ii, 1465.

PREMATURE CANITIES

Premature canities may be defined as greying of the hair beginning before the age of 20 in Caucasoids or 30 in Negroids [10]. Although greying has been reported in gross malnutrition and cachectic states of any origin, it is doubtful whether true canities occurs under these circumstances; the suggestion that correcting gluten-sensitive enteropathy causes reversal of greying requires proof. The pigmentary changes of nutritional and chemical origin are described below on p. 2024.

Autoimmune disease. Premature greying is significantly correlated with a number of disorders associated with organ-specific autoantibodies. It is possible that an autoimmune mechanism is responsible for greying in some of the other syndromes mentioned below, and perhaps also for the physiological canities of old age. However, it could represent pleiotropy of this gene.

Pernicious anaemia. Premature greying is significantly more frequent in pernicious (Addison's) anaemia, and may be an early sign of this disease [2].

Hyperthyroidism. The incidence of premature canities is increased in hyperthyroidism and in other thyroid disorders.

Rapid whitening of the hair [3, 8, 9]. Rapid greying or whitening of the hair after severe emotional stress has been reliably recorded on many occasions, and need no longer be regarded as the dramatic creation of the popular novelist. Hair which already appears grey from the presence of many white hairs is whitened over the course of a few days or weeks when the surviving pigmented hairs are preferentially shed in alopecia areata of rapid onset [10]. Other cases in which the whitening has developed more slowly have subsequently proved to have vitiligo.

Cardiovascular disease [6]. The association of premature canities with an increased incidence of cardiovascular disease, as manifested by angina or myocardial infarction, peripheral arterial disease, hypertension or left bundle-branch block, has been claimed.

Other workers report an association between canities and biological age [4] or mortality, but the findings remain inconclusive.

Hereditary premature canities. Premature canities is a feature of several hereditary syndromes, but may also occur as an apparently isolated defect determined by an autosomal dominant gene [5] in individuals who are otherwise normal or, indeed, exceptionally long lived. The first white hairs appear during the second decade, or occasionally earlier, and conspicuous greying of scalp and body hair develops within a few years, but does not affect eyebrows or eyelashes. In some pedigrees the premature greying is confined to the temples.

Böök's syndrome [1]. In this rare syndrome, which is also determined by an autosomal dominant gene, premature canities is associated with palmoplantar hyperhidrosis and hypodontia of the premolar region—the bicuspids are partially or totally lacking.

Progeria (p. 0000). The hair is very sparse as well as prematurely grey, and other cutaneous attributes of ageing are conspicuous from the second year.

Rothmund syndrome (p. 151). Canities is an inconstant feature, sometimes appearing in adolescence and progressing rapidly. Spastic paresis (progressive), vitiligo and a distinctive facial appearance have been described in association with premature greying of hair [7].

Werner's syndrome (p. 1816). Canities beginning in childhood or adolescence is present in the majority of cases and is often the earliest manifestation.

Dystrophia myotonica. Premature canities in the second or third decade may precede or accompany the myotonia and severe muscle wasting. Male pattern alopecia also develops early.

Waardenburg's syndrome (p. 1588). Premature canities may develop in the third decade in many patients with a white forelock and in a small proportion of those without; the most constant features are lateral displacement of the medial canthi, hypertrophy of the nasal root and perceptive deafness.

REFERENCES

1 Böök J.A. (1950) *Am J Hum Genet* **2**, 240.
2 Dawber R.P.R. (1970) *Br J Dermatol* **82**, 221.
3 Ephraim A.J. (1959) *AMA Arch Dermatol* **79**, 228.
4 Flügel B. (1971) *Z Alternforsch* **23**, 397.
5 Hare H.J.H. (1929) *J Hered* **20**, 31.
6 Lebon J., *et al* (1957) *Alger Med* **61**, 871.
7 Lison M., *et al* (1982) *Am J Med Genet* **9**, 351.
8 Tournaine A. (1945) *Prog Med* **73**, 47.
9 de Villez R.L. & Buchanan J.M. (1982) *Int J Dermatol* **2**, 344.
10 Waring J.J., *et al* (1940) *Arch Intern Med* **65**, 763.

ACCIDENTAL DISCOLORATION

The hair may be accidentally discoloured by occupational exposure to chemicals [4] or by the use of inappropriate ingredients in topical applications to the scalp. In most cases the cause of the discoloration is obvious to patient and doctor, but occasionally the exposure is unsuspected.

In industry the metals, especially copper, are the main offenders. In copper workers the hair may be stained a brilliant green colour. Tap water with a

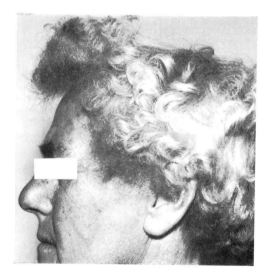

FIG. 53.60. Accidental discoloration of the hair by tobacco tars. This condition is very common in white-haired cigarette smokers but is seldom recognized. The yellow-brown discoloration is most marked in the frontal region and along the scalp margins (Addenbrooke's Hospital).

high content of copper produced green discoloration [3, 6] of the light blonde hair of girls who had used it for frequent shampoos [5]. Bright blue hair occurs in cobalt workers and a deeper blue has been seen in those handling indigo [2]. Picric acid stains the hair yellow, and in TNT workers the skin is yellow but the hair is reddish-brown. Spectroanalysis may sometimes be necessary to identify the metal for medicolegal purposes. Chinoform application may colour hair red [1].

Yellow or yellow–brown discoloration of white or grey hair by cigarette smoke is very common, yet the patient is rarely aware of its cause.

The main offender among topical medicaments is resorcin, which stains black or white hair yellow or yellowish-brown. Chrysarobin produces an impressive tint of rich mahogany brown. The careless use of cosmetic colorants alone or in conjunction with medicaments may produce bizarre effects.

REFERENCES

1 BANDMANN H.J. & SPAER U. (1984) *Contact Dermatol* **10**, 113.
2 BEIGEL H. (1867) *Arch Pathol Anat Physiol* **83**, 324.
3 GOLDSCHMIDT H. (1979) *Arch Dermatol* **115**, 1285.
4 JIRNECKE H. (1938) *Dermatol Wochenschr* **106**, 212.
5 NORDLUND J.J., *et al* (1977) *Arch Dermatol* **113**, 1700.
6 ROOMANS G.M. & FORSLIND B. (1980) *Ultrapathology* **1**, 310–18.

COSMETIC HAIR COLOURINGS
[1, 3, 4, 9, 11, 12, 13]

Hair colouring has been practised by women and sometimes, though with greater circumspection, by men since at least the days of the Pharaohs. Its primary purpose has been to conceal the onset of greying, but the development of sophisticated and simple techniques in modern society has encouraged the practice of changing the hair colour, often at frequent intervals, as an expression of personality or in pursuit of an ideal or fashion.

The skill of the cosmetic chemists has devised processes which, when correctly carried out, involve very little risk of damaging the hair or of inducing dermatitis [2]. It is because hair colourants are used on such an extensive scale that accidents occur, for they are sometimes applied carelessly and without regard to the manufacturer's recommendations, usually by the patient herself or by a friend but occasionally by a hairdresser. The consequences may be distressing to the patient and are sometimes a source of litigation [2].

Vegetable dyes [1, 10]. The development of synthetic chemicals which are easier to use has largely supplanted the vegetable dyes in westernized countries, but they are of historic importance and are still in common use in many parts of the world.

Henna is derived from the powdered leaves of *Lawsonia alba*. The active principal is 2-hydroxy-1, 4-naphthoquinone, which in acid solution will penetrate and dye keratin a reddish-auburn shade. It is messy to use and stains the finger nails but involves no significant dematitis risk. It is seldom used as such in Britain, but henna extract is incorporated in some hair rinses.

Camomile is extracted from the flowers of *Anthemis nobilis* or *Matricaria chamomilla*, The yellow dyestuff 1,3,4-trihydroxyflavone coats the surface of the cuticle but does not penetrate the keratin. It is safe but ineffective.

Metallic dyes [5, 6]. The mode of action of the metallic dyes is uncertain. Metallic salts in aqueous solution are deposited as sulphides in the cortex.

Lead is commonly used, often as lead acetate [6]. The coloration of the hair is progressive with repeated applications and gives a series of shades of brown and black. Bismuth dyes are also progressive and produce various shades of brown.

Synthetic organic dyes [4, 5]. The oxidation dyes, which are more or less permanent, have been commercially available for over 50 yr and are still of great importance, but in Britain changing fashions and the growing popularity of self-treatment have given less permanent and safer preparations large sales.

Temporary dyes. The temporary dyes are applied as simple rinses. They are substances of high molecular weight which are deposited on the surface of the hair. A wide variety of dyestuffs may be employed in their formulation to give numerous different shades. The dyes used in Britain are selected from those appearing in the E.E.C. Council Directive Relating to Cosmetics, 1976, and sensitization reactions are extremely uncommon. The dye is removed by shampooing. Sometimes the hair is pretreated with a cationic detergent to increase the amount of dye taken up. These dyes are used in setting aids which are usually dilute aqueous or alcoholic solutions of resin fixatives such as copolymers of vinyl pyrrolidone–vinyl acetate.

Semipermanent dyes. The semipermanent dyes, which are now the most popular in Britain, have small molecules which penetrate keratin without drastic pretreatment and persist for six to ten shampoos. Chemically these dyes are a heterogeneous group including the nitro dyes, such as 2-nitro-*p*-phenylenediamine, 2-amino-4-nitrophenol, picramic acid and 4-nitro-*o*-phenylenediamine, and various anthraquinones. Azo dyes are commonly used [11]. Many proprietary preparations contain a mixture of dyestuffs formulated as a liquid cream. Some formulations have a special affinity for hair permanently waved with thioglycollates.

Allergic reactions to the semipermanent dyes are rare [2].

Permanent dyes [10, 11]. The oxidative dyes *para*phenylenediamine, *para*toluendiamine and related compounds are mixed with hydrogen peroxide to form benzoquinone imines which are deposited in the cortex. The imines rapidly react with 'couplers' or an unoxidized *para* dye to produce indo dyes. The couplers most frequently used are 2,4-diaminoanisole, resorcinol, *meta*-aminophenol and 1-naphthol. Couplers increase the range of shades which can be obtained.

Allergic reactions to *para* dyes were formerly a serious problem [2], but now occur less frequently than once in 100,000 applications. This improvement is due partly to technological advances and partly to the declining incidence of sensitivity to other aromatic benzenes such as sulphonamides and certain local anaesthetics. Under E.E.C. regulations, the use of *para*phenylenediamine in concentrations up to 6% is permitted.

Exceptionally, allergic contact dermatitis has occurred in the partner of a woman whose hair has recently been dyed [14] and on the arm of a dental hygienist from contact with a patient's recently dyed hair [8].

Bleaches. Hydrogen peroxide is the most popular bleach and is often applied at home. During bleaching the melanin of hair undergoes irreversible chemical changes and the keratin is altered by the oxidation of combined cysteine. The cysteic acid residues formed cause a significant change in the distribution of electrostatic cross-links [15]. After repeated or prolonged applications the hair may become brittle and fluffy or woolly in appearance. Small nodules may be detectable with the naked eye on many hairs, and trichorrhexis nodosa and other shaft defects (p. 2006) may be seen under the microscope. Such hair may break on exposure to cold-waving agents or, though less often, to semipermanent or permanent dyes [2].

The 'platinum' blonde shade is produced by rinsing the bleached hair in methylene blue 1:100,000.

Ammonium persulphate is often used to accelerate peroxide bleaching. It may cause contact dermatitis, or irritation, wealing, faintness or asthma [7].

Removal of dyes. A hairdresser's mistake or a customer's sudden change of mind results in a demand that the dye be removed. Hasty and ill-considered attempts to remove a dye are the cause of a large proportion of cases of serious damage to the hair. It is easy to cover a light shade with a dark one, but if a semipermanent or permanent dye is used the additional insult to keratin already damaged by bleaching or cold waving may sometimes lead to extensive loss of hair. Hair which has recently received such treatment and has lost its normal texture is best left alone or treated only with a temporary dye which merely coats the hair shafts.

Metallic dyes cannot be removed without risk of serious injury to the hair and must be allowed to grow out. Semipermanent dyes are not usually difficult to remove with a shampoo to which ammonia may be added, but some penetrate keratin too effectively to be rapidly washed out.

The oxidative dyes are difficult to remove, but treatment with 5% sodium formaldehyde, sodium sulphoxylate or 5% sodium hydrosulphite may be useful.

REFERENCES

1 BALSAM M.S. & SAGARIN E. (1972) *Cosmetics: Science and Technology.* Vol. 2, 2nd edn. New York, Wiley.
2 BROWN K. (1982) *J Soc Cosmet Chem* **33**, 375.
3 BERGFELD W.F. (1979) In *Hair Research.* Eds. Orfanos C. & Montagna W. Springer, Berlin, p. 507.
4 BURNETT C.M. & CORBETT J.F. (1977) In *Cutaneous Toxicity.* Eds. Drill V.A. & Lazar P. New York, Academic Press, p. 203.
5 CORBETT J.F. (1976) *J Soc Dyers Colour* **92**, 285.
6 EDWARDS E.K. JR. & EDWARDS E.K. (1982) *Cutis* **30**, 629.
7 FISHER A.A. & DOOMS-GOOSSENS A. (1976) *Arch Dermatol* **112**, 1407.
8 HINDSON C.C. (1975) *Contact Dermatitis* **1**, 333.
9 REDGRAVE H.S. & BARI-WOOLLSS J. (1939) *Hair Dyes and Hair Dyeing*, London, Heinemann.
10 SCHWARTZ L. (1953) *South Med J* **46**, 769.
11 SIDI E. & ZVIAK C. (1966) *Problems Capillaires.* Paris, Gauthier-Villars.
12 SPOOR H.J. (1976) *Cutis* **18**, 341.
13 THULLIEZ M. (1970) *Arch Belg Dermatol Syphiligr* **26**, 73.
14 WARIN A.P. (1976) *Clin Exp Dermatol* **1**, 283.
15 WOLFRAM L.J., *et al* (1970) *J Soc Cosmet Chem* **21**, 875.

HAIR SETTING

Temporary setting involves the application of constraint to wet hair, and allowing the hair to dry before the constraint is removed. Setting lotions leave on the fibres a film which helps to retain the configuration by interfibre bonding and possibly by increasing fibre-to-fibre bonding [1, 2].

Wet hair takes up to 30% of its weight of water and swells 10% diametrically but only 1–2% longitudinally. Popular modern film formers are water-soluble or dispersible materials such as polyvinylmethyl ether, maleic acid copolymers, and polyvinylpyrrolidone and its copolymers with vinyl acetate. Setting lotions usually contain ethanol as a wetting agent, and to increase the rate of drying they also contain plasticizer, antistatic agents such as polyethylic glycols and emollients such as lanolin derivatives.

Hair sprays contain similar resins but in different formulations. They hold a coiffure by forming inter-fibre welds.

REFERENCES

1 CORBETT J.F. (1976) *J Soc Dyers Colour* **92**, 285.
2 PRICE V.H. (1979) In *Hair Research*. Eds. Orfanos C. & Montagna W. Berlin, Springer, p. 501.

HAIR WAVING

Principles and techniques [6–8]. Permanent waving has been defined as the process of changing the shape of the hair so that the new shape persists through several shampoos. The degree of permanence varies from a few weeks to several months. The techniques are essentially similar whether their object is to impose a wave on straight hair or to straighten tightly coiled hair. All procedures involve three distinct stages; the hair must first be softened, then shaped and then hardened in the new form.

Current practices and hazards

Hot waving. Locks of hair are wound round rollers and covered by strips of absorbent material saturated in an alkaline solution. Many different alternatives may be used; either a combination of 20·0% ammonium hydroxide and 2.0% potassium sulphite or triethanolamine are often favoured. Heat is then applied for about 10 min; then the rollers are removed and the lotion is washed out. Hot waving demands skill and judgement. Excess application of heat or alkali can damage the keratin, which becomes brittle.

Cold waving [2–4, 6]. In the popular cold-waving process the hair is wetted with a thiol solution before and after it is wound round the curlers. The solution contains 5–9% of thioglycollic acid and 1.3–1·8% of pure ammonia or monoethanolamine. The weaker solutions are usually provided for home use. To obtain the right degree of softening the lotion is allowed to remain on the hair for 10–49 min, according to its concentration. 'Neutralization' is achieved with 1·5% hydrogen peroxide or, in 'home processes', with sodium perborate or potassium bromate.

Accidents are rather rare [1, 9]. The waving solution is an irritant and, if carelessly applied or allowed to remain too long in contact with the scalp, may produce a burn-like lesion; this is usually small and heals rapidly. The patient may notice a burning sensation during the waving procedure and within a few hours develops a circumscribed red oedematous patch, often along the frontal hair line or above or behind the ear.

Damage to the hair itself is more frequent. It occurs most commonly in hair which was previously abnormal from a developmental defect or from too recent waving or bleaching, but may be produced in normal hair by excessive and too prolonged application of the waving lotion. Electron microscopy shows damage to the cuticular cells, many of which may be shed, denuding areas of cortex [10]. The hair may appear woolly and lifeless and may break at once, or progressively over a period of days, with the trauma of ordinary brushing or combing. Patchy loss and breakdown may be the result of winding the locks too tightly [5].

Sensitization dematitis is extremely uncommon. Perfumes, emulsifying agents, dyes and so-called 'conditioners', often lanolin, are ingredients of many proprietary cold-wave lotions and more likely to be responsible than the thioglycollate.

REFERENCES

1 BERGFELD W.F. (1979) In *Hair Research*. Ed. Orfanos C. Berlin, Springer, p. 507.
2 BORELLI S. (1956) *Hautarzt* **7**, 337.
3 BORELLI S. (1957) *Hautarzt* **8**, 159, 211, 247, 411, 498, 540.
4 BRAUN W. (1963) *Hautarzt* **14**, 468.
5 BRUNNER M.J. (1952) *AMA Arch Dermatol Syphilol* **65**, 316.
6 FREYTAG H. (1962) *Aesthetic Med* **11**, 278.
7 FREYTAG H. (1964) *J Soc Cosmet Chem Br Edn* **15**, 667.
8 MCLAUGHLIN T.P. (1963) In *Handbook of Cosmetic Science*. Ed. Hibbott H.W. Oxford, Pergamon, p. 284.
9 NORRIS J.A. (1965) *Food Cosmet Toxicol* **3**, 93.
10 SELZLE D. & WOLFE H.H. (1976) *Hautarzt* **27**, 452.

MEDICAL AND MEDICOLEGAL ASPECTS OF HAIRDRESSING PROCEDURES

The relationship between a woman and her hairdresser is often ambivalent, and complex psychological factors may motivate the not infrequent complaints against hairdressers and the manufacturers of colouring and waving preparations. The complaints are sometimes frivolous and without foundations, but are justified when it can be established that the operation has not received a reasonable degree of skill and care. The majority of the cases in which negligence is compensated by an award of damages in court or, more commonly, by settlement out of court fall into two categories— allergic reactions to *para* dyes and cumulative physical and chemical injury to the hair.

Reactions to dyes. The risk of severe allergic reactions to the *para* dyes has been widely recognized by special legislation, but has now been considerably reduced by technical advances so that these dyes may now be sold in E.E.C. countries in concentrations of up to 6%. In most countries, including Britain and the U.S.A., these and related dyes must carry a warning label and the hairdresser is expected to patch test his client before using them. The *para* dyes are contained in almost all the permanent dyes and many of the semipermanent types. Allergic reactions occur because the hairdresser fails to patch test before each application and does not appreciate that allergic sensitization may be acquired at any time and is not excluded by a series of previous negative results. In many cases hairdressers do not apply or interpret the tests correctly. Repeated testing, unfortunately, itself involves a risk of producing sensitization, but the legal implications of this hazard have not been clarified.

Many women who develop dermatitis dye their own hair using special home kits and claim compensation from the manufacturers. The dermatologist consulted in a case of alleged dye dermatitis should record a detailed history of the attack and the findings on examination. He must also enquire into previous exposure, with or without reactions, to related aromatic benzenes. He must patch test, after the acute stage has subsided, with *para*phenylenediamine, *para*toluenediamine and with the actual preparation employed by the hairdresser or the patient. In his report he will state whether his patient is allergic to the dye and whether the reaction in question is compatible with an allergic reaction to such a substance.

Physical and chemical injury to the hair. In our experience cases of cumulative physical and chemical injury to the hair are increasing in number and now form the majority of those in which litigation against hairdressers is contemplated. Surprisingly, the history often follows the same pattern; the customer's hair was waved and dyed but she was dissatisfied with the effect and persuaded the hairdresser to repeat the procedure 1 or 2 days later. At once, or after a short interval, the hairs broke off just above the level of the scalp. Sometimes the patient has herself applied a 'home perm' or a bleach shortly before her visit to the hairdresser. Sometimes she has demanded the removal of a rashly chosen dye and the immediate application of another. In all cases the hair has been subjected to a succession of treatments which disrupt and distort the keratin.

The distribution and extent of the broken hairs must be determined, and representative hair stumps and apparently intact hairs should be plucked and examined under the microscope. The nature and degree of any defects in the shaft must be recorded. The possibility that the hair was in some way abnormal before any treatment was applied must be considered and the common structural defects of the shaft (p. 2006) excluded. If a defect of a type likely to increase the vulnerability of the hair is present, the court will require an opinion as to whether the hairdresser could reasonably have been expected to detect it.

Systemic effects of hair dyes. Many investigations have suggested, but not proved, that certain hair dyes may cause systemic abnormalities such as chromosome damage [3, 4], breast and other carcinomas [2] and aplastic anaemia [1].

REFERENCES

1 BURNETT C.M., *et al* (1978) *Drug Chem. Toxicol* 1, 45.
2 HENNEKRENS C.H. (1979) *Lancet* i, 1390.
3 KIRKLAND D.J., *et al.* (1978) *Lancet* ii, 124.
4 KIRKLAND D.J., *et al* (1978) *Lancet* ii, 271.

SHAMPOOS

The purpose of all shampoos [2] is to remove grease and dirt trapped within the hair and to do so without leaving the hair or scalp uncomfortably dry or provoking irritation or allergic sensitization. The literature has been well reviewed [1, 4].

Liquid shampoos account for a large proportion of the market. In the U.K. these are based largely on sodium alkyl ether sulphates and the alkalonin salts of alkyl sulphates, and in the U.S.A. on trie-thanolamine lauryl sulphate. Such shampoos have three main types of constituent. These are (i) primary surfactants to provide foam and detergency, (ii) secondary or auxiliary surfactants to enhance detergency and stabilize foam, and (iii) miscellaneous adjuncts such as antidandruff agents, setting agents, conditioning agents, perfumes and dyes.

The so-called medicated shampoos may contain liquid tars, selenium disulphide [3], zinc pyrithione or Irgasen DP 300. Allergic reactions to shampoos, other than certain medicated preparations, are uncommon. A physical phenomenon known as 'matting' is occasionally produced (see below).

REFERENCES

1 Anon (1977) *Soap Perfum Cosmet* **50**, 47.
2 Balsam M.S. & Sagarin E. (1972) *Cosmetics: Science and Technology.* Vol. 2, 2nd edn. New York, Wiley.
3 Chetty G.N., et al (1981) *Int J Dermatol* **20**, 119.
4 Robbins C.R. (1979) *Chemical and Physical Behaviour of Human Hair.*

MATTING OF THE HAIR

The term *plica neuropathica* has been applied to an uncommon state in which the hair is compacted into numerous irregularly twisted, irreversibly entangled plaits. The condition is induced by the repeated manipulation of the hair by psychologically disturbed women [4]. Densely tangled 'bird's nest' hair has followed the use as a shampoo of cetrimide, a cationic detergent [3]. The process of matting is probably similar to the 'felting' of fibres familiar in the wool and textile industries and which is due to the compaction of contiguous fibres exposed to friction in a liquid medium [1]. Other factors relevant in shampoo matting may be viscous fluid welding and the formation of lipotrophic liquid crystal phases [2, 3].

REFERENCES

1 Bogaty H. & Dunlap F.E. (1970) *Arch Dermatol* **101**, 348.
2 Dawber R.P.R. (1984) *Clin Exp Dermatol* **9**, 209.
3 Dawber R.P.R. & Calnan C.D. (1976) *Clin Exp Dermatol* **1**, 135.
4 Simpson M.H. & Mullins J.F. (1969) *Arch Dermatol* **100**, 456.

DISEASES OF THE SCALP

The presence of a profuse growth of terminal hair and of large and active sebaceous glands are the principal factors influencing the surface biology of the scalp and determining the incidence and course of many of the disorders which afflict it. Apart from abnormalities of the hair itself, pityriasis capitis is the most characteristic disorder resulting from the special conditions prevailing at the scalp surface. These conditions also favour the development of seborrhoeic dermatitis and provide a suitable habitat for the head louse and certain ringworm fungi.

The large number of cutaneous appendages explains the relative frequency of naevi derived from them.

There are many other conditions, notably psoriasis, lichen planus and lupus erythematosus, which not infrequently involve the scalp, although no satisfactory explanation for this predilection can yet be put forward. Lichen planus and lupus erythematosus may give rise to cicatricial alopecia. Psoriasis is usually considered not to affect hair growth, but careful investigation [1] shows that temporary partial hair loss is relatively common in psoriatic plaques, and on examination by electron microscopy, keratinization of the hair shafts is seen to be abnormal [3, 4]. Very rarely, pustular psoriasis of the scalp may lead to extensive non-cicatricial alopecia [2].

Most diseases affecting the scalp also occur in other regions of the body, and are considered fully in the appropriate chapters.

Here we shall describe pityriasis capitis, pityriasis amiantacea and two rare disorders characterized by diffuse overgrowth of the scalp, i.e. cutis verticis gyrata and lipoedematous alopecia.

Acne necrotica and perifolliculitis of the scalp are considered on p. 746. Certain other conditions involving the scalp are briefly considered here as problems in differential diagnosis: pruritic syndromes, cysts, naevi and tumours.

REFERENCES

1 Braun-Falco O. & Rassner B. (1966) *Arch Klin Exp Dermatol* **225**, 42.
2 Eisenmann H.T. & Mikhail G.R. (1969) *Arch Dermatol* **100**, 598.
3 Orfanos C., et al (1970) *Arch Klin Exp Dermatol* **236**, 107.
4 Wyatt E., et al (1872) *Br J Dermatol* **87**, 368.

Pruritic syndromes. Pruritus of the scalp may occur as an isolated symptom in the absence of any objective changes. The patient is often middle-aged, the pruritus is spasmodic and may be intense, and exacerbations are frequently related to periods of stress or fatigue.

Pruritus is also the predominant manifestation of

acne necrotica (p. 746) in which scattered vesicles followed by small crusts are a source of severe discomfort. Dermatitis herpetiformis (p. 1651) may involve the scalp. Grouped papules and vesicles in recurrent crops are associated with similar lesions of the trunk and limbs.

Lichen simplex (p. 412) is a frequent cause of pruritus of the nape and occipital region in women, and may also be localized above one or both ears. The scalp in the affected region is thickened and scaly.

The protection provided by the hair accounts for the rarity of contact dermatitis, and even reactions to hair dyes and other hair cosmetics more commonly involve the ears, neck, forehead or face than the scalp itself. However, intense irritation of the scalp is sometimes the initial symptom of a sensitization reaction and, rarely, eczematous changes may affect the whole or part of the scalp. Apart from hair cosmetics and medicaments, hair nets and hats should be suspected.

Seborrhoeic and atopic dermatitis and other inflammatory disorders may be pruritic, but pruritus is seldom a presenting symptom. Psoriasis is not usually pruritic but may occasionally be so.

In children and in women of any age, pediculosis should be excluded no matter what the social status of the patient. Multiple insect bites are sometimes a puzzling source of irritation in children, and are usually rapidly complicated by infection as a result of excoriation. In infants and in old age scabies may cause scalp irritation.

Naevi, cysts and tumours [4, 8]. In the child epithelial naevi, especially those of sebaceous and apocrine gland origin, are relatively frequent in the scalp. Melanocytic naevi, often warty, and vascular naevi are also common. Dermoid cysts, often above the ears but sometimes in other parts of the scalp, may be present at birth or develop in early childhood. Osteomas may also be present at birth [6]. A solitary superficial lipomatous naevus has been reported in a young adult [7].

In adolescence epidermal and pilar cysts increase in frequency. They may be multiple. The soft fibrous nodules of neurofibromatosis may also appear at this age.

In adult life cylindromas—turban tumours—may give rise to single or multiple firm nodules (p. 2411). Basal cell epitheliomas may develop in epithelial naevi or arise independently. Squamous epithelioma is uncommon, except in solar keratosis arising in the bald areas of the scalp. Carcinoma of sweat gland origin is less uncommon in the hairy scalp. Melanoma of the scalp is rare, and the correct diagnosis is often delayed with serious consequences.

Multiple globular tumours, superficially resembling cylindromas but histologically granulomas of foreign-body type, may be induced by the trauma of hot irons and combs in hair straightening [3].

The commonest tumour in the older patient is the seborrhoeic keratosis (p. 2388), a circumscribed, rather greasy, warty and pigmented nodule or plaque.

The rapid development of solitary or multiple hard nodules or an irregular scirrhous plaque in an elderly patient should suggest the possibility of metastatic carcinoma, particularly from the breast, kidney or prostrate [1].

Among the rare tumours of the scalp are dermatofibrosarcoma (p. 2461), which presents as a firm dermal nodule, and osteogenic sarcoma, which arise in Paget's disease of the skull [2]. Mixed tumours of salivary gland origin involve the scalp in about 10% of cases. Lymphangiosarcoma of the scalp [5] occurs mainly in the very elderly and presents as irregular nodules which may ulcerate.

Multiple bluish-red nodules may develop in the scalp in malignant reticuloses and in monocytic and lymphocytic leukaemia.

REFERENCES

1 BAUM E.M., *et al* (1981) *J Am Acad Dermatol* **4**, 588.
2 FEINERMAN L.K. & SHAPIRO L. (1970) *Int J Dermatol* **9**, 96.
3 HELFMAN R.J. (1965) *Arch Dermatol* **91**, 345.
4 PAGES A. & MARTY M. (1960) *Montpellier Med* **58**, 223.
5 REED R.J., *et al* (1966) *Arch Dermatol* **94**, 396.
6 TRITSCH H. (1965) *Arch Klin Exp Dermatol* **221**, 336.
7 WEITZNER S. (1968) *Arch Dermatol* **97**, 540.
8 WINKELMANN R.K. (1979) In *Hair Research*. Eds. Orfanos C. & Montagna G. Springer, Berlin, p. 363.

Lumpy scalp syndrome [1]. The inheritance of this syndrome is determined by an autosomal dominant gene of variable expressivity. Raw areas are present in the scalp at birth. They heal to leave irregular nodules of connective tissue, which on histological examination are not cheloidal in structure. The pinnae are deformed; the tragus, antitragus and lobule are small or rudimentary. The nipples are rudimentary or absent, and only areolae are present.

REFERENCE

1 FINLAY A.Y. & MARKS R. (1978) *Br J Dermatol* **99**, 423.

Lipoedematous alopecia [1, 2]. This syndrome has been recognized only in Negro women, in whom an increase in thickness of the subcutis of the scalp, affecting particularly the subcutaneous fat, is associated with atrophy and fibrous replacement of many hair follicles. Clinically there is slowly progressive diffuse alopecia and obvious thickening of the scalp.

REFERENCES

1 COSKEY R.J., *et al* (1961) *Arch Dermatol* **84**, 619.
2 CURTIS J.W. & Heising R.A. (1964) *Arch Dermatol* **89**, 819.

CUTIS VERTICIS GYRATA
SYN. PACHYDERMIE PLICATURÉE (FR.)

Definition and terminology. Cutis verticis gyrata is a morphological syndrome characterized by hypertrophy and folding of the skin, usually of the scalp. The term has been wrongly applied to syndromes, especially pachydermoperiostosis, of which cutis gyrata is merely one component.

Aetiology and pathology. The essential abnormality is overgrowth of the scalp in relation to the underlying skull. It occurs in such a very low proportion of cases of the conditions with which it may be associated, that the existence of some predisposing defect, probably developmental, may be postulated. The pathological picture varies with the provocative factor from apparently normal skin to simple hy-

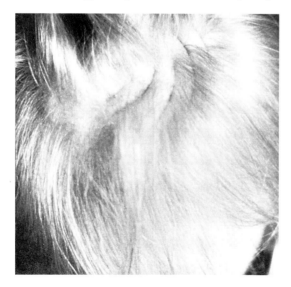

FIG. 53.61. Cutis verticus gyrata (Dr Allan Highet, York District Hospital).

pertrophy of epidermis and dermis, neurofibromatous hyperplasia or severe chronic inflammatory changes. The circumscribed naevoid forms usually prove to be melanocytic naevi.

The so-called primary form is emerging as a well-defined syndrome which is probably genetically determined, perhaps by an autosomal recessive gene often lethal in the female, for almost all cases occur in males. The syndrome accounts for 1–2% of severely retarded males [4]. Sex-linked recessive inheritance has been claimed for a much rarer syndrome in which thyroid aplasia is an additional feature [4].

Developmental syndromes and systemic diseases
Primary cutis verticis gyrata. The folding of the scalp begins at puberty. The IQ is rarely over 35, and epilepsy and cerebral palsy are frequent [2,3,5]. Some patients diagnosed in childhood as exhibiting the Lennox–Gastaut syndrome—mental retardation and a distinctive EEG pattern—subsequently develop cutis verticis gyrata [10].

Pachydermoperiostosis [157]. This is usually of the primary form. Skin changes are uncommon in the secondary form associated with intrathoracic neoplasms.

Acromegaly [1, 13, 15]. Mild and moderate degrees of cutis gyrata are frequent, but the severe forms are rarely seen.

Other associations [11]. Association with myxoedema, cretinism and other endocrine states has been reported infrequently and may be fortuitous. At least six cases have been attributed to syphilis, but without modern diagnostic criteria. Other associated conditions include dystrophia myotonica [7], acute myelogenous leukaemia [6] and mental retardation [7].

Local inflammatory disorders [11]. Inflammatory disorders have been incriminated as the cause of cutis verticis gyrata, but their significance is difficult to evaluate. The grossly seborrhoeic scalp in primary cutis verticis gyrata is highly susceptible to pyogenic infection, and the inflammatory changes are in many cases probably the result, rather than the cause, of the abnormality. However, in some reported cases localized hypertrophy and folding appear to have followed trauma or infection. Some of these patients probably had dissecting cellulitis (p. 2005). Chronic rotational traction was the cause of cutis verticis gyrata in one case [9].

Naevi [8]. Naevi involving the scalp may be associated with hypertrophy and folding, which may simulate the convolutions of the brain.

Clinical features and diagnosis. In pachydermoperiostosis and primary cutis verticis gyrata the scalp changes begin soon after puberty, and are almost always restricted to males. Folding produces a corrugated, gyrate or convoluted pattern of firm ridges and furrows, usually roughly symmetrical and often most marked in the occipital region. The changes usually become slowly more severe for 5–10 yr and then remain stationary. The conditions are differentiated by the associated abnormalities. In acromegaly the scalp involvement tends to be less severe, and the age of onset and the associated manifestations of pituitary excess establish the diagnosis.

These three forms of cutis gyrata must be excluded before any inflammatory changes present are accepted as causative. In the true secondary forms the process is usually localized and asymmetrical.

In the naevoid forms the folding may be associated with pigmentation, but may be the only obvious change. From a small localized area of folding present at birth or appearing in early childhood a large part of the scalp may be covered over a period of a few years, but the affected area remains sharply demarcated from surrounding normal tissues. Exceptionally, naevoid cutis gyrata has occurred in sites other than the scalp—the sides of the neck [14] and the abdominal wall [12].

Treatment. In the primary and systemic forms there is no treatment possible, other than relief of the associated disease where this is practicable. The naevoid forms, and occasionally the systemic forms [1], can be improved by plastic surgery.

REFERENCES

1 ABU-JAMRA F. & DIMICK D.F. (1966) *Am J Surg* 111, 274.
2 AKESSON H.O. (1964) *Acta Med Scand* 175, 115.
3 AKESSON H.O. (1965) *Acta Med Scand* 177, 459.
4 AKESSON H.O. (1965) *Rev Int Genet Med Gemell* 14, 200.
5 BERG J.M. & WINDRATH-SCOTT A. (1961) *J Ment Defic Res* 6, 75.
6 CHESON B.P. & CHRISTIANSEN R.M. (1980) *Am J Hematol* 8, 415.
7 GARCOVICH A., et al (1979) *G Ital Dermatol Minerva Dermatol* 114, 139.
8 HAMMOND G. & RANSOM H.K. (1937) *Arch Surg* 35, 309.
9 KHARE A.K. & SINGH G. (1984) *Bri J Dermatol* 110, 125.
10 PAULSON G.W. (1974) *Dev Med Child Neurol* 16, 196.
11 POLAN S. & BUTTERWORTH T. (1953) *Am J Ment Defic* 57, 613.
12 RUDBERG S. (1939) *Acta Paediatr Scand* 27, 67.
13 SERFLING H.J. & FOELSCHE W. (1959) *Zentralbl Chir* 84, 473.
14 WEBER G. (1955) *Dermatol Wochenschr* 131, 49.
15 ZEISLER E.P. & WIEDER L.M. (1940) *Arch Dermatol Syphilol* 42, 1092.

PITYRIASIS CAPITIS
SYN. DANDRUFF

Definition and nomenclature. Pityriasis (simplex) capitis consists of the desquamation of small flakes of scale from an otherwise normal scalp. The scales may be dry or trapped in a film of sebum. The term pityriasis steatoides has been applied to a mild form of seborrhoeic dermatitis (see p. 375).

Aetiology and pathology [4]. Pityriasis of the scalp is a physiological state which is elevated to the status of a 'disease' solely on cosmetic grounds. Horny scales are continuously shed over the entire surface of the skin at a rate which varies from one region to another but is normally constant in each site. Friction ensures the regular loss of horny scales, and if this is prevented by the application of an occlusive cap [5] a greasy mass of scales soon accumulates. On the scalp the hair interferes with the normal shedding process and flakes of keratin are retained amongst the hair shafts.

Pityriasis is uncommon in infancy and early childhood, but becomes gradually more frequent between the ages of 5 and 10 and rapidly so between 10 and 20, when it reaches its highest incidence and affects some 50% of Caucasoids of both sexes. Comparable figures for other races are not available. Over 40% of Caucasoids are affected in some degree from the age of 30 onwards.

The age incidence suggests that androgenic stimulation may play some permissive role and a certain level of sebaceous activity is presumably a necessary factor. Wide individual variation in severity cannot yet be convincingly explained. A genetic factor may be concerned.

The role of micro-organisms in pityriasis is still uncertain [4, 9, 10, 11]. Both *Pityosporon ovale* and *P. orbiculare* are more abundant in patients with pityriasis than in controls. It has been believed that these and other changes in the scalp flora are secondary to the pityriasis, but experiments with antibiotics and resistant strains of *P. ovale* [6] suggest that this organism may play a part in causing pityriasis [10, 11]. Antibody to *P. ovale* was detectable in high titre in some affected individuals, but also in some controls [3]. Yeast inhibitors produced greater reduction in pityriasis than did bacteria inhibitors [13], but it is possible to reduce the microflora without affecting the pityriasis [1]. The virtual disappearance of the anaerobic *Corynebacterium acnes* during the transition from pityriasis to seborrhoeic dermatitis could be secondary to the increased blood flow [7]. Is the increase in the yeast population also a secondary phenomenon?

Histologically, the scalp shows a loose parakeratotic horny layer, usually fewer than 10 cells thick as compared with the compact 25–35 cell layers of normal scalp [1]. Autoradiographic studies demonstrate increased epidermal turnover [9].

Clinical features. Small silvery-grey scales, lamellar or branny, accumulate first on the vertex, upper parietal and temporal regions of the scalp. They may be confined to one or more usually symmetrical patches or may involve the whole scalp. If male-pattern alopecia is present pityriasis is conspicuously absent from the bald areas. The scales may be more or less adherent and become detached only after brushing or combing, or may separate freely to drift among the hair shafts and be shed on the clothing. In early childhood the pityriasis is rarely sufficiently obvious to be troublesome, but during the second and third decades reaches its greatest severity. In some individuals it remains an embarrassment until the fifties, but more often slowly subsides. Quantitative studies fully confirm the clinical impression that short- and long-term variations in severity occur without obvious cause. In childhood the pityriasis is always dry, and this form persists after puberty in many patients who suffer a greater cosmetic disability than those in whom the development of seborrhoea at puberty binds the scales to the surface in a greasy paste.

Patients with pityriasis and seborrhoea show an increased susceptibility to seborrhoeic dermatitis. In the mild form of the latter, sometimes known as pityriasis steatoides, the scales become larger, thicker and more adherent. If they are forcibly removed the underlying scalp is moist and red.

Diagnosis. The presence of more than a mild degree of pityriasis in a young child is sufficiently unusual to throw doubt on the diagnosis. Severe scaling may accompany some forms of ichthyosis (p. 1416). Localized scaling with broken hairs is characteristic of *Microsporon* ringworm. The hair shafts should be examined microscopically, and if Wood's light is available the presence of greenish fluorescence must

be excluded. Persistent heavy scaling should suggest the possibility of psoriasis, even in the absence of the characteristic changes in this disease.

In traumatic alopecia the hairs are broken and twisted but of normal texture. Severe localized scaling may accompany the inflammatory changes induced by scratching.

Profuse sticky asbestos-like scales occur in pityriasis amiantacea (see below).

Treatment [11]. The treatment of pityriasis is unsatisfactory and control rather than cure must be the objective. In mild cases 2% salicylic acid in emulsifying ointment may be rubbed into the affected areas and removed after 1 or 2 h with a detergent shampoo. Tar shampoos [2, 3] have been shown to be more effective than the vehicle alone, and their weekly use often gives a satisfactory result.

Many proprietary preparations are pleasant to use and are reasonably effective. Some contain selenium disulphide or zinc pyrithione which exert a cytostatic effect and reduce epidermal turnover [8]. Others are claimed to control the yeast flora, and may owe their efficacy to other actions.

Those who believe that pityrosporon species are important often recommend imidazole therapy particularly during bad spells (e.g. topical miconazole or ketoconazole); relapse is common even after successful 'cure'. Oral ketoconazale is no longer used because of the risk of hepatic toxicity.

REFERENCES

1 ACKERMAN A.B. & KLIGMAN A.M. (1969) *J Soc Cosmet Chem* **20**, 81.
2 ALEXANDER S. (1967) *Br J Dermatol* **79**, 92.
3 ALEXANDER S. (1967) *Br J Dermatol* **79**, 549.
4 BRAUN-FALCO O. & HEILGEMEIR G.P. (1978) *Hautarzt* **29**, 245.
5 GOLDSCHMIDT H. & KLIGMAN A.M. (1964) *Archs Dermatol* **88**, 709.
6 GOSSE R.M. & VANDERWYCK R.W. (1969) *J Soc Cosmet Chem* **20**, 603.
7 McGINLEY K.J., *et al* (1975) *J Invest Dermatol* **64**, 401.
8 PLEWIG G. & KLIGMAN A.M. (1970) *Arch Klin Exp Dermatol* **236**, 406.
9 PRIESTLEY G.L. & SAVIN J.A. (1976) *Br J Dermatol* **94**, 469.
10 SHUSTER S. (1984) *Br J. Dermatol* **111**, 235.
11 VAN ABBE H.J., *et al* (1979) In *Hair Research*. Eds. Orfanos C. & Montagna W. Springer, Berlin, p. 582.
12 VANDERWYCK R.W. & HECHEMY K.E. (1967) *J Soc Cosmet Chem* **18**, 629.

PITYRIASIS AMIANTACEA
SYN. TINEA AMIANTACEA

Aetiology. Pityriasis amiantacea is a morphological entity presenting a distinctive pattern of reaction of the scalp to infection or to trauma. It is not a specific manifestation of the seborrhoeic state and can occur at any age but is most frequent in children and young adults. It may be observed as a complication or sequel of streptococcal infection or lichen simplex and it also occurs in psoriasis [4], of which it may be the first clinical manifestation.

Pathology [6]. The histological features are essentially eczema with conspicuous spongiosis and considerable parakeratosis.

Clinical features [1, 2, 3, 5, 6]. Masses of sticky silvery scales, overlapping like tiles on a roof, adhere to the scalp and to the hairs. The underlying scalp is red and moist in those cases secondary to an infective process. The asbestos-like scales cling firmly to the hair shafts and extend some distance along them. The underlying or associated disease is usually obvious but may not be apparent until the pityriasis amiantacea has been treated. Commonly, only a small area of scalp is affected, but the condition can be extensive.

A common form complicates chronic or recurrent fissuring behind the ears in young girls, the sticky scales extending several centimetres into the neighbouring scalp and overlying and concealing the infective eczematoid dermatitis. The same site or the nape may be affected in women with lichen simplex. Hair casts of large dimensions may be present.

Diagnosis. The clinical appearance is so distinctive that confusion with other conditions is unlikely. Psoriasis, seborrhoeic dermatitis and tinea are possible sources of difficulty and may coexist.

Treatment. Those cases secondary to an infective dermatitis respond quickly to a broad spectrum antibiotic ointment or to a preparation such as Fucidin H.C. In the many cases secondary to psoriasis or lichen simplex, the treatment appropriate for those conditions should be prescribed. However, the mass of scale may first be removed by applications

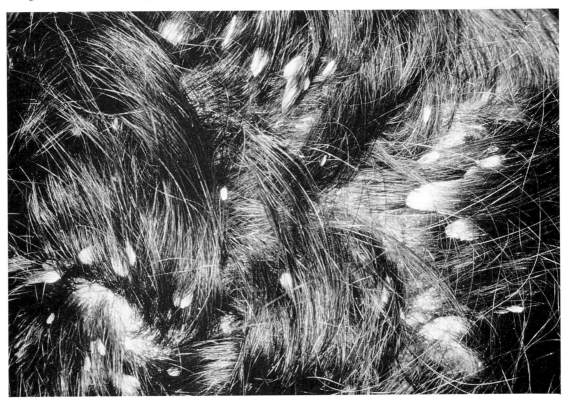

FIG. 53.62. Pityriasis amiantacea (Dr Allan Highet, York District Hospital).

of a tar/keratolytic agent washed out after 4 or 5 h with a detergent shampoo. Relapses are frequent.

REFERENCES

1 BECKER S. & MUIR K. (1929) *Arch Dermatol Syphiligr* 20, 45.

2 DUBREUILH W. (1930) *Ann Dermatol Syphilol* 1, 61.

3 GSCHWANDTNNER W.R. (1974) *Hautarzt* 25, 134.

4 HIRSLE K., *et al* (1979) *Dermatologica* 159, 245.

5 JORDAN P. & NOLTING S. (1971) *Schr Marchionini Stift* 2, 55.

6 KNIGHT A.G. (1977) *Clin Exp Dermatol* 2, 137.

CHAPTER 54

The Nails

R. P. R. DAWBER & R. BARAN

The major part of the nail apparatus develops *in utero* from the primitive epidermis; consequently it has many similarities both in health and disease to the hair and stratum corneum. In generalized integumentary diseases such as psoriasis, the nail apparatus, the hair follicle and the epidermis may all be structurally and functionally affected, presumably because of their common tissue of origin.

The main function of the nail apparatus is to produce a strong, relatively inflexible, keratinous nail plate over the dorsal surface of the end of each digit. The nail plate acts as a protective covering for the fingertip; by exerting counter pressure over the volar skin and pulp, the flat nail plate adds to the precision and delicacy of both, the ability to pick up small objects and many other subtle finger functions [1]. Finger nails typically cover approximately one-fifth of the dorsal surface, whilst on the great toe the nail may cover up to 50% of the dorsum of the digit.

REFERENCE

1 BARAN R. & DAWBER R.P.R. (Eds.) (1984) *Diseases of the Nail and Their Management*. Oxford, Blackwell Scientific.

STRUCTURE

Gross anatomy [12, 13]. The component parts of the nail apparatus are shown in Fig. 54.1. The rectangular nail plate is the largest structure, resting on and firmly attached to the nail bed; the bone is less firm proximally, apart from the posterolateral corners. Approximately one-quarter of the nail is covered by the proximal nail fold whilst a narrow margin of the sides of the nail plate is often occluded by the lateral nail folds. Underlying the proximal part of the nail is the white lunula (syn. half-moon, lunule); this area represents the most distal region of the intermediate (distal) matrix. The reason for the white colour is not clearly known though many researchers have written on the subject [1, 4, 5]. The natural shape of the free margin of the nail is the same as the contour of the distal border of the lunula. The nail plate distal to the lunula is usually pink due to its translucency which allows the redness of the vascular nail bed to be seen through it. The proximal nail fold has two epithelial surfaces, dorsal and ventral; at the junction of the two the cuticle projects distally onto the nail surface. The lateral nail folds are in continuity with the skin on

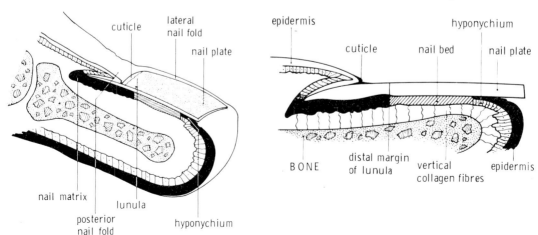

FIG. 54.1. Longitudinal section of a digit showing the dorsal nail apparatus.

the sides of the digit laterally, and medially they are joined by the nail bed. Some authorities term the lateral nail fold and adjacent tissue lateral to the nail fold the nail wall.

The nail matrix (Fig. 54.2) can be subdivided into dorsal and intermediate sections, the latter underlying the nail plate to the distal border of the lunula; some texts prefer the terms proximal and distal matrix respectively. It is now generally considered that the nail bed contributes to the deep surface of the nail plate (ventral matrix). At the point of separation of the nail plate from the nail bed, the proximal part of the hyponychium may be modified as the solehorn [16]. Beyond the solehorn region the hyponychium terminates at the distal nail groove; the tip of the digit beyond this ridge assumes the structure of the epidermis elsewhere.

When the attached nail plate is viewed from above several distinct areas may be visible: the proximal lunule and the larger pink zone. On close examination two further distal zones can often be identified, the distal yellowish-white margin and immediately proximal to this the onychodermal band [18]. This band is a barely perceptible narrow transverse band 0·5–1·5 mm wide; it is more prominent in acrocyanosis. The exact anatomical basis for the onychodermal band is not known but it appears to have a different blood supply than the main body of the nail bed; if the tip of the finger is pressed firmly, the band and an area just proximal to it blanch, and if the pressure is repeated several times the band reddens. Many changes in colour have been described in the onychodermal band in health and disease [18].

granular layer. From the distal area of the proximal nail folds the cuticle reflects onto the surface of the nail plate; it is composed of modified stratum corneum and serves to protect the structures at the base of the nail, particularly the germinative matrix, from environmental insults such as irritants, allergens and bacterial and fungal pathogens.

Nail matrix (intermediate and dorsal; syn. distal and proximal, respectively). This is the area which produces the major part of the nail plate (Fig. 54.2). As in the epidermis of the skin, the matrix possesses a dividing basal layer producing keratinocytes which differentiate, harden, die and contribute to the nail plate, which is thus analogous to the epidermal stratum corneum. The nail matrix keratinocytes mature and keratinize without keratohyalin (granular layer) formation. Apart from this, the detailed cytological changes seen in the matrix epithelium under the electron microscope are essentially the same as in the epidermis [9, 10].

The nail matrix contains melanocytes in the lowest two cell layers and these donate pigment to keratinocytes [11]. Under normal circumstances pigment is not visible in the nail plate of Caucasoid individuals but many Negroid subjects show patchy melanogenesis as linear longitudinal pigmented bands.

Nail bed. This consists of an epidermal part (ventral matrix) and the underlying dermis closely apposed to the periosteum of the distal phalanx. There is no subcutaneous fat in the nail bed although scattered dermal fat cells may be visible microscopically.

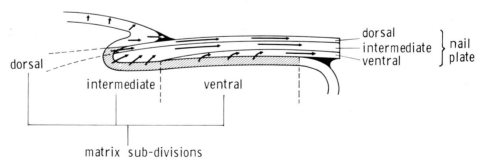

FIG. 54.2. Diagram to show the direction of differentiation and cell movement within the nail apparatus.

Microscopic anatomy
Nail folds. The proximal and lateral nail folds are similar in structure to the adjacent skin but are normally devoid of dermatoglyphic markings and pilosebaceous glands. Keratinization within the nail folds proceeds via keratohyalin formation in the

The nail bed epidermal layer (ventral matrix) is usually no more than two or three cells thick, and the transitional zone from living keratinocyte to dead ventral nail plate cell is abrupt, occurring in the space of one horizontal cell layer—in this regard it closely resembles the *Henle* layer of the internal root sheath of the epidermis [2]. As the cells differentiate they are incorporated into the ventral surface of the nail plate and move distally with this layer [19]. The process of nail bed keratinization has been likened to that seen in rat tail epidermis, possibly being effected by pressure changes.

The nail bed dermal collagen is mainly oriented vertically, being directly attached to phalangeal periosteum and the epidermal basal lamina. Within the connective-tissue network lie blood vessels, lymphatics, a fine network of elastic fibres and scattered fat cells; at the distal margin eccrine sweat glands have been visualized [15].

Nail plate. The nail plate comprises three horizontal layers: a thin dorsal lamina, the thicker intermediate lamina and a ventral layer from the nail bed. Microscopically, it is composed of flattened squamous cells closely apposed owing to tortuous and interlocking plasma membranes [9, 10]. At high magnifications, the contents of each cell show a uniform fine granularity similar to the hair cuticle.

In older age groups, acidophilic masses are occasionally seen, the so-called pertinax bodies [14].

The nail plate contains significant amounts of phospholipid, mainly in the dorsal and intermediate layers, which contributes to its flexibility. The detectable free fats and long-chain fatty acids may be of extrinsic origin. For further details of these and other histochemical and histoenzymological changes in the component parts of the nail apparatus, the reader is referred to more detailed texts [4, 17].

The nail plate is rich in calcium, found as the phosphate in hydroxyapatite crystals; it is bound to phospholipids intracellularly [6]. The relevance of other metals which are present in smaller amounts, including copper, manganese, zinc, iron and others, is not exactly known [20]. Calcium exists in a concentration of 0·1% by weight, 10 times greater than in hair. It is possible that calcium is not an intrinsic part of the nail but is incorporated from extrinsic sources. Calcium does not significantly contribute to the hardness of the nail [7].

Nail keratin analysis shows essentially the same fractions as in hair:
  1. α-fibrillar, low sulphur protein;
  2. globular, high sulphur matrix protein;
  3. high glycine–tyrosine–rich matrix protein.
Amino acid analytical studies show higher cysteine, glutamic acid and serine and less tyrosine in nail compared with hair and wool [3, 8]. The hardness of nail is due to the high sulphur matrix protein, which contrasts with the relatively soft keratin of

the epidermis. The normal transverse curvature of the nail relates to the shape of the underlying phalangeal bone.

REFERENCES

1 ACHTEN G. (1963) *Dermatologica* **126**, 229.
2 ACHTEN G. (1968) In *Handbuch der Haut und Geschlechtskrankheiten*. Ed. Jadassohn J. Berlin, Springer, Vol. 1, p. 339.
3 BADEN H.P., *et al* (1973) *Biochem Biophys Acta* **322**, 269.
4 BARAN R. & DAWBER R.P.R. (Eds.) (1984) *Diseases of the Nails and Their Management*. Oxford, Blackwell Scientific.
5 BURROWS M.T. (1917) *Anat Rec* **12**, 161.
6 CANE A.K. & SPEARMAN R.I.C. (1967) *J Zool (Lond)* **153**, 337.
7 FORSLIND B., *et al* (1976) *J Invest Dermatol* **67**, 273.
8 GILLESPIE J.M. & FRENKEL M.J. (1974) *Comp Biochem Physiol* **47B**, 339.
9 HASHIMOTO K. (1971) *J Invest Dermatol* **56**, 235.
10 HASHIMOTO K. (1971) *J Ultrastruct Res* **36**, 391.
11 HIGASHI N. (1968) *Arch Dermatol* **97**, 570.
12 LEWIN K. (1965) *Br J Dermatol* **77**, 421.
13 LEWIS B.L. (1954) *Arch Dermatol* **70**, 732.
14 LEWIS B. L. & MONTGOMERY H. (1955) *J Invest Dermatol* **24**, 11.
15 MARICQ H.R. (1967) *J Invest Dermatol* **48**, 399.
16 PINKUS F. (1927) In *Handbuch der Haut und Geschlechtskrankheiten*. Ed. Jadassohn J. Berlin, Springer.
17 SAYAG J. & JANCOVICI E. (1980) In *Précis de Physiologie Cutanée*. Ed. Meynadier J. Paris, Editions de le Porte Verte, p. 121.
18 TERRY R.B. (1955) *Lancet* i, 179.
19 ZAIAS N. (1967) *J. Invest Dermatol* **48**, 402.
20 ZAIAS N. (1980) *The Nail in Health and Disease*. New York, Spectrum Press.

Development and comparative anatomy. The nail apparatus develops and matures from the primitive epidermis between the ninth and 20th weeks of intra-uterine growth. At 20 weeks, the matrix cells show postnatal-type cell division, differentiation and keratinization and the nail plate begins to form and move distally [5, 6]; the nail bed loses its granular layer at this stage [1]. By 36 weeks the complete nail plate reaches the tip of the digit and is surrounded by prominent lateral nail folds and a well-formed cuticle.

The structure of claws and hooves and their evolutionary relationship to man has been well reviewed [4]. In higher primates, nails have evolved with the acquisition of manual dexterity; other mammals do not possess such flattened claws from which nails have evolved. Claws and talons are harder than human nails, probably because of their high content of calcium phosphate as crystalline hydroxyapatite within keratinized cells compared with human nails [2]. The hard 'soft plate' under hooves is produced from an area equivalent to the subungual part of the claw. In some animals, cloven hooves have only developed on the 'digits' that touch the floor; in horses, the single large hoof is produced from the third digit. The keratin biochemistry of the human nail has many similarities to that of the anteater or pangolin [3].

REFERENCES

1 BREATHNACH A.S. (1971) *An Atlas of the Ultrastructure of Human Skin*. London, Churchill.
2 PAUTARD F.G.E. (1964) In *Progress in the Biological Sciences in Relation to Dermatology*. Eds. Rook A.J. and Champion R.H. Cambridge, Cambridge University Press.
3 SPEARMAN R.I.C. (1967) *J Linn Soc Zool* **46**, 267.
4 SPEARMAN R.I.C. (1978) In *The Physiology and Pathophysiology of the Skin*. Ed. Jarrett A. New York, Academic Press, Vol. 5, p. 1827.
5 ZAIAS N. (1963) *Arch Dermatol* **87**, 37.
6 ZAIAS N. (1980) *The Nail in Health and Disease*. New York, Spectrum Press.

Blood supply. There is a rich arterial blood supply to the nail bed and matrix derived from paired digital arteries. The main supply passes into the pulp space of the distal phalanx before reaching the dorsum of the digit. An accessory supply arises further back on the digit and does not enter the pulp space [1]. There are two main arterial arches (proximal and distal) supplying the nail bed and matrix, formed from anastomoses of the branches of the digital arteries. In the event of damage to the main supply in the pulp space, such as may occur with infection or scleroderma, there may be sufficient blood from the accessory vessels to permit normal growth of the nail.

There is a capillary loop system to the whole of the nail fold, but the loops to the roof and matrix are flatter than those below the exposed nail [3] (see p. 97 for observations on capillaries of the posterior nail fold). There are many arteriovenous anastomoses below the nail, glomus bodies, which are concerned with heat regulation. Glomus bodies are important in maintaining acral circulation under cold conditions—arterioles constrict with cold but glomus bodies dilate. The nail bed of fingers and toes contain 93–501 such bodies per square centimetre. Each glomus is an encapsulated oval organ 300 µm long, made up of a tortuous vessel uniting an artery and venule, a nerve supply and a capsule; also within the capsule are many cholinergic muscle cells [2].

REFERENCES

1 FLINT M.H. (1955) *Br J Plast Surg* **8**, 186.
2 RYAN T.J. (1973) In *The Physiology and Pathophysiology of the Skin*. Ed. Jarrett A. London, Academic Press, Vol. 2, p. 612.
3 SAMMAN P.D. (1959) *Br J Dermatol* **71**, 296.

NAIL DYNAMICS

Clinicians used to observing the slow rate of clearance of diseased or damaged nails are apt to view the nail apparatus as a rather inert structure although it is in fact the centre of very marked kinetic and biochemical activity.

Cell kinetics. Unlike the hair matrix which undergoes a resting or quiescent (telogen) phase every few years, the nail matrix germinative layers continue to undertake DNA synthesis, to divide and to differentiate throughout life, akin to the epidermis in this respect. Exactly which parts of the nail apparatus contribute to the nail plate has attracted much attention [25, 31]: it is now usually accepted that the three-layered nail plate is produced from the dorsal matrix, the intermediate matrix and the ventral (nail bed) matrix (Fig. 54.2). Some authorities have suggested that a further contribution is made by the proximal hyponychial area, the solehorn [31]; the latter contribution is probably more significant in diseases typically producing distal subungual hyperkeratosis such as pityriasis rubra pilaris.

Cell kinetics studies on human nails have been limited by the difficulty of obtaining tissues, since many of the techniques used to study DNA synthesis, mitotic cycle and transit times in skin require serial observations on biopsy tissue. Mitotic activity can certainly be seen in the basal area of the dorsal, intermediate and ventral matrices. Labelled thymidine and glycine studies have shown that, of the dorsal, intermediate and nail bed (ventral) matrices, the intermediate matrix has the fastest mitotic rate and the ventral matrix the slowest; also, the nail bed defininitely contributes a ventral layer to the nail plate [27, 37, 40].

Why the nail grows flat, rather than as a heaped up keratinous mass, has generated much thought and discussion [2, 19, 20, 33]. Several factors probably combine to produce a relatively flat nail plate: the orientation of the matrix rete pegs and papillae; the direction of cell differentiation [15]; and the fact that since keratinization takes place within the confines of the nail base, limited by the proximal nail fold dorsally and the terminal phalanx ventrally [18], the differentiating cells can only move distally

Faster	Slower	Faster	Slower
Daytime	Night	Psoriasis [22]	Finger immobilization [9]
Pregnancy [17]	First day of life [36]	(i) 'normal' nails [6]	
Minor trauma/nail biting [13, 14]		(ii) pitting	Fever [38]
Right-hand nails	Left-hand nails [28]	(iii) onycholysis [10]	
Youth Increasing age	Old age [6, 23]		Beau's lines [39]
		Pityriasis rubra pilaris [8, 34]	Methotrexate
Fingers	Toes [30]		
Summer [5]	Winter or cold environment [11, 32]	Etretinate—rarely [3]	Azathioprine [6]
			Etretinate [3]
Middle, ring and index	Thumb and little [21, 24, 28, 30]	Idiopathic onycholysis of women [10]	Denervation [16]
Men	Women [14, 24]	Bullous ichthyosiform erythroderma [35]	Poor nutrition [13]
			Kwashiorkor [1]
		Hyperthyroidism [28]	
		L-dopa [26]	Hypothyroidism [28]
		A–V shunts [28]	Yellow nail syndrome [35]
			Relapsing polychondritis [12]
(a)		(b)	

FIG. 54.3. (a) Physiological and environmental factors affecting nail growth; (b) pathological factors affecting nail growth.

and form a flat structure—by the time they leave the confines of the proximal nail fold all the cells are hardened and keratinized.

Linear nail growth. Over the last century very many studies have been carried out on the linear growth of the nail plate in health and disease; these have been well reviewed [4, 34] and are listed in Fig. 54.3 Most of these studies have been carried out by observing the distal movement of a reference mark etched on the nail plate over a fixed period of time; this may well correlate with matrix germinative cell kinetics but there is no direct proof that it does. However, the studies on nail growth in psoriasis, and its inhibition by cytostatic drugs [6, 7] suggest that cell kinetics and linear growth rate do have a direct correlation.

Finger nails grow at approximately 1 cm per 3 months and toe-nails at one-third of this rate.

REFERENCES

1 BABCOCK M.J. (1955) *J Nutr* **55**, 323.
2 BARAN R. (1981) *J Am Acad Dermatol* **4**, 78.
3 BARAN R. (1982) *Ann Dermatol Vénéréol* **109**, 367.
4 BARAN R. & DAWBER R.P.R. (Eds.) (1984) *Diseases of the Nail and Their Management*. Oxford, Blackwell Scientific.
5 BEAN W.B. (1974) *Arch Intern Med* **134**, 497.
6 DAWBER R.P.R. (1970) *Br J Dermatol* **82**, 454.
7 DAWBER R.P.R. (1970) *Br J Dermatol* **83**, 680.
8 DAWBER R.P.R. (1980) *Arch Derm Res* **269**, 197.
9 DAWBER R.P.R. (1981) *Clin Exp Derm* **6**, 1.
10 DAWBER R.P.R., *et al* (1971) *Br J Dermatol* **85**, 558.
11 DONOVAN K.M. (1977) *Br J Dermatol* **96**, 507.
12 ESTES S. A. (1983) *Cutis* **32**, 471.
13 GILCHRIST M.L. & BUXTON L.H.D. (1939) *J Anat* **73**, 575.
14 HAMILTON J.B., *et al* (1955) *J Geront* **10**, 401.
15 HASHIMOTO K. (1971) *Arch Dermatol Forsch* **240**, 1.
16 HEAD H. & SHERRIN J. (1905) *Brain* **28**, 116.
17 HEWITT D. & HILLMAN R.W. (1966) *Am J Clin Nutr* **19**, 436.
18 KELIKIAN H. (1974) *Congenital Deformities of the Hand and the Forearm*. Philadelphia, Saunders, p. 210.
19 KLIGMAN A.M. (1961) *Arch Dermatol* **84**, 181.
20 KLIGMAN A.M. (1981) *J Am Acad Dermatol* **4**, 82.
21 KNOBLOCH V.H. (1953) *Dtsch Med Wochenschr* **78**, 743.
22 LANDHERR G., *et al* (1982) *Hautarzt* **33**, 210.
23 LAVELLE C.E. (1981) *Curr Probl Dermatol* **9**, 102.
24 LE GROS-CLARK W.E. & BUXTON L.H.D. (1938) *Br J Dermatol* **50**, 221.
25 LEWIS B.L. (1954) *Arch Dermatol* **70**, 732.
26 MILLER E. (1973) *N Engl J Med* **288**, 916.
27 NORTON L. A. (1971) *J Invest Dermatol* **56**, 61.
28 ORENTREICH N., *et al* (1979) *J Invest Dermatol* **73**, 126.
29 PFISTER R. (1955) *Z. Haut Geschlechtskr* **18**, 132.
30 PFISTER R. & HENEKA J. (1965) *Arch Klin Exp Dermatol* **223**, 263.
31 PINKUS F. (1927) In *Handbuch der Haut und Geschlechtskrankheiten*. Ed. Jadassohn J. Berlin, Springer, p. 267.

32 ROBERTS D. F. & SANDFORD M.R. (1958) *J Appl Physiol* 13, 135.
33 RUNNE U. (1980) *Hautarzt* 31, 344.
34 RUNNE U. & ORFANOS C.E. (1981) *Curr Probl Dermatol* 9, 102.
35 SAMMAN P.D. (1978) *The Nails in Disease*. 3rd ed. London, Heinemann, p. 14.
36 SCHNCK B. (1908) *Säuglings Jahro Kinderh* 67, 146.
37 SCHMIEGELOW P., et al (1983) *Aktuelle Dermatol* 2, 62.
38 SIBINGA M. S. (1959) *Pediatrics* 24, 225.
39 WEISMANN K. (1977) *Br J Dermatol* 97, 571.
40 ZAIAS N. & ALVAREZ J. (1968) *J Invest Dermatol* 51, 120.

THE NAIL IN CHILDHOOD AND OLD AGE

Childhood. In early childhood, the nail plate is relatively thin and may show temporary koilonychia; because of the shape of the matrix, some children show ridges which start laterally, by the proximal nail fold, and join at a central point just short of the free margin. In one study [5], 92% of normal infants between 8 and 9 weeks of age showed a single transverse line (Beau's line) on the fingernails. One child demonstrated a transverse depression through the whole nail thickness on all 20 digits [6].

Old age. In the elderly, elastic tissue changes diffusely affecting the nail bed epidermis are often seen histologically [1]; these changes may be due to the effects of UV radiation, although it has been stated that the nail plate is an efficient filter of UV light [4]. The whole subungual area in old age may show thickening of blood vessel walls with vascular elastic tissues fragmentation. Pertinax bodies are often seen in the nail plate; they are probably remnants of nuclei of keratinocytes. Nail growth is inversely proportional to age [2]; related to this slower growth, corneocytes are larger in old age [3].

The nail plate becomes paler, dull and opaque with advancing years and white nails similar to those seen in cirrhosis, uraemia and hypoalbuminaemia may be seen in normal subjects. Longitudinal ridging is present to some degree in most people after 50 years of age and this may give a 'sausage links' appearance.

For details of the common traumatic abnormalities and changes due to inadequate pedicure or neglect, detailed texts should be consulted [2].

REFERENCES

1 BARAN R. (1982) *Curr Med Res Opin* 7(2), 96.
2 BARAN R. & DAWBER R.P.R. (Eds) (1984) *Diseases of the Nail and Their Management*. Oxford, Blackwell Scientific.
3 GERMAIN H., et al (1980) *J Invest Dermatol* 74, 115.
4 PARKER S.G. & DIFFEY B.L. (1983) *Br J Dermatol* 108, 11.
5 TURANO A. F. (1968) *Pediatrics* 41, 996.
6 WOLF D., et al (1982) *Cutis* 29, 141.

NAIL DISORDERS ASSOCIATED WITH DERMATOLOGICAL DISEASES AND MISCELLANEOUS ACQUIRED NAIL DISORDERS

Psoriasis. Psoriasis is probably the disease which most often produces nail deformities. Not only is the nail very often involved in the presence of psoriasis on other parts of the body, but not infrequently the nail is affected in the complete absence of psoriasis at other sites, or with only minimal changes elsewhere, e.g. in the scalp, on the genitalia or in the ear and external auditory canal. It is possible that almost every patient with psoriasis has nail involvement some time during the course of his disease. If only a single careful inspection of the nails is made, 15–25% of all cases show nail involvement. Finger nails are said to be involved more often than toe nails, but this may be apparent rather than real, as toe nail involvement is seldom a cause for complaint. In children, nail changes are less common [2].

Nail changes in psoriasis are very varied and diagnosis can at times be difficult. There are three characteristic patterns of nail involvement: pitting, onycholysis and grosser abnormalities, notably discoloration and thickening. Pitting (Fig. 54.4) is the best known of the nail deformities in psoriasis and probably the most frequent, although onycholysis occurs almost as often. Pits may vary in frequency from a few small, irregularly spaced depressions on the surface of one or more nails to regular uniform pitting of all nails. The pits are usually quite small, about the size of a pin-head (under 1 mm in diameter), but much larger depressions, and even isolated punched-out areas, are seen occasionally. The pits are formed during the process of keratinization of the nail and are undoubtedly due to an intermittent defect in the matrix, presumably the most proximal part of the matrix as the upper surface of the nail is affected. The pits may be seen first as they emerge from below the cuticle and move forward with the growth of the nail. A mottling in the half-moon is often seen in psoriasis, and less often with pitted nails from other causes. Alkiewicz [1] claims that the pits are due to the retention of nuclei in parts of the nail keratin; these areas, being weaker, are shed and the pits form when the surface is lost. Zaias [10] has shown more exactly how

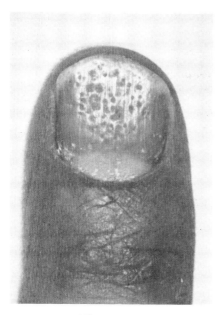

FIG. 54.4. Psoriasis—diffuse pitting.

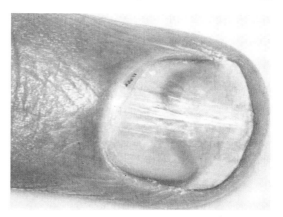

FIG. 54.5. Psoriasis—onycholysis with proximal inflammatory margin.

this occurs and also how nail bed psoriasis is responsible for onycholysis and coloured patches on the nail plate. A scanning electron microscopy study [8] of normal and psoriatic nails has shown that the surface of normal nails is made up of overlapping flat cells with the overlap opposite to the direction of nail growth. The cell surfaces are generally flat and closely opposed. A few micropits are visible. The pits of psoriatic nails differ from normal nails in that the cells of the surface are smaller and do not have the overlapping pattern. They appear to be heaped up and growing, in a haphazard way and are more on edge, as if crowded together. There are spaces between the poorly interdigitated cells. Numerous micropits are also seen.

Nail pitting is not always due to psoriasis. A similar, although rather finer, pitting may be seen in alopecia areata. A coarser more irregular pitting is often seen in eczema or dermatitis and is then often accompanied by cross-ridging. Less common causes of pitting are fungal infections, chronic paronychia and lichen planus. A few isolated small pits may be found without other evidence of skin disease and, rarely, uniform pitting of the whole nail plate appears to be a developmental anomaly in its own right.

Onycholysis occurs in many diseases but psoriasis is probably its most frequent cause (Fig. 54.5). It usually starts at the edge or free margin of one or more nails and may progress until much of the nail

is separated from the nail bed. Intervening between the separated area of the nail, which appears white in colour, and the pink of the attached nail there is often a yellow or brown band. This band is only occasionally seen in onycholysis due to other causes. Less often, the separation starts in the centre of the nail plate with the formation of a small area of yellow which may extend until a white spot is seen surrounded by a yellow margin. Several such yellow spots may be present on one nail. Onycholysis can come on very suddenly, several nails being affected simultaneously. There is often some slight discomfort during its formation.

There seems little doubt that onchyolysis in psoriasis is due to the development of psoriasis in the nail bed and is in no way due to a defect in the matrix.

A complication of onycholysis which is seen occasionally in severe cases is the development of a ridge on the proximal part of the nail bed, which lifts the separated area of the nail plate so far from the bed that the patient is forced to keep the nail cut very short for comfort. The reason for the development of the ridge is unknown.

The grosser changes, though less common, are more disfiguring. Discolouration of a yellow or brown hue is seen to start as it emerges from below the cuticle and moves forward with the growth of the nail until the whole nail is involved. The nail becomes opaque, loses its lustre and may become rough and softer than normal. Slight thickening is common. Usually many nails are affected, although not necessarily all to the same extent, but, as in fungal infections of the nail, one nail may be completely spared when all other nails are involved. This condition can mimic fungal infections very closely, but can be distinguished by the absence of typical mycelia in a potash preparation. Very seldom are dermatophytes found in combination with nail psoriasis, although yeasts and bacteria are commonly present in the subungual debris [10] and it has been pointed out that chronic paronychia is common in association with nail psoriasis [6]. The colour is said to be due to large amounts of a serum-like exudate containing glycoprotein which is found in the affected nails [10].

Great thickening of the nail is another occasional feature of psoriasis (Fig. 54.6). The nail changes are

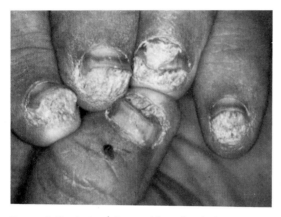

FIG. 54.6. Psoriasis—subungual hyperkeratosis.

similar to those described in the previous paragraph, except that the nail is greatly thickened by the incorporation of material from the nail bed into the nail (ventral nail). A very similar change is seen occasionally in Darier's disease and pachyonychia congenita. The associated findings should make the differential diagnosis easy.

Hyperkeratosis of the nail bed is another feature of psoriasis; this may distort the nail by upward curvature at the free margin.

A light microscopy study [7] has shown that psoriasis of the finger nail produces metaplastic changes of the matrix and nail bed so that they resemble skin epithelium, and the subsequent histological changes are the same as those of psoriasis of the skin.

Arthropathic psoriasis occurs more often in patients with nail psoriasis than in those whose nails are normal. There is no direct relationship, however, between arthritis of the distal interphalangeal joint and psoriasis of the corresponding nail [3].

Treatment of nail psoriasis is very unsatisfactory. Many cases clear spontaneously or during treatment of the skin. When methotrexate is given the nails usually return to normal. Some cases persist indefinitely. The application of fluorinated topical steroids with polyethylene occlusion at night is sometimes helpful but should only be used for a few weeks at a time. Skilful manicure can greatly improve the appearance of many affected nails. Temporary improvement can be obtained by injections of triamcinolone into the nail matrix using a jet injector. This treatment is not recommended for routine use, however, as there is a theoretical possibility of transferring viral infections from one patient to the next because the apparatus is very difficult to sterilize completely and relapse is common. Fredriksson [5] claims considerable improvement from the topical application of 1% 5-fluorouracil solution without occlusion over a period of 6 months. About 25 ml of the solution was used each month. The possible value of PUVA (p. 1505; see also Ref. 4) and aromatic retinoids [9] remains to be clarified.

REFERENCES

1 ALKIEWICZ J. (1948) *Br J Dermatol* **60**, 195.
2 ASBOE-HANSEN G. (1961) In *Psoriasis: Proc Int Symp Stanford University*. Eds. Farber E.M. & Cox A.J. Stanford, Stanford University Press.
3 BAKER H., *et al* (1964) *Br J Dermatol* **76**, 549.
4 BARAN R. (1982) *Ann Dermatol Vénéréol* **109**, 367.
5 FREDRIKSSON T. (1974) *Arch Dermatol* **110**, 735.
6 GANER S. (1975) *Br J Dermatol* **92**, 685.
7 LEWIN K., *et al.* (1972) *Br J Dermatol* **86**, 555.
8 MAURO J., *et al* (1975) *NY State J Med* **75**, 339.
9 RABINOVITZ H.S., *et al* (1983) *Arch Dermatol* **119**, 627.
10 ZAIAS N. (1969) *Arch Dermatol* **99**, 567.

Pustular psoriasis and acrodermatitis continua [1]. The nail changes in these two conditions closely simulate the grosser changes described under psoriasis and are probably basically the same. In some cases complete disruption of the nail occurs, especially when pustules form below the nail plate (Fig. 54.7). Occasionally the nail is permanently lost.

REFERENCE

1 BARAN R. (1979) *Arch Dermatol* **115**, 815.

Dermatitis and eczema. The nails become involved in any form of eczema or dermatitis affecting the hands, and especially the posterior nail folds. They are more often affected in atopic dermatitis than in other forms. The changes are usually dystrophic, leading to a roughening of the nail surface, coarse pitting and some discoloration. Irregular cross-

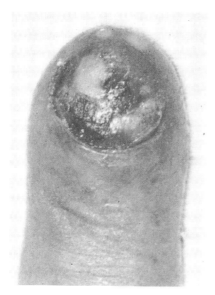

FIG. 54.7. Psoriasis—pustular.

associated with inflammation around the cuticle. Dermatitis of the finger tips may be accompanied by onycholysis of one or more nails.

Dermatitis affecting the nails is generally easily diagnosed by the associated changes in the skin and the history of dermatitis. It has to be distinguished from fungal infections, chronic paronychia (which may, however, also be present) and from psoriasis (Table 54.1). It should be realized that dermatitis occasionally precipitates nail psoriasis in psoriatic subjects, when the nail alone may be involved. At times the nails are severely affected in the presence of a minimal pompholyx, presumably because there is an associated eczematous change in the nail fold.

Treatment. No specific treatment is required; the nail changes will slowly clear when the dermatitis is controlled.

Parakeratosis pustulosa [3]. This is a disorder mainly confined to young children, especially girls. The condition lasts a long time, often several years. The lesions begin close to the free margin of the

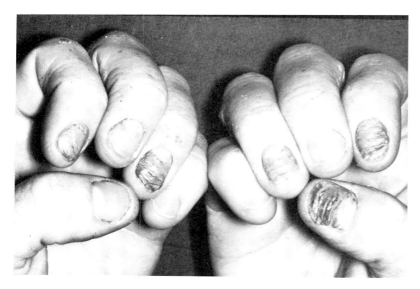

FIG. 54.8. Polymorphic nail plate dystrophy—chronic eczema.

ridging appears on many of the affected nails (Fig. 54.8) and some of the ridges may be quite deep; some may penetrate deeply enough to lead to temporary loss of the nail. The cuticle is often partly or wholly destroyed. The onset of generalized dermatitis or erythroderma may be marked by a deep ridge on several nails followed by roughnesss and discoloration of the nail behind the ridge. In place of these dystrophic changes a greatly thickened nail may, much less often, be formed; this is likely to be

nail, and in 25% of cases a few isolated pustules or vesicles can be seen in the initial phase. These soon clear and eczematoid changes cover the skin immediately adjacent to the free margin of the nail. The area is pink or skin-coloured and covered with fine scales. It may extend to the dorsal nail fold or to the sides of the finger or toe. The most striking and characteristic changes result from hyperkeratosis under the free margin of the nail. The nail itself is lifted and deformed, and sometimes thick-

TABLE 54.1. Differential diagnosis between four common nail disorders: fungal infections, psoriasis, chronic paronychia and dermatitis

	Colour	Onycholysis	Pitting	Filaments or spores in potash preparations	Cross-ridging	Other
Fungal infections	Often yellow or brown; part or whole of nail	Frequent	Infrequent	Filaments, usually abundant	Absent	Associated fungal infections elsewhere
Psoriasis	May be normal or yellow or brown	Frequent	Often present and fine	Absent	Uncommon	Associated psoriasis elsewhere or family history of psoriasis
Chronic paronychia	Edge of nail often discoloured brown or black	Usually absent	Uncommon	May be spores in edge of nail; filaments and spores in scrapings from nail fold	Frequent	Usually women; wet work and cold hands
Dermatitis	May be normal	Confined to tip or absent	Coarse pits frequent	Absent	Frequent	Recent history of dermatitis on hands

ened. The hyperkeratosis rarely extends more than 1–2 mm into the nail bed. The condition is often not symmetrical but limited to one corner of the nail. There may be pitting and, rarely, cross-ridging. The condition is more common on the hands and usually is limited to one digit, less often two, rarely more. Thumb and index finger are most often affected on the hands and great toes on the feet. The condition may recur after apparent cure and may then involve a different digit.

Although the nail changes are more like psoriasis than eczema, Hjorth & Thomsen [3] consider the condition to be an independent eczematoid eruption.

Other writers believe it is a symptom of various disorders including psoriasis [1, 2].

REFERENCES

1 BOTELLA R., *et al* (1973) *Actas Dermo-Sifiliogr* **64**, 579.
2 DULANTO F., *et al* (1974) *Acta DermVenereol (Stockh)* **54**, 365.
3 HJORTH N. & THOMSEN K. (1967) *Br J Dermatol* **79**, 527.

Darier's disease [1–5]. The nails are often affected in this rare condition. Several types of change are seen. The most characteristic is a white streak or streaks extending longitudinally through the nail, and which may be seen crossing the half-moon. This is an early change, and later the streaks are of a darker colour (Fig. 54.9). Where the streaks meet the free edge of the nail, V-shaped notches may be

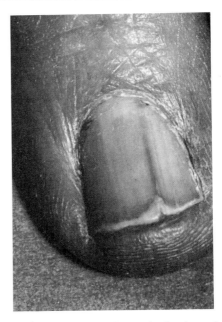

FIG. 54.9. Darier's disease—longitudinal red streak with distal notching.

present. Excess ridging and a rough nail surface may also be found. Occasionally, marked thickening of the nail plate occurs. It is probable that the nail is sometimes affected in the absence of disease elsewhere [1].

REFERENCES

1 RONCHESE F. (1965) *Arch Dermatol* **91**, 617.
2 SAVIN J.A. & SAMMAN P.D. (1970) *Med Biol Illus*, **20**, 85.
3 SCHUBERT H. (1966) *Z Haut Geschlechtskr* **41**, 239.
4 ZAIAS N. (1973) *Arch Dermatol* **107**, 193.
5 ZAIAS N. & ACKERMAN A.B. (1973) *Arch Dermatol* **107**, 193.

Syphilis [1, 2]. Older texts attribute a great many nail disorders to syphilis. Whether or not this is justified it is impossible to say, but syphilis affecting the nails is now very rare, and the only lesion of any importance is the primary chancre.

A chancre may occur on the finger and present as a paronychia, but with very little pain. If allowed to progress untreated it may cause partial or complete loss of the nail, with atrophy, but if treated early should cause little permanent deformity.

REFERENCES

1 ADAMSON H.G. & MCDONAGH J.E.R. (1911) *Br J Dermatol* **23**, 68.
2 STARZYCKI Z. (1983) *Brit J Vener Dis* **59**, 169.

Bacterial paronychia. Acute paronychia is a common complaint and is usually due to the staphylococcus. It may result from local injuries, e.g. splits, splinters or nail biting, or there may be no preceding injury. It also occurs frequently as a complication of chronic paronychia, when other organisms may be involved, including streptococci, *Pseudomonas pyocyanea*, coliform organisms and *Proteus vulgaris*.

The condition presents as a painful swelling of the nail fold. If quite superficial it may point close to the nail and can easily be drained by incision with a sharp-pointed scalpel, without anaesthesia. Deeper lesions are best treated by antibiotics in the first place, but if they do not improve rapidly incision under general or local anaesthesia will be required. A broad spectrum antibiotic is preferred, because it is unlikely that the organism can be identified in advance. Some authorities recommend removing the proximal one-third of the nail plate to aid drainage and speed healing.

Chronic paronychia. This is one of the commonest nail complaints met with in dermatological practice. It ranks in importance with fungal infections and psoriasis as a cause of nail disease, but presents more commonly and is often misdiagnosed and mistreated. It occurs in persons whose hands are much exposed to water, and especially in persons with cold hands [3, 5]. It is common in diabetics [5]. It is much more common in women than in men. It may occur at any age, but the majority of cases are in patients between 30 and 60 years of age [3]. It is occasionally seen in children, especially as a result of finger- or thumb-sucking [10]. It is predominantly a disease of housewives and of people involved in certain occupations such as bar-tenders and canteen workers. Among affected men the chief occupations are chef, barman and fishmonger [4].

Any finger may be involved, but those most often affected are the index and middle fingers of the right hand and the middle finger of the left [4]. These fingers may be more subject to minor trauma than the remainder. The condition begins as a slight swelling at the base of one or more nails (Fig. 54.10), which is tender, but much less so than in acute paronychia. The cuticle is soon lost and pus may form below the nail fold. The condition appears

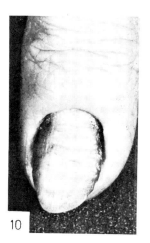
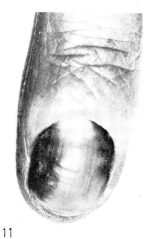

10   11

FIG. 54.10. Chronic paronychia (St John's Hospital).

FIG. 54.11. Chronic paronychia with *Ps. pyocyanea* infection at the edge of the nail (Westminster Hospital).

to be due largely to infection with *Candida* species, usually *Candida albicans* [6]. Spores and mycelia can always be found in the bead of pus when it forms, and they can usually be found if the keratin of the posterior nail fold is gently scraped. Stone & Mullins [9] showed that chronic paronychia can be produced by nonviable *C. albicans* introduced into a relatively sterile nail fold. Foreign material passes through the epidermis of the roof of the nail fold and sets up a chronic inflammation in the dermis. The foreign material may well be derived from *Candida*. This reaction initiates the rounding off of the dorsal nail fold and accounts for the chronicity of the infection. Once the foreign material has penetrated the epidermis, it is very difficult to remove. Acute exacerbations occur from time to time and are due to secondary bacterial infection. Various organisms may be found, including *Staphylococcus aureus* or *albus*, *Proteus vulgaris*, *Escherichia coli* and *Pseudomonas pyocyanea*. Barlow *et al.* [2] believe *Staph. aureus* plays a more active part in initiating the process by penetrating the keratin at the base of the nail and opening up the nail fold. Darkening and irregularity of the edge of the nails are frequent (Fig. 54.11). There is some evidence that the darkening is due to the pigment from *Pseudomonas* infection entering the nail [7]. Cross-ridging of the nail similar to that seen in dermatitis and, less often, greater distortion of the nail may occur. In long-standing cases the size of the nail may be reduced, and this reduction is exaggerated by the great bolstering of the fold all around the nail. Most of the nail deformity is due to the inflammation interfering with the formation of the nail, but a true Candida infection of the nail plate is seen occasionally.

Treatment. Miconazole nitrate cream is a useful application in the early stages. Barlow *et al.* [2] suggest using gentamicin ointment during the day and nystatin ointment at night. When redness and tenderness are present they recommend a course of erythromycin by mouth, because they found pathological staphylococci sensitive to this antibiotic were always present under these circumstances. Later, 15% sulphacetamide in 50% spirit (alcohol) or Castellani's paint may be more useful. A vasodilator in suitable dosage should be given to patients with cold hands; tolazoline hydrochloride (Priscol) 12.5 mg 6-hourly may be effective. Perhaps the most important part of treatment, but the one most difficult to achieve, is to keep the hands dry. For all wet work the patients should be advised to wear cotton gloves under rubber gloves. They should be advised to avoid further damage from fiddling with the nails and to take care with their personal toilet

by protecting the affected fingers first. Covering the affected fingers with a porous surgical tape may afford some protection, but normal occlusion aggravates. Incision is never indicated, and removal of the nail only if there is extensive *Candida* infection of the nail plate. In very long-standing cases it may be worth trying to produce an acute inflammation chemically [8] by inserting a sharpened orange stick dipped in pure phenol into the space between the surface of the nail and the roof of the nail fold. This may have to be repeated two or three times weekly for a few weeks. It should not be used unless local circulation is adequate, or gangrene may be produced. More conservative treatment is continued subsequently. Attempting to clean out the nail fold with a sharpened orange stick is not recommended. If there is obvious candidal infection elsewhere this must also be treated. Wilson says that no aqueous solution, cream or ointment should be used in treatment, and recommends 4% thymol in chloroform inserted into the groove with a dropper [11]. Cryosurgery, using liquid nitrogen spray to the nail folds, or surgical removal of the proximal nail fold and adjacent part of the lateral nail folds may cure recalcitrant cases [1].

REFERENCES

1 BARAN R. & BUREAU H. (1981) *J Dermatol Surg Oncol* 7, 106.
2 BARLOW A.J.E., *et al* (1970) *Br J Dermatol* 82, 448.
3 ESTEVES J. (1959) *Dermatologica* 119, 229.
4 FRAIN-BELL W. (1957) *Trans St John's Hosp Dermatol Soc* 38, 29.
5 HELLIER F.F. (1955) *Br Med J* ii, 1358.
6 MARTEN R.H. (1959) *Br J Dermatol* 71, 422.
7 STONE O.J. & MULLINS J.F. (1963) *J Invest Dermatol* 41, 25.
8 STONE O.J. & MULLINS J.F. (1964) *Arch Dermatol* 89, 455.
9 STONE O.J. & MULLINS J.F. (1965) *Arch Dermatol* 91, 70.
10 STONE O.J. & MULLINS J.F. (1968) *Clin Pediatr* 7, 104.
11 WILSON J.W. (1965) *Arch Dermatol* 92, 726.

Herpetic whitlow [1,2]. Uncommon, and probably usually overlooked, this condition is encountered most often among nurses and in orderlies of neurosurgical units. It is due to primary inoculation of the herpes simplex virus and presents as single or grouped blisters close to the nail; it may give a honeycomb appearance. Clear at first, the blisters soon become purulent and may break and be replaced by crusts. It may be very painful and takes about 3 weeks to resolve, but the pain usually subsides in 10 days. Lymphangitis sometimes occurs.

Diagnosis may be established by recovering the virus from a recent blister and by cytological examination of the blister floor. Contact cases may occur.

Treatment does little to shorten the course of the disorder, but cleaning with 1/6000 potassium permanganate, followed by the application of a bland cream, is recommended. Relapse may occur as with other primary herpetic infections. The value of thymidine analogues such as 5% topical idoxuridine and oral or topical acyclovir remains unproven at this site.

REFERENCES

1 CHANG T. & GORBACH S.L. (1977) *Int J Dermatol* **16**, 752.
2 STERN H., *et al* (1959) *Lancet* ii, 871.

Dystrophia unguis mediana canaliformis (Heller) [1, 3, 6] (median nail dystrophy). This is an uncommon and curious condition in which a split or true canal develops in one or more nails, usually the thumbnails. The split may be observed as it emerges from below the cuticle and moves forward with the growth of the nail. It is usually just off centre. Extending from the split there are often a few fine cracks projecting towards, but not reaching, the edges of the nail on each side (Fig. 54.12).

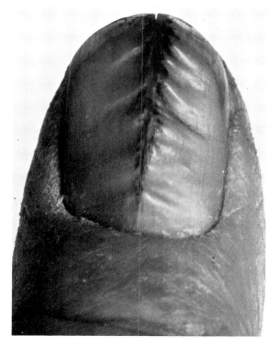

FIG. 54.12. Median canaliform nail dystrophy.

The whole appearance has been likened to an inverted fir tree. After a period of months or years the nails return to normal, but relapse may occur [5]. With healing, a ridge often replaces the split in the nail. The cause of this disorder is unknown, but it is certainly due to some temporary defect in the matrix interfering with nail formation. As most of the patients with this disorder have a large lunula on the affected nail, it is possible that the condition is traumatic in nature, as less of the matrix than usual lies under the protection of the posterior nail fold. Some cases give a definite history of trauma [2]. Familial cases have been recorded. Sutton [4] describes a case on a toe nail in which a flabby filament of fleshy tissue was present in the canal. The only important differential diagnoses are splits in association with dystrophies (e.g. nail–patella syndrome), the damage caused by playing with the nails as a habit tic, punctate matrix scars from microtrauma and split nail deformity. Treatment is unnecessary, but the patient should be advised to apply an emollient cream to the nail fold.

REFERENCES

1 HELLER J. (1928) *Dermatol Z* **51**, 416.
2 RONCHESE F. (1953) *Ind Med Surg* **22**, 45.
3 SELLER J. (1974) *Hautarzt* **25**, 456.
4 SUTTON R.J. JR. (1965) *South Med J* **58**, 1143.
5 SWEET R.D. (1951) *Arch Dermatol Syphil* **64**, 61.
6 ZELGER J., *et al* (1974) *Hautarzt* **25**, 629.

Onycholysis (idiopathic). This is a painless separation of the nail from its bed which occurs without apparent cause. Overzealous manicure, frequent wetting and cosmetic 'solvents' may be the cause and they may not be admitted by the patient. There may, however, be a minor traumatic element, as the condition occurs rather more often in persons who keep their nails abnormally long. Maceration with water may also be a factor [2]. It must be distinguished from other causes of onycholysis (see below). The affected nails grow very quickly [2].

The condition usually starts at the tip of one or more nails and progresses until one-third of the affected nails are loose (Fig. 54.13). The separated area is pale owing to the loss of light reflection from the nail bed. The nail bed is at first normal in appearance, but it is difficult to remove dirt which accumulates below the nail. Pain occurs only if there is further extension as a result of trauma or if active infection supervenes. More often there is a silent infection of a mixed nature, including *C. albicans* and several bacteria, of which *Ps. pyocyanea* is perhaps the most important. If the condition

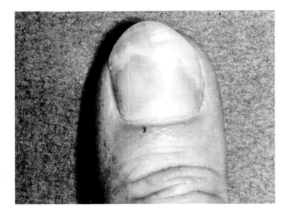

FIG. 54.13. Onycholysis of a thumbnail.

persists for several months the nail bed becomes dark and irregularly thickened.

The condition is almost confined to women and many cases return to normal after a few weeks or months. The longer it lasts the less likely is the nail to become reattached.

Treatment. The patient should be advised to cut away as much as possible of the loosened nail and to apply 15% sulphacetamide in 50% spirit (alcohol) [7] or a topical steroid preparation containing antibiotics and nystatin, e.g. Triadcortyl (Mycolog) ointment, to the nail bed two or three times daily, or to use miconazole hydrocortisone cream (Daktacort) b.d. Re-attachment is slow, and the loosened nail should be recut several times if necessary. The object of treatment is to prevent infection becoming established below the loosened nail, because this leads to thickening of the nail bed and prevents re-attachment. Four per cent thymol in chloroform has been recommended as a means of preventing infection and further maceration of the nail bed [10]; 2% thymol is often as strong as the patient can tolerate, however, and is usually effective.

Onycholysis (secondary). There are many other causes of onycholysis which is one of the commonest nail symptoms [1]. They may be grouped as follows.

(a) Dermatological disorders: psoriasis, fungal infections and dermatitis are all common causes; congenital ectodermal defect is a rare one.

(b) General medical conditions: impaired peripheral circulation, hypothyroidism [4], hyperthyroidism [6], hyperhidrosis, yellow nail syndrome (p. 2066) and shell nail syndrome (p. 2067).

(c) Trauma: minor trauma is a common cause and many occupational cases are due to trauma [3, 5]. Immersion of the hands in soap and water may be considered traumatic, as also may be the use of certain nail cosmetics (p. 2062). It has also been described after the application of 5% 5-fluorouracil to the fingertips [9].

(d) Hereditary partial onycholysis associated with hard nails is described by Schultz [8].

(e) Drugs.

REFERENCES

1 BARAN R. & DAWBER R.P.R. (Eds.) (1984) *Diseases of the Nails and Their Management.* Oxford, Blackwell Scientific, p. 62.
2 DAWBER R.P.R., *et al* (1971) *Br J Dermatol* **85**, 558.
3 FORCK G. & KASTNER N. (1967) *Hautartzt* **18**, 85.
4 FOX E.C. (1940) *Arch Dermatol Syphil* **41**, 98.
5 HEIMANN H. & SILVERBERG M.G. (1941) *Arch Dermatol Syphil* **44**, 426.
6 LURIA M.N. & ASPER S.P. (1958) *Ann Intern Med* **42**, 102.
7 RAY L. (1963) *Arch Dermatol* **88**, 181.
8 SCHULTZ H.D. (1966) *Dermatol Wochenschr* **152**, 766.
9 SHELLEY W.B. (1972) *Acta Derm Venereol (Stockh)* **52**, 320.
10 WILSON J.W. (1965) *Arch Dermatol* **92**, 726.

***Pseudomonas pyocyanea* infection.** This is almost always a complication of oncholysis or chronic paronychia and is usually restricted to one or two nails. The nail plate takes on a very characteristic bluish-black or green colour [1–3] and there is often considerable malodour. This colour is due to accumulation of debris below the nail and the pigment pyocyanin which may remain after the organism has been removed. In some cases the nail plate appears to be invaded by the bacillus [2]. Treatment [4] is with sulphacetamide as described for onycholysis or with gentamicin cream or ointment. Blackening of the edge of the nail in chronic paronychia is also probably due to *Pseudomonas* infection [5].

REFERENCES

1 BAUER M.F. & COHEN B.A. (1957) *Arch Dermatol* **75**, 394.
2 CHERNOSKY M.E. & DUKES C.D. (1963) *Arch Dermatol* **88**, 548.
3 GOLDMAN L. & FOX H. (1944) *Arch Dermatol* **49**, 136.
4 SAMMAN P.D. (1982) *Clin Exp Dermatol* **7**, 189.
5 STONE O.J. & MULLINS J.F. (1963) *J Invest Dermatol* **41**, 25.

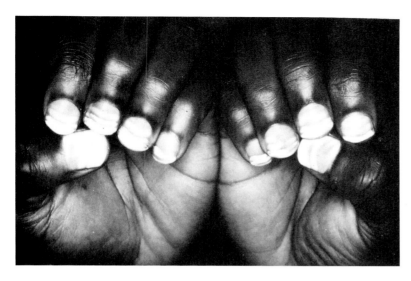

FIG. 54.14. Hereditary striate
leukonychia (Col. S. Salache,
San Antonio).

Leukonychia [2, 3]. Leukonychia may be congenital
or acquired. In each type total, partial or striate
forms (Fig. 54.14) have been described and among
the acquired forms there is in addition punctate
variety, which is by far the commonest. The congenital forms are inherited as autosomal dominants.
Congenital leukonychia is uncommon; in youth all
nails are strikingly white, but the keratin is poor
and when exposed to trauma is very liable to damage, so that in adult life the free edges of the nails
tend to become brown and rough. The condition
may be associated with congenital epidermal cysts.
Koilonychia and leukonychia have been reported as
being inherited together [4].

The acquired forms may occasionally be the result of illness, e.g. Mees' stripes in chronic arsenical
poisoning and the numerous other instances reported of leukonychia associated with general disease [1]. The great majority of cases, however, show
no such association, and the whitening appears to
be either spontaneous or due to minor trauma, e.g.
manicure.

A number of explanations have been offered for
the white colour, but none is completely satisfactory. It is generally held that the colour is due to
incomplete keratinization, so that nuclei or nuclear
debris are retained in the nail plate. In several sections of leukonychial nails the writers have been
unable to confirm this, nor is there consistent evidence of air spaces in the nail plate.

Leukonychia must be distinguished from whitening due to other causes, e.g. fungal infection and
pallor of the nail bed in hypoalbuminaemia. Longitudinal white streaks are found in Darier's disease.

REFERENCES

1 ALBRIGHT S.D. & WHEELER C.E. (1964) *Arch Dermatol*
90, 392.
2 BARAN R. & DAWBER R.P.R. (Eds.) (1984) *Diseases of the
Nails and Their Management.* Oxford, Blackwell Scientific,
p. 77.
3 DANIEL C.R. & OSMENT L.S. (1982) *J Am Geriat Soc.* 30,
734.
4 GRACIANSKY P. DE & BOULLE S. (1961) *Bull Soc Fr Dermatol Syphiligr* 68, 15.

Other causes of nail discoloration [4, 5]. These may be
grouped as follows:

(a) Staining from external factors.

(b) Degenerative changes in a nail growing very
slowly.

(c) Partial destruction after formation.

(d) Abnormal formation.

(e) Incorporation of a stain in the nail during
formation.

(f) Miscellaneous causes.

(a) Under this heading should be included dyes
encountered at work or elsewhere, such as hair
dyes, nicotine, medicaments applied by the patient
to himself or others (mercury, vioform, resorcin, picric acid, etc.) and tints leaking out of nail lacquer.

(b) This is seen in old age, congenital ectodermal
defect and the yellow nail syndrome. In all these
the nail becomes yellow or greenish in hue.

(c) Fungal and candidal infections of the nail
plate will cause browning of the nail, but occasionally a chalky appearance is produced. Discoloration
of the edge of the nail is common in chronic paronychia.

(d) Severe psoriasis is the most important condition under this heading, and the nail is often yellow or brown. Much less common causes are pityriasis rubra pilaris, pachyonychia congenita and alopecia areata. Excess ionizing radiation may so affect the nail matrix that the nail is discoloured and rough.

(e) Many drugs may cause discoloration of the nails (see below).

(f) Black streaks in the nails are very common in the coloured races and are probably the result of very minor trauma and of no significance in most cases. They have been attributed to malnutrition, however, in Indians [3]. They may also occur in Addison's disease [1]. A single dark black band on the nail may be evidence of an active junctional naevus in the matrix, and, as mentioned later, this may progress to a melanoma. A subcutaneous haemorrhage is the commonest cause of blackening of part of the nail. The nail lunulae may have a bluish hue in Kinnier Wilson disease or be red in cardiac failure.

Baran & Gioanni [2] describe the various colour changes seen in the nails. They also show how the onychodermal band of Terry [8] may on occasion become wider to form the lilac arc of syphilis described by Milian [7] and the unusual colour change of azotaemia described by Lindsay [6].

REFERENCES

1 ALLENBY C.F. & SNELL P.L. (1966) *Br Med J* i, 1582.
2 BARAN R. & GIOANNI T. (1969) *Hôpital, Paris* 57, 101.
3 BISHT D.B. & SINGH S.S. (1962) *Lancet* i, 507.
4 DANIEL C.R. & OSMENT L.S. (1982) *Cutis* 30, 348.
5 JEANMOUGIN M. & CIVATTE J. (1983) *Int J Dermatol* 22, 279.
6 LINDSAY P.G. (1967) *Arch Intern Med* 119, 583.
7 MILIAN G. (1936) In *Nouvelle Pratique Dermatologique*. Paris, Masson, Vol. VII, p. 298.
8 TERRY R.B. (1955) *Lancet* i, 179.

Abnormalities of the nails due to drugs [1]. Loss or partial loss of the nail may result from a bullous eruption affecting the tips of the digits. The loss is due to actual destruction of the nail matrix. Temporary loss has also been described due to large doses of cloxacillin and cephaloridine, during the treatment of two anephric patients [3]. Onycholysis may occur during treatment with demethylchlortetracycline [6] (p. 1262) and rarely other antibiotics

There are a number of colour changes which are due to drugs. Yellowing of the nail is a rare occurrence in prolonged tetracycline therapy. The whole nail is affected and returns to normal when the

drug is discontinued. A similar effect, but of a bluish colour, is seen with mepacrine (atebrin) and the nails will fluoresce yellow–green or white if viewed under Wood's light. Normal nails show slight fluorescence of violet–blue colour.

Chloroquine may produce blue–black pigmentation of the nail beds [9], whilst other antimalarials may produce longitudinal or vertical bands of pigmentation on the nail bed or in the nail [2, 5]. The fixed drug eruption of phenolphthalein, if it occurs on the nail bed, will produce a dark blue colour [10]. Argyria may discolour the nails slate blue, whilst inorganic arsenic may produce longitudinal bands of pigment or white stripes (Mees' stripes) across the nail.

Hyperpigmentation due to an increase of melanin pigment in the nail and nail bed has been noted in children after 6 weeks of treatment with doxorubicin (Adriamycin) [7]; other similar drugs may cause a variety of patterns of increased pigmentation [1].

REFERENCES

1 BARAN R. & DAWBER R.P.R. (Eds.) (1984) *Diseases of the Nails and their Management*. Oxford, Blackwell Scientific, p. 248.
2 COLOMB D., *et al* (1975) *Bull Soc Fr Dermatol Syphiligr* 82, 319.
3 EASTWOOD J.B., *et al* (1969) *Br J Dermatol* 81, 750.
4 FRANKS S.B., *et al* (1971) *Arch Dermatol* 103, 520.
5 MAGUIRE A. (1963) *Lancet* i, 667.
6 ORENTREICH N., *et al* (1960) *Arch Dermatol* 83, 730.
7 PRATT C.B. & SHANKS E.C. (1974) *JAMA* 228, 460.
8 RAMELLI G., *et al* (1972) *Cutis* 10, 155.
9 TUFFANELI D., *et al* (1963) *Arch Dermatol* 88, 419.
10 WISE F. & SULZBERGER M.B. (1933) *Arch Dermatol Syphil* 27, 549.

SURGERY OF THE NAIL APPARATUS

In general, dermatologists seem averse to undertaking nail surgery. This is very surprising in view of the good blood supply and the well-recognized rapid healing of the nail apparatus after injury. One reason for it appears to be that the consequences of poor case selection or poor technique are great because of the importance of a normal nail to the efficient functioning of each digit.

The major objectives in carrying out nail surgery are (i) to obtain diagnostic, therapeutic or prognostic information by nail biopsy, (ii) the treatment of nail tumours, (iii) for pain relief, (iv) for infections and (v) to repair or correct congenital and traumatic deformities. The majority of these are described in the appropriate sections with each disease, but it is necessary here to consider the principal biopsy methods.

Most biopsy techniques are quick, are simple to carry out and cause no greater functional impairment or scarring than any other skin biopsy technique [2]. The type of biopsy selected will depend on the information required [1]. For the diagnosis of fungal infection, it is useful to take specimens that include a portion of the distal nail plate and hyponychium. A 3-mm punch biopsy limited to the nail plate can be performed when suspected mycotic infection is proximal or deep. Periodic acid–Schiff or silver methenamine staining is necessary to identify fungal elements.

Nail bed biopsy. A 3- to 4-mm punch biopsy (Fig. 54.15) should reach the periosteum before it is withdrawn. Fine scissors are then used to release the specimen. If the nail is thinned before biopsy, the operation will be easier to perform. It may be advisable to avulse the nail plate fully or partially

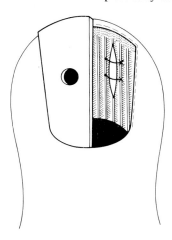

FIG. 54.15. Nail bed biopsy.

for the diagnosis of a tumour or any unusual lesion. The removal of a longitudinal elliptical wedge of tissue down to the bone is then carried out. After removal, the edges of the ellipse are undermined to facilitate primary closure with 4–0 dexon. Relaxing incisions may be useful at the lateral margins of the nail bed.

Nail matrix biopsy. It is cosmetically important to maintain the normal contour of the distal margin lunula. The visualization of the matrix is accomplished by a proximal incision at the junction of the proximal and lateral nail folds bilaterally (Fig.

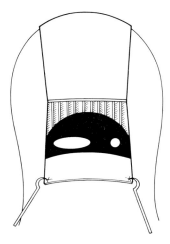

FIG. 54.16. Nail matrix biopsy.

54.16). This enables the proximal nail fold to be reflected back. Nail matrix biopsy is crucial to define the histological characteristics of longitudinal pigmented streaks.

Longitudinal melanotic streak biopsy. Simple examination of nail clippings allows one to locate the proximal end of the band before biopsy. When the pigment appears in the upper layers of the nail, it is produced by the most proximal part of the matrix. Staining of the deeper layers of the nail means that the pigment is originating from the distal portion of the matrix.

When a longitudinal melanotic streak is accompanied by periungual pigmentation, this phenomenon, known as Hutchinson's sign, has proved to be a valuable clue to the clinical diagnosis of malignant melanoma in the subungual location.

A longitudinal melanotic streak may be examined by one of three means, depending on its width and location:

(1) If it is less than 3 mm wide, a punch biopsy is performed at the proximal end of the band, through the nail plate, down to the bone.

(2) When the band is 3 mm or wider, the proximal portion of the nail plate is removed and the remaining band in the nail plate will serve as a guide, enabling the widest portion of the crescent or fusiform-shaped matrix biopsy to be placed on the same axis.

(3) If the longitudinal melanotic streak is asymmetrical, the technique recommended for the lateral–longitudinal biopsy is more suitable.

Lateral–longitudinal nail biopsy. This elliptical biopsy may be on either side of the nail plate and proximal nail fold (Fig. 54.17). For the most part the incisions parallel the lateral edge of the nail plate and should include a segment 3–4 mm long

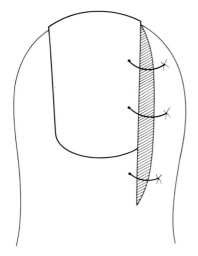

FIG. 54.17. Lateral–longitudinal nail biopsy.

reaching to the bone. This ensures that a whole thickness fragment of the matrix, with its lateral horn, is obtained. Slightly curved iris scissors are useful for this procedure. The incision should begin at the tip of the finger, proceed proximally and keep in contact with the bony phalanx.

REFERENCES

1 BARAN R. & DAWBER R.P.R. (Eds.) (1984) *Diseases of the Nails and Their Management.* Oxford, Blackwell Scientific, p. 356.
2 BARAN R. & SAYAG J. (1976) *J Dermatol Surg Oncol* **2**, 322.

TUMOURS UNDER OR ADJACENT TO THE NAIL

Tumours of the nail apparatus and adjacent structures are relatively common. Neoplasms of the nail area can be divided into benign, benign but aggressive lesions (e.g. keratoacanthoma, recurring digital fibrous tumours of childhood and some warts) and malignant tumours.

Clinical diagnosis is often difficult because of traumatic factors, infection and the presence or absence of pigmentation, and because the translucent nail plate masks physical signs in the nail bed. Also common tumours, well recognized at other sites, may behave differently in the nail apparatus. An X-ray investigation should be carried out on all swellings in or around the nail apparatus, particularly those affecting a single digit.

Benign tumours
Warts. By far the commonest tumour adjacent to the nail is the common wart. It presents as a roughening at the edge of the nail which, in the early stages, amounts to little more than a hardening of the cuticle. It enlarges and may grow until it completely surrounds the covered part of the nail. The nail is usually unaffected, but at times the surface becomes rough and there may be cross-ridges. Less often, linear depressions are formed. Periungual warts are often found in nail biters or cuticle pickers so that the nail may show changes due to these habits. Warts under the free edge of the nails are much less common but may displace the nail from its bed.

Treatment. Periungual warts may be treated by destruction using curettage and cautery or diathermy, or with liquid nitrogen spray. Many cases, however, respond very well to monochloroacetic acid and 40% salicylic acid plasters [1]. A nearly saturated aqueous solution of the acid is used. The results are best when the solution has been freshly prepared and there are crystals present with the fluid. The solution is applied with an orange stick covered by a wisp of cotton wool. It is applied sparingly, as keratin will take up a large quantity of the acid if allowed to do so and this will lead to much pain after 48 h. The solution is allowed to dry—there is no whitening of the surface as with trichloroacetic acid. The wart is then covered with 40% salicylic acid plaster cut to the size of the wart and held in place with two or three layers of zinc oxide adhesive tape. The dressing is left in place for 3 days and is then replaced by a strip dressing. The patient is seen again after 7–14 days, when many of the warts may be picked out or the procedure repeated if necessary. Although the nail fold may be much deformed when the wart comes away, especially if pus forms, it regrows with little or no scarring or deformity.

Warts below the nail may be treated similarly after the overlying nail has been cut away.

X-ray and radium treatments are obsolete. Shumer and O'Keefe [2] have recommended intralesional bleomycin fortnightly, but this requires further study.

REFERENCES

1 HALPERN L.K. & LANE C.W. (1953) *Missouri Med* **50**, 765.
2 SHUMER S.M. & O'KEEFE E.J. (1983) *J Am Acad Dermatol* **9**, 91.

Myxoid cyst (syn. mucous cyst, synovial cyst). The so-called myxoid or synovial cyst is not primarily connected with the distal interphalangeal joint but is really a degenerative change in the connective tissue of the distal phalanx. It forms a small, cystic lesion with a smooth, shiny surface, almost translucent and situated between the distal interphalangeal joint and the base of the nail. If it is situated over the nail matrix it gives rise to a depression on the nail, usually about 1–2 mm across and extending throughout the length of the nail (Fig. 54.18).

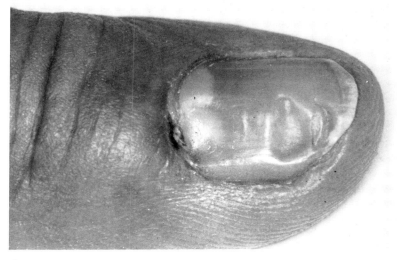

It presents as a firm swelling below the nail, which usually displaces the tip and is often mistaken for a wart. It is most commonly found in the great toes. X-ray examination will establish the diagnosis with certainty.

Whether subungual osteochondroma is a different entity remains unclear [2].

REFERENCES

1 EVISON G. (1966) *Br J Radiol* **39**, 451.
2 NORTON L.A. (1980) *J Am Acad Dermatol* **2**, 451.

Enchondroma [1]. This is a rare tumour which, if it occurs in the distal phalanx, will lead to enlargement of the fingertip, giving the appearance of finger clubbing. It may present as a chronic paro-

FIG. 54.18. Nail plate groove due to a myxoid cyst.

The cyst varies in size from time to time and the reduction in size may be accompanied by the escape of a drop of glairy fluid from below the cuticle down the depression in the nail. Occasionally, haemorrhage occurs into the cyst, which then becomes black.

Treatments are many and various including repeated pricking, dissection with excision (and grafting if necessary), cryosurgery, aspiration of the contents and injection of triamcinolone, and removal of the proximal nail fold and associated cyst [1].

REFERENCE

1 SALASCHE S.J. (1984) *J Dermatol Surg Oncol* **10**, 35.

Subungual exostosis [1]. This lesion is not a true exostosis but an outgrowth of normal bone tissue.

nychia [2] or there may be greater distortion of the nail [3].

X-ray examination will show a radiolucent defect associated with expansion of the distal phalanx.

Treatment is by removal of the chondroid tissue and by filling in of the cavity so formed, by bone graft if necessary [2].

REFERENCES

1 NORTON L.A. (1980) *J Am Acad Dermatol* **2**, 451.
2 SHELLEY W.B. & RALSTON E.I. (1964) *Arch Dermatol* **90**, 412.
3 YAFFEE M.A. (1965) *Arch Dermatol* **91**, 361.

Keratoacanthoma [1, 2]. When occurring below the nail, this tumour is quite unlike the classical lesion. It presents as erythema and swelling of the tip of the digit with increasing pain. After a time part of the nail separates from its bed and a crusted nodule appears at the edge. For the first few weeks progress is rapid; it may mimic a chronic paronychia. X-ray examination shows extensive bone destruction of the distal phalanx. The histology is the same as when the lesion occurs in one of its more usual sites and can easily be mistaken for a squamous cell epithelioma. Treatment is by total excision after removal of the overlying nail, but partial amputation is not required.

REFERENCES

1 NORTON L.A. (1980) *J Am Acad Dermatol* **2**, 451.
2 STOLL D.M. (1980) *Am J Dermatopath* **2**, 265.

Pigmented naevus [1–3]. Although rather uncommon, a junctional naevus in the matrix is an important lesion. It may give rise to a dense band of pigment in the nail plate. Pigmented bands in the nails are very common in coloured persons and are of little or no significance, but a single band in a white person may indicate the presence of increased melanocytic activity or a junctional naevus in the matrix. The spill of pigment into the nail plate may start at any age, but once it begins it tends to persist indefinitely. The importance lies in the potential of these lesions to become malignant. The number likely to become malignant may be quite small but is certainly real.

Treatment must depend, to some extent, on the importance of the nail affected. In the case of lesions under toe nails, the affected area of the matrix should be removed after avulsion of the nail. This applies also to some finger nails, but in the case of the index fingers a policy of waiting may be justified.

REFERENCES

1 COSKEY R.J. & MAGNELL T.D. (1984) *J Am Acad Dermatol* **9**, 747.
2 HARVEY K.M. (1960) *Lancet* **ii**, 848.
3 NOBLE J.F., *et al* (1952) *Arch Dermatol Syphil* **65**, 49.

Pyogenic granuloma. A classical pyogenic granuloma near the nail is somewhat rare and should be treated by removal with curettage and diathermy. Overgrowth of granulation tissue simulating a pyogenic granuloma is much more common, especially in association with an ingrowing toe nail. It should be treated as described under that heading. As a malignant melanoma can simulate a pyogenic granuloma, this possibility must be con-

sidered and the lesion after removal should therefore be sent for histological examination.

Pseudo pyogenic granuloma (p. 2144): one case, a woman aged 40 years, presented with nodules of the fingertip, lateral nail folds and nail bed [1].

REFERENCE

1 VERRET J.L., *et al* (1983 *Ann Dermatol Vénéréol* **110**, 251.

Subungual epidermoid inclusions [1]. These develop as bulbous proliferations at the tips of the rete ridges of the nail bed. Usually microscopic in size, they occasionally become large enough to give rise to symptoms and must be considered in the differential diagnosis of nail bed swellings. They are found in finger clubbing, but may occur without this. Trauma is a possible cause.

REFERENCE

1 LEWIN K. (1969) *Br J Dermatol* **81**, 671.

Other benign tumours are fibromata and glomus tumours. Fibromata may be single or multiple. They are most common in association with adenoma sebaceum (p. 123), but may occur independently of that condition. They usually lie outside the nail, projecting from below the cuticle, but occasionally are under the nail plate and extend from the base of the nail to the tip as a narrow thread causing few or no symptoms but visible through the nail and below the tip of the nail.

Treatment for these lesions is usually unnecessary, but they may be excised.

The so-called garlic clove fibroma has been described as a small lump which grows away from the nail bed projecting from the cuticle over the dorsum of the nail of fingers or toes. It is loosely attached by a pedicle. The tumour is either a benign fibroepithelial polyp or an irritation fibroma of the nail bed. Histological examination shows that it is covered, except at its base, by a layer of hyperkeratotic, stratified squamous epithelium. The core is composed of interlacing bundles of dense collagenous tissue with capillary channels. The lesion is painless and does not recur after removal [4, 5].

Glomus tumours [3] are rare but may occur under the nail, when they present as a painful, slightly blue discoloration of part of the nail. They are exquisitely tender and should be excised after removal of the nail. X-ray examination may be helpful in diagnosis [1].

Tender subungual tumours consisting of pseudo-epitheliomatous hyperplasia and bone destruction of the distal phalanges have been described in association with incontinentia pigmenti [2].

REFERENCES

1 CAMIRAND P. & GIROUX J.N. (1970) *Arch Dermatol* **102**, 677.
2 MASCARO J., *et al* (1985) *J Am Ac Dermatol* **13**, 740.
3 RETTIG A.C. & STRICKLAND J.W. (1977) *J Hand Surg* **2**, 261.
4 STEEL H.H. (1965) *JAMA* **191**, 1082.
5 UNDEUTSCH W. & SHRIEFERSTEIN G. (1974) *Dermatologica* **149**, 110.

Malignant tumours

Squamous epithelioma of the nail apparatus. This is a rare condition but may present in one of several ways. It may present like a pyogenic granuloma [3], as a chronic paronychia affecting a single nail and increasingly painful, as an outgrowth from below the edge of the nail, or superimposed on Bowen's disease of the nail bed [2, 5, 6, 7]. The only way to establish the diagnosis with certainty is by biopsy. Once the diagnosis has been established treatment should be either by partial amputation of the digit or by removal of the tumour using Mohs' chemosurgical technique [1, 5].

Secondary carcinoma in the bone of the distal phalanx [4] is also rare. X-ray examination will show rarefaction of the bone. In the presence of a known primary carcinoma the diagnosis may be accepted without biopsy, but otherwise biopsy will be required.

REFERENCES

1 ALBOM M.S. (1975) *J Dermatol Surg* **1**, 43.
2 BARAN R., *et al* (1979) *Ann Dermatol Vénéréol* **106**, 227.
3 DRIBAN N.E. & LACAGNATAC (1975) *Dermatologica* **150**, 186.
4 HÖDL S. (1980) *Aktuelle Dermatol* **6**, 249.
5 MIKHAIL G.R. (1984) *J Am Acad Dermatol* **11**, 291.
6 MIKHAIL G.R. (1981) *J Med Esthet* **8**, 216.
7 RUBIN L. (1973) *J Am Podiatry Assoc* **63**, 195.

Malignant melanoma (melanotic whitlow) [1, 2]. This also is rare but is more important than the other malignant tumours. There are four ways in which this may present. Following the development of a pigmented band in the nail, granulation tissue may appear some years later at the edge of the nail, and the pigment band may become wider (Fig. 54.19). The second method of presentation is by a recalcitrant chronic paronychia affecting a single nail; the presence of a developing melanoma should be sus-

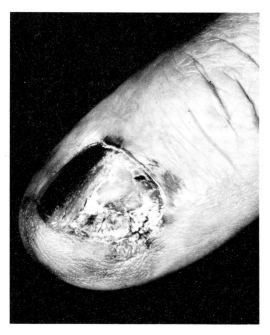

FIG. 54.19. Subungual malignant melanoma with spread to adjacent tissues and nail dystrophy (courtesy Drs U. Runne and C. Orfanos).

pected if there is any appearance of pigment on the neighbouring skin (Hutchinson's sign). The third method of presentation is by the development of a warty growth of the nail bed accompanied by shedding of the nail. An amelanotic lesion may present in the form of a pyogenic granuloma. Unfortunately the diagnosis is often overlooked for months or years [3].

If a melanoma is suspected, a biopsy should be carried out (p. 2055). A section should be examined urgently and if the diagnosis is confirmed the digit should be amputated immediately. The draining glands should be removed later if there is any suggestion of secondary spread to this site.

REFERENCES

1 DUPERRAT B. & CINTRACT M. (1974) *Ann Dermatol Syphiligr* **7**, 235.
2 FEIBLEMAN C.E., *et al* (1980) *Cancer* **46**, 2492.
3 LEPPARD B., *et al* (1974) *Br Med J* **i**, 310.

NAIL DEFORMITIES OF TRAUMATIC ORIGIN

The nails may be damaged by trauma in a number of ways. The injury may be single, occasional, or often repeated (as in nail biting).

Single or occasional injuries may result in haematomas, splits or, if sufficiently severe, total loss of the nail.

Haematoma. This is probably the commonest occasional injury to the nail. Depending on the point of injury and the severity of damage, the haemorrhage will appear immediately or after a few days. Thus a minor injury over the posterior nail fold will be followed by the appearance of haemorrhage under the nail a few days later. The blood will later be incorporated into the nail plate [2]. In most other cases the haemorrhage appears immediately, and temporary partial loss of the nail will usually follow. The only treatment that can be offered is to relieve the pressure, and if seen soon after the injury this can be done by puncturing the nail, e.g. with a hot pointed implement, a cautery or a small drill. This procedure will relieve pain and may save the nail. The possibility of an underlying fracture must be considered [1].

REFERENCES

1 FARRINGTON H. (1964) *Br Med J* i, 742.
2 STONE O.J. & MULLINS J.F. (1963) *Arch Dermatol* **88**, 186.

Splits [1]. These occur when the nail matrix is injured, usually by a straight cut with a sharp instrument. If seen early enough, the nail may be removed and the cut edges sutured, when a ridge will replace the split.

Ridges are due to an injury of the same type as that causing a split, but less severe.

Repeated injuries are often more subtle, and the patient may be unaware of them. A few distinctive types will be described.

REFERENCE

1 HOFFMAN S. (1973) *Arch Dermatol* **108**, 568.

Nail biting (onychophagia). This is an extremely common habit, and several members of a family may be nail biters. The patient is usually restless and the family background may be insecure. Normally the biting is at the tip of the nail and a short irregular nail results. All finger nails are often bitten, but occasionally one or more is spared. The nail is often bitten right back to its point of separation from its bed. Fine spicules may be left at the edge, which cause splits and mild paronychia. Concurrently with the biting of the nail the cuticles are often bitten, and so become irregular and broken. Periungual warts are common in nail biters. Treatment is unsatisfactory, because the patient can seldom be persuaded to give up the habit. Psychotherapy may be useful with some patients.

Deformities similar to nail biting can be caused by constant rubbing of the fingertips with a nail from the other hand or by close trimming of the nails with an instrument such as a razor blade, instead of nail scissors or a file. This is a common habit in Nigeria.

REFERENCE

1 BALLINGER B.R. (1970) *Br J Psychol* **117**, 445.

Habit tic deformity [2]. Under this heading is described the less common deformity caused by playing with the nails. The deformity usually consists of a depression down the centre of one nail with numerous horizontal ridges extending across the nail from it (Fig. 54.20). The depression is sometimes missing. The deformity is usually confined to

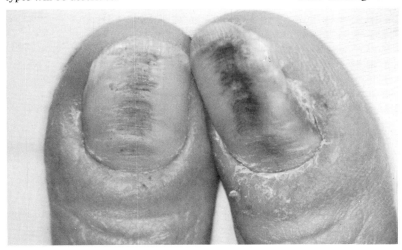

FIG. 54.20. Multiple transverse lines and central nail depression of the thumbs, self induced.

one or both thumb nails and is caused by the patient picking at the cuticle [1] or stroking the nail of the affected digit with a finger of the same hand. Like nail biting, this habit is difficult to break once established. It should be distinguished from the true median dystrophy.

REFERENCES

1 MacAuley W.L. (1966) *Arch Dermatol* **93**, 421.
2 Samman P.D. (1963) *Arch Dermatol* **88**, 895.

Onychotillomania [1]. This is essentially similar to the habit tic, but is more closely allied to parasitophobia as the patient picks off pieces of nail fold and may claim that they contain parasites. A rough and irregular nail and nail fold result. Many finger nails are involved.

Pimozide may be beneficial [2].

REFERENCES

1 Combes F.C. & Scott M.J. (1951) *Arch Dermatol Syphil* **63**, 778.
2 Hamann K. (1982) *Acta Derm Venereol (Stockh)* **62**, 364.

Nail artefacts [1]. These are due to deliberate trauma and may take various forms. When the nail is pierced with a sharp instrument over the lunula, the growth of the nail is distorted locally, and sepsis and the formation of granulation tissue may result. Nail artefacts are rare.

REFERENCE

1 Hurley P.T. & Balu V. (1982) *Arch Dermatol* **118**, 956.

Hang nails. These are due to hard pieces of epidermis breaking away from the lateral nail folds. Although often due to nail biting, they may result from many other minor injuries. The splits may penetrate to the underlying dermis when they will be painful, otherwise they are painless. They should be removed with very sharp pointed scissors.

Nutcracker nails. Under this heading Cohen *et al.* [1] describe splitting and onycholysis in a patient who was in the habit of separating the two halves of cracked walnuts over a period of 10 years.

REFERENCE

1 Cohen B.H., *et al* (1975) *Cutis* **16**, 141.

Splitting into layers (lamellar dystrophy, onychoschizia). This is a more subtle form of injury. The tips of the nails split into layers so that small pieces may flake (Fig. 54.21). It is almost always confined to women. Probably many forms of minor injury contribute, but the most important appears to be the constant uptake and drying out of water, which causes repeated softening and hardening of the nail. After a time splits develop, and dirt and moisture enter the cracks and aggravate the damage.

The patient should be advised to keep the hands as dry as possible and the nails as short as she can tolerate. An emollient hand cream should be used regularly, preferably one containing glycerine. Nail varnish should not normally be forbidden, as this does cover the defect to some extent. However, in a few cases varnish appears to be an aggravating factor. Sometimes a nail cosmetic containing a plas-

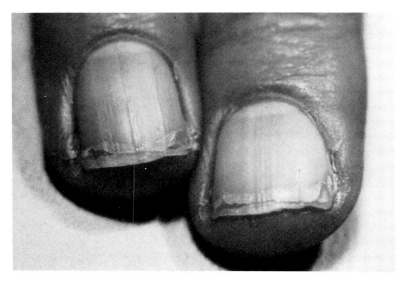

Fig. 54.21. Lamellar nail splitting (Professor L. Juhlin, Uppsala).

tic which fills in the cracks and artificially thickens the edge of the nail is helpful.

Very occasionally a single nail is split into two layers throughout its length as a result of a single injury splitting the matrix tangentially. Graham-Brown and Holmes described lamellar dystrophy in polycythaemia vera [2].

Splitting and ridging of nails are very common findings, often without apparent cause, but many cases of splitting of this type probably have the same cause as lamellar dystrophy. Other causes of this change are ageing, impaired peripheral circulation, lichen planus and Darier's disease (p. 1438).

Brittle nails [1], again, are often due to the same type of trauma, namely constant immersion of the hands in water, especially if alkaline [4]. Treatment is the same as for lamellar dystrophy. Other common causes are iron deficiency anaemia and impaired peripheral circulation. A rare cause is disturbance of arginine metabolism, when it is associated with diffuse alopecia [3].

REFERENCES

1 BARAN R. (1978) *Cutis* **2**, 457.
2 GRAHAM-BROWN R.A.C. & HOLMES R. (1980) *Clin Exp Dermatol* **5**, 209.
3 SHELLEY W.B. & RAWNSLEY H.M. (1965) *Lancet* **ii**, 1327.
4 SILVER H. & CHIEGO B. (1940) *J Invest Dermatol* **3**, 357.

Damage caused by nail cosmetics [2, 9]. Most nail cosmetics are well tolerated and cause little damage to the nail or its surrounds, even when they occasionally cause dermatitis elsewhere. However, a few patients are seen where damage has been caused. Onycholysis [6] may be due to nail hardeners containing free formalin. The separation is usually limited to a small area near the fingertip and is probably due to direct irritation. Most patients admit to using the hardener more often than recommended by the suppliers. Yellow staining of the nail plate has been encountered in a number of persons using nail varnish of a pink or rose colour. It is due to one of the dyes in the varnish leaking out and penetrating the nail plate. The colour can be removed only by allowing it to grow out after discontinuation of the use of the varnish.

Many years ago cases of onycholysis were reported from the use of a base coat which contained synthetic resins [3, 5, 7, 8]. Experiments showed that, some time after application of the base coat to the nail surface, phenol could be detected on the undersurface [7]. It was probable, therefore, that the resin penetrated the nail and irritated the nail bed, possibly by an allergic mechanism.

More recently synthetic stick-on nail dressings were marketed for a short time in the U.S.A. and in Britain. They had numerous advantages over nail polish, e.g. the speed and ease of application, but it was soon found that they caused damage to the nail in many ways, in particular by pulling small pieces off the surface of the nail, which led to greater deformity and breaking of the nail [1]. The damage was probably due to interference with the free exchange of moisture between the atmosphere and the nail [10].

Recently several cases of nail damage have been encountered where materials used in the manufacture of dentures have been used to 'improve' and strengthen the nails. The patient will usually be found to be sensitive to one of the materials and improvement follows their withdrawal. The condition was described in 1957 in the U.S.A. [4], but only recently have cases been encountered in this country.

Artificial finger nails may also irritate the nail bed and disrupt the nails. Removal of the cuticle either by chemical or mechanical means may cause distortion of the nails.

REFERENCES

1 CALNAN C.D. (1958) *Trans St John's Hosp Dermatol Soc* **41**, 66.
2 CRONIN E. (1980) *Contact Dermatitis*. Edinburgh, Churchill Livingstone, p. 792.
3 DOBES W.L. & NIPPERT P.H. (1944) *Arch Dermatol Syphil* **49**, 183.
4 FISHER A.A., *et al* (1957) *J Allergy*, **28**, 84.
5 LAYMON C.W. & RUSTEN E.M. (1949) *Minn Med* **31**, 1218.
6 LAZAR P. (1966) *Arch Dermatol* **94**, 446.
7 MITCHELL J.H. (1949) *Med Clin North Am*, **33**, 95.
8 REIN C.R. & ROGIN J.R. (1950) *Arch Dermatol Syphil.* **61**, 971.
9 RYCROFT R. & BARAN R. (1984) In *Diseases of the Nail and Their Management*. Eds. Baran R. & Dawber R.P.R. Oxford, Blackwell Scientific, p. 283.
10 SAMMAN P.D. (1961) *Trans. St John's Hosp Dermatol Soc* **46**, 48.

Damage caused by weedkillers and insecticides. The weedkillers Paraquat and Diquat can cause a number of changes in the nails if the nails are allowed to come into contact with concentrated or even with dilute solutions [2, 3]. The changes range from a white band across the nail to total loss of the nail. Similar changes have been recorded following contamination with 5% dinitro-orthocresol used as an insecticide [1].

REFERENCES

1 BARAN R.L. (1974) *Arch Dermatol* **110**, 467.
2 HEARN C.E.D. & KEIR W. (1971) *Br J Ind Med* **28**, 399.
3 SAMMAN P.D. & JOHNSTON E.N. (1969) *Br Med J* i, 818.

Microwave injury. Two cases of nail loss due to exposure to microwaves have been reported by Brodkin & Bleiberg [1].

REFERENCE

1 BRODKIN R.N. & BLEIBERG J. (1973) *Acta Derm Venereol (Stockh)* **53**, 50.

Trauma from footwear

Onychogryphosis and nail hypertrophy [2–4]. Not all cases of onychogryphosis or hypertrophied toe nails are due to injury, but there is no doubt that many are so caused. At one time onychogryphosis was known as ostlers' nail, owing to the fact that some cases could be traced to injury caused by a horse trampling on the foot of the ostler whilst he was stabling it. The injury once sustained is aggravated by footwear and as the nail becomes longer and thicker the damage from the footwear becomes progressively more important. Nail hypertrophy implies thickening and increase in length, whilst onychogryphosis implies curvature also.

Some cases of nail hypertrophy are intrinsic, and this applies especially to toe nails other than the nail of the great toe; the nail becomes thick and circular in cross-section instead of flat, and comes thus to resemble a claw. There are two possible explanations for this formation: the first is that there is insufficient matrix under cover of the posterior fold to exert a flattening effect, and the second is that the nail bed is contributing a greater quantity of keratin to the nail than usual. In some patients sebaceous cysts were also present. Hypertrophy of finger nails is usually traumatic in origin and is often the result of a single injury.

In onychogryphosis (Fig. 54.22) one or more nails become greatly thickened and with neglect are permitted to increase in length, becoming curved like a ram's horn. The nails of the great toes are most often involved, but no toe nail is exempt. In extreme cases, the free edge may press on or even re-enter the soft tissues of the foot.

Treatment of onychogryphosis and nail hypertrophy is either radical or palliative. Radical treatment consists of surgical removal of the nail and matrix and is recommended in young persons with good circulation. Palliative treatment requires regular paring and trimming of the affected nails, usually by a chiropodist using nail clippers and file or mechanical burr. The thickened nails are extremely hard and trimming is difficult. Not infrequently the nail is invaded by granulation tissue from the nail bed, and incision of this during trimming will result in pain and haemorrhage.

Other causes of thickened nails are psoriasis, pityriasis rubra pilaris, Darier's disease, fungal infections, pachyonychia congenita, congenital ectodermal defects, and congenital mal-alignment of the great toe nails [1].

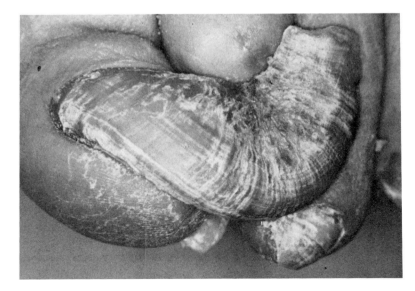

FIG. 54.22. Onychogryphosis, limited to the great toe nail.

REFERENCES

1 BARAN R. & BUREAU H. (1983) *Clin Exp Dermatol* **8**, 619.
2 DOUGLAS M.A. & KRULL E.A. (1981) In *Current Therapy*. Ed. Conn W.B., Philadelphia, Saunders, p. 712.
3 GILCHRIST A.K. (1979) *Geriatrics* **34**, 67.
4 LUBACH D. (1982) *Hautarzt* **33**, 331.

Ingrowing toe nail. The soft tissue of the side of the nail (lateral nail fold) is penetrated by the edge of the nail plate, resulting in pain, sepsis and, later, the formation of granulation tissue [1]. Penetration is usually caused by spicules of nail at the edge of the nail plate which have been separated from the main portion of the nail. The great toes are those most often affected. The main cause for the deformity is compression of the toe from the side due to ill-fitting footwear, and the main contributory cause is cutting of the toe nails in a half-circle instead of straight across. Anatomical features such as an abnormally long great toe and prominent lateral nail folds are important in some cases. In recent years the condition has been caused in a minority of cases by the successful therapy of fungal infections of the nails with griseofulvin. A nail which has been infected for a long time is reduced in size, and the nail bed shrinks around it. When the infection is even partly overcome the nail plate is increased in size; the nail bed is no longer large enough to accommodate the whole of the new nail, and the lateral nail fold may be penetrated on each side.

In infancy, ingrowing toe nail most commonly occurs before shoes are worn, associated with crawling, 'pedalling' or wearing undersized 'jumpsuits' [2]; acute paronychia may be associated [3].

The first symptoms are pain and redness, soon followed by swelling and pus formation. Granulation tissue then forms and adds to the swelling and discharge. More severe infection may follow. There is seldom any difficulty about diagnosis.

Treatment may be difficult and prolonged [1]. The first essential is to insist on the patient wearing shoes sufficiently wide and pliable to remove lateral pressure. The patient must also be instructed to cut the nail straight across instead of in a semicircle. The nail must be allowed to grow until its edges are clear of the end of the toe before it is cut; this prevents the further formation of marginal spicules. In the early stages the infection may be overcome by the application of antiseptic paints such as aqueous gentian violet and by inserting a pledget of cotton wool under the edge of the nail. Twice-daily warm water baths followed by careful drying and powdering are helpful. If the infection is more severe and there is local cellulitis, a systemic antibiotic should be administered. When granulation tissue forms this should be destroyed by cauterization with a silver nitrate stick. If these conservative measures fail, operation—which may be carried out under digital block—will be required. The granulation tissue should be excised and the nail fold may have to be removed at the same time. In some cases avulsion of the nail will be required, and indications for this are continuing cellulitis, severe pain and failure to improve with less radical treatment. The time-honoured removal of part of the nail is not now considered satisfactory treatment. It is important, however, to remove the spicule, which may be quite large, from its embedded site.

If recurrence occurs after simple avulsion, then removal of the nail and matrix is required. This operation is suitable for young persons, but in the elderly and especially in association with diabetes or impaired peripheral circulation, conservative treatment employing a skilled chiropodist is recommended.

REFERENCES

1 LATHROP R.G. (1977) *Cutis* **20**, 119.
2 VERBOV J. (1978) *Br Med J* ii, 1087.
3 WALKER S. (1979) *Clin Pediatr* **18**, 247.

Shedding of the nails. Periodic shedding of nails may be a developmental anomaly when one or more nails may be shed repeatedly. Although the nails are replaced, regrowth may be incomplete or defective. The condition is inherited as an autosomal dominant character. Repeated shedding, however, may be the result of trauma. The nails of the great toes are those most often involved, and the condition usually occurs in persons taking part in some sporting activity. The trauma is inflicted by wearing shoes or boots which are too small, whether soft (such as canvas) or firmer (e.g. football boots). The injury may be quite painless and the period of exposure quite short (a few minutes to an hour or more). In many cases, but not all, the nail loss is preceded by subungual haematoma. The condition is more often seen in those with some underlying instability. Oliver [2] describes the condition in three members of a family. Like ingrowing toe nails, it may at times be partly due to anatomical deformities such as an abnormally long great toe, so that it is difficult to obtain shoes which fit satisfactorily. The shedding is temporary and a new nail replaces the one lost. No special treatment is required in most cases, but the cause should be explained to the patient so that he may take precautions to prevent recurrence.

Many cases of haemorrhage below the great toe nail with or without nail loss have been seen since platform shoes became fashionable [1].

REFERENCES

1 ALMEYDA J. (1973) *Br Med J* i, 176.
2 OLIVER W.J. (1927) *Br J Dermatol* **39**, 297.

Overcurvature of the nails (pincer nail deformity). This is another condition often due to ill-fitting foot-wear, but occasionally it occurs apparently as a result of psoriasis and occasionally without obvious cause [1]. The nails of the great toes are those most often affected, but no nail is exempt. The curvature is in the long axis of the nail, so that the edges press deeply into the lateral nail folds (Fig. 54.23). If the epidermis is penetrated the condition will resemble an ingrowing nail, but at times great pain will be caused by partial strangulation of the soft tissues without penetration of the epidermis.

For treatment, removal of the nail is required; if the condition repeats itself, removal of both the nail and the nail matrix may be needed.

Occasionally, excess curvature of several nails is seen and this appears to be a developmental anomaly. The affected nails may resemble claws and look rather like the nail in pachyonychia. No special treatment is required, unless they are causing pain, but the nail substance is very hard and regular chiropody may be required to keep the nails trimmed.

REFERENCE

1 BARAN R. (1974) *Arch Dermatol* **110**, 639.

NAIL DISORDERS ASSOCIATED WITH GENERAL DISEASE

Nail changes associated with impaired peripheral circulation. The blood supply to the nail is excellent under normal circumstances but, being in an exposed situation, the nails are very subject to the effects of cold. The digital arteries readily go into spasm, inducing Raynaud's phenomenon. Under these circumstances, the nails may be deprived of an adequate blood supply for many hours at a time. The nails may react in various ways.

The most frequent change noted in the nails in patients with severe Raynaud's symptoms is a rather characteristic one [3]. The nail is thin, brittle and ridged longitudinally, and splits may occur along the ridges (Fig. 54.24). The thinning may result in flattening of the nail plate, or even koilonychia. Parts of the nail show onycholysis and appear white. This contrasts markedly with other parts of the nail which may be redder than normal; thus the even, pink colour of the nail is lost. Owing to the tendency to splitting, the patient keeps the nails cut rather short.

In contrast with the thin nail, impaired circulation, especially in older persons, may be accompanied by thickening of the nail plate. These patients usually have onycholysis of several nails and the corresponding nail beds are thick and roughened. Secondary contamination with bacteria or *Candida* give the nail a dark colour and there may be true invasion of the nail plate with *C. albicans*. This is particularly liable to occur in uncontrolled diabetics.

Acute digital ischaemia may cause the 'blue toe'

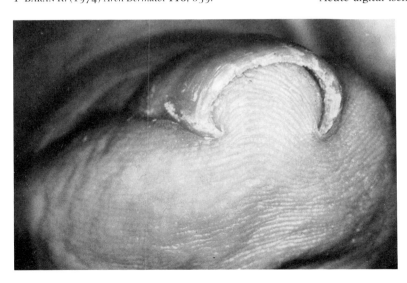

FIG. 54.23. Pincer nail deformity.

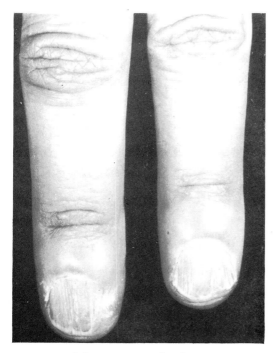

FIG. 54.24. Nail changes associated with impaired peripheral circulation (St John's Hospital).

syndrome, due to microemboli from a more proximal source in the arterial tree—major peripheral pulses may feel normal [2].

Another less common change in impaired circulation is pterygium formation [1] (Figure 54.25). This is due to partial destruction of the matrix and fusion of the epithelium of the dorsal nail fold and the nail bed. In extreme cases the nail is completely destroyed and replaced by scarring.

Although arterial spasm appears to be the main cause of nail damage associated with impaired circulation, similar changes may occur as a result of digital arterial occlusion from any cause. In these cases there is often some associated soft tissue damage and not infrequently partial or total loss of one or more nails is noted. The various causes of Raynaud's phenomenon and the technique of digital arteriography are described by Strickland & Urquhart [4].

Treatment should be directed at the underlying disease when present and the patient should be advised to keep her hands warm at all times; vasodilators are sometimes helpful.

REFERENCES

1 EDWARDS E.A. (1948) *N Engl J Med* **239**, 362.
2 KARMODY A.M., *et al* (1976) *Arch Surg* **111**, 1263.
3 SAMMAN P.D. & STRICKLAND B. (1962) *Br J Dermatol* **74**, 165.
4 STRICKLAND B. & URQUHART W. (1963) *Br J Radiol* **36**, 465.

Nail changes associated with lymphoedema. In the yellow nail syndrome (Samman's syndrome) there is a highly characteristic nail change, often accompanied by lymphoedema [6, 7]. The patient notices that the nails have ceased, or almost ceased, to grow and some time later the colour change is noted. The nails do in fact continue to grow but at a greatly reduced rate: 0·1–0·25 mm per week for finger nails compared with the lowest normal 0·5 mm per week. The nails themselves usually remain

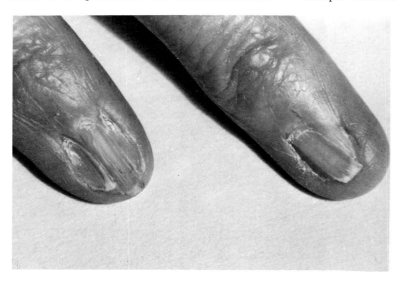

FIG. 54.25. Dorsal pterygium.

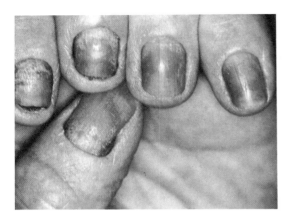

FIG. 54.26. Yellow nail syndrome.

smooth; they are slightly thicker than normal and are excessively curved on their long axis. The cuticles are lost. The colour is a pale yellow or greenish yellow, but the edges may have a darker hue (Fig. 54.26). Onycholysis affects one or more nails and may be so extensive that the nail is lost and is only very slowly replaced. Some of the loosened nails may show a distinct hump. All nails, finger and toe, are affected in most cases.

The oedema most frequently affects the legs but may not be seen for some months after the nail change has been noted. Less often it affects the face or hands and occasionally is universal. Recurrent pleural effusions have been noted in a few cases [3, 5]. Chronic bronchitis and bronchiectasis may also occur [2]. The oedema has been shown to be due to abnormalities of the lymphatics, either atresia, or varicosity in some cases [5]. As some cases seem to have normal lymphatics it seems possible that a functional rather than an anatomical defect may be present, or perhaps only the smallest lymph vessels are defective. Although the nail changes may draw attention to the underlying lymphatic abnormality, they are found only in a minority of patients with congenital abnormality of the lymphatics. This condition may be associated with an increased incidence of malignant neoplasms [5]. Other associations include D-penicillamine therapy [4], nephrotic syndrome [1] and hypothyroidism.

The condition is most often seen in middle age, but a similar condition has been described in young children. Although the nail changes, once established, are usually permanent, complete reversion to normal may occur at times, and is probably independent of treatment.

REFERENCES

1 COCKRAM C.S. & RICHARDS P. (1979) *Br J Dermatol* **101**, 707.
2 DILLEY J.J., *et al* (1968) *JAMA* **204**, 122.
3 EMERSON P.A. (1966) *Thorax* **21**, 247.
4 ILCHYSHIN A., *et al* (1983) *Acta Derm Venereol (Stockh)* **63**, 554.
5 MILLER E., *et al* (1972) *Chest* **61**, 452.
6 SAMMAN P.D. & WHITE W.F. (1964) *Br J Dermatol* **76**, 153.
7 VENENCIE P.Y. & DICKENS C.H. (1984) *J Am Acad Dermatol* **10**, 187.

Shell nail syndrome associated with bronchiectasis. Under this title Cornelius & Shelley [1] report a patient who, following whooping cough at the age of 4 years, developed bronchiectasis; when aged 5 years changes in the finger nails were noted. All finger nails showed longitudinal curvature and there were dystrophic fingertips, resulting from atrophy of the distal nail bed. X-ray examination of one finger showed thinning of the distal phalanx and complete loss of tufting. The nail plate could be seen to be separated from the nail bed.

It seems possible that this is a variant of the yellow nail syndrome.

REFERENCE

1 CORNELIUS C.E. III & SHELLEY W.B. (1967) *Arch Dermatol* **9**, 694.

Koilonychia. This is a common deformity of the nail in which the normal contour of the nail is lost, becoming flat or truly concave, so that in severe cases it may be able to hold one or two drops of fluid. The nail is usually thin and often brittle.

Koilonychia is most often associated with hypochromic anaemia; the reason for this is obscure, but it is not due to iron deficiency *per se* [4]. The cystine content of spoon-shaped nails is lower than normal [5]. The nails of children in the first year or two of life are not infrequently spoon shaped. In a few cases this condition may persist into adult life without any other evidence of disease—familial cases have been recorded [3]. Inheritance is determined by a single autosomal dominant gene [1, 2]. The thin nails of impaired circulation may be spoon-shaped, as may the separated halves of the nails in the nail–patella syndrome may each be spoon shaped.

Treatment consists of attention to the underlying disease when present, but the nail takes a long time to return to normal.

REFERENCES

1 BURGERON J.R. & STONE O.J. (1967) *Arch Dermatol* **95**, 351.
2 HANDA Y., *et al* (1960) *Acta Genet Med Gemell* **9**, 309.
3 HELLIER F.F. (1950) *Br J Dermatol* **62**, 213.
4 HOGAN G.R. & JONES B. (1970) *J Pediatr* **77**, 1054.
5 JALILI M.A. & AL-KASSAB S. (1959) *Lancet* **ii**, 108.

Finger clubbing (Hippocratic nails). Clubbing of the fingers is another common abnormality encountered more often by the physician than the dermatologist [1]. In the earliest phase the condition may be difficult to recognize, as it consists only of the loss of the normal angle between the nail and the posterior nail fold. Later the distal phalanx becomes enlarged and there may be an increase in the size of the nail (Fig. 54.27). In the most severe cases

The factors involved in the formation of finger clubbing are obscure and a number of theories have been put forward [3]. Arteriograms show that there is an abundant blood supply to the digits. The fault may be due to the loss of the detoxicating action of the lungs on venous blood. When clubbing is present mixed arterial and venous blood is shunted past normal lung tissue [2]. It has been suggested that the shape is due to angulation of the nail matrix secondary to connective-tissue changes below the nail [4].

REFERENCES

1 BLUMSOHN D. (1981) *Heart and Lung* **10**, 1069.
2 HALL G.H. (1959) *Lancet* **i**, 750.
3 Leading articles (1959) *Lancet* **ii**, 390; (1975) *Lancet* **i**, 1285.

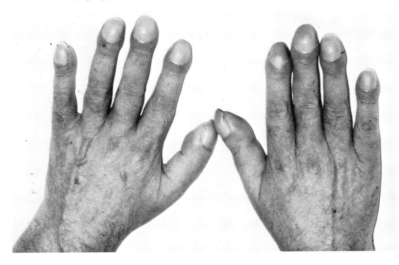

FIG. 54.27. Clubbing, associated with hypertrophic pulmonary osteoarthropathy (carcinoma of the bronchus).

(hypertrophic pulmonary osteoarthropathy) there is much periosteal change affecting the metacarpals, the two proximal rows of phalanges and the terminal few centimetres of ulna and radius in the hands and arms, and the corresponding bones in the feet and legs.

Most cases of finger clubbing occur in patients with chronic lung disease (especially carcinoma of the bronchus) or cyanotic heart disease, but it is also seen in patients with diseases of the thyroid gland and in some abdominal diseases, including biliary cirrhosis, sprue and ulcerative colitis. It has been suggested that it only occurs in disease of the organs supplied by the vagus nerve. Some support for this is supplied by observations on patients with ulcerative colitis, as only part of the colon is supplied by the vagus [5]. In a few cases it is present from birth with no underlying disease.

4 STONE O.J. & MABERRY J.D. (1965) *Tex State J Med* **61**, 620.
5 YOUNG J.R. (1966) *Br Med J* **i**, 278.

Beau's lines [1]. Transverse depressions on the nails are known as Beau's lines (Fig. 54.28) [2]. They are due to temporary interference with nail formation and become visible on the nail surface some weeks after the disease which caused the condition. They appear first at the cuticle and move forward with the growth of the nail. In many cases they may be seen on all twenty nails.

Many diseases, including coronary thrombosis, measles, mumps and pneumonia, may produce Beau's lines, provided they are sufficiently severe. The growth of the nail is temporarily depressed but returns to normal during convalescence from the disease. Recently it has been shown that Beau's

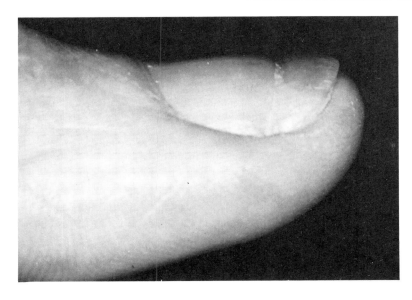

FIG. 54.28. Beau's line, lateral view.

lines may be associated with zinc deficiency. They were seen in two cases of acrodermatitis enteropathica and in one patient on total parenteral nutrition [1]. Exposure to severe cold and the carpel tunnel syndrome may produce a similar depression on isolated nails. A traumatic injury may also produce a depression on the affected nail. Depressions may occur on the nail when the adjacent skin is affected by dermatitis, but the nail behind the depression is roughened.

REFERENCES

1 BEAU J.H.S. (1846) *Arch Générales Med* **11**, 447.
2 RUNNE V. & ORFANOS C.E. (1981) *Curr Probl Dermatol* **9**, 102.
3 WEISMANN K. (1977) *Acta Derm Venereol (Stockh)* **57**, 88.

Colour changes. Various colour changes in the nails or nail bed have been described in connection with systemic disease. Those associated with drugs are described elsewhere (p. 2054), and leukonychia is described independently (p. 2053).

White nails have been described in association with cirrhosis of the liver. The colour change is apparently in the nail bed and not in the nail plate. In severe cases all finger nails are affected and there is a ground-glass-like opacity of nearly the whole of the nail bed, but a zone of normal pink may remain near the distal edge of the nail [12]. In some cases, the white area may have a peak distally [10].

Paired, narrow, white bands have been described in patients with hypoalbuminaemia [11]. The bands are parallel to the lunula and are separated from one another and from the lunula by areas of normal pink nail. They do not move forward with the growth of the nail and are therefore not in the nail plate; they disappear when the serum albumin level returns to normal [3].

The half-and-half nail is a condition described by Lindsay [8] in renal disease and azotaemia in which the proximal nail bed is white and the distal half red, pink or brown. The colour of the distal half is thought by Bussels *et al.* to be due to capillary changes and is probably reversible [2]. The condition may remain static despite haemodialysis [9].

Azure half-moons may be seen in hepatolenticular degeneration (Kinnear Wilson disease) [1]. Red half-moons may occur in congestive heart failure [13] and rheumatoid arthritis [6].

In addition to these rather specific colour changes, it should be remembered that the nails may look pale in any severe anaemia.

Splinter haemorrhages below the nails are common and are most often the result of minor trauma, as shown by the fact that they are more common in patients recently admitted to hospital than in patients who have been in hospital for some weeks [4]. Splinter haemorrhages also occur frequently in many general medical conditions [5], including subacute bacterial endocarditis, trichinosis (when they are said to be horizontal), severe rheumatoid arthritis and, much less often, in uninfected mitral stenosis, peptic ulceration, hypertension and malignant neoplasms [5]. In dermatological practice they are often found in association with psoriasis, dermatitis and fungal infection of the nails. As they occur under so many conditions, their importance as a symptom of disease is often exaggerated.

REFERENCES

1 BEARN A.G. & McKUSICK V.A. (1958) *JAMA* **186**, 904.
2 BUSSELS L., *et al* (1972) *Arch Belg Dermatol* **28**, 363.
3 CONN R.D. & SMITH R.H. (1965) *Arch Intern Med* **116**, 875.
4 GROSS N.J. & TALL R. (1963) *Br Med J* ii, 1496.
5 HEATH D. & WILLIAMS D.R. (1978) *Br Heart J* **40**, 1030.
6 JORIZZO J.L., *et al* (1983) *J Am Acad Dermatol* **8**, 711.
7 KUSKE H. VON (1961) *Dermatologica* **123**, 219.
8 LINDSAY P.G. (1967) *Arch Intern Med* **119**, 583.
9 LUBACH D., *et al* (1982) *Hautarzt* **33**, 303.
10 MOREY D.A.J. & BURKE J.O. (1955) *Gastroenterology* **29**, 259.
11 MUEHRCKE H.C. (1956) *Br Med J* i, 1327.
12 TERRY R. (1954) *Lancet* i, 757.
13 TERRY R. (1954) *Lancet* ii, 842.

Ridging and beading. These have been described as occurring more often than normal in patients with rheumatoid arthritis [1]. These signs are common, however, in patients with no evidence of rheumatoid arthritis and are probably not of great significance. They tend to become more prominent with increasing age.

REFERENCE

1 HAMILTON E.D.B. (1960) *Ann Rheum Dis* **19**, 167.

DEVELOPMENTAL ANOMALIES

Compared with the number of acquired nail disorders, developmental anomalies of the nail are rare [3]. Some of these are described in other parts of this book: pachyonchia congenita (p. 155); congenital ectodermal defect (p. 129); leukonychia (p. 2053); supernumerary digits (p. 222); koilonychia (p. 2067). The remainder are described here. For detailed analysis of the nail in congenital and hereditary diseases, further reading is suggested [3].

Anonychia. Absence of the nails from birth is a rare congenital anomaly. It may occur as an isolated symptom or be accompanied by other defects of the digits and other structures. Littman & Levin [5] described a girl with seven nails missing, and reported that her brother was similarly affected; it was suggested that this was a recessive trait. The mode of inheritance of most of these disorders has not yet been established with certainty. The condition described as anonychia with ectrodactylia [4] has

been investigated more fully, however, and has been shown to be inherited as a dominant without sex-linkage. In this condition there is usually complete absence of the nails on the index and middle fingers, and when there is any nail on the thumb it is often present on the proximal lateral corners of the nail fold. On the ring fingers the radial half of the nail is often absent, but the nail of the little finger is usually normal. The toes are usually affected in a similar way to the fingers. When the nail is absent, the nail bed is also missing. In a minority of affected individuals there are striking and bizarre defects of the digits, sometimes restricted to one hand or foot. The defects usually take the form of omission of one or more digits. Two sisters in a sibship of five, whose parents were first cousins, are recorded as having rudimentary nails associated with congenital deafness. The parents showed neither abnormality [2]. Bart *et al.* [1] describe a family with congenital absence of areas of skin, blistering of skin and mucous membranes and absence or deformity of the nail inherited as an autosomal dominant gene. Verbov [6] describes a case with bizarre flexural pigmentation and anonychia and considers that it is an autosomal dominant condition.

REFERENCES

1 BART B.J., *et al* (1966) *Arch Dermatol* **93**, 296.
2 FEINMESSER M. & ZELIG S. (1962) *Arch Otolar* **74**, 507.
3 JUHLIN L. & BARAN R. (1984) In *Diseases of the Nails and Their Management*. Eds. Baran R. & Dawber R.P.R. Oxford, Blackwell Scientific, p.303.
4 LEES D.H., *et al* (1957) *Ann Hum Genet* **22**, 69.
5 LITTMAN A. & LEVIN S. (1964) *J Invest Dermatol* **42**, 177.
6 VERBOV J. (1975) *Br J Dermatol* **92**, 469.

Nail–patella syndrome (see p. 154). This uncommon condition is of special interest because it involves abnormalities of ectodermal and mesodermal structure. It is inherited as an autosomal dominant, with linkage between the locus controlling the syndrome and that of the ABO blood groups [8]. In the typical case the nails are grossly defective, only one-third or one-half the normal size and never reaching the free edge of the nail [6]. In other cases the thumb nails alone may be defective or only the ulnar half of each may be missing [4] (Fig. 54.29). In every case the thumb nails are most affected and the remaining nails, if involved, are progressively less damaged from index to little finger. The half-moons may be triangular [2]. Even when the nail is completely missing the nail bed is present. In

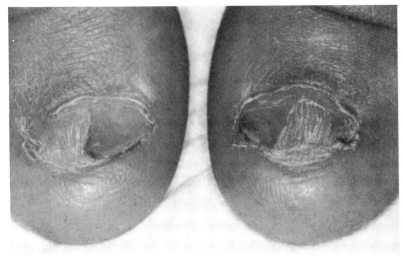

FIG. 54.29. Nail–patella syndrome—hemionychia.

addition to the nail changes the patellae are smaller than normal and may be rudimentary so that the knees are unstable. There are also bony spines arising from the posterior aspect of the iliac bones visible on X-ray examination.

Other features which have been recorded are over-extension of the joints, laxity of the skin, hyperhidrosis [5] and renal abnormalities. The ultra-structure of the renal changes has been described [1, 3].

In 1965 there were 255 patients with this syndrome known to be living in the U.K., and the prevalence is estimated at 1 per 22 million. The mutation rate is estimated at 1 per 1·9 per million alleles per generation [7].

The condition must be distinguished from congenital ectodermal defect and pachyonychia congenita.

REFERENCES

1 BEN BASSAT M., *et al* (1971) *Arch Pathol* 92, 350.
2 DANIEL C.R., *et al* (1980) *Arch Dermatol* 116, 448.
3 GOODMAN R.M. & COPPAGE F.E. (1967) *Arch Intern Med* 120, 68.
4 LEVAN N.E. (1961) *Arch Dermatol Syphil* 83, 938.
5 PECHMAN K.J. & BERGFIELD W.F. (1980) *J Am Acad Dermatol* 3, 627.
6 RENWICK J.H. (1956) The genetics of the nail–patella syndrome. *Thesis*, London.
7 RENWICK J.H. & IZATT M.M. (1965) *Ann Hum Genet* 28, 369.
8 RENWICK J.H. & LAWLER S.D. (1955) *Ann Hum Genet* 19, 312.

Congenital onychodysplasia of the index fingers [1].
In this condition the nail of the index finger is absent, small or represented by two nails of unequal size. Although the change is present at birth, it does not appear to be familial. It is very rare outside Japan [2].

REFERENCES

1 KIKUCHI I., *et al* (1974) *Arch Dermatol* 110, 243.
2 BARAN R. (1980) *Ann Derm Vénéréol* 107, 431.

Racket nail (nail en raquette). This condition is much more common but is seldom a cause for complaint. It is really an abnormality of the thumbs in which the distal phalanx is shorter and wider than normal. The nail is correspondingly short and wide and the normal curvature in the nail is lost (Fig. 54.30). It may occur on one or both thumbs. It is inherited as a dominant trait and is commoner in women than men [3]. Basset [1] distinguished this from two similar conditions, one of which the racket shape affects all the fingers and the other in which the nails are short without the corresponding shortening of the distal phalanx.

Tertiary hyperparathyroidism produces a racket nail appearance due to the underlying bone erosion [2].

REFERENCES

1 BASSET M.R.H. (1962) *Bull Soc Fr Dermatol Syphiligr* 69, 15.
2 FAIRRIS G.M. & ROWELL N.R. (1984) *Clin Exp Dermatol* 9, 267.
3 RONCHESE F. (1951) *Arch Dermatol Syphil* 63, 565.

Regular pitting of the nail [5]. Many cases of regular pitting of the nail may be attributed to psoriasis [3] or alopecia areata [6], but when both

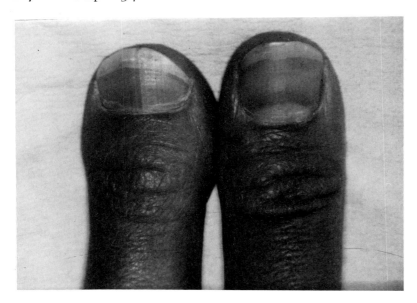

FIG. 54.30. Racquet thumb (on the left).

these diseases have been excluded some unexplained cases remain. Several examples have been seen in more than one member of a family so that some congenital abnormality exists [1]. The pits may appear in early life or become manifest years later. In some cases they are present for a short time only; in others they persist for years. One or, more often, many fingers or toes may be affected. The cause appears to be an incomplete and intermittent defect in the matrix so far unexplained.

As variants of this may be considered excess ridging, when the pits are produced rapidly at no appreciable interval in time (trachyonychia or vertical striated 'sand-papered' nails), and rippling when the pits are very close together in the transverse axis of the nail (see Figs 54.31, 54.32 and 54.33).

Excess ridging is also the principal feature of a condition which has been given the name 'twenty nail dystrophy of childhood' [2]. The condition is not present at birth but appears in early childhood. There is a very slow return to normality and the condition is not seen in adults. All 20 nails are affected. It is better to consider this as a physical sign that may be seen as an isolated defect [1, 7], or in diseases such as lichen planus [4] and alopecia areata.

REFERENCES

1 ARIAS A.M., *et al* (1982) *J Am Acad Dermatol* **7**, 349.
2 HAZELRIGG D.E., *et al* (1977) *Arch Dermatol* **113**, 73.
3 KLINGMULLER G. & REEH E. (1955) *Arch Klin Exp Dermatol* **210**, 574.
4 PERSON J.R. (1984) *Arch Dermatol* **120**, 437.
5 SAMMAN P.D. (1978) *The Nails in Disease*. London, Heinemann, p. 122.
6 STUHMER A. (1957) *Arch Klin Exp Dermatol* **204**, 1.
7 WILKINSON J.D., *et al* (1979) *Br J Dermatol* **100**, 217.

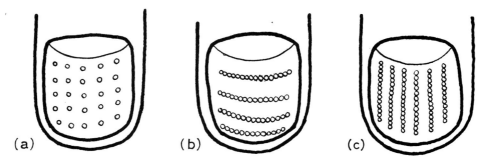

FIG. 54.31. Diagram to show how regular pitting might cause various nail dystrophies: (a) pitting; (b) rippling; (c) ridging.

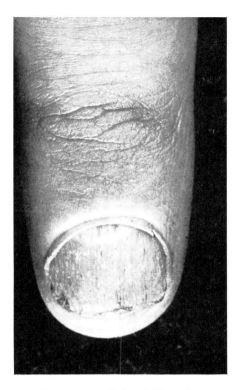

FIG. 54.32. Excess ridging (St John's Hospital).

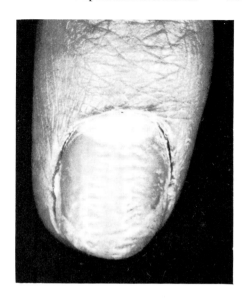

FIG. 54.33. Rippling (St John's Hospital).

REFERENCE

1 SAMMAN P.D. (1969) *Br J Dermatol* **81**, 746.

Pterygium unguis. This condition may result from lichen planus (p. 1672) or impaired circulation (p. 2065), but in some cases both these diseases may be excluded and the condition appears to be developmental but not familial. One or more nails are partly or wholly destroyed and replaced by a scar. It may occur with other changes in the condition named idiopathic atrophy of the nail [1]. In this condition the nails are normal at birth but after a few years one or more nails become deformed, and the deformity ranges from excess ridging and opacity to total loss with scarring. Finger nails are more often affected than toe nails.

Familial subungual pterygium [1, 3]. In this condition there appears to be a forward extension of the nail bed epithelium dislocating the hyponychium. The condition is painful. The cases recorded were of mother and daughter and affected fingers of both hands. Isolated acquired cases under the diagnosis of pterygium inversum unguis have also been recorded [2, 4]. A very similar change may occur in systemic sclerosis [5].

REFERENCES

1 AMBLARD P. & REYMOND J.L. (1980) *Ann Dermatol Vénéréol* **107**, 949.
2 CAPUTO R. (1973) *Arch Dermatol* **108**, 817.
3 CHRISTOPHERS E. (1975) *Hautarzt* **26**, 543.
4 DRAKE L. (1976) *Arch Dermatol* **112**, 255.
5 PATTERSON J.W. (1977) *Arch Dermatol* **113**, 1429.

CHAPTER 55

Disorders of the Oral Cavity and Lips

J. J. PINDBORG

THE HISTOLOGY OF THE NORMAL ORAL MUCOSA

The normal histology of the oral mucosa shows striking regional variations which are adaptive in origin [3]. A broad classification differentiates three main types. The frictional mucosa of the gingiva and hard palate is well keratinized. There appears to be a spectrum of degrees of keratinization rather than distinct types, and the degree of keratinization is reflected in the degree of packing and orientation

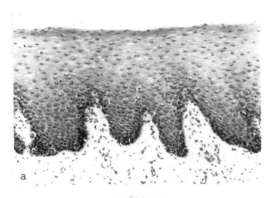

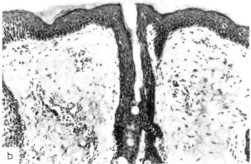

FIG. 55.1. Comparison between epithelial thickness in oral mucosa and skin in the same patient (Royal Dental College, Copenhagen): (a) mucosal area of the labial commissure (×84); (b) cutaneous area of the labial commissure (×84).

of tonofilaments [1]. The dermis, properly referred to as the lamina propria, is dense and is firmly attached to underlying bone or tooth. The lining mucosa typically seen in the buccal region or the lips and in the floor of the mouth is not keratinized and lies on looser connective tissue not firmly attached to bone. Finally there is highly specialized mucosa such as that of the dorsum of the tongue.

The epithelium is thicker than that of the skin (Fig. 55.1) and the rete ridges extend more deeply in the underlying connective tissue. The cells of the basal layer are cuboidal or columnar with large darkly staining nuclei. The wide prickle cell layer consists of polyhedral cells with paler nuclei. The stratum granulosum may be inconspicuous or several cells thick. In most regions there is a recognizable stratum corneum; it is well developed in the frictional mucosa (Fig. 55.2) and virtually absent under normal conditions in some regions of lining mucosa.

A fibrillar basement membrane [3] separates the epithelium from the underlying connective tissue or lamina propria. The density of the texture of the connective tissue varies with the region of the mouth.

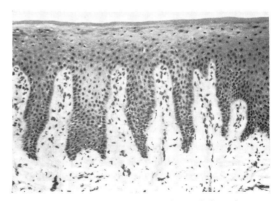

FIG. 55.2. Slight orthokeratosis in the epithelium from marginal gingiva (×91).

Salivary glands are found all over the oral mucosa but are most numerous over the palate and lips; most of the glands have mucous acini.

Saliva [1, 2]. The mucosa is constantly bathed in saliva, which is of complex and variable composition. It certainly plays an important role in maintaining the health of the mucosa, as is evident from the dystrophic changes which occur when salivary secretion is grossly diminished, but the mechanism of its action on the epithelium has not been established. Apart from its digestive and lubricating functions saliva has antibacterial effects, assists wound healing and influences dental caries. Severe congenital xerostomia from aplasia of the parotid glands or from irradiated glands is associated with extensive caries.

REFERENCES

1 ADAMS D. (1976) *Ann R Coll Surg Engl* **53**, 351.
2 *JENKINS G.N. (1966) *The Physiology of the Mouth*, 3rd ed. Oxford, Blackwell.
3 MEYER J. *et al* (1984) *The Structure and Function of Oral Mucosa*, Oxford, Pergamon Press.

ORAL NAEVI

Naevi are relatively uncommon on the oral mucosa. Accurate figures for the incidence of naevi of different types are not available, for small lesions are often overlooked. The natural history of oral naevi closely parallels that of comparable naevi in the skin (see Chapter 6) and will not be described here. Vascular, lymphangiomatous and melanocytic naevi all may present special problems in diagnosis and treatment, and certain epithelial naevi are peculiar to the oral mucosa whilst others show special features.

Vascular naevi. The common haemangiomatous naevi (p. 201) often involve the lips or oral mucosa. They may be present at birth or first appear during early infancy. As in the skin they enlarge for some months and then slowly regress. They vary greatly in size and may be red or bluish-grey in colour (Fig. 55.3). During the phase of active growth they may bleed with slight trauma and may interfere with feeding. If possible, treatment should be avoided, since spontaneous resolution can be expected. If treatment is essential, surgical excision or the injection of sclerosing agents should be preferred to radiotherapy.

Oral haemangiomas, developing in later childhood or early adult life, may occur in Maffucci's syndrome (p. 209).

In the Sturge–Weber syndrome (see p. 196) of

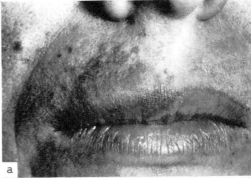
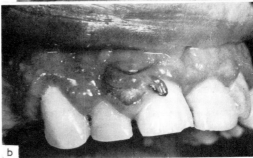

FIG. 55.3. Vascular naevus of (a) lips and (b) gingivae (University Hospital, Copenhagen).

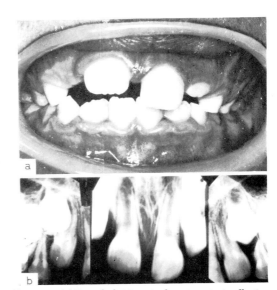

FIG. 55.4. (a) Encephalotrigeminal angiomatosis affecting the upper gingiva. (b) Advanced tooth eruption and formation on the affected side. Note the difference in apical area of the central incisors. (University Hospital, Copenhagen.)

encephalotrigeminal angiomatosis, the lips, buccal mucosa and gingiva may be extensively involved (Fig. 55.4). The gingival mucosa may show slight vascular hyperplasia or large nodules which may prevent closure of the mouth. The soft purple gingival enlargement reaches the midline of the maxilla, whereas the facial naevus stops at the outer margin of the philtrum [1]. When the gingiva is involved the teeth erupt prematurely and there may be accelerated tooth formation leading to malocclusion (Fig. 55.4(b)).

REFERENCE

1 *GORLIN R.J., *et al* (1976) *Syndromes of the Head and Neck*, 2nd ed. New York, McGraw-Hill.

Lymphangioma (see p. 1237) [2]. Lymphangiomas may develop anywhere on the oral mucosa as grouped superficial vesicles or as deep poorly circumscribed nodular masses. They may be present at birth or may first appear in childhood or later.

Involvement of the tongue (Fig. 55.5) gives rise to macroglossia, which may be asymmetrical. On the surface are irregular clusters of deep red or pink vesicles, fancifully described as resembling frog spawn. Characteristic but not invariable are recurrent episodes of pain and swelling. Cystic hygroma of the neck may be associated—the lymphangioma then involves the tongue, submandibular region and neck [1].

Small lymphangiomas require no treatment. If the macroglossia is of such a degree as to impair speech or if the inflammatory episodes are frequent and disabling, hemiglossectomy or wedge resection may be attempted. The results may be excellent.

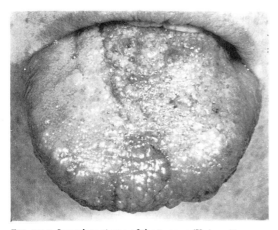

FIG. 55.5. Lymphangioma of the tongue (University Hospital, Copenhagen).

REFERENCES

1 FARMAN A.G., *et al* (1978–79) *Br J Oral Surg* 16, 125.
2 KOOP C.E. & MOSCHAKIS E.A. (1961) *Pediatrics* 27, 800.

Oral pigmented naevi. Up to 1979 the total number of well-documented cases of oral pigmented naevi reported in the literature was 75. Then a series of 32 was published from the U.S.A. [1]. According to this investigation more than one-third of the naevi are found in the palate. The rest were equally divided between buccal mucosa, vermilion border, labial mucosa and gingiva.

Classified according to histological type 66% were intramucosal, 25% blue, 6% compound and 3% junctional naevi. 78% were in women and 22% in men. When a blue spot of the oral mucosa is located close to the gingiva an amalgam tattoo should be considered as a diagnostic possibility.

REFERENCE

1 BUCHNER A. & HANSEN L. (1979) *Oral Surg* 48, 131.

DEVELOPMENTAL EPITHELIAL DISORDERS OF THE ORAL MUCOUS MEMBRANE

Keratotic lesions of the oral mucous membrane are a constant or occasional feature of several hereditary disorders of keratinization (Table 55.1). At least three forms of isolated epithelial dysplasia of developmental origin can also be differentiated. Whilst many of these syndromes are readily identified and classified on the basis of their extra-oral lesions, the interrelationships of the oral lesions themselves have not been adequately studied and any conclusion must be tentative.

Hereditary benign intraepithelial dyskeratosis [1, 2]. This syndrome has been found in many members of a large pedigree of mixed ancestry in North Carolina, U.S.A., in which it is determined by an autosomal dominant gene. Histologically the oral and ocular lesions show marked acanthosis with numerous large vacuolated cells in the middle and upper part of the epithelium. Throughout these layers and continuing to the surface are many eosinophilic cells which appear to be engulfed by normal cells.

The oral lesions, which vary greatly in extent, appear in infancy or childhood and reach full development at adolescence. They involve the mucosal surface of the commissure, the buccal and labial mucosa, the floor of the mouth and the ventral surface of the tongue. In their mildest form the

TABLE 55.1. Oral lesions in hereditary disorders of keratinization

	Age of onset of oral lesions	Sites	Histology	Associated features	Prognosis
Hereditary, benign intraepithelial dyskeratosis	Infancy	Buccal and labial mucosa, floor of mouth, underside of tongue	Acanthosis, vacuolated cells, engulfed eosinophilic cells, parakeratosis and hyperkeratosis	Eye lesions	Benign
Pachyonychia congenita	From second decade	Buccal mucosa, tongue, larynx, anal mucous membrane	Parakeratosis and hyperkeratosis, acanthosis	Thickened nails, palmoplantar keratoderma	Carcinoma frequent
Dyskeratosis congenita	From second decade	Buccal mucosa, tongue, anorectal	Parakeratosis and hyperkeratosis, acanthosis	Nails dystrophic, shed; reticulate pigmentation	Carcinoma frequent
Darier's disease	From childhood	Posterior buccal mucosa, lips	Acanthosis, suprabasal lacunae and dyskeratosis	Extensive skin lesions	Benign
White sponge naevus	Any age from infancy	Buccal and labial mucosa, floor of mouth	Acanthosis, vacuolated cells, parakeratosis and hyperkeratosis	Lesions of anal and vaginal mucosa	Benign

plaques are smooth and opalescent; thicker lesions are creamy-white and folded. There are no symptoms.

The eye lesions also appear in early infancy. They range from small pingueculae to large raised foamy gelatinous plaques overlying the intensely injected conjunctiva. Photophobia and lachrymation are sometimes severe, especially in the summer months.

Both ocular and oral lesions are entirely benign.

REFERENCES

1 SALLMANN L. & VON PATON D. (1960) *Arch Ophthalmol* 63, 421.
2 WITKOP C.J., *et al* (1960) *Arch Pathol* 70, 696.

White sponge naevus (syn. white folded gingivo-stomatitis [1.2.5]; hereditary leukokeratosis [3]; leuko-oedema exfoliativum mucosae oris [1]). This epithelial irregularity is often familial and is determined by an autosomal dominant gene [1]. Histologically the epithelium is acanthotic and shows irregular, if any, keratosis. Many of the prickle cells may be vacuolated.

The lesions may be present at birth or may appear during childhood or adolescence. The affected mucous membrane is white, thickened and irregularly folded, and feels soft and spongy. The buccal mucosa, labial mucosa and gingiva are most frequently involved, but the greater part of the oral mucosa may be affected in some degree. Similar

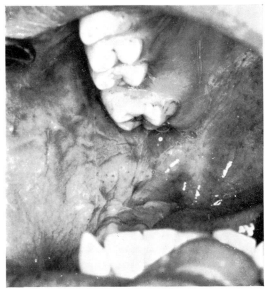

FIG. 55.6. White sponge naevus of the buccal mucosa (University Hospital, Copenhagen).

changes are sometimes found in the anal canal or the vagina. The condition appears to be benign.

The differentiation from hereditary benign intra-epithelial dysplasia is at present based on the involvement of the conjunctiva, but not of the anal and vaginal mucosa, in the latter condition. Clinically the oral changes are similar and the possible histological differences [4] are of questionable significance.

REFERENCES

1 *Bánóczy J., et al (1973) *Swed Dent J* **66**, 481.
2 Cooke B.E.D. & Morgan J. (1959) *Br J Dermatol* **71**, 134.
3 Scott C.R. (1966) *J Pediatr* **68**, 768.
4 Witzkop C.J. & Gorlin R.J. (1961) *Arch Dermatol* **84**, 762.
5 Zegarelli E.V., et al (1959) *Arch Dermatol* **80**, 59.

Fordyce spots (syn. Fordyce's disease). Fordyce's spots are a physiological variant of oral sebaceous gland development, elevated to the status of a disease by the anxiety they sometimes arouse in patients who become aware of their presence. Clinically, they present as small discrete slightly elevated yellowish or white granules.

In adults the prevalence level is about 80% for prolabial and about 95% for oral sebaceous glands. The prevalence reaches a peak at the age of 20–29 yr. Size increases in males up to the age of 50–59. Oral sebaceous glands occur in adults most often in the buccal mucosa and thereafter with decreasing frequency in the contact zone of the lips, the pterygomandibular fold, the lower alveolobuccal sulcus, the upper labial mucosa, the maxillary alveolar mucosa and the mandibular retromolar area [1]. The extent of the glands is greater, the density higher and the size larger in males than in females.

The importance of the condition is exclusively in differential diagnosis.

REFERENCE

1 *Sewerin J. (1975) *Acta Odontol Scand* **33**, (Suppl. 68).

Congenital fistula of the lower lip. This genetically determined defect is one component of a triad which also includes cleft upper lip and palate. A single dominant gene of variable expressivity is probably responsible [2]. In some 60% of patients with labial fistulae a cleft lip is associated, but in some families the fistulae are inherited as an isolated defect [1]. Symmetrical pits on the vermilion border of the lower lip are situated on each side of the midline. Sinuses extend downwards for 5–25 mm to end blindly in the orbicularis oris muscle. Mucus may exude from the orifices. Occasionally only a single paramedian or median fistula may be present [3]. If the lesion is disfiguring the fistula may be excised surgically. Intra-orally, bilateral blind epithelium-lined tracts may be formed on the alveolar mucosa in proximity to the interior lateral frenium [2].

REFERENCES

1 Koechlin H. (1950) *Praxis* **39**, 918.
2 Stalker W.H. & Allen G.W. (1983) *Oral Surg* **55**, 173.
3 Van Der Wonde A. (1954) *Am J Hum Genet* **6**, 244.

Angular fistulae. Rarely, fistulae at the angles of the mouth, also determined by a dominant gene and sometimes associated with aural sinus, may present clinically as recurrent or refractory angular cheilitis [2]. Asymptomatic pits are found in 12% of Caucasians and 20% of Negroes [1].

REFERENCES

1 Baker B. (1966) *Oral Surg* **21**, 56.
2 Essner H. (1959) *Dermatol Wochenschr* **140**, 1192.

Epidermoid cysts [1]. Epidermoid cysts are rare in the floor of the mouth. They often become clinically apparent between the ages of 15 and 35. A circum-

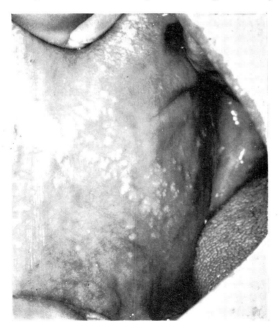

Fig. 55.7. Fordyce spots in the buccal mucosa (University Hospital, Copenhagen).

scribed midline swelling may enlarge to fill the floor of the mouth and displace the tongue. Treatment is by surgical excision.

REFERENCE

1 MEYER I. (1955) *Oral Surg* **8**, 1149.

Idiopathic gingival fibromatosis and hypertrichosis [2,3]. Idiopathic gingival fibromatosis is a hereditary disorder determined by an autosomal dominant gene [4] and characterized by gross enlargement of the gingivae. Histologically the hyperplastic tissue consists of thick bundles of hyalinized collagen fibres with few fibroblasts or capillaries and little or no inflammatory infiltrate.

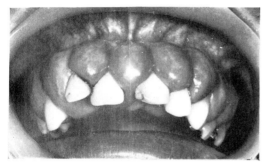

FIG. 55.8. Idiopathic gingival fibromatosis in a young woman who also suffered from hypertrichosis. (University Hospital, Copenhagen).

Clinically, overgrowth of the gingivae, especially in the anterior maxillary region, begins between infancy and the ninth year. The fibromatosis gradually increases and the teeth may be completely covered by thick firm resilient gingiva. The surface may be stippled or smooth and shining according to the degree of inflammatory change caused by bacterial invasion from the gingival pseudo-pockets. The swelling may be so pronounced that the lips cannot be closed.

In some families gingival fibromatosis is apparently an isolated defect, but in others it is associated with other abnormalities of which the most striking is hypertrichosis of variable degree. The hypertrichosis may be evident from infancy but it becomes more severe and extensive. The eyebrows are wide and bushy, and hair growth is particularly prolific on the forehead, back and arms. Some cases have shown mental retardation and cranial deformities, gynaecomastia and in one girl [1] massive enlargement of the breasts in adolescence from giant fibroadenomata. Related to the gingival fibromatosis is bilateral fibrous enlargement of the max-

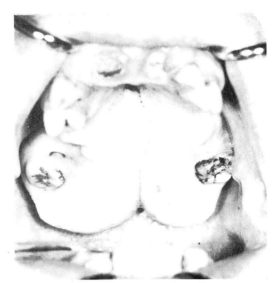

FIG. 55.9. Idiopathic fibromatosis of maxillary tuberosities (University Hospital, Copenhagen).

illary tuberosities (Fig. 55.9). In both conditions recurrences are common even after extensive surgery. The simultaneous occurrence of gingival fibromatosis and cherubism has also been reported [4].

In differential diagnosis the gingival hyperplasia induced by hydantoin derivatives must be excluded (p. 2092).

REFERENCES

1 BYARS L.T. & JURKIEWICZ M. (1961) *Plast Reconstr Surg* **27**, 608.
2 *FORET J. (1964) *Acta Stomatol Belg* **61**, 161.
3 GORLIN R.J., *et al* (1976) *Syndromes of the Head and Neck* 2nd ed. New York, McGraw-Hill.
4 RANOM Y., *et al* (1967) *Oral Surg* **24**, 435.

Papillon–Lefèvre syndrome (see p. 1457 [1]. This syndrome, determined by an autosomal recessive gene, combines palmoplantar keratoderma with destruction of the supporting tissues of both primary and secondary dentitions.

The eruption of the primary teeth proceeds normally but the gingivae later swell and become soggy and foetor develops. Destruction of the periodontium almost immediately follows the eruption of the last molar. By the age of 4 nearly all the primary teeth have been lost. The inflammatory changes then subside and the gingiva appears normal. The process is repeated when the permanent teeth erupt, but the third molars are spared.

REFERENCE

1 GORLIN R.J., *et al* (1976) *Syndromes of the Head and Neck*. 2nd ed. New York, McGraw-Hill.

ORAL PIGMENTATION

Endogenous pigmentation—melanin

Physiological [3,4]. Pigmentation in the mouth is most marked on the gingiva, the buccal mucosa, the hard palate, the tongue and the soft palate. In intensity and extent it parallels the degree of pigmentation of the skin, but increases from childhood to adult life. Racial variation is described on p.48, 1554. Pigmentation may increase in pregnancy.

Smoker's melanosis. A large number of Caucasian patients with melanin pigmentation of the oral mucosa, especially of the gingivae, may have acquired this pigmentation through tobacco smoking. In a series of Swedish patients it was found that all with pigmentation proved to be tobacco smokers. Patients with smoker's melanosis had a significantly higher tobacco consumption than smokers without pigmentation [5].

Addison's disease (p. 1566). In Addison's disease, as in other conditions in which the output of MSH is raised, mucosal pigmentation is increased, darkening in areas already pigmented and extending to new sites. The distribution is an accentuation of the physiological pattern (Fig. 55.10).

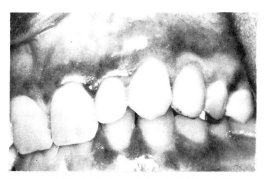

FIG. 55.10. Gingival pigmentation in Addison's disease (University Hospital, Copenhagen).

Peutz–Jeghers syndrome (p. 1556) [6]. Round, oval or irregular greyish-brown macules develop on and around the lips and on the oral mucosa (Fig. 55.11). The tongue and the floor of the mouth are usually spared. Pigmented macules may also be present on the hands and feet.

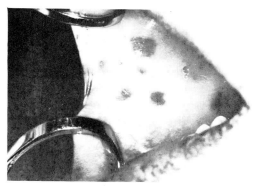

FIG. 55.11. Mucosal pigmentation of the buccal mucosa in Peutz–Jeghers syndrome (University Hospital, Copenhagen).

Albright's syndrome—polyostotic fibrous dysplasia (p. 1562). Oral pigmentation may be found, but the extensive cutaneous plaques dominate the clinical picture.

Acanthosis nigricans (p. 1460). Mucosal pigmentation is most conspicuous in the malignant form, where it is associated with warty papillomatosis.

Other pigments. Mucosal pigmentation, consisting of both haemosiderin and melanin, may be seen in *haemochromatosis* (p. 2334) and *Cooley's anaemia*.

Yellowish-green discoloration by bile pigments is detectable in *jaundice*, especially at the junction of the hard and soft palate.

Exogenous pigmentation

Amalgam tattoo [7]. The most frequent type of exogenous pigmentation in the oral cavity is caused by deposits of silver amalgam which enter the subepithelial connective tissues during the filling of a

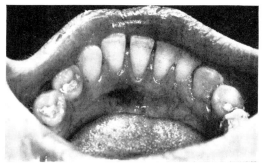

FIG. 55.12. Amalgam tattoo on the alveolar mucosa (University Hospital, Copenhagen).

tooth with amalgam or the extraction of a filled tooth. An epidemiological survey of 20,333 Swedes has shown an astonishingly high prevalence of 8% [1]. The granules are grouped along the collagen fibres and rarely provoke the formation of foreign body granulomas. Clinically they present as small well-defined bluish-black spots, usually on the alveolar mucosa, and must be differentiated from pigmented naevi.

Lead and bismuth poisoning. Despite advances in industrial hygiene, lead poisoning still occurs. Deposits of lead sulphide in capillary walls and macrophages in the gingivae give rise to the lead line, which may be seen early in the disease, especially if the patient has pre-existing gingivitis and calculus. It is rare in children in whom the metal is more readily deposited in the bones [3]. The lead line, greyish in colour and consisting of discrete granules, is near the gingival margin (Fig. 55.13).

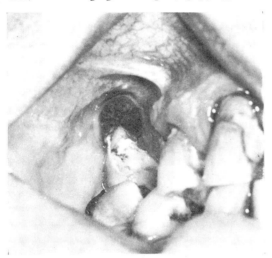

FIG. 55.13. Heavy deposits of lead sulphide on the gingiva of the maxillary first molar revealed after calculus was removed (University Hospital, Copenhagen).

Bismuth poisoning is now rarely seen, but some clinics are strangely reluctant to abandon this drug. The bismuth line is darker in colour than the lead line but cannot be reliably differentiated clinically. It may be limited to the interdental papillae.

Heavy metal lines can be effectively treated by removing the calculus and massaging the gingivae with hydrogen peroxide 30% which oxidizes the sulphide to colourless sulphate.

Argyria (p. 1600). Diffuse oral pigmentation occurs but is overshadowed by the cutaneous changes.

Antimalarial drugs. The prolonged administration of certain antimalarial drugs induces mucosal pigmentation. Pigmentation, especially on the palate, has been observed in association with cutaneous changes (p. 1601) in troops receiving mepacrine. Similar mucosal changes were produced by amodiaquine hydrochloride [2], the incidence increasing with the length of exposure to 66% of adults after 2 yr but only 12% of children after 3 yr. Chloroquine may also cause pigmentation of the palate and of the skin, but does so relatively rarely [8].

REFERENCES

1 AXÉLL T. (1976) *Odontol Rev* **27** (Suppl. 36).
2 CAMPBELL C.H. (1960) *Med J Aust* **47**, 956.
3 COHEN G.J. & AHRENS W.E. (1959) *J Pediatr* **54**, 271.
4 DUMMETT C.O. & BARENS J. (1967) *J Periodontol* **38**, 369.
5 HEDIN C.A. (1977) *Arch Dermatol* **113**, 1533.
6 *KLOSTERMANN G.F. (1960) *Pigmentfleckenpolypose.* Stuttgart, Thieme.
7 ORBAN B. (1946) *J Periodontol* **17**, 55.
8 TUFANELLI D., *et al* (1963) *Arch Dermatol* **58**, 419.

INFECTIOUS DISEASES INVOLVING THE ORAL MUCOSA

Virus infections. The virus infections involving the oral mucosa have been fully considered in other chapters. Here the clinical features of the oral lesions are recapitulated with emphasis on their differential diagnosis. Virological diagnostic techniques are described in Chapter 20.

Herpes simplex (p. 685). Primary infection with *Herpesvirus hominis* may give rise to herpetic gingivostomatitis, which is the commonest form of stomatitis in children between the ages of 1 and 6. Fever, headache and malaise are soon followed by vesicles 2–5 mm in diameter on the lips, gingiva and oral mucosa. The vesicles are soon broken to leave erosions. The gingiva is diffusely red and swollen and very tender, and the appearance is sometimes similar to that of an acute necrotizing gingivitis, although destruction of the gingiva rarely occurs.

Recurrent infections with the virus occur almost exclusively on the lips. The vesicles, which are about 1–3 mm in diameter, are closely grouped. There are no constitutional symptoms. Recurrent intraoral herpes simplex lesions have been reported [4].

Herpes zoster (p. 680). Oral lesions may occur when the second or third division of the trigeminal nerve is involved. Grouped vesicles on the buccal mucosa, tongue (Fig. 55.15), palate and gingiva develop uni-

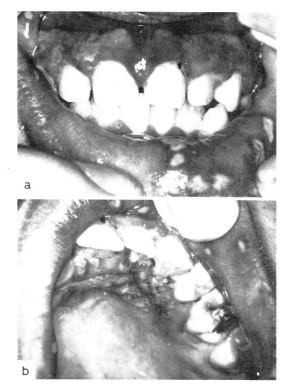

FIG. 55.14. Herpetic gingivostomatitis: (a) acute gingivitis and vesicles on the lips; (b) palatal lesions in the same patient (University Hospital, Copenhagen).

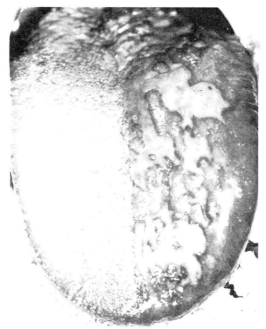

FIG. 55.15. Herpes zoster affecting the left side of the tongue (University Hospital, Copenhagen).

laterally in association with skin lesions and usually preceded by pain.

Varicella (p. 680). A few scattered vesicles on the oral mucosa often accompany the skin eruption but are not an important or troublesome manifestation.

Hand, foot and mouth disease (p. 663). Stomatitis is usually the presenting feature of this Coxsackie infection, especially in childhood. Rather few large vesicles are irregularly distributed over the palate, buccal mucosa, gingiva and tongue. Fever is slight. The inconstant skin lesions are pearly-grey 5 mm vesicles on the fingers and toes.

Herpangina (p. 662). Herpangina, also a Coxsackie infection of childhood, commonly begins with fever of 38–40°C, soon followed by sore throat and abdominal pain. Up to 15 or 20 minute vesicles are scattered over the pharynx, palate and tonsils.

Vesicular stomatitis (p. 706) *and foot and mouth disease* (p. 665). These are both rare in man, but are included in Table 55.2.

Vaccinia (p. 693). Accidental vaccinia of the lip was not uncommon, but was rare on the oral mucosa. The usually solitary large vesicles were surrounded by intense oedema [5].

Orf (p. 695): *Milker's nodes* (p. 695). Very rarely, lesions have occurred on the lips.

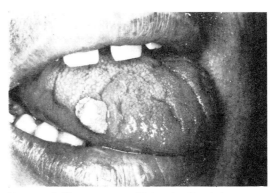

FIG. 55.16. Wart on tongue (University Hospital, Copenhagen).

TABLE 55.2. Virus infections of the oral mucosa

	Age	Morphology	Distribution	Systemic symptoms
Herpetic gingivostomatitis	Usually 1–6	Scattered vesicles 2–5 mm	Lips, gingiva and oral mucosa	Fever and malaise precede onset
Recurrent herpes	Children or adults	Grouped vesicles c. 1 mm, usually one group	Lips or oral mucosa	None
Herpes zoster	Children or adults	Unilateral grouped vesicles	Buccal mucosa, palate, tongue, gingiva	Pain, malaise, skin lesions
Hand, foot and mouth disease	Children	Few scattered large vesicles	Irregularly distributed over oral mucosa	Slight fever, vesicles of fingers and toes
Herpangina	Children	Scattered tiny vesicles	Pharynx, palate, tonsils	Onset with fever to 38–40°C
Foot and mouth disease (very rare in man)	Adults in contact with infected animals	Ragged, painful vesicles, burning pain	Buccal mucosa, tongue, lips	Preceded by fever, malaise, vesicles of palms and soles
Vesicular stomatitis (mainly South America)	In contacts of infected cattle and horses	Mild stomatitis, adenitis	Irregularly distributed over oral mucosa	Mild fever and malaise; vesicles on fingers

Infectious warts (p. 668) (syn. verruca vulgaris). Warts are not uncommon on the lips or oral mucosa at any age. They may be associated with warts on the hands. The horn is macerated by saliva and appears white, but the surface remains warty or granular. The lesions are superficial and there is no surrounding induration (Fig. 55.16).

Focal epithelial hyperplasia [6]. The term 'focal epithelial hyperplasia' was introduced in 1965 [1] to

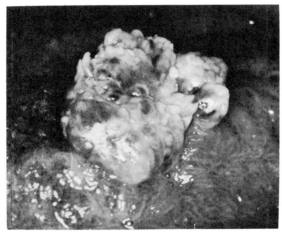

FIG. 55.17. Condyloma acuminatum on the margin of the tongue of a man whose partner had vulval condylomas (Dental Department, University Hospital, Copenhagen).

signify certain multiple nodular elevations of the oral mucosa observed among American Indians in New Mexico, U.S.A., and the Mato Grosso district in Brazil. The condition has also been described among Indians in El Salvador, Guatemala, Venezuela, Colombia, Peru and Paraguay. In Colombia the focal epithelial hyperplasia was found in a family of half-breed Indians with a possible Negro influence [3]. Focal epithelial hyperplasia has been found in 19.4% of 460 inhabitants of an Eskimo population in south-west Greenland (Nanortalik). Small series of cases have been reported from Egypt, Israel and South Africa, and isolated cases from a number of other countries [7]. The condition is characterized by circumscribed sessile soft elevated nodules which either are rounded and with a surface like the adjoining normal mucosa or have a flat whitish surface located on the oral mucosa of the lips, the buccal mucosa, the gingiva, the hard and soft palate and the tongue (Fig. 55.18). Histologically, the focal epithelial hyperplasia is characterized by epithelial hyperplasia with acanthosis, elongation and anastomosing of rete ridges, increased cellular density of the epithelium, enlarged epithelial nuclei and multinucleated cells (Fig. 55.19). Recently, evidence of a viral infection has been found, based on microscope, electron microscope and immunofluorescence examinations [2]. Possible influence of a genetic factor as well cannot be excluded, however.

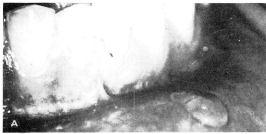

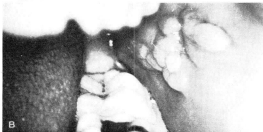

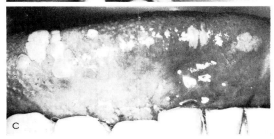

FIG. 55.18. Focal epithelial hyperplasia in a Greenlandic Eskimo (from Clausen *et al* [2]).

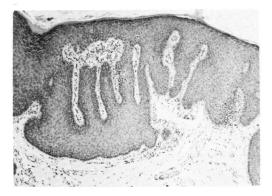

FIG. 55.19. Epithelial hyperplasia with Thor's hammer configuration of rete ridges in an Eskimo with focal epithelial hyperplasia (× 90) (Royal Dental College, Copenhagen).

REFERENCES

1 ARCHARD H.O., *et al* (1965) *Oral Surg* **20**, 201.
2 CLAUSEN F.P. (1969) *Tandlægebladet* **73**, 1013.
3 GOMEZ A., *et al* (1969) *J Am Dent Assoc* **79**, 663.
4 GRIFFIN J.W. (1965) *Oral Surg* **19**, 209.
5 PINDBORG J.J. (1985) *Atlas of Diseases of the Oral Mucosa* 4th ed. Copenhagen, Munksgaard.
6 *PRETORIUS-CLAUSEN F. (1972) *Oral Surg* **34**, 604.
7 VAN WYK C.W., *et al* (1977) *J Oral Pathol* **6**, 1.

Bacterial infections. Bacterial infections of the oral mucosa are uncommon. Apart from Vincent's infection, the pathogenesis of which is complex and obscure, only tuberculosis and syphilis are of real importance.

Acute necrotizing gingivitis (syn. *Vincent's stomatitis; ulceromembranous gingivitis; acute ulcerative gingivitis*). Acute necrotizing gingivitis, formerly common in schools and military establishments [9], is now generally relatively rare in Western countries. The annual incidence in Harvard students was estimated [2] at 0·9%. It is quite common among children in South East Asia and Africa [10]. Most cases occur in adolescents, and although poor dental hygiene and smoking may be factors [8], and stress, malnutrition and systemic disease sometimes appear to predispose, the pathogenesis remains mysterious. Acute necrotizing gingivitis is commonly regarded as an endogenous infection caused by the combined influence of several microorganisms. *Borrelia vincenti* and *Bacillus fusiformis* usually predominate in smears from diseased tissue [3]. Several observations indicate that the effects of endotoxins are more predominant in necrotizing gingivitis than in chronic gingivitis [5].

Clinically the essential changes are punched-out lesions of the marginal gingiva and interdental papillae, which usually destroy the gingiva rapidly if treatment is not instituted. Necrotic areas along the gingival margin are covered by a yellowish pseudomembrane. Pain and bleeding may be troublesome and foetor is characteristic. The palatal and lingual marginal gingiva is less frequently affected [5]. The disease continues indefinitely but without serious consequences in the healthy, apart from destruction of the osseous supporting apparatus of the teeth. The acute necrotizing process may spread to other parts of the oral mucosa.

Vincent's angina, an uncommon fusospirochaetal pharyngitis, may be associated with the gingivitis or may occur alone.

The diagnosis must be made on clinical grounds for there are no specific bacteriological findings.

Herpetic gingivostomatitis is vesicular and is not confined to the marginal gingiva.

Underlying systemic disease should be sought and treated. The treatment consists in cleaning the ulcerations. In several studies metronidazole has been shown to be effective in the initial treatment of acute ulcerative gingivitis [6]. Systemic penicillin should be given only when fever is present.

Gonorrhoea (p. 753). Gonococcal stomatitis [12] is very rarely reported, but may result from cunnilingus or fellatio. The stomatitis is acute but superficial. The oral mucosa as a whole is fiery red and multiple erosions are covered by a yellowish pseudomembrane.

Tuberculosis (p. 798) [1]. Primary tuberculosis of the oral mucosa is excessively rare. A nodule at the site of inoculation soon ulcerates and is associated with enlargement of the regional lymph nodes which may break down.

Secondary tuberculosis ulcers on the tongue are not uncommon in patients with extensive laryngeal, pulmonary or gastrointestinal infection [4,7]. The rounded or irregularly linear ulcer, usually at the base of the tongue with an overhanging edge and with purulent exudate on its floor, may be very painful. Lupus may rarely first involve or later extend to the mucosa. The granulomatous nodules tend to become eroded.

Tuberculosis cutis orificialis occurs in poorly-nourished patients with active pulmonary infection (see p. 809).

The diagnosis of oral tuberculosis is established histologically (see p. 803).

Syphilis (p. 839). Oral lesions are seen at all stages of syphilis. In a Finnish study [11] of 254 congenital syphilitics, 45% showed abnormal incisors and 22% abnormal molars. The mesial and distal surfaces of the crown of the incisors taper and converge towards the incisal edge, which is concave apically—Hutchinson's teeth. The deformed first molars are descriptively termed 'mulberry molars', because their multiple cusps are poorly developed. Scars may radiate from the angles of the mouth.

The chancre of acquired primary syphilis is relatively common on the lips and is occasionally seen on the oral mucosa. A small papule soon forms a painless ulcer with an indurated margin. The regional lymphatic glands are enlarged.

In secondary syphilis the oral mucosa is usually involved but the changes may be limited to a simple pharyngitis. More characteristic are the eroded papules which form *mucous patches*. They may occur on the tongue, at the angles of the mouth, on the palate or anywhere on the oral mucosa (Fig. 55.20). They may be inconspicuous, like small areas of leukoplakia. The whitish membrane can easily be scraped off to leave a raw erosion. In areas frequently traumatized the patches may be large, diffuse and ulcerated but are usually painless.

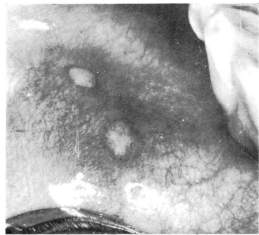

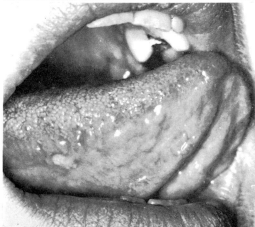

FIG. 55.20. Mucous patches on the oral mucosa in secondary syphilis (University Hospital, Copenhagen).

In the tertiary stage gummata are classically situated on the palate, which may perforate. Interstitial glossitis, the result of syphilitic endarteritis, is characterized by shrinkage of the tongue, which may become lobed and by loss of lingual papillae. Later, leukoplakia and carcinoma may develop (Fig. 55.21).

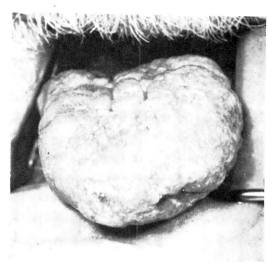

FIG. 55.21. Lobed tongue with leukoplakia and carcinoma in a man with tertiary syphilis (University Hospital, Copenhagen).

REFERENCES

1 *DARLINGTON C.C., *et al* (1937) *Ann Rev Tuberc* **35**, 147, 180.
2 GIDDON D.R., *et al* (1964) *J Am Dent Assoc* **41**, 674.
3 HADI A.W. & RUSSELL C. (1968) *Arch Oral Biol* **13**, 1371.
4 *KATZ F.L. (1940) *Q Bull Seaview Hosp* **6**, 239.
5 KRISTOFFERSON T. & LIE T. (1983) In *Textbook of Clinical Periodontology*. Ed. Lindhe J. Munksgaard, Copenhagen, pp. 202–218.
6 LORDAN J., *et al* (1971) *Br Dent J* **130**, 294.
7 DE MONTIGNY G. (1945) *J Can Dent Assoc* **11**, 334.
8 PINDBORG J.J. (1947) *J Dent Res* **26**, 261.
9 PINDBORG J.J. (1951) *J Am Dent Assoc* **42**, 517.
10 PINDBORG J.J., *et al* (1960) *J Periodontol* **37**, 14.
11 PUTKONEN P. (1962) *Acta Derm Venereol (Stockh)* **42**, 44.
12 SCHMIDT H., *et al* (1961) *Acta Derm Venereol (Stockh)* **41**, 324.

Mycotic infections

Candidiasis. The mycology and ecology of *Candida albicans* are considered fully on p. 946. Here only the differential diagnosis of oral infections will be discussed.

Candida infections of the oral mucosa are much

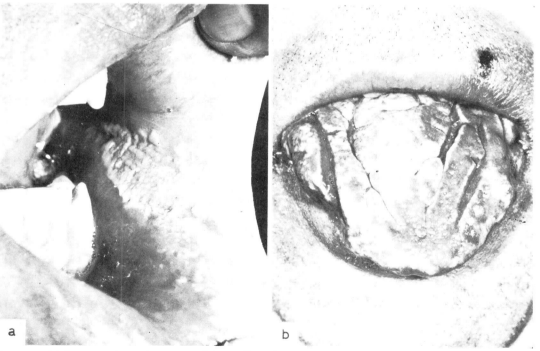

FIG. 55.22. (a) Acute pseudomembranous candidiasis of buccal mucosa and (b) candidal granuloma of the tongue (University Hospital, Copenhagen).

more common than hitherto thought. The reason for misdiagnosis is partly because candidiasis may present with completely different clinical manifestations. A rather simple classification (somewhat modified after Lehner [2]) divides oral candidiasis into acute (comprising a pseudomembranous and an atrophic type) and chronic (comprising a hyperplastic and an atrophic type).

Thrush, the acute pseudomembranous type, is common in infancy; the incidence has been established in a survey in Israel [4] as 149 ± 34 per 1,000 live births. The onset is commonly at the end of the first week, with the appearance of creamy-white patches which can be scraped off to leave an erythematous base. The patches may be small or may form extensive plaques (Fig. 55.22).

Thrush in an older child or adult should always suggest the possibility of underlying systemic disease (p. 948) including AIDS, which must be carefully sought.

Acute atrophic candidiasis, where the oral mucosa has a fiery red colour, is most often caused by the use of antibiotics. In contrast with the other types of candiasis, the acute atrophic form is very painful and is the seat of small ulcerations.

In chronic hyperplastic candidiasis the white patches are rather more adherent and occasionally are surrounded by a zone of pronounced erythema. The most common site is the retrocommisural mucosa (see also p. 2108). In a number of cases, however, the retrocommissural lesions are associated

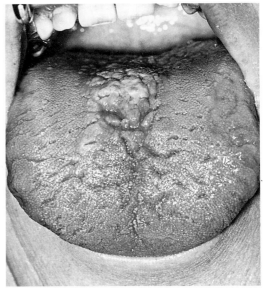

FIG. 55.23. Chronic hyperplastic candidiasis in the area where median rhomboid glossitis usually occurs (University Hospital, Copenhagen).

with lesions in the palate and dorsum of the tongue [1,3]; the latter manifestation is often erroneously called median rhomboid glossitis (Fig. 55.23). In these cases, and also in isolated cases, the cessation of tobacco smoking may improve the lesion considerably.

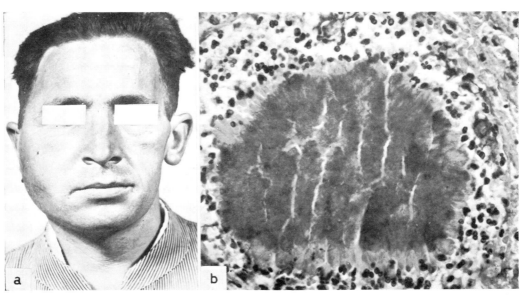

FIG. 55.24. Cervicofacial actinomycosis: (a) clinical appearance; (b) colony of *Actinomyces* (× 264) (University Hospital, Copenhagen).

The white patches, which are relatively easily removed, suggest the diagnosis, which must be confirmed by biopsy or by smear. After early infancy the isolation of *Candida* from clinically appropriate lesions should not be considered to establish a final diagnosis but to initiate detailed investigation of predisposing local and systemic disorders.

The chronic atrophic type may manifest itself as either denture sore mouth (see below) or angular cheilitis (p. 2123).

A very rare type of candidiasis is the candidal granuloma (p. 959), where the tongue is persistently involved (Fig. 55.22b).

Treatment is considered on p. 961.

Actinomycosis (p. 982). The classical form of actinomycosis occurs in the cervicofacial region in about 70% of cases but is a relatively rare disease in Western Europe. The subcutaneous swelling later breaks down to form abscesses discharging through multiple sinuses. 'Sulphur granules' representing colonies of the microorganism may be detected in the purulent exudate.

More commonly *Actinomyces israelii* is isolated from cystic swellings of the cheek over the openings of sinuses from dental abscesses.

Actinomycosis may also involve the tongue, usually as a solitary abscess.

Treatment is considered on p. 984.

REFERENCES

1 *Cernea P., *et al* (1965) *Rev Stomatol* **66**, 103.
2 Lehner T. (1962) *Dent Practnr Dent Rev* **17**, 209.
3 Pindborg J.J. (1985) *Atlas of Diseases of the Oral Mucosa*, 4th ed. Copenhagen, Munksgaard.
4 Rosenweig K.A. & Karov S. (1964) *Alpha Omega* **57**, 126.

CANCRUM ORIS
SYN. NOMA; INFECTIVE GANGRENE OF THE MOUTH

Aetiology [1,2,4]. Malnutrition, especially protein deficiency, is the principal predisposing factor, but chronic infections, such as malaria, or recurrent acute infections, such as acute herpetic gingivostomatitis, often contribute. The organisms isolated are the normal bacteriological flora of the mouth. Most cases occur in children between 1 and 7 yr old.

Clinical features [2,4]. Ulcerative stomatitis of the gingiva of maxilla or mandible extends rapidly to adjacent soft tissue, producing gross destruction which may involve the whole thickness of the cheek. In the worst cases there is little fever and no leukocytosis. The prognosis is generally poor but the milder forms may recover with early treatment.

Treatment [5]. High protein diet and vitamin supplements, antibiotics to control infection and skilful nursing will save the less severe cases. Plastic surgery will be required to lessen the residual deformity.

REFERENCES

1 Eckstein A. (1940) *Am J Dis Child* **59**, 219.
2 Emslie R.D. (1963) *Dent Practnr Dent Rec* **13**, 781.
3 Jelliffe D.B. (1952) *Pediatrics* **9**, 544.
4 Luder J. (1955) *Gt Ormond St J* **9**, 22.
5 Raynaud P., et al (1961) *Bull Soc Méd d'Afrique Noire* **6**, 416.

DENTURE STOMATITIS

Aetiology. The inflammatory changes seen beneath an upper denture have been called 'stomatitis prosthetica', 'denture sore mouth' or 'denture stomatitis', of which the last-mentioned term seems to have gained universal acceptance.

Denture stomatitis is a clinical syndrome of multiple causation and with variable physical signs occurring mainly in middle-aged or elderly women, but occasionally seen in men or women of any age. More than one factor can often be incriminated in the individual patient.

Systemic disease. Iron-deficiency anaemia and other nutritional deficiencies may increase the vulnerability of the oral mucous membrane.

Trauma. This is an important factor. If the denture fits badly, repeated minor traumata may be transmitted to certain areas of the palate or gingiva.

Infection. Most probably, the majority of cases of denture stromatitis are caused by *Candida albicans* [2]. Most cases are easily treated, but recurrences are frequent and the infection often spreads to involve other parts of the oral mucosa such as the tongue and the angles of the mouth [1].

A mycological study of two patients with denture stomatitis identified eight yeast species: five *Candida*, two *Torulopsis* and one *Kluyveromyces* [3].

Clinical features. Usually the condition is classified into three types: (1) a localized simple type of inflammation which includes both pinpoint hyperaemia and diffuse inflammation of a limited area of the palatal mucosa, (2) a generalized type of inflammation and (3) a granular papillary type [1]. The first type is due to trauma. The second and third types are associated with a *Candida* infection.

Allergic reactions present as diffuse erythema and oedema, mainly on the palate (pp. 2091 and 510).

Diagnosis. Close collaboration between dental surgeon and dermatologist is a great advantage. Each case must be carefully evaluated and the possible role of systemic factors assessed, bearing in mind

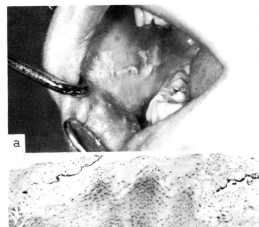

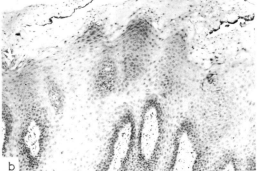

FIG. 55.26. Cheek biting: (a) clinical appearance; (b) histology (University Hospital and Royal Dental College, Copenhagen).

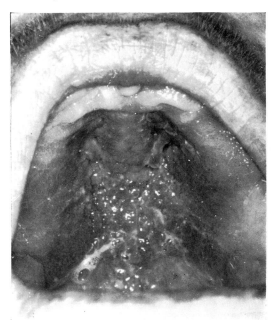

FIG. 55.25. Denture stomatitis (type 3) under a full upper denture (University Hospital, Copenhagen).

that trauma and infection are the common causes. The use of *Candida*-infected saliva in patch tests for allergy to denture materials gives rise to false positive reactions [4].

Treatment. Remodelling of the denture is usually the solution for type 1 denture stomatitis. Fungistatic drugs are required for types 2 and 3, but if recurrences are to be avoided the dentures should be removed and carefully cleaned each night.

REFERENCES

1 *BUDTZ-JÖRGENSEN E. (1974) *Scand J Dent Res* **82**, 151.
2 NIEL D.J., *et al* (1965) *Dent Practnr Dent Res* **16**, 135.
3 *OLSEN I. (1976) *Studies on oral yeast infection with emphasis on denture stomatitis*. Thesis, Oslo.
4 SALO G.P. & HIRVONEN M.-L. (1969) *Br J Dermatol* **81**, 338.

CHEEK BITING [1,2]

In cheek biting (morsicatio buccarum), a common habit, a fold of buccal mucosa is sucked in between the teeth and chewed. The traumatized areas show superficial erosions and shreds of macerated epithelium. Histologically the damaged epithelium is thickened and hyperkeratotic with large, sometimes vacuolated, cells, and may be not unlike white sponge naevus (p. 2078). The history and the site differentiate leukoplakia, lupus erythematosus, lichen planus and white sponge naevus.

The lesions heal when the biting tic ceases, but the habit may be difficult to break.

REFERENCES

1 HJÖRTING-HANSEN E. & HOLST E.(1970) *Scand J Dent Res* **78**, 492.
2 OBERMEYER M.E. (1964) *Arch Dermatol* **90**, 185.

IRRITANT AND ALLERGIC STOMATITIS

Aetiology. Inflammatory changes of the oral mucosa induced by primary irritants or allergic sensitizers are surprisingly rare if the severe reactions to caustic chemicals ingested accidentally or suicidally are excluded. Many published case reports of allergic stomatitis are of doubtful reliability. The rarity of chemical stomatitis is no doubt partly the result of the normally very short periods of contact with the mucosa but other factors may be concerned. Many patients who give positive patch tests on the skin fail to show any reactions to mucosal patch tests. Dentrifices and mouthwashes may cause cheilitis without stomatitis.

True allergic stomatitis is occasionally seen. Dental medicaments are the main offenders. The essential oils of cassia and cloves [5], antibiotics such as streptomycin and penicillin, mercury and nickel have all been incriminated. The flavourings used in dentifrices and chewing-gums have also sometimes caused reactions [4].

Chewing the leaves of poison ivy has caused a severe stomatitis in sensitized subjects [6].

Allergic reactions to denture materials [1,2] were relatively common when dentures were made of vulcanized rubber. Most dentures are now made of acrylic resins, usually methylmethacrylate. The fully heat-cured resin rarely causes trouble but is still occasionally reliably incriminated. Self-curing acrylics, especially when used for amateur repairs to broken dentures, are most likely to contain free monomer.

Clinical features. The essential features are erythema and oedema but in severe reactions there may be vesiculation or even necrosis. The distribution of these changes depends on the sites of greatest contact with the irritant or sensitizer. Local reactions to metals or resins in prostheses contrast with the generalized reactions to lozenges, mouthwashes or disinfectants.

Reactions to denture materials are characterized by erythema and oedema, especially of the palate.

Candidiasis may complicate chronic or recurrent chemical stomatitis.

Diagnosis. The history and the distribution of the lesions will usually establish the diagnosis. Patch testing may be helpful, but a negative skin test should be supplemented by a mucosal patch test [3] if the circumstantial evidence justifies the inconvenience to the patient.

Shavings of denture material should be used for testing, as the use of the denture itself produces misleading traumatic reactions.

Treatment. Symptomatic measures and avoidance of further contact will usually suffice. Intensely severe reactions require hospital treatment, antibiotics and even tracheotomy.

REFERENCES

1 CRISSEY J.T. (1965) *Arch Dermatol* **92**, 45.
2 FISHER A.A. (1954) *JAMA* **156**, 238.
3 GOLDMAN L. & GOLDMAN B. (1944) *Arch Dermatol Syphilol* **50**, 79.
4 KERR D. A., *et al* (1971) *Oral Surg* **32**, 402.
5 PINDBORG J.J. (1985) *Atlas of Diseases of the Oral Mucosa*. 4th ed. Copenhagen, Munksgaard.
6 SASSAMAN D. (1945) *Am J Orthol* **31**, 695.

STOMATITIS MEDICAMENTOSA
ORAL INVOLVEMENT IN SYSTEMIC REACTIONS TO DRUGS

Changes in the oral mucosa may occur in a very large number of reactions to drugs, usually in association with skin lesions but sometimes as the only visible evidence of the reaction. The mucosal changes in reactions to many drugs receive incidental mention in Chapter 34. The possibility of a drug reaction should always be considered in the presence of bullous or erosive stomatitis or of an otherwise unexplained inflammatory or hyperplastic lesion of the oral mucosa.

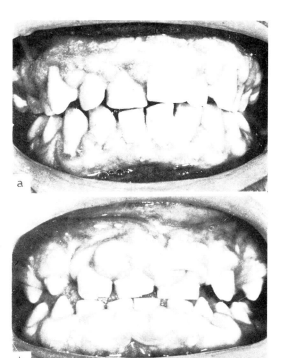

FIG. 55.27. Gingival hyperplasia caused by diphenylhydantoin: (a) confined to interdental papillae; (b) gross hyperplasia also involving attached gingiva (University Hospital, Copenhagen).

Certain drug reactions in which the oral lesions are distinctive or of special diagnostic significance will be considered here.

Gingival hyperplasia from diphenylhydantoin [1]. Gingival hyperplasia is a characteristic reaction to hydantoin (Fig. 55.27). The incidence is related to the daily dose and is relatively higher in children. The degree of hyperplasia is also influenced by the standard of oral hygiene. Histologically there is a massive increase of collagen fibres with moderate epithelial hyperplasia and non-specific inflammatory changes from secondary infection. The hyperplasia begins at the tips of the interdental papillae which enlarge progressively. Ultimately the teeth may be almost concealed by the masses of fibrous tissue.

Treatment is by gingivectomy but recurrences are frequent unless high standards of hygiene can be maintained.

Gold stomatitis. The stomatitis usually accompanies the skin changes (p. 1258) but may precede them. Extensive erythema with superficial erosions involves mainly the buccal mucosa, the palate and the lower surface of the tongue (Fig. 55.28). Sub-

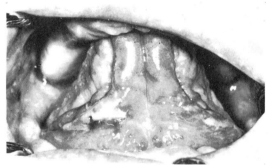

FIG. 55.28. Gold stomatitis, involving predominantly the sublingual area (University Hospital, Copenhagen).

jective symptoms are mild but the lesions run a protracted course and are resistant to topical therapy. In a few cases there may be a faint blue or purple pigmentation of the gingivae.

Oral changes caused by antibiotics. Four types of reaction, induced by different mechanisms, may be seen in patients receiving antibiotics:

(1) black hairy tongue (p. 2118);

(2) a generalized stomatitis with a tender atrophic glossitis, acute atrophic candidiasis; gradual recovery occurs when the antibiotic is stopped;

(3) acute pseudomembranous oral candidiasis (p. 951);

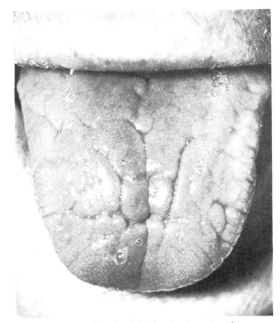

FIG. 55.29. Atrophic glossitis after treatment with chloramphenicol (University Hospital, Copenhagen).

(4) an allergic stomatitis, sometimes bullous, as part of a general allergic reaction.

Stomatitis caused by cytotoxic drugs. The increasing use of antimetabolites such as 6-mercaptopurine and the folic acid antagonists such as methotrexate (Fig. 55.30) has made the recognition of this form of stomatitis a matter of great practical importance. We have seen stomatitis develop in a

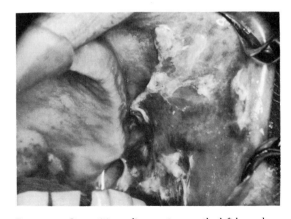

FIG. 55.30. Stomatitis medicamentosa on the left buccal mucosa in a woman receiving treatment with methotrexate (University Hospital, Copenhagen).

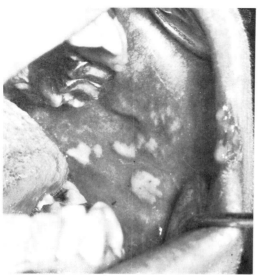

FIG. 55.31. Lesions in the buccal mucosa caused by aminopterin (University Hospital, Copenhagen).

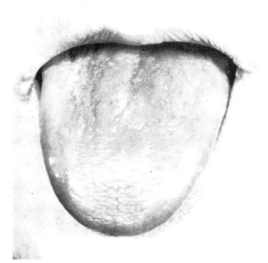

FIG. 55.32. Atrophy of tongue papillae in iron-deficiency anaemia (University Hospital, Copenhagen).

third of a group of patients with psoriasis treated with aminopterin, usually after a week's treatment (Fig. 55.31). The drug disturbs the maturation of oral epithelium and nuclear abnormalities may be seen histologically [2].

The stomatitis begins on the vermilion border, in the buccal mucosa or less often elsewhere as yellowish plaques which soon ulcerate. They are often surrounded by a zone of erythema.

REFERENCES

1 *AAS E. (1963) *Acta Odont Scand* **21**, (Suppl. **34**).
2 DREIZE S. (1978) *J Prosthet Dent* **40**, 650.

ORAL CHANGES IN SYSTEMIC DISEASE

Blood dyscrasias. A wide variety of blood dyscrasias produce changes in the oral mucous membranes, which may sometimes be an early, or indeed the only, clinical manifestation of their presence.

Anaemias

Iron-deficiency anaemia. The patient may complain of a dry mouth and a burning tongue before any visible mucosal changes develop. Later, the tongue becomes smooth and devoid of papillae (Fig. 55.32) (see p. 2116).

In the *Paterson–Kelly* or *Plummer–Vinson* syndrome [2], now sometimes called sideropenic dys-

phagia, which predominantly afflicts middle-aged women, the changes in the tongue are associated with dysphagia and nail changes. The iron deficiency is severe and prolonged, and the mucosa is pale and atrophic. The vermilion border of the lips appears abnormal and there is often angular cheilitis. Leukoplakia and multiple oral carcinomas may develop in the atrophic mucosa (Fig. 55.33), but intensive iron therapy has reduced the incidence in recent years.

Pernicious anaemia [1]. The oral symptoms may precede changes in the peripheral blood at a stage when study of bone marrow and serum vitamin B_{12} can establish the presence of pernicious anaemia. Burning of the tongue is associated with atrophy of the papillae and the mucosa is deep red in colour. There may be lobulation of the surface or a 'cobblestone' appearance (Fig. 55.34). Superficial oral erosions are not uncommon. The glossitis responds promptly to vitamin B_{12}.

Leukaemias. In the acute leukaemias [3] the oral changes are often dramatic. Gingival hyperplasia is characteristic and may be extensive. The hyperplastic gingiva is flabby and often ulcerated and may almost cover the teeth. In addition to necrosis from infarction of small vessels there may be a superadded acute necrotizing gingivitis. Spontaneous bleeding occurs from the gingiva and from other regions of the oral mucosa in which petechiae, ecchymoses and ulcers are frequent (Fig. 55.35).

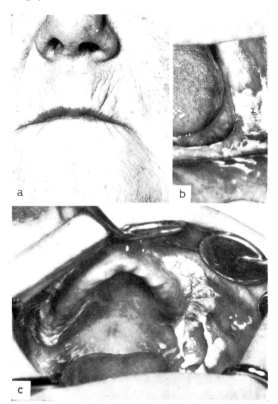

FIG. 55.33. Woman with sideropenic dysphagia:
(a) narrow vermilion border and circumoral fissures;
(b) extensive leukoplakia in the mandible; (c) carcinoma
in the leukoplakia in the maxillary left buccal groove
(University Hospital, Copenhagen).

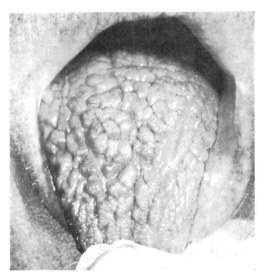

FIG. 55.34. Cobblestone tongue in a man with pernicious
anaemia (University Hospital, Copenhagen).

In the chronic leukaemias there may be ulceration of oral mucosa, but gingival hyperplasia is less usual.

Polycythaemia. The mucosa is deep red and congested and bleeds easily. The gingivae are oedematous.

Neutropenia. In *agranulocytosis* the mucosal changes reflect the severity of the fall in the leukocyte count. There may be an acute gingivitis, multiple superficial erosions or a deep punched-out necrotic ulcer of the buccal, palatal or pharyngeal mucosa with large foul-smelling sloughs. Fever is usual (Fig. 55.36).

Periodic or cyclic neutropenia [4]. This is a rare disorder characterized by recurrent attacks of fever, headache, malaise, oral ulceration and cervical lymphadenopathy. The attacks, which may begin in

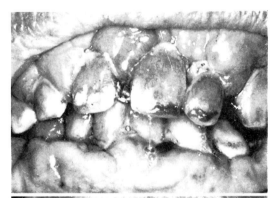

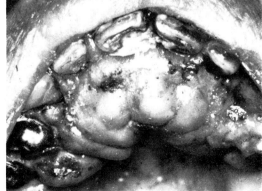

FIG. 55.35. Enlargement of the gingivae in acute
leukaemia (University Hospital, Copenhagen).

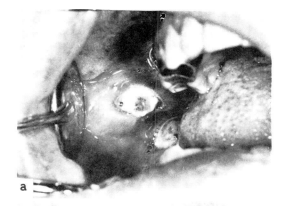

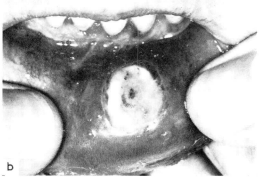

FIG. 55.36. Agranulocytosis: ulceration of (a) the right buccal mucosa and (b) the lower lip (University Hospital, Copenhagen).

childhood and continue at intervals of about 3 weeks, coincide with cyclic reduction in the polymorphonuclear count.

Ulceration and bleeding occur on the gingiva and elsewhere on the oral mucosa. Figure 55.37 illustrates the desperate periodontal condition of a man aged 17 afflicted since infancy.

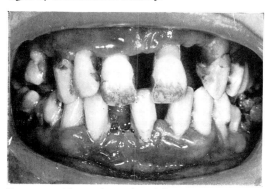

FIG. 55.37. Advanced periodontal destruction in a man aged 17 years with periodic neutropenia (University Hospital, Copenhagen).

REFERENCES

1 HJORTING-HANSEN E. & BERTRAM U. (1968) *Br Dent J* **125**, 266.
2 JONES R.F.M. (1961) *J Laryngol Otol* **75**, 529.
3 MICHAUD M., *et al* (1977) *J Am Dent Assoc* **75**, 932.
4 REIMANN H.A. & DE BERARDINIS C.T. (1949) *Blood* **4**, 1109.

'COLLAGEN DISEASES'

The oral mucosa may be extensively involved in the collagen diseases [4] and in some cases is the site of the presenting manifestations.

Lupus erythematosus [1,3]. The frequency of oral lesions in lupus erythematosus is uncertain. An estimate of 25% is probably too low since they are not always carefully sought.

In chronic discoid lupus erythematosus lesions on the vermilion border of the lips may occur alone or in association with skin lesions (Fig. 55.38). The sites of predilection are the buccal mucosa, the vermilion border and the gingiva. Lesions on the vermilion border and the oral mucosa are alike except for the presence of scaling on the former. The typical lesion is a plaque of depressed dull-red atrophic epithelium, sometimes with puncta or striae, surrounded by a white elevated zone 2–4 mm wide fading into white parallel lines at its outer margin (Figs. 55.38 and 55.39). Old lesions may simulate leukoplakia (Fig. 55.40) but hyperaemic radiating vessels may be recognized around the margins. Some lesions simulate lichen planus. The diagnosis may be confirmed histologically (p. 1287) and by immunofluorescence techniques; deposits of IgG and IgM may be found on the upper part of the

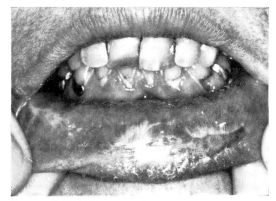

FIG. 55.38. Discoid lupus erythematosus of the vermilion border. Note the radiating white striae. (University Hospital, Copenhagen.)

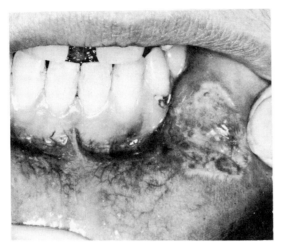

FIG. 55.39. Characteristic lesion on the labial mucosa in a woman with discoid lupus erythematosus. Note the radiating white lines. (University Hospital, Copenhagen.)

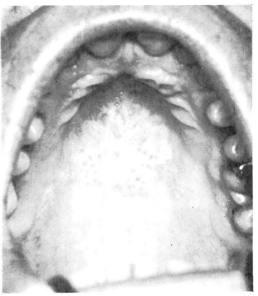

FIG. 55.40. Discoid lupus erythematosus of the palate (University Hospital, Copenhagen).

lamina propria. In a number of cases the oral lesions are the first indication of lupus erythematosus.

In systemic lupus erythematosus the oral lesions are of three types: erythematous lesions, discoid lesions and non-specific ulcers, most often on the palate.

Scleroderma (see p. 1347). The oral mucosa is affected in a large proportion of cases of systemic scleroderma in which the face is involved. The rigidity and induration of the skin around the lips may interfere with speech and feeding. The buccal

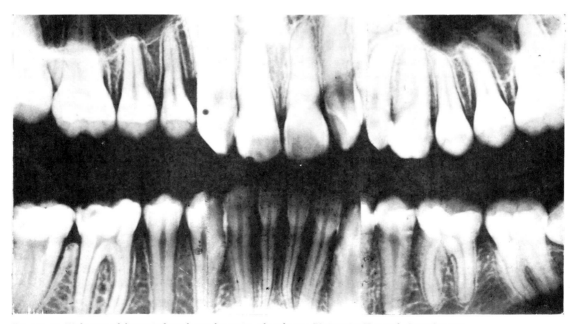

FIG. 55.41. Widening of the periodontal membrane in scleroderma (University Hospital, Copenhagen).

mucosa feels hard, the epithelium may be atrophic and the margin of the palate may be obliterated. The tongue may at first be enlarged by oedema but is later shrunken and fibrotic.

In some cases widening of the periodontal membrane [4] may cause extrusion of the teeth, sometimes resulting in painful traumatic occlusion (Fig. 55.41).

Circumscribed scleroderma may rarely involve the lips or oral mucosa [2].

REFERENCES

1 ANDREASEN J.O. & POULSEN H.E. (1964) *Acta Odontol Scand* **22**, 389.
2 BARBER H.W. (1944) *Proc R Soc Med* **37**, 73.
3 SCHIODT M., *et al* (1978) *Int J Oral Surg* **7**, 85.
4 STAFNE E.C. & AUSTIN L.T. (1944) *Am J Orthod* **30**, 25.

CROHN'S DISEASE

The oral manifestations of Crohn's disease vary greatly. The main features are thickening of the oral mucosa, mostly affecting the vestibule, in a linear form (Fig. 55.42) or with a cobblestone-like appearance, 'denture granuloma' in edentulous patients, linear ulcers, marked swellings, swollen boggy gingivae and widespread 'aphthous' ulcerations [1,2].

In one series of 100 patients with Crohn's disease, nine had oral manifestations of the disease [1].

The striking clinical and microscope resemblance between the oral manifestations in Melkersson–Rosenthal syndrome and the oral changes observed in Crohn's disease may suggest a possible relationship between the two diseases [4]. A series of 16 patients with Melkersson–Rosenthal syndrome were examined thoroughly for Crohn's disease [5], and no relationship was demonstrated. However, a recent study of a girl of 15 with chronic granulomatous cheilitis revealed an asymptomatic Crohn's disease of the lower gastrointestinal tract [3] (see also granulomatous cheilitis, p. 2127).

REFERENCES

1 BASU M.K., *et al* (1975) *Gut* **16**, 249.
2 BERNSTEIN M.L. & McDONALD J.S. (1978) *Oral Surg* **46**, 234.
3 BROOK I.M., *et al* (1983) *Oral Surg* **56**, 405.
4 TYLDESLEY W.R. (1979) *Br J Oral Surg* **17**, 1.
5 WORSAAE N., *et al* (1980) *Br J Oral Surg* **18**, 254.

METABOLIC DISORDERS

The oral cavity is involved in many metabolic disorders, and oral lesions may occur early in the course of the disease and cause the patient to seek advice.

Lipoid proteinosis (p. 2312). Hoarseness in early infancy is a characteristic finding. Later, recurrent or persistent ulceration of the oral mucosa may occur.

Primary amyloidosis (p. 2303). The tongue is enlarged and yellowish nodules may develop, especially along its margins. Purpuric macules and large

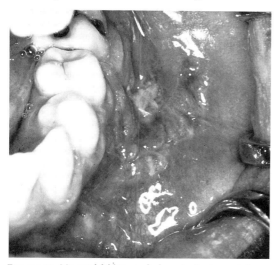

FIG. 55.42. Mucosal folding and ulcers in the lower left buccal vestibule in a patient with Crohn's disease (University Hospital, Copenhagen).

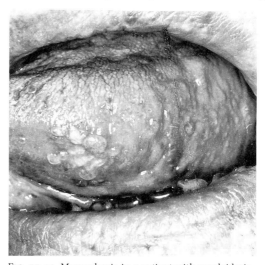

FIG. 55.43. Macroglossia in a patient with amyloidosis. The thickness of the tongue is characteristically increased. (University Hospital, Copenhagen.)

ecchymoses are not uncommon. The thickness of the tongue is increased (Fig. 55.43).

Hand–Schuller–Christian disease (p. 1703). Loosening of teeth may occur at an early stage. As the granulomatous infiltrate extends to the gingivae the teeth may be shed. The maxilla and mandible may be severely involved. Sometimes, ulceration of the oral mucosa is observed.

Eosinophilic granuloma (ulcer). Eosinophilic granuloma of the tongue (Fig. 55.44) is now agreed to be a distinct entity [1,2]. It is a benign, probably self-limited, lesion, usually with an ulcerated surface. Histologically, the lesion is dominated by eosinophil leukocytes.

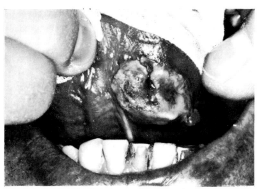

FIG. 55.44. Eosinophilic granuloma on the inferior surface of the tongue (University Hospital, Copenhagen).

Diabetes. Periodontal disease is frequent in diabetes, particularly in children. Marginal gingivitis is most commonly seen but there may be severe gingival inflammation with resorption of alveolar bone. The incidence of periodontal abscesses is also increased. Injuries to the mucosa show delayed healing.

REFERENCES

1 HJØRTING-HANSEN E. & SCHMIDT H. (1961) *Acta Derm Venereol (Stockh)* **41**, 235.
2 SHAPIRO L. & JUHLIN E.A. (1979) *Dermatologica* **140**, 242.

RECURRENT APHTHAE
SYN. APHTHOSIS; MIKULICZ APHTHAE; CANKER SORES; RECURRENT APHTHOUS ULCERATION

Definition. Recurrent aphthae is a common disorder characterized by recurrent ulceration of the oral mucosa. Very rarely, there is a simultaneous occurrence of ulceration on the genital mucosa.

Aetiology. The cause of recurrent aphthae is unknown. The herpes simplex virus is not responsible and there is no certain evidence incriminating any other microorganism, although recently a possible association with transitional L-forms of bacteria has been suggested. There is some evidence that hypersensitivity to bacteria, as demonstrated by skin tests, may be implicated [8]. Recent studies have shown that cell-mediated immunity against *Streptococcus* 2A and adult human oral mucosa is significantly increased in relation to exacerbations of recurrent aphthae [3]. An autoimmune background has also been suggested [9].

In many cases emotional stress appears to precipitate recurrences [11], but often no obviously significant factor can be elicited.

Among 130 patients with recurrent aphthae in Glasgow [15] 18% had deficiencies of vitamin B_{12}, folic acid and iron. The majority of these patients showed complete remission of ulcerations after replacement therapy. An association between jejunal mucosal abnormalities and recurrent aphthae has also been suggested [6].

The familial occurrence of unusually severe cases of recurrent aphthae has been recorded [7], and in one series of cases 45% of patients gave a positive family history [4] but this figure may merely reflect the prevalence of the condition.

The prevalence rates have been determined in a questionnaire survey [5]. The lifetime prevalence was 39% in men and 50% in women. A study of hospital patients in Sheffield [12] suggested that some 20% of the population are affected at some time during their lives, but a Philadelphia enquiry amongst students [11] showed a prevalence of over 50%. Recurrent aphthae are rare in early childhood but the frequency increases slowly during the first decade and rapidly during the second, to reach a peak in the third. Before puberty the sexes are equally affected but in adult life females predominate.

Touraine [13], amongst other authorities, regards the various types of aphthous ulceration (recurrent aphthae, Sutton's aphthae and Behçet's syndrome) as manifestations of the same disease process.

Pathology. In the early stages there is an inflammation below the epithelium with migration of inflammatory cells through the epithelium. Later, the lesion is that of a non-specific ulceration with loss of epithelium and a mixed inflammatory infiltrate essentially limited to the lamina propria. No vesicle formation is found [14].

Clinical features. Aphthae first appear as small red macules from 1 to 10 mm in diameter; within a few hours the surface whitens and then rapidly breaks down to form a shallow ulcer with a greyish-yellow base. Healing normally occurs in 7–10 days without scarring. A burning sensation often precedes or accompanies the initial changes and the fully developed ulcer is usually tender, and sometimes acutely so. The ulcers may occur anywhere but are most common on the movable mucous membranes—lips (Fig. 55.45), buccal mucosa, tongue and particularly in the mucobuccal fold. The

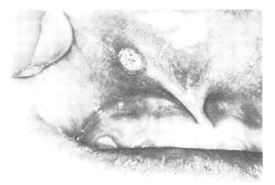

FIG. 55.45. Aphthous ulceration of the upper labial mucosa (University Hospital, Copenhagen).

frequency of recurrences is infinitely variable. Commonly, one to three ulcers develop at irregular intervals of weeks or months, but attacks may occur at short, more or less regular, intervals so that the patient is seldom free from discomfort.

Prognosis. A reliable prognosis is usually impossible. In most, but not all, patients the recurrences cease in the fourth decade; some continue into the fifth or sixth. More severe and frequent attacks are likely in the tense individual under continual stress.

Diagnosis. Recurrent herpes simplex of the oral mucous membrane has often been confused [14]. The lesions are clusters of small superficial erosions. The diagnosis may be confirmed by isolation of the virus.

Reliable differentiation from Behçet's syndrome may be difficult, and is particularly so if the lesions also involve the genitalia. The diagnosis is established only by the addition of ocular changes or cutaneous pustulation.

The bullous eruptions involving the oral mucous membrane often present as ragged erosions. They are discussed on p. 2101.

Traumatic ulcers are usually irregular and are obviously related to local dental trauma.

Opaque vesicles forming shallow erosions are seen in 6–10% of patients with Reiter's disease.

Treatment. There is no specific treatment. In severe cases an attempt should be made to reduce stress, and occasionally sedatives may be indicated.

The most effective topical treatment is a suspension of tetracycline 250 mg/5 ml held in the mouth for 5 min four or five times daily and then spat out. It is of benefit in about 70% of patients [8]. Discomfort may be reduced and healing encouraged with a steroid in a base such as Orabase, which should be applied every 2 or 3 h. Silver nitrate or phenol is often prescribed, but although they may relieve pain they do not encourage healing and are best avoided.

Very large or very painful ulcers may be infiltrated with triamcinolone or hydrocortisone suspension. The injection of 0·1–0·5 ml into the base of the lesion is often dramatically effective.

Levamisole, an anthelmintic known to increase immune responses, has been used successfully in treatment [10].

A chlorhexidine gel has been reported to reduce the duration and severity of the ulcers but had no effect on the incidence of ulcers [1].

REFERENCES

1 ADDY M., *et al* (1976) *Br Dent J* **141**, 118.
2 BARILE M.F., *et al* (1963) *Oral Surg* **16**, 1395.
3 DONATSKY O. (1976) *Acta Pathol Microbiol Scand* **84**, 270.
4 DRISCOLL E.J., *et al* (1959) *Ann Intern Med* **50**, 1475.
5 EMDIL J.A., *et al* (1975) *Can Med Assoc J* **113**, 627.
6 FERGUSON R., *et al* (1976) *Br Med J* **i**, 11.
7 FORBES I.J. & ROBSON H.N. (1960) *Br Med J* **1**, 599.
8 *GRAYKOWSKI E.A. (1966) *JAMA* **196**, 637.
9 LEHNER T. (1968) *Proc R Soc Med* **61**, 515.
10 OLSON J.A., *et al* (1976) *Oral Surg* **41**, 588.
11 *SHIP I.I., *et al* (1962) *Am J Med* **32**, 32.
12 *SIRCUS W., *et al* (1957) *QJ Med* **26**, 235.
13 *TOURAINE A. (1941) *Bull Soc Franc Dermatol Syphiligr* **48**, 61.
14 WEATHERS D.R. & GRIFFIN J.W. (1976) *J Am Dent Assoc* **81**, 81.
15 WRAY D., *et al* (1975) *Br Med J* **ii**, 490.

PERIADENITIS MUCOSA NECROTICA RECURRENS
SYN. SUTTON'S APHTHAE

Periadenitis mucosa necrotica recurrens [1,2] is also a clinical variant of recurrent aphthae. The onset is usually in childhood or early adult life. The lesions differ from those of typical aphthosis in that they are initially nodular, but after 3 or 4 days a necrotic plug separates to leave a crateriform ulcer. Rarely, the vulva may also be affected. The main characteristic of the periadenitis is the formation of marked scars on the oral mucosa, which is not seen in recurrent aphthae.

Pathology. The earliest lesions show a lymphocytic infiltrate usually around the lobules and duct of a minor salivary gland. The duct epithelium is disrupted. As tissue destruction proceeds, the infiltrate, more pleomorphic but still predominantly lymphocytic with few eosinophils or plasma cells, extends more deeply. Primary vascular changes are not detectable.

REFERENCES

1 HJØRTING-HANSEN E. & SIEMSSEN S.O. (1961) *Odontol Tidskr* 69, 294.
2 MONTELEONE L. (1967) *Oral Surg* 23, 586.

BEHÇET'S SYNDROME

Definition. Behçet's syndrome is a chronic, often progressive disease, characterized by recurrent ulceration of the mouth and genitalia associated with iritis.

Aetiology. There is suggestive but as yet inconclusive evidence that Behçet's syndrome may be caused by a virus. A virus cultured from the eye, blood and urine has provoked somewhat similar symptoms in rabbits [5]. Antibodies against mucous membrane were demonstrated in 17 of 40 patients [12] but their significance cannot yet be evaluated.

This rare syndrome, which has been reported from many parts of the world, usually begins between the ages of 10 and 30 but onset in early childhood and middle age has been reported. Males are affected five to ten times more frequently than females.

Pathology. [2]. The oral and genital ulcers usually show only non-specific inflammatory changes, although there may be infiltration of the grossly thickened walls of thrombosed arterioles.

When the central nervous system is involved [13,14] there are widely distributed small foci of necrosis which are most numerous in the brain stem basal ganglia, diencephalon and optic tracts and are associated with a low-grade inflammatory meningo-encephalomyelitis.

Changes in other organs [15] may include extensive atrophy of the gastrointestinal tract and pulmonary and myocardial fibrosis.

Clinical features [1,4,6,8]. The full syndrome comprises oral and genital ulceration, ocular lesions and a characteristic pyoderma; in many cases the clinical picture is ultimately dominated by changes in the central nervous system or, less commonly, by pulmonary or cardiac involvement.

The first manifestation is usually oral or genital ulceration, which is followed after an interval of days or months by iritis and then by involvement of other organs, but the course is a very variable and some cases present with ocular or other changes.

The mouth ulcers are rounded or oval and are sharply demarcated with a yellowish floor and a bright red areola (Fig. 55.46). They may increase

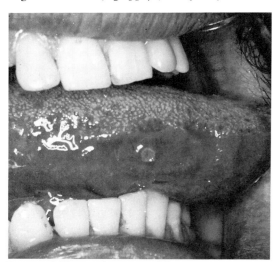

FIG. 55.46. Ulcer on the margin of the tongue in a patient with Behçet's syndrome (University Hospital, Copenhagen).

in size for weeks and heal only after several months. They occur most often on the labial mucous membrane but may develop anywhere in the mouth or may extend to the oesophagus. Pain and tenderness may be severe and dysphagia may be a serious problem.

The genital ulcers, which tend to be smaller, occur mainly on the scrotum, around the root of the penis or on the labia majora.

Skin lesions [11] are present at some stage in 80% of cases. Small follicular and non-follicular pustules develop irregularly on the trunk or limbs but tend to favour the genitocrural flexures and may involve the genitalia. Acneiform papules and pustules may also be present. Very characteristically, when the disease is active sterile pustules develop at the sites of skin punctures, as for example for therapeutic injections. Crops of small dermal nodules, resembling erythema nodosum, may appear at intervals, mainly on the legs but occasionally elsewhere. Recurrent cellulitis after minor trauma has also been recorded [3].

The earliest ocular changes [7] are photophobia and irritation, and in some cases only conjunctivitis develops in successive attacks. More commonly it is followed by uveitis, often with loss of vision from vitreous opacification, and eventually by hypopyon. Sometimes posterior uveitis and optic neuritis may occur at an early stage.

Fever and constitutional symptoms are variable, but may be moderate or severe during periods of activity. Arthralgia, often with joint swelling, may accompany each recrudescence. Episodes of thrombophlebitis are present in some 20% of cases [6].

Involvement of the central nervous system [5,11,13,14] may occur at any stage. The clinical manifestations are extremely variable: they may be meningoencephalitic, or a well-defined brain-stem syndrome or may simulate disseminated sclerosis or an organic confusional state.

Rare manifestations follow pulmonary or cardiac involvement [9].

The laboratory findings are also variable. Most constant is hypergammaglobulinaemia. There may be a leukocytosis, occasionally with pronounced eosinophilia.

Course and prognosis. During the early stages a reliable prognosis is impossible but Behçet's syndrome is always a potentially dangerous disease. Orogenital or ocular lesions at long and irregular intervals, ceasing after 5–10 yr, may cause the patient little more than intermittent discomfort. Other cases are soon severely disabling and some patients die from involvement of the nervous system or heart. Progression in one organ system may continue after other manifestations are quiescent.

Diagnosis. Some causes of ulceration of the oral mucosa are listed in Table 55.2. Recurrent aphthae cannot always be differentiated with certainty, but if the ulcers involve the genitalia the possibility of Behçet's syndrome should be considered. The diagnosis is established by the development of ocular lesions, bizarre patterns of skin sepsis or neurological signs.

Treatment. There is no specific treatment. Our own experience confirms that of others [10] that systemic steroids are of very limited value. Symptomatic and supportive measures must be prescribed.

Malignant granuloma and Wegener's granulomatosis (see p. 1178). This may begin with nasal obstruction or with ulceration of the mouth, especially the palate. The ulceration later extends to the soft tissue and bones of the middle third of the face.

REFERENCES

1 BERLIN C. (1960) *Arch Dermatol* **82**, 73.
2 CABRÉ J. & BREHM G. (1964) *Dermatol Wochenschr* **150**, 566.
3 CARR G.R. (1957) *Lancet* **ii**, 358.
4 *CURTH H.O. (1956) *Ann Dermatol Syphiligr* **83**, 130.
5 EVANS A.D., *et al* (1957) *Lancet* **ii**, 349.
6 *FRANCE R., *et al* (1951) *Medicine (Baltimore)* **30**, 335.
7 *FRANCESCHIETTI A., *et al* (1946) *Arch Ophthalmol* **35**, 469.
8 *KATZENELLENBOGEN I. & FENNMANN E.J. (1965) *Hautarzt* **16**, 13.
9 LEWIS P.D. (1964) *Br Med J* i, 1026.
10 MAMO J.G. & BAGHDASSARIAN A. (1964) *Arch Ophthalmol* **71**, 4.
11 MONACELLI M. & NAZZARO P. (1966) *Behçet's Disease.* Basel, Karger.
12 OSHIMA Y., *et al* (1963) *Ann Rheum Dis* **22**, 36.
13 RUBINSTEIN L.J. & URICH H. (1963) *Brain* **86**, 151.
14 *STROUTH J.C. & DYKEN M. (1964) *Neurology* **14**, 794.
15 SULHEIM O., *et al* (1959) *Acta Pathol Microbiol Scand* **45**, 145.

BLISTERING LESIONS OF THE MOUTH

Bullae may involve the oral mucous membrane in any of the major bullous diseases (Chapter 41). Of some they are a characteristic and dominant symptom and may at some stages be the only manifestation, whilst in others they are a rare incidental feature. They may be of considerable importance in differential diagnosis.

Bullae within the mouth, particularly intra-epithelial bullae, tend to rupture as soon as they are formed and are commonly seen as fibrin-covered erosions irregularly covered or surrounded by shreds of epithelium. The patient complains of soreness or dysphagia and of an unpleasant taste.

The clinical diagnosis will be based on the mode of onset and duration of the lesions, their distribution within the mouth and the presence or absence of scarring. Lesions should be sought on other mucous membranes and on the skin.

The examination of cells gently scraped from the

bulla floor—Tzanck test (p. 79)—is often informative. If a biopsy is performed a recent bulla should be selected and the specimen taken across its edge.

Erythema multiforme (p. 1085). Oral lesions, usually mild, are frequent in the common forms of erythema multiforme and may be found in some 40% of cases. They usually appear shortly after the skin eruption but may precede it and are occasionally the only manifestation of the disease. In a number of cases the disease is drug induced [1].

Small red plaques are soon followed by bullae which rupture and become confluent, forming shallow erosions covered by necrotic epithelium which, with the exudate, forms a pseudomembrane. They may become secondarily infected. The lesions occur typically on the lips where they may form characteristic crusts. They also occur more or less symmetrically on the buccal and gingival mucosa, the tongue, and the hard and soft palate. If the gingiva is involved a combination of catarrhal and necrotic gingivitis may result.

Diagnosis and systemic treatment are considered on p. 1087. Topical steroids in ointment or lotion may benefit the oral lesions, particularly those on the lips.

Pemphigus (p. 1631). In *pemphigus vulgaris* [8] oral lesions are almost constantly present and are the presenting manifestation in 60–70% of cases. They may precede the development of lesions elsewhere by many months, often with uncharacteristic features. They occur anywhere in the mouth but with a predilection for sites exposed to trauma, i.e. the buccal mucosa and the tongue. There are often large denuded areas with only shreds of epithelium, and discomfort may be severe. Either direct or indirect immunofluorescence will disclose the presence of antigens on the surface of the supra-basal-cell layers [10]. The Tzanck test is also valuable in diagnosis.

In *pemphigus vegetans* the bullae are seldom seen as such. The picture is soon dominated by the masses of hyperplastic epithelium.

In *pemphigus foliaceus* and *erythematosus* (p. 1635) oral lesions are usually absent and, if they occur, are mild.

Pemphigoid (p. 1639). In bullous pemphigoid, bullae on the mucous membranes occur in only 20% of cases and usually late in the course of the disease. They are more liable to remain discrete than those of pemphigus vulgaris. The diagnosis is established by the direct or indirect immunofluorescence tech-

niques. Antibodies to the basement membrane of stratified squamous epithelium are found both in serum and in tissue bound *in vivo* to tissue [10]. The lack of pemphigus cells in the Tzanck test differentiates from pemphigus but not from benign mucous membrane pemphigoid. Extensive and persistent oral involvement in pemphigoid should suggest the possibility of systemic malignant diseas.

Benign pemphigoid of the mucous membranes (p. 1644). The oral lesions are a distinctive and almost constant feature but may be preceded by ocular involvement. The bullae are often extensive and occasionally haemorrhagic. They are most often seen on the palate (Fig. 55.47) tongue and buccal

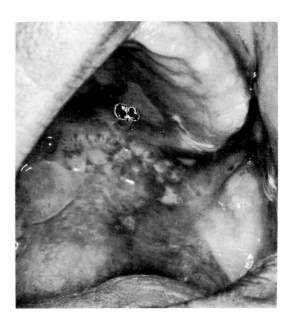

FIG. 55.47. Bullae and ulcerations in the palate of a woman with benign mucous membrane pemphigoid (University Hospital, Copenhagen).

mucosa. Repeated recurrence at the same site leads to the formation of irregularly linear scars in which carcinoma may later develop [6].

Diffuse involvement of the gingiva is possibly one of the causes of the so-called desquamative gingivitis [9].

Treatment is considered on p. 1646).

Acquired non-dystrophic epidermolysis bullosa. Haemorrhagic bullae of the palate or labial gingivae, occurring mainly in middle-aged patients and induced by trauma, have been described as a distinct entity (p. 1647).

Dermatitis herpetiformis (p. 1651). Oral lesions are relatively uncommon and usually mild; they tend to appear after the skin lesions have been present for some time. Exceptionally they may be the first manifestation of the disease [13]. They are small and grouped as on the skin and may occur anywhere in the mouth. After rupture they may be painful. In the absence of skin lesions diagnosis can be made by immunofluorescence techniques. In the upper part of the lamina propria IgA deposits may be found.

Benign familial pemphigus (p. 1629). Erosions of the lips and buccal mucosa have occurred in this hereditary disease [5], but the mucous membranes are not usually involved.

Epidermolysis bullosa [4,7,14]. The group of hereditary disorders commonly classified together as epidermolysis bullosa is fully considered elsewhere (p. 1620). The oral lesions seldom present a diagnostic problem as the distinctive cutaneous lesions are invariably associated. In the simple form traumatic bullae of the oral mucosa are inconstant and rarely troublesome.

In the polydysplastic form recurrent bulla formation in the mouth (Fig. 55.48), pharynx and oesophagus may be present from early infancy and may materially increase the patient's distress. There may be numerous milia formed from detached islands of epithelium at the sites of former bullae [2]. Severe scarring obliterates the labial sulci and immobilizes the tongue; it may eventually be followed by carcinoma [12]. Tooth formation may be disturbed. The changes in the enamel somewhat

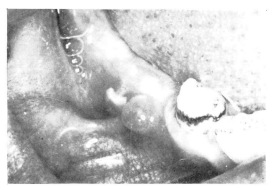

FIG. 55.48. Bulla on the alveolar ridge in a child with dystrophic epidermolysis bullosa (University Hospital, Copenhagen).

resemble those found in some types of amelogenesis imperfecta [11]. Both dentitions are affected. The surfaces of the teeth are usually heavily pitted. Histologically the enamel matrix of unerupted teeth is hyaline, lamellar or sometimes globular. The outer enamel epithelia show intense proliferation and metaplasia of the ameloblasts to a stratified squamous epithelium at the onset of mineralization [3].

Other causes of oral blisters. Bullae may be found in drug eruptions involving the mouth (p. 1246). They may occur incidentally and irregularly in lichen planus.

Small vesicles of the buccal mucosa and palate are also seen in submucous fibrosis (p. 2111).

Vesicles are also a feature of certain virus infections—herpes simplex and herpes zoster.

REFERENCES

1 AL-UBARDY S.S. & NALLY F.F. (1976) *Oral Surg* **41**, 601.
2 ANDREASEN J.O., *et al* (1965) *Acta Pathol Microbiol Scand* **63**, 37.
3 *ARWILL T., *et al* (1965) *Oral Surg* **8**, 723.
4 DELAIRE J., *et al* (1960) *Rev Stomatol* **61**, 189.
5 FISCHER H. & NIKOLOWSKI W. (1962) *Arch Klin Exp Dermatol* **214**, 261.
6 JAMIESON W.J. (1964) *Aust J Dermatol* **7**, 129.
7 KASLICK R.S. & BRUSTEIN H.C. (1961) *Oral Surg* **14**, 1315.
8 KATZENELLENBOGEN I. & SANDBACH M. (1959) *Hautarzt* **10**, 363.
9 MCCARTHY P.L. & SHKLAR G. (1964) *Diseases of the Oral Mucosa.* New York, McGraw-Hill.
10 NISENGARD R.J. (1975) *Oral Surg* **40**, 365.
11 PINDBORG J.J. (1970) *Pathology of the Dental Hard Tissues.* Copenhagen, Munksgaard.
12 SCHILLER F. (1960) *Arch Klin Exp Dermatol* **209**, 643.
13 SCHIMPF A. (1964) *Arch Klin Exp Dermatol* **226**, 250.
14 WEINSTOCK D. (1962) *Br J Dermatol* **4**, 431.

LICHEN PLANUS [1]

Oral involvement is reported in from 10% to 50% of patients with lichen planus. Of 611 patients in Copenhagen with oral lichen planus lesions, only 32% exhibited skin lesions. Two-thirds of the patients were women, and the majority arose in the 50–75 yr age group. Oral lichen planus is not rare. Epidemiological studies in India [6] and Sweden [2] have revealed prevalences of 1·5% and 1·9% respectively. Oral lichen planus involves, in decreasing order of frequency, the buccal mucosa, gingiva, tongue, lower lip, floor of mouth and palate. The diagnosis of oral lichen planus should be made only in the presence of Wickham's striae.

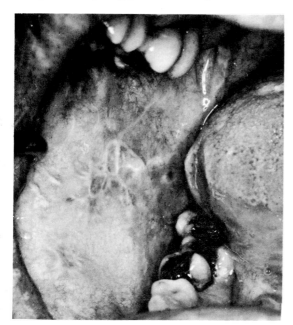

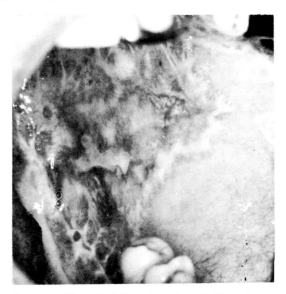

FIG. 55.50. Ulcerative lichen planus in the left buccal mucosa. Note Wickham's striae at the periphery of the lesion. (University Hospital, Copenhagen.)

FIG. 55.49. Reticular lichen planus in the right buccal mucosa with criss-crossing Wickham's striae (University Hospital, Copenhagen).

Most frequent are *linear* or *reticular* patterns, in which irregular streaks or an extensive delicate network of bluish-white elevations (the so-called Wickham's striae) may adorn the buccal mucosa (Fig. 55.49) or involve other sites. In the *papular* pattern there are few or many well-defined small white papules which are discrete or confluent. On close scrutiny minute striae may be detected at the periphery of the papules. Another manifestation is the plaque type consisting of homogeneous patches in connection with the Wickham's striae. One study [5] has shown that the frequency of smoking is higher in patients with the plaque type. Therefore it can be assumed that in many cases the plaque type is a leukoplakia superimposed upon lichen planus lesions. *Atrophic* or *ulcerative* lesions occur mainly in patients over 40; on a dry red shiny mucosa are irregular superficial erosions (Fig. 55.50). *Bullous* forms are uncommon; the bullae usually develop on reticular or linear lesions and rupture to leave erosions which may become secondarily infected.

The complaint of symptoms from oral lichen planus lesions shows considerable variance ranging from 28% to 91% of the patients. The atrophic and ulcerative forms are painful.

The prognosis of the oral lesions is difficult to assess in the individual patient. In general they are more persistent than the cutaneous lesions and may continue indefinitely. Malignant change was formerly considered exceptional, but carcinoma is now known to develop, particularly in the atrophic and erosive forms [7], and the incidence estimated at 1% may prove to be too low when more cases have been followed for long periods [4, 8]. It has been demonstrated that in 1% of cases oral lichen planus is associated with erythroplakia [6].

In diagnosis skin changes should be sought. Biopsy is often helpful but basal liquefaction and the saw-toothed epithelial pattern are less striking than in the skin lesions.

Oral lichen planus seldom requires treatment. If the patient complains of pain or discomfort Adcortyl-A in Orabase—known as Kenalog in the U.S.A.—or intralesional injections of steroids may give some relief.

REFERENCES

1 ANDREASEN J.O. (1968) *Oral Surg* **25**, 31, 158.
2 AXÉLL T. (1976) *Odontol Rev* **27** (Suppl. 36).
3 HOLMSTRUP P. & PINDBORG J.J. (1979) *Acta Derm Venereol (Stockh)* **59** (Suppl. **85**), 77.
4 MARDER M. & DEESEN K.C. (1982) *J Am Dent Assoc* **105**, 55.
5 NEUMANN-JENSEN B., *et al* (1977) *Oral Surg* **43**, 410.
6 PINDBORG J.J., *et al* (1972) *Acta Derm Venereol (Stockh)* **52**, 216.
7 POGREL M.A. & WELDON L.L. (1983) *Oral Surg* **55**, 62.
8 SILVERMAN G., *et al* (1985) *Oral Surg* **60**, 30.

PSORIASIS [1, 2]

The mucous membranes are very rarely involved in psoriasis, and some alleged examples appear to be other lesions fortuitously associated. There appears to be four types of oral manifestations of psoriasis. The first type consists of minute well-defined grey to yellowish-white lesions which are round or oval. The second type is characterized by white elevated lacy circinate lesions on the oral mucosa; these eruptions parallel those of the skin. The third type consists of a fiery red erythema of the oral mucosa which is mostly seen in the acute forms of psoriasis. The fourth type of oral lesion described in psoriasis is a geographic tongue.

The diagnosis should be made only reluctantly and after biopsy to demonstrate intra-epithelial abscesses.

REFERENCES

1 Cataloo E., *et al* (1977) *Cutis* 20, 705.
2 Pindborg J.J. (1985) *Atlas of Diseases of the Oral Mucosa.* 4th ed. Copenhagen, Munksgaard.

GRANULOMATOUS LESIONS OF THE MOUTH

Three entities present epithelioid non-caseating giant cell granulomas: sarcoidosis (p. 1755), Melkersson–Rosenthal syndrome (p. 2127) and Crohn's disease (Fig. 55.42) (see granulomatous cheilitis (p. 2127)).

REFERENCE

1 Basu M.K., *et al* (1975) *Gut* 16, 249.

BENIGN TUMOURS AND TUMOUR-LIKE LESIONS

Epulides [1]. The term epulis, coined by Virchow, literally means from the gingiva. Current usage is inconsistent. Some authorities apply it to many different types of swelling arising from the gingiva, whereas others restrict it to the so-called fibrous epulis, the giant-cell epulis, and the telangiectatic epulis which are in all probability reactions to trauma.

The most common form is the *peripheral fibroma*, the so-called *fibrous epulis* [2]. Histologically the fibroma consists of bundles of interlacing collagen fibres with small numbers of fibroblasts. There may be small foci of calcification or ossification. The overlying epithelium is slightly hyperkeratotic. Most cases occur in women aged 20–45.

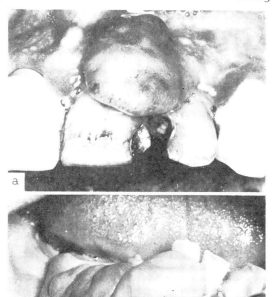

FIG. 55.51. Peripheral fibromas, clinically termed epulides: (a) fibroma probably caused by the sharp edges of carious teeth; (b) extensive fibroma partially covering the teeth (University Hospital, Copenhagen).

Clinically the fibroma is a hard nodule attached to the gingiva by a broad base and covered by normal mucosa. The majority are small and circumscribed but show a tendency to proliferate around the teeth, which may sometimes be completely covered (Fig. 55.51).

Next in frequency is the *giant-cell epulis* [3], which in childhood affects the sexes equally but in adults occurs mainly in women. Histologically the lesion is characterized by the presence of numerous multinucleate giant cells and a very cellular stroma of ovoid or spindle-shaped young connective-tissue cells grouped in granuloma-like structures. The lesion is very vascular and haemorrhage is often seen. This epulis was formerly considered a true tumour but is now regarded as a peripheral giant-cell granuloma, a response to injury. Clinically the lesion is a soft nodule bluish in colour.

The *pyogenic granuloma* (p. 2466) on the gingiva is also known as a telangiectatic epulis. It may occur in any part of the oral cavity but is most frequent in sites exposed to trauma [1]. Rarely it

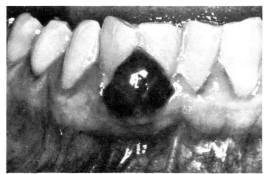

FIG. 55.52. Pyogenic granuloma—telangiectatic epulis (University Hospital, Copenhagen).

may develop from the maxillary sinus through an infected socket, usually that of the first molar. Clinically the lesion is a deep red pedunculated or sessile nodule. The surface may be ulcerated and bleeding may be troublesome (Fig. 55.52).

All three types of epulis should be excised. Great care should be taken to remove all abnormal tissue as there is a tendency to recurrence. When pyogenic granuloma of the maxillary sinus is removed the oro-antral fistula should be closed.

The so-called 'pregnancy tumour' has a histolog-

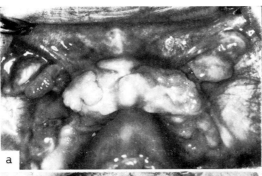

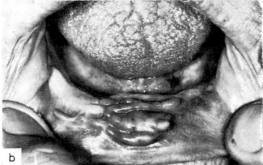

FIG. 55.53. Irritation hyperplasia caused by ill-fitting dentures: (a) maxilla; (b) mandible (University Hospital, Copenhagen).

ical appearance very similar to pyogenic granuloma.

REFERENCES

1 BHASKAR S.N. & JACOWAY J.R. (1966) *J Oral Surg* **24**, 391.
2 BHASKAR S.N. & JACOWAY J.R. (1966) *J Am Dent Assoc* **73**, 1312.
3 DOP F.V. (1967) *De Epulis*. Graduation Thesis, Groningen.

Irritation hyperplasia [1]. This lesion, which is caused by ill-fitting dentures, is also known as inflammatory hyperplasia, 'epulis fissuratum' and granuloma fissuratum. Histologically the reaction is characterized by excessive relatively acellular collagen with chronic inflammatory changes, especially underlying the epithelium.

The lesion occurs mostly in the buccolabial sulcus. The hyperplastic tissue is always elongated and of soft flabby consistency (Fig. 55.53).

REFERENCE

1 NORDENRAM Å. & LANDT H. (1969) *Acta Odontol Scand* **27**, 481.

Mucous cysts (syn. Mucocele) [1–4]. These are frequently traumatic in origin. Mucus or saliva escapes into surrounding tissues and a lining of granulation or connective tissue is formed. This is an extravasation type of mucocele. Most are not lined by epithelium. Some are caused by blockage of the excretory duct. This is a retention type of mucocele.

Young adults are usually affected but the cysts are not uncommon in children and have occurred in early infancy.

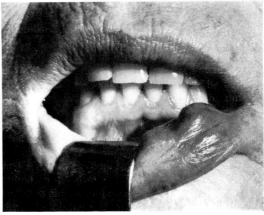

FIG. 55.54. Mucous cyst of the lower lip (Addenbrooke's Hospital).

The cyst forms a smooth fluctuant swelling, often with a bluish tinge, up to 2 cm in diameter (Fig. 55.54). Most occur on the lips, particularly the lower, but they are also seen on the floor of the mouth (in this region they are called ranulae) and on the gingiva, buccal mucosa and tongue. They may occasionally resemble a haemangioma.

The cyst should be excised by careful dissection.

REFERENCES

1 BADEN E. (1955) *J Oral Surg* **13**, 331.
2 EHLERS G. (1963) *Z Haut Geschlkrankh* **34**, 77.
3 *ORMEA F. & PORZIO P.A. (1966) *Minerva Dermatol* **35**, 471.
4 ROBINSON L. & HJRTING-HANSEN E. (1964) *Oral Surg* **18**, 191.

Fibroma (syn. fibropithelial polyp). The fibroma is the most frequent tumour of the oral mucosa and is seen mainly in adults, affecting the sexes equally. It may occur in any site but is commonest in sites exposed to trauma. Both histologically and clinically it is almost impossible to differentiate a fibroma from a fibromatous reaction to trauma. The tumour is a pedunculated or sessile nodule, the surface of which may be ulcerated or hyperkeratotic (Fig. 55.55).

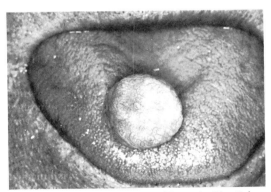

FIG. 55.55. Fibroma of the tongue (University Hospital, Copenhagen).

REFERENCE

1 COOKE B.E.D. (1952) *Br Dent J* **93**, 305.

Lipoma [1,3]. Oral lipomas form 1–4% of all benign tumours of the oral cavity, according to most authors, but it has been suggested that they are indeed common [2]. One-third of the oral lipomas

occur on the buccal mucosa; next in frequency are the floor of the mouth, the buccal sulcus, the retromolar area and the tongue. The yellowish colour of the soft non-painful compressible nodule shows clearly through the thin epithelium in the floor of the mouth.

REFERENCES

1 BRAUNSTEIN L.E. (1949) *JAMA*, **140**, 155.
2 CANNELL H., *et al* (1976) *J Maxillofac Surg* **4**, 116.
3 SIMPSON H.E. (1959) *Oral Surg* **17**, 349.

Haemangioma. The distinction between haemangiomatous naevi (p. 201) and acquired haemangiomas is not clearly definable. Solitary haemangiomas developing in patients over 40 are relatively common, especially on the buccal mucosa and lower lip, but also on the tongue and in other sites. They present as reddish-purple or bluish lobulated compressible nodules. They may be excised or injected with sclerosing agents. Usually they are of the cavernous type in contrast with the haemangiomatous naevi which are of the capillary type.

REFERENCE

1 *SHKLAR G. & MANGER I. (1965) *Oral Surg* **19**, 335.

Leiomyoma [1]. Leiomyomas are uncommon in the oral cavity, but most often seen on the tongue and palate. They are circumscribed firm tumours, sometimes pedunculated, bluish or red in colour. On the palate they are presumed to arise from the smooth muscle fibres in the large palatal arteries since they often show a vascular component. Recurrences after surgical removal are rare.

REFERENCE

1 GILES A.D. (1982) *Br J Oral Surg* **20**, 142–46.

Granular cell myoblastoma (p. 2475). This tumour is uncommon in the oral cavity but may occur at any age. Although the majority are on the tongue, especially its margins, they can be found anywhere. Clinically the myoblastoma presents as a circumscribed smooth whitish plaque or nodule.

The histology is discussed on p. 2475. The degree of associated pseudoepitheliomatous hyperplasia may be such as to lead to the misdiagnosis of squamous carcinoma. There is no tendency to recurrence after excision.

REFERENCE

1 WORSAAE N., *et al* (1979) *Int J Oral Surg* **8**, 133.

Infectious warts (p. 668). Infectious warts in the oral cavity are usually referred to as papillomas. They, and focal epithelial hyperplasia, are described on p. 2084.

Salivary gland adenoma. Salivary gland adenomas are not uncommon. Histologically most of them are pleomorphic, showing wide variation in the appearance of both the glandular elements and the connective-tissue stroma. They are seen mainly on the palate but may occur anywhere in the mouth. They are circumscribed slow-growing tumours, often mistaken for chronic abscesses or infected lymph nodes. They are easily enucleated but show some tendency to recur. Most of these tumours are pleomorphic adenomas, but monomorphic adenomas and muco-epidermoid tumours are also seen.

Neurofibromatosis [2–5] (see p. 119). Oral lesions are not unusual. The tongue is most commonly involved [1]. There may be macroglossia, enlargement of the papillae or solitary or multiple nodules, usually on the dorsum or around the margins. Nodules or tags, sessile or pedunculated, may also occur on the lips, palate and buccal mucosa. Extreme involvement of the parotid and submandibular regions and of half the tongue is illustrated in Fig. 55.56. Solitary neurofibromas are very rare.

Neurilemmoma (syn. neurinoma; Schwannoma) (see p. 2473). This benign tumour derived from the Schwann cells is usually seen in adults. It may develop anywhere in the oral cavity but is commonest on the tongue and the floor of the mouth. It presents as a sessile nodule, softer than a fibroma but harder than a haemangioma. Recurrence after excision is unusual.

REFERENCE

1 *Hatziotis J.C. & Asprides H. (1967) *Oral Surg* **24**, 510.

LEUKOPLAKIA [10]

Leukoplakia is the most common and the most important disturbance of oral keratinization. In this chapter leukoplakia is defined as a persistent white patch not attributable to any known specific disease process. The term may therefore provide a tentative clinical diagnosis which must be supplemented by a description of the histological features.

Leukoplakia can be regarded as a somewhat variable and non-specific response of the oral mucosa to external stimuli, which is sometimes influenced by the pre-existing state of the mucosa and its underlying connective tissue stroma. Most cases occur in men aged 40–70. Tobacco smoking is the

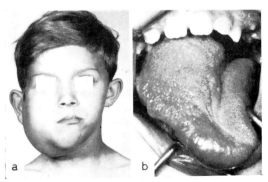

FIG. 55.56. Neurofibromatosis: (a) swelling since birth of the submandibular region; (b) involvement of the tongue. (After Christensen E. & Pindborg J.J. (1956) *Acta Odontal Scand* **14**, 1.)

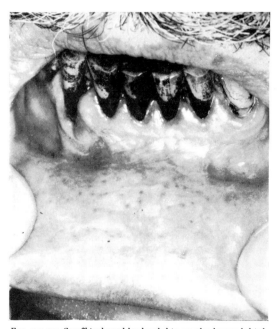

FIG. 55.57. Snuff-induced leukoplakia on the lower labial mucosa, groove and gingiva (University Hospital, Copenhagen).

REFERENCES

1 *Baden E., *et al* (1955) *Oral Surg* **8**, 263.
2 Christensen E. & Pindborg J.J. (1956) *Acta Odontol Scand* **14**, 1.
3 Rappaport H.M. (1953) *Oral Surg* **6**, 599.
4 Stillman F.S. (1952) *J Oral Surg* **10**, 112.
5 Toto P.D. (1954) *Oral Surg* **7**, 423.

most important external factor, but a special form may be induced by snuff (Fig. 55.57). Mechanical irritation, from toothbrushing or chewing upon the edentulous alveolar ridge, may also cause white patches. However, such lesions should be called frictional keratosis rather than leukoplakia. Syphilis is a significant factor only in leukoplakia of the tongue which may complicate an atrophic glossitis. In the so-called idiopathic leukoplakias no local factor can be demonstrated. This group includes the leukoplakia seen, for example, in some patients with sideropenic dysphagia. Here the mucosal atrophy must be considered the essential predisposing factor.

In recent years a number of studies have been concerned with the association of *Candida albicans* invasion in oral leukoplakias [3,4,7,8]. These lesions are known as chronic hyperplastic candidiasis or candidal leukoplakia. Undoubtedly, hyperkeratosis is a prerequisite for *Candida* infections as *Candida* is a keratophilic microorganism. The favourite location of candidal leukoplakia is the labial commissure, from where the lesion may extend to the buccal mucosa. In a recent British study [1] it was found that all patients with candidal leukoplakias were smokers and wore their dentures continuously day and night. Approximately half of the candidal leukoplakias were described as 'speckled'

(nodular) (see p. 2110), which may be the reason why the percentage of dysplastic lesions was as high as 45%.

Candidal leukoplakia may also be part of a chronic multifocal candidiasis. In a series of 32 Danish patients, all were smokers and 21 were denture wearers [6]. The patients were treated with antimycotics; the median length of treatment was 45 days. Nodular lesions became homogeneous, and less marked lesions disappeared.

Histology. The histological changes are inconstant. Most characteristic are hyperorthokeratosis or hyperparakeratosis occasionally associated with acanthosis (Fig. 55.58). The mitotic activity has been shown to be four times greater in lesions showing hyperparakeratosis than in hyperorthokeratotic lesions. The lamina propria may show little inflammatory change or, in cases of a superimposed *Candida* infection, a pleomorphic infiltrate in which lymphocytes, plasma cells and histiocytes predominate, with micro-abscesses in the upper layer of the epithelium (Fig. 55.59(b)).

In about 10–20% of cases of leukoplakia the epithelium shows epithelial dysplasia from mild to severe and carcinoma *in situ*—disturbed maturation, increased mitotic activity and cellular pleomorphism.

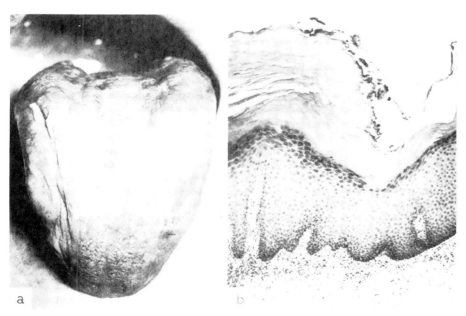

FIG. 55.58. Leukoplakia on the tongue: (a) clinical appearance; (b) histology (note the hyperorthokeratosis and microabscesses) (× 40) (University Hospital and Royal Dental College, Copenhagen).

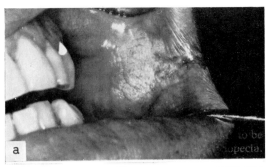

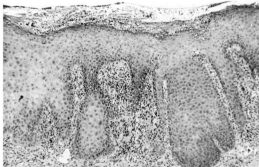

FIG. 55.59. Leukoplakia in the labial commissure:
(a) clinical appearance; (b) histology (note the
hyperparakeratosis) (× 105) (University Hospital and Royal
Dental College, Copenhagen).

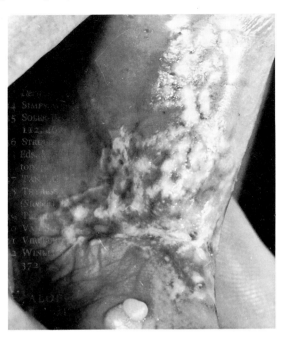

FIG. 55.60. Nodular leukoplakia on the left commissure
and buccal mucosa (University Hospital, Copenhagen).

Clinical features [5]. In order of decreasing frequency leukoplakia involves the buccal mucosa, the retrocommissural mucosa (Fig. 55.59(a)), the edentulous alveolar ridge, the tongue (Fig. 55.58(a)), the labial mucosa, the hard palate, the sublingual area and the gingiva. On the buccal and retrocommissural mucosa the lesions are often bilaterally symmetrical and in the commissures frequently associated with a *Candida* infection (Fig. 55.59(b)). It is very rare to observe true leukoplakias on the vermilion border. In that location a crusty lesion is found.

The clinical appearance and extent of the leukoplakia are very variable. The lesions may be small well-defined white patches like drops of candlewax. There may be extensive plaques, leathery in consistency or like a fine opalescent membrane. Other lesions may be irregularly thickened and nodular. Ulceration may follow repeated local trauma. There are usually no symptoms but some patients complain of burning or irritation.

Whilst there is no constant correlation of clinical and histological features, speckled white nodular thickening on an atrophic red background is characteristic of lesions with epithelial dysplasia [9] and

show a high degree of malignant transformation [10]. Figure 55.60 illustrates such a lesion.

Many leukoplakias are reversible if the external irritation be discontinued. Some long-standing lesions will not regress. The incidence of malignant change has been exaggerated. Recent studies in several countries have demonstrated an incidence rate of malignancy between 4% and 6% [8].

Diagnosis [2]. Other white lesions of the oral mucous membrane are described on pp. 2077 and 2111.

Histological examination is essential.

Treatment. Most leukoplakias do not require treatment. Caustics must never be employed. Dental hygiene should be improved and smoking forbidden. Regular examination is advisable at intervals of not more than a year or until the lesion has regressed. If the leukoplakia exhibits epithelial dysplasia and fails to regress, surgical excision should be considered. A large number of tobacco-associated leukoplakias will disappear if smoking is stopped.

REFERENCES

1 ARENDORF T.M., *et al* (1983) *Br Dent J* **155**, 340.
2 CAWSON R.A. (1969) *Proc R Soc Med* **62**, 610.

3 CAWSON R.A. & LEHNER T. (1968) *Br J Dermatol* **80**, 9.
4 CERNEA P., *et al* (1965) *Rev Stomatol* **66**, 103.
5 COOKE B.E.D. (1956) *Br J Dermatol* **68**, 151.
6 HOLMSTRUP P. & BESSERMAN (1983) *Oral Surg* **56**, 388.
7 JEPSEN A. & WINTHER J.E. (1965) *Acta Odontol Scand* **23**, 239.
8 PINDBORG J.J. (1980) *Oral Cancer and Precancer*. Bristol. John Wright.
9 PINDBORG J.J., *et al* (1963) *Acta Odontol Scand* **21**, 407.
10 WALDRON C.A. & SHAFER W.G. (1975) *Cancer* **36**, 1021.

Smokers' keratosis of the palate [3,4] (syn. stomatitis nicotina). This condition is commonly caused by the excessive smoking of pipes or cigars and is therefore seen mainly in men aged 40–50. It may also occur in those who smoke cheroots with the lighted end in the mouth [2]. The palatal mucosa is studded with white umbilicated papules with a red central punctum (Fig. 55.61(a)). If the palate is partially protected by a denture only the area directly exposed to smoke is affected (Fig. 55.61(b)).

Histologically [1,4] hyperkeratosis surrounds the orifices of the mucous glands. The ducts may become obstructed with the formation of retention cysts and there may be intense dermal fibrosis.

The keratosis is usually reversible when smoking is stopped. Malignant change is a possibility if exposure is continued but appears to be extremely uncommon.

REFERENCES

1 DUPERRAT B., *et al* (1962) *Sem Hôp Paris* **38**, 321.
2 MEHTA F.S., *et al* (1969) *Cancer* **24**, 832.
3 TAPPENER J. (1966) *Hautarzt* **17**, 152.
4 VAN WYCK C.W. (1967) *J Dent Assoc S Afr* **27**, 106.

'Hairy' leukoplakia. 'Hairy' leukoplakia on the lateral border of the tongue is a unique finding in homosexual men and its presence indicates a past contact with the HTLV-III-virus. In c. 20% of the patients AIDS will develop. The 'hairy' leukoplakia is asssociated with a human papilloma virus, Epstein–Barr virus and Candida. It has a unique histological structure [1].

REFERENCES

1 GREENSPAN J., *et al* (1985) *New Engl J Med* **313**, 154.

Erythroplakia (see p. 2199). Erythroplakia is a rare superficial lesion, more often seen on the genital than the oral mucosa, presenting as a fiery red sharply demarcated plaque (Fig. 55.62). Erythroplakia in the mouth has been classified into three types: homogeneous, red with white patches and granular [5]. The sites of predilection are the floor of the mouth, the retromolar area and the buccal mucosa [4]. Histologically the changes are those of epithelial dysplasia or carcinoma *in situ* or frank squamous cell carcinoma. Excision is the treatment of choice.

Submucous fibrosis. Submucous fibrosis is a relatively common condition in South East Asia, where it is attributable to a hypersensitive reaction to chewing the areca (betel) nut. Histologically a densely sclerotic lamina propria underlies the atrophic epithelium. Any area of the oral mucosa may be affected, but the first changes are often seen on the palate or buccal mucosa. Vesicles may be found at an early stage but are later followed by the appearance of fibrous bands, especially in buccal,

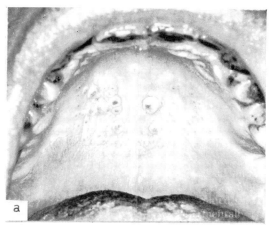
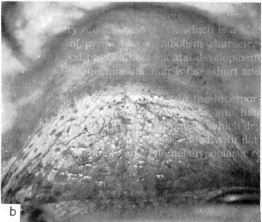

FIG. 55.61. Leukokeratosis nicotina palati in (a) an unprotected palate (note the red dots in the small papules) and (b) a hard palate protected by a denture (University Hospital, Copenhagen).

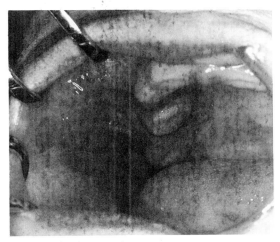

FIG. 55.62. Erythroplakia on the right buccal mucosa. Three independent carcinomas are developing inside the erythroplakia (University Hospital, Copenhagen).

labial and palatal mucosa, which is the most outstanding clinical feature of the condition [1]. Also present may be hypopigmentation or patches of irregularly mottled pigmentation. Later the progressive fibrosis may lead to difficulty in eating and speaking.

The condition is precancerous [2,3].

REFERENCES

1 PINDBORG J.J. & SIRSAT S.M. (1966) Oral Surg 22, 764.
2 *PINDBORG J.J., et al (1970) Br J Cancer 24, 253.
3 PINDBORG J.J., et al (1984) Scand J Dent Res 92, 224.
4 SHAFER W.G. & WALDRON C.A. (1975) Cancer 36, 1021.
5 SHEAR M. (1972) Int Dent J 22, 460.

MALIGNANT TUMOURS

Intraepithelial carcinoma (syn. carcinoma *in situ*). The point at which a premalignant lesion, leukoplakia or erythroplakia (see pp. 2108 and 2111) becomes an intraepithelial carcinoma may not be clinically identifiable. Histologically the transition is marked by the addition of atypical mitotic figures to the existing epithelial dysplasia and changes throughout the epithelium. Figure 55.64(a) illustrates an intraepithelial carcinoma clinically simulating a benign leukoplakia. Histological examination revealed the presence of tripolar mitosis (Fig. 55.64(b)).

Carcinoma [6]. The incidence of oral cancer shows striking geographical variation. Figure 55.65 gives examples of such differences based upon the incidence of cancer in five continents [7]. Fig. 55.65(a) shows the incidence of oral cancer in males in European countries. It is surprising that an area of

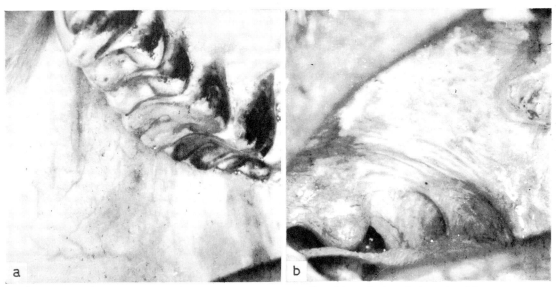

FIG. 55.63. Diffuse oral submucous fibrosis: (a) right buccal mucosa affected (note the loss of pigment and the occurrence of perpendicular fibrous bands); (b) soft palate affected with scar-like fibrous bands and loss of pigment (University Hospital, Copenhagen).

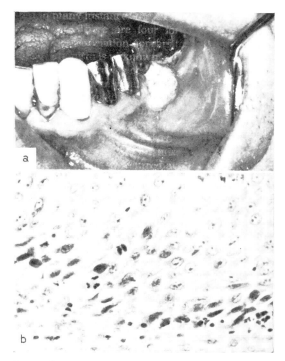

FIG. 55.64. Carcinoma *in situ*: (a) clinical appearance of the leukoplakia-like lesion; (b) histology. Note the irregularity of the basal cell layer, the increased mitotic activity and a tripolar mitosis (× 230). (University Hospital and Royal Dental College, Copenhagen.)

France has an oral cancer rate six times higher than that of an area in England. The shaded areas of the columns represent the rates for intra-oral cancer, and the unshaded areas represent cancer of the vermilion border. It is interesting to note that intra-oral cancer dominates in the wine-growing countries (France, Italy and Switzerland). Fig. 55.65(b) shows the few figures available from Asia. Not surprisingly India shows the highest incidence rate. The rate is also high in the triracial population of Singapore, comprising Chinese, Malays and Indians. The Chinese and Malays have much lower rates than the Indians because the Indians continue with the habit of their motherland, i.e. chewing areca (betel) nuts with tobacco.

The relative importance of predisposing factors varies with the site. Gross iron-deficiency anaemia, syphilitic glossitis and alcoholic cirrhosis are all significant. Oral carcinoma is 10 times more frequent in heavy spirit drinkers than in abstainers [8]. Erythroplakia, leukoplakia, oral lichen planus and submucous fibrosis are all associated with an increased cancer incidence. Among eliciting factors tobacco is the most important. Chewing tobacco is responsible for the high incidence of carcinoma in South East Asia. In the U.S.A. cigar and pipe smoking carry a heavier risk than cigarette smoking. The role of other local irritants is controversial.

Cancer of the lower lip is induced primarily by prolonged light exposure and complicates actinic cheilitis. It occurs prodominantly in white males, in whom it is the commonest form of oral cancer. The relatively rare carcinoma of the upper lip is more frequent in women. The situation of other oral cancers also shows geographical variation, in accordance with the predisposing and eliciting factors concerned. In India, where the quid of tobacco is usually held in the lower buccal sulcus, most cancers are seen in the commissural or buccal mucosa. In the Scandinavian countries cancer of the tongue is more frequent than elsewhere, perhaps because of a higher incidence of severe iron-deficiency anaemia.

Histologically the vast majority of oral carcinomas are of squamous cell type, showing varying degrees of differentiation, though usually highly differentiated with epithelial pearl formation. The more posterior is the location of the tumour in the mouth the more anaplastic it tends to be. Attempts to correlate clinical behaviour with the degree of histological differentiation have been inconclusive.

Rarely, oral carcinomas are derived from the salivary glands [2], and are histologically of adenoid cystic type.

A distinct entity has been described, especially among tobacco chewers; this is the so-called verrucous carcinoma or Ackerman tumour [3], which has a characteristic growth pattern and is more benign in its behaviour (Fig. 55.66 on p. 2115).

Clinically oral cancer presents few disturbing symptoms during its early stages [5]. The cardinal features are induration and ulceration (Fig. 55.67 on p. 2115), often in existing areas of leukoplakia (Fig. 55.68 on p. 2115). The appearance of red areas (erythroplakic patches), usually within a leukoplakia, should always be regarded as an early sign of malignancy [4]. Growth is usually in depth. Oral cancers readily involve the regional lymph nodes, a tendency which is particularly evident in the case of carcinoma of the tongue.

Salivary gland tumours may present as indurated nodules, usually in the posterior part of the palate.

Any indurated lesion, the diagnosis of which is not beyond any possible doubt, and any ulcer which does not heal with 2 weeks' treatment must be regarded as suspect and submitted to biopsy.

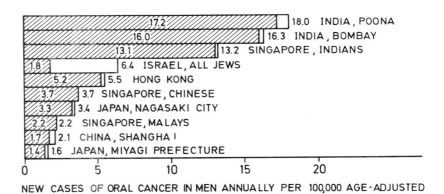

FIG. 55.65. (a) Histogram illustrating the incidence rates of oral cancer in men in Europe annually per 100,000, (age adjusted). The columns give the rate for vermilion border cancer (lip cancer) plus intra-oral cancer, and the white part represents lip cancer. (b) Histogram illustrating the incidence rates of oral cancer in men in Asia annually per 100,000 (age adjusted). (From Waterhouse J., *et al* (1982) *Cancer Incidence in Five Continents*. Lyons, International Agency for Research on Cancer.)

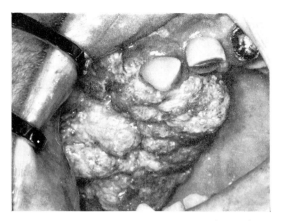

FIG. 55.66. Verrucous carcinoma originating from either palate or alveolar ridge (University Hospital, Copenhagen).

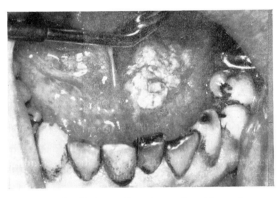

FIG. 55.67. Small ulcerated carcinoma in sublingual region (University Hospital, Copenhagen).

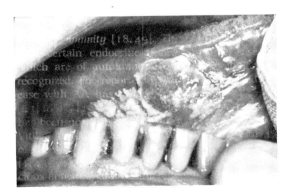

FIG. 55.68. Development of carcinoma in leukoplakia (University Hospital, Copenhagen).

Treatment. The treatment of oral cancer is not within the province of the dermatologist. The patient should be referred without delay for oncological consultation.

Malignant melanoma [1]. Malignant melanoma of the oral cavity occurs in men more than women and usually over the age of 40. About 30% are said to arise in pre-existing melanocytic naevi. The hard palate, the alveolar mucosa and the soft palate are the most frequent sites, but the tumour may occur elsewhere. The clinical appearance is variable. A raised nodule, soft at first but soon becoming indurated and ulcerated, may be red or lightly or heavily pigmented.

The prognosis is very poor for metastasis occurs early.

REFERENCES

1 *CHAUDHRY A.P., et al (1958) Cancer 11, 923.
2 CHRISTENSEN R.W. & BLOSSOM R.A. (1955) Oral Surg 8, 130.
3 JACOBSON S. & SHEAR M. (1972) J Oral Pathol 1, 66.
4 MASHBERG A., et al (1973) Cancer 32, 1436.
5 NEIDERS M.E. (1972) Int Dent J 22, 441.
6 PINDBORG J.J. (1980) Oral Cancer and Precancer. Bristol, John Wright.
7 WATERHOUSE J., et al (1982) Cancer Incidence in Five Continents. Lyons, International Agency for Research on Cancer.
8 WYNDER L.E., et al (1957) Cancer 10, 923.

THE TONGUE

Development and surface anatomy [5,6]. The anterior two-thirds of the tongue are formed by the fusion of the two external tubercles, derived from the first branchial arch, with the central tuberculum impar. The posterior third is formed from the hypobranchial eminence which is derived from the second arch, with a contribution from the third.

The dorsal surface of the tongue is covered by filiform papillae, 1–3 mm long, closely set in rows parallel to the V-shaped terminal sulcus. These papillae give the tongue a velvety white appearance. Irregularly scattered over the tongue are the larger red round fungiform papillae which are very vascular. Occasionally, these are darkly pigmented in Negroes. The circumvallate papillae, 7–11 in number, are arranged in a line anterior to the terminal sulcus; each is surrounded by a small depression. The so-called foliate papillae are parallel folds of mucous membrane along the lateral margins of the posterior part of the tongue. Salivary glands are present over the entire surface of the root of the tongue and extend forward some way along the lateral margins, in the sulci around the circumvallate papillae and laterally in the region of the foliate papillae. The anterior lingual glands open on the lower surface of the tongue near the apex.

The basic mucosal pattern of the tongue is determined by the relative numbers, size and arrangement of filiform and fungiform papillae and by the presence or absence of fissuring. There are wide variations in normal individuals. The patterns are possibly genetically determined [2,8].

When the normal tongue is examined under Wood's light fluorescence can be seen at the tips of the filiform papillae of the posterior three-quarters of the tongue [9]. Absence of fluorescence is normal in children and young adults, but it is found in 50% of elderly individuals. Fluorescence is temporarily abolished by some antibiotics and is perhaps related to the presence of bacteria. It is reduced or absent when the tongue is smooth.

The furred tongue. Furring is the clinical manifestation of hypertrophy of the filiform papillae or failure of normal desquamation. There is wide individual variation in the normal pattern and the less mobile posterior half is always more heavily furred than the tip. The traditional association between furring and constipation or other gastrointestinal disturbances has no scientific basis. Furring may be increased in fevers and especially in oral or upper respiratory infections. It is also increased by smoking.

The smooth tongue [3]. Atrophy of the filiform papillae gives the tongue a smooth appearance, and diminution or loss of fluorescence under Wood's light. There may be a real or apparent increase in the prominence of the fungiform papillae. The mechanism by which the filiform papillae are lost is uncertain. It is suggested [4] that they may be very sensitive to oxygen deficiency. Smooth tongue is classically associated with iron-deficiency anaemia, ariboflavinosis, pellagra and the malabsorption syndrome, but it may also occur in uncomplicated cardiac failure. It may be found in pernicious anaemia and has preceded changes in the peripheral blood in patients with achlorhydria and megaloblastic bone marrow [1].

In pernicious anaemia the atrophy may be accompanied by *Hunter's glossitis* (syn. Möller's glossitis) in which there are painful vivid red patches at the sides and tip of the tongue.

When a specific nutritional deficiency is corrected the filiform papillae may be regenerated in as little as 5–7 days [7].

REFERENCES

1 ADAMS J.F. (1957) *Lancet* i, 1120.
2 DI PALMA J.R. (1946) *Arch Intern Med* 78, 405.
3 *FABER M. (1945) *Acta Med Scand* 121, 179.
4 FRANTZELI A., et al (1945) *Acta Med Scand* 122, 207.
5 KAPLAN B.J. (1961) *Lancet* i, 1094.
6 *SCHAFFER J. (1951) *Oral Surg* 4, 1287; (1952) *Oral Surg* 5, 87.
7 SCHIEVE J.F. & RUNDLES R.W. (1949) *J Lab Clin Med* 34, 439.
8 SQUIRES A.T. (1955) *Lancet* i, 647.
9 TOMASZEWSKI W. (1951) *Br Med J* i, 117.

Scrotal tongue (syn. fissured tongue, lingua fissuratum, lingua plicata). The scrotal tongue is a developmental defect, which in lesser degrees is of common occurrence. In a general population of 20,333 Swedes above the age of 15, the prevalence is 6·5% [1]. It may be present in infancy but may not be manifest until later life. An American study [3] showed prevalence of 0·4% in the first decade rising to 14·3% in the seventh. In some families it is inherited as an apparently isolated defect, determined by an autosomal dominant gene. It occurs in some 80% of mongoloids and is a characteristic though inconstant feature of the Melkersson – Rosenthal syndrome.

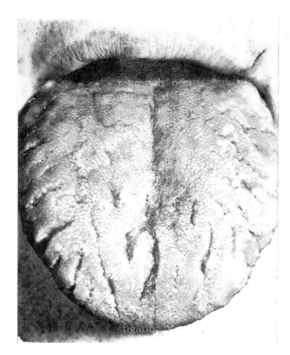

FIG. 55.69. Scrotal tongue (University Hospital, Copenhagen).

Clinically the scrotal tongue has a deep longitudinal groove with more or less deep radiating grooves dividing the tongue in a transverse cerebriform or irregular configuration (Fig. 55.69). In a South African study (Europeans and Xhosa Negroes) six distinct patterns of tongue fissuring have been observed [2]. The papillae usually extend into the mucosa of the fissures, but if the latter are deep their lowest portions may be denuded of papillae, when there may be chronic inflammatory changes of the subepithelial connective tissue. In the great majority of cases of scrotal tongue there are no symptoms.

REFERENCES

1 Axéll T. (1976) *Odontol Rev* **27** (Suppl. 36).
2 Farman A.G. (1976) *J Biol Buccale* **4**, 349.
3 Halperin V., *et al* (1953) *Oral Surg* **6**, 1072.

Oral–facial–digital syndrome (p. 140). The tongue is bifid or multilobed. The palate is cleft and the teeth are widely spaced.

Ankyloglossia (syn. tongue tie) [1]. Ankyloglossia is a developmental defect characterized by an abnormally short lingual frenum, either fibrous or muscular. Its importance as a cause of speech difficulty has been exaggerated, but it may cause periodontal defects [2]. Correction by Z-plasty is possible if the function of the tongue is significantly impaired.

REFERENCES

1 McEnery E.T. & Gaines F.P. (1941) *J Pediatr* **18**, 252.
2 Pindborg J.J. (1985) *Atlas of Diseases of the Oral Mucosa*. 4th ed. Copenhagen, Munksgaard.

Macroglossia [2]. Macroglossia describes a tongue excessively large in relation to the size of the mouth and jaws.

Primary macroglossia. The tongue is normal apart from its increased dimensions. The abnormality may be present as an isolated defect, in association with exomphalos and other developmental abnormalities [5], or as one feature of mongolism (see p. 114) in which the tongue may also be fissured.

Haemangiomatous and lymphangiomatous macroglossia. The tongue is asymmetrically enlarged. The haemangiomatous lesion is betrayed by its colour and consistency (p. 202). The lymphangioma may be studded with small vesicles and may be subject to recurrent episodes of pain and swelling (p. 1237).

Neurofibromatous macroglossia (pp. 119 and 2108). The tongue is asymmetrically enlarged. Other signs of neurofibromatosis should be sought.

Hypothyroid macroglossia. The tongue may be symmetrically enlarged in cretinism and myxoedema.

Oedematous macroglossia. Enlargement of the tongue may occur in angioneurotic oedema, and in wasp or bee stings of the tongue itself.

Oedema of the tongue manifest as increased dental marking may occur in superior vena cava obstruction, and also in cardiac and renal disease and in acute glossitis of any origin.

Amyloid macroglossia. Enlargement of the tongue occurs in 30–40% of patients with primary amyloidosis (p. 2303). In multiple myelomatosis the macroglossia may be associated with gingival ulceration and haemorrhage from amyloid or plasma cell infiltration [3].

Rare causes. These include actinomycosis, thyroglossal duct cysts, gummata and sarcoidosis [4].

Treatment [1]. The treatment of primary lymphangiomatous, haemangiomatous or neurofibromatous macroglossia is surgical. The timing and extent of any necessary surgery should be planned in consultation with an orthodontist.

REFERENCES

1 Bell H.G. & Millar R.G. (1948) *Surgery* **24**, 125.
2 Nathanson I. (1948) *Oral Surg* **1**, 547.
3 Pickle D.E., *et al* (1966) *Oral Surg* **21**, 347.
4 Tillman H.H. (1966) *Oral Surg* **21**, 190.
5 Wiedemann H.-R. (1964) *J Génét Hum* **13**, 223.

Median rhomboid glossitis (syn. glossite lozangique médiane) [3]. This condition, said to occur in 0·3% of the population, is usually regarded as a developmental defect, a persistent tuberculum impar [2], but as it seldom becomes clinically manifest until the third or fourth decade, and often later, other factors may be implicated. A substance has been found in the saliva of these subjects which provokes a cutaneous reaction and is destroyed by heat [4]. Its significance is unknown.

Histologically there is epithelial hyperplasia with a non-specific chronic inflammatory infiltrate (Fig. 55.70(b)).

The patient is usually a middle-aged man who has accidentally noticed the lesion and is anxious about cancer. The affected area in the midline of the base of the tongue is about 1 cm × 2 cm (Fig. 55.70(a)), is devoid of papillae and may be smooth or elevated and irregularly nodular.

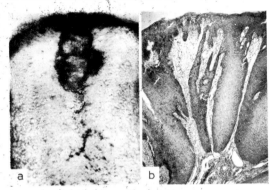

FIG. 55.70. Median rhomboid glossitis: (a) clinical appearance; (b) histology (× 22) (University Hospital and Royal Dental College, Copenhagen).

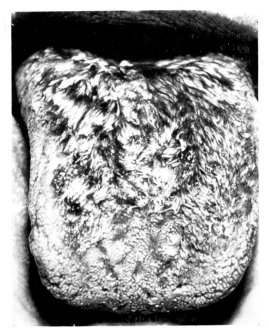

FIG. 55.71. Marked case of hairy tongue. Note the extremely elongated filiform papillae (University Hospital, Copenhagen).

A similar, if not identical, lesion has been called central papillary atrophy [1] and is found in 17% of diabetics.

The condition is not premalignant and no treatment is necessary. Biopsy may be required if carcinoma cannot be excluded. This is a very rare site for carcinoma. Recent studies (p. 2088) have demonstrated the presence of *Candida albicans* in a number of cases of the type usually labelled as median rhomboid glossitis and the lesion has responded favourably to antimycotic treatment.

REFERENCES

1 FARMAN A.G. (1976) *J Oral Pathol* 5, 255.
2 MARTIN H.E. & HOWE M.E. (1938) *Ann Surg* 107, 39.
3 ROXER R.Q. & BRUCE K.W. (1952) *Oral Surg* 5, 1287.
4 SIDI E., *et al* (1964) *J Invest Dermatol* 42, 145.

Black hairy tongue (syn. lingua villosa nigra). Black hairy tongue is a hyperplasia of the filiform papillae [3] which may be as long as 2 cm (Fig. 55.71). This elongation is the result of a disturbance of normal epithelial desquamation but its pathogenesis remains a mystery. Associated with the papillary, hyperplasia is increased pigmentation attributed to the activities of pigment-producing bacteria. The degree of hyperplasia and of pigmentation vary independently.

The condition occurs only in adults. In some there is a clear relationship to the administration of topical or systemic antibiotics [2]. Poor dental hygiene, excessive smoking and rinsing with chlorhexidine are also sometimes incriminated, but in some patients no provocative factor can be established.

The formation of 'hair' begins posteriorly on the dorsum of the tongue and extends forwards and laterally. The colour of the elongated papillae varies from yellow or brown to grey or black (Fig. 55.72(a)). There are usually no symptoms but some patients complain of tickling of the palate or of retching. The condition may persist for many months or even for years. If treatment is required the most effective procedure is regular gentle brushing with a soft tooth brush (Fig. 55.72(b)). The response is more rapid if this is done a few minutes after the application of a 40% solution of urea [1].

REFERENCES

1 PEGUM J.S. (1971) *Br J Dermatol* 84, 602.
2 TOMAZEWSKI W. (1953) *Br Med J* i, 1249.
3 WINN L.H. (1958) *Arch Dermatol* 77, 97.

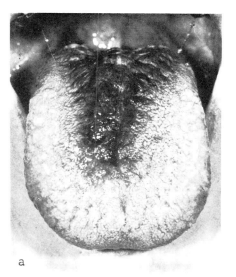
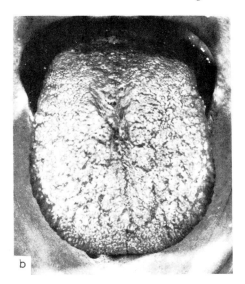

FIG. 55.72. Black hairy tongue: (a) typical appearance; (b) after 1 week of tongue brushing (University Hospital, Copenhagen).

Geographical tongue (syn. erythema migrans; benign migratory glossitis; exfoliatio arcata linguae). Geographical tongue is a benign inflammatory disorder of unknown origin. The prevalence in a general population in Scandinavia has been found to be 9% [1], but it was found in 15% of 8,000 children in Israel [4]. Children under the age of 4 are most commonly affected. In a sample of 70 patients with the disease 13% had a familial background [2]. An association with fissured tongue has been demonstrated, the latter sometimes developing some years later [3,4]. An association with seborrhoeic dermatitis or psoriasis has been noted but not statistically evaluated.

Histologically [3] there is an acute inflammatory infiltrate with many polymorphonuclear leukocytes in the lamina propria. Many cells invade the spongiotic epithelium after forming microabscesses in the upper part of the epithelium.

Multiple smooth red patches on the dorsum of the tongue are outlined by a slightly elevated greyish-yellow or white margin. The configuration of the patches, which are formed by the desquamation of the filiform papillae, is constantly changing to form map-like patterns. The rapidity of the change in pattern is illustrated by Fig. 55.73 which records observations over an interval of 9 days. Very rarely similar lesions may develop on the lip and soft palate [3]. There are usually no symptoms. The condition continues, often with remissions, for months or years.

The same lesions as seen on the tongue may, in

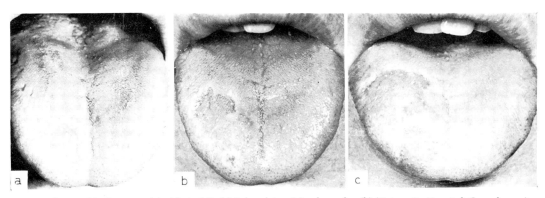

FIG. 55.73. Geographical tongue: (a) at first visit; (b) 6 days later; (c) 3 days after (b) (University Hospital, Copenhagen).

rare instances, occur on other parts of the oral mucosa—stomatitis areata migrans [5].

Treatment is seldom needed but if the lesions are painful the discomfort may be relieved with 5% carbolfuchsin or 0·5% gentian violet paints.

REFERENCES

1 AXÉLL T. (1976) *Odontol Rev* **27** (Suppl. 36).
2 BÁNÓCZY J., et al (1975) *Oral Surg* **39**, 113.
3 COOKE B.E.D. (1955) *Oral Surg* **8**, 164.
4 *RAHAMIMOFF P. & MUHSAM H.V. (1957) *Am J Dis Child* **93**, 519.
5 SAPIRO S. & SHKLAR G. (1973) *Oral Surg* **36**, 28.

Glossodynia (syn. burning tongue) [1–5]. This syndrome occurs almost exclusively in middle-aged or elderly women. It is usually accepted as psychosomatic in origin.

The patient complains of burning sensations which are most intense when she is tired but do not usually interfere with eating, although very hot or highly seasoned foods may cause increased discomfort. Some patients also complain of an unpleasant taste and some insist that the tongue is asymmetrical or that they can see or feel a tumour.

On examination the tongue either appears normal or presents the changes of some fortuitously associated disorder, eg candidiasis and poor denture construction.

In all cases a detailed physical examination is essential. The burning mouth syndrome may be an initial stage of anaemia. Since any pathological conditions discovered can rarely be related to the glossodynia the persistence of the patient's symptoms is not surprising. Reassurance is often unavailing. If the symptoms persist and are clearly seriously distressing the patient the help of a psychiatrist must be enlisted. Treatment of emotional disorders has led to relief of symptoms.

REFERENCES

1 BASKER R.M. (1978) *Br Dent J* **145**, 9.
2 HANEKE E. (1978) *Dtsch Med Wochenschr* **103**, 1302.
3 HANEKE E. (1980) *Zungen und Mundschleimhautbrennen.* Munich, Hauser.
4 MAIN D.M.G. & BASKER R.M. (1983) *Br Dent J* **154**, 206.
5 ZISKIN D.E. & MOULTON R. (1946) *J Am Dent Assoc* **33**, 1422.

Sublingual varicosis [1]. Prominence and tortuosity of the sublingual veins is present in 7–10% of patients over 40. The phlebectasia is not reliably proved to be associated with any systemic disease and is significant only as a source of anxiety to the patient who discovers it and fears cancer. The condition has also been called caviar tongue.

REFERENCE

1 RAPPAPORT I. & SHIFFMAN M.A. (1964) *Oral Surg* **17**, 263.

Inflammation of the foliate and circumvallate papillae [1]. The fungiform papillae are most frequently involved. The patient complains of burning and stinging on the tip and sides of the tongue. On careful examination the fungiform papillae are seen to be engorged and prominent. Avoidance of smoking, hot drinks and other irritants usually produces a cure.

The foliate papillae, which consist largely of lymphoid tissue, are situated at the sides of the tongue near its base. They are liable to be irritated by sharp broken tooth or ill-fitting loose dentures. When they are inflamed they become red and swollen and may cause considerable discomfort. Dental hygiene and bland applications are curative.

If the tender area feels indurated biopsy is essential since carcinoma may occur in this site.

Histologically the lesions comprise lymphoid tissue with germ centres, emphasizing that they are parts of Waldeyer's ring.

REFERENCE

1 SCHOLTZ M. (1935) *Arch Dermatol Syphilol* **32**, 801.

THE TEETH IN HEREDITARY ECTODERMAL DISORDERS

Many hereditary syndromes involving the skin are associated with dental anomalies, which are sometimes a constant and characteristic feature [1].

In *anhidrotic ectodermal dysplasia* (p. 130) there is a saddle nose and frontal bossing. The teeth are few and their eruption is often retarded. The consequent loss of vertical dimension causes the lips to protrude. The incisors, canines and bicuspids, when present, are often conical and peg shaped in crown form. The dental changes are an important diagnostic feature of the syndrome. The labial and buccal mucous glands are poorly developed or absent.

In *incontinentia pigmenti* (p. 1559) both the primary and permanent dentitions are abnormal. There is marked hypodontia, delayed tooth eruption and the crowns are peg shaped.

Some of the syndromes in which dental anomalies occur frequently are listed in Table 55.3.

TABLE 55.3. Dental changes in hereditary syndromes

Polydysplastic, epidermolysis bullosa	Amelogenesis disturbed; teeth discoloured and pitted
Anhidrotic ectodermal dysplasia	Teeth few; peg shaped, conical
Incontinentia pigmenti	Teeth small; eruption delayed; crown peg shaped
Oculodentaldigital dysplasia	Amelogenesis disturbed
Chondro-ectodermal dysplasia	Small, peg-shaped teeth; teeth few; incisors premolar shaped

REFERENCE

1 PINDBORG J.J. (1970) *Pathology of the Dental Hard Tissues.* Copenhagen, Munksgaard.

DISCOLORATION OF THE PRIMARY DENTITION

The primary dentition may be discoloured from a variety of causes, some of which are of importance to the dermatologist.

Developmental defects. In hereditary dentinogenesis imperfecta the teeth are brown or grey–blue. The condition may be an isolated defect but may be associated with osteogenesis imperfecta (p. 1845).

In amelogenesis imperfecta the teeth are brown. The enamel is hypomineralized or hypoplastic.

Acquired staining—systemic. In neonatal jaundice the teeth may be green and may also show enamel hypoplasia. Tetracycline administration (see below) causes yellow–brown staining. In fluorosis the enamel is mottled.

External. A variety of medicaments produce external staining, usually temporary but rarely permanent, if the drug, e.g. nitrofurantoin, is incorporated into the tooth substance.

REFERENCES

1 *BALLS J.S. (1964) *Clin Pediat* 3, 394.
2 PINDBORG J.J. (1970) *Pathology of the Dental Hard Tissues.* Copenhagen, Munksgaard.

TETRACYCLINE DISCOLORATION OF THE TEETH

The tetracyclines are localized in actively mineralizing structures. In man dental mineralization continues from the fifth fetal month until the age of 12. Tetracyclines prescribed in therapeutic dosage may cause yellow or yellow–brown discoloration of those primary or permanent teeth at the critical stage of their development during the period of administration. The widespread use of tetracycline is demonstrated in a study from Belfast which revealed that more than half of a group of children aged 3–15 yr had had tetracyclines some time during their first decade of life [2]. The affected teeth show light yellow fluorescence under UV light. The types of colour can be divided into three groups [3]: (1) a grey–brown colour, usually caused by chlortetracycline (Aureomycin®), (2) a yellow colour, often caused by oxytetracycline (Terramycin®), demethylchlortetracycline (Ledermycin®) and tetracycline (Achromycin®), and (3) a brownish colour. It has been suggested that a level of 21 mg/kg body weight of tetracycline per day is required to cause discoloration. With increasing age the yellow-brownish colour tends to fade away [1]. In the last decade there has been a reduction in the number of children with tooth discoloration due to tetracyclines.

REFERENCES

1 PINDBORG J.J. (1970) *Pathology of the Dental Hard Tissues.* Copenhagen, Munksgaard.
2 STEWART D.J. (1968) *Br Dent J* **124**, 318.
3 WEYMAN J. (1965) *Br Dent J* **118**, 289.

DENTAL ABSCESSES AND SINUSES

Aetiology and pathology [2]. A chronic periapical dental abscess frequently perforates a surface of the alveolar bone by continued resorption to form a sinus discharging into the mouth. Less commonly, after perforating the bone the pus tracks beneath the mucoperiosteum and discharges externally. The bacteriological findings are usually not specific, but occasionally *Actinomyces israeli* may give rise to distinctive changes [1].

External abscesses and sinuses may occur at any age. Although usually related to clinically evident dental disease they may first develop many years after dental extraction [6].

Clinical features [3,4,8]. Abscesses and sinuses within the mouth will rarely be encountered in dermatological clinics. The tender swelling or discharging sinus surrounded by hyperplastic epithelium may be seen on the gingiva or the palate.

External abscesses and sinuses may present in a variety of forms. Most common is a vascular nodule or papule, simulating pyogenic granuloma or lupus vulgaris. Sometimes epithelial hyperplasia may be considerable and the nodule may resemble a carcinoma [6]. The opening of the sinus may be obvious but is more often concealed. In some cases, notably those in which *Actinomyces* is isolated, the lesion is an indolent fluctuant mass which is easily mistaken for a sebaceous cyst.

The site, on the cheeks or chin or below the angle of the jaw, depends on the situation of the periapical infection but need not overlie it [5]. Rarely the pus may track some distance and a dental sinus draining to the inner canthus of one eye has been recorded [7]. There are often no dental symptoms.

The diagnosis is established radiologically.

Treatment. If the abscess or sinus is related to demonstrable periapical infection, it may heal after extraction of the offending tooth. Rarely a chronic sinus may require excision.

If *Actinomyces* is present without persistent dental disease systemic penicillin may be curative.

REFERENCES

1 CARON G.A. & SARKANY I. (1964) *Br J Dermatol* **76**, 421.
2 FARMER E.D. & LAWTON F.E. (1966) *Stones' Oral and Dental Diseases.* 5th ed. Edinburgh, Livingstone.
3 *GURDIN M. & PANGMAN W.J. (1953) *Plast Reconstr Surg* **11**, 444.
4 KOHN S.I. (1940) *Am J Orthod* **26**, 797.
5 McCLUER C.F.A. & BURNS R.G. (1961) *Arch Dermatol* **83**, 941.
6 RUCH M. (1960) *Arch Dermatol* **82**, 639.
7 SMITH E.L. & PETTY A.H. (1962) *Br J Dermatol* **74**, 450.
8 WINSTOCK D. (1959) *Proc R Soc Med* **52**, 749.

THE LIPS

ARTHUR ROOK & J.L. BURTON (p. 2122–2129)

CONTACT CHEILITIS

Definition and aetiology. Contact cheilitis is an inflammatory reaction of the lips, provoked by the irritant or sensitizing action of chemical agents in contact with them. A very large number of substances have been incriminated, but most cases are caused by lipsticks or lip salves.

Lipsticks. Lipsticks are composed of mineral oils and wax which form the stick, castor oil as a solvent for the dyes, lanolin as an emollient, preservatives, perfumes and colour [3]. The colours include azo dyes and eosin, which is a bromofluorescein derivative. An impurity in the eosin used to be an important

sensitizer, but the use of purer eosin in recent years has led to a marked decrease in the incidence of lipstick allergy. Other ingredients which are occasionally incriminated include the azo dyes, carmine, oleyl alcohol, lanolin, perfumes, azulene and propyl gallate [3].

Lipsalves and other medicaments. Lipsalves containing lanolin are frequently applied for dryness or chapping. Phenyl salicylate and antibiotics have also been incriminated as a cause of cheilitis [8].

Mouthwashes and dentrifices [6]. Essential oils, such as peppermint, cinnamon, cloves and spearmint, and bactericidal agents can cause cheilitis.

Dental preparations. Mercury and eugenol, both much used in dentistry, may cause cheilitis in the absence of stomatitis. Allergy to epimine-containing materials used for crowns and bridges can cause cheilitis [5]. The subject of allergy to dental preparations has been reviewed by Kulenkamp [9].

Foods. Oranges, artichokes and mangoes are among the food plants which occasionally cause an allergic cheilitis and dermatitis of the skin around the lips. The oil on the peel of citrus fruits is irritant to the skin, but in addition some sweet oranges contain a weakly phototoxic agent which can cause a reaction in pale-skinned people [11].

Miscellaneous objects. Common causes are various objects favoured by obsessional suckers of all ages— metal hair clips, metal pencils, the cobalt paint on blue pencils, etc. Allergy to nail varnish can also cause cheilitis [4]. The wooden and nickel mouthpieces of musical instruments are a rare cause. Clarinettists' cheilitis due to prolonged playing of reed instruments has also been reported, but this is thought to be due to mechanical factors rather than allergy [7].

Pathology. See contact dermatitis (p. 466).

Clinical features [1,2]. *Lipstick cheilitis* is sometimes confined to the vermilion border but more often extends beyond it. There may be persistent irritation and scaling or a more acute reaction with oedema and vesiculation. The offending lipstick may have been adopted only recently or may have been in regular use for many years. Exacerbations develop a few hours or over a day after the application. In some cases a lipstick may be well tolerated unless there is also exposure to sunlight.

The other forms of cheilitis vary greatly in their

clinical appearance. Those caused by foods commonly also involve the skin around the mouth. If a small sucked object is responsible the reaction may be confined to one part of the lips.

Diagnosis. If acute eczematous changes are obviously present the diagnosis of contact cheilitis presents no difficulty. If the changes are confined to irritation and scaling the various forms of exfoliative cheilitis must be excluded (see p. 2125).

If an allergic reaction is suspected patch tests should be carried out as described in Chapter 14 using the appropriate concentrations of the substances concerned.

Treatment. Topical steroids will give symptomatic relief but the offending substance must be traced and avoided.

REFERENCES

1 *CALNAN C.D. & SARKANY I. (1957) *Trans Rep St John's Hosp Dermatol Soc Lond* **39**, 28.
2 CALNAN C.D. & SARKANY I. (1960) *Trans Rep St John's Hosp Dermatol Soc Lond* **44**, 47.
3 CRONIN E. (1980) *Contact Dermatitis.* Edinburgh, Churchill Livingstone, p. 141.
4 CRONIN E. (1980) *Contact Dermatitis.* Edinburgh, Churchill Livingstone, p. 154.
5 DUXBURY A.J. (1979) *Br Dent J* **147**, 331.
6 *FISHER A.A. (1973) *Contact Dermatitis.* 2nd ed. Philadelphia, Lea & Febiger, p. 320.
7 HINDSON T.C. (1978) *Br Med J* **ii**, 1295.
8 HINDSON C. (1980) *Contact Dermatitis* **6**, 216.
9 KULENKAMP D., *et al* (1977) *Hautarzt* **28**, 353.
10 MARCHAND B., *et al* (1982) *Arch Dermatol Res* **272**, 61.
11 VOLDEN G., *et al* (1983) *Contact Dermatitis* **9**, 201.

Drug-induced cheilitis. Cheilitis is a feature of the Stevens–Johnson syndrome (p. 1086), but it can also occur as an isolated feature of a drug reaction, either as a result of allergy or as a pharmacological effect. The aromatic retinoids, etretinate and isotretinoin, cause dryness and cracking of the lips in most patients, and the effect is dose related. Beta blockers can also cause cheilitis as the initial manifestation of a drug reaction [2]. The effect of systemic drugs in producing reactions of the oral mucosa has been reviewed by Duxbury [1].

REFERENCES

1 DUXBURY A.J. (1980) *Oral Manifestations of Systemic Disease.* Saunders, London, Chapter 16.
2 TANGSRUD S.E. & GOLF S. (1977) *Br Med J* **ii**, 1385.

ANGULAR CHEILITIS

Definition and aetiology [3,6,7]. Angular cheilitis is an acute or chronic inflammation of the skin and contiguous labial mucous membrane at the angles of the mouth, of variable and usually mixed aetiology. The term perlèche is often used as a synonym but is sometimes restricted to those cases, usually in children, in which an infective agent appears to be concerned.

Angular cheilitis is a clinical syndrome in which four main groups of factors are implicated, but in differing combinations and degree.

Mechanical factors [1]. In the edentulous patient who does not wear a denture and also as a normal consequence of the ageing process, the upper lip overhangs the lower at the angles of the mouth, producing an oblique curved fold and keeping a small area of skin constantly macerated. Prognathism may give rise to a similar state of affairs in the young.

Systemic disorders which may increase the vulnerability of the mucous membrane [4,5,7]. Nutritional deficiencies, in particular deficiencies of riboflavine and iron and general protein malnutrition, have often been incriminated but frequently mechanical and other factors are also concerned.

Diseases of the skin. Atopic dermatitis involving the face is often associated with angular cheilitis. The incidence appears also to be increased in seborrhoeic dermatitis but the association with other skin diseases is probably fortuitous.

Infective agents. A microbiological study of 100 cases [2] showed *Staph. aureus* in 79%, *Candida* species in 44% and beta haemolytic streptococci in 15%.

Oral candidiasis, particularly common in those wearing dentures, may be associated with a persistent or recurrent angular cheilitis. Permanent cure can be achieved only by eliminating the growth of *Candida* beneath the upper denture. Candidiasis was probably responsible for some of the cases of cheilitis attributed to allergy to denture materials since contamination of denture material by *Candida* may cause false positive patch test reactions [6].

Outbreaks of acute pustular and fissured cheilitis may occur in children, particularly if they are ill-nourished, and in some such streptococci or staphylococci have appeared to be causative.

Other factors. Hypersalivation from any cause may ensure the continued maceration of the angles of

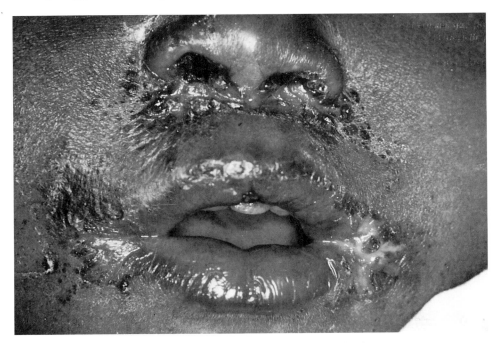

FIG. 55.74. Severe cheilitis in a South African child with nutritional deficiency (kwashiorkor).

the mouth. Cheilitis is common in Down's syndrome, the large tongue and the constant dribbling being contributory factors.

A rare cause is the presence of fistulae of developmental origin at the angles of the mouth.

Clinical features. All forms of angular cheilitis present as a roughly triangular area of erythema and oedema at one, or more commonly both, angles of the mouth. Additional changes reflect the influence of other factors (Fig. 55.74).

The commonest form is certainly largely mechanical in origin and the patients are often elderly. Recurrent exudation and crusting are frequent. A smooth tongue may indicate an associated nutritional deficiency. An eczematous dermatitis may extend some distance onto the cheek or chin as an infective eczematoid reaction (p. 373) or as a reaction to topical medicaments.

In all cases in denture wearers *Candida* should be sought not only in the lesions but also beneath the denture.

In atopic dermatitis, especially in children and adolescents, dry scaling and thickening, and sometimes hyperpigmentation, are combined with crusted radial fissures. Licking, as a nervous tic, often perpetuates the changes.

Diagnosis and treatment. Each case must be carefully assessed. The presence of atopic dermatitis elsewhere on the face or in other regions, together with the distinctive appearance of the cheilitis, will establish the diagnosis. The licking habit is often difficult to break. A steroid/antibiotic/nystatin ointment gives symptomatic relief.

If there is an obvious mechanical factor, dental treatment may increase the vertical dimension of the bite.

The treatment of candidiasis is considered on p. 961.

If the cause of the cheilitis is not apparent, underlying systemic disease must be sought and treated.

REFERENCES

1 CHERNOVSKY M.E. (1966) *Arch Dermatol* **93**, 332.
2 MACFARLANE T.W. & HELNARSKA S.J. (1976) *Br Dent J* **140**, 403.
3 *MARCUSSEN P.V. (1943) *Acta Derm Venereol (Stockh)* **24**, 83.
4 MURPHY N.C., *et al* (1979) *J Am Dent Assoc* **99**, 640.
5 ROSE J.A. (1968) *Br Dent J* **125**, 67.
6 SALO O.P. & HIRVONEN M.-L. (1969) *Br J Dermatol* **81**, 338.
7 SCHOENFELD R.J., *et al* (1977) *Cutis* **19**, 213.
8 SPRAFKE H. (1965) *Dermatol Wochenschr* **151**, 359.

ACTINIC CHEILITIS

An eczematous cheilitis may be induced by the photo-sentitizing action of certain ingredients of lipstick or oranges (p. 513).

Intense and prolonged exposure to sunlight may give rise to an acute and recurrent erosive cheilitis without the mediation of chemical agents [1]. In differential diagnosis herpes simplex must be considered, for attacks of the latter may sometimes be induced by light.

Under tropical conditions actinic cheilitis may at first be the only manifestation of a polymorphic light eruption (see below) and may be an early manifestation of a genetically abnormal susceptibility to light damage, as in xeroderma pigmentosum (p. 144).

Chronic actinic cheilitis [7] is common on the lower lip (Fig. 55.75), especially in seamen and

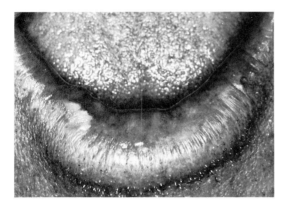

FIG. 55.75. Chronic actinic cheilitis. Note the unclear border between the labial mucosa, the vermilion border and the skin. On the right-hand side there is a small area of leukoplakia on the mucosa. (University Hospital, Copenhagen).

agricultural workers. It has also occurred in arc-welders [9]. It first develops after many years of exposure as dryness and fine scaling. Later the epithelium becomes visibly and palpably thickened with small greyish-white plaques. Vertical fissuring and crusting occur increasingly readily, particularly in cold weather. Later still, warty nodules may form. At first they may drop off or be knocked off and may vary in size with fluctuation in the degree of oedema and inflammatory change surrounding them, but eventually one or more may undergo malignant change. Histologically [6] there is some superficial ulceration of a flattened epithelium, beneath which is a band of inflammatory infiltrate in which plasma cells may predominate. The collagen

often shows basophilic (elastotic) degeneration. In the differential diagnosis of chronic actinic cheilitis, lupus erythematosus (p. 1293) and lichen planus (p. 1665) must be considered.

Treatment of actinic cheilitis. Protection from further exposure by a sun-screening lipstick is required. Since the condition is premalignant, surgical treatment by a 'lip-shave' operation may be advisable [2,4]. Radiotherapy has also been used [8], but this may compound the problem in the long run. The application of 5% fluorouracil solution causes considerable discomfort, but the long-term results are relatively good [5].

Actinic cheilitis in hereditary polymorphous light eruption [3]. This condition affects Indians in North, Central and South America. It produces a photosensitive facial rash, with erythema, papules, exudation and crusts, and is often associated with an acute or chronic exudative cheilitis of the lower lip. The histology shows a dense mixed infiltrate throughout the dermis, and the lymphocytes may be clustered in dense aggregates with reactive centres. This type of actinic cheilitis due to enhanced sensitivity is distinguished from the type described above, which is due to prolonged and excessive exposure to UV irradiation, by the relative absence of epidermal dysplasia and solar elastosis.

REFERENCES

1 BIELICKY T. (1965) *Hautarzt* **16**, 25.
2 BIRT B.D. (1977) *J Otolaryngol* **6**, 407.
3 BIRT A.R., et al (1979) *Arch Dermatol* **115**, 699.
4 COTALDO E., et al (1981) *J Dermatol Surg Oncol* **7**, 289.
5 EPSTEIN E. (1977) *Arch Dermatol* **113**, 906.
6 KOTEN J.W., et al (1967) *Dermatologica* **135**, 465.
7 NICOLAU S.G. & BALUS L. (1964) *Br J Dermatol* **76**, 278.
8 SZABO P. (1979) *Hautarzt* **30**, 257.
9 VERNON S. (1949) *JAMA* **140**, 1333.

EXFOLIATIVE CHEILITIS
SYN. FACTITIOUS CHEILITIS: LE TIC DE LÈVRES

Exfoliative cheilitis is a chronic superficial inflammatory disorder of the vermilion borders of the lips characterized by persistent scaling (Fig. 55.76). The diagnosis is now applied rather uncommonly to the few patients presenting this clinical syndrome whose lesions cannot be attributed to contact sensitization or to light (see actinic cheilitis, above). Many of these cases are now thought to be factitious, owing to repeated lip sucking or other manipulation of the lips [1,2,4,5]. Most cases occur in

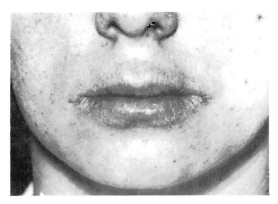

FIG. 55.76. Exfoliative cheilitis in a girl with atopic dermatitis (Addenbrooke's Hospital).

girls or young women, and the majority have a personality disorder. The process, which often starts in the middle of the lower lip and spreads to involve the whole of the lower or both lips, consists of scaling and crusting more or less confined to the vermilion border and persisting in varying severity for months or years. The patient often complains of irritation or burning and can be observed frequently biting or sucking the lips.

Contact cheilitis (p. 2122) must be carefully excluded. Reassurance and topical steroids are helpful in some cases, but others require psychotherapy or tranquillizers. Chronic cheilitis is readily contaminated by *Candida* but may also sometimes be caused by candidiasis. In such cases the clinical features are very variable and may simulate epithelioma [3,4], lichen planus or discoid lupus erythematosus.

REFERENCES

1 CARTEAUD A. (1967) *Presse Méd* **75**, 2763.
2 CROTTY C.P., *et al* (1981) *Arch Dermatol* **117**, 338.
3 DELACRETAZ J., *et al* (1970) *Dermatologica* **140**, 107.
4 FINNERTY E.F. (1976) *Cutis* **18**, 236.
5 SAVAGE J. (1978) *Br J Dermatol* **99**, 573.

ORODYNIA (BURNING MOUTH)
(SEE ALSO GLOSSODYNIA (p. 2120))

Patients with orodynia complain of a feeling of burning or discomfort in the mouth, which may be localized on the tongue, buccal mucosa or lips. The burning feeling may be exacerbated by acids such as fruit juice or vinegar. There are many possible causes, not all of which are well substantiated [1]. These include problems with dentures, diabetes mellitus and various deficiency states such as lack of iron, vitamins B_2, B_6 and B_{12}, folic acid, etc. It may also occur as a manifestation of oesophageal reflux [3] and following antibiotic therapy. It is also commonly seen as a manifestation of neurosis, and some of these patients suffer from cancer phobia. Some cases will respond to oral pimozide therapy [4], and oestrogen replacement therapy is sometimes helpful in menopausal females [2].

REFERENCES

1 BASKER R.M., *et al* (1978) *Br Dent J* **145**, 9.
2 FERGUSON M.M., *et al* (1981) *J R Soc Med* **74**, 492.
3 GARRETTS M. (1960) *Lancet* ii, 1376.
4 SNEDDON I.B. (1979) *Acta Derm Venereol* (Suppl. **85**) (*Stockh*) **59**, 177.

GLANDULAR CHEILITIS

Aetiology. Glandular cheilitis is an uncommon disorder characterized by enlargement and secondary inflammatory changes of heterotopic salivary glands in the lips [1, 4, 5]. The various forms, eponymously labelled, are regarded as different degrees of severity of a single process. The cause is unknown, but in some cases the condition has apparently been hereditary [6]. The onset is in childhood or early adult life.

Pathology [2]. In the simple form there is some sclerosis surrounding the hyperplastic salivary glands. In the rare suppurative forms there is also a dense chronic inflammatory infiltrate.

Clinical features [3]. In simple glandular cheilitis the lower lip is slightly enlarged and bears numerous pinhead orifices from which saliva can readily be squeezed.

In the suppurative form (syn. Volkmann's cheilitis) the lip is considerably and permanently enlarged, but is subject to episodes of pain, tenderness and increased enlargement. The surface is covered by crusts and scales, beneath which the duct orifices may be discovered.

Treatment. The only effective measure is plastic excision of an elongated ellipse of tissue containing the hyperplastic glands [2].

REFERENCES

1 BALUS L. (1965) *Hautarzt* **16**, 364.
2 DOKU H.C., *et al.* (1965) *Oral Surg* **20**, 563.
3 *MICHALOWSKI R. (1946) *Acta Derm Venereol* (*Stockh*) **27**, 31.
4 STULLER C.B., *et al* (1982) *Oral Surg* **53**, 602.

5 THIELE B., *et al* (1983) *Hautarzt* **34**, 232.
6 WEIR T.W. & JOHNSON W.C. (1971) *Arch Dermatol* **103**, 433.

MULTIPLE MUCOSAL NEUROMA SYNDROME

Familial syndromes of multiple endocrine neoplasia (MEN) occur in at least three separate clinical patterns [4]. The type 3 MEN syndrome is characterized by medullary carcinoma of the thyroid and phaeochromocytoma in association with a marfanoid habitus and multiple mucosal neuromas. By 1975, 41 cases of type 3 MEN syndrome had been reported in the literature [2].

The facial appearance is striking, with thick slightly everted lips which usually have a slightly bumpy surface. The eyelids are thickened, and multiple neuromas produce an irregular lumpy appearance of the eyelids, lips and tongue. They are less frequently seen on the buccal mucosa, gingivae, palate and pharynx.

Intestinal ganglioneuromatosis may also occur in about one-third of patients [3]. There may be absence of the axon flare when histamine is injected intradermally, suggesting that there may be a widespread defect in neural structure in this syndrome [1].

REFERENCES

1 BA███████ ████ ██72) *Arch Ophthalmol* **87** 574.█████████████
2 BROWN ███ ████ (1975) *J Pediatr* **86**, 77.
3 KHAIRI M.R.A. (1975) *Medicine* **54**, 89.
4 SCHIMKE R.N. (1976) *Adv Intern Med* **21**, 249.

PLASMA CELL CHEILITIS

This entity [1,2] appears to be the counterpart of Zoon's plasma cell balanitis (p. 2189), with which it shows many clinical and pathological similarities. The cause and nosological status of the condition are unknown; it may be a variant of actinic cheilitis.

REFERENCES

1 LUGER A. (1966) *Hautarzt* **17**, 244.
2 MOLDENHAUER E. (1966) *Dermatol Wochenschr* **152**, 636.

GRANULOMATOUS CHEILITIS
(MELKERSSON–ROSENTHAL SYNDROME)

Nomenclature [5]. Melkersson, in 1928, described recurrent facial palsy in association with labial oedema. Rosenthal, in 1930, emphasized the role of genetic factors and added scrotal tongue to the syndrome which for some years has been eponymously linked with the names of both researchers. The full syndrome however, had been described by Rossolino in 1901 [14].

Granulomatous cheilitis, frequently associated with Miescher's name, is generally accepted as a monosymptomatic form of the same syndrome [10].

Aetiology. There may be a genetic predisposition to the syndrome [5]. Siblings have been affected and a scrotal tongue may be present in otherwise normal relations. The possibility that an infective agent may be implicated has been repeatedly raised, but without convincing evidence. So many different infective agents have been held responsible that the possibility must be considered that the syndrome is a non-specific pattern of reaction.

The condition has been reported from many parts of the world and affects the sexes equally. The earliest manifestations usually develop in childhood or adolescence, but may be delayed until middle or old age.

Pathology [1,5,11,15,19]. Biopsy of the swollen lip or facial tissues during the early stages of the disease shows only oedema and perivascular lympho-

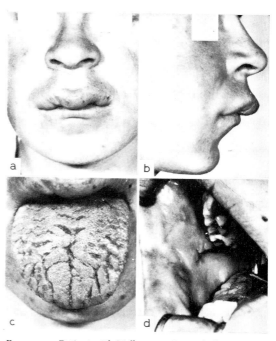

FIG. 55.77. Patient with Melkersson–Rosenthal syndrome. Note the oedema of the upper lip and buccal mucosa and the scrotal tongue (University Hospital, Copenhagen).

cytic infiltration. In some cases of long duration no other changes are seen, but in others the infiltrate becomes more dense and pleomorphic and small focal granulomas are formed. They may be indistinguishable from sarcoidosis or Crohn's disease. Similar changes may be present in cervical lymph nodes.

Clinical features [1,5,8,18,19]. The earliest cutaneous manifestation is sudden diffuse swelling, simulating angio-oedema, and most commonly involving the upper lip, the lower lip and one or both cheeks in decreasing order of frequency. Less commonly the forehead, the eyelids or one side of the scalp may be involved. The attacks are sometimes accompanied by fever and mild constitutional symptoms. At first the oedema subsides completely in hours or days, but after recurrent attacks at irregular intervals the swelling persists and slowly increases in degree. At first soft, it becomes firmer and eventually acquires the consistency of hard rubber. After some years the swelling may very slowly regress [13]. The regional lymph nodes are enlarged in 50% of cases [5] but not usually very greatly.

The fissured or scrotal tongue, which has been regarded as a key feature of the syndrome, may not in fact be so. It is certainly present from birth in some cases and may indicate genetic susceptibility, but it has been confused with furrowing of the tongue, secondary to its enlargement by the granulomatous process.

Facial palsy occurs in some 30% of cases. It may precede the attacks of oedema by months or years, but more commonly develops later. Intermittent at first, it may become permanent. Other cranial nerves (the olfactory, auditory, glossopharyngeal and hypoglossal) may occasionally be involved. Involvement of the central nervous system is frequent [4], but the significance of the resulting symptoms is easily overlooked as they are very variable, sometimes simulating disseminated sclerosis but often a poorly defined association of psychotic and neurological features. Autonomic disturbances may dominate the picture.

Diagnosis. The essential feature of the syndrome is the granulomatous swelling of lip or face. In the early attacks confident differentiation from angio-oedema is impossible in the absence of either scrotal tongue or facial palsy. Persistence of the swelling between attacks should suggest the diagnosis, which can sometimes be confirmed by biopsy. In some cases the histological changes are, however, inconspicuous and non-specific.

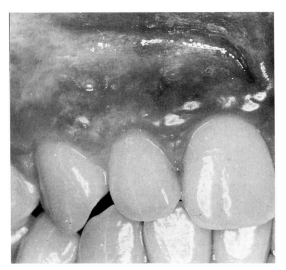

Fig. 55.78. Distinct irregular bluish-red oedematous swellings of the marginal and alveolar gingiva in the Melkersson–Rosenthal syndrome. (From Worsaae N. & Pindborg J. J. (1980) *Oral Surg* **49**, 131).

In the established cases other causes of macrocheilia (see Table 55.4) must be excluded. Ascher's syndrome is likely to cause confusion—here the

Table 55.4. Macrocheilia: acute or chronic enlargement of one or both lips

Acute	Chronic
Traumatic	Developmental
	Familial idiopathic
Infective	Double lip
Pyococcal	Ascher's syndrome
Anthrax	Lymphangioma
Diphtheria	Haemangioma
Primary syphilis	Neurofibroma
Trichophytosis	
Leishmaniasis	Acquired
Herpes simplex	Post-traumatic
Trichiniasis	Postinfective
	on basis of developmental lymphatic defect
Angio-oedema	Infective
	Tuberculosis
	Leprosy
	Rhinoscleroma
	South American leishmaniasis
	Neoplastic
	Melkersson–Rosenthal syndrome
	Cheilitis glandularis
	Sarcoidosis
	Crohn's disease

swelling of the lip is caused by redundant salivary tissue and is present from childhood. Blepharochalazia is associated.

The condition can also be difficult to distinguish from labial Crohn's disease which can precede the onset of regional ileitis by several years [2,6,16].

Treatment. Surgery alone is relatively unsuccessful [17], but the repeated injection of triamcinolone into the lips every few weeks may be effective [3]. The injections have to be repeated every 4–6 months once a plateau has been reached. This treatment has also been combined with surgical reduction (cheiloplasty) [7]. The injections must be continued periodically after the surgery or there may be an exaggerated recurrence of the condition.

Treatment with dapsone has been reported to be of value [12].

In our experience systemic corticosteroids have failed to reduce the swelling and have prevented further attacks only as long as their administration was continued.

REFERENCES

1 *BAZEX A. & DUPRÉ A. (1957) *Toulouse Med* **58**, 89.
2 CARR D. (1974) *Br Med J* **iv**, 636.
3 EISENBUD L., *et al* (1971) *Oral Surg* **32**, 384.
4 GOTTWALD W. (1972) *Z Haut Geschl Krankh* **47**, 19.
5 *HORNSTEIN O.P. (1973) *Curr Probl Dermatol* **5**, 117.
6 KINT A., *et al* (1977) *Hautarzt* **28**, 319.
7 KRUTCHKOFF D. & JAMES R. (1978) *Arch Dermatol* **114**, 1203.
8 LAYMON C.W. (1960) *Arch Dermatol* **83**, 112.
9 LOPEZ GONZALEZ J., *et al* (1972) *Med Cutan Iber Lat Am* **6**, 21.
10 MIESCHER G. (1945) *Dermatologica* **91**, 57.
11 RHODES E.L. & STIRLING G.A. (1965) *Arch Dermatol* **92**, 40.
12 RODRIGUEZ O., *et al* (1973) *Dermatol Rev Mex* **17**, 5.
13 ROOK A.J. & MOFFATT J.L. (1956) *Proc R Soc Med* **49**, 818.
14 ROSSOLINO G.J. (1901) *Neurol Zentralbl* **20**, 744.
15 *SCHUPPEINER H.J. (1956) *Dtsch GesundhWes* **11**, 1598.
16 VERBOV J.L. (1973) *Trans Rep St John's Hosp Dermatol Soc Lond* **59**, 30.
17 VISTNES L. & KERNOHAN D. (1971) *Plast Reconstr Surg* **48**, 126.
18 WHITE I.R., *et al* (1981) *Clin Exp Dermatol* **6**, 391.
19 *WORSAAE N., *et al* (1982) *Oral Surg* **54**, 404.

CHAPTER 56

Diseases of the External Ear

J.D. WILKINSON

Anatomy and physiology [5, 8–11]. The external ear consists of the auricle, the external auditory canal and the outer layer of the tympanic membrane. The *auricle*, or *pinna*, is a convoluted, elastic and cartilaginous plate covered by skin which is continuous medially with the lining of the external auditory canal. Except on the lobe and at the back of the ear, the skin is bound firmly to the cartilage. The pinna is attached to the head by fibrous ligaments and three vestigial auricularis muscles. In man the auricle is largely functionless and motionless.

The epidermis of the ear has a complex dermo-epidermal junction, a conspicuous stratum granulosum and a thick compact stratum corneum [10]. The dermis contains abundant elastic tissue. Sebaceous glands are numerous, particularly on the tragus and lobe, and fine vellus or terminal hair occurs over the entire surface but is especially prominent on the helix and tragus. Coarser terminal hair is seen in some men as a Y-linked and androgen-dependent inherited trait [5]. Eccrine sweat glands are sparsely and irregularly distributed except in the external auditory canal which has, instead, a large number of modified apocrine or ceruminous glands. The pinna has a variably thick fatty layer which extends between perichondrium and reticular dermis and which also forms the main fibro-fatty core of the lobe of the ear.

The blood supply to the auricle is provided by anastomosing branches of the superficial temporal and posterior auricular arteries, which drain via posterior auricular and superficial temporal veins into the external jugular vein and via the superficial temporal, maxillary and facial veins into the internal jugular vein. Lymphatic drainage is to the superficial parotid, retro-auricular and superficial cervical lymph nodes. Embryonic fusion planes and minute deficiencies in the cartilaginous portion of the external auditory canal provide potential pathways for the spread of infection and tumours.

There is a complex nerve supply to the ear involving elements of the Vth, VIIth, IXth and Xth cranial nerves as well as cervical branches of the greater and lesser auricular nerves. The back of the ear is supplied by the greater auricular nerve (C2, 3), the concha by the auricular branch of the vagus (X) and the anterior part of the ear by the auriculo-temporal branch of the Vth cranial nerve. Intercommunicating branches of the VIIth, IXth and Xth supply the deeper parts of the ear. With this complicated nerve supply, otalgia is more commonly due to referred pain than to disease in the ear itself [2]. Within the epidermis the nerve supply is abundant, especially around hair follicles where there are complicated basket-like networks of acetyl- and butyl-cholinesterase nerve fibres [10]. Free nerve endings are also present but there are no organized nerve endings, as occur on glabrous skin elsewhere [12].

The *external auditory canal* extends upwards and backwards in an S-shaped curve from the concha to the tympanic membrane. The angle of curvature varies between races and individuals, being more marked in Caucasoids than in Negroes or Polynesians. This has a bearing on trauma, infection and the retention of moisture. The length of the canal is 2·5 cm as measured from the concha to drum. The outer third of the canal is cartilaginous and is lined by a thin layer of epithelium. Subcutaneous tissue is scanty and the epithelium is firmly bound to the perichondrium. Sebaceous glands are plentiful and open into the follicles of extremely fine vellus hairs. Occasionally, larger terminal hairs (tragi) arise in the canal or around the meatus and these, if they become matted with wax or debris, may interfere with normal epidermal 'migration' and ventilation of the ear and hence may play a part in the development of 'hot-weather ear'.

Eccrine sweat glands are not present in the auditory canal but modified apocrine (ceruminous) glands are numerous. They increase in size and activity at puberty. There is great individual and racial variability, and, although concentrated in the cartilaginous part of the canal, they may also occur, albeit sparsely, in the osseous portion.

The inner osseous part of the acoustic canal constitutes two-thirds of its total length. The skin is firmly bound to the periosteum, subcutaneous tissue being nearly absent. The epidermis in this situation is thin and easily traumatized and rete ridges are absent [11]. The skin of the external auditory canal and tympanic membrane is unique in that there is no frictional squame loss; cerumen (wax) and epithelial debris has therefore to be removed by a special 'migratory' property of the external ear canal epithelium [1]. A slight narrowing of the canal, the isthmus, occurs at or just medial to the junction of the two parts. When marked, it may impede the flow of cerumen to the exterior. Just medial to the isthmus, inferiorly and anteriorly, is the tympanic sulcus. Debris often collects here, especially in patients with chronic external otitis.

The surface pH of the auditory canal varies [4] from 5·6–5·8 at the concha to 7·3–7·5 at 5–10 mm within the canal. With inflammation the pH becomes slightly more acid.

Cerumen is the combined product of sebaceous and apocrine glands. It contains both squalene and insoluble fatty acids. Its extrusion is aided by mastication and by the peripheral movement and desquamation of the epithelial cells of the canal and is impeded if the ear canal is too narrow or tortuous or when inflammation interferes with the normal process of 'migration'.

There are two varieties of cerumen: a dark, hard variety more common in males and a soft, lighter variety normally found in females. Though not bactericidal, cerumen does not actually encourage bacterial or fungal growth. An increased secretion of cerumen occurs with excessive sweating, stress or inflammation and has also been reported in patients treated with aromatic retinoids [3, 7]. If wax becomes impacted or adherent it may be removed either manually or by syringing. Both its presence and its removal may cause inflammation due to trauma, infection or contact dermatitis from medicaments or irritant cerumenolytics [6]. Inflammation interferes with normal epidermal migration and tends therefore both to induce and to encourage the retention of scale. The pruritus associated with excess cerumen, and the low grade inflammation that often accompanies this, frequently leads to a persistent form of low grade neurodermatitis.

REFERENCES

1 ALBERTI P.W.R.M. (1964) *J Laryngol Otol* **78**, 808.
2 AL SHEIKHLI A.R. (1980) *J Laryngol Otol* **94**, 1433.
3 BURGE S.M., *et al* (1981) *Br J Dermatol* **104**, 675.
4 FABRICANT N.D. (1957) *Arch Otolatolaryngol* **65**, 11.
5 HAMILTON J.B. (1958) In *The Biology of Hair Growth.* Eds. W. Montagna & R.A. Ellis. New York, Academic Press.
6 HOLMES R.C., *et al* (1982) *J R Soc Med* **75**, 27.
7 KRAMER M. (1981) *Acta Derm Venereol (Stockh)* **62**, 267.
8 MATSUNGUA E. (1962) *Ann Hum Genet* **25**, 273.
9 MAWSON S.R. & LUDMAN H. (1979) *Diseases of the Ear: A Textbook of Otology.* 4th ed. London, Arnold.
10 MONTAGNA W. & GIACOMETTI L. (1969) *Arch Dermatol* **99**, 757.
11 PERRY E.T. (1957) *The Human Ear Canal.* Springfield, Thomas.
12 SINCLAIR D.C., *et al* (1952) *J Anat* **86**, 402.

Developmental defects [2, 3, 6, 8]. Developmental defects of the ear are considered in detail on p. 218. Only those defects which are sufficiently common to constitute a part of general dermatological practice are therefore considered here, together with some general principles relating to congenital ear abnormalities and their more important medical and otological associations.

Pre-auricular pits, sinuses, tags and other malformations of the pinna are relatively common, with an incidence of approximately 1% [6, 8]. Abnormal or low-set ears occur as an inconstant feature in many genetically determined and congenital syndromes. Minor variations in size and shape of the pinna are common and are not usually associated with any other abnormality. These include 'bat ear', 'lop ear', a prominent Darwin's tubercle and variations in the shape or contour of the helix or antihelix as in 'Mozart's ear' and 'Wildermuth's ear'. Accessory auricles occur as small firm elevations of skin and cartilage just anterior to the tragus or ascending crus of the helix. They may be single or multiple and may occur anywhere in a line from the tragus to the angle of the mouth. Accessory auricles, congenital fistulae and other external ear manifestations may occur alone or may be associated with more widespread first and second branchial arch abnormalities [3, 6, 8] or with developmental abnormalities of the genito-urinary tract [7].

Sebaceous cysts, often multiple, occur on the lobe and on the posterior auricular skin, and epidermoid cysts and haemangiomas are also fairly common.

Congenital ear abnormalities exhibit great variability, even within syndromes or families, and any one aetiological factor may be associated with a variety of ear malformations. Syndromic external ear malformations usually account for less than 10% of all external ear abnormalities; isolated cases of ear malformation may therefore be either non-genetic in origin or associated with poor gene penetrance [8].

The dermatological associations of external ear malformation include haemangiomas, pigmented naevi, café-au-lait spots and leucoderma. External ear malformations are also commonly associated with hearing loss, usually conductive [4], which may in some instances involve the 'non-affected' rather than the 'affected' side.

Many syndromes are associated with small ears (microtia) [1] including Down's syndrome, the Treacher–Collins syndrome (p. 216), oculo-auriculo-vertebral dysplasias (p. 217) and Apert's syndrome (p. 160). More severe degrees of microtia may be associated with atresia [5] of the ear canal.

A distinctive 'railroad track' abnormality with marked prominence of the crus of the helix is said to occur in up to 30% of children with foetal alcohol syndrome [1] and a protruding auricle may, rarely, be a sign of neuromuscular disease [10]. Hypertrichosis of the ears may occur in infants born of diabetic mothers [9, 11].

REFERENCES

1 AASE J.M. (1980) In *Birth Defects: Original Article Series*, March of Dimes Birth Defects Foundation. New York, Alan R. Liss Vol. XVI, p. 289.

2 ANSON B. J. & DONALDSON J. A. (1973) In *Surgical Anatomy of the Temporal Bone and Ear*. Part II. *The Ear: Developmental Anatomy*. 2nd ed. Philadelphia, W. B. Saunders.

3 BELLUCCI R. J. (1981) *Congenital Aural Malformations: Diagnosis and Treatment: Symp on Congenital Disorders in Otolaryngology*. In *Otolaryngol Clin North Am* **14**, 95.

4 JAFFE B. F. (1976) *Pediatrics* **57**, 332.

5 JAHRSDOERFER R. A. (1978) *Laryngoscope* **88** (Suppl. 13), No. 9, Part III.

6 MELNICK M. (1980) In *Birth Defects: Original Article Series*, March of Dimes Birth Defect Foundation. New York, Alan R. Liss, Vol. XVI, No. 4, p. 303.

7 MELNICK M. (1980) In *Birth Defects: Original Article Series*, March of Dimes Birth Defect Foundation. New York, Alan R. Liss, Vol. XVI, No. 7, p. 59.

8 MELNICK M. & MYRIANTHOPOULOS N. C. (1979) In *Birth Defects: Original Article Series*, March of Dimes Birth Defect Foundation. New York, Alan R. Liss, Vol. XV, No. 9.

9 RAFAAT M. (1981) *Pediatrics* **68**, 745.

10 SMITH D. W. & TAKASHIMA H. (1978) *Lancet* i, 747.

11 WOODS D. L., *et al* (1980) *S Afr Med J* **58**, 441.

DISEASES AFFECTING THE PINNA, EXTERNAL AUDITORY CANAL AND ADJACENT SKIN [1, 4, 8, 12]

Trauma. The exposed position of the ear makes it particularly vulnerable to trauma. Bruises, cuts and lacerations are common. Deep haematomas—occurring between the perichondrium and cartilage—may lead to cartilaginous necrosis and distortion ('cauliflower ear') if not managed correctly or if the trauma is frequent or repeated, as in boxers, rugby football players, etc. Subperichondrial haematomas must therefore be incised and drained early and a pressure dressing applied if permanent damage is to be avoided. Full aseptic technique is necessary in view of the risk of secondary perichondritis; prophylactic antibiotics are also sometimes given.

Perichondritis can occur as a result of injury or trauma. It may follow haematomas, lacerations or surgery or result from pressure by tightly fitting headphones or headgear. It has also been described as an industrial hazard from irritant chemicals [7].

The ears are extremely susceptible to cold and the pinna may be affected by chilblains in winter. Extreme cold will cause frostbite (see p. 624). This may result in vesiculation, blisters and ischaemic necrosis of both skin and cartilage. Ears that have been affected by cold should be allowed to warm slowly and gently (38–42 °C). Analgesics are often required. Cold is also a provoking factor in patients with 'juvenile spring eruption', nodular chondrodermatitis helicis, chilblain lupus erythematosus and in those with cryoglobulinaemia. Ears that have previously been damaged by cold may subsequently become calcified. 'Frostbite' has also been reported as a consequence of using excessive amounts of ethyl chloride spray for ear piercing [10].

Most other forms of trauma to the external ear tend to be either artefactual or iatrogenic. Ear piercing may lead to infection, cheloid formation or contact dermatitis due to nickel studs or 'sleepers'. Complications occurred in 34% of people who had had their ears pierced in one survey [2] and a new spring-gun technique has recently been reported to have caused embedding of the studs in the ear lobe in some patients [3]. Rupture of the tympanic membrane and acquired atresia of the external auditory canal are usually the result of surgery, trauma [6], injudicious 'fiddling' or over-zealous attempts to remove foreign bodies or impacted cerumen [13]. Contractures of the external auditory meatus may also follow burns [11].

Foreign bodies in the ear are more common in children. If external to the isthmus they may be recovered by hook or forceps or by syringe or sucker. This is generally best performed by a specialist in the field. Insects can be first killed by drowning or by the installation of ether, chloroform or spirit and then removed by forceps or syringe [14]. Flies may even deposit their eggs in the ear and the resulting myiasis will lead to pain and inflammation and, occasionally, more severe complications [9]. Impacted cerumen is a frequent cause of irritation; conversely, too little cerumen, especially in women, may also cause pruritus. Recently [11] attention has been drawn to the problems arising from excessive use of cotton buds for cleaning or scratching the ear. The use of matches or nickel clips may cause a continuing contact dermatitis (p. 2137).

Loose hairs in the ear canal have been reported as a cause of noise in the ear [5] and foreign bodies should always be looked for whenever there is pain, inflammation or infection of the external auditory canal.

REFERENCES

1 *BALLENTYNE J. & GROVES J. (Eds.) (1982) *Scott-Brown's Diseases of the Ear, Nose and Throat.* 4th ed. London, Butterworth.
2 BIGGAR R.J. & HAUGHIE G.E. (1975) *NY State J Med* **75**, 1460.
3 COCKIN J., *et al* (1977) *Br Med J* ii, 1631.
4 *CODY D.T.R., *et al* (eds.) (1981) *Diseases of the Ears, Nose and Throat: A Guide to Diagnosis and Management.* Chicago, Year Book Medical Publishers.
5 GOLDMAN G. & TOHER L. (1982) *N Engl J Med* **306**, 1553.
6 HABERMAN R.S. & WERTH J.L. (1981) *Am J Otol* **2**, 269.
7 LIVERLSLEY B. & LAMBALLE J. (1967) *J Laryngol Otol* **81**, 1063.
8 MAWSON S.R. & LUDMAN H. (1979) *Diseases of the Ear: A Textbook of Otology.* 4th ed. London, Arnold.
9 MENDIVIL J.A. & EL SHAMMAA N.A. (1979) *Milit Med* **144**, 261.
10 NOBLE D.A. (1979) *Br Med J* i, 125.
11 ROBERTSON M.S. (1977) *NZ Med J* **86**, 102.
12 *SENTURIA B.H., *et al* (1981) *Diseases of the External Ear: An Otologic—Dermatological Manual.* 2nd ed. New York, Grune-Stratton.
13 SILVERSTEIN H., *et al* (1973) *Trans Am Acad Ophthalmol Otolaryngiol* **77**, 125.
14 SUCHARIT S. (1981) *J Med Assoc Thai* **64**, 96.

Chondrodermatitis nodularis helicis (painful nodule of the ear) [4, 14]. This not uncommon and painful condition of the pinna affects mainly middle-aged or elderly men.

Aetiology [2, 12, 15]. The principal factors in its pathogenesis are pressure and a compromised local blood supply [19]. It is more common in patients who habitually sleep on one side at night but can be triggered off by other factors including cold or pressure from headgear [18]; women are normally protected by their longer hair [3]. The age of onset is over 40 in 70% of cases. We have only once

encountered it in a patient under 20, a boy whose father and uncle were similarly affected. Once started, the condition tends to recur following even the slightest trauma [4]. The changes in the cartilage are probably secondary to foci of degeneration and inflammation of the dermis.

Pathology [7, 10, 15]. A typical lesion of chondrodermatitis nodularis helicis consists of a nodule of degenerate, homogeneous collagen surrounded by vascular granulation tissue [9, 12] with an overlying acanthotic epidermis and a central ulcer through which the damaged dermal collagen is extruded [6, 9]. The glomus-like proliferation of vascular tissue that occurs in this condition explains the exquisite tenderness of many lesions [14]. Many researchers now regard chondrodermatitis nodularis helicis as a perforating dermatitis with transepidermal elimination of damaged collagen or as the inflammatory reaction to a penetrating corn or callus [16].

Clinical features. The patient, usually a middle-aged to elderly man, seeks advice on account of pain. The more stoical may postpone consultation until lesions interfere with sleep. The pain, which is sometimes severe, is initiated by pressure and occasionally by cold. It may be brief but can persist and throb for an hour or more. Occasionally, and particularly in women, there is little discomfort. The lesion is a globular or oval nodule, about 0·5–2 cm in diameter, raised above the often hyperaemic surrounding skin (Fig. 56.1). The surface is frequently scaly or crusted, concealing a small ulcer.

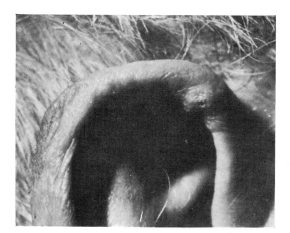

FIG. 56.1. Chondrodermatitis nodularis, showing the typical nodule on the rim of the helix (Addenbrooke's Hospital).

In men nearly 90% of nodules are situated on the helix, usually at the upper pole and more frequently on the right [3], but they may occur on the anti-helix, tragus, concha and antitragus, in order of decreasing frequency. Occasionally, there are multiple nodules. In women, the left and right ears are affected equally and the proportion of lesions on the antihelix and tragus is greater [18]. The nodules attain a maximum size in a few months and then remain unchanged indefinitely.

Diagnosis. Although the associated pain and tenderness are characteristic, this lesion is often surprisingly misdiagnosed. The degree of epithelial hyperplasia may lead to an erroneous biopsy report of a squamous cell carcinoma.

Treatment [2, 8, 19, 20]. Excision, with a margin of normal skin, is the treatment of choice [1, 15] and is easily carried out under local anaesthetic. It should be carried out carefully and gently, for the trauma of operation may induce the formation of a new nodule. A narrow ellipse of skin containing the lesion allows the nodule and the affected subjacent cartilage to be 'scalloped out' with ease. In more severe or recurrent cases a larger section of the helix may have to be removed. Early lesions may be successfully treated with intralesional steroids [16]. In all patients efforts must be made to reduce pressure or trauma to the helix.

Perichondritis of the tragus [11]. Coarse terminal hairs which develop on the tragus in some middle-aged men may give rise to an irritative perichondritis.

REFERENCES

1 BARKER L.P., *et al* (1960) *Arch Dermatol* **81**, 53.
2 COHEN E.L. (1966) In *Modern Trends in Dermatology*, Series 3. Ed. Mackenna R.M.B. London, Butterworth.
3 Cutrone P. (1970) *G Ital Dermatol Minerva Dermatol* **45**, 576.
4 FORSTER O.H. (1925) *Arch Dermatol Syphil* **11**, 149.
5 GARCIA E., *et al* (1980) *J Dermatol Surg Oncol* **6**, 582.
6 GOETTE D.K. (1980) *J Am Acad Dermatol* **2**, 148.
7 HABER H. (1960) *Hautarzt* **11**, 122.
8 KINGERY F.A.J. (1966) *JAMA* **197**, 137.
9 LEONFORTE J.E. (1979) *Ann Dermatol Vénéréol* **106**, 577.
10 LEVER W.F. & SCHAUMBERG-LEVER G. (1983) *Histopathology of the Skin*. 6th ed. Philadelphia, Lippincott oo.
11 MARURI C.A. (1954) *Actas Dermo-Sifilogr* **44**, 194.
12 NEWCOMER V.D., *et al* (1953) *Arch Dermatol Syphil* **68**, 241.
13 POTH D.O. (1937) *Tex State J Med* **33**, 19.
14 SANTA CRUS D.J. (1980) *J Cutan Pathol* **7**, 70.
15 SHUMAN R. & HELWIG E.B. (1954) *Am J Clin Pathol* **24**, 127.
16 WADE T.R. (1979) *Cutis* **24**, 406.
17 WINKLER M. (1916) *Arch Dermatol Syphil* **121**, 278.
18 YAFFEE H.S. (1963) *Arch Dermatol* **87**, 735.
19 ZIMMERMAN M.C. (1958) *Arch Dermatol* **78**, 41.
20 ZIMMERMAN M.C. (1977) In *Skin Surgery*, Ed. Epstein E. 4th ed. Springfield, Thomas.

Infections. The anatomy of the ear with its many folds and the semioccluded nature of the external auditory canal make it particularly susceptible to intertriginous infection, especially with Gram-negative organisms. The close anatomical relationship between the middle and external ear means that infections can pass relatively easily from one to the other and the ear drum should always be examined.

Acute infections of the pinna are relatively uncommon. *Staphylococcus pyogenes*, alone or in association with group A β-haemolytic *streptococcus*, may cause *impetigo contagiosum* of the ear or, more frequently, a retro-auricular bacterial intertrigo, furunculosis or otitis externa. Secondary bacterial infection also frequently complicates ear piercing. *Furunculosis*, when it occurs in the external auditory canal, is extremely painful since the epidermis is bound down tightly to the perichondrium and there is thus little room for expansion. Gram-negative infections, especially those due to *Pseudomonas aeruginosa*, are a particular problem among swimmers [6] and divers [1]. Otitis externa is discussed in more detail on p. 2139.

Cracks and fissures around the auricle are often the portal of entry for acute or recurrent attacks of cellulitis of the face. Fissuring of the auriculofacial notch is common in children. Some are atopics, others obligate staphylococcal carriers, but the condition can occur in the absence of either of these conditions. Fissures may become secondarily eczematized or infected.

Treatment consists of careful washing and drying to prevent the retention of excess soap or moisture and the application of a suitable antibacterial, antibiotic or steroid-antibacterial cream or ointment. *Infective eczematoid dermatitis* commonly affects the postauricular fold and is often associated with fissures. It occurs in atopics and in those suffering from seborrhoeic dermatitis but may occur in a localized form on its own. Patients with recurrent staphylococcal problems should have their urine checked for sugar and both they and their family should have nasal and skin swabs taken to try to identify and eradicate occult staphylococcal carriage.

Streptococcal cellulitis, typically, is ushered in by

rigors and fever and the ear becomes hot, red, swollen and painful. There is often associated lymphadenopathy and infection may spread to involve the ipsilateral eyelid and cheek. Recurrent attacks of cellulitis lead to tissue fibrosis and lymphoedema. Treatment is as for streptococcal cellulitis elsewhere; antibiotics must be given early (preferably intramuscularly or intravenously initially) and in sufficient dosage if lymphoedema is to be avoided. Management of infective eczematoid dermatitis involves treatment of both the infection and the eczema. Steroid-antibacterial preparations are commonly used. Antiseptic wet compresses and systemic antibiotics may be required in the acute phase.

Otomycosis is common in the tropics and subtropics because of the high humidity and the warm moist environment. It should also be suspected in cases of chronic or 'resistant' otitis externa, especially when these have been treated with multiple antibiotics [5]. The principal symptom is usually itching without much evidence of inflammation and the ear may be plugged with white debris (*Candida*) or a matt of mycelium (*Aspergillus fumigatus*, *Aspergillus niger*, *Penicillium* or *Mucor*). Treatment consists of good ear toilet and measures to try to improve the ventilation and reduce the maceration of the external auditory canal. Specific treatment consists of either nystatin drops or powder, aniline dyes or one of the newer imidazole preparations.

Herpes simplex ('scrum-pox') [4] occasionally involves the ear. It is often transmitted during contact sports such as rugby and wrestling. A bullous or haemorrhagic otitis externa or myringitis also sometimes occurs as a complication of acute viral or influenzal illnesses. The tympanic membrane, however, may become non-specifically inflamed and thickened in any upper respiratory tract infection.

Herpes auricularis (*Herpes Zoster otiticus*; *Ramsay Hunt's syndrome*; *Geniculate herpes*) may present as an isolated herpetiform eruption of the external ear or may be associated with ipsilateral facial palsy and auditory symptoms. The condition usually begins with pain and may initially be mistaken for erysipelas. Vesicles usually appear on about the fifth day and involve the auricle, the external auditory meatus and, rarely, the tympanic membrane. There is usually malaise, pyrexia and lymphadenopathy. Facial palsy, when it occurs, is usually transient but more severe and persistent cases do occur. Taste and lacrimation may also be affected. Compression damage to the VIIIth cranial nerve may lead to tinnitus, vertigo, nystagmus, nausea and deafness. Symptomatic treatment with or without topical idoxuridine is all that is required in mild cases. In cases where there is compression of the VIIth or VIIIth cranial nerves, prednisolone may be given. The role of acyclovir in this condition remains to be determined but, if given early, it would no doubt hasten resolution and might reduce the incidence of neuralgic and post-herpetic complications.

The ears are nearly always involved in lepromatous leprosy and are the site of choice for bacterial examination and biopsy. Lupus vulgaris, although now rare in the Western World, also affects the ears. Fungal diseases [3, 8], which may at times mimic perichondritis [2], and syphilis, gonorrhoea [7] and many other infectious conditions may, incidentally, affect the pinna. These are considered in more detail elsewhere.

REFERENCES

1 ALCOCK S.R. (1977) *J Hyg (Cambridge)* **78**, 395.
2 BISHOP M. & RIST T.E. (1979) *Cutis* **23**, 638.
3 COX R.L. & RELLER L.B. (1979) *Arch Dermatol* **115**, 1229.
4 CUTLER T.P. (1980) *Br Med J* **281**, 808.
5 GREGSON A.E.W. & LA TOUCHE C.J. (1961) *J Laryngol Otol* **75**, 45.
6 HOADLEY A.W. & KNIGHT D.E. (1957) *Arch Environ Health* **30**, 445.
7 PAREEK S.S. (1979) *N Engl J Med* **300**, 1490.
8 VERBOV J. (1973) *Br J Dermatol* **89**, 212.

Chondritis and perichondritis. Acute perichondritis of the auricle is an occasional consequence of trauma to the pinna or external auditory canal. It may follow burns (both thermal and chemical) [2], frostbite or surgery, or develop as a late consequence of haematoma. It has also been reported following acupuncture [3]. Perichondritis sometimes follows superficial infections of the ear such as furunculosis or otitis externa, which can spread deeply to affect the perichondrium. Cartilage which has become exposed is particularly vulnerable. The most common infecting organism is usually *Ps. aeruginosa* although *Staphylococcus aureus* and other organisms may at times be responsible, e.g. *Pseudomonas pyocyanea* and *Proteus* sp., etc.

Clinically, the condition usually presents as a hot, painful, swollen ear with loss of normal contour due to oedema and accumulation of pus in the subperichondrial layer. The affected ear may appear protruberant as a result of oedema and inflammation. Constitutional symptoms are common. The condition must be differentiated from cellulitis of the auricle, which usually affects the lobe as well as the cartilaginous portions of the ear, and from relapsing polychondritis (p. 1856), which normally affects cartilage elsewhere and is usually recurrent.

Treatment. Treatment should not be delayed. Broad spectrum antibiotics or those with potential activity against Gram-negative organisms should be given until specific sensitivities are known. Frequent wet dressings are helpful and incision and drainage may be necessary if a subperiosteal abscess develops. Tubal drainage and irrigation are also then helpful [1]. In spite of these measures cartilaginous necrosis often occurs and necrotic or infected cartilage may then need to be excised. The overall cosmetic prognosis is poor.

REFERENCES

1 BASSIOUNY A. (1981) *Laryngoscope* **91**, 422.
2 LIVERSLEY B. & LAMBALLE J. (1967) *J Laryngol Otol* **81**, 1063.
3 TRAUTERMANN H.G. & TRAUTERMANN H. (1981) *HNO* **29**, 312.

Miscellaneous conditions

Relapsing polychondritis [1, 2, 7] (p. 1856). This rare disease is characterized by recurrent inflammation and destruction of cartilage and in most cases by pain and swelling of the pinnae with fever, arthralgia and a high ESR. The condition can usually be differentiated from perichondritis (p. 2136) by its relapsing course and the fact that cartilaginous structures elsewhere are usually involved. Anaemia, thrombophlebitis and toxic erythema may also occur [9]. In contrast with cellulitis and erysipelas of the ear (p. 2135), the lobes are spared. Recurrent attacks eventually give a characteristic floppiness to the ear [4]. Immunological factors are thought to be important in its pathogenesis [5, 7, 10, 11] and the disease may possibly represent an immunological sensitivity to native type II collagen [3, 8].

REFERENCES

1 *ATKIN C.R. & MASAI A.T. (1975) *Semin Arthritis Rheum* **5**, 41.
2 FOIDART J.M. & KATZ S.I. (1979) *Am J Dermatopathol* **1**, 257.
3 FOIDART J.M., *et al* (1978) *N Engl J Med* **299**, 1203.
4 GANGE R.W. (1976) *Clin Exp Dermatol* **1**, 261.
5 HASHIMOTO K., *et al* (1977) *Arthritis Rheum* **20**, 91.
6 LE CHARPENTIER Y., *et al* (1981) *Semin Hôp Paris* **17–18**, 879.
7 *McADAM L.P., *et al* (1976) *Medicine* **55**, 193.
8 McCUNE W.J., *et al* (1982) *Arthritis Rheum* **25**, 266.
9 ROWELL N.R. & COTTERILL J.A. (1973) *Br J Dermatol* **88**, 387.
10 SHANE S.R. & SCHUMACHER H.R. (1975) *Arthritis Rheum* **18**, 617.
11 VALENZUELA R., *et al* (1980) *Hum Pathol* **11**, 19.

Eczema, psoriasis and *acne* are three common conditions which frequently involve the pinna and external auditory meatus. The ear appears to be a favoured site, certainly as far as psoriasis and seborrhoeic dermatitis are concerned. In its mildest form *seborrhoeic dermatitis* simply causes a little scaling and inflammation at the entrance to the external auditory meatus, in the concha or in the auricular folds. When severe, the whole pinna may be affected and there may be infective eczematoid dermatitis both in and around the ear or postauricularly. The relationship between seborrhoeic dermatitis and otitis externa has already been discussed on p. 2135. *Psoriasis* may similarly affect the concha and distal part of the external auditory canal but usually its colour, the nature of the scaling and the presence of psoriasis elsewhere allow it to be differentiated. Sometimes both conditions appear to coexist. *Comedonal acne* frequently involves the concha and *acne cysts* may be found on the lobe, at the entrance to the external auditory canal and postauricularly. When in the external auditory canal they are often painful. Large cysts can be lanced and phenolized.

The ears may also be involved in *atopic eczema*. Retro-auricular infective eczematoid dermatitis or infected eczema of the tragal notch is a common finding in atopics; sometimes the ear may be diffusely involved. An eczematous rash in the superior retro-auricular area has also recently been reported to be a reliable sign of atopy in about 30% of children and occurs even in the absence of a previous history of atopic or seborrhoeic dermatitis or ichthyosis [30]. The external ear is commonly affected by allergic *contact dermatitis*: the lobe by nickel from earrings [12, 31], the helix and posterior aspects of the ear from hair dyes and the constituents of hairsprays and shampoos [7] and the concha by nail varnish.

Bathing caps, hair-nets, headgear, hearing-aids [14], glasses and telephone ear-pieces are less frequent but occasional causes of contact dermatitis. The problem of occult allergic contact dermatitis in patients with otitis externa is discussed on p. 2139). Topical medicaments in eardrops are a frequent cause of trouble [9]. The pinna is also involved in several *photodermatoses*. Actinic prurigo (Hutchinson's summer prurigo and spring eruption) commonly affects the ear (especially in the helical margins) in boys (p. 644) and photodermatitis and porphyria cutanea tarda (p. 2280) may also affect the exposed parts of the ear. Atrophy of the rims of the ear has been noted in patients with erythropoietic protoporphyria. *Lupus erythematosus* and *lymphocytic infiltration* may involve the pinna. Pits and scarring of the concha occur in lupus erythematosus [24, 26] and there may be atrophy of the lobe and even perforation of the pinna [18]. A particularly indolent form of scarring lupus erythematosus is sometimes seen peri-orificially on the face and this may affect the ear. Jessner-like infiltrations of the ear lobe and isolated lymphocytoma cutis-like lesions have also been reported [21].

Other miscellaneous conditions affecting the external ear include gouty tophi, now rare in Great Britain, and ochronosis which gives a characteristic slate-grey discoloration of the cartilage. '*Mudi-chood*' is a peculiar and persistent dermatosis affecting the nape of the neck and upper shoulders of girls and young women in the Kerala State of South India. It is thought to be the result of the frictional and occlusive effects of moist oily hair in a hot and humid environment. It has also been reported to occur on the ears [27]. Other reactive conditions include *ear lobe cheloids* (usually a consequence of ear piercing), split ear lobes [20], elephantiasis nostras verrucosa of the ears [13] and spectacle frame acanthomas [28] (p. 598).

Degenerative changes occur with age and include venous lakes and elastosis and calcification of the pinna and helix. *Elastotic nodules* of the antihelix and helix may also occur as a result of actinic damage [5, 32] and may at times be confused with chondrodermatitis nodularis helicis or basal cell carcinoma. *Pseudocysts of the auricle* have been reported in the Chinese [10].

The external ear may, rarely, act as a marker of *systemic disease*. Acrokeratosis paraneoplastica (Bazex' syndrome) commonly affects the ears and is a good indicator of internal malignancy [2]. *Diagonal ear lobe creases* are purported to be more common in patients with coronary artery disease [15, 17, 22, 23, 34]. *Ossification* of the auricular cartilage may occur in association with long-standing hypoadrenalism [6, 35] and the ears may be involved in *epidermolysis bullosa acquisita*.

Hypertrophy of the retro-auricular folds has also been reported as a consequence of diphenylhydantoin therapy [29]. *Ear lobe cheloids*—a common complication of ear piercing—are probably best treated by a combination of intralesional steroids and surgery [33]. The postoperative use of a pressure earring has been suggested to reduce the risk of recurrence [3].

Due to the complicated nerve supply to the ear (p. 2131) *referred pain* is commoner than pain due to lesions in the ear itself [25]. Non-otological causes of such pain include the otomandibular syndrome [1] due to dysfunction of the temporomandibular joint, cervical arthritis with involvement of the cervical nerve, tonsillitis and carcinoma of the pharynx. Psychogenic otalgia has also been reported [8].

REFERENCES

1 ARLEN H. (1978) *Ear Nose Throat J* **57**, 56.
2 BAZEX A. & GRIFFITHS W.A. (1980) *Br J Dermatol* **103**, 301.
3 BRENT B. (1978) *Ann Plast Surg* **1**, 579.
4 CALNAN C.D., *et al* (1958) *Br Med J* ii, 544.
5 CARTER V.H., *et al* (1969) *Arch Dermatol* **100**, 282.
6 CHADWICK J.M. & DOWNHAM T.F. (1978) *Int J Dermatol* **17**, 799.
7 CRONIN E. (1980) In *Contact Dermatitis*. Edinburgh, Churchill Livingstone, pp. 54, 153, 752, 761.
8 DIGHT R. (1980) *Med J Aust* i, 76.
9 DOOMS-GOOSENS A., *et al* (1979) *Acta Otorhinolaryngol Belg* **33**, 474.
10 ENGEL D. (1966) *Arch Otolaryngol* **83**, 29.
11 FRANK S.T. (1973) *N Engl J Med* **289**, 327.
12 GAUL C.E. (1967) *JAMA* **200**, 176.
13 GRANT J.M. (1982) *Cutis* **29**, **441**.
14 GUILL M.A. & ODOM R.B. (1978) *Arch Dermatol* **114**, 1050.
15 HAINES S.J. (1977) *N Engl J Med* **297**, 1181.
16 HINTER H., *et al* (1982) *Hautarzt* **33**, 310.
17 KAUKOLA S., *et al* (1979) *Lancet* ii, 1372.
18 LUCKY P.A. (1983) *Cutis* **32**, 554.
19 MARKS M.B., *et al* (1981) *J Am Acad Dermatol* **4**, 519.
20 MUNRO-ASHMAN D., *et al* (1975) *Contact Dermatitis* **1**, 393.
21 ODEHNAL F., *et al* (1981) *Cesk Otolaryngol* **30**, 366.
22 PASTERNAC A. & SAMI M. (1982) *Can Med Assoc J* **126**, 645.
23 PETRAKIS N. & KOO L. (1980) *Lancet* i, 376.
24 REBORA A. (1982) *Br J Dermatol* **106**, 122.
25 SHEIKHI A.R. (1980) *J Laryngol Otol* **94**, 1433.
26 SHUSTER S. (1981) *Br J Dermatol* **104**, 350.
27 SUGATHAN P. (1976) *Br J Dermatol* **95**, 197.
28 TENNSTEDT D. & LACHAPELLE J.M. (1979) *Ann Dermatol Vénéréol* **106**, 219.
29 TRUNNELL T.M. & WAISMAN M. (1982) *Cutis* **30**, 207.
30 VON MOSS M., *et al* (1982) *Dermatol Monatsschr* **168**, 394.
31 WAHT L. & BANMANN R.R. (1968) *Arch Dermatol* **98**, 155.
32 WEEDON D. (1981) *J Cutan Pathol* **8**, 429.
33 WEIMAR V.M. & CEILLEY R.I. (1979) *J Dermatol Surg Oncol* **5**, 522.
34 WYRE H.W. (1979) *Cutis* **79**, 328.
35 ZILLESSEN E., *et al* (1978) *Dtsch Med Wochenschr* **103**, 698.

EXTERNAL OTITIS [2, 26, 29, 30, 40]

Otitis externa is a loose term that embraces more than one disease process. Aetiologically, it is rarely unifactorial [30] and constitutional, traumatic, environmental and microbial factors usually coexist. The condition is characterised by scaling, thickening and oedema of the canal epithelium and by varying degress of pain, itch, deafness and discharge [28, 37].

Pathogenesis [30]. Otitis externa can be divided, for convenience, into two main groups [29]: a 'reactive' group consisting of patients suffering from eczema, psoriasis or seborrhoeic dermatitis and a predominantly 'infective' group in which either bacteria or fungi are involved; the two components often, however, coexist. Furunculosis (p. 2135), acute pyococcal infection (p. 2135) and viral infections (p. 2136) have already been dealt with elsewhere. The following predisposing factors appear to be important [30, 35]:

Genetic and constitutional. There are significant racial and individual differences in susceptibility to otitis externa. This may be due to anatomical differences in the curvature of the external auditory canal or narrowing of the isthmus—natives of New Guinea with wide, straight canals only rarely suffer from external otitis [38]—or, possibly, to differences in the type, amount or composition of cerumen [27, 33]. Abundant tragal hair or plugs of wax and debris increase the relative humidity and reduce ventilation of the external auditory canal so that the canal epithelium becomes macerated and more susceptible to infection. Dental abnormalities and poor mastication [13, 17] may also retard expulsion of wax and epithelial squames.

The atopic and seborrhoeic states predispose to external otitis not only by interfering with the integrity of the auricular epithelium but also by encouraging scratching and secondary infection [27]. Both too much and too little [3, 10, 31] cerumen and alterations in skin pH [37] have at times been held responsible.

Environmental. Heat, humidity and moisture are undoubtedly important in 'hot-weather ear' or 'swimmers' ear' [7, 48]. This condition is common, especially among Caucasians, in tropical and subtropical regions. High temperature, high relative humidity and swimming all encourage maceration and secondary bacterial or fungal infections of the canal epithelium. Failure to dry the ears completely after swimming, shampooing or showering may also be a factor in some cases.

Traumatic. Trauma, in the opinion of many investigators [27, 30, 43, 47], is one of the prime factors in both the initiation and the persistence of many cases. In one series of 113 patients, 58 admitted using wool-tipped matches, two admitted using bare matches and seven used hairgrips to relieve itching [30]. Patients suffering from eczema or those with neurodermatitis tend to scratch, rub or 'fiddle' with their ears; other patients appear obsessed about cleaning their ears and by doing so excessively they interfere with the normal homeostatic and self-cleaning properties [1]. Impacted cerumen may cause irritation, which is often increased by inexpert attempts to remove it; so may pressure from hearing-aids and transistor ear-pieces and, especially with the newer type of 'internal' hearing-aid, a combination of pressure and occlusion often leads to the development of external otitis.

Pyococcal and myotic infection. The epidermis of the external auditory canal is normally fairly resistant to infection and the bacterial flora, although varying with race, geography and season, usually resembles that of the skin [4, 42]. Potential pathogenic organisms are few and are found in only 5–30% of isolates [4, 26]. In hot humid environments, however, and particularly among swimmers, whose ears are habitually wet, the incidence of *Ps aeruginosa* and other Gram-negative infections rises substantially [21, 28, 38] as does the frequency with which *Aspergillus* or *Candida* is isolated [47]. An outbreak of *Pseudomonas* otitis has been reported in association with contaminated pool water [44] but a source has rarely been found in other series [28]. In tropical countries mycotic infections of the external ear canal are relatively common [3, 49]. *Aspergillus* [9, 19, 20, 24, 45, 48], *Candida* [12, 17, 19], *Penicillium* [20] and *Mucor* [9] are the species most often incriminated, most cases being due to either *A. niger* or *Candida albicans*. There is some debate, however, as to whether these fungi are pathogenic, opportunistic, saprophytic or simply commensal [19, 20, 26, 41, 49].

In more temperate climates *Staph. pyogenes* is the most common pathogen isolated [27, 30]. This may be associated with evidence of skin disease elsewhere or with staphylococcal carriage. Certainly, recurrent cases of staphylococcal otitis externa should have nasal and perianal swabs; occasionally it may be necessary to swab and 'destaph' the whole family. In other cases there may be an underlying tympanic perforation or coexistent otitis media. The ear drums should therefore always be examined, especially in patients with unilateral or recurrent disease. Occasionally, infection spreads out from the ear canal and causes impetigo or infective eczematoid dermatitis of the auricle and surrounding skin.

In non-tropical countries the incidence of *Candida* infection is usually less then 20% [19, 23] but more than 80 of 180 'selected' patients were found to be suffering from fungal infection in one series [19]. Many of these had been treated with repeated courses of antibiotics and the diagnosis should therefore be considered in any chronic or apparently 'resistant' case of otitis externa.

Histopathology [26, 34, 35]. In most cases of external otitis there is acanthosis, elongation of the rete ridges and an increase in orthokeratosis and parakeratosis. Spongiosis occurs in eczematous and seborrhoeic forms. The nature of the dermal infiltrate varies with both cause and chronicity of the lesion. The histopathology is seldom diagnostic except when fungal mycelia are seen.

Clinical features. Otitis externa may be localized, as in furunculosis, limited to the lateral or distal portion of the external auditory canal, as in uncomplicated eczema or psoriasis, or diffuse as in 'swimmers' ear' or 'hot-weather ear'. The condition can be acute, subacute or chronic. In patients seen at hospital it tends to be severe, chronic or chronic relapsing, but in the community it is less severe and recalcitrant [28, 36]. Mild attacks may present with pain or itching without discharge and with a minimally congested or swollen meatus. The degree of irritation or discomfort is often out of all proportion to the appearance. This stage probably represents early damage to the meatal skin [47]. Most cases of this type will resolve with simple therapeutic measures but a minority, perhaps due to trauma, secondary infection or failure to keep the ear dry and clean, progress to more chronic disease.

Diffuse otitis externa has been given many names including 'swimmers' ear', 'Hong Kong ear', 'Aden ear', etc. Once established, the condition tends to affect the whole length of the auditory canal and *Pseudomonas* or fungal infection is common, especially in the tropics and subtropics and in those whose meatal epithelium has become macerated from swimming. Hot climatic conditions, sand, dust, trauma and high relative humidity may all be important. 'Swimmers' ear' is particularly prevalent during the summer months [28]. The condition is often bilateral. In unilateral cases, or in severe and recurrent disease, the ear should always be checked for the presence of tympanic perforation or underlying middle ear disease. A particularly heavy and malodorous discharge raises the possibility of cholesteatoma (p. 2147). Diffuse otitis may be associated with fever, malaise and localized abscess formation as well as cervical and preauricular and postauricular lymphadenopathy.

In patients with external otitis the canal epithelium may show all changes, from a mild erythema with desquamation to gross oedema, exudation and granulation, with bleeding at the slightest trauma. In *furunculosis* and *acute otitis*, owing to the close approximation of skin and perichondrium, the pain may be such as to prohibit full examination. Infection of the pinna and surrounding skin may also be present. Patients with multiple or recurrent furunculosis should have their urine checked for sugar.

Seborrhoeic dermatitis, atopic dermatitis and psoriasis usually occur only at the meatus but may sometimes extend further into the canal. *Seborrhoeic otitis externa* is extremely common and has been regarded by some dermatologists as the basis for most cases of otitis externa. The symptoms and signs, however, are normally mild unless complicated by secondary factors and usually consist of no more than superficial scaling and a little discomfort or itching. Signs of pityriasis capitis or of seborrhoeic dermatitis elsewhere are usually present. The condition may deteriorate at times of stress or fatigue. Secondary bacterial infection is common. In this 'reactive' group the appearance is often that of of a dermatitis 'spreading into the ear' in contrast with those cases with a primarily 'infective' aetiology where infection and/or inflammation often appears to be 'spreading out from the ear' and where the entire length of the canal is often affected. The clinical appearance, however, is often non-diagnostic.

In *infective eczematoid dermatitis* there is usually intense pruritus associated with exudative dermatitis. The condition may complicate both otitis media and otitis externa and is usually associated with some degree of otorrhoea. In others it appears to develop from seborrhoeic dermatitis which has become secondarily infected. The condition may affect the meatus, concha, lobe and periauricular skin and often spreads widely. The postauricular fold is commonly affected. The symptoms and signs are those of eczema with an accompanying or preceding aural discharge. In seborrhoeic individuals other areas may be involved at the same time. Fissures and cellulitis are common complications.

Contact dermatitis is often occult [22] and easily overlooked. Sensitivity to topically applied medicaments is common in chronic otitis externa. Occlusion, the recurrent nature of the disease and frequent usage of antibiotics on an already damaged skin probably account for the high incidence of contact dermatitis at this site. Other sensitivities include nickel from hair pins, metal implements, etc., chromate [16, 30] and phosphorus sesquisulphide [25, 30] in matches, and nail varnish [11]. It is characteristic that the degree of itching and burning is often markedly out of proportion to the amount of erythema and oedema present. Clinically, it is often difficult to differentiate neurodermatitis from contact dermatitis.

Lichen simplex (neurodermatitis) may be localized to one area of the meatus or may occur more diffusely over the tragus, triangular fossa and adjoining skin. The condition is usually diagnosed by the history rather than the signs. Itching is intense, though often intermittent. The need to scratch or rub is compulsive, though often denied. Signs of inflammation are often minimal, although some degree of oedema and scaling is common. Complications from trauma, infection and sensitization are frequent. Intermittent itching of the external auditory canal—*non-specific external otitis* [26]—can also occur, irregularly and over a long period, without any obvious cause and with minimal signs of disease.

Whatever the primary aetiology, with the passage of time chronic external otitis becomes an increasingly complex diagnostic and therapeutic problem.

Differential diagnosis. The part played by trauma, environment, infection, sensitization and altered physiology and anatomy must be assessed and evaluated as accurately as possible. Difficulties often arise in the interpretation of bacteriological and mycological findings. 'Hearing-aid dermatitis' is more often due to traumatic and physical factors than to allergic sensitivity. Antibiotics, especially when prescribed in combination with corticosteroids, may cause occult sensitivity and are one cause of chronicity. The importance of perineal and nasal transfer of infection should not be underestimated and mechanical interference with the external auditory canal in patients with otitis externa tends to be the rule rather than the exception.

External otitis is unlikely to be confused with any other condition except perhaps psoriasis and eczema and these, of course, may coexist. Middle ear disease, past and present, should always be excluded.

Swabs should always be taken for bacteriological culture and epithelial debris examined and sent for mycological culture. Potassium hydroxide preparations showing evidence of epithelial invasion with hyphae are probably more important in this respect than a positive culture, which may simply indicate commensal or saprophytic infection. In any long-standing or 'resistant' case, patch testing with a special 'ear battery' [22] should be undertaken to rule out unsuspected contact dermatitis. If there is excess granulation, middle ear disease should be ruled out, and if the patient is diabetic, debilitated, very young, elderly or immunosuppressed then *malignant otitis externa* must also be excluded.

Complications. In 'resistant' cases, otomycosis, contact dermatitis (especially to medicaments), neurodermatitis and secondary traumatization must be excluded. Recurrent otitis externa may also develop into hypertrophic otitis externa or *localized elephantiasis nostras* [18] of the ears as a result of the effects of chronic lymphatic obstruction. The resultant narrowing of the external acoustic canal coupled with the underlying lymphoedema makes recurrent and repeated infections even more likely.

Secondary trauma. Once an irritable focus occurs in the canal, energetic attempts to remove wax or debris or to satisfy the urge to rub or scratch the infected area often intensify the inflammation. Cotton buds, although frequently regarded as safe, are a common cause of tympanic perforation [39].

Secondary sensitization. This is usually a consequence of treatment or a reaction to objects placed in the ear to alleviate itching. Therapeutic agents may therefore enhance and perpetuate the condition for which they were prescribed. Penicillin, neomycin, framycetin (Soframycin) and chloramphenicol are all well-known topical sensitizers but even gentamicin, Vioform (chinoform), polymyxin and bacitracin may sensitize at times [11, 22]. Sensitivity to nail varnish may be misconstrued as lichen simplex and, in women who are nickel sensitive, otitis externa may be aggravated by using metal objects to alleviate itching or to clear the ear. Otoscopes themselves may release nickel. Another source of contact dermatitis is chromate [16, 30] or phosphorus sesquisulphide [25, 30] in match-heads which some people use to scratch their ears.

Allergic and 'ide' reactions [5, 26]. A few well-documented cases have been reported in which recurrent pruritus, oedema and scaling of the ear canal have occurred with or without involvement of the hands or other areas in response to fungal infections elsewhere or with food or drug allergies.

Treatment. The general principles of treatment are to relieve pain, to reduce itching, to prevent trauma and to avoid known or potential sensitizers. Significant infective components should be identified and treated appropriately. Many mild cases of otitis externa will respond to simple aural toilet, antiseptic wicks and the use of appropriate antiseptic or antibiotic drops. When there is coexistent eczema, combined steroid-antiseptic or steroid-antibiotic drops or wicks can be used. It should be noted, however, that many of the common infecting organisms are frequently antibiotic resistant and swabs for culture and sensitivity should therefore be taken before prescribing topical or systemic antibiotics. In chronic cases a great variety of treatments will already have been given and medicament contact dermatitis will therefore be more likely. Since this is often 'occult', patch testing should be done in all patients with chronic disease.

Pain is often severe, especially with furunculosis and acute staphylococcal infections, and strong analgesics may be required. Local heat also often helps. Bed rest and daily wicks or dressings may be needed in the more severe case. Oral antibiotics may be given if necessary once sensitivities are known.

Topical treatment. This is the essential part of therapy and the most difficult to carry out satisfactorily. Eardrops are of less value than regular cleaning of the ear, and this initially needs to be done daily by a doctor or an experienced nurse. Less severe cases may be treated once a week. Having cleaned the ear of debris and wax, a wick may be inserted or the patient instructed to apply eardrops regularly. When the cartilaginous portion of the canal alone is involved, the patient can be shown how to apply the prescribed medicament by holding a loose wool-tipped orange stick 2·5 cm from its end and inserting this until his fingers touch the tragus.

If wax is impacted this can be softened with oil, glycerine or sodium bicarbonate eardrops (BPC) and then removed either manually or by syringing as long as the drum can be visualized and there is no perforation. Obstinate cases should be referred to an otologist. Some proprietary cerumenolytics are irritant and should be left in the ear for only 15–30 min before syringing.

In most chronic or complicated cases, treatment must be continued regularly for some weeks after apparent cure. Care must be taken to prevent cross-infection from other body sites, especially the anterior vestibule of the nose and the perineum, and the ear should be kept as dry and as clean as possible. A very large number of medicaments have been used in the treatment of otitis externa. Alcohol 70–85% (isopropyl alcohol), 1–2% acetic acid, aluminium subacetate solution and 2% salicylic acid in 60% spirit [14] are all safe and useful. Wicks

with 8–13% aluminium acetate, $\frac{1}{4}$–$\frac{1}{2}$% silver nitrate or glycerine and ichthyol are used to treat hypertrophic otitis externa. Wicks may also be impregnated with corticosteroids. Although the use of corticosteroids in the form of lotions, paints, creams and ointments is a common practice, the choice of an associated bacterial agent is more difficult. Neomycin, framycetin (Soframycin), gentamicin and polymyxin are probably acceptable as short-term treatments for acute otitis externa but the risk of sensitization and cross-sensitization increases with more protracted usage. For patients with chronic or chronic relapsing otitis externa, iodochlohydroxyquinoline (Vioform, chinoform) can be used alone or in combination with corticosteroids (Remotic, Locorten-Vioform). This has a broad range of action but sensitivity can still occur and a recent study found it effective in only 66% of patients [8]. Old remedies such as the aniline dyes 0·5–1% in 70% spirit (e.g. gentian violet) are still very useful.

The imidazoles have largely replaced nystatin and amphotericin as antifungal agents since they are active against *Aspergillus* as well as *Candida* but acetic acid, boric acid and 25% *m*-cresyl acetate may still at times be useful: 2% salicylic acid in spirit [14] is a useful prophylaxis. 2·5% ammonium mercury ointment is still occasionally used and is both antibacterial and antifungal but there is a risk of both sensitization and nephrotoxicity.

Several eardrops, e.g. the aminoglycosides, chlorhexidine, polymyxin and chloramphenicol, are potentially ototoxic [6, 32] and should be avoided in the presence of tympanic perforation.

Wright [46] has recently reviewed the choice of antimicrobial agents. Eardrops containing polymyxin or colistin in combination with neomycin [15] will cover most of the common infecting organisms but regular ear toilet and antiseptic drops or wicks are preferred for those with chronic disease.

In all cases of external otitis, treatment should be prolonged beyond the time of apparent recovery and patients should be advised how best to avoid recurrence and about the dangers of indiscriminate or prolonged self-medication. There appears to be little indication for the use of preparations containing topical antihistamines or local anaesthetics.

REFERENCES

1 ALBERTI P.W.R.M. (1964) *J Laryngol* **78**, 808.
2 *BALLANTYNE J. & GROVES J. (Eds.) (1982) *Scott-Brown's Diseases of the Ear, Nose and Throat*. 4th ed. London, Butterworth.
3 BEANEY G.R.E. & BROUGHTON A. (1967) *J Laryngol Otol* **81**, 987.

4 BROOK I. (1981) *Acta Otolaryngol (Stockh)* **91**, 285.

5 BROWN W.H. (1948) *Br J Dermatol* **60**, 81.

6 BRUMMETT R.E., *et al* (1976) *Laryngoscope* **82**, 1177.

7 CALDERON R. & MOOD E.W. (1982) *Arch Environ Health* **37**, 300.

8 CASSISI N., *et al* (1977) *Ann Otol Rhinol Laryngol* [*Suppl.* 39] **86**, 1.

9 CHISHOLM J.J. & SUTTON A.C. (1925) *Arch Otolaryngol* **2**, 543.

10 CONLEY J.J. (1948) *Arch Otolaryngol* **47**, 721.

11 CRONIN E. (1980) *Contact Dermatitis*. Edinburgh, Churchill Livingstone, p. 153.

12 DAGGETT W.I. (1942) *J Laryngol Otol* **57**, 427.

13 DUNN B. (1962) *J Laryngol* **76**, 981.

14 ELLIOTT D.H. & HEAD P.W. (1974) *Br Med J* **iii**, 523.

15 FAIRBANKS D.N.F. (1981) *Ear Nose Throat J* **60**, 64.

16 FREGERT S. (1962) *Acta Derm Venereol (Stockh)* **42**, 473.

17 GORDON A.T. (1948) *Bull US Army Med Dept* **8**, 245.

18 GRANT J.M. (1982) *Cutis* **29**, 441.

19 GREGSON A.E.W. & LA TOUCHE C.J. (1961) *J Laryngol* **75**, 45.

20 HALEY L.D. (1950) *Arch Otolaryngol* **52**, 208.

21 HOADLEY A.W. & KNIGHT D.E. (1975) *Arch Environ Health* **30**, 445.

22 HOLMES R.C., *et al* (1982) *J R Soc Med* **75**, 27.

23 HURLEY R. & WINNER H.I. (1966) *Dermatol Int* **5**, 151.

24 ISMAIL H.K. (1962) *J Laryngol* **76**, 713.

25 IVE F.A. (1967) *Trans St John's Hosp Dermatol Soc* **53**, 135.

26 *JONES E.H. (1965) *External Otitis*. Springfield, Thomas.

27 KEOGH C. & RUSSELL B. (1956) *Br Med J* **i**, 1068.

28 LAMBERT I.J. (1981) *J R Coll Gen Pract* **31**, 291.

29 *MAWSON S.R. & LUDMAN H. (Eds.) (1979) *Diseases of the Ear*. 4th ed. London, Arnold.

30 *McKELVIE M. & McKELVIE P. (1966) *Br J Dermatol* **78**, 227.

31 McLAURIN J.W., *et al* (1965) *Laryngoscope* **75**, 1699.

32 MITTLEMAN H. (1977) *Trans Am Acad Ophthalmol Otolaryngol* **76**, 1432.

33 ONO T., *et al* (1981) *J Dermatol* **8**, 75.

34 PERRY E.T. (1957) *The Human Ear Canal*. Springfield, Thomas.

35 PETERKIN G.A.G. (1974) *J Laryngol* **88**, 15.

36 PRICE J. (1976) *J R Coll Gen Pract* **26**, 610.

37 PULLEN F.W. (1964) *Eye Ear Nose Throat Mon* **43**, 38.

38 QUAYLE A.F. (1944) *Med J Aust* **2**, 228.

39 ROBERTSON M.S. (1977) *NZ Med J* **86**, 103.

40 SENTURIA B.H., *et al* (1981) *Diseases of the External Ear: An Otologic-dermatological Manual*. 2nd ed. New York, Grune-Stratton.

41 SMYTH G.D.L. (1964) *Br J Dermatol* **76**, 425.

42 STEWART J.P. (1951) *J Laryngol* **65**, 24.

43 SYLVERTON J.J., *et al* (1946) *Arch Otolaryngol* **43**, 213.

44 WEINGARTEN M.A. (1977) *J R Coll Gen Pract* **27**, 359.

45 WOLF F.I. (1947) *Arch Otolaryngol* **46**, 361.

46 WRIGHT D.J.M. (1978) In *Recent Advances in Otolaryngology*, No. 5. Eds. Bull T.R., Ramsone and Holden. Edinburgh, Churchill Livingstone, p. 211.

47 WRIGHT D.N. & ALEXANDER J.M. (1974) *Arch Otolaryngol* **99**, 15.

48 YASSIN A., *et al* (1964) *J Laryngol* **8**, 591.

49 YOUSSEF Y.A. & ABDOU M.H. (1967) *J Laryngol Otol* **81**, 401.

INVASIVE EXTERNAL OTITIS [*5] ('MALIGNANT' EXTERNAL OTITIS [*2])

This severe, progressive and destructive otitis [9] usually presents with pain, tenderness and purulent discharge and with excessive granulation tissue at the junction of the cartilaginous and osseous parts of the external auditory canal. The condition characteristically occurs in elderly diabetics [2] but has also been reported in children [4, 7], in association with diabetes insipidus [6] and in the immuno-suppressed [17]. Abnormalities of cellular immunity and polymorphonuclear function have been described [3, 16]. The infecting organism is usually *Ps. pyocyanea* but predisposing factors are obviously important [15]. It is now thought that in most cases acellular necrosis of cartilage rather than infection by opportunistic organisms is the primary event [10]. Many patients are diabetics with long-standing disease, and microangiopathy of the skin of the external auditory canal may well be the initial pathogenetic factor [5]. The resultant infective and destructive granuloma invades widely, involving adjacent soft tissue and bone, and often leads to parotitis, mastoiditis, cranial nerve palsies, meningitis and death [11]. Neurological complications are associated with a grave prognosis [5].

Differential diagnosis. This includes necrotizing otitis media due to β-haemolytic streptococcal or *Str. pneumoniae* infection and, in the tropics, *Corynebacterium diphtheriae* infection [1].

Treatment. Treatment is with systemic antibiotics in full dosage, as for osteomyelitis. Drugs with presumed activity against *Pseudomonas* should be used initially until culture and sensitivities are known. The initial use of an aminoglycoside and a semi-synthetic penicillin appears to be better than one antibiotic alone [5]. In the early stages local curettage [14] and antibiotic or antiseptic wicks may prove helpful but effective treatment generally requires early diagnosis, prompt antibiotic therapy and good control of diabetes, if this is an aetiological factor [13]. Local surgical debridement or wide surgical ablation may be necessary [12]. In 'resistant' cases hyperbaric oxygen [8] and ascorbic acid [3] have been used as adjunctive therapy and to improve granulocyte function.

REFERENCES

1 BALLENGER J.J. (1977) *Disease of the Nose, Throat and Ear.* 12th ed. Philadelphia, Lea & Febiger.
2 *CHANDLER J.R. (1968) *Laryngoscope* **78**, 1257.
3 CORBERAND J., *et al* (1982) *Arch Otolartyngol* **108**, 122.
4 COSER P.L., *et al* (1980) *Laryngoscope* **90**, 312.
5 *DOROGHAZI R.M., *et al* (1981) *Am J Med* **71**, 603.
6 GIGUERE P. & ROUILLARD G. (1976) *J Otolaryngol* **5**, 159.
7 JOACHIMS H.Z. (1976) *Arch Otolaryngol* **102**, 236.
8 MADER J.T. & LOVE J.T. (1982) *Arch Otolaryngol* **108**, 38.
9 MELTZER P.E. & KELEMEN G. (1959) *Laryngoscope* **69**, 1300.
10 OSTFELD E., *et al* (1981) *Laryngoscope* **91**, 965.
11 PETROZZI J.W. & WARTHAM T.L. (1974) *Arch Dermatol* **110**, 258.
12 RAINES J.M. & SCHINDLER R.A. (1980) *Laryngoscope* **3**, 369.
13 RESOULY A., *et al* (1982) *Lancet* i, 805.
14 SESAL S. & MAN A. (1981) *Am J Otol* **2**, 223.
15 WILSON D.F., *et al* (1971) *Arch Otolaryngol* **93**, 419.
16 YUST I., *et al* (1980) *Acta Otolaryngol (Stockh)* **90**, 398.
17 ZAKY D.A., *et al* (1976) *Am J Med* **61**, 298.

Granulomas. Infective and non-infective granulomas of the ear are not uncommon. *Sarcoidosis* [18, 21], especially *lupus pernio* and other granulomas, including *granuloma faciale* [6], occur both in isolation and by extension from neighbouring skin. Metastatic Crohn's disease may, rarely, involve the ear [16]. *Granuloma annulare, lupus vulgaris* (p. 809), fungal disease [23], syphilis [25], cutaneous leishmaniasis (p. 1021) and leprosy (p. 823) may all affect the ear [21]. The ear is a useful site for diagnostic smears or biopsy in patients with lepromatous leprosy (7, 14).

Wegener's granulomatosis may present with serous or suppurative otitis and conductive or sensorineural deafness [11, 15], and Bentley-Phillips and Bayles have reported a slowly progressive and destructive allergic granulomatosis affecting both ears in a young Negro who died from glomerulonephritis [2].

Granuloma (Acanthoma) fissuratum [5] is a chronic fissured lesion occurring behind or on top of the ear, at the junction of the pinna and scalp, caused by ill-fitting spectacles, and is often mistaken for basal cell carcinoma (p. 598).

Cholesterol granulomas may occasionally involve the external auditory canal [13].

Angiolymphoid hyperplasia with eosinophilia [1, 3, 17, 22], which frequently involves the head

and neck, occurs both in a dermal [27] and in a subcutaneous [24] form, predominantly in young adults. The dermal form, *pseudopyogenic granuloma* [27], commonly affects the ears and scalp and, rarely, the face. The external auditory meatus, pinna and retro-auricular fold are particularly affected (Fig. 56.2). The patients may present with bleeding or pruritus [12]. The lesions consist of persistent angiomatous nodules, less than 1 cm in size and usually sessile and multiple, and have a characteristic histology with abnormal capillaries and swollen endothelial cells showing greatly reduced alkaline phosphatase activity and a fairly dense and predominantly perivascular lymphohistiocytic and eosinophilic infiltrate. The subcutaneous nodules, also known as *subcutaneous angiolymphoid hyperplasia* [24] or *Kimura's disease* [9], are larger with more prominent lymphoid follicles. The two forms are now usually regarded as variants of the same condition [10, 17, 19].

The condition has to be differentiated from ordinary *pyogenic granuloma*, rare in this site and consisting of a polypoid mass of exuberant but

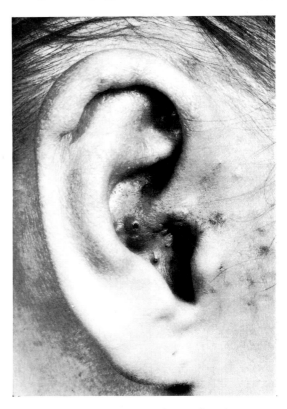

FIG. 56.2. Pseudopyogenic granuloma—clinical appearance (St. John's Hospital).

normal-looking vascular tissue arising from the upper dermis [4], and from angiosarcoma [20, 26] which is, in general, a disease of the elderly.

REFERENCES

1 BALER G.R. (1981) *J Dermatol Surg Oncol* 7, 229.
2 BENTLEY-PHILLIPS, B. & BAYLES M.A.H. (1980) *Int J Dermatol* 19, 336.
3 COLOMB D., *et al* (1981) *Dermatologica* 163, 94.
4 DAVIES M.G., *et al* (1980) *J Am Acad Dermatol* 2, 132.
5 EPSTEIN E. (1965) *Arch Dermatol* 91, 621.
6 FOSS M.H. (1957) *Acta Derm Venereol (Stockh)* 37, 471.
7 GIDEON H. & JOB C.K. (1965) *Leprosy in India* 37, 74.
8 HORI Y. (1981) *J Dermatol Surg Oncol* 7, 130.
9 INADA S., *et al* (1977) *J Dermatol* 4, 207.
10 KANDIE E. (1970) *Br J Dermatol* 83, 405.
11 KORNBLUT A.D., *et al* (1982) *Laryngoscope* 92, 713.
12 LEONARD J.N., *et al* (1981) *Clin Exp Dermatol* 6, 215.
13 MANASSE P. (1894) *Virchows Arch* 136, 245.
14 MANSFIELD R.E., *et al* (1968) *Arch Dermatol* 100, 407.
15 McCAFFREY T.V., *et al* (1980) *Otolaryngol Head Neck Surg* 88, 586.
16 McCALLUM D.I. & GRAY W.M. (1976) *Br J Dermatol* 95, 551.
17 MEHREGAN A.H. & SHAPIRO L. (1971) *Arch Dermatol* 103, 50.
18 NORA S. (1981) *Ear Nose Throat J* 60, 387.
19 REED R.J. & TERAZAKIS N. (1972) *Cancer* 29, 489.
20 REED R.J., *et al* (1966) *Arch Dermatol* 94, 396.
21 SWENSSON-BECK H., *et al* (1982) *Hautarzt* 33, 115.
22 THOMPSON J.W., *et al* (1981) *Arch Otolaryngol* 107, 316.
23 VERBOV J. (1983) *Br J Dermatol* 89, 212.
24 WELLS G.C. & WHIMSTER I.W. (1969) *Br J Dermatol* 81, 1.
25 WILCOX J.R. (1981) *Br J Vener Dis* 57, 30.
26 WILSON JONES E. (1964) *Br J Dermatol* 76, 21.
27 WILSON JONES E. & BLEEHEN S.S. (1969) *Br J Dermatol* 81, 804.

TUMOURS OF THE PINNA AND EXTERNAL AUDITORY CANAL [8, 16]

Benign tumours [10, 18] of the external ear include papillomas, adenomas, seromas [24], lipomas, myomas, chondromas, osteomas, fibromas [37], neurofibromas [36], haemangiomas, lymphangiomas [18], neurilemmomas [15], choristomas [6], trichoepitheliomas [14] and trichofolliculomas [31, 35]. For many of these the diagnosis is made only on histology, although some have the characteristic features of similar tumours elsewhere on the body. In general, diagnosis and treatment are by local excision. Sebaceous cysts may at times be confused. Cheloids occur on the lobe of the ear, usually as a result of ear piercing. Other reactive lesions with which these tumours may be confused

include exostoses, *keratosis obturans*, viral warts and molluscum contagiosum.

Glandular tumours of the external auditory canal (ceruminomas) are rare [1] and comprise benign and pleomorphic adenomas, locally malignant muco-epidermoid carcinomas, malignant adenocarcinomas and adenoid cystic carcinomas (cylindromas) [33]. Isolated cases of syringocystadenoma papilliferum, apocrine cystadenoma, benign eccrine cylindroma and hidradenoma papilliferum have also been reported (12, 30). Pain is the usual presenting feature of the more malignant adenomas and prompt and radical surgery is required if death from local spread or distant metastasis is to be avoided [33]. The benign adenomas usually present with obstructive symptoms and local excision is then usually all that is required. Ceruminomas have been reported in association with other sweat gland tumours elsewhere [19].

Malignant and premalignant tumours of the external ear [5, 8, 32]. Because of its constant exposure, especially in men [21], the auricle is a common site for malignant and premalignant skin lesions. Carcinoma of the auricle accounts for nearly 6% of all cutaneous tumours [13]; two-thirds of these involve the pinna and one-third (including glandular tumours) involve the external auditory canal [26]. Squamous cell carcinoma (55%) and basal cell carcinoma (40%) account for the majority [8]. The ear is known to be a high risk site [23, 25] and once there is spread of the tumour the prognosis is poor [26]. There is also a high rate of recurrence if the tumour is not treated definitively at the first attempt [5, 29]. For this reason even *solar keratosis, Bowen's disease* and *cutaneous horns* (which usually arise on a dysplastic base) must be treated throughly once the diagnosis is made. These lesions commonly occur on the helix, antihelix and posterior border of the ear. Frequently multiple, they may progress to squamous cell carcinoma, malignant transformation occurring earlier and with greater frequency on the ear than elsewhere on sun-damaged skin [5, 26]. *Keratoacanthomas* [3] on the ear, especially when large or in the very old, may at times fail to resolve and develop into squamous cell carcinoma.

Squamous cell carcinoma usually arises from a pre-existing lesion, as described above. The same areas are predominantly affected, although very occasionally the concha, tragus, intertragal notch and external auditory canal may be involved [10]. Ulcerative, fungating or hard, infiltrating lesions may occur and, in advanced cases, much of the ear is

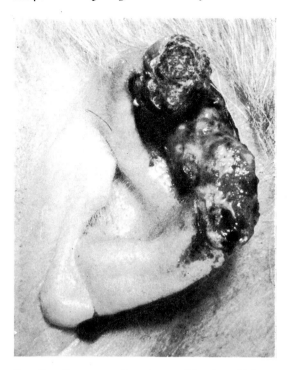

FIG. 56.3. Squamous cell carcinoma of the pinna (Stoke Mandeville Hospital).

destroyed by the tumour (Fig 56.3). Spread is often through perichondrial, periosteal and neurovascular planes [4]. These carcinomas accounted for 45% of all tumours of the external and middle ear in one recent study [10]. The prognosis appears to be worse for those with lesions of the external auditory canal [10]. Involvement of the auricle from a carcinoma of the neighbouring skin is also fairly common.

Basal cell carcinomas [5, 23, 25] frequently involve the preauricular and postauricular skin but may also be found on the helix, antihelix and posterior surface of the ear [4]. They occur much less frequently on the tragus, lobe and concha. Those arising close to the external auditory canal are unpredictable and may infiltrate deeply [29]. High risk lesions include all tumours larger than 1 cm, morphoeic basal cell carcinomas and any multiply recurrent tumour [5]. Tumours of long duration or those that have had previous unsuccessful treatment are the most likely to invade bone or cartilage [23, 34]. Small lesions may be relatively inconspicuous and may be misdiagnosed as keratoses or chondrodermatitis nodularis helicis. The skin frequently has to be stretched to show the character-

istic pearly edge. Basal cell carcinomas arising in front of or behind the auricle may also involve it by extension. Since these tumours remain symptomless for months or years, quite extensive spread or erosion may occur and in all cases the surface appearance of the lesion belies its true extent.

Treatment. Smaller squamous and basal cell carcinomas can often be adequately treated by simple excision [32] or by curettage and cautery or electro-desiccation [38]. Extensive or recurrent tumours, however, are probably best treated by Mohs' technique [4, 7, 8, 28], although conventional plastic surgery [32] and radiotherapy [2, 19] are still successful in eradicating most of them. Megavoltage electron beam therapy has therapeutic and cosmetic advantages over conventional orthovoltage X-ray treatment [22]. Premalignant lesions can usually be treated by cryotherapy, curettage and trichloroacetic acid, or by a combined cryosurgical and chemotherapeutic approach [20] (Chapter 68.). Although both cryotherapy [17] and chemotherapy (5-fluorouracil) [27] have been used in the primary treatment of cancers of the ear, it seems preferable to use major modalities whenever possible in view of the high recurrence rates for tumours at this site [5, 7, 8]. Histological confirmation and control are particularly important in managing neoplastic and pre-neoplastic lesions.

Other tumours [8, 16]. Other tumours occurring on the external ear or in the external auditory canal such as melanoma [9], paragangliomas (chemodectomas, glomus jugulare tumours) [11], sarcomas and other rare tumours are not considered further since they are more the province of the ear, nose and throat or plastic surgeon.

REFERENCES

1 ARATI J., et al (1980) *J Otolaryngol* **9**, 482.
2 AVILA J., et al (1977) *Cancer* **40**, 2891.
3 BAER R.L. & KOPF A.W. (1900) In *The Year Book of Dermatology* (1962–63). Eds. Baer R.L. & Kopf A.W. Chicago, Year Book Medical Publishers, p. 7.
4 *BAILIN P.L.,et al (1980) *Arch Otolaryngol* **106**, 692.
5 BLAKE G.B. & WILSON J.S.P. (1974) *Plast Surg* **27**, 67.
6 BRAUN G.A., et al (1978) *Arch Otolaryngol* **104**, 467.
7 *BUNSTED R.M. & CEILLEY R.I. (1982) *Arch Otolaryngol* **108**, 225.
8 *BUNSTED R.M., et al (1981) *Arch Otolaryngol* **107**, 721.
9 BYERS R.M., et al (1980) *Am J Surg* **140**, 518.
10 *CHEN K.T.K. & DEHNER L.P. (1978) *Arch Otolaryngol* **104**, 247.
11 *CHEN K.T.K. & DEHNER L.P. (1978) *Arch Otolaryngol* **104**, 253.

12 *DEHNER L.P. & CHEN K.T.K. (1980) *Arch Otolaryngol* **106**, 13.

13 DRIVER J.H. & COLE H.N. (1942) *AJR* **48**, 66.

14 FERLITO A., *et al* (1981) *J Laryngol Otol* **95**, 835.

15 FODOR R.I., *et al* (1977) *Laryngoscope* **87**, 1760.

16 *FRIEDMAN I. (1974) *Pathology of the Ear*. Oxford, Blackwell Scientific, p. 145.

17 GAGE A.A. (1977) *J Dermatol Surg Oncol* **3**, 417.

18 GRABB W.C., *et al* (1980) *Plast Reconstr Surg* **66**, 509.

19 HABIB M.A. (1981) *J Laryngol Otol* **95**, 415.

20 HEISING R.A. (1979) *Cutis* **24**, 271.

21 HILLSTROM L. & SWANBECK G. (1970) *Acta Derm Venereol (Stockh)* **50**, 129.

22 HUNTER R.D., *et al* (1982) *Clini Radiol* **33**, 341.

23 JACKSON R. & ADAMS R.H. (1973) *J Surg Oncol* **5**, 431.

24 LAPINS S.A. & ODOM R.B. (1982) *Arch Dermatol* **118**, 503.

25 LEVINE H.C. & BAILIN P.L. (1980) *Laryngoscope* **90**, 955.

26 LEWIS J. (1966) *Laryngoscope* **70**, 551.

27 LITWIN M.S. & KREMENTZ E.T. (1971) *Laryngoscope* **81**, 840.

28 MOLIS F.E. (1947) *Surgery* **21**, 605.

29 MULLER D. (1955) *Laryngoscope* **65**, 448.

30 NISSIM F., *et al* (1981) *J Laryngol Otol* **95**, 843.

31 O'MAHONY J.J. (1981) *J Laryngol Otol* **95**, 623.

32 PLESS J. (1976) *Scand J Plast Reconstr Surg* **10**, 147.

33 *PULEC J.L. (1977) *Laryngoscope* **87**, 1601.

34 ROBINSON J.K., *et al* (1980) *J Am Acad Dermatol* **2**, 499.

35 SRIVASTAVA R.N. & AJWANI K.D. (1979) *Ear Nose Throat J* **58**, 159.

36 TREVISANI T.P., *et al* (1982) *Plast Reconstr Surg* **70**, 217.

37 VARLETZIDES E., *et al* (1980) *Panminerva Med* **22**, 37.

38 WILSON R.S. & JOHNSON J.T. (1980) *Laryngoscope* **90**, 379.

Acquired atresia of the external auditory canal is rare but may be a consequence of trauma [1] or inflammation [7] or secondary to a tumour. Cholesteatoma has been reported as a complication of acquired canal atresia [4].

Keratosis obturans and external auditory canal *cholesteatoma* are often regarded as being synonymous although there is some evidence to suggest that keratosis obturans may be due to the localized accumulation of large amounts of desquamated keratin in the ear canal, whereas external auditory canal cholesteatoma occurs when squamous tissue accumulates adjacent to or under the periosteum [6]. Whilst conservative debridement is the treatment of choice for keratosis obturans, external auditory canal cholesteatoma may require surgical intervention.

Exostoses [3] are usually bilateral, symmetrical, multiple, diffuse, broad-based growths of bone arising from the tympanic bone in the external auditory canal. Frequent exposure to cold water is an aetiological factor in nearly all cases [2]. *Osteomas* can usually be differentiated by their solitary and unilateral distribution. Both conditions are normally asymptomatic unless they enlarge sufficiently to block the external auditory canal [5].

REFERENCES

1 BONDING P. & TOS M. (1975) *Acta Otolaryngol* **79**, 115.

2 DiBARTOLOMEO J.R. (1979) *Ann Otol Rhinol Laryngol* **88**, Suppl. **61**, 2.

3 GRAHAM M.D. (1979) *Ann Otol Rhinol Laryngol* **88**, 566.

4 HABERMAN R.S. & WERTH J.H. (1981) *Am J Otol* **2**, 269.

5 KENRICK J.L. & GRAHAM M.D. (1982) *J Laryngol* **11**, 101.

6 PIEPERSERDES M.C., *et al* (1980) *Laryngoscope* **90**, 383.

7 PROUD G.O. (1966) *Arch Otolaryngol* **83**, 436.

8 SHEEHY J.L. (1982) *Otolaryngol Head Neck Surg* **90**, 337.

CHAPTER 57
The Skin and the Eyes

ARTHUR ROOK and J. L. BURTON

Many of the structures of the eye share, with the skin, a common ectodermal origin, and in numerous syndromes parallel changes involve both skin and eye. Like the skin, the conjunctiva and cornea are directly exposed to environmental influences. The eyelids form part of the skin, but are so modified in many respects that dermatoses involving them often show distinctive features. The eyebrows are sometimes involved in disorders of the scalp or beard, but may be the first or only site affected.

The variety of dermatoses which may involve the ocular adnexa and the external eye, and the number of systemic diseases which may involve both skin and eyes, is so large that only certain selected aspects can be considered here as a guide to differential diagnosis. The conditions mentioned in this chapter have been included because they may present as such in dermatological clinics or because they have some special practical or theoretical interest for the dermatologist. The references listed refer to the large amount of literature on oculocutaneous syndromes.

The diagnostic changes in the ocular fundus in tuberous sclerosis and pseudoxanthoma are described in the accounts of these disorders.

REFERENCES

1 CASANOVAS J. & VILANOVA X. (1967) Dermato-Oftalmologia. Barcelona, Alhacan.
2 *DUKE-ELDER SIR STEWART & MACFAUL P. A. (1974) System of Ophthalmology. London, Kimpton, Vol. XIII.
3 GEERAETS W.J. (1976) Ocular Syndromes, 3rd ed. Philadelphia, Lea & Febiger.
4 GIVNER I. (1952). Trans Am Acad Ophthal Oto-lar 56, 751.
5 KORTING G.W. (1969) Haut und Auge. Stuttgart, Thieme.
6 KORTING G.W. (1978) The Skin and the Eye. Philadelphia, W. B. Saunders.

THE EYEBROWS

Histologically, the skin of the eyebrow region shows special features [2]. The large follicles are so richly vascularized that they are comparable with the vibrissae of other primates, but about half the follicles produce vellus hairs only. There are few or no eccrine sweat glands. It has been observed that in some patients receiving leukocyte A interferon such a marked degree of trichomegaly develops after about 4 months of treatment that the lashes need to be trimmed regularly [1].

The most distinctive characteristics of the eyebrows are the direction of growth of the hairs and their distribution, variations in which give rise to the wide range of forms. Inheritance of the form of the eyebrows is polygenic [3]. Specific genes control direction of growth, density, distribution and colour.

Many of the hereditary variations are of no known clinical significance, but others are associated with other developmental defects or are one component of recognized syndromes [4].

Hypertrophy and fusion of the eyebrows (synophrys)
    Isolated familial characteristic
    Hypertrichosis lanuginosa
    Cornelia de Lange syndrome

Hypoplasia or aplasia of the eyebrows
    Isolated familial characteristic
    Anhidrotic ectodermal dysplasia
    Polydysplastic epidermolysis bullosa
    Keratosis pilaris atrophicans (including ulerythema oöphryogenes)
    Oculomandibular dysostosis
    Oculovertebral dysplasia
    Monilethrix
    Pili torti
    Progeria
    Atrichia congenita

The eyebrows may be shed in alopecia areata, and are sometimes the only site affected. They may also be involved in follicular mucinosis. Thinning of the eyebrows, especially of the outer half, is seen in hypothyroidism, in secondary syphilis and in leprosy. Plucking of the eyebrows is an uncommon variant of trichotillomania. Fusion of the eyebrows has been reported in kwashiorkor.

Post-inflammatory cicatricial alopecia may involve the eyebrows. It may follow lupus erythematosus, or specific infections such as lupus vulgaris or tertiary syphilis, but is occasionally seen in such conditions as folliculitis decalvans.

The eyebrows share in the hypopigmentation of albinism, and may be affected in piebaldism, in Waardenburg's syndrome and in vitiligo.

The eyebrows are often affected in seborrhoeic dermatitis, and sometimes in psoriasis.

REFERENCES

1 FOON K.A. & DOUGHER G. (1984) *N Engl J Med* **311**, 1259.
2 MONTAGNA W. (1970) *Arch Dermatol* **101**, 257.
3 *ROZPRÝM F. (1934) *J R Anthrop Inst* **64**, 353.
4 *WAARDENBURG P.J. (1961) In *Genetics and Ophthalmology*. Ed. Waardenburg P.J., *et al*. Oxford, Blackwell.

THE EYELIDS

Numerous developmental defects affect the configuration of the palpebral aperture or the size and shape of the eyelids. Some are associated with the complete branchial arch syndromes (p. 216). Some are a component of other syndromes of interest to the dermatologist, to whom they may provide a valuable diagnostic clue. The presence of structural abnormalities of the eyelids should therefore be noted and an ophthalmologist consulted concerning their significance.

A divided naevus is a melanocytic naevus in adjacent areas of the upper and lower eyelids which appears to be a single lesion when the lids are closed. The precursor cells must have been present at the time when the lids were fused, between the ninth and the 20th weeks of gestation [1].

The eyelids are involved in many hereditary dermatoses. In ichthyosiform erythroderma the development of ectropion as early as the first decade is a characteristic and troublesome feature. Scarring and tumour formation occur in xeroderma pigmentosum. The histology and cytochemistry of the normal eyelid have been described in some detail [2].

REFERENCES

1 HAMMING M. (1983) *Pediatr Dermatol* **1**, 51.
2 MONTAGNA W. & FORD D.M. (1969) *Arch Dermatol* **100**, 328.

Oedema of the eyelids. The dermatologist encounters oedema of the eyelids mainly in angio-oedema and in allergic contact dermatitis. These are usually readily differentiated by the presence of erythema, exudation, scaling or other evidence of epidermal change in the latter. However, angio-oedema or eyelid oedema of other origin may be complicated by epidermal changes induced by rubbing, or by topical medicaments.

Eyelid oedema related to other local or systemic disease is often referred to dermatological departments. The principal causes are listed in Table 57.1.

TABLE 57.1 Oedema of the eyelids

Local lesions (often unilateral)	Systemic processes
Stye	Angio-oedema
Chancre	Blepharochalasis
Chalazion	Trichiniasis
Dacrocystitis	Filariasis
Orbital cellulitis	Onchocerciasis
Orbital tumours	Acute bacterial and
Cavernous sinus	protozoal infections—
thrombosis	may be an early sign—
Intra-ocular infections	scarlatina,
diphtheria, typhoid,	trypanosomiasis,
Erysipelas	malaria
Trauma (may be self-	Nephritis
inflicted)	Cardiac failure
Insect bites	Hyperthyroidism
Contact dermatitis	Hypothyroidism
Myiasis	Dermatomyositis
Anthrax	Hypoproteinaemia
Accidental vaccinia	Anaemia
Cat-scratch disease	Leukaemia
Primary herpes simplex	
Herpes zoster	
Chronic lymphoedema	
of any origin	

In some patients who complain of recurrent puffiness of the eyelids, often middle-aged women, no convincing cause can be established.

Loss or fenestration of the orbital septum with age gives the appearance of lid oedema, but is in fact prolapsed fat.

Pigmentation of the lids

Hereditary [1, 3]. Hyperpigmentation of the eyelids may occur as an apparently isolated defect, determined by an autosomal dominant gene. It is first noticed in childhood.

Naevoid [2]. Melanocytic naevi may involve either or both eyelids. If both eyelids are involved the configuration of the naevus when the eyelids are closed suggests that it arose from a single focus.

Endocrine. Hyperpigmentation of the eyelids is often marked in MSH-induced melanosis of any origin (p. 1550).

Metabolic. In ochronosis the conjuctiva as well as the eyelids may show brownish pigmentation.

Chemical. The prolonged use of mercurial eye ointments or silver preparations may produce permanent hyperpigmentation, greyish brown in colour. Hypermelanosis may be induced by cosmetics containing phototoxic agents, usually psoralens (p. 512).

Lichen planus [4]. Lichen planus on the eyelids may present as violaceous papules, sometimes in annular configuration, or as reticulate brown pigmentation.

Melanoacanthoma [5]. Minute shining black papules may develop in the ciliary margin.

REFERENCES

1 AGUILERA DIAZ L. (1972) *Ann Dermatol Syphiligr* **99**, 43.
2 HARRISON R. & OKUN M. (1960) *Arch Dermatol* **82**, 235.
3 HUNZIKER N. (1962) *J Génét Hum* **11**, 16.
4 MICHELSON H.E. & LAYMON C.W. (1938) *Arch Dermatol Syphil* **33**, 27.
5 SPOTT D.A. (1972) *Arch Dermatol* **105**, 898.

Eyelashes. The eyelashes may be shed in alopecia areata, and in rare cases the condition remains confined to them. The diagnosis in such cases is difficult. Very rarely trichotillomania involves the eyelashes.

Eczema [1, 2]. The skin of the eyelids is thin, and it is commonly touched by the fingers many times each day. It is therefore a frequent site of contact dermatitis, and may indeed be the only region involved.

The substances most often incriminated are cosmetics, especially nail varnish, ophthalmic medicaments, including antibiotics, atropine and mercurial preparations, plants, especially *Primula obconica*, and occupational hazards. The changes are those of an acute eczema (p. 370). The cause, often unsuspected because the substance is believed by the patient not to come in contact with the eyelids, must be confirmed by patch testing.

Nickel dermatitis may be associated with secondary eczematous changes of the eyelids.

The eyelids are also involved in some cases of atopic dermatitis.

Chronic eczema of the eyelids, with scaling and thickening, sometimes occurs, mainly in middle-aged women, without discernible cause. The condition is often referred to as neurodermatitis of the eyelids, but it is probable that many such cases are due to unrecognized contact dermatitis.

REFERENCES

1 BORRIE P. (1956) *Br J Ophthal* **40**, 742.
2 KAALUND-JORGENSEN O. (1951) *Acta Derm Venereol (Stockh)* **31**, 1

Infections

Styes, syn. hordeoli [1]. Styes are furuncles of the eyelash follicles, and are caused by *Staphylococcus pyogenes*. Over 90% of patients with recurrent styes were found to carry the staphylococcus in the anterior nares. In treatment an antibiotic ointment, selected after sensitivity testing, should be regularly applied to both eyelids and nares.

The glands of Moll were involved in a patient with hidradenitis suppurativa [2].

REFERENCES

1 COPEMAN P.W.M. (1958) *Lancet*, ii, 728.
2 SACHS D.D. & GORDON A.T. (1967) *Arch Dermatol Ophthal NY* **77**, 635.

Viral infections. The viral infections listed in Table 57.2 are often associated with a conjunctival follicular reaction. The lesions, especially those of molluscum, are modified if they occur at the lid margins and are moistened with tears, sometimes making diagnosis difficult.

Ocular vaccinia [1] occurred mainly after a primary vaccination, which it followed in about 10 days. In most patients eyelids or conjunctiva were involved but corneal changes probably developed in at least 10% of cases.

REFERENCE

1 RUBEN F.L. & LANE J.M. (1970) *Arch Ophthal NY* **84**, 45.

Blepharitis. This occurs in many clinical forms, of which one is frequently encountered in dermatological clinics.

Seborrhoeic blepharitis. This is a distinct clinical entity, but its relationship to the seborrhoeic state is

TABLE 57.2 Other infections which may involve the eyelids

Mycotic	Viral	Bacterial and protozoal
Actinomycosis	Infectious wart	Anthrax
Sporotrichosis	Molluscum contagiosum	Primary tuberculosis
Blastomycosis	Herpes zoster	Syphilitic chancre
Dermatophytosis	Herpes simplex	Leishmaniasis
Aspergillosis	Cat-scratch disease	Impetigo
	Vaccinia	Chancriform pyoderma
	Adenovirus infection	Granuloma venereum
		Chancroid
		Rhinoscleroma

controversial, although it is certainly more common in adolescents with seborrhoeic dermatitis. It is more frequent in boys than in girls, but may begin early in childhood before there is any evidence of sebaceous activity.

The margins of the eyelids are red, with small adherent scales. Crusts may form, especially in the early morning. Irritation and soreness may be troublesome. In severe cases there may be destruction of the eyelash follicles by scar tissue. Persistent or recurrent attacks may continue for some years before ceasing spontaneously.

In differential diagnosis psoriasis of the eyelid margins, which is uncommon, may cause confusion. Lupus erythematosus may also involve the eyelids. The crusts should be removed gently with warm water, and an antibiotic eye ointment with hydrocortisone applied each night.

Demodectic blepharitis [1, 2]. Demodectic blepharitis is not universally accepted as a distinct entity, for *Demodex folliculorum* can be found in normal eyelash follicles. Some authorities maintain that irritation, burning and inflammatory changes in the eyelash follicles in adults aged 30–80 may be caused by the *Demodex*. Objective changes are slight; there may be some redness but no scaling and some eyelashes may be shed. Frequent bathing with boric acid or with benzalkonium 1/7,000 is said to be curative.

Phthiriasis (p. 1049). This may involve the lashes and cause a pruritic blepharitis.

REFERENCES

1 MORGAN R.J. & COSTON T.O. (1964). *South Med J* 57, 694.
2 POST C.F. & JUHLIN E. (1963) *Arch Dermatol* 88, 298.

Xanthelasma (p. 2288). The yellow plaques on the eyelids may be an isolated finding or associated with other signs of xanthomatosis.

Amyloidosis (p. 2306). Amber-coloured papules of the eyelids have been reported as an early sign of systemic amyloidosis [1].

Lipoid proteinosis (p. 2312). Pearly nodules of the lid margins are a distinctive feature.

REFERENCE

1 NATELSON E.A., *et al* (1970) *Arch Intern Med* 125, 304.

Tumours of the eyelids and orbital skin [2, 6]. A wide variety of benign and malignant tumours may occur on the eyelids or orbital skin.

Some 10% of all basal cell carcinomas of the face involve the eyelids, usually the lower lid. Early diagnosis is important. Radiotherapy or plastic excision are usually the preferred treatments [1, 3].

An uncommon, but important, tumour is a squamous carcinoma derived from the Meibomian glands [4]. It favours the upper lid and is potentially dangerous.

The intra-epidermal carcinoma of the ciliary margin may be warty and misleadingly innocent in appearance. An adequate biopsy must include one entire lash follicle [5].

Other tumours, tumour-like lesions and cysts occurring on the eyelids and orbital skin are listed in Table 57.3.

REFERENCES

1 BELISARIO J.C. (1959) *Hautarzt,* 10, 68.
2 BONIUK M. (1964) *Ocular and Adnexal Tumours.* St Louis, Mosby.

TABLE 57.3 Tumours, tumour-like lesions and cysts of the eyelids and orbital skin

Cysts of sweat gland origin
    Hidrocystoma—usually multiple
    Cysts of Moll's glands on eyelid
        margins—usually solitary
Cysts of sebaceous gland origin
    Sebaceous cysts
    Milia
    Meibomian cysts—in the eyelid
    Dermoid cysts
Basal cell carcinoma
Kerato-acanthoma (Fig. 57.1)
Squamous cell carcinoma
Intra-epidermal carcinoma
Benign calcifying epithelioma
Cylindroma
Tricho-epithelioma (usually multiple)
Senile keratosis
Seborrhoeic keratosis
Inverted follicular keratosis
	Adenoma sebaceum
	Syringoma
	Lipoma
	Vascular naevus
	Haemangio-endothelioma
	Kaposi's sarcoma
	Pyogenic granuloma
	Melanocytic naevus
	Melanoma
	Metastatic carcinoma
	Lymphomas—the eyelids may be
	    incidentally involved
	Neurofibroma
	Mucosal neuroma

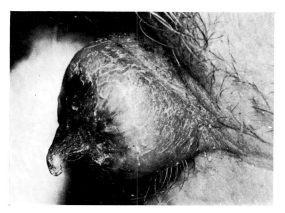

FIG. 57.1. Kerato-acanthoma of the eyelid (Addenbrooke's Hospital).

3 DOMONKOS A.N. (1965) *Arch Dermatol* **91**, 369.
4 GINSBERG J. (1965) *Arch Ophthal NY* **73**, 271.
5 McCALLUM D.I., *et al* (1975) *Br J Dermatol* **93**, 239.
6 WELCH R.B. & DUKE J.R. (1958) *Am J Ophthal* **45**, 415.

Fibrillary neuroma syndrome. Multiple soft lipoma-like fibrillary neuromas developed in childhood on the lips, tongue and eyelids of a woman who subsequently failed to mature sexually [1]. The association may represent a distinct syndrome, but is probably the same as mucosal neuroma syndrome (see p. 2349).

REFERENCE

1 MICHALOWSKI R. (1967) *Arch Klin Exp Dermatol* **231**, 20.

THE CONJUNCTIVA

Diseases of the conjunctiva are now relatively uncommon in hospital practice in Britain, but are frequent in countries where trachoma is prevalent. Most of the common disorders of the conjunctiva are inflammatory. Many affect only the conjunctiva but some also involve other mucous membranes and the skin. Vernal conjunctivitis is often associated with seasonal rhinitis.

Ocular lesions may occur early, or even as the presenting manifestation of some bullous eruptions. Those that involve the conjunctiva are listed in Table 57.4.

Redness and soreness of the eyes are often early and conspicuous manifestations of Sjögren's syndrome (p. 1389).

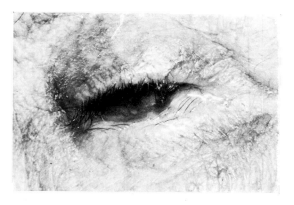

FIG. 57.2 Severe conjunctival shrinkage in mucous membrane pemphigoid (Addenbrooke's Hospital).

TABLE 57.4. Bullous eruptions involving the conjunctiva

	Age	Clinical features	Associated lesions
Bullous erythema multiforme (syn. Stevens-Johnson syndrome)	Children; young adults	Acute onset; intense oedema; large bullae	Bullae of mouth, genital skin
Benign mucous membrane pemphigoid (Fig. 57.2)	Usually over 60, F > M	Insidious onset; soreness; scarring	Erosions and scarring in mouth; skin bullae few, inconstant
Pemphigus vulgaris	40–60, often Jewish	Eyes involved infrequently	Erosions of oral mucous membrane; skin bullae
Recessive dystrophic epidermolysis bullosa	Children	Onset from birth; eyes involved infrequently; bullae and scarring	Extensive bullae of skin and mucous membranes
Dermatitis herpetiformis	Adults	Ocular involvement rare; vesicles and erosions of conjunctiva have been reported	Irritable papules and vesicles of limbs and trunk
Hydroa vacciniforme	Children	Vesiculo-ulcerative or hypertrophic conjunctivitis in 20%	Vesicles on light-exposed skin

Conjunctivitis may result from allergic sensitivity to thiomersol in the solution in which soft contact lenses are stored and cleaned [3].

Conjunctival lesions occur in many other dermatoses, notably sarcoidosis, rosacea and Reiter's disease, but are commonly an incidental finding rather than a dominant or presenting symptom. Duke-Elder [1] provides a detailed review of the literature.

Melanocytic naevi in malignant melanoma can occur in the conjunctiva and presents similar problems in diagnosis to those in the skin [2].

REFERENCES

1 DUKE-ELDER SIR STEWART (1965) *System of Ophthalmology*. London, Kimpton, Vol **VIII**, Part 1.
2 JAY B. (1965) *Br J Ophthal* **49**, 169.
3 RIETSCHEL R.L. & WILSON L.A. (1982) *Arch Dermatol* **118**, 147.

THE CORNEA

Congenital corneal dystrophy [2]. Corneal dystrophy occurs in many hereditary syndromes which involve the skin.

Corneal changes are a characteristic and almost invariable feature of the following:

Epidermolysis bullosa of the polydysplastic type
Sex-linked recessive ichthyosis vulgaris [5]
Keratoderma palmoplantaris of the circumscribed type
Keratosis follicularis spinulosa [3]

Corneal dystrophies are inconstant in

Rothmund's syndrome
Pityriasis rubra pilaris
Darier's disease
Xeroderma pigmentosum
Anhidrotic ectodermal dysplasia
Angiokeratoma corporis diffusum
Hurler's syndrome

Keratoconus [1]. Keratoconus is a conical deformity of the cornea. It occurs 10 times more frequently among patients with atopic eczema than in controls. It is probable that there is a defect of the stromal collagen, and rubbing the eye may account for the high incidence in patients with eczema and hay fever.

A brittle cornea prone to spontaneous perforation has occurred in Marfan's syndrome and Ehlers–Danlos syndrome. It has been reported in twins as an isolated defect associated with red hair [6].

REFERENCES

1 COPEMAN P.W.M. (1965) *Br Med J* **ii**, 977.
2 *FRANCESCHETTI A. & THIER C.J. (1961) *Albrecht von Graefes Arch Ophthal* **162**, 610.
3 FRANCESCHETTI A., et al (1957) *Ophthalmologica, Basel*, **135**, 259.
4 *GRAYSON M. & KEATES R.H. (1969) *Manual of Diseases of the Cornea*. London, Churchill.
5 SEVER R.J., et al (1968) *JAMA* **206**, 2283.
6 TICHO U., et al (1980) *Br J Ophthal* **64**, 175.

Rosaceal keratitis (p. 1608). Corneal vascularization is followed by keratitis and ulceration. The keratitis may precede or follow the skin changes, and progresses independently. Non-specific blepharitis and conjunctivitis may be associated.

Scleritis in connective-tissue disorders. Scleritis may be the presenting manifestation of systemic and active tissue disease [2], including polychondritis [1].

REFERENCES

1 McKay D.A.R., *et al* (1974) *Br J Ophthal* **58**, 600.
2 Watson P.G. & Hazelman B.L. (1976) *Sclera in Systemic Disorders*. Philadelphia, W. B. Saunders.

THE LENS

Cataract [2, 6, 7]. The occurrence of cataracts in many complex hereditary syndromes, which also involve the skin, is believed to be due to the presence of a common, but as yet unknown, defect of lens and skin.

Cataract occurs with some frequency in the following syndromes:

Werner's syndrome
Rothmund's syndrome
Incontinentia pigmenti
Conradi's syndrome
Hallermann–Streiff syndrome
Pachyonychia congenita

Cataracts may be induced by drugs such as triparanol, which block the synthesis of cholesterol and disturb keratinization of skin and hair.

The incidence of cataracts is increased in alopecia areata universalis, but the mechanism is not understood.

In atopic dermatitis the incidence of cataract is also considerably increased. The cataracts, which tend to develop during adolescence or early adult life, are shield shaped and pathognomonic. The incidence of cataract in reported series [1, 5] varies from 3% to over 10% of the more severe adolescent and adult cases, varying according to the criteria for the selection of cases. Keratoconus is also present in some cases [3].

The demonstration [4] that, in the dog, two apparently identical antigens are shared by skin and lens capsule may be relevant.

REFERENCES

1 Brunsting L.A., *et al* (1957) *Arch Derm* **76**, 779.
2 *Carleton A. (1943) *Br J Dermatol* **83**, 98.
3 Francois J. (1961) *Ann Dermatol Syphiligr* **88**, 397.
4 Gingrich R.E. & Fusaro R.M. (1964) *J Invest Dermatol* **43**, 235.
5 *Kornerup T. & Lodin A. (1959) *Acta Ophthal.* **37**, 508.
6 *Kugelberg I. (1934) *Klin. Monatsbl Augenheilkd* **92**, 484.
7 *Muller S.A. & Brunsting L.A. (1963) *Arch Dermatol* **88**, 330.

CHAPTER 58

The Breast

ARTHUR ROOK & J. L. BURTON

Although most of the more serious diseases of the breast come within the province of the surgeon, the gynaecologist or the endocrinologist, there are many which affect only the breast skin and are wholly the concern of the dermatologist, and others which may involve the skin and present difficult problems in differential diagnosis [1, 3, 4].

The breasts are traditionally regarded as modified apocrine sweat glands but they show no histological or histochemical similarities [2, 5]. The skin of the breast does not differ structurally from that of the neighbouring chest wall, but the skin of the nipple and areola is very highly specialized. The under-surface of the epidermis covering the tip of the nipple resembles that found on tactile surfaces. The nipple is glabrous. Lactiferous ducts, sebaceous glands and apocrine glands open only at its tip. Sensory nerve end organs are also confined to the tip of the nipple. The areola is almost glabrous; there are a few vellus follicles, a few eccrine glands, clusters of large sebaceous glands and the so-called tubercles of Montgomery. These are the ducts of the the glands of Montgomery, which are identical in structure with the glands opening at the nipple and form an integral part of the mammary organ [6].

The normal proliferation of the primitive mammary ducts in the girl at puberty is induced by oestrogen but is also dependent on corticosteroids and some somatotrophin. These hormones, together with prolactin and progesterone, bring about further proliferation of the lobule-alveolar system during pregnancy.

Here we shall describe only certain conditions which occur exclusively on the breast or are significantly modified in their morphology or course when they affect the breast and which are not fully described elsewhere.

REFERENCES

1 *ANDERSON N.P. (1952) South Med J **45**, 896.
2 GIACOMETTI G. & MONTAGNA W. (1962) Anat Rec **144**, 191.
3 *HAAGENSEN C.D. (1971) Disease of the Breast. 2nd ed. Philadelphia, Saunders.
4 *LEIS H.P. (1970) Diagnosis and Treatment of Breast Lesions. London, Lewis.
5 MONTAGNA W. (1970) Br J Dermatol **83**, 2.
6 MONTAGNA W. & YUN J.S. (1972) Br J Dermatol **86**, 126.

SUPERNUMERARY BREASTS (POLYMASTIA) OR NIPPLES (POLYTHELIA)

Supernumerary breasts and the far more common supernumerary nipples usually develop along the course of the embryological milk lines, which run from the anterior axillary folds to the inner thighs; in 10% of cases they occur in other sites [4, 5]. They have been reported on the posterior aspect of the thigh in a man [1]. A familial incidence is sometimes noted. They have been found in association with ectodermal dysplasia [2] and also with a wide variety of anomalies including unilateral renal agenesis and carcinoma [3].

The accessory nipple is usually easily recognized if the diagnosis is considered, but is otherwise often confused with a pigmented naevus. If functional breast tissue is present, enlargement at puberty or in pregnancy may be embarrassing or painful. Simple excision is advisable, as carcinoma may occur.

Supernumerary areolae have occurred as an isolated abnormality [1].

REFERENCES

1 CAMISA C. (1980) J Am Acad Dermatol **3**, 467.
2 HAY R. J. & WELLS R.S. (1976) Br J Dermatol **94**, 227.
3 KHAN S.A. & WAGNER R.F. (1982) Cutis **30**, 225.
4 SHEWMAKE S.W. & IZUMO G.T. (1977) Arch Dermatol **113**, 523.
5 TOW S. H. & SHANMUGARANTHAM K. (1962) Br Med J ii, 1236.

RUDIMENTARY NIPPLES

Absence or maldevelopment of the nipples may be present as an isolated congenital defect. The association of absent or rudimentary nipples with congenital abnormality of the scalp and external ears has been reported in 10 members of one family. The condition was thought to be inherited as an autosomal dominant trait [1].

REFERENCE

1 FINLAY A.Y. & MARKS R. (1978) *Br J Dermatol* **99**, 423.

HYPERKERATOSIS OF THE NIPPLE [2, 3, 4, 5]

Hyperkeratosis of the nipple and areola occurs in either sex in ichthyosiform erythroderma and in some cases of ichthyosis. It is seen also in some lymphomas, in acanthosis nigricans, in Darier's disease [1] and in men with carcinoma of the prostrate treated with oestrogens [4, 6].

All forms are rare but the most frequent develops in women in the second or third decade as an isolated naevoid defect [1, 2, 7]. The skin of the nipple is diffusely thickened and hyperpigmented and covered with filiform or papular warty excrescences. In other cases only the nipple or only the areola is affected.

REFERENCES

1 DUPRÉ A., *et al* (1980) *Ann Dermatol Vénéréol* **107**, 303.
2 MAYCOCK P.M. (1978) *Arch Dermatol* **114**, 1245.
3 MEHREGAN A.H. & RAHBARI H. (1977) *Arch Dermatol* **113**, 1691.
4 MOULD DE JEGASUTHY B.L. (1980) *Cutis* **26**, 95.
5 OBERSTE-LEHN H. (1950) *Z Haut GeschlKrankh* **8**, 388.
6 SCHWARTZ R.A. (1978) *Arch Dermatol* **114**, 1245.
7 SODEN C.E. (1983) *Cutis* **32**, 69.

PEAU D'ORANGE

This term describes a circumscribed area of dimpled indurated skin and should lead to an intensive search for underlying carcinoma. Rarely, it occurs in the absence of any clinically palpable tumour.

It has also been reported as a complication of anasarca, nephrotic syndrome and cardiac failure [2].

PAGET'S DISEASE

This condition, which is a marker of an underlying breast carcinoma, is discussed on p. 2437.

ECZEMA OF THE NIPPLE

Eczema of the nipple occurs mainly in young women between the ages of 15 and 30, and is usually bilateral. It was formerly most common during lactation and was induced by infection and the medicaments applied to combat it, but in Britain it is now seen more often in non-pregnant girls. In every case the presence of scabies must be carefully excluded. Often no cause can be established, particularly in atopic subjects in whom the condition is more frequently found than in non-atopic controls.

The intermittent course, indefinite margin and lack of distortion of the nipple help the important differentiation from Paget's disease (p. 2437). If the diagnosis is doubtful, biopsy should not de delayed.

Irregular patches of eczema on the breasts should suggest a contact dermatitis to nail varnish.

Intensely irritable papules on the areola in young women are a feature of Fox–Fordyce disease (p. 1895).

Psoriasis of the nipple may be provoked by the trauma of suckling.

JOGGER'S NIPPLES [1]

Long-distance runners of either sex may suffer from irritation of the nipples caused by prolonged friction against a shirt. The problem is more pronounced in women who do not wear a bra, or in men who wear a string vest. The condition is self-healing and can be prevented by the application of tape to the nipples before running.

REFERENCE

1 LEVIT F. (1977) *N. Engl J Med* **297**, 1127.
2 MCELLIGOTT G & HARRINGTON M.G. (1986) *Br Med J* **292**, 446.

EROSIVE ADENOMATOSIS OF THE NIPPLE [1–5]

SYN. BENIGN PAPILLOMATOSIS OF THE NIPPLE; FLORID PAPILLOMATOSIS

The adenoma of the nipple is a benign naevoid tumour, usually considered to be derived from the apocrine sweat ducts of the nipple epithelium but probably of lactiferous duct origin [4]. It consists of tubules with an inner layer of columnar cells and an outer layer of cuboidal myoepithelial cells.

The clinical features are rather variable. Women aged 25–70 are usually affected; exceptionally, the condition has occurred in an elderly man [4]. There may be a small nodule on the nipple, or crusting and superficial ulceration. There may be a bloody discharge or eczema.

Certain clinical differentiation from Paget's disease may not be possible. Excision of the nipple is the treatment of choice.

REFERENCES

1 HANDLEY R.S. & THACKRAY A.C. (1962) *Br J Cancer* **16**, 187.
2 LEWIS H.M., *et al* (1976) *Arch Dermatol* **112**, 1427.
3 ROBERT H., *et al* (1963) *Prev Med* **71**, 2713.
4 SHAPIRO L. & KARPES C.M. (1965) *Am J Pathol* **44**, 155.
5 SMITH E.J., *et al* (1970) *Arch Dermatol* **102**, 330.

MAMILLARY FISTULA

This is a relatively common inflammatory disease of the breast resulting from obstruction to a lactiferous duct. It affects adult women and presents as a discharging sinus of the areola. Sometimes there are recurrent subcutaneous abscesses. Treatment is surgical [1].

REFERENCE

1 ATKINS H.J.B. (1955) *Br Med J* ii, 1473.

BASAL CELL CARCINOMA OF THE NIPPLE [1]

This is an extremely rare lesion. It can occur in either men or women, usually in old age. It presents as a red eczema-like patch of the nipple and of the areola. It runs a long indolent course. Biopsy is essential to differentiate it from Paget's disease.

REFERENCE

1 SAUVEN P. & ROBERTS A. (1983) *J R Soc Med.* **76**, 699.

ADNEXAL POLYP OF NEONATAL SKIN

This is a small, usually solitary, tumour which occurs mainly on the areola of the neonate. The tumour becomes dry and brown and falls off within a few days of birth. Histologically, it contains hair follicles, eccrine glands and vestigial sebaceous glands. A survey of newborn infants in Tokyo showed that the condition occurred in 4% of 3,257 infants.

REFERENCE

1 HIDANO A. & KOBAYISHI T. (1975) *Br J Dermatol* **92**, 659.

PAINFUL NIPPLES

This symptom is common, especially if fissures develop during early lactation, but in other circumstances it can occur as a form of localized mastalgia [2]. The pain tends to be worse in cold weather and the patient can often accurately localize it to the nipple or subareolar area. The condition may be associated with duct ectasia or periductal mastitis, and the mammogram may show coarse calcification. The condition may respond to excision of a wedge of the areola [2], and bromocryptine and danazol have each had a 70% success rate in cyclical mastalgia [1]. Some cases will also respond to oral contraceptives, which abolish the mid-cycle increase in breast sensitivity which occurs in most normal women [3].

REFERENCES

1 MONTGOMERY A.C.V., *et al* (1979) *J R Soc Med* **72**, 489.
2 PREECE P.E., *et al* (1976) *Lancet* ii, 670.
3 ROBINSON J.E. & SHORT R.V. (1977) *Br Med J* i, 1188.

GYNAECOMASTIA [2, 9, 11, 23]

Gynaecomastia, a potentially reversible enlargement of the male breast, may occur as an isolated defect or as a manifestation of a wide range of different pathological states in which it may be a valuable diagnostic sign. The multiplicity of syndromes associated with gynaecomastia reflects the complexity of the hormonal mechanisms concerned in breast enlargement.

The histopathological changes [15] are related to the duration of gynaecomastia and not to its cause. At early stages there are active proliferating ducts in a vascular fibroblastic stroma. Later, there is progressive fibrosis and hyalinization, and the number of ducts is reduced.

Incidence and aetiology. Palpable asymptomatic gynaecomastia is common, and can be found in 30–40% of normal men [2].

Gynaecomastia may result from an imbalance between the stimulatory effect of oestrogens on mammary tissue and the inhibitory effect of androgens. Defective androgen receptors, as found in testicular feminization and related syndromes, may also contribute. The role of prolactin is less clear, though it may play a part by its indirect effect on gonadal, and possibly adrenal, function [7].

Physiological gynaecomastia [2, 4, 16]. Some enlargement of the breast occurs at puberty in about

60% of normal boys. Serum oestradiol is increased in relation to testosterone in boys with gynaecomastia, and the gynaecomastia regresses as the ratio reverts to normal adult values [13]. The peak incidence is around the age of 14, but the onset may be at any age between 10 and 20. The degree of enlargement is usually slight but may be sufficient to cause embarrassment and anxiety. Spontaneous regression usually takes place within a few months, but the enlargement persists for over 2 years in 5% of boys.

Gynaecomastia also occurs in some elderly men as a result of testicular failure, and obesity can also produce gynaecomastia by increasing the peripheral aromatization of androgens to oestrogens [2].

Gynaecomastia in endocrine disorders [2, 9]. Gynaecomastia occurs in a very wide range of endocrine disorders. Primary or secondary reduction of testicular androgen production is of special importance. Leprous orchitis may be associated with marked gynaecomastia. Some tumours of the testis are associated with gynaecomastia, notably seminoma, interstitial cell tumour, Sertoli cell tumour and certain teratomas. These tumours often produce human chorionic gonadotrophin, which stimulates the normal Leydig cells to secrete excessive amounts of oestradiol [6, 19].

Gynaecomastia occurs in most men with Klinefelter's syndrome, and there is an increased risk of breast cancer in this syndrome [17].

In other endocrine disorders, gynaecomastia is less common, but may occur in tumours or hyperplasia of the adrenal gland, in pituitary tumours and in hyperthyroidism. It is a rare manifestation of bronchial carcinoma.

Gynaecomastia in nutritional , metabolic, renal and hepatic disease [2, 8, 9, 14, 22]. Gynaecomastia may occur during starvation or on resumption of a more adequate diet after prolonged starvation. The endocrine basis of the breast enlargement is inconstant, depending in varying degree on impaired liver function, testicular atrophy and disturbed pituitary function [18].

In 40–50% of patients receiving maintenance haemodialysis for renal failure, gynaecomastia develops after 2–9 months [8]. It resembles the so-called refeeding gynaecomastia mentioned above.

Impaired liver function in cirrhosis, carcinoma of the liver or haemochromatosis may also be associated with gynaecomastia. Several mechanisms are involved, including decreased testosterone production, excessive oestrogen production from circulating precursors, changes in sex-hormone-binding globulin levels and increased progesterone [2, 5].

The gynaecomastia occasionally observed in patients with mycosis fungoides, extensive erythroderma and other severe widespread and persistent diseases of the skin is presumed to be of nutritional or hepatic origin.

Gynaecomastia in diseases of the nervous system [9]. Gynaecomastia may occur in paraplegia as a result of unexplained testicular changes, and is also present in some cases of dystrophia myotonica.

Drug-induced gynaecomastia [2]. Drugs which can produce gynaecomastia are shown in Table 58.1.

TABLE 58.1 Drugs which produce gynaecomastia

Amphetamines	Isoniazid
Androgens	Ketoconazole
Cimetidine	Marijuana
Cytotoxic agents	Methyldopa
Diazepam	Oestrogens
Diethylpropion	Penicillamine
Digitalis	Phenothiazines
Domperidone	Reserpine
Human chorionic gonado-	Spironolactone
trophin	Tricyclic antidepressants

Some of these, such as spironolactone and cimetidine, are anti-androgens, and others, such as isoniazid, may act by the 'refeeding' mechanism. Cytotoxic drugs may damage the testes, but gonadotrophins and oestradiol were also increased in five out of six cases due to cytotoxic drugs [20, 21]. Some drugs which act on the central nervous system increase prolactin and thus induce a secondary hypogonadal state. Testosterone might act through its conversion to oestrogens.

Gynaecomastia can also be due to the topical application of oestrogen-containing creams [3].

Management of gynaecomastia. Clinical examination may rarely reveal areas of local firmness or irregularity which may suggest the possibility of breast cancer, and this should lead to biopsy. It should be noted though that gynaecomastia is often asymmetrical, and biopsy is rarely required. Careful examination for other underlying disease and a full drug history are required, particularly if the gynaecomastia is symptomatic or of recent onset in an adult, but it should be remembered that a large proportion of otherwise normal men have some slight gynaecomastia.

In suitable cases screening tests may include

measurements of serum human chorionic gonadotrophin, plasma testosterone, oestrogen, prolactin
and urinary steroid excretion.

For cases with considerable breast discomfort, or
if the condition is severe enough to cause embarrassment, treatment with tamoxifen, clomiphene or
danazol may be considered [1, 2, 10]. The prolonged
application of topical dihydrotestosterone cream has
also been suggested [12]. In extreme cases reduction mammoplasty may be performed by a plastic
surgeon.

REFERENCES

1 Beck W., *et al* (1982) *Horm Metab Res* **14**, 653.
2 *Carlson H.E. (1980) *N Engl J Med* **14**, 795.
3 Cimmorra G.A., *et al* (1982) *Br J Plas Sur3* **35**, 209.
4 *Decourt J., *et al* (1962) *Sem Hôp* **38**, 1266.
5 Farthing M.J.G., *et al* (1982) *Gut* **23**, 276.
6 Forest M.G., *et al* (1979) *J Clin Endocrinol Metab* **49**,
   284.
7 Franks S., *et al* (1978) *Clin Endocrinol* (Oxf) **8**, 277.
8 Freeman R.M., *et al* (1968) *Ann Intern Med* **69**, 67.
9 *Hall P.F. (1959) *Gynaecomastia* Monograph 2, Fed-
   eral Council Medical Association of Australia.
10 Jeffreys D.B. (1979) *Br Med J* i, 1119.
11 Korting G.W. (1961) *Hautarzt* **12**, 529.
12 Kuhn J.M., *et al* (1983) *Presse Med* **12**, 21.
13 Large D.M. & Anderson D.C. (1979) *Clin Endocrinol*
   (Oxf) **11**, 505.
14 Morley J.E., *et al* (1979) *Metabolism* **28**, 1051.
15 Nicole G.L., *et al* (1971) *J Clin Endocrinol Metab* **32**,
   173.
16 Nydick M., *et al* (1961) *J Am. Med. Assoc.* **178**, 455.
17 Scheike O., *et al* (1973) *Acta Pathol Microbiol Scand*
   81, 352.
18 Smith S.R., *et al* (1975) *J Clin Endocrinol Metab* **41**,
   60.
19 Stephanas A.V., *et al* (1978) *Cancer* **41**, 369.
20 Trump D.L., *et al* (1982) *Arch Intern Med* **142**, 511.
21 Turner A.R., *et al* (1982) *Arch Intern Med* **142**, 896.
22 Wheeler C.E., *et al* (1953) *Arch Dermatol Syphilol* **68**,
   685.
23 Wheeler C.E., *et al* (1954) *Ann Intern Med* **40**, 985.

MONDOR'S DISEASE
SYN. SCLEROSING PERIPHLEBITIS OF THE CHEST WALL

Mondor's disease has been regarded as an obliterative phlebitis usually affecting the thoracoepigastric,
lateral thoracic or superior epigastric vein. However, there is evidence [2] that it might be primarily
a lymphangitis. It occurs mainly between the ages

of 30 and 60 and affects women three times as
frequently as men. There may be a history of
trauma, accidental or surgical, or of contact dermatitis near the affected vessel. However, often no
cause is apparent. Rarely, the condition is bilateral
[7]; it has accompanied a lupus erythematosus-like
syndrome apparently induced by procainamide.

There may be some tenderness or discomfort, but
there are often no symptoms until the patient discovers a red linear cord running from the lateral
margin of the breast, crossing the costal margin and
extending to the abdominal wall. The cord is 2–
3 mm in diameter and is attached to the skin but
not to the deep fascia. It is usually only a few centimetres long, but may extend for 30–40 cm. The
symptoms subside in a few weeks, and there are no
known complications.

REFERENCES

1 Bircher J.B., *et al* (1962) *Proc Staff Meet Mayo Clin* **37**,
   651.
2 Heede G. (1968) *Dermatol Wochenschr* **154**, 337.
3 *Hogan G.F. (1964) *Arch Intern Med* **113**, 881.
4 *Hughes E.S.R. (1952) *Aust NZ J Surg* **22**, 17.
5 Legar L. (1947) *Presse Med* **55**, 849.
6 Rossman R.E. & Freeman R.G. (1963) *Arch Dermatol*
   87, 475.
7 Sivula A. & Somer T. (1973) *Ann Chir Gynaecol Fenn*
   62, 361.
8 Skipworth G.B., *et al* (1967) *Arch Dermatol* **95**, 95.

HAIR SINUS OF BREASTS

Hair sinus of the peri-areolar area of the breast has
been observed in women engaged in sheep shearing
(roustabout's breast) and also in hairdressers [1].
The lesions are similar to the interdigital pilonidal
sinuses which occur in barbers [2].

REFERENCES

1 Bowers P.W. (1982) *Clin Ex Dermatol* **7**, 445.
2 Price S.M. & Popkin G.L. (1976) *Arch Dermatol* **112**,
   523.

COWDEN'S DISEASE

This hereditary syndrome, which is characterized
by multiple hamartomas, is described elsewhere
(p. 128). In some cases fibrocystic disease may lead
to massive bilateral hyperplasia of the breasts.

CHAPTER 59

Diseases of the Umbilical, Perianal and Genital Regions

F. A. IVE & D. S. WILKINSON

A number of common diseases affect the genitalia and genitocrural folds only incidentally, while others present here with unusual features. These will be dealt with briefly or by cross-reference to their full description elsewhere. However, there are some conditions that are entirely or predominantly confined to these regions, and they are discussed in more detail.

The chapter is divided into five sections:

(i) the umbilicus—included for convenience
(ii) the genitocrural region
(iii) the perineal and perianal regions
(iv) the male genitalia
(v) the female genitalia

THE UMBILICUS

Though the umbilicus is not strictly part of the genital apparatus, its evolution and connections link it to the pelvic region.

Anatomy and embryology. At birth the umbilical cord contains two arteries and a vein, the rudimentary arachus (allantois) and the vitelline (omphalo-mesenteric) duct enveloped in Wharton's jelly. After separation and retraction of the stump an umbilicus of variable depth is formed. Persistence of the urachal or vitelline ducts at this 'carrefour embryologique' [11] may cause trouble in early or later life. A deeply retracted umbilicus may be the seat of infection or foreign body.

The umbilicus in the newborn. Haemorrhages may occur from slipped ligatures. The cord normally separates within a week of birth and the raw surface is epithelized by 15 days. During this time the umbilicus is obviously prone to infection, especially in maternity hospitals and nurseries. Impetigo (pemphigus neonatorum) or, fortunately very rarely, more severe bacterial infections occur (see below). Talc granulomas are a particular hazard.

A giant pigmented naevus of this area extended up the umbilical cord [24].

The 'absent navel' syndrome has been described as a sign of dystrophic epidermolysis bullosa [21].

Omphalocoele. This form of abdominal hernia appears to be more common in Africans. Thirty-three cases were seen in 5 yr in Ibadan [19]. The minor form is due to herniation of the umbilical cord; a major form is probably due to a fault of embryonic folding of the fetus.

Developmental errors and congenital anomalies [20]. These are all rare, more common in males and usually due to failure of obliteration of the omphalo-mesenteric duct or urachus. They present as fistulae, cysts or polypoid tumours.

Patent urachal duct. The umbilical opening is lined by skin or a pouting mucous membrane. Urine may be seen to escape from it, particularly in the elderly, when an obstruction to micturition exists. It is rare.

Persistent vitelline duct and polyp. If a connection with the intestine persists it may become inflamed or cause a faecal umbilical discharge. More commonly, the remains of the duct give rise to a polyp in later life [15]. This may be accompanied by intermittent bleeding or a more persistent mucoid discharge, sometimes profuse. A symptomless sterile umbilical discharge should always cause suspicion. The histopathological features are those of intestinal or gastric mucosa. It may be mistaken for a pyogenic granuloma.

Peri-umbilical 'choristia'. Under this title (meaning dysgenetic translocation of tissue) Bellone *et al* [1] described extending crusted erythematous peri-umbilical plaques in which islands of intestinal mucosal cells were found in the epidermis.

Perforating pseudoxanthoma elasticum. It has occurred here [23] and was the only site involved in six black females [16].

Granulomas [17]. The following granulomas may present as such or with an associated discharge, infection, bleeding or profuse sterile purulent exudate.

Granuloma pyogenicum. This is a dull-red fleshy polypoid lesion, often pedunculated. Bleeding readily takes place from trauma. If it occurs early in life, it may be confused with a capillary haemangioma.

Talc granuloma (Fig. 59.1). This lesion, which is probably more frequent than is recognized, occurs

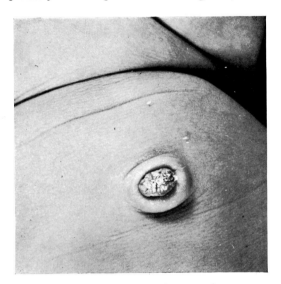

FIG. 59.1. Talc granuloma. Note talc scattered over umbilicus and abdomen. (Dr D.I. McCallum, General Hospital, Nottingham.)

in infants and very young children. It is distinguished histologically from a pyogenic granuloma (on which it may supervene) by the doubly refractile talc crystals [17].

A pilonidal sinus may occur here [12].

Ileo-umbilical fistulae may follow laparatomy for Crohn's disease, rarely spontaneously [25].

Omphalith. In deeply set umbilici an accumulation of sebum and keratin may lead to the gradual formation of a hard stone-like mass which may remain unnoticed for many years until discovered accidentally or revealed by secondary infection or ulceration.

A spontaneously regressing warty condition of the umbilicus in a youth defied accurate diagnosis [33].

Infections. Infection of the umbilicus in the newborn used to carry a high mortality. It still occurs in some countries. A number of bacterial organisms may be responsible, but staphylococcal, pseudomonal and clostridial species [14] are the most important. Minor forms consist of oozing and crusting but a spreading oedematous erythema, progressing to gangrene, is of very serious import. Liver abscess, portal vein thrombosis or osteomyelitis can supervene [2]. At any time in later life, but usually after middle age, the umbilicus may be the seat of intertrigo or candidal infections. This is more common in the obese or in those with poor personal hygiene. Foreign bodies, inserted by children or psychotics, may be overlooked as a cause of purulent infection in a deeply set umbilicus. The peri-umbilical skin is a common site of bilharziasis when it affects the skin [7].

Eczematous and other conditions. Contact dermatitis is usually due to medicaments. Irritant reactions to soap and quaternary ammonium compounds also occur. The umbilicus is not infrequently involved in pemphigoid and cicatricial pemphigoid, and may be the site of presentation of the latter (Chapter 41).

Peri-umbilical *staining* (Cullen's sign) occurs in acute pancreatitis, and occasionally in ruptured ectopic pregnancy or with duodenal ulcer perforation [13].

Umbilical haemorrhage has been described [10] as a complication of cirrhosis, following gross ulceration of the umbilical vein.

Tumours and implantations. The umbilicus is not an uncommon site of implantation of endometriomas [27], which may clinically resemble melanomas [34]. A unique case of post-operative endosalpingiosis has also been reported [9]. Colonic mucosa was implanted in an infant after colostomy for Hirschprung's disease [22]. A single case of carcinoid of the umbilicus has been noted [5]. Paget's disease has also been recorded [32]. Skin metastases from neoplasms of the digestive tract occurred in only 3% of 2187 cases [31] but the umbilicus is a characteristic site, especially from cancers of the stomach (Sister Joseph's nodule) [27] (Fig. 59.2) which was the primary source in 33 out of 40 cases [31]. The ovary and colon are responsible for most of the others [28, 35], though the pancreas has also been a rare primary site [29]. The lesions usually present as firm irregular nodules but can occasionally infiltrate diffusely or ulcerate with a foetid discharge. Such metastases were the presenting symptom in 18 out of 40 cases and a major diagnostic

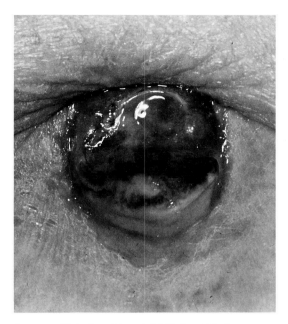

FIF. 59.2. 'Sister Joseph's nodule' (Dr Janet Marks, Freeman Hospital, Newcastle-upon-Tyne.)

feature in 28 cases [30]. The prognosis is always bad though not entirely hopeless [6]. After histological confirmation, surgical intervention is obligatory since it is occasionally the earliest and only metastasis [28].

Umbilical artery catheterization. Unilateral skin necrosis of the buttock has been reported following indwelling umbilical artery catheterization [3, 4, 8, 18], probably due to thrombosis leading to occlusion of the inferior gluteal artery. A rather similar case was due to misdirection of the tip of the arterial catheter [26]. However, 'spontaneous gangrene' can also occur without catheterization, possibly owing to minor trauma to the umbilicus [3]. Very rarely, the bladder and kidney may also be involved.

REFERENCES

1 BELLONE A.G., *et al.* (1978) *Ann Dermatol Vénéréol* **105**, 601.
2 BINGHAM E.A. & BEARE J.M. (1979) In *Modern Topics in Paediatric Dermatology.* Ed Verbov J. London, Heinemann, pp. 43–44.
3 BONIFAZI E. & MENEGHINI C. (1970) *J Am Acad Dermatol* **3**, 596.
4 BOOK I.S., *et al* (1978) *J Pediatr* **92**, 793.
5 BRODY H., *et al* (1978) *Arch Dermatol* **114**, 570.
6 CHATTERJEE S.N. & BAUER H.M. (1980) *Arch Dermatol* **116**, 984.
7 COLIN M., *et al* (1980) *Ann Dermatol Vénéréol* **107**, 759.
8 CUTLER V.E. & STRETCHER G.S. (1977) *Arch Dermatol* **113**, 61.
9 DORÉ N., *et al* (1980) *Arch Dermatol* **116**, 909.
10 DOUGLAS J.G. (1981) *Postgrad Med* **57**, 461.
11 DUPERATT M.B. & DUPERATT-NOURY G. (1968) *Bull Soc Fr Dermatol SyphilIgr* **75**, 638.
12 EBY C.S. & JETTON R.L. (1972) *Arch Dermatol* **106**, 893.
13 EVANS D.M. (1971) *Br Med J* i, 154.
14 GORMLEY D. (1977) *Arch Dermatol* **113**, 683.
15 HEJAKI N. (1975) *Dermatologica* **150**, 111.
16 HICKS J., *et al* (1979) *Arch Dermatol* **115**, 300.
17 McCALLUM D.I. & HALL G.F.M. (1970) *Br J Dermatol* **83**, 151.
18 MANN P.N. (1980) *Arch Dis Child* **55**, 815.
19 NIVABUEZE I. & HEKWABA F. (1981) *Postgrad Med J* **57**, 635.
20 NIX T.E. & YOUNG C.J. (1964) *Arch Dermatol* **90**, 160.
21 PASLIN D. (1978) *Br J Dermatol* **98**, 584.
22 PEACHEY R.R.G. (1974) *Br J Dermatol* **90**, 108.
23 PREMALATHA P., *et al* (1982) *Int J Dermatol* **21**, 604.
24 REED W.B., *et al* (1973) *Acta Derm Venereol (Stockh)* **53**, 318.
25 REUTZ T.W. (1979) *Digest Dis* **24**, 316.
26 RUDOLPH N., *et al* (1974) *Paediatrics* **53**, 106.
27 SAMITZ M.H. (1975) *Arch Dermatol* **111**, 1478.
28 SHARAKI M. & ABDEL-KADER M. (1981) *Clin Oncol* **7**, 351.
29 SHVILI D., *et al* (1983) *Cutis* **31**, 555.
30 STECK W.D. & HELWIG E.B. (1965) *Cancer* **18**, 907.
31 TEXIER L., *et al* (1978) *Ann Dermatol Vénéréol* **105**, 913.
32 UCKI H. & KOHDA M. (1979) *Hautartz* **30**, 267.
33 WHITE S.W. (1983) *J Am Acad Dermatol* **8**, 421.
34 WILLIAMS H.E., *et al* (1976) *Arch Dermatol* **112**, 1435.
35 ZELIGMAN I. & SCHWILM A. (1974) *Arch Dermatol* **110**, 911.

THE GENITOCRURAL REGION

This section deals with conditions affecting the genitocrural region, irrespective of the sex of the patient. It is a region of the body that is particularly prone to mycotic and pyococcal infections and flexural forms of common dermatoses. Moisture and friction lead to maceration and fissuring. Vegetating reactions are often very resistant to treatment.

Diffuse lymphangiomas or angiomas may cause irregular subcutaneous swellings. Epidermal naevi are not uncommon. Papilliferous moles and skin tags often become large and pedunculated on the inner aspect of the thighs. Dystrophic forms of epidermolysis bullosa may cause separation of the skin during delivery or, if less severe, bullae and erosions at these sites of friction.

The reticulate pigmented anomaly of the flexures (Dowling–Degos) involved the flexures in 8 out of 10 patients [9].

Infestations. Pediculosis pubis is sometimes overlooked as a cause of pruritus in the female. In the hirsute male, the infestation may be widespread. Oxyuriasis has caused localized urticaria as well as pruritus [2]. Scabies in children is diffuse and the inguinal glands are often enlarged from secondary infection. Seabathers' eruptions and 'seaweed dermatitis' affect the bathing trunk area.

Schistosomiasis (p. 1005) causes phagedaenic necrosis, fistulae and pseudo-elephantiasis and may also give rise to granulomas and condylomatous masses. Onchocerciasis causes depigmentation, nodules, atrophy, lymphadenopathy and a 'hanging groin' infection and lichenification [5].

Infections. Bacterial or candidal infections complicate eczema, scabies, intertrigo, napkin erythema and many tropical diseases. Vincent's organism, *Pseudomonas aeruginosa* and a wide variety of Gram-negative organisms are commonly found. Giant condylomata acuminata may infiltrate the groin [4].

Gangrenous ecthyma of infants (pp. 770, 785) may, very rarely, affect the inguinocrural area and gangrene has followed operations for inguinal hernia [1].

Erythrasma of the groins (p. 759) is symptomless and is very often overlooked. Lesions are usually also found in the axillae or toe-webs. It may coexist with *Trichophyton rubrum* [7].

Candidiasis is extremely common either as a primary infection, particularly in infants, pregnancy and diabetes, or supervening on other dermatoses. It is a frequent cause of genitocrural pruritus. A glazed erythematous sheet extends from the genitalia, anus or inguinal folds and is bordered by a thin, vesicular or slightly macerated edge (Fig.

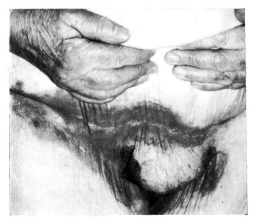

FIG. 59.3. Candidal intertrigo in an obese 'latent' diabetic (Stoke Mandeville Hospital).

59.3). Outlying papules rapidly develop small erosions with a collarette edge. In bacterial infections scaling, crusting or oozing are more usual, or folliculitis is present.

Tinea cruris (p. 921) is much more frequent in the male, though females are affected more commonly in hot climates. Spread occurs onto the thighs and pubis. *Epidermophyton floccosum* infections are usually symmetrical or more marked on the side on which the patient dresses. There is a fine peripheral scaling (eczema marginé of Hebra). Cases have been described in infants [6]. *T. rubrum* infections are often deceptive or atypical, with irregular or polycyclic margins and extension to the pubis, perianal area and buttocks. When corticosteroids have suppressed scaling and reduced the erythema the clinical diagnosis may be in doubt. *Trichomycosis* presents with malodour and discoloured broken hairs [8], which should be distinguished from those of trichorrhexis nodosa, caused by repeated scratching [3]. Blastomycosis, actinomycosis and other deep fungal infections (Chapter 25) simulate tuberculosis but are more prone to form fissures, sinuses and vegetating or exuberant granulomatous lesions. They are distinguished by histological and bacteriological examination.

Among chronic infections, tuberculosis, tertiary syphilis and leishmaniasis are diagnosed by their characteristics, which are described elsewhere. In tropical countries tuberculous inguinal lymphadenopathy may be a cause of genitocrural lymphoedema. Amoebiasis (p. 1013) involves the groins and perineum by extension from the anus. Hidradenitis suppurativa (p. 785) usually involves the area widely, though localized lesions are sometimes seen.

Venereal diseases. These are fully discussed in Chapter 21 and 24. Granuloma inguinale affects the genitalia only in less than half the cases, causing coalescing nodules, serpiginious ulcers and fungating masses. The buboes and fistulae of lymphogranuloma venereum are characteristic (p. 710). In both diseases vulval (rarely scrotal) lymphoedema and elephantiasis may occur.

REFERENCES

1 AUDEBERT C. (1981) *Ann Dermatol Vénéréol* **108**, 451.
2 BIAGHI F. & MAETUSCELLI Q. (1963) *Dermatol Trop* **2**, 129.
3 CHERNOSKY M.E. & OWEN D.W. (1966) *Arch Dermatol* **94**, 577.
4 ENG A.M., *et al* (1979) *Cutis* **24**, 203.
5 NELSON G.S. (1958) *Trans R Soc Trop Med Hyg* **52**, 272.
6 PARRY E.L., *et al* (1982) *A, J Dis Child* **136**, 273.
7 SCHLAPPNER O.L.A., *et al* (1979) *Br J Dermatol* **100**, 147.
8 WHITE S.W. & SMITH J. (1979) *Arch Dermatol* **115**, 444.

9 WILSON JONES E. & GRICE K. (1978) *Arch Dermatol* **114**, 1150.

Genitocrural dermatitis. The main features in differential diagnosis are as follows.

Contact dermatitis (Chapter 14). This may present suddenly with pruritus, oedema and erythema or insidiously as a gradual intensification of a pre-existing dermatitis. Sensitization to applied medicaments, contraceptives or, in men, industrial or other contact agents transferred by hand may be responsible, especially if the scrotum and thighs are also affected.

Constitutional eczema. Infantile napkin erythemas are discussed in Chapter 7. The distinction of von Jacquet's erythema from congenital syphilis and from the exuberant plaques and nodules of infantile gluteal granuloma [2, 8] is important. Candidiasis may be overlooked as a common cause of genitocrural inflammation, and Letterer–Siwe disease as a rare cause.

In the adult, the genitocrural and lower abdominal folds are likely to be involved in any form of seborrhoeic or intertriginous dermatitis. Psoriasis and lichen planus are recognized by their special characteristics, though the diagnosis may be difficult when the former arises in an exclusively flexural distribution. The alternation of flexural seborrhoeic dermatitis and psoriasis or of psoriasis and lichen planus may pose diagnostic difficulties.

Acrodermatitis enteropathica and the acquired zinc deficiency syndrome may well be overlooked as causes of genitocrural dermatitis.

Intertrigo

Definition. Intertrigo is a generic name for an inflammatory dermatosis involving the body folds, notably those of the submammary and genitocrural regions.

Pathogenesis. There is no clear distinction between constitutional and infective causes. Physical factors such as obesity, sweating, friction, incontinence and soiling by excreta may cause erythema or fissuring and render the skin vulnerable to the effect of other agents. Initially, it is marked by soreness or slight itching and a superficial mild erythema of the opposed surfaces. Secondary infection occurs rapidly and the condition is then perpetuated as an infective dermatitis. In eczematous subjects this will take on the physical characteristics of eczema; in others the infection may progress to crusting, pustular or vegetating lesions. The organisms concerned are *Staphylococcus pyogenes*, rarely the haemolytic streptococcus, *Escherichia coli*, *Proteus species* and, occasionally, *Pseudomonas aeruginosa*. In infants, diabetics and the obese, yeasts are often present. Latent diabetes should be borne in mind when the disease is refractory (Fig. 59.3).

Overtreatment readily induces further irritation or a sensitization dermatitis.

Diagnosis. Candidiasis and contact dermatitis are differentiated by the history, the appearance and microscope examination. The diffuse macerated erythema, often with fissures at the apex of the fold and without a sharply defined edge, distinguishes intertrigo from psoriasis and fungal infections, though scrapings and culture should always be undertaken. Mistakes in diagnosis arise from failure to recognize that two or more aetiological factors may coexist [6].

Treatment. In the early stages the condition can be controlled by avoidance of friction and pressure, and restriction of movement and tight clothing. Driving or sitting for long periods should be avoided. In severe cases the patient must rest in bed, preferably with groins unclothed and bedclothes lifted by a cradle, the opposed skin surfaces being kept apart with appropriate dressings [10]. Obesity, diabetes and incontinence should receive attention. Wet dressings, applied properly, are often useful initially in acute cases and may be followed by bland or mild antibacterial creams or lotions. The aniline dyes and magenta paints still have a place in therapy. In general, lotions, paints and powders are more acceptable than creams. Nystatin, hydroxyquinoline and the newer imidazoles can be applied, alone or with hydrocortisone.

Bullous and vegetating lesions. Bullous impetigo occurs in childhood, often secondary to scabies. All forms of pemphigus and pemphigoid (especially pemphigus vegetans [11] and pyodermite végétante [3]) affect this region, and juvenile pemphigoid and herpes gestationis affect it selectively and sometimes exclusively (p. 1655). Benign familial pemphigus (Fig. 59.4) affected the groins or genitalia in 14 out of 21 patients in one series [4]. It is easily mistaken for intertrigo, especially when a family history is lacking. Seasonal exacerbations over many years should arouse suspicion and compel a biopsy. Subcorneal pustular dermatosis (p. 1659) extends outwards from the inguinal folds as flaccid pustules, rapidly rupturing to form gyrate and circinate crusted lesions. Epidermal necrolysis (p. 1658) may present as desquamation, sometimes involving the

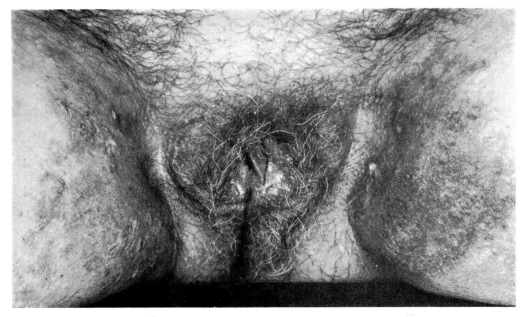

Fig. 59.4. Benign familial chronic pemphigus. Note the involvement of frictional areas. (St John's Hospital.)

whole region. Severe erythema multiforme involves the genital or anal mucosa in half the cases. Necrolytic migratory erythema also extends in waves from this area [9].

Pemphigus vegetans must be distinguished from vegetating forms of pyoderma (p. 1639), which are not uncommon in the groins, and from blastomycosis and other mycoses, verrucous forms of tuberculosis and granuloma inguinale. Careful histological examination and culture are usually essential unless diagnostic lesions are present elsewhere.

Other conditions likely to involve diagnostic problems. Changes in the pattern of pubic hair are dealt with on p. 1992. Acanthosis nigricans (p. 1460) invariably affects the groins. Pseudo-acanthosis nigricans can present as a macerated intertrigo and secondary infection. These can be separated from each other and from lichenification in pigmented skins by a rubber silicone impression technique [5].

Impetigo herpetiformis (p. 1526) frequently starts in the groin with small angry inflammatory yellowish-green pustules which rupture to produce scabs and crusts.

Calcinosis involving the upper inner thighs may resemble pseudoxanthoma elasticum [1].

In the 'short-bowel syndrome' kwashiorkor-like changes include an 'enamel paint skin' [7].

REFERENCES

1 COCHRAN R.J. & WILKINSON J.K. (1983) *J Am Acad Dermatol* **8**, 103.
2 HAMADO T. (1975) *Arch Dermatol* **111**, 1072.
3 NEUMANN H.A.M. & FABER W.R. (1980) *Arch Dermatol* **116**, 1169.
4 RAASCHOU-NIELSEN W. & REYMANN F. (1959) *Acta Derm Venereol (Stockh)* **39**, 280.
5 SARKANY I. (1962) *Br J Dermatol* **74**, 254.
6 SCHLAPPNER O.L.A., *et al* (1970) *Br J Dermatol* **100**, 147.
7 SMITH S.R. (1977) *Ann Dermatol* **113**, 657.
8 TAPPEINER J. & PFLEGER L. (1971) *Hautarzt* **22**, 383.
9 WILKINSON D.S. (1973) *Trans Rep St John's Hosp Dermatol Soc* **59**, 244.
10 WILKINSON D.S. (1977) *The Nursing and Management of Skin Diseases*, 4th ed. London, Faber.
11 WINKELMANN R.K. & SU W.P.D. (1979) *Arch Dermatol* **115**, 446.

Pruritus and lichenification. Genitocrural pruritus may be unusually predominant in psoriasis and infective conditions in this area. Lice, oxyuris infestation and diabetes must always be excluded as primary causes. Diffuse or localized pruritus, often severe and spasmodic, occurs with lichen simplex. The psychological mechanisms involved are similar to those discussed in relation to pruritus vulvae (p. 2217) and pruritus ani (p. 2177).

Lichenification occurs readily, either as lichen

simplex or superimposed on a pre-existing dermatitis. In women, vulval lichenification may spread to involve the thighs and lower belly or the perianal region. In men, the perianal region, scrotum, the root of the penis and pubis are chiefly affected, though a localized area on the inner thigh may alone be involved. Lichenification occurs commonly in atopic patients and in those of an anxious or obsessional nature. The 'giant' form of lichenification described by Pautrier [1] may resemble dermatitis vegetans and be extremely resistant to treatment.

Diagnosis. The appearances are characteristic even when rubbing is denied. It is important to determine any primary underlying organic cause. To label a disease 'psychosomatic' because an anxious patient has the ability to lichenify a pre-existing organic dermatosis does him a disservice and delays correct treatment.

Treatment. If no primary cause is evident and if diabetes and infestations have been excluded, a careful history may disclose relevant psychogenic factors, or a state of extreme tension, anxiety or conflict requiring discussion and reassurance.

Local treatment with corticosteroid applications is supplemented by reassurance, rest and sedation. All factors provoking local itching must, as far as possible, be removed. A short period of complete bed rest, preferably away from home, is often more successful than local therapy.

REFERENCE

1 PAUTRIER L.M. (1936) In *Nouvelle Pratique Dermatologique*. Ed Darier J. Paris, Masson, Vol. 7, p. 497.

DISEASES PARTICULARLY AFFECTING INFANTS

These usually involve part or all of the napkin area. They are discussed in this Chapter on p. 2115 and more fully in Chapter 7.

THE PERINEAL AND PERIANAL REGIONS

Anatomy and physiology. The central part of the pelvic floor, bounded posteriorly by the coccyx and anococcygeal raphe and anteriorly by the perineal body and its attachment to the genital organs, encloses one mucocutaneous junction and adjoins another. The natal cleft is deep and firmly fixed to underlying fibrous and fascial tissues, and its sides are steep and closely opposed. Mucous discharges, excreta and moisture are retained easily within it. Proximity to the genital organs and anus give it a special physical and psychological importance.

The perineum is endowed with numerous eccrine sweat glands whose function is retained after lumbar and thoracolumbar sympathectomies. Sweating may be due to an alternative parasympathetic sudomotor pathway from the fourth sacral anterior root. Apocrine glands are present but many are functionless.

A variable number of sebaceous glands are present both in pilosebaceous units and as individual 'free' sebaceous glands at the transitional part of the anal canal.

Developmental anomalies. Gross anomalies will only be seen incidentally by the dermatologist because of skin complications. Minor abnormalities such as haemangiomas, skin tags and papilliferous acanthomas are common on the inner sides of the thighs and infragluteal region. Pigmented hairy naevi may involve one or both buttocks.

Developmental cysts, fistulae and sinuses. They are not uncommon and frequently become infected. They may be mistaken for hidradenitis suppurativa or furuncles. Dermoid cysts occur on or adjacent to the perineal raphe and scrotum. Cloacal sinuses form fistulae from the anus to the adjoining skin; others involve the urethra and perineum.

Pilonidal cyst and sinus [9]. This common midline lesion may present as a cyst, often with a pigmented or hairy surface which ruptures and quickly becomes infected. The sinus usually extends to the sacrum and causes sacrococcygeal fistulae with deep ramifications. This heals if the track is thoroughly cleaned. It may be successfully dealt with on an out-patient basis [8].

Since the perineum is at the cross-roads of the anogenital area, it is often involved in conditions primarily involving the perianal skin, groins and scrotum or vulva. These will not be described separately.

PERIANAL INFLAMMATION

The causes of perianal inflammation in infants are dealt with on p. 2215. In older children oxyuris infestation causes irritation and excoriations at night. Physical agents, tight underclothes or moisture from discharges are also sources of local inflammation.

In the adult, inflammation may result from the

coexistence of several factors: haemorrhoids, anal discharge, proctitis, the presence of fissures or the effect of scratching. Oxyuris infestation is sometimes postulated but seldom confirmed. Pediculosis pubis must be excluded. Traumatic lesions are seen in male homosexuals.

Contact dermatitis results chiefly from antipruritic or antibiotic applications. In 43 suspected cases, neomycin (27%) and 'caine mix' (24%) were the most frequent offenders; quinolines (7%), lanolin (7%) and ethylenediamine (5%) were less common [15]. Fixed drug eruptions may produce striking pigmentation. Lichen planus involving the buttocks and perianal region is extremely irritable and may become excoriated or hypertrophic. In elderly, delibitated or bed-ridden patients a persistent patch of erythema on the sacral or ischial region is a sign of impending ulceration.

Five common conditions cause diagnostic difficulties; seborrhoeic dermatitis, psoriasis, contact dermatitis, lichen simplex and mycotic infections. The lesions of seborrhoeic dermatitis are brownish-red with branny or rather larger greasy scales towards the edge, extending beyond and outside the fold and involving other areas of the body. Psoriasis has a smooth rather glazed surface and a dull-red hue, often fissured; other signs of the disease are nearly always present. Contact dermatitis is highly irritable, usually eczematous and has an ill-defined spreading border. When due to a medicament the hand may be involved. Gross lichenification simulates psoriasis but is usually unilateral except when it involves the perianal area. It may occur as a small intensely irritable area, localized to the edge of the anus in one area which is indicated exactly by the patient. Mycotic infections are dealt with below. The prior use of topical corticosteroids frequently confuses the issue.

Treatment. This should be bland. The strength of added active ingredients should be less than that used elsewhere on the skin. Humidity, natural occlusion of the area and the presence of fissures, cracks and excoriation increase the risk of sensitization. Wet dressings, cool bathing, bland or mildly astringent packs and simple creams are indicated in acute stages. Antibacterials should be chosen with care. Hydroxyquinolines, though reasonably safe, are being displaced by imidazoles. Betadine cleansing preparations are useful. Prosiasis and lichenification call for more vigorous measures. Tar pastes, dithranol and steroid ointments are tolerated if applied carefully and in an appropriate strength. Prolonged use of strong topical corticosteroids causes a dusky erythema, atrophy or ulceration.

In all cases of perianal and perineal inflammation, the urine should be tested for sugar, and swabs and scrapings examined. A vaginal or rectal examination is mandatory. Any irregularity of the bowels which causes straining or soiling should be corrected.

SUPERFICIAL INFECTIONS OF THE PERIANAL SKIN

Though the high temperature and humidity of this area, combined with pressure [4] and friction, encourages colonization by staphylococci, primary pyococcal infections are now uncommon in countries with cultural or aquired habits of cleanliness. The perineal carriage of staphylococci [11] may not cause local lesions in the host but is especially important in acting as a reservoir from which *Staphylococcus aureus* may be disseminated to other sites or to eczematous lesions elsewhere. In adults the carriage rate is of the order of 13–22%; in neonates it may be higher. Some persons are better 'dispersers' of the staphylococcus than others and the organisms may remain (and even increase) after washing. The risk of dispersion of staphylococci from this site is of obvious importance in hospital operating theatres, where attempts have been made to minimize it by the provision of special clothing [10]. Gram-negative organisms are seldom pathogenic unless the balance of the skin is grossly disturbed (p. 725). *Ps aeruginosa* may be found in deep ulcers and fissures.

The presence of an infective condition in this area may overlie and disguise a more important lesion of the colon or rectum [6].

Viral infections. In infants, Coxsackie A infections commonly cause a transient papular or papulovesicular eruption of the perianal area and buttocks. Both herpes simplex and accidental vaccinia may occur. Anogenital zoster [2], involving S2-4, or, less commonly, the ileo-inguinal segment of L1-2, may cause acute cystitis or urinary or faecal retention [5, 13, 14]. Vaccinia, usually by indirect transmission [2], is now seen only rarely. Acquired immunodeficiency syndrome (AIDS) has presented as an anogenital herpes zoster [12].

Condylomata acuminata. These are distinguished without difficulty from the moist flat syphilitic condylomata (Figs 59.5 and 59.6). Although they occasionally occur in infants and young children, they are normally seen in young adults and are not always venereal. They may be extraordinarily profuse, extending into the anal canal, especially in

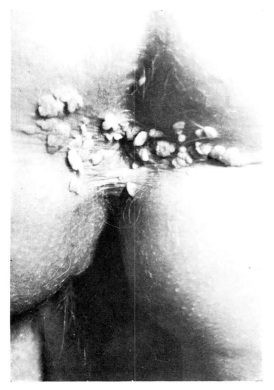

FIG. 59.5. Condylomata acuminata which extended into the anal canal (Stoke Mandeville Hospital).

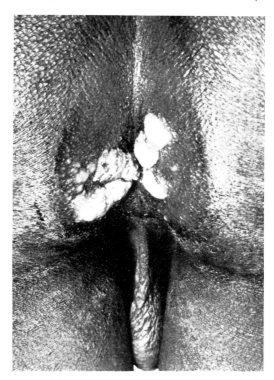

FIG. 59.6. Condylomata lata (Makerere College Medical School).

homosexuals or in immunodeficient subjects. They may sometimes be associated with other lesions of the gastrointestinal tract [7].

The giant condyloma of Buschke–Lowenstein (see p. 2183). Only five cases have been reported in the anal area [1].

Mycotic infections. These are common. Candidiasis causes a bright-red glazed area, often with outlying pustulettes, and may spread to the groins or natal cleft. Microscopy and culture distinguish it from other fungal infections and from psoriasis and pyococcal infections. Erythrasma, present also in other sites, was found in 15 of 81 patients examined using Wood's light [3]. All were males. In our experience it is less common. The well-marked scaly circinate edge, the spread and the chronicity of *T. rubrum* infections offer a clue to diagnosis, which is easily verified in the usual way. However, prior treatment with corticosteroids may so disguise the appearance as to trap the unwary. All unusual forms of perianal dermatitis should therefore be

examined with fungal infections in mind. Histoplasmosis, blastomycosis and other forms of mycotic infection have also been recorded in this area.

REFERENCES

1 ALEXANDER R.M. & KAMINSKY D.B. (1979) *Dis Colon Rectum* **22**, 561.
2 BESSIÈRE L., *et al* (1979) *Ann Dermatol Vénéréol* **105**, 339.
3 BOWYER A. & McCOLL L. (1971) *Acta Derm Venereol (Stockh)* **5**, 444.
4 FELMAN Y.M. & NIKITAS J.A. (1980) *Cutis* **26**, 347.
5 FUNGELSO P.D., *et al* (1973) *Br J Dermatol* **89**, 285.
6 GROSSHANS E., *et al* (1979) *Ann Dermatol Vénéréol* **106**, 25.
7 LIBESKIND M., *et al* (1980) *Rev Fr Gastroenterol* **160**, 33.
8 LORD P.H. & MILLAR D.M. (1965) *Br J Surg* **52**, 298.
9 MILLAR D.M. (1970) *Proc R Soc Med* **63**, 126.
10 MITCHELL N.J. & GAMBLE D.R. (1974) *Lancet* ii, 1133.
11 NOBLE W.C. & SOMERVILLE D.A. (1974). *Microbiology of Human Skin*. Vol. 2. *Major Problems in Dermatology*. Ed. Rook A.J. London, Saunders.
12 THUNE P., *et al* (1983) *Acta Derm Venereol (Stockh)* **63**, 540.

13 WAUGH M.A. (1974) *Br J Dermatol* **90**, 235.
14 WEAVER S.M. & KELLY A.P. (1982) *Cutis* **29**, 611.
15 WILKINSON J.D., *et al* (1980) *Acta Derm Venereol (Stockh)* **60**, 245.

Effects of corticosteroids. The prolonged use of potent topical corticosteroids for inflammatory conditions of the groins or perianal area can produce misleading appearances. Tinea incognito [1] is well recognized but a persistent deep livid erythema of the perianal skin may be regarded as primarily infective. Striae occur readily on the thighs. Multiple *perianal comedones* followed the application of a topical corticosteroid for 3 yr [3]. The 'infantile gluteal granuloma' [4] (p. 244) usually affecting infants of 4–6 months may also occur in incontinent elderly patients [2].

REFERENCES

1 IVE F.A. & MARKS R. (1968) *Br Med J* iii, 149.
2 MACKAWA Y., *et al* (1978) *Arch Dermatol* **114**, 382.
3 OLIER E.J. & ESTES S.A. (1982) *J Am Acad Dermatol* **7**, 405.
4 ORTONNE J.P., *et al* (1980) *Ann Dermatol Vénéréol* **107**, 631.

Danthron erythema [3, 4]. This form of contact irritant dermatitis *per rectum* is due to the use of a laxative containing danthron in situations where there is retention of faeces. It is seen in mentally backward children, in those with Hirschprung's disease or encopresis and sometimes in aged incontinent patients [1, 2, 4]. Danthron (1,8-dihydroxyanthroquinone) is reduced in the large bowel to 1,8-dihydroxyanthron which is the active agent [4]. This is chemically identical with dithranol and the lesions produced by faecal incontinence are equivalent to dithranol 'burns'.

A bizarre livid erythema in the perianal area, groins, thighs and buttocks, with sharp outlines, corresponds to the areas of contact with the faeces and is easily differentiated from other causes of perianal or inguinocrural lesions.

REFERENCES

1 BARTH J.H., *et al* (1984) *Clin Exp Dermatol* **9**, 95.
2 BROHOLM K.A. (1973 *Gerontol Clin (Basel)* **15**, 25.
3 BUNNEY M.H. & NOBLE I.M. (1974) *Br Med J* ii, 731.
4 IPPEN H. (1959) *Dermatologica* **119**, 211.

Hidradenitis suppurativa (p. 785). This can give rise to all degrees of inflammation and scarring. Friction and pressure accentuate the inflammatory changes which invade the fat and cause further granulomatous changes extending widely over the buttocks and thighs. Persistent perineal sinuses are frequent and deep lesions cause anal fistulae. In mild cases only a few isolated lesions are present. Secondary bacterial invasion, often from the gut [1], is an important complicating factor.

Differential diagnosis. This is not difficult when the condition is well established. The advanced case, with its fluctuant abscesses, burrowing sinuses, epithelial 'bridges', scarring and fibrosis can scarcely be mistaken (Fig. 59.7). Regional ileitis may cause anal fistulae (see below).

Mild or localized forms are frequently misdiagnosed as furunculosis or 'infected cysts', and

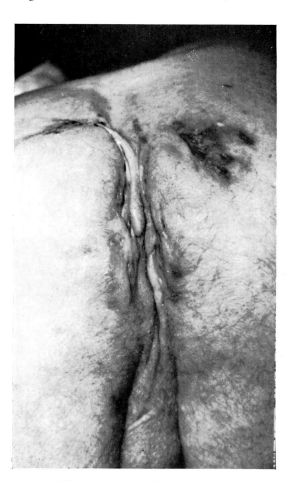

FIG. 59.7. Hidradenitis suppurativa in a man aged 55. Hypertrophic and bridged scarring and a recently active lesion on the buttock can be seen (Stoke Mandeville Hospital.)

confusion occurs with severe acne, developmental fistulae and lymphogranuloma venereum (p. 710). The relative painlessness, recurrences in the same or other sites and oblique sinuses that end in soft swollen inflamed nodules are characteristic.

Treatment [4]. Small localized sinuses may be phenolized successfully and early lesions may respond to intralesional corticosteroids. However, this may have to be repeated and recurrent or extensive lesions require a more radical approach. Marsupialization (as with pilonidal sinuses) and diathermy destruction of the affected tissue has been very successful in some of our cases, even those involving the scrotum. The use of Silastic foam dressing allowed easier healing [2]. Otherwise, plastic surgery with complete excision of all the involved skin is required. Long-term antibiotics are often given 'blind' but are seldom of lasting value though elimination of specific secondary invaders such as *Streptococcus milleri* [1] has given good results. Recently, cyproterone acetate and 13-*cis*-retinoic acid have been used [3]. Results are still being evaluated but both approaches merit consideration.

Lichen sclerosis et atrophicus. The perianal skin is rarely affected alone but is involved in two-thirds of the cases in which the vulva is affected [6], forming a characteristic 'figure-of-eight' distribution. One case of carcinoma has been reported [5].

REFERENCES

1 HIGHET A.S., *et al* (1980) *Br J Dermatol* 103, 375.
2 MORGAN W.P., *et al* (1980) *Br J Surg* 67, 277.
3 MORTIMER P.S., *et al* (1986) *Br J Dermatol* in Press.
4 MOULY M.R. (1969) *Bull Soc Fr Dermatol Syphiligr* 76, 723.
5 SLOAN P.J.M. & GOEPEL J. (1981) *Clin Exp Dermatol* 6, 399.
6 WALLACE H.J. (1971) *Trans Rep St John's Hosp Dermatol Soc* 57, 9.

Anosacral cutaneous amyloidosis. Fourteen cases of a new type of cutaneous amyloidosis have been reported in elderly Japanese [1, 2]. Pigmented macules and glossy hyperkeratotic lesions fan out in lines from the anus. Moderate pruritus was present in eight patients [3]. There are no systemic changes. Amyloid deposits are seen in upper reticular dermis and around hair follicles. It is thought to represent an ageing process [1].

REFERENCES

1 YAMAMOTO T. & MUKAI H. (1981) *Jpn J Dermatol* 91, 398.

2 YANAGHIHARA M. & MORI S. (1981) *Jpn J Dermatol* 91, 463.
3 YANAGHIHARA M., *et al* (1982) *16th Congress on Dermatology, 1982*. Tokyo, Tokyo University Press, p. 922.

FISSURED AND ULCERATING LESIONS OF THE PERIANAL SKIN

Non-specific. Non-specific anal and perianal fissures occurring as a result of chronic constipation in young people may be painless but intensely pruritic. They are usually situated posteriorly. If lateral, a primary lesion in the anal canal should be sought. An oedematous 'sentinel tag' is usually present if the fissure arises in the anus itself. Small erosions and fissures may occur in the sulcus beneath oedematous haemorrhoids or in an area of dermatitis. Proctoscopy is mandatory if the aetiology is in doubt and especially if the fissure extends to the anal margin or within. Benign fissures are superficial and not indurated, but when persistent they may be painful and cause bleeding, especially in the elderly. Unless they heal quickly under treatment, a biopsy should always be performed to exclude malignancy.

The presence of even a small fissure in an area of dermatitis maintains the pruritus and prolongs the course.

Behçet's disease occasionally presents with multiple, shallow ulcers and fissures of the anal margin [5]; psoriasis, lichen simplex and lichen sclerosus et atrophicus may cause splits in the skin folds.

Anorectal carcinoma may present as an ischiorectal abscess [3, 7, 11].

Specific
Syphilis (p. 845) [9]. Anal chancres are often mistaken for fissures; at the anal margin their significance may not be appreciated. Pain on defaecation or at night may be severe, but is often absent. The posterior midline is the site of election. Bilateral lymphadenopathy is extremely rare with other perianal ulcers. Dark-ground examination is useless if a lubricant or ointments have been used.

Gonorrhoea. This causes anal inflammation and discharge or an oedematous perianal dermatitis with multiple fissures and erosions. Chancroid can cause extremely painful anal lesions instead of multiple soft chancres.

Tuberculosis (Chapter 22). This is still seen where tuberculosis is common [10]. A primary chancre is exceptional; the accompanying unilateral lymphadenopathy is very suggestive. Indolent irregular painful ulcers, fistulae and abscesses may be difficult to distinguish from those accompanying Crohn's disease [6, 8]. Lupus vulgaris and verrucous tuberculosis may spread widely over the buttock and postanal region or assume a fungating and vegetating appearance.

Histiocytosis X has caused ulceration in this area [4].

Schistosomiasis has presented as pruritic papules in the genital, umbilical and perineal regions in countries where it is endemic [1]. It is usually preceded by rectal or intestinal symptoms. Viable or calcified ova are found in the dermis. The lesions mimic those of subcutaneous tuberculosis. Bilharziasis also occurs as papules or lichenified plaques in endemic areas [2].

Ischiorectal abscesses are common in Crohn's disease (see below) but may on occasion herald an underlying anal or rectal carcinoma [3].

Treatment. The patient is often apprehensive and after a full examination must be reassured that the lesion is benign, when this is so. Small erosions and excoriations frequently heal with treatment for anogenital pruritus (p. 2177). If they are hidden between haemorrhoids or anal tags, protective pastes are helpful. Fissures in psoriasis and seborroeic dermatitis are difficult to heal, particularly in the postnatal fold. If the underlying disease is satisfactorily controlled, the crack will heal without special attention. Intralesional corticosteroids may be effective in non-infective inflammatory conditions.

REFERENCES

1 ADEYEMI-DORU F.A.B., *et al* (1979) *Br J Vener Dis* **55**, 446.
2 COHN M., *et al* (1980) *Ann Dermatol Vénéréol* **107**, 759.
3 DRUMM M., *et al* (1982) *Br Med J* **285**, 1393.
4 GENIAUX B., *et al* (1973) *Bull Soc Fr Dermatol Syphiligr* **80**, 380.
5 *LOCKHART-MUMMERY H.E. (1963) *Br J Vener Dis* **39**, 15.
6 LORD P.H. (1975) *Dis Colon Rectum* **18**, 661.
7 MCCONNELL E.M. (1970) *Br J Surg* **57**, 89.
8 MORSON B.C. (1968) *Proc R Soc Med* **61**, 79.
9 SAMENIUS B. (1966) *Proc R Soc Med* **49**, 629.
10 STRESCOBICH D., *et al* (1969) *Prensa Med Argent* **56**, 1622.
11 TAIT W.F. & SYKES P.Z. (1982) *Br Med J* **4**, 1742.

GRANULOMATOUS, VEGETATING AND STENOSING LESIONS [2, 3]

Many banal conditions take on a vegetating appearance in this area, especially in hot humid climates and in the presence of infection. For these the term 'dermatitis vegetans' can be used.

Elephantiasis forms of progressive tuberculosis [1] and syphilis are now seldom seen but deep fungal infections must not be overlooked.

Benign mucosal pemphigoid (p. 1644) [4]. This may affect the groin, perineum and perianal skin and may cause anal stenosis. The drug clonidine may have been responsible in one case [5]. Pyodermite végétante (p. 1639) can be distinguished by the histology and by immunofluorescent studies. Ulcerative colitis may be present [2]. A peri-orificial form of eosinophilic granuloma may cause ulcerating and vegetating lesions around and within the anal canal.

In the differentiation of these rare proliferative and granulomatous lesions, repeated biopsies and tissue cultures are usually necessary.

Lymphogranuloma venereum (p. 710). When unrecognized or undiagnosed this disease causes widespread vegetating and scarring lesions of the genitoperineal area. The Frei and complement fixation tests distinguish it from hidradenitis suppuritiva.

REFERENCE

1 DELACRETAZ J. & CHRISTELER A. (1969) *Dermatologica* **139**, 313.
2 FORMAN L. (1966) *Trans Rep St John's Hosp Dermatol Soc* **52**, 139.
3 GOLDBERG J. & BERNSTEIN R. (1963) *Br J Vener Dis* **40**, 137.
4 *LEVER W.F. (1965) *Pemphigus and Pemphigoid*. Springfield, Thomas.
5 VAN JOOST T.H., *et al* (1980) *Br J Dermatol* **102**, 715.

Regional ileitis (syn Crohn's disease) [2, 5, 10, 11]. The cutaneous manifestations of Crohn's disease are as follows:

(i) erythema nodosum (p. 1156)
(ii) anal and perianal lesions
(iii) spreading ulceration of perineum and buttocks after colectomy
(iv) skin changes around ileostomies and colostomies
(v) 'sarcoid'-type lesions in remote sites
(vi) pyoderma gangrenosum
(vii) granulomatous cheilitis
(viii) epidermolysis bullosa acquisita (p. 1647)
(ix) non-specific changes due to malabsorption

Crohn's disease affects any part of the gastrointestinal tract but particularly the terminal ileum.

A sarcoid-like granulomatous histology is found in about 60% of cases. Anal or perianal lesions have occurred in a high proportion of all those affected [2, 4, 14] and may precede other signs by months or years; therefore they are of considerable diagnostic importance (Fig. 59.8). In one recent series of

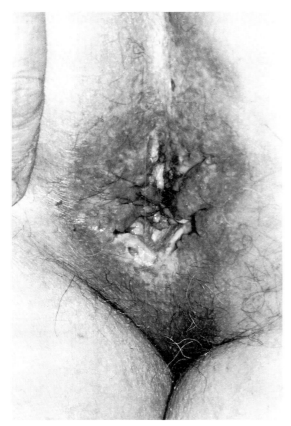

FIG. 59.8. Crohn's disease: perianal lesions (York District Hospital).

151 consecutive patients, 23 had ulcers and 26 had abscesses or fistulae [4]. In another series [8], 112 out of 329 patients were affected and in nearly all cases the colon was involved. Suspicion should be aroused whenever the anal margin or perianal skin is the site of pronounced maceration or inflammatory swellings, fistulae or ischiorectal abscesses, multiple ulcers or florid, 'juicy' skin tags. If there is any doubt about the causation, biopsy of the edge of a lesion and sigmoidoscopy is obligatory.

Similar though less extensive lesions occur, although much less commonly, in ulcerative colitis and only very rarely in diverticulitis [2]. Syphilis,

florid condylomata acuminata [13] and anorectal carcinoma presenting with an ischiorectal abscess [12] must be excluded.

Resection of the affected segment of bowel does not always cure the lesions or prevent their recurrence, especially at the ileostomy or colostomy sites.

Actinomycosis and mycetomas. Ulcerating and vegetating lesions, often unrecognized and of long duration, have followed trauma in patients with actinomycosis [3]. Correct diagnosis depends on histological confirmation but the yellow or red grain pus should arouse suspicion [9]. Mycetoma has also occurred on this site [6, 7].

Amoebiasis of the perianal skin [1, 6] (p. 1013). This is usually associated with bowel infections, but where the disease is endemic direct inoculation of abraded skin or operation wounds can occur.

Abscesses and fistulae may at first be indolent and symptomless. Ulcers typically extend slowly with serpiginous outlines, firm cord-like edges and a whitish slough [1, 11]. Sometimes, however, progression is rapid and remorseless until a phagadaemic ulcer completely destroys the perianal and sacral tissues. A black foul-smelling eschar is surrounded by a violaceous edge resembling pyoderma gangrenosum. The patient is extremely ill. Vegetating or condyloma-like lesions of intermediate severity occur less frequently.

Amoebiasis should be suspected when such a lesion occurs unexpectedly in the course of 'ulcerative colitis' or in a prolonged mild undiagnosed colitis. Cases have been described in infants [14]. The diagnosis is made by finding the *Entamoeba* in a biopsy specimen from the edge of a lesion (which is always secondarily infected) or by examination, while warm, of a fresh high sigmoidoscopy swab. Treatment with metronidazole (p. 2518) may be dramatically effective but in severe cases surgery may also be required.

Granuloma inguinale (p. 775). The initial rapidly ulcerating papule may occur in the perianal region in homosexuals. It is soft, painless and bleeds easily on trauma. It may be hypertrophic, sclerotic or phagadaenic. There is normally no regional adenopathy but a 'pseudobubo' may be present. In the anal canal the lesion never extends beyond the stratified epithelium and strictures do not occur, but anal stenosis or, rarely, epitheliomatous change can supervene.

REFERENCES

1 CAPETANAKIS J. & DOXIADES TH. (1966) *Am J Proctol* 17, 58.
2 *CROHN N.N. & YARNIS H. (1958) *Regional Ileitis*. 2nd ed. New York, Grune & Stratton.
3 GRIGORIU D. & DELECRETAZ J. (1981) *Ann Dermatol Vénéréol* 108, 159.
4 HOBBISS J.H. & SCHOFIELD P.F. (1982) *J R Soc Med* 75, 414.
5 *LOCKHART-MUMMERY H.E. (1963) *Br J Vener Dis* 39, 15.
6 LORD P.H. & SAKELLARIADES P. (1973) *Proc R Soc Med* 66, 677.
7 MARIAT F., *et al* (1977) *Contrib Microbiol Immunol* 4, 1.
8 MARKS C.G., *et al* (1981) *Br J Surg* 68, 525.
9 MILLET P., *et al* (1982) *Ann Dermatol Vénéréol* 109, 789.
10 *RANKIN G.B. *et al* (1979) National Co-operative Crohn's Disease Study *Gastroenterology* 77, 914.
11 SMITH J.N. & WINSHIP D.H. (1980) *Med Clin North Am* 64, 1161.
12 TAIT W.F. & SYKES P.A. (1982) *Br Med J* iv, 1742.
13 THOMSON J.P.S. & GRACE R.H. (1978) *J R Soc Med* 71, 181.
14 WYNNE J.M. (1980) *Arch Dis Child* 55, 234.

Epidermolysis bullosa acquisita and bowel disease [4]. A connection has been recognized in recent years between epidermolysis bullosa acquisita and inflammatory bowel disease. There have been several reports of association with Crohn's disease [1–3] and we have been able to confirm this.

REFERENCES

1 CHOUVET B., *et al* (1982) *Ann Dermatol Vénéréol* 109, 53.
2 LIVDEN J.K., *et al* (1978) *Acta Derm Venereol (Stockh)* 58, 241.
3 PEGUM J.S. & WRIGHT J.T. (1973) *Proc R Soc Med* 66, 234.
4 RAY T.L., *et al* (1982) *J Am Acad Dermatol* 6, 242.

NECROTIZING AND GANGRENOUS LESIONS

A number of closely associated and overlapping severe gangrenous or necrotizing lesions may affect the anorectal, perineal and scrotal skin and subcutaneous tissues. Although they are often a result of surgery or trauma and thus are primarily of surgical importance they are mentioned here because of the great importance of their early recognition and treatment (see also Chapter 21). These conditions are described under several names [2]:

Clostridial and non-clostridial [1, 2, 10] gangrene
Streptococcal cellulitis and myositis
Synergistic necrotizing cellulitis
Necrotizing fasciitis [3, 6, 8]
Meleney's progressive bacterial synergistic gangrene [5]
Synergistic gangrene [3]
Fournier's gangrene, etc.

Clinical features [2, 6, 8]. Although middle-aged and elderly subjects are most often affected, the conditions can follow trauma in young adults and the prognosis in these, given vigorous early treatment, is good [2]. They have also been described in children [7]. The infection may present as a primary perirectal abscess in the perineum or on the scrotum or labia. Pain is generally the first symptom and may be severe. A distinct black spot may appear on the scrotum or labium and is of ominous significance. Tenderness and a dusky erythema extends with extreme rapidity to involve wide areas and all the perirectal and perineal spaces (hence the terms 'fasciitis' and 'myositis'). Crepitus is an important feature, as is the presence of a dark brown turbid fluid without pus. Many patients have been diabetic [2, 6] or leukaemic; in these, the overall mortality of 12–25% is vastly increased [6]. A perianal distribution, old age and delay in treatment also greatly reduce the survival rate.

Bacteriology. Swabs should be taken from the outer margin of the lesion [4]. An immediate Gram stain will distinguish clostridial infections by the finding of large Gram-positive rods. *Clostridium perfringens* was the most common organism in one series [2], but other clostridia, aerobic and anaebic streptococci and *Pseudomonas* [7] have all been isolated. Anaerobics may easily be missed. A wide variety of secondary organisms are commonly cultured.

Treatment [2]. Early recognition and immediate and aggressive treatment are essential in this devastating condition. An electrolyte and fluid balance must be established and high dosage antibiotic therapy started without waiting for the result of culture. This will normally consist of intravenous penicillin (24–30 million units/day [2] together with a broad-spectrum antibiotic, usually an aminoglycosuride or cephalosporin; this can be modified later.

However, the most important single therapeutic manœuvre is rapid and extensive debridement of all affected tissue. Other surgical procedures, such as colostomy, may also be necessary. The value of hyperbaric oxygen [9] is disputed but it should probably be used if available.

REFERENCES

1 BESSMAN A.N. & WAGNER W. (1975) *JAMA* **233**, 958.
2 *BUBRICK M.P. & HITCHCOCK G.R. (1979) *Surgery* **86**, 655.
3 FISHER J.R., *et al* (1979) *JAMA* **241**, 803.
4 FLANIGAN R.C., *et al* (1978) *J Urol* **119**, 369.
5 MELENEY F.L. (1924) *Arch Surg* **9**, 317.
6 OH C., *et al* (1982) *Surgery* **91**, 49.
7 RABINOWITZ R. & LEWIN E.B. (1980) *J Urol* **124**, 43.
8 ROSENBERG P.H., *et al* (1978) *Ann Surg* **187**, 430.
9 SCHWEIGEL J.F. & SHIM S.S. (1973) *Surg Gynecol Obstet* **136**, 969.
10 SKILES M.S., *et al* (1978) *Surg Gynecol Obstet* **147**, 65.

PRURITUS ANI

The very common symptom of itching localized to the anus or the close perianal skin is seen especially in middle-class middle-aged Caucasian males. It occurs less frequently in females, either alone or with pruritus vulvae (p. 2217). It can be associated with most forms of anal disease and with skin conditions involving the perianal area. The factors are complex and may complement or perpetuate each other.

Anal itching occurs, to a variable degree, with any inflammatory or eczematous condition of the skin of that area, with anal fissures, whatever their aetiology, and with malignant tumours (p. 2179). Mycotic infection often causes intense pruritus and diabetes must be excluded in all severe or persistent candidal infections. Threadworm infestations are a well-recognized cause in childhood and occasionally in adults.

We are concerned here with anal itching in which there is no obvious primary dermatological cause. Changes secondary to rubbing and scratching are, of course, evident, as may be a contact dermatitis arising from treatment.

Pathogenesis. The common factor linking most forms of pruritus ani is faecal contamination [1, 6]. In addition to potential allergens and bacteria, faeces contain enzymes of bacterial origin known as endopeptidases [5, 9]. In the presence of pre-existing skin disease, e.g. seborrhoeic dermatitis or flexural psoriasis, or even in the absence of visible disease, these enzymes are capable of inducing both itching and inflammation.

The causes of faecal contamination are as follows. More than one factor may be operative.

Difficulty in cleansing the area. This may be due to the following factors.

(i) Simple obesity: poor ventilation and maceration play an additional role.
(ii) Frequency of defaecation: patients with a colostomy never suffer from perianal itching, whilst patients with pruritus ani are rarely constipated although they may sit long at stool owing to faulty training techniques with resultant prolapse or haemorrhoids and soiling [1, 2, 4]. Patients frequently admit to two or more motions a day. These are often tense individuals in whom everyday problems induce a profound colonic reflex, resulting in defaecation and soiling.
(iii) Anatomical factors: it is often noted that the anus is deeply placed. The association of this 'funnel anus' with marked hirsutism causes mechanical problems in the maintenance of hygiene.

Anal leakage. This may be due to the following factors.

(i) Local causes such as active haemorrhoids, perianal tags or fissures which interfere with the efficient functions of the anus.
(ii) Primary anal sphincter dysfunction: anal canal manometry studies [2] have shown that in one common group of patients the sphincter relaxes in response to rectal distension in a more rapid and profound manner than in a control group. The arrival of faeces or flatus in the rectum may then regularly result in reflex faecal soiling.

Bacterial contamination is frequently a secondary cause, but rarely a primary cause by itself. However, cross-infection of staphylococci may occur between the anus and the ears for example.

Food and drink: the role of ingested metabolites or food chemicals in inducing pruritus ani is still uncertain and virtually unexplored, but anecdotal evidence in individual cases is sometimes compelling.

Psychological factors are often involved as causes of pruritus ani, particularly where the itching appears to be out of proportion to the changes observed. However, as Whitlock [10] points out in a careful review, the evidence is unsatisfactory, except perhaps in primary lichen simplex. Psychosexual connotations of suppressed homosexuality certainly do not withstand critical assessment. It is quite understandable, however, that prolonged pruritus ani can lead to tension, irritability or depression and the treatment of this is an important part of the management of the condition.

Clinical features. These vary somewhat according

to the factors responsible but are all complicated by the effects of rubbing, secondary infection or contact dermatitis.

(i) *Lichen simplex* may be present in a 'pure' form, often localized to a small area at the edge of the anus or slightly away from it. The perception of itch from 'easily alerted' nerve endings is more acute in those of anxious temperament or at times of psychic trauma or fatigue.

(ii) A more general area of *maceration, lichenification* and *fissuring*—the 'mossy bank' anus—may be present. The architecture of the anal margin may be distorted by haemorrhoids, tags, oedema and infection. There is usually a gross degree of discharge [4].

(iii) Features of acute eczema may be due to secondary infection of possibly minimal seborrhoeic dermatitis or psoriasis, or to contact dermatitis. This should always be suspected when there has been any sudden change of pattern or intensity of rash. The fingers may also be involved. One of the commonest offenders is the 'caine' group of drugs [11], often self-prescribed.

(iv) Intense *erythema* with no obvious features of eczema may occur. This tends to vary in intensity over short periods and probably represents the pruritic stage of the next group.

(v) There may be *no visible abnormality* at the time of examination. These patients may have noticed erythema at times of intense itch and commonly give a story of intermittent sensation of wet anal margins and slight faecal soiling. It is in this group that dyskinesia of the sphincter appears to be a primary factor.

Diagnosis. A full history, including that of bowel habits, is essential and a search for underlying disease must be carried out. A rectal examination will prevent the occasional serious error and will always reassure the patient. Sigmoidoscopy may be indicated if there is marked bowel upset. In the young, threadworms should be sought with nocturnal 'Sellotape' swabs.

Treatment [1]. Time is well spent in dealing in detail with all aspects of hygiene. Patients should be encouraged to limit evacuation to once daily or less and to situations where they can wash the area gently with wool or soft toilet tissue afterwards. Long sitting should be corrected. Underwear should be loose and preferably cotton.

Certain foods such as nuts are probably best excluded from the diet, but bran and a high fibre diet should be encouraged if there is any history of constipation or haemorrhoids [3].

When active pathology such as fissures, haemorrhoids or anal spasm are present, surgical help will be needed. Lord's stretch procedure [7] has proved helpful. The long-term results are particularly satisfactory in those patients with strong ultra-low-pressure waves [3]. However, it may not always relieve the pruritus [8].

Local applications should be mild and soothing. If infection is present or suspected, antibacterials may be combined with mild corticosteroid preparations. Considerable relief from nocturnal itching can be achieved with corticosteroid suppositories. A wick of bandage impregnated with hydrocortisone 1% and silicone 10% inserted within the natal cleft is anti-inflammatory and lubricating. The anal skin is 'quasi-occluded' and is easily damaged by fluorinated corticosteroids. We have found the application of zinc paste with 1–2% phenol a safe and useful antipruritic and protective application if used both before and after bowel movement and again at night.

REFERENCES

1 *Alexander-Williams J (1983) Br Med J **287**, 159.
2 Eyers A.A. & Thomson J.P.S. (1979) Br Med J ii, 1549.
3 Hancock B.D. (1981) In *The Haemorrhoid Syndrome*. Ed. Kaufman H.D. Tunbridge Wells, Abacus, pp. 93–104.
4 Kaufman H.D. (1981) *The Haemorrhoid Syndrome*. Tunbridge Wells, Abacus, p. 61.
5 Keele C.A. (1957) *Proc R Soc Med* **50**, 477.
6 Kocsard E. (1981) *Cutis* **27**, 518.
7 Lord P.H. (1973) *Dis Colon Rectum* **16**, 180.
8 Ortiza H., *et al* (1978) *Br J Surg* **65**, 281.
9 Shelley W.B. & Arthur R.P. (1957) *Arch Dermatol* **76**, 296.
10 Whitlock F.A. (1976) *Psychophysiological Aspects of Skin Disease*. London, Saunders, pp. 118–121.
11 Wilkinson J.D., *et al* (1980) *Acta Derm Venereol (Stockh)* **60**, 245.

CHRONIC PERIANAL PAIN AND THE 'PERINEAL SYNDROME' [4, 5]

A number of names have been given to sensations of pain localized to the anogenital region in the absence of evident organic cause. Proctalgia fugax affects young adult males and occurs chiefly at night in the form of a sudden cramp-like pain which resolves in a few minutes. 'Coccygodynia', 'descending perineum syndrome' and 'chronic idiopathic anal pain' chiefly affects females. This pain is described as dull and throbbing. In 35 such patients it was noted that the pain was precipitated by sitting and that these three conditions differed from proctalgia fugax [4]. Electrophysiological studies gave inconstant results. There was a high incidence of previous sciatica and damage to the pelvic floor musculature. Treatment was disappointing.

Such patients will present to surgeons or gynaecologists. However, dermatologists may be confronted by a similar problem in which a patient complains of short-lived episodes of intense burning, which may be accompanied by sweating, limited to the perineum or occasionally the scrotum. Attacks occur without warning, though they they may be brought about by a full rectum. In one patient the attacks were severe enough to cause him to stop walking for some minutes. The patients tend to be stressful individuals, as are those with proctalgia fugax [5]. The skin is entirely normal.

The mechanism is unknown. Two patients appeared to have been helped by propantheline, suggesting a cholinergic mechanism [3]. However, the condition may also fall into the group of 'dermatological non-disease' [1] in which the perineum was affected in 8 out of 28 patients.

In women a similar condition ('vulvodynia') may be comparable (p. 2217). It has also been reported in children suffering from intrafamilial stresses [2].

REFERENCES

1 COTTERILL J.A. (1980) *Br J Dermatol* **103** (Suppl. **18**), 13.
2 LARK B. (1982) *J R Soc Med* **75**, 370.
3 MONRO P.A.G. (1959) *Sympathectomy*. Oxford, Clarendon Press, p. 146.
4 NEILL M.E. & SWASH M. (1982) *J R Soc Med* **75**, 96.
5 PARKS A.G., *et al* (1966) *Proc R Soc Med* **59**, 477.

MISCELLANEOUS CONDITIONS

Pregnancy, Addison's disease and other pigmentary disorders increase the pre-existing pigmentation. Acanthosis nigricans causes acanthotic and papillomatous lesions in the perineum. The anus is involved in about 5% of cases of Stevens–Johnson syndrome (p. 1086). Leukoplakia is rare and is usually superimposed on lichen sclerosus et atrophicus.

Anal manifestations of intestinal diseases. These have been well documented recently [5]. Though they are usually non-specific, the particular skin manifestation of tuberculosis, amoebiasis, bilharziasis and Crohn's disease may lead to diagnosis of the underlying disease by their typical histology.

Anal and perianal lesions in homosexuals [2, 6]. This has become a subject of great importance in recent years, particularly in view of the increasing prevalence of AIDS [1, 5, 8]. The brief summary given here will obviously be overtaken by further advances in the subject which is also dealt with on p. 719. Whatever condition the patient presents with, it is imperative to recognize that other infections may coexist. Herpes simplex and gonorrhoea were the most common infections found in 52 subjects in the U.S.A. [6]. However, *Giardia lamblia*, *Entamoeba histolytica* and *Chlamydia trachomatis* were also isolated and multiple infections were present in six patients. Syphilis, found in seven patients, presented atypically with anorectal pain or discomfort, changes in bowel habit or tenesmus; perianal lesions were not always present. The importance of primary rectal syphilis has been emphasized [3]. Dark-ground examination, cultures and a search for ova are obligatory. If no pathogenic agents are recovered but polymorphs are abundant in smears, a rectal biopsy is indicated.

In the immunodeficiency syndrome herpes simplex may be severe, extensive and ulcerative [8]. Amoebiasis [7] may be overlooked. Repeated stool specimens, properly examined, are often required for diagnosis [2]. Anorectal gonorrhoea may present with a bloody mucous discharge, or may be asymptomatic. Anal warts are five to ten times as common as penile warts in homosexual men [9].

Such is the complexity, atypicality and potential severity of infections in homosexual men that all dermatologists to whom they present must not only be aware of the range of such infections but must either have the facilities for full and accurate identification of pathogens or refer them to those who have.

REFERENCES

1 Centres for Disease Control (1982) MMWR, U.S.A.
2 *FELMAN Y.M. & NIKITAS J.A. (1982) *Cutis* **30**, 706.
3 GLUCKMAN J.B., *et al* (1974) *NY State J Med* **74**, 2210.
4 GOTTLIEB M.S., *et al* (1981) *N Engl J Med* **305**, 1425.
5 GROSSHANS E., *et al* (1979) *Ann Dermatol Vénéréol* **106**, 25.
6 QUINN T.C., *et al* (1981) *Am J Med* **71**, 395.
7 ROBERTSON D.H.H. (1982) *J R Soc Med* **75**, 564.
8 SIEGAL F.P., *et al* (1981) *N Engl J Med* **305**, 1439.
9 WAUGH M. (1972) *Br Med J* ii, 527.

MALIGNANT AND PREMALIGNANT LESIONS

RONA M. MACKIE

The anogenital area is not exposed to solar radiation, the chief cutaneous carcinogen. Treatment of pruritus with such agents as radiotherapy or tar preparations, and the use of radiotherapy for gynaecological malignancy carry theoretical hazards and can occasionally be incriminated. They do not, however, appear to have influenced greatly the frequency of perineal tumours. Post-granulomatous scarring is an important background to perianal malignancy in areas where the venereal granulomas are common and other scarring processes, such as lichen sclerosus, are a potential hazard. There are a small number of cases where condyloma acuminatum precedes squamous cell carcinoma of the anal canal or perianal skin [10, 11].

Anal tumours are uncommon and are mainly squamous cell carcinomas. The perianal skin may give rise to a variety of tumours: basal-cell carcinomas and malignant melanoma are uncommon and show no special features requiring comment here; other malignant tumours are rare. In a recent survey of 71 patients the female-to-male ratio was 4:1 [8].

Bowen's disease. Bowen's disease of the perianal skin has no particularly special features. In the recent past it has been confused with pigmentary multicentric Bowen's disease [7], but this is now by convention called Bowenoid papulosis (p. 2196) and can occur on the genitals as well as the perineum [12]. It is regarded as a distinct disorder of uncertain prognosis [1]. True Bowen's disease of the perianal skin varies in its appearance on the degree of moistness of the involved area. It may present as a dry scaling erythematous or ulcerating plaque, or be erythematous, moist and velvety rather like erythroplasia of Queyrat (p. 2199). There is a greater than normal risk that a woman with anogenital Bowen's disease will have a carcinoma *in situ* or invasive malignancy elsewhere in the genital tract [3], and a full gynaecological examination is thus obligatory in such cases.

Squamous cell carcinoma

Incidence and aetiology. Although the sexes are equally affected, there is a difference in the anatomical distribution. Tumours of the anal margin are three times more common in males [13] and are usually well differentiated, whereas in females the tumour is more likely to be anaplastic and situated in the anal canal. Some tumours arise in an area of Bowen's disease, but the aetiological factors in most are obscure [9].

Clinical features. The appearance and natural history of the tumour in this site are similar to those of squamous cell carcinoma. Induration is the most important sign in a lesion, which may be an ulcer, a warty nodule or a plaque. Maceration and secondary infection are common. Examination of the anal canal should be carried out as part of the investigation of any patient with symptoms in this area.

Diagnosis. The commonest tumours of the anal margin are virus warts, which are distinguished by their multiplicity, their lack of induration and ulceration and their rapid evolution. Syphilitic condylomata are also multiple and not indurated. A syphilitic chancre of the anal margin or canal may be more easily mistaken for carcinoma. Amoebiasis is considered on p. 2175 and tuberculosis on p. 2173.

Treatment. Surgical excision of the tumour, and of the inguinal lymph nodes when these are involved, is the treatment of choice. In small well-differentiated tumours, particularly adenocarcinomas, a local excision and repair is ideal. Small squamous and basal cell carcinomas also respond well to irradiation. More extensive lesions require abdomino-perineal excision. In all cases obsessive follow-up is necessary to detect lymph node metastases before they become fixed. Tumours that are too advanced for surgery may respond to palliative radiotherapy. A number of different regimes have been suggested, mostly using a combination of methotrexate and/or bleomycin, particularly in well-differentiated squamous cell tumours. 5-Fluorouracil alone will sometimes cause temporary regression of adenocarcinomas.

Extramammary Paget's disease (p. 2438). In extramammary Paget's disease there is disagreement on how often a careful search will reveal an underlying cancer. Two recent reviews of the literature revealed only a 25% association [1, 8]. Despite this, a search for a primary adenocarcinoma of underlying secretory glands should be carried out in perianal Paget's disease. In some cases the primary tumour is an anorectal, or even more distant, carcinoma [6]. The primary tumour and the Paget cells in the epidermis are usually mucus secreting. In some cases electron microscopy shows the Paget cells to be squamous in character [2]. In all cases of perianal Paget's disease a careful search for the primary source, particularly by proctoscopy, must be made. Anorectal carcinomas may arise from rectal mucosa or from the intramuscular glands. In the latter case the malignant cells may track to the buttock through the ischiorectal fossa and the Paget's plaque may begin at a distance from the anal margin, rather like an ischiorectal abscess. Recent topographic studies have shown that the plaque of Paget's disease is much larger than the visible lesion [5]. Any attempt at removal must be radical and histologically controlled.

The pattern of the intramuscular glands and of the wide range of tumours that arise from them ('cloacogenic' carcinoma) resemble genito-urinary rather than intestinal endothelium [4]. The carcinoma may spread to involve the anorectal mucosa or through the perianal tissue to produce a chronic fistula-in-ano [14].

REFERENCES

1 BREEN J.L., *et al* (1978) *Clin Obstet Gynecol* 21, 1107.
2 FETHERSTON W.C. & FRIEDRICH E.G. (1972) *Obstet Gynecol* 39, 735.
3 FRANKLIN E.W. & RUTLEDGE F.D. (1972) *Obstet Gynecol* 39, 165.
4 GRENVALSKY H.T. & HELWIG E.B. (1956) *Cancer (NY)* 16, 387.
5 GUNN R.A. & GALLAGHER S. (1980) *Cancer* 46, 590.
6 HELWIG E.B. & GRAHAM J.H. (1963) *Cancer (NY)* 16, 387.
7 LLOYD K.M. (1970) *Arch Dermatol* 101, 48.
8 MOHS F.E. & BLANCHARD L. (1979) *Arch Dermatol* 115, 706.
9 SINGH R., *et al* (1981) *Cancer* 48, 411.
10 SOUTH L.M., *et al* (1977) *Clin Oncol* 3, 107.
11 STURM J.T., *et al* (1975) *Dis Colon Rectum* 18, 147.
12 WADE T.R., *et al* (1979) *Arch Dermatol* 115, 306.
13 WOLFE H.R.I. & NUSSEY H.J.R. (1968) *Br J Surg* 55, 295.
14 ZEINBERG V.H. & KAY S. (1957) *Ann Surg* 145, 344.

THE MALE GENITALIA

Introduction. The difference between the circumcised and uncircumcised penile skin causes differences in the incidence and appearance of dermatoses of the glans and corona. A long prepuce and poor hygiene predispose to infection and carcinoma, particularly in the elderly. Psoriasis of the exposed glans is easily recognized but loses its habitual scaling when covered. The deep fold formed by the junction of the prepuce and the penis behind the corona is subject to maceration from epithelial debris and glandular secretion, and is a common site of infection.

Pilosebaceous units are absent on the penis except, sparsely, at the proximal part of the body. On the corona and in its sulcus, modified sebaceous glands—the preputial glands—secrete a fatty substance wrongly believed to be the chief source of smegma, which is mostly derived from desquamating epithelial cells. Free sebaceous (Tyson's) glands open directly onto the surface. Apocrine and eccrine glands are abundant, but there is great variation in the amount of their secretion. The median raphe may be the site of infections, notably gonococcal [1, 2].

The rugose and apparently thick skin of the scrotum in fact allows excellent penetration of topical agents, Carcinogens such as soot and tar (p. 2378) also penetrate more readily.

The penile and scrotal skin easily become contaminated by urinal and urethral discharges; contact with the female genitalia allows cross-infection of viral or venereal disease.

The proximity of deep skin folds encourages moisture and maceration. The influence of social customs such as tight clothing and contraceptives add hazards in sophisticated races. The unique freedom from photodermatitis is occasionally of diagnostic value.

REFERENCES

1 JOHNSON H.D. & THIN R.N.T. (1972) *Br J Vener Dis* 49, 467.
2 SOWMINI C.N., *et al* (1972) *Br J Vener Dis* 49, 469.

DEVELOPMENTAL AND CONGENITAL LESIONS

The more severe embryological and developmental defects will not present to the dermatologist. However, he sees minor abnormalities affecting the median raphe [6]. Cysts of various types occur here, particularly at the peno-scrotal junction or arising from the dysembryonic diverticula of the urethra. These canals may be lined with non-keratinizing clear cells [3]. If they become infected in later life, they are apt to be misdiagnosed [5]. Angiomas, lymphangiomas [7] and lipomas occasionally occur. Unduly profuse or enlarged sebaceous glands of the shaft are often a cause of anxiety to the patient. Ectopic pilosebaceous elements causing naevus comedonicus on the glans have been reported [1]. Syringiomas, rare on the genitalia, presented as papular lesions limited to the penis [8]. Nodular hidradenoma (apocrine hidrocystoma) has occurred as a slow-growing tumefaction of the prepuce [2, 4].

REFERENCES

1 ABDEL-A'AL H. & ABDEL-AZIZ A.H.M. (1975) *Acta Derm Venereol (Stockh)* 55, 78.
2 AHMED A. & JONES A.W. (1969) *Br J Dermatol* 81, 899.
3 CIVATTE J. *et al* (1982) *Ann Dermatol Vénéréol* 109, 84.
4 DE DULANTE F., *et al* (1973) *Ann Dermatol Syphiligr* 100, 417.
5 DUPRÉ A., *et al* (1982) *Ann Dermatol Vénéréol* 109, 81.
6 SOWMINI C.N., *et al* (1972) *Br J Vener Dis* 49, 469.

7 TSUR H., *et al* (1981) *Cutis* **28**, 642.
8 ZALLA J.A. & PERRY H.O. (1971) *Arch Dermatol* **103**, 215.

TRAUMATIC LESIONS

The more bizarre forms of self-inflicted or experimental traumatic lesions of the penis are unlikely to be seen. However, unusual or unexpected manifestations or artefacts may deceive the unwary. Recurrent or necrotic lesions without evident cause should always be suspect. Ecchymosis may be marked, sometimes tracking back down the median raphe [7]. Traumatic urethral diverticula may be present as soft compressible nodulocystic lesions at the site of the penile shaft [8]. They must be distinguished from inclusion cysts, lipomas, lymphangiomas and epithelial tumours. Penile nodules due to the self-insertion of glass beads [3, 9] may be mobile and inert, but the injection of silicone or oil often causes granulomas [4, 11].

'Hair coil strangulation' of the penis owing to the mother's hair encircling the penis (usually after circumcision) [1] causes fistulae or gangrene. Mechanical avulsion—as in the scalp—has been noted [10]. Fracture of the penis occurs, with a loud crack, during intercourse. Over 80 cases have been reported in the English literature [5, 6].

Zip fastener and vacuum cleaner injuries are less common than previously. The role of trauma in penile thrombosis and non-venereal sclerosing lymphangitis is discussed below.

'Penile venereal oedema'. This occurs within a few hours of intercourse, and affects the shaft and the mucosal surface of the prepuce of circumcised patients. It is attributed to 'non-cooperating partners' with no vaginal secretion. Twenty-five cases were seen in 5 years [2]. (See p. 1395).

REFERENCES

1 BASHIR A.Y. & EL-BARBARY M. (1979) *J R Coll Surg Edinb* **25**, 47.
2 CANBY J.P. & WILDE H. (1973) *N Engl J Med* **289**, 108.
3 COHEN E.L. & KIM S.-W. (1982) *J Urol* **127**, 135.
4 DATTA N.S. & KERN F.B. (1973) *J Urol* **109**, 840.
5 DAVIES D.M. & MITCHELL I. (1978) *Br J Urol* **50**, 426.
6 GOH S.H. & TRAPNELL J.E. (1980) *Br J Surg* **67**, 680.
7 JOHNSON H.W. & THIN R.N.T. (1972) *Br J Vener Dis* **49**, 467.
8 MAGED A. (1969) *Br J Urol* **37**, 560.
9 NITIDANDHAPRABHAS P. (1975) *Br J Urol* **47**, 463.
10 SERRANO ORTEG S. (1980) *Actas Dermo sifilogr* **71**, 381.
11 STEWART R.C., *et al* (1979) *Plast Reconstr Surg* **64**, 108.

PENILE MANIFESTATIONS OF COMMON DISEASES [1]

Fixed drug eruptions cause recurrent erythematous or bullous lesions. Their rapidity of onset and cyclical pattern are characteristic. Other drugs produce severe erythema-multiforme-like eruptions of the genital and oral mucosae. Lichen planus (Fig. 59.9) affects the shaft or glans as multiple or papular or annular lesions. Lichen nitidus involved the penis in 9 out of 43 cases [2]. Psoriasis in the uncircumcised may resemble erythroplasia or plasma cell balanitis. However, confirmatory lesions elsewhere or nail pitting are usually present. The tumid papules of scabies are diagnostic and occur in no other disease. They may persist after other lesions have been eradicated.

The penis is involved in flexural and seborrhoeic forms of eczema, though less markedly than the

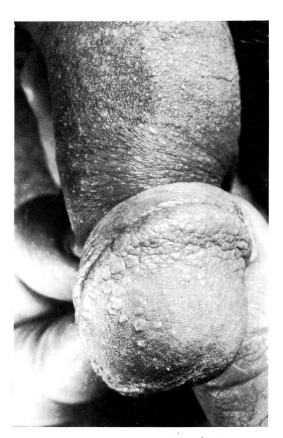

FIG. 59.9. Lichen planus. This presentation is difficult to distinguish from lichen nitidus, but the shining. polygonal confluent papules on the glans are more characteristic of lichen planus. (St John's Hospital.)

scrotum and groins. Patches of exudative discoid and lichenoid dermatitis (p. 387) may affect the shaft or glans in middle-aged or elderly Jews and are sometimes the initial presentation.

Overtreatment of common conditions with powerful topical corticosteroids may produce a dusky erythema of the glans and prepuce ('purple penis') or atrophic striae and increased visibility of blood vessels of the shaft [3].

REFERENCES

1 *CALLOMON F.T. & WILSON J.F. (1956) *The Non-venereal Diseases of the Genitals*. Springfield, Thomas.
2 LAPINS N.A., *et al* (1978) *Cutis* **21**, 634.
3 STANKLER L. (1982) *Br J Dermatol* **107**, 371.

INFECTIVE CONDITIONS OF THE PENIS

Early primary syphilis in the pre-chancre stage (p. 845) and the erythematous and papular forms of secondary syphilis, though rare, must not be overlooked. Condylomata lata may occur with fissures and erosions of the coronal sulcus or the free margin of the prepuce, or with papulosquamous lesions of the shaft. The late annula syphilide resembles sarcoidosis and is differentiated only by histology. Gonococcal lesions may confuse the unwary.

Condylomata acuminata (p. 675). They affect the coronal sulcus, the preputial border and the ureth-

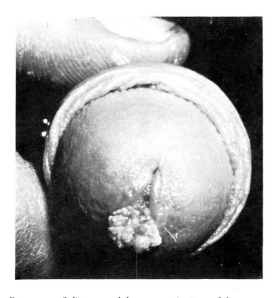

FIG. 59.10. Solitary condyloma acuminatum of the urethral orifice (Stoke Mandeville Hospital).

ral orifice, sometimes extending within the urethra (Fig. 59.10). They present as soft velvety hyperplastic or sessile lesions at sites that are probably determined by microtrauma. The incubation period in 332 patients who developed condylomata after intercourse was 2–3 months [12]. Genital warts are designated as HPV 6, although two other 'anogenital' HPV types may exist [13]. 1–2% resemble common warts and may be HPV1 [10]. In common with other sexually-related diseases, with which they may coexist, their incidence has risen in recent years [2]. In a large survey of 478 patients attending a Special Treatment Centre with genital warts, 61% of the women and 32% of the men had another genital infection [6]. The author stressed the importance of recognizing and dealing with such infections to reduce the moist conditions favourable for wart proliferation, especially *C. vaginale*, *Neisseria gonorrhoeae* and *Trichomonas vaginalis*.

Despite its toxicity and potential oncogenicity, podophyllin, applied carefully and sparingly, probably remains the first choice of treatment, except in any woman suspected of being pregnant. However, 50% or more patients failed to respond in one trial [7] and only 22% cleared in another [15]. 5-FU (1% in ethanol) is an alternative [8]. Colchicine has also been used [9]. Cryotherapy or electrocautery may be required in severe or resistant cases. A new technique of cutting off the condylomata to skin level is becoming favoured as it destroys less normal tissue. Four-fifths of 75 patients treated in this way cleared with one operative procedure and had little postoperative discomfort [16]. Anal lesions may be concealed and were the main cause of recurrences. Laser therapy may eventually be a method of choice [10].

Giant condyloma acuminatum (Buschke–Loewenstein) (p. 2199). This form of condyloma pursues a relentless growth and is resistant to topical therapy such as podophyllin. The surface is hard, unlike the exuberant 'cauliflower-like' form of a large condyloma [11]. Though more common in the perianal area or groin [4], it may affect the coronal sulcus, especially in the uncircumcised. Infiltration and penetration are characteristic, producing fistulae and sinuses. Histologically, the very acanthotic epithelium forms club-shaped rete ridges. Epidermal cells may show perinuclear halos or hyperchromasia. Viral bodies are not seen, but this may be because the viral material becomes incorporated into the genetic material of the cell [3].

Though metastases are rare, the invasive nature of the lesions has prompted some workers to regard it as a true carcinoma. Others have compared it to verrucous carcinoma and florid oral papillomatosis [5, 11].

Treatment is usually surgical, though aggressive cryotherapy [5] and bleomycin [14] have been used with success. Irradiation is to be avoided.

The whole subject of 'pre-neoplastic papillomatosis' is discussed by Barrière [1].

REFERENCES

1 BARRIÈRE H., et al (1973) *Bull Soc Fr. Dermatol Syphiligr* **80**, 388.
2 CATTERALL R.D. (1981) *Lancet* i, 315.
3 DOUTRÉ M.-S., et al (1979) *Ann Dermatol Vénéréol* **106**, 1031.
4 ENG A.M., et al (1979) *Cutis* **24**, 203.
5 HUGHES P.S.H. (1979) *Cutis* **24**, 43.
6 KINGHORN G.R. (1978) *Br J Dermatol* **99**, 405.
7 VON KROGH G. (1978) *Acta Derm Venereol (Stockh)* **58**, 163.
8 VON KROGH G. (1978) *Sex Trans Dis* **5**, 137.
9 VON KROGH G. & RUDÉN A.-K. (1980) *Acta Derm Venereol (Stockh)* **60**, 87.
10 LUGER A. & GSCHUART F. (1981) *Wien Klin Wochenschr* **93**, 746.
11 MARGHESCU S., et al (1975) *Bull Soc Fr Dermatol Syphiligr* **83**, 293.
12 *ORIEL J.D. (1971) *Br J Vener Dis* **47**, 1.
13 *ORIEL J.D. (1982) *Clin Exp Dermatol* **7**, 361.
14 PUISSANT A., et al (1975) *Bull Soc Fr Dermatol Syphiligr* **79**, 9.
15 SIMMONS P.D., et al (1981) *Br J Vener Dis* **57**, 273.
16 THOMSON J.P.S. & GRACE R.H. (1978) *J R Soc Med* **71**, 180.

Fungal infections. These are rare on the penis but are well documented [1, 3]. The lesions, affecting the shaft, were unusual but the inguinal or pubic areas were also involved in all cases. Pityriasis versicolor is more common, especially if looked for under Wood's light [1]. Here also the infection is more widespread than is at first apparent. Candidal infections are dealt with in the section on balanitis (p. 2186).

Molluscum contagiosum. This affects the genital and paragenital areas of infants and young adults. Solitary lesions can be confused with lymphangiomas and multiple lesions with furuncles. Central umbilication is a characteristic distinguishing feature.

Tuberculosis. This was once a common complication of circumcision [2], but is now rare. Orificial tuberculosis occurs as multiple shallow crusted ulcers. Papulonecrotic tuberculides may involve the penis. If successive crops occur the eventual scarring leads to a remarkable 'worm-eaten' appearance. A persistent indolent chancriform lesion

occurs very rarely at the coronal sulcus secondary to tuberculosis in the spouse. It lacks the induration of a syphilitic chancre. The inguinal glands enlarge, soften and sometimes ulcerate. A case of 'anonymous' mycobacterial infection of the glans has been reported [4].

REFERENCES

1 AVRAM A., et al (1973) *Bull Soc Fr Dermatol Syphiligr* **80**, 607.
2 MINKIN W., et al (1972) *Arch Dermatol* **106**, 756.
3 PILLAI K.G., et al (1975) *Dermatologica* **100**, 252.
4 SCHNITZLER L., et al (1972) *Bull Soc Fr Dermatol Syphiligr* **79**, 571.

Herpes progenitalis [4, 7, 13, 16]. This infection is fully discussed in Chapter 21 and genital infections in the female are dealt with on p. 2211. The incidence of genital herpes has increased in the U.K. from 19·7 per 100,000 in 1976 to 27·1 per 100,000 in 1980 [20] and is now a very important cause of genital infection in women [1, 9, 19]. In the U.K. most cases are caused by HSV 2 strain, though an increasing number, particularly in women, are due to HSV 1. The finding of HSV 2 antibody in young children in Nigeria has led to the suggestion that the virus may survive on fomites in hot humid climates [12, 21]. However, this must be rare.

Clinical manifestations. The primary infection usually occurs within a week of sexual exposure (including oral or anal intercourse), but occasionally after a longer period. Asymptomatic attacks may occur in as many as half the cases [13]. Otherwise they are usually more severe than recurrent attacks that may follow. The eruption may be preceded by the usual prodromal symptoms, localized or general, which are often misdiagnosed as influenza [16]. Clustered tiny papules on an erythematous base develop into vesicles and rapidly break down to form superficial erosions or painful ulcers. The glans, prepuce and fraenum are usually involved; the shaft is rarely involved. The attack lasts 2–3 weeks but may be complicted [4, 6] by recrudences, infections or viraemic spread. Severe or anomalous forms may cause difficulty in diagnosis, especially in the immunosuppressed patient.

Neurological complications include meningeal involvement and sacral radiculitis [17].

Recurrent attacks occur in 30–70% of those affected [16]. These are usually less severe and shorter lived than the primary infection. They involve the same or an adjacent area and may be preceded by prodromal malaise, aching or odd pricking sensations, or paraesthesiae of the thighs or perineum. Subsequent attacks may involve the buttock [4]. The frequency of attacks varies but tends to become less in time. They may be precipitated by trauma, stress and diverse other events [5]. However minor, they cause great anxiety and depression to those affected and must be treated seriously.

Diagnosis. In the early stages the clustered vesicular eruption is characteristic. However, later stages or anomalous manifestations invite errors. The patient must be screened for other coexistent disease, including chancroid and candidiasis. Confirmation of the virus can be obtained by electron microscopy, immunofluorescence or tissue culture (see p. 660). It is vital that the correct transport medium is used. The examination of a Papanicolaou-stained slide is less accurate [14]. Neutralizing or complement-fixing antibodies rise to a peak in about 3 weeks and may be of value in doubtful primary infections.

Treatment [16, 18]. Symptomatic measures include potassium permanganate or similar soaks and mild antibacterial agents, e.g. collodial iodine paint. 'Folk' remedies—ice-bags, tea-bags, etc.—should not be disregarded and have a certain logic.

The search for a specific remedy continues. Idoxoridine (5–40% in dimethyl sulphoxide) is of value in shortening the healing time if applied early and may even abort attacks in those who recognize the prodromal signs. Cytarabine, given as a bolus of 3–4 mg/kg per day for 3–4 days, cuts down the time of viral shedding [7] but is toxic if given by infusion. Acyclovir, however, must be given intravenously (5 mg/kg 8-hourly for 5 days) and is the treatment of choice for severe primary infections [11] or for immunocompromised patients, although it does not prevent recurrences. Orally, it has also been of some value [15] but this has yet to be fully assessed. The same reservation applies to its topical use [3, 4, 10].

At one time photoinactivation with neutral red or proflavine was fashionable but the results were not impressive [8] and the procedure may be carcinogenic [2].

In all cases the patient must be counselled about sensible precautions with regard to avoiding intercourse at the time of attacks.

REFERENCES

1 BARTON I.G., *et al* (1981) *Lancet* ii, 1108.
2 BERGER R.S. & PATA C.M. (1977) *JAMA* 238, 133.
3 COREY L., *et al* (1982) *N Engl J Med* 305, 1356.
4 *FELMAN Y.M. & NIKITAS J.A. (1982) *Cutis* 30, 442.
5 HILL J. & BLYTH W.A. (1976) *Lancet* i, 397.
6 *JEANSSON S. & MOLIN L. (1974) *Proc Symp on Genital Infections and their Complications.* Eds. Danielsson D., *et al.* Stockholm, Almquist & Wickesell (p. 189).
7 *JUEL-JENSON B. (1982) *Clin Exp Dermatol* 7, 355.
8 KAUFMAN R.H., *et al* (1978) *Am J Obstet Gynecol* 132, 861.
9 KAWANA T., *et al* (1976) *Lancet* ii, 964.
10 LUBY J. (1982) *N Engl J Med* 306, 1356.
11 MINDEL A., *et al* (1982) *Lancet* i, 697.
12 MONTEFIORE D., *et al* (1980) *Br J Vener Dis* 56, 49.
13 *NAHMIAS A.J., *et al* (1981) *The Human Herpesviruses.* New York, Elsevier.
14 NAIB Z.M. (1981) In *The Human Herpesviruses.* New York, Elsevier, p. 381.
15 NILSEN A.E. (1982) *Lancet* ii, 571.
16 *OATES J.K. (1983) *Br J Hosp Med* 29, 13.
17 OATES J.K. & GREENHOUSE P.R. (1978) *Lancet* i, 691.
18 OXFORD J.S., *et al* (1977) *Chemotherapy of Herpes Simplex Virus Infections.* London, Academic Press.
19 PEUTHERER J.F., *et al* (1981) In *The Human Herpes Viruses.* New York, Elsevier, p. 595.
20 *Report, Department of Health and Social Security* (1981–1982). London, HMSO.
21 SOGBETUN A.O., *et al* (1979) *Br J Vener Dis* 55, 44.

UNCOMMON AND MISCELLANEOUS CONDITIONS

Several non-venereal diseases affect the penis uniquely or in a distinct fashion. Mention should be made briefly of Fordyce's disease (p. 2079), which simulates lichen planus on the glans, granular cell myoblastoma, which characteristically has the appearance of a truncated dome [6], neurinoma of the glans [9], and congenital os penis [1]. The term 'penile horn' has been given [4] to a compact tapered keratinous mass arising on areas of acanthosis or condylomas, often after excision. Though histologically benign, wide excision is advocated. In pellagra the penile skin may be grossly excoriated. Crohn's disease may very rarely affect the penis as well as the scrotum [2].

Pigmentary anomalies. Both vitiligo and occupational leukoderma can involve the scrotum [8]. Wood's light examination may reveal 'hidden' cases. Of 54 patients with occupational vitiligo, the penis or scrotum were affected in 38 [5]. Chemicals in condoms and pessaries have also been incriminated and hypopigmented macules on the glans followed recurrent gonococcal infection, presumably as a post-inflammatory phenomenon [3].

Bullous eruptions. *Pemphigus vulgaris* (p. 1631) may develop first on the penis, with the flaccid bullae rupturing readily to form erosions and crusts. The diagnosis may sometimes be confirmed cytologically. Pemphigoid (p. 1639) is less common and typical lesions will be present elsewhere. Pemphigus vegetans is exceedingly rare.

Benign mucosal pemphigoid (p. 1644) is rare in males but may involve the corona or glans in association with ocular and oral lesions. The combination of bullae and irregular cicatrization is well shown in Fig. 59.11. Meatal stricture may eventually occur.

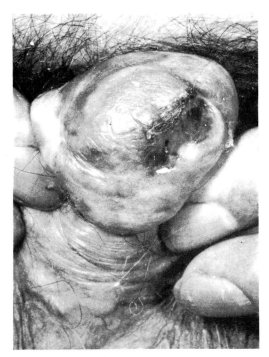

FIG. 59.11. Benign mucosal pemphigoid. Bullae and synechial scarring are shown together. (St John's Hospital.)

Bullous drug reactions, notably fixed eruptions, are suggested by acute recurrent lesions and residual pigmentation.

Erythema multiforme exudativum (p. 1086) frequently involves the penis. Bullae are common.

Haemorrhagic thick-roofed bullae may occur in the ivory-white plaques of lichen sclerosus et atrophicus (p. 2190).

Vegetating lesions. Condylomata acuminata become exuberant in the presence of a urethral discharge. An extensive tumour-like form of tuberculosis has been described [7]. Chronic forms of pyoderma are less common than elsewhere on the genitalia, but a fungating and vegetating response to a mixed or fusopilliary infection is seen in the uncircumcised under conditions of poor hygiene or debility. If rapid resolution does not occur under appropriate treatment a carcinoma must be suspected (p. 2200). Bowen's disease may cause difficulty in diagnosis.

REFERENCES

1 CHAMPION R.H. & WEGRZYN J. (1964) *J Urol* **91**, 663.
2 COCKBURN A.G., *et al* (1980) *Urology* **15**, 596.
3 GAFFOOR P.M.A. (1983) *Cutis* **31**, 214.
4 HASSAN A.A., *et al* (1967) *J Urol* **97**, 315.
5 JAMES O., *et al* (1977) *Lancet* **ii**, 1217.
6 KERN A.B., *et al* (1950) *Arch Dermatol Syphilol* **62**, 109.
7 MENZEL E. (1966) *Z Urol Nephrol* **59**, 287.
8 MOSS J.R. & STEVENSON C.J. (1981) *Br J Vener Dis* **57**, 145.
9 VON PARRA C.A. (1968) *Dermatologica* **137**, 150.

BALANITIS

Definition. Inflammation of the penile skin. Properly, the condition is called 'balanoposthitis, from 'balanitis' referring to inflammation of the glans and 'posthitis' referring to that of the mucous surface of the prepuce.

'Balanitis' is used here to describe acute and chronic forms of inflammation of the glans penis and prepuce owing to traumatic, irritant or infective causes.

Pathogenesis. There are obvious predisposing factors such as irritation by smegma, urine, alkalis and external contacts, susceptibility to clothing, friction and trauma, a long foreskin combined with poor hygiene, and exposure to venereal and vaginal pathogens. Bacteria, yeasts and fusospirillary organisms flourish in the moist covered preputial sac and saprophytes may become pathogens under conditions of lowered local or general resistance. In humid climates, especially, balanitis is far commoner in the uncircumcised. A mixed pathogenesis is thus common, and recurrences of seemingly simple infections are often due to continuing non-specific causes of inflammation. In such cases circumcision may effect a cure.

Irritants and pathogens are normally extraneous in origin but occasionally derive from infected urine, faeces or perineal foci of infection or carriage. The part played by *Clamydiae* [4, 10] and *Mycoplasmas* [13] is receiving increasing attention.

Histopathology. There is no specific histological picture. In infective and superficial erosive forms the features are those of inflammation, with spongiosis and a more or less intense dermal inflammatory infiltrate. Bacteria, spirochaetes, acid-fast bacilli and other pathogens are found by appropriate methods of examination or staining.

Clinical varieties of balanitis. All morphological forms of acute superficial balanitis may be grouped together, despite aetiological differences.

Acute superficial balanoposthitis

(a) *Traumatic.* Accidental wounds and frictional trauma cause erosions, fissures or localized areas of erythema and oedema. Postcoital fraenal erosions are not uncommon. 'Zip fastener' injuries lacerate the prepuce and cause haemorrhage and oedema.

(b) *Irritant.* Retained smegma, poor hygiene and retained soap, detergent or inadequate drying may cause an irritant dermatitis. Contact dermatitis affects the shaft rather than the glans, except when medicament or contraceptives are involved.

Syphilophobia may lead to the use of antiseptics in irritant strength. Occasionally, bizarre forms of inflammatory reaction follow sexual experimentation.

(c) *Infective.* This is the common cause of balanitis.

Infective forms of balanitis. Erythema of the glans, the coronal sulcus and the inner surface of the prepuce may arise suddenly with irritation or develop insidiously and unnoticed by the patient (Fig. 59.12).

In more acute infections, or as a result of treatment, the erythema and oedema extend widely and phimosis may result. The involved area is red and moist. The edge is usually ill-defined. Maceration and exudation are marked in the uncircumcised. Acute infections are accompanied by offensive creamy purulent discharge. Secondary invasion by Vincent's organism and Gram-negative bacteria leads to erosion and ulceration. A great variety of organisms are found on culture; some are obviously pathogenic, and others are doubtfully so. In resistant or recurrent cases the partner should always be examined.

Circinate erosive balanitis. A variety of balanitis that occurs in two forms. One is an early short-lived mucosal presentation of Reiter's disease (p. 1537). The second is a persistently recurring form of balanitis with a circinate or polycyclic edge extending onto the glans and prepuce, which cannot be distinguished aetiologically from the more common form.

Candidal balanitis [9, 14]. *C. albicans* can be recovered from both the vagina and, less commonly, the coronal sulcus in the absence of clinical infec-

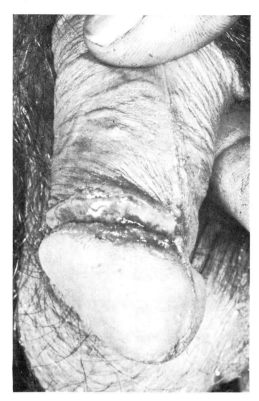

FIG. 59.12. Infective balanitis confined to the coronal sulcus (St John's Hospital).

tion. The strains are usually the same in both partners, but it is not always possible to determine whether the source is exogenous or endogenous from the rectum, anus or mouth. Though candidal balanitis most frequently follows intercourse with an infected partner [1, 11], the pathogenicity of the organism also depends upon host factors, of which diabetes is the most important. It should be looked for in any severe persistent or unexplained case, as the balanitis may be a presenting symptom of the disease. In the elderly, it may be associated with cachexia or malignancy.

The distinguishing features include a glazed non-purulent surface, a slightly scaling edge (in the circumcised) and satellite eroded pustules. The groins may be affected. An acute fulminating oedematous type occurs, though the typical case is mild. Microscopy and culture confirm the diagnosis and should be taken from both partners and from the anal as well as the genital areas. It is wise to examine the blood as well as the urine for sugar. A glucose-tolerance test is indicated when there is a family history of diabetes.

An allergic reaction to *Candida* infection in the partner may account for some cases of recurrent balanitis in which burning and erythema of the glans and prepuce occurs shortly after intercourse [1, 9]. Cultures are negative or non-contributory in the subject but yeasts are found in the partner.

Recurrent candidal balanitis causes fissuring of the prepuce, fibrosis and sclerosis.

Treatment. Specific remedies are available for this specific form of balanitis. Both partners, if affected, should be treated concurrently. There is now a large variety of effective anticandidal agents of the polyene or imidazole type. Ketaconazole is an oral alternative for severe cases. However, none of these achieve more than a 90% cure rate [9] and it is probable that intestinal or urethral reservoirs—as well as re-infection—contribute to the failure rate in the refractory 10%.

Amoebic balanitis [3]. A severe amoebic infection leading to rupture of the prepuce and erosion of the shaft has been found in New Guinea. *Antamoeba histolytica* was found in direct smears. Emetine or circumcision cured the patients, whose infection was thought to have been contracted through anal intercourse.

Micaceous and keratotic pseudo-epitheliomatous balanitis [2]. This is a curious condition, apparently not very rare, in which coronal balanitis gradually

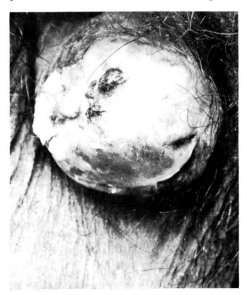

FIG. 59.13. Micaceous and keratotic pseudo-epitheliomatous balanitis (Dr H.T.H. Wilson, Royal Northern Hospital, and St John's Hospital).

takes on a silvery-white appearance, and mica-like crusts and keratotic horny masses form on the glans (Fig. 59.13). There is a loss of elasticity of the prepuce and the general appearance is atrophic.

Histologically, there is extreme hyperkeratosis and pseudo-epitheliomatous hyperplasia with elongation of the rete ridges and acanthosis. It has been regarded as a form of pyodermatitis or a pseudo-epitheliomatous response to infection, possibly even a variant of Reiter's syndrome. It is not considered to be malignant. Circumcision does not cure. Topical cytotoxic agents have been used [6].

Trichomonal balanitis. This is receiving increasing recognition. It occurs as a superficial or an erosive balanitis in young subjects with trichomaniasis [8] with or without urethritis. It is more common in those with a long prepuce. Phimosis may occur but it responds rapidly to metronidazole. Occasionally, more severe lesions of chancriform type or with penile abscesses [5] are seen.

Mycoplasma balanitis [12]. Although not yet widely recognized by dermatologists, it has been suggested that a balanitis may accompany mycoplasma urethritis, either as a primary infection or secondary to gonorrhoea. Swabs should be carbon tipped to avoid inhibition. It responds to tetracyclines in high dose.

Chlamydial infections [10]. The D–K serotypes of *Chlamydia trachomatis* are now recognized as the cause of the commonest genital infections in the Western world [4]. L_1–L_3 serotypes are the cause of lymphogranuloma venereum. The clinical spectrum is still expanding. In the female, especially, they may give rise to a variety of clinical diseases—salpingitis, Bartholinitis, abacterial urethritis, etc. In the male, by far the most common manifestation is non-gonococcal urethritis, of which over 70,000 cases are diagnosed annually in the U.K. [10]. In homosexual men it is a cause of proctitis. The importance of this organism lies in the importance of its recognition and treatment in a patient presenting, perhaps, with a non-specific but associated irritant balanitis. The characteristic penile lesions of Reiter's syndrome (p. 1539) may also be an indicator of this infection.

Syphilitis balanitis (Follmann) [7]. This rare condition follows a primary chancre (p. 845). The glans shows a whitish coalescent surface on an oedematous background. Histologically, multilocular pustules are full of polymorphs and *T. pallidum* is abundant in epidermal scrapings.

Differential diagnosis. Fixed drug eruptions, contact dermatitis and psoriasis are most likely to be confused, particularly in the uncircumcised. Aphthae and herpetic lesions are usually characteristic. Porokeratosis of Mibelli is sometimes mistaken when localized to the penis. Erythroplasia (p. 2199) is distinguished by its fixed appearance, the impression of thickness on palpation and its velvety surface.

Complications. Venereal disease may become superimposed on a damaged and eroded surface. Treatment may increase the extent of the inflammation if too vigorous or cause sensitization if prolonged. Phimosis is common. The peculiar effect of quaternary ammonium derivatives is dealt with separately (p. 2192).

Necrosis and gangrene may develop in infections complicated by fusospirillary organisms.

All forms of balanitis may become chronic or relapse frequently, especially in the elderly. When this happens, the glans and prepuce gradually undergo sclerotic and fibrotic changes. The final picture is that of an obliterative balanitis.

Carcinoma may complicate long-standing irritative lesions in the uncircumcised (p. 2200).

Treatment. Mild forms of balanitis respond to repeated cool bathing with permanganate or Burow's solution and the application of mild antibacterial creams, with or without weak corticosteroids. Hydroxyquinolines are widely used in the U.K. but are conveniently replaced in many cases, even those not due to yeast infections, by the newer imidazoles, e.g. miconazole, with or without hydrocortisone. Gentamicin is sometimes of value. In persistent cases, circumcision may be curative.

REFERENCES

1 CATTERALL R.D. (1966) In *Symposium on Candida Infections*. Eds. Winner H.L. & Hurley R. Edinburgh, Livingstone, p. 113.
2 CIVATTE J. & LORTAT-JACOB E. (1966) *Bull Soc Fr Dermatol Syphiligr* **68**, 164.
3 COOKE R.A. & RODRIGUEZ R.B. (1964) *Med J Aust* **5**, 114.
4 DUNLOP E.N.C. (1983) *Br J Hosp Med* **29**, 6.
5 DUPERRAT B. & CARTON F.-X. (1969) *Bull Soc Fr Dermatol Syphiligr* **76**, 345.
6 FLECK F. & FLECK M. (1974) *Organische w. funktionelle Sexualer krankrungen*. Berlin, Verlag und Gesundheit.
7 LEYJMAN K. & STARZYCKI Z. (1975) *Br J Vener Dis* **51**, 138.
8 MICHALOWSKI R. (1981) *Ann Dermatol Venereol* **108**, 731.
9 ODDS F.C. (1982) *Clin Exp Dermatol* **7**, 345.
10 ORIEL J.D. & RIDGWAY G.L. (1982) *Current Topics in Infection—Genital Infections by Chlamydia trachomatis*. London. Arnold.
11 ROHATINER J.J. (1966). In *Symposium on Candida Infections*. Eds. Winner H.L. & Hurley R. Edinburgh, Livingstone, p. 118.
12 SIBOULET A., *et al* (1975) *Bull Soc Fr Dermatol Syphilol* **82**, 419.
13 TAYLOR-ROBINSON D. & McCORMACK W.M. (1980) *N Engl J Med* **302**, 1063.
14 WINNER H.L. & HURLEY R. (Eds.) (1966) *Symp. on Candida Infections*. Edinburgh, Livingstone.

Plasma cell balanitis [1, 7, 9] ('Pseudo-erythroplasic balanitis' [5]). Despite the paucity of case reports, this distinctive condition is not excessively rare. Its characteristic features allow ready recognition. It presents in middle-aged or elderly men as one or more indolent circumscribed plaques, almost always on the glans [7], which remain localized indefinitely. The surface is shiny and smooth, occasionally eroded, in contrast with the velvety appearance of erythroplasia, with which it may be confused. The surface is slightly moist, giving the impression of 'incompletely dried varnish' [5] and is stippled with minute red specks—the 'cayenne pepper' spots. It is important to verify the diagnosis by biopsy.

Histologically, the changes are also distinctive [3, 7]. The epidermis is attenuated, and the horny and granular layers are absent. Individual suprabasal keratinocytes are diamond shaped ('lozenge keratinocytes' [8]). Occasional dyskeratotic cells are seen but no atypia is present. The intercellular spaces are widened ('watery spongiosis'). The dense band-like mixed dermal infiltrate usually contains more than 50% plasma cells, though these are sometimes less numerous [8]. Vertical or obliquely oriented vascular proliferation, haemosiderin deposition and free extravasated erythrocytes complete the characteristic pattern.

Dupré *et al* [2] have described a variant showing fleshy buds and erosions. A rare vegetating form also occurs. Jonquières and de Lutsky [5], who also include variants with marked dermal oedema and a predominantly lymphocyte infiltrate, prefer to avoid the name 'plasma cell' for what they consider to be a spectrum of different stages of the same process [4].

The aetiology of this condition remains unclear. It is best regarded as a persistent chronic form of balanitis. Immunological studies [3] in four cases suggested that IgA found in the lesions might be secreted by the infiltrate as a reflection of its mucosal situation.

Topical corticosteroids are not very helpful. Gentamycin may be helpful. Circumcision is often curative [6, 7].

REFERENCES

1 Bureau Y., *et al* (1962) *Ann Dermatol Syphiligr* **89**, 271.
2 Dupré A., *et al* (1976) *Bull Soc Fr Dermatol Syphiligr* **83**, 62.
3 Dupré A., *et al* (1981) *Ann Dermatol Vénéréol* **108**, 691.
4 Jonquières E.D.L. (1971) *Arch Argent Dermatol* **21**, 85.
5 Jonquières E.D.L. & de Lutzky F.K. (1980) *Ann Dermatol Vénéréol* **107**, 173.
6 Sonnex T.S., *et al* (1982) *Br J Dermatol* **106**, 585.
7 Souteyrand P., *et al* (1981) *Br J Dermatol* **105**, 195.
8 Wong E., *et al* (1981) *Br J Dermatol* **105** (Suppl. 19), 28.
9 *Zoon J.J. (1952) *Dermatologica* **105**, 1.

LICHEN SCLEROSUS ET ATROPHICUS
[12, 13]
SYN. BALANITIS XEROTICA OBLITERANS

The old term 'balanitis xerotica obliterans' is probably best discarded since it merely refers to an anatomical situation, similar to 'kraurosis vulvae'. It is still used, however, as a descriptive term by surgeons and others. We believe that almost all cases are due to lichen sclerosus et atrophicus, although we concede that very occasionally other fibrosing or synechial pathological entities such as severe mucosal pemphigoid or very chronic balanoposthitis may lead to a similar picture (Fig. 59.14). We would prefer to use the term 'cicatricial balanitis' for these.

Definition and aetiology. This is dealt with fully elsewhere (p. 1368). Females are affected far more frequently than males [13], though many cases in men are unrecorded or undiagnosed. There is some evidence that the disease has an autoimmune basis. Patients have an increased incidence of autoimmune disorders [6, 7]; vitiligo or alopecia areata were or had been present in 5 out of 25 males in a recent study [9], and a higher than expected incidence of autoantibodies is found in patients and their relatives [6, 7, 9]. However, the results of two recent studies on HLA typing have been conflicting. In one series of 50 females, HLA B40 was found to have an increased frequency [8], but in a larger series of 120 patients [10] there was no statistical difference from the frequencies found in 8,837 random individuals typed in the U.K. This suggests that the relationship may not be very strong, at least in males.

Histopathology (see p. 1369). In a recent biochemical ultrastructural and immulogical study [5], the

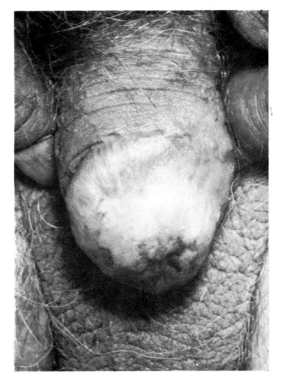

Fig. 59.14. Balanitis xerotica obliterans. Scarring of the glans, obliteration of the dorsal sulcus and meatal stenosis. (Stoke Mandeville Hospital.)

few elastic fibres present in the superficial dermis were abnormal and there was a loss of antigenicity of macromolecules in the homogenized zone of collagen. There were no significant biochemical abnormalities. It was not possible to demonstrate a supposed overactivity of elastase.

Clinical features. Though usually a disease of young adult men, it may occur in childhood and adolescence rather more frequently than is recognized, as its early stages are readily overlooked. Our own experience agrees with the findings of Chalmers *et al* [3] that it is not an uncommon cause for circumcision in boys of 5–11 yr and above. There are three forms of presentation. The patient may recognize typical ivory-white macules or confluent plaques on the glans (Fig. 59.15) or become alarmed at the appearance of a haemorrhagic bulla (often after intercourse) sometimes leading to blood-stained urine if it is situated on the meatus. Alternatively, the condition may be confined to the meatus itself and the adjacent perimeatal mucosa (Fig. 59.16), leading him to present to the surgeon because of difficulty in micturition. The smooth white appear-

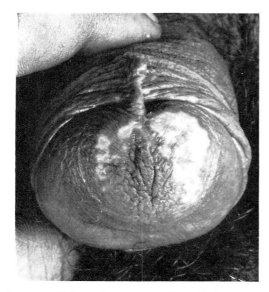

FIG. 59.15. Lichen sclerosus et atrophicus. Early stage showing individual and confluent ivory-white papules. (St John's Hospital.)

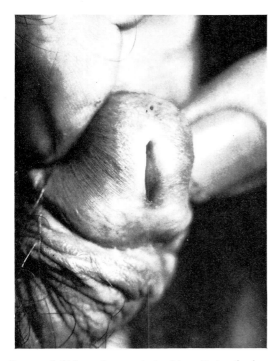

FIG. 59.16. Lichen sclerosus et atrophicus. Periurethral involvement. (Wycombe General Hospital.)

ance of the contracted meatal orifice and, often, the surrounding atrophic meatal collar are distinctive. In other cases the changes preferentially involve the preputial area, leading to progressive stenosis and eventually phimosis. The shaft is rarely involved.

In Wallace's large series [13], half the patients had been circumcised. The glans was ultimately affected in all; only two cases involved the shaft alone. Meatal lesions were present in half the cases but meatal strictures were uncommon.

Lesions of lichen sclerosus et atrophicus elsewhere are less frequent than in the female but should be sought.

Course and prognosis. In most cases the condition appears to reach a certain stage and then 'burn out' and cease to extend further. However, phimosis is common and is frequently the cause of initial presentation. Meatal strictures may continue to be troublesome over several years. Leukoplakia is less common than in women [14] and has seldom been a problem in a series extending over 15 yr. Squamous cell carcinoma is rare [2, 14], but is highly invasive when it occurs. In a personal case death occurred at an early age from invasion of the inguinal glands and femoral artery haemorrhage. These complications may proceed unnoticed in the uncircumcised.

Treatment. Weak corticosteroids will usually be sufficient for mild forms not involving the meatus. Powerful corticosteroids should only be used for limited periods. However, meatal involvement may respond to strong corticosteroids inserted by means of a nozzle-headed tube [4] or to repeated dilatation or meatotomy [12, 16]. Testosterone proprionate 2·5% ointment is advocated by some [11]. Leukoplakic areas respond to cryotherapy [1], but careful follow-up is essential. The condition may recur on excised or grafted sites [15]. Circumcision (or a dorsal slit) is advisable when it is impossible to retract the foreskin, as leukoplakic or early neoplastic changes may otherwise be missed.

REFERENCES

1 AUGUST R.J. & MILWARD T.M. (1980) *Br J Dermatol* **103**, 667.
2 BART R.S. & KOPF A.W. (1978) *J Dermatol Surg Oncol* **4**, 556.
3 CHALMERS R.J., *et al* (1982) *Br J Dermatol* **107** (Suppl. 22), 29.
4 CROW K.D. (1983) personal communication.
5 FRANCES C., *et al* (1981) *Ann Dermatol Vénéréol* **108**, 209 (Abstract).
6 GOOLAMALI S.K., *et al* (1974) *Br Med J* iv, 78.

7 HARRINGTON C.I. & DUNSMORE I.R. (1981) *Br J Dermatol* **104**, 563.

8 HARRINGTON C.I. & GELSTHORPE K. (1981) *Br J Dermatol* **104**, 561.

9 MEYRICK THOMAS R.H., *et al* (1983) *Br J Dermatol* **109**, 661.

10 MEYRICK THOMAS R.H., *et al* (1984) *Clin Exp Dermatol* **9**, 290.

11 PASIECZNY T.A.H. (1977) *Acta Derm Venereol (Stockh)* **57**, 277.

12 *STAFF W.G. (1970) *Br J Urol* **47**, 234.

13 *WALLACE H.J. (1971) *Trans Rep St John's Hosp Dermatol Soc* **57**, 9.

14 WEIGAND D.A. (1980) *J Dermatol Surg Oncol* **6**, 45.

15 WHIMSTER I.W. (1973) *Trans Rep St John's Hosp Dermatol Soc* **59**, 195.

16 WILLIAMS J.L. & CRAWFORD B.H. (1968) *Br J Urol* **40**, 712.

PENILE ULCERATION AND NECROSIS

Traumatic. Zip fastener and other traumatic ulcers are usually easily recognized. However, self-inflicted lesions may be bizarre and unacknowledged. Extravasation of material injected into the dorsal vein by a heroin addict caused local necrosis [18]. Condom catheter drainage systems in paraplegic and geriatric patients may be attached by tapes applied too tightly, causing painless necrosis or gangrene of the glans or shaft [6, 16].

Venereal infections. Syphilis must be considered and excluded in any case of penile ulceration, however strongly the possibility is refuted; chancre redux and pseudochancre are rare but may be overlooked [5]. Chancroid (p. 764) is also a trap for the unwary [12] as it may present in unusual forms—especially in tropical countries—and may coexist with other viral or bacterial infections [17]. Granuloma venereum (p. 710) may also present with ulceration. Multiple erosions with ragged edges result from contamination with *N. gonorrhoeae* [8, 10]. Discrete pustules or ulcers may also occur without urethritis. Careful and accurate smear and culture techniques are important in differentiating this group of diseases [12].

Other infections. Primary tuberculosis [3] may simulate a syphilitic chancre but lymphadenopathy is more marked. Orificial tuberculous ulcers are multiple with shallow ragged edges; bacilli abound. Papulonecrotic tuberculides have involved the penis (p. 815) and acne scrofulosorum has also been reported [1]. Fusospirillary infections are now uncommon in Western Europe. Deep sloughing necrotic lesions and even gangrene develop with great rapidity (p. 2193). Histoplasmosis and varicella oc-

casionally ulcerate, sometimes deeply. HSV 2 infections have caused necrotic lesions of the glans and shaft [15], and amoebriasis [14] gross tissue loss.

Other causes. Gummas and epitheliomas may ulcerate especially if neglected. Severe aphthosis sometimes causes quite deep painful lesions. In Behçet's syndrome, genital ulceration is said to occur in over 90% of cases [7].

Although vasculitis seldom involves the penis, erythema multiforme may produce ulcerative lesions, especially in the Stevens–Johnson form (p. 1086). Curiously, there have also been reports of Wegener's granulomatosis causing penile necrosis [9, 13].

Dequalinium necrosis [2]. An outbreak of 'necrotizing ulcers of the penis' (Fig. 59.17) was found to be due to the quaternary ammonium antibacterial agent decamethylenebis(4-aminoquinaldinium). This was

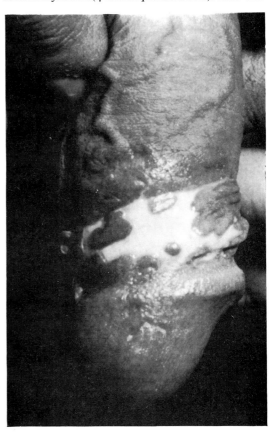

FIG. 59.17. Dequalinium necrosis. A late stage showing the well-marked necrotic ulcer with irregular sharply cut edges. (Stoke Mandeville Hospital.)

well tolerated in most parts of the body but caused a necrotic reaction in some subjects in occluded areas of the body. A similar effect has been noted from other quaternary ammonium products [4] and from needles sterilized in these.

The treatment of all forms of penile necrosis lies first in identifying the cause. In fulminant necrotic organgrenous lesions, excision of all necrotic tissue may be life-saving. In milder cases antibacterial dressings and applications may be sufficient. Recently, dextran polymer particles have been advocated [11]. We feel that further experience of this modality is required.

PENILE GANGRENE

Gangrene of the penis is rare in Western Europe. It usually presents to surgeons and dermatologists will see few cases. Many of the cases of penile necrosis, especially those due to trauma, may extend to gangrene. Known predisposing factors are diabetes, old age and intravascular coagulation syndromes.

Particular causes include varicella in infants, and haemolytic streptococcal, post-operative, malignant and leukaemic diseases.

Among rare causes are tuberculosis, syphilis, penile thrombosis (p. 2195) and dermatitis artefacta.

Gangrenous balanitis (phagedaenic balanitis). This occurs as an occasional complication of venereal infection and super-added (usually fusospirillary) infection. Operative procedures, such as a dorsal slit, extend the infection.

In the form originally described by Fournier, oedema, blisters and rapidly extending sloughs spread over the penis and scrotum of young men after trivial injury. Severe constitutional symptoms are present and the condition is sometimes fatal (see p. 2198).

Treatment must be immediate and thorough. Complete excision of all the affected area is combined with antibiotic therapy and attention to any underlying disease or venereal infection.

REFERENCES

1 BREATHNACH S.M. & BLACK M.M. (1981) *Clin Exp Dermatol* 6, 339.
2 COLES R.B. & WILKINSON D.S. (1965) *Trans Rep St John's Hosp Dermatol Soc* 51, 46.
3 DELZOTTO L. & TENTARELLI T. (1967) *Urologica* 34, 171.
4 DUPRÉ A. & CHRISTOL B. (1973) *Bull Soc Fr Dermatol Syphiligr* 80, 194.
5 *EVANS A.J. & SUMMERLY R. (1964) *Br J Vener Dis* 40, 222.
6 FAVER R. & MORROW J.W. (1978) *Urology* 11, 180.
7 HAIM S. (1974) *Acta Derm Venereol (Stockh)* 54, 299.
8 HAIM S. & MERZBACH D. (1970) *Br J Vener Dis* 46, 336.
9 KALIS B.J. (1982) *16th Inter Congr on Dermatology, Tokyo*, Case Presentations, Univ of Tokyo Press, Tokyo, p. 841.
10 *LANDERGREN G. (1961) *Acta Derm Venereol (Stockh)* 41, 321.
11 LASSUS A., et al (1977) *Acta Derm Venereol (Stockh)* 57, 361.
12 MARGOLIS R.J. & HOOD A.F. (1982) *J Am Acad Dermatol* 6, 493.
13 MATSUDA O., et al (1976) *Tohuku J Exp Med* 2, 118, 145.
14 PARKASH S. (1982) *Postgrad Med J* 58, 375.
15 PEUTHERER J.F., et al (1979) *Br J Vener Dis* 55, 48.
16 STEINHARDT J. & McROBERTS W. (1980) *JAMA* 244, 1238.
17 TAN T., et al (1977) *Asian J Infect Dis* 1, 27.
18 WHITE W.B. & BARRETT S. (1981) *Cutis* 29, 62.

GRANULOMATOUS LESIONS

Although many infections may develop granulomatous forms, three conditions in particular are properly referred to as granulomas.

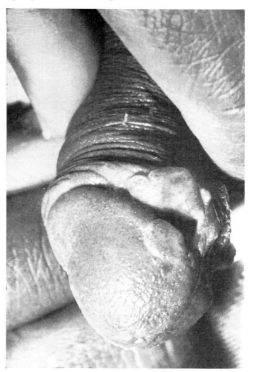

FIG. 59.18. Granuloma inguinale showing the early plaque-like 'cobblestone' lesion (Stoke Mandeville Hospital).

Lymphogranuloma venereum (p. 710). This is still an important tropical venereal disease, and it became endemic in Finland between 1925 and 1940. Its penile manifestation in 37 patients in that country has been recorded [3]. It may present as lymphangitis, preputial infiltration or small granulomatous or fistulous lesions. Late complications in the male are unusual; elephantiasis of penis and scrotum is the most common.

Granuloma inguinale (p. 775). The button-like lesion (Fig. 59.18) develops after an incubation period of about 15 days. A painful inguinal adenitis due to secondary infection may be present [2]. Syphilis may coexist [1]. A mutilating and cicatricial form has been described. Streptomycin cured 91% of 122 patients in India but resistance and side effects occurred [4]. Tetracyclines in high dose are effective.

Eosinophilic granuloma. This is always rare in the genital area, and is more common in the perivulval and perianal regions, but has been described on the penis [5].

REFERENCES

1 DAVIS C.M. (1970) *JAMA* **211**, 632.
2 DUPERRAT B. & LABOUCHE F. (1975) *Bull Soc Fr Dermatol Syphiligr* **102**, 241.
3 HOPSU-HAVU V.K. & SONCK C.E. (1973) *Br J Vener Dis* **49**, 193.
4 *LAL S. (1970) *Br J Vener Dis* **46**, 461.
5 ROUSSELOT M., *et al* (1975) *Bull Soc Fr Dermatol Syphiligr* **82**, 44.

SCLEROSING LIPOGRANULOMA OF PENIS AND SCROTUM

This was originally named to describe a local reaction to injury of adipose tissue, but it is now felt admissable to narrow the definition to 'a local reactive process following injection of exogenous lipids into the subcutaneous tissues' [5].

Pathogenesis. It follows from this that the condition is to be regarded as factitial [1, 2, 5] despite lack of admission by the patient. Paraffin hydrocarbons may be found by IR spectrophotometry [5] and severe psychological problems may be present [3]. Several cases have followed operations [4].

Histopathology. A hyaline necrosis in the fat lobules and intracellular septa leads to disruption of fat cells and a granulomatous reaction. This is followed by a proliferative phase leading to dense hyaline scar tissue. Ultrastructural studies showed a histiocyte-like cell infiltrate with numerous intracytoplasmic vacuoles [2].

Clinical features. The granuloma affects the shaft of the penis or scrotum. The skin is frequently attached to the tumour, which may become tethered down or ulcerated, softening and discharging liquified adipose tissue. As they evolve, the tumours frequently become cystic, though smaller ones may fibrose. The condition is resistant and spontaneous healing does not readily occur.

Treatment. Surgical excision is advocated, though recurrences are usual.

REFERENCES

1 CARLSON H.E. (1968) *J Urol* **100**, 656.
2 CLAUDY A., *et al* (1981) *Br J Dermatol* **105**, 451.
3 FORSTROM L. & WINKELMANN R.K. (1974) *Arch Dermatol* **110**, 747.
4 FOUCAR E., *et al* (1983) *J Am Acad Derm* **9**, 103.
5 *OERTEL Y.C. & JOHNSON F.B. (1977) *Arch Pathol* **101**, 321.

PEARLY PENILE PAPULES [2, 5]
SYN. HIRSUTOID PAPILLOMAS OF THE PENIS; HAIRY PENIS

Definition and aetiology. Pearly penile papules are small smooth dome-shaped or hair-like papules invoving the penile corona. They appear to be a physiological variant, symptomless and without functional significance. They occur at any age after puberty but are chiefly detected between the ages of 20 and 50. An incidence of 10% has been reported [5].

Histopathology. The lesions consist of a core of normal connective tissue covered by epidermis that is thinned centrally and acanthotic at the periphery [4]. The body of the lesion contains a rich, vascular network surrounded by dense connective tissue and a mild lymphocytic infiltrate. They are best considered as angiofibromas [1].

Clinical features [3–5]. The patient complains of 'warts' which are situated on the corona, particularly the anterior border, in one to three irregular rings partly or completely encircling the glans. The individual papules, which are flesh-coloured, white or red are from 1 to 3mm broad and anything up to 3 mm or more in height. Longer filiform lesions also occur.

Treatment. Reassurance alone is required.

REFERENCES

1 Ackerman A.B. & Kornberg R. (1973) *Arch Dermatol* 108, 673.
2 Buschke A. (1909) *Med Klin (Munich)* , 1621.
3 Glickman J.M. & Freeman R.G. (1966) *Arch Dermatol* 93, 56.
4 *Johnson B.L. & Baxter D.L. (1964) *Arch Dermatol* 90, 166.
5 *Tannebaum M.H. & Becker S.W. (1965) *J Urol* 93, 39.

THROMBOSIS OF THE PENIS [4]

Only a few cases of this condition have been described [2]. It is said to be more common in Negroes. The cause is unknown. Of nine cases [3], it followed strenuous intercourse in three and was traumatic in one. Another case has been described with gout [1], and one with thrombophlebitis migrans after resection of the colon for thrombosis of the mesenteric vein [2]. It may also occur in leukaemia and other blood diseases. In granulomatous phlebitis the veins of the sphincter are affected, but not those of the penis itself [5]. Priapism is the chief symptom.

REFERENCES

1 Aubertin E., *et al* (1960) *J Rev Bordeaux* 137, 1486.
2 Grossman A., *et al* (1965) *JAMA* 192, 329.
3 Harrow B.R. & Sloane J.A. (1963) *J Urol* 89, 81.
4 Leading article (1965) *Br Med J* i, 401.
5 Nesbitt R.M. & Hodgson N.W. (1959) *Trans Am Assoc Genito-urin Surg* 51, 92.

PENILE VENEREAL OEDEMA [2]

This uncommon but not rare condition accounted for 1·7 per 1,000 male visits to a clinic for sexually transmitted diseases [3]. In almost all cases other venereal diseases were present.

The condition consists of a self-limiting painless boggy oedema involving the prepuce and distal penile shaft seen in sexually active males. There may be some difficulty in separating this condition from non-venereal sclerosing lymphangitis (though this is partly semantic). The two sometimes coexist. They are both related to previous sexual intercourse and both run a benign course after sexual abstinence. One case has been reported in a 2-yr-old boy with gonorrhoea [1].

This acute rapidly developing oedema must be distinguished from angioedema and from penoscrotal or penile lymphoedema (p. 2198).

REFERENCES

1 Fleisher G., *et al* (1980) *Ann Emerg Med* 9, 314.

2 Wilde H. & Canby J.P. (1973) *Arch Dermatol* 108, 263.
3 Wright R.A. & Judson F.N. (1979) *JAMA* 241, 157.

NON-VENEREAL SCLEROSING LYMPHANGITIS OF THE PENIS
MONDOR'S PHLEBITIS OF THE PENIS [1]

The apparent rarity of this condition is probably misleading [2, 5] as it is painless and symptomless. It affects males aged 20–40 yr, appearing 24–48 h after intercourse. It appears as single or grouped doughy purplish cord-like lesions arising from or around the coronal sulcus (Fig. 59.19). It may extend to the dorsal lymphatic. Ulceration is rare and the lesion is self-limiting in a matter of weeks.

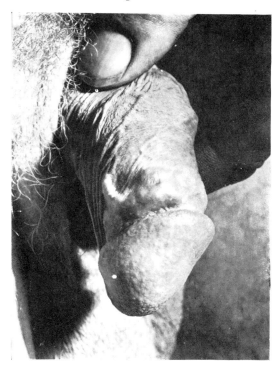

Fig. 59.19. Sclerosing lymphangitis of the penis. Note the thickened lymphatic on the left. (Finsen Institute, Copenhagen.)

Histologically, it has always been believed that the lymphatic vessels were thickened and sclerosed, but a good case has been made recently [1] for regarding the early changes as affecting the veins with occlusion of the lumina by a clot invaded by disintegrating polymorph neutrophils and granulation tissue in the vein wall, similar to Mondor's phlebitis.

The aetiology is unknown but the role of trauma

[2, 3, 5] is obviously important. Cases have been reported following herpes simplex [7] and coincidental with chlamydial infections [4], gonorrhoea and urethritis [6]. The condition can coexist with and be concealed by penile venereal oedema (see below).

REFERENCES

1 FINDLAY G.H. & WHITING D.A. (1977) *Clin Ex Dermatol* **2**, 65.
2 GREENBURG R.D. & PERRY T.L. (1972) *Arch Dermatol* **105**, 728.
3 KANDIL E. & AL-KASHLAN I.M. (1970) *Acta Derm Venereol (Stockh)* **50**, 309.
4 KRISTENSEN J.K. & SCHEIBEL J. (1981) *Acta Derm Venereol (Stockh)* **61**, 455.
5 LASSUS A., *et al* (1972) *Br J Vener Dis* **48**, 545.
6 STOLZ E., *et al* (1974) *Hautarzt*, **25**, 231.
7 VAN DE STAAK W.J.B.M. (1977) *Br J Dermatol* **96**, 679.

PLASTIC INDURATION OF THE PENIS
[1, 4, 5]
SYN. PEYRONIE'S DISEASE

This is a chronic fibrous induration of the intercavernous septa of the penis. More than 1,500 cases have been reported. The peak incidence occurs at or after middle age [4], but cases occur in the third decade.

One or more fibrous masses occur, usually on the dorsum or sides of the penile shaft. Multiple lesions feel like grains of lead. The patients present with curvature on erection, pain on intercourse or impotence. The condition is to be distinguished from penile thrombosis, which is short lived and painful. Urethritis may also be present.

The cause is unknown, but there is a well-recognized association with Dupuytren's contracture [4] which may be present in up to 50% of cases.

Many forms of treatment have been advocated; success is rarely obtained. Invasive measures are often counterproductive. Ultrasound has been tried. Spontaneous resolution may occur over a period of years.

Calcinosis cutis of the penis. Dystrophic calcification of the male genitalia is very rare but may follow trauma or Peyronie's disease or accompany diffuse connective tissue disease or cytotoxic therapy [3]. Metastatic calcinosis from renal hyperparathyroidism is exceptiona. Idiopathic calcinosis in a healthy boy has been recorded [2].

REFERENCES

1 GALLIZIA F. (1966) *Urologia* **33**, 233.
2 HUTCHINSON I.F., *et al* (1980) *Br J Dermatol* **102**, 341.
3 IHDE D.C., *et al* (1975) *Cancer Chemother Rep* **59**, 1039.
4 LEPONAY B. & MEYER M.J. (1974) *Bull Soc Fr. Dermatol Syphiligr* **81**, 468.
5 *UMBELHOR R. (1966) *Urologia* **33**, 213.

BOWENOID PAPULOSIS
SYN. MULTIFOCAL INDOLENT PIGMENTED PENILE PAPULES
MULTICENTRIC PIGMENTED BOWEN'S DISEASE

Definition and aetiology. This recently recognized condition was first described in the groin by Lloyd [6] but was recognized as an entity by Kopf and colleagues a few years later [5, 12, 13]. It consists of indolent and usually symptomless fleshy papules, which are usually pigmented, involving the genitalia or perigenital areas of both sexes (but chiefly young men). The histological features suggest a pre-invasive carcinoma *in situ* but the course is almost certainly benign, although one case progressing to true Bowen's disease (in an older man) has been reported [11]. The aetiology remains unknown, though a pre-existing herpes simplex infection or condylomata have occurred in a significant proportion of patients. However, a viral aetiology has not yet been proved.

Histopathology. This shows the changes of Bowen's disease, with acanthosis, atypical keratinocytic hyperplasia, a moderate degree of nuclear dysplasia and atypical crowded mitotic activity. Pigment is usually prominent in the basal-cell layer and pigment-laden macrophages are present in the dermis [3]. The overall appearance is that of carcinoma *in situ*. Electron microscopy studies have not usually shown any sign of viral inclusion [3, 12], though viral-like intranuclear particles were reported in one study [4]. The epidermal cells displayed marked interdigitation of plasma membranes, numerous desmosomes and condensed tonofilaments [3]. The nuclei of many cells had irregular invagination and dilatation of the nuclear envelope. The basement membrane was intact though occasionally tortuous. A decrease in intact desmosomes and aggregation of tonofilaments around intracellular vacuolation were found in another study [2].

Clinical features (See p. 2226). The lesions present in young patients as multiple papules, often grouped, 2–20 mm in diameter and with a verrucous or smooth surface, more commonly on the shaft than the glans. Their colour usually ranges from brown–

red to violaceous or black but they may be rosy [10] or pale. At times they may show a lichenoid or psoriasiform appearance. The patients have usually been circumcised [12], in contrast with those with true Bowen's disease or erythryplasia.

Differential diagnosis [7, 9]. The lesions may be confused with condylomata, verrucae vulgares (on the shaft), sebborrhoeic warts, epithelial naevi or lichen planus. The presence of pigmented papules in the penile shaft of a young man should be a pointer to the correct diagnosis.

Treatment. Although Bowenoid papulosis appears to remain a benign condition, it has not been followed long enough to be certain of this [1]. Local excision of solitary lesions enables the diagnosis to be confirmed [8]. Electrocoagulation, electrodesiccation, cryotherapy or 5-fluorouracil have been employed successfully [1, 7, 9]. However, close follow-up is essential. Spontaneous regression has occasionally occurred.

REFERENCES

1 Cutler T.C. (1980) *Clin Exp Dermatol* **5**, 97.
2 Faber M. & Hagedorn M. (1981) *Acta Derm Venereol (Stockh)* **61**, 397.
3 Katz H.I., *et al* (1978) *Br J Dermatol* **99**, 155.
4 Kimura S., *et al* (1978) *Dermatologica* **157**, 229.
5 Kopf A.W. & Bart R.S. (1977) *J Dermatol Surg Oncol* **33**, 265.
6 Lloyd K.M. (1970) *Arch Dermatol* **101**, 48.
7 Mascaro J.M., *et al* (1980) *Actas Dermosifilogr* **71**, 119.
8 Peters M.S. & Perry H.O. (1981) *J Urol* **126**, 482.
9 Taylor D.R. Jr. (1981) *Cutis* **27**, 92.
10 Toribio J., *et al* (1981) *Actas Dermosifilogr* **72**, 545.
11 de Villez R.L. & Stevens C.S. (1980) *J Am Acad Dermatol* **3**, 149.
12 Wade T.R., *et al* (1978) *Cancer* **42**, 1890.
13 Wade T.R., *et al* (1979) *Arch Dermatol* **115**, 306.

CONDITIONS PARTICULARLY INVOLVING THE SCROTUM

Cavernous haemangiomas in infants habitually ulcerate, healing spontaneously after some weeks. Angiokeratoma (syn. of Fordyce) selectively involves the scrotal skin (p. 213); the lesions seldom require treatment, though they are easily destroyed by electrodesiccation. The punctate spots of angiokeratoma corposis diffusum (p. 2309) are smaller and less hyperkeratotic and are present elsewhere. Epidermal naevi are distinguished by their usual features (p. 169). Cutaneous horns and lipomas occur as occasional curiosities. A pendulous fibroma [8] can be troublesome to the patient. Sebocystomas (Fig. 2406) arise in early life as multiple firm yellow-white nodules, to be distinguished from the lesions of idiopathic calcinosis (see p. 2198), which sometimes break down and extrude chalky contents.

Acanthosis nigricans, pemphigus vegetans and pyodermite végétante affect the scrotum; benign familial pemphigus may easily be overlooked as the cause of an erosive dermatitis which is refractory to treatment.

Absorption of topical medicaments is greatly enhanced through the scrotal skin. Corticosteroids should be used sparingly [7]. Hexachlorophane concentrate in baths has caused burns [25]. Straw-coloured cysts, cometimes itchy or becoming inflamed, occur in chloracne [4].

Infections and infestations. Condylomata acuminata do not commonly involve the scrotal skin, except in the presence of maceration, infection or discharge.

The scrotum is involved in genitocrural infective dermatitis, when fissuring and superficial ulcerations of the penoscrotal junction may be a marked feature. Infection secondary to scabies, pruritus or eczema is occasionally seen. It is a common site of lichen simplex (p. 410).

Infestation with *Phthirius pubis* is common in hirsute patients, and scabetic lesions occur, though less frequently than on the penis. Though the scrotum may appear to be spared in *fungal infections*, it is not infrequently affected, though the epidermal reaction is poor [16] and may be completely absent in patients treated with corticosteroids [11].

Schistosomiasis causes fistulae, sinuses, phagadaenic ulceration and pseudoelephantiasis. A chronic papular dermatitis has also been recorded [24]. True elephantiasis, often extraordinary in extent, is caused by *Wucheria bancrofti* (p. 1001). Calcified nodules may result from encysted forms of this or of filariae of *Onchocerca volvulus* [1].

Erythematous and eczematous conditions. The scrotal skin is frequently involved in seborrhoeic and intertriginous eczemas. Eczema confined to the scrotum suggests an exogenous cause, usually industrial. Lichen simplex is most frequent at the scroto-perineal junction, where it is sustained by rubbing through trouser pockets. The pruritus often has a particular 'burning quality'.

Scrotal dermatitis and pigmentation, often with scaling and superficial ulceration, formed a characteristic part of an 'oculogenital' syndrome seen in 75% of 8,000 American prisoners of war fed on an inadequate diet of rice [12]. Intense burning and itching accompanied the condition, in which conjunctivitis and stomatitis were also present. The patients recovered on a full diet. Riboflavin and to some extent nicotinic acid deficiencies have been blamed for a syndrome of scrotal dermatitis, seborrhoeic dermatitis, angular stomatitis and fissuring of the alae nasi. This was reproducible experimentally on a diet low only in riboflavin [10]. However, since these features are seen without any evidence of riboflavin deficiency, it seems likely that local inflammatory factors lead to an increased demand for the vitamin.

The scrotum may be involved in the 'perineal syndrome' (p. 2178).

Increased pigmentation is seen with steatorrhoea and malabsorption syndromes.

Scrotal gangrene [6, 8, 23]. Fournier's 'idiopathic' gangrene continues to be seen and carries a high mortality. It occurs explosively and progresses rapidly [2]. Although the patients are often diabetic [5, 6, 14], the essential cause remains obscure. It has been regarded as a synergistic necrotizing cellulitis, a form of disseminated intravascular coagulation [6, 18] or equivalent to necrotizing fasciitis [17]. An immunological deficit, e.g. myeloma, was present in one case [9] and may play a part in others. It has followed vasectomy [21] and lower gut resection [2]. Organisms are not always found but *Bacteroides fragilis* has sometimes been recovered. Extensive debridement of all affected tissue is essential [19], in conjunction with supportive measures and agressive therapy.

Juvenile gangrenous vasculitis of the scrotum [20]. A less severe form of gangrene, healing in 15–45 days, is preceded by fever and burning. Polycyclic vasculitis lesions with histological features of angiitis follow. It may also be related to aphthosis. Rickettsial infection may also cause scrotal gangrene.

Other conditions. Lymphangiectases may follow filiarial infection or be due to lymphangioma circumscription. A milky discharge may seep from the scrotum after rupture ('weeping scrotum') [13]. Lipgranuloma may involve the scrotum (p. 1870). Crohn's disease does so rarely, and causes boggy oedema and fistulae [3].

Penoscrotal lymphoedema [22] must be distinguished from transitory penile venereal oedema (p. 2195). It occurs as a manifestation of primary hypoplastic lymphatics or following infection, with a secondarily compromised lymphatic channel. This may unexpectedly follow local operative procedures.

Acute haemorrhagic oedema (p. 254) affects the newborn [15].

REFERENCES

1 BROWNE S.G. (1962) *Br J Dermatol* **74**, 136.
2 CABRERA H.N. (1973) *Med Cutan Iber Lat Am* **1**, 145.
3 COCKBURN A.G., *et al* (1980) *Urology* **15**, 596.
4 CROW K.D. (1981) *Clin Exp Dermatol* **6**, 243.
5 DOOTSON G.M., *et al* (1982) *J R Soc Med* **75**, 916.
6 *FEINGOLD D.S. (1982) *J Am Acad Dermatol* **6**, 289.
7 FELDMANN R.T. & MAIBACH H.L. (1967) *J Invest Dermatol* **48**, 181.
8 FLECK F. & FLECK M. (1974) *Organische W. funktionelle Sexualerkrankungen.* Berlin, Verlag Volk und Gesundheit.
9 FRIER B.M. & HOWIE A.D. (1972) *Br Med J* **iv**, 26.
10 HILLS O.W., *et al* (1951) *Arch Intern Med* **87**, 682.
11 IVE F.A. & MARKS R. (1968) *Br Med J* **iii**, 149.
12 JACOBS E.C. (1951) *Ann Intern Med* **35**, 1409.
13 JOHNSON W.T. (1979) *Arch Dermatol* **115**, 464.
14 KATSAS A.G. (1982) *J R Soc Med* **75**, 988.
15 LAMBERT D., *et al* (1979) *Ann Dermatol Syphiligr* **106**, 975.
16 LA TOUCHE C.J. (1967) *Br J Dermatol* **79**, 339.
17 OH C., *et al* (1982) *Surgery* **91**, 49.
18 PANDE S.K. & MEWARA P.C. (1976) *Br J Surg* **63**, 479.
19 PARDY B. & EASTCOTT H.H.G. (1982) *Proc R Soc Med* **75**, 829.
20 PIÑOL AGUADE J., *et al* (1974) *XIVe Congrès de l'Association des Dermatologistes et Syphiligraphes de Langue Française, Genève, 1973. II Vascularites*, p. 112. Geneva, Ed. Médecine et Hygiène, 1974.
21 PRYOR J.P., *et al* (1976) *Br Med J* **i**, 272.
22 SAMSOEN M., *et al* (1981) *Ann Dermatol Vénéréol* **108**, 541.
23 SMODA A., *et al* (1980) *J Dermatol* **7**, 371.
24 WALKER R.R. (1979) *Arch Dermatol* **115**, 869.
25 WILKINSON D.S. (1978) *Contact Dermatitis* **4**, 172.

Idiopathic calcinosis of the scrotum [2, 3, 5]. Multiple asymptomatic nodules develop in childhood or early adult life [5] as greyish or white firm nodules scattered in the scrotal skin. As they increase in size, they may break down to discharge their chalky contents. They are frequently misdiagnosed as cysts. Blood calcium and phosphorus levels are normal, in contradistinction to metastatic calcinosis which only rarely affects the skin but which carries a poor prognosis [4]. Histologically, these amorphous deposits may be surrounded by a granulomatous epithelinoid cell and a foreign body giant cell reaction.

True secondary dystrophic calcinosis follows tissue injury, local chronic infection or connective tissue disease. Cases have been reported following onchocerciasis [1].

Surgical treatment should be limited to the removal of large or discharging lesions. Healing of scrotal skin is often slow.

REFERENCES

1 BROWNE S.G. (1962) *Br J Dermatol* **74**, 136.
2 FISHER B.K. & DVORETSKY I. (1978) *Arch Dermatol* **114**, 957.
3 MOSS R.L. & SHEWMAKE S.W. (1981) *Int J Dermatol* **20**, 134.
4 PUTKONEN T. & WANGEL G.A. (1959) *Dermatologica* **118**, 127.
5 *SHAPIRO L., et al (1970) *Arch Dermatol* **102**, 199.

PREMALIGNANT AND MALIGNANT LESIONS OF THE PENIS AND SCROTUM

RONA M. MACKIE

Giant condylomata acuminata (Buschke–Lowenstein). This condition occupies an uncertain position on the borderline of malignant disease. These rare but dramatic tumours have many similarities to florid oral papillomatosis of the oral mucosa and epithelioma cuniculatum in that, while all three conditions have the cytological appearance of a benign condition, they are locally extremely aggressive and tend to recur repeatedly and extensively even after apparently adequate surgery.

Pathology. The lesion has none of the obvious hallmarks of malignancy. There is obvious and extreme acanthosis of the epidermis or mucosa but little or no cellular atypia or mitotic figures. It has long been suspected that the human papilloma virus (HPV) is an aetiological agent, and modern methods of identification of the HPV have recently confirmed the presence of human papilloma virus DNA (HPV6) in these lesions [1, 2].

Clinical features. Giant condylomata are found on both the male and female genitalia. Initially they may appear as no more than a cluster of genital warts, but the lesion expands relentlessly causing gross local tissue destruction (Fig. 59.20).

Treatment. Because of the extreme frequency of local recurrence early and effective therapy is essential. Surgical excision and cryotherapy are effective, but topical wart preparations tend to be ineffective. Even with apparently adequate surgery the lesion may recur, and in some cases partial penile amputation is necessary.

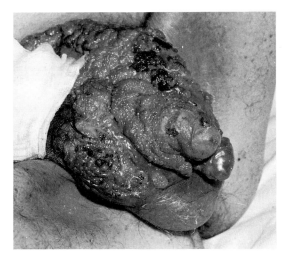

FIG. 59.20. Gross condylomata of Buschke–Lowenstein on the genitalia. Ten years after amputation this patient is alive with no recurrence. (Professor R.M. Mackie, Department of Dermatology, Glasgow University.)

REFERENCES

1 GISSMAN L., et al (1982) *Int J Cancer* **29**, 143.
2 ZOCHOW K.R., et al (1982) *Nature* **300**, 771.

Erythroplasia of Queyrat. This can be defined as a barely raised, sharply outlined, bright red, glistening and velvety plaque occurring on mucous membranes, particularly the penis, which is refractory to treatment and eventuates in malignancy [6]. The use of the term should be restricted to an intraepidermal carcinoma, histologically similar to Bowen's disease. Erythroplasia is not associated with Bowen's disease elsewhere, nor with an increase in incidence of internal cancer [7].

Incidence. It is an uncommon condition. On the penis it does not occur in men circumcised in infancy and is not confined to the elderly [17]. It has been described on the mucous membranes of the mouth and tongue and on the vulva. In the last site British and American authorities tend to prefer the diagnosis of Bowen's disease rather than erythroplasia.

Pathology. The surface may be denuded of stratum corneum and crusted or covered by parakeratosis. The epidermis is thickened, particularly in the interpapillary ridges, which may become bulbar and extend quite deeply into the dermis. The acanthosis is similar to Bowen's disease in the variety of abnormal cells in the prickle-cell layer, large and hyperchromatic nuclei, multinucleate cells, increased mitoses, premature keratinization and disturbance of polarity. The dermis may be infiltrated by inflammatory cells.

Clinical features [6]. The penile lesions are situated on the glans, beginning under the foreskin as a red, glazed, barely raised well-circumscribed and rather irregularly shaped plaque which typically has a lacquered appearance. It is soft and supple, Crusting or erosion may occur later. Advanced lesions may spread from the mucous membrane to the skin. Invasive change is indicated by induration, verrucosity or ulceration. Metastasis can occur [3].

Diagnosis. Most of the common inflammatory conditions of the glans or foreskin are less sharply circumscribed and respond to application of a steroid and antimicrobial agent. Biopsy should be performed in cases of doubt.

Treatment. Erythroplasia response to the local application of antimitotic agents such as 5-fluorouracil cream [13] or thiocolciran cream. A radium mould can be used [14]. If there is evidence of invasion it must be treated as squamous cell carcinoma.

Squamous carcinoma of the penis and scrotum

Incidence and aetiology [22, 23]. Carcinoma of the penis and scrotum are caused by differing environmental factors but both are preventable malignancies. Scrotal cancer, which is commoner in those of lower socio-economic status [16], appears to be caused by contact with mineral oils and tars. It is thus an industrial disease and with appropriate protective clothing could be prevented. Men who survive scrotal cancer appear to have a higher incidence of other primary malignancies [11]. However, a recent study of 12 scrotal cancers, nine squamous cell carcinomas and three basal cell carcinomas suggested that poor hygiene and chronic irritation may also be important [18].

Penile cancer is very rare in the circumcised male [20], and here the association with poor hygiene is well established. Unlike scrotal cancer, however, there is no association with socio-economic status. There are studies reporting a high incidence of carcinoma of the cervix in the wives of men with carcinoma of the penis, suggesting a common, probably viral, aetiologic factor [19, 24].

There are a few reports of carcinoma of the penis developing after lichen sclerosus et atrophicus and a recent study reports two such cases in 44 cases of lichen sclerosus et atrophicus [5].

Clinical features [10, 25]. The initial lesion on the penis is almost always within the preputial sac. It may be preceded by erythroplasia, leukoplakia or a warty excrescence which is frequently misdiagnosed as a wart. Lesions may occasionally be multiple and closely resemble condyloma acuminatum [15, 21]. The majority of tumours are histologically well differentiated and are at first vegetating rather than ulcerative. Despite this, metastases are present in the inguinal glands in about half the cases when first seen [19]. The general characteristics of squamous cell carcinoma are described on p. 2431.

Diagnosis [9]. Biopsy of any suspicious warty, leukoplakic, reddened or ulcerated area should give a definite diagnosis. A low-grade carcinoma may show only epithelial hyperplasia microscopically for a considerable time before invasion becomes apparent [9].

Treatment. Radiotherapy can be used in cases where the regional nodes are not involved [12], but it is not effective in the verrucous cancer [15]. Most authorities recommend partial or complete amputation, depending on the extent of the spread, with removal of involved nodes. Combination chemotherapy can be used in advanced cases.

Other malignant tumours. Extramammary Paget's disease, basal cell carcinoma and malignant melanoma are uncommon on the male genitalia. They are described elsewhere. A variety of connective tissue tumours of the penis have been reported, including malignant haemangio-endothelioma, Kaposi's sarcoma, fibrosarcoma, leiomyosarcoma, undifferentiated sarcoma angiosarcoma and dermatofibrosarcoma protuberans [1, 2, 4, 6, 8].

REFERENCES

1 ARMIYO M., *et al* (1978) *Ann Dermatol Vénéréol* **105**, 267.
2 ASHLEY D.J.B. & EDWARDS E.C. (1957) *Br J Surg* **45**, 170.
3 AVRACH W.W. & CHRISTENSEN H.E. (1976) *Acta Derm Venereol (Stockh)* **56**, 409.
4 BELAICH S., *et al* (1978) *Ann Dermatol Vénéréol* **105**, 331.
5 BINGHAM J.S. (1978) *Br J Vener Dis* **54**, 350.
6 BLAU S. & HYMAN A.B. (1955) *Acta Derm Venereol (Stockh)* **35**, 341.
7 DEHNER L.P., *et al* (1970) *Cancer (NY)* **25**, 1431.
8 GHANDUR-MNAYMNEH L. & GONZALEZ M.S. (1981) *Cancer* **47**, 1318.
9 GRAHAM J.H. & HELWIG E.B. (1964) *Tumours of the Skin.* Chicago, Yearbook Medical Publishers, p. 209.
10 HANASH K.A., *et al* (1970) *J Urol* **104**, 291.
11 HOLMES J.G., *et al* (1970) *Lancet* **ii**, 214.

12 HOPE-STONE H. (1975) *Proc R Soc Med* **68**, 777.

13 HUESER J.N., *et al* (1969) *J Urol* **102**, 595.

14 KAPLAN C. & KATOH A. (1973) *J Surg Oncol* **5**, 281.

15 KRAUS F.T. & PEREZ-MESA C. (1966) *Cancer* (NY) **19**, 26.

16 LEE W.R., *et al* (1972) *Br J Ind Med* **29**, 188.

17 McANINCH J.W., *et al* (1970) *J Urol* **104**, 287.

18 McDONALD M.W. (1982) *Urology* **19**, 269.

19 MARTINEZ I. (1969) *Cancer* (NY) **24**, 777.

20 MELMED E.P. & PAYNE J.R. (1967) *Br J Surg* **54**, 729.

21 ORANJE A.P., *et al* (1976) *Dermatologica* **152**, 47.

22 POINTON R.C.S. (1975) *Proc R Soc Med* **68**, 779.

23 SCHREK R. & LENOWITZ H. (1947) *Cancer Res* **7**, 180.

24 SMITH P.G., *et al* (1980) *Br J Cancer* **41**, 422.

25 STAUBITZ W.J., *et al* (1955) *Cancer* (NY) **8**, 371.

Genital malignancy and hypercalcaemia [1, 4]. Of about 30 sporadic case reports of hypercalcaemia in patients with non-parathyroid neoplasms without bone disease, about half were of genito-urinary origin [2, 3]. This curious finding has been noted in a case of squamous cell carcinoma of the penis in which the serum calcium fell to normal within 24 h of removal.

The mechanism is entirely unknown. It has been suggested [5] that the tumour may elaborate a parathormone-like or vitamin-D-like substance, causing excessive absorption of calcium from the gut and bone, or a substance that binds calcium and carries it in this form. An extract of the tumours has shown antigenic reactions with specific antiparathyroid hormone antibody. The calcium level drops if steroids are administered.

REFERENCES

1 ANDERSON E.E. & GLENN J.F. (1965) *JAMA* **192**, 328.

2 Case records of Massachusetts General Hospital (1963) *N Engl J Med* **269**, 801.

3 Case records of Massachusetts General Hospital (1964) *N Engl J Med* **270**, 1302.

4 KRONFIELD S.J. & REYNOLDS T.B. (1964) *N Engl J Med* **271**, 399.

5 PLIMTON C.H. & GELLHORN A. (1956) *Am J Med* **21**, 750.

THE FEMALE GENITALIA

Introduction. Mention should be made at the outset of three authoritative and excellent accounts of this subject, which can necessarily be dealt with only briefly below. The reader is referred to them for further information. They are as follows.

1 GARDNER H.L. & KAUFMAN R.H. (1969) *Benign Diseases of the Vulva and Vagina*. St Louis, Mosby.

2 BEILBY J.O.W. & RIDLEY C.M. (1986) *Pathology of the Vulva* In *Hailes and Taylors Obstetric and Gynaecological Pathology* Ed Fox H. Churchill Livingstone. Edinburgh

3 *RIDLEY C.M. (1976) *The Vulva*. London, Saunders.

In order to save space, these will be referred to subsequently in the text as references 1–3.

Anatomy [1–3]. The female external genitalia extend between the pubis and the posterior commisure. The labia majora are equivalent to the scrotum and the clitoris is the homologue of the penis. The labia majora are endowed with abundant subcutaneous fat and loose connective tissue, allowing considerable oedema to take place in inflammation with minimal residual damage or scarring. The skin is thick, rugose and hairy on the outer aspect, and smooth and moist on the inner aspect where it takes on the character of a mucosal surface. Pilosebaceous units and 'free' sebaceous glands are abundant on the labia majora but only the latter are found on the labia minora. Small mucous glands occur on the skin of the vestibule. Nerve endings are numerous, especially on the clitoris. Apocrine glands, twice as abundant as in the male, are found on the mons veneris and labia majora.

Bartholin's glands, a homologue of Cowper's glands, are compound branching tubular glands secreting a clear alkaline mucus into a duct lined deeply by columnar cells and superficially by transitional and then stratified epithelium. They lie between the superficial and deep layers of the urogenital diaphragm, opening by a duct 2 cm long at the posterior aspect of the labium minus. The acini are lined by a single layer of columnar or cuboidal cells.

The vagina is lined by stratified epithelium. The cells are stimulated by oestrogen and mature keratinized cells are shed just before ovulation. The pH in reproductive life is in the region of 3·8–4·2 but is higher at menstruation.

In pregnancy pigmentation increases, varicosities may develop and the pH falls. At the menopause the vasculature declines and becomes less regular [8]; the sebaceous glands become less active.

Congenital and developmental conditions. Malformations will not be discussed. An admirable summary is available [3]. Accessory mammary tissue may become active in pregnancy and give rise to fibroadenomas [2]. Dermoid cysts at the perineal raphe and para-urethral cysts are both rare but may present when infected. Cavernous haemangiomas ulcerate readily, as on the scrotum. Angiokeratomas may cause intermittent bleeding or increase in size in pregnancy [6]. All other forms of angiomatous dysplasia, including angiokeratoma corporis diffusum occur, though rarely. Local or general dysplasia of the lymphatic system may manifest itself in childhood or young adult life as lymphangiectasia or as recurrent attacks of cellulitis. Perineal as well as axillary freckling may occur in neurofibromatosis [5].

Special characteristics of common vulval dermatoses [7].

The normal characteristics of common diseases are modified. The lax tissues of the vulva encourage oedema rather than vesiculation. Psoriasis loses its characteristic scaling, bullous lesions become erosive or vegetating, intertriginous lesions spread from the inguinal or abdominal folds and secondary infection is common in the obese middle-aged or elderly patient. Lichenification frequently complicates and may mask any pruritic skin lesion.

Urticaria and angio-oedema affecting the vulva give rise to considerable oedema and discomfort though only rarely to difficulty in micturition [3]. Hereditary angio-oedema, however, may involve the urethra [9]. Atopic eczema seldom affects the vulva though lichen simplex is common. Seborrhoeic dermatitis and psoriasis are easily confused in this area but other stigmata are usually present. Erythrasma may affect the labia majora and is often overlooked unless Wood's light examination is carried out.

Fixed drug eruptions, less common now than previously, appear to have a predilection for the genital region. Residual pigmentation must be distinguished from general causes of pigmentation.

Vitiligo commonly involves the vulval area. Cytotoxic drugs may cause loss of pubic as well as scalp hair.

Contact dermatitis.

The vulva has been shown to be significantly more susceptible than forearm skin to irritants [4]. Irritant contact dermatitis is most commonly seen in overscrupulous ladies whose enthusiastic use of soap and water may be combined with a rather guilty conscience ('I'm going to wash that man right out of my hair'). Other culprits may be corrosive chemicals, disinfectants or deodorant sprays applied too closely. Friction, trauma, moisture or the proximity of infective discharges play a role and are considered below. Allergic contact dermatitis may present as oedema or be mistaken for angio-oedema. It is usually the result of medicaments, especially local anaesthetic and antihistamine creams. Other less common causes are nail varnish, perfumes in sprays and sanitary napkins, contraceptives, clothing dyes, etc. A full battery of patch tests may reveal unsuspected sensitivities. This diagnosis should be considered whenever a pruritic vulval dematosis fails to respond adequately to treatment.

REFERENCES

1–3 As cited on p. 2201.
4 BRITZ M.B. & MAIBACH H.I. (1979) *Contact Dermatitis* **5**, 375.
5 CROWE F.W. (1964) *Ann Int Med* **61**, 1142.
6 JOOSSE L.A., et al (1964) *Ned Tijdschr Verlosk Gynaecol* **64**, 179.
7 KLOSTERMANN G.F. (1972) In *Handbuch der Speziallen pathologischen Anatomie and Histologie* Berlin, Springer.
8 RYAN T.J. (1973) In *Physiology and Pathophysiolology of the Skin.* New York, Academic Press, Vol. 2.
9 WARIN R.P. & CHAMPION R.H. (1974) *Urticaria*. London, Saunders, p. 114.

Miscellaneous conditions [1–9].

Varicosities of the labial veins may occur unilaterally in association with limb varicosities or appear in pregnancy. Though usually symptomless they may cause pruritus or discomfort. Pediculosis, scabies or even insect bites may be an unexpected cause of pruritus.

Vulval oedema accompanies acute infections and is a feature of Crohn's disease. Urticaria, angio-oedema and hereditary angio-oedema may involve the vulva, sometimes predominantly, and can occasionally be associated with immediate type hypersensitivity to seminal plasma [4]. Lymphoedema may be primary or secondary to repeated streptococcal infections [11], lymphogranuloma venereum, filariasis, tuberculosis and other chronic infections or neoplasms.

Accidental or purposeful traumatic lesions [1] are seldom seen by dermatologists and may therefore be overlooked in differential diagnosis.

Darier's disease affecting the vulva forms brownish crusts which break down and become malodorous; the vagina may be involved [9]. Acanthosis nigricans and seborrheic dermatitis may be simulated [3]. Ehlers–Danlos syndrome causes trouble at delivery. Pseudoxanthoma elasticum also affects the vulva and sometimes the vagina [7].

Non-effective granulomas are uncommon. Midline granuloma has been reported [6]. Eosinophilic granuloma involving the vulval or perianal skin usually affects women aged 15–59, presenting as papules, vesicles or pustules, often painful or pruritic. Diabetes insipidus was present in 24 of 25 cases [14]. Vaginal extension was rare.

Bullous diseases.

Rapidly developing bullae may occur in erythema multiforme. Epidermolysis bullosa may affect the vulva [3], but seldom affects the vagina. In two of three recent personal cases of herpes gestationis the vulva was especially affected. Juvenile dermatitis herpetiformis also has a predilection for the genital area [8], as have pemphigus vulgaris and vegetans. The vagina, usually spared in other chronic bullous diseases, may be involved and the cervix has also been affected [5, 12]. Familial benign chronic pemphigus [13] is easily induced here by friction, infection and irritants, and may escape recognition. Benign mucosal pemphigoid not infrequently involves the vulva, which has also been implicated at some stage in all reported cases of necrolytic erythema [10].

All secondarily infected chronic bullous diseases may be mistaken for intertrigo.

REFERENCES

1–3 As cited on p. 2201.
4 CHANG T.-W. (1976) *Am J Obstet Gynecol* **126**, 442.
5 FRIEDMAN D., *et al* (1971) *Am J Obstet Gynecol* **110**, 1023.
6 FRIEDMAN I. (1964) *Proc R Soc Med* **57**, 289.
7 GOODMAN R.M. (1963) *Medicine* (Baltimore) **42**, 297.
8 GRANT D.W. (1968) *Trans Rep St John's Hosp Dermatol Soc* **54**, 128.
9 KLOSTERMANN G.F. (1972) In *Handbuch des Speziellen Pathologischen Anatomie und Histologie* Berlin, Springer.
10 MALLINSON C.N., *et al* (1974) *Lancet* **ii**, 1.
11 NORBURN L.M. & COLES R.B. (1960) *J Obstet Gynaecol Br Commonw* **67**, 279.
12 SAGHER F., *et al* (1974) *Br J Dermatol* **90**, 407.
13 THIERS H., *et al* (1968) *Bull Soc Fr Dermatol Syphiligr* **75**, 352.
14 VALLET C.H. (1974) *Thesis*. Paris.

Disorders of the sweat glands

[1, 2, 3, 6]. Fox–Fordyce disease involves the mons pubis and labia and is exquisitely pruritic. The pink follicular papules may be obscured by secondary infection or lichenification. The itching distinguishes this condition from syringomas, but apocrine or miliarial retention cysts [2] may cause difficulty. Rarely, chromidrosis and trichomycosis cause discoloration of the pubic hair and must be distinguished from pediculosis [5].

Hidradenitis suppurativa

(p. 785). This is less common than in men in this area. The aetiology is obscure but secondary inflammation in occluded apocrine glands may be responsible for the symptoms. Distortion, sinus formation and fistulae develop, often continuously and remorselessly, involving ever wider areas as the post-inflammatory scarring induces further disorganization. Carcinoma has developed in the affected area [4]. Early lesions are often mistaken for boils, and later ones for lymphogranuloma venereum or Crohn's disease.

Small local lesions respond well to phenolization, cryotherapy or injections of corticosteroids. More advanced lesions may be helped by appropriate antibiotics but will require surgery—either plastic excision and grafting or marsupialization and diathermy, a technique that has proved very effective in personal cases. Spontaneous regression of activity usually occurs as scarring destroys gland tissue, or with the advent of the menopause.

Tumours of apocrine origin are discussed below.

REFERENCES

1–3 As cited on p. 2201.
4 HUMPHREY L.J., *et al* (1960) *Arch Dermatol* **100**, 59.
5 WHITE S.W. & SMITH J. (1979) *Arch Dermatol* **115**, 444.
6 WINKELMANN R.J. & MONTGOMERY H. (1965) *Arch Dermatol* **75**, 63.

Benign tumours of the vulva

[1–3]. These are relatively rare [1]. Epidermal naevi, seborrhoeic warts and especially fibroepithelial polyps, often of considerable size, are not uncommon, though usually in the pubic area or genitocrural folds rather than on the vulva itself. They are probably more common in the male on the inner thighs, but form part of the spectrum of 'pseudo-acanthosis nigricans' in the middle-aged female.

Epidermal cysts are seen on the labia majora and in the region of the clitoris. They are especially common in tribal societies who practice female circumcision [8] and may become inflamed or present because of increasing size. Obstruction of the duct of a Bartholin gland occurs in the reproductive years, causing cysts in the posterior part of the labia majora. Marsupialization [1] may be performed if the cyst is troublesome, unless there is suspicion of malignancy when an excision–biopsy is to be preferred.

Eccrine syringomas are asymptomatic and rarely involve the vulva [13] but hidradenoma papilliferum is seen almost exclusively in this region [7], especially in the labium majus. It presents as a solitary firm or soft nodule, up to 4 cm in diameter [3], showing histological features of apocrine-type papillary epithelium similar to the intraduct papillomas of the breast. Over 200 cases had been reported up to 1973 [7].

Angiokeratoma of the vulva is probably more common than is recognized [4]. The lesions, which are solitary or multiple, may cause bleeding in pregnancy. They may correspond to the lesions called 'senile haemangiomas' [1]. They must be distinguished from the more important lesions of angiokeratoma corporis diffusum in which other regions—particularly the umbilical area—will be involved.

Numerous types of benign tumours may occasionally occur on the vulva as elsewhere on the body: moles, angiomas, capillary naevi and neurofibromas [11]. Granular-cell myoblastoma [5], presenting as flesh-coloured occasionally pedunculated or ulcerated lesions is likely only to be diagnosed histologically. Pseudo-epitheliomatous hyperplasia must be distinguished from the true malignancy that occasionally occurs [10].

The rare but troublesome leiomyoma presents as a solitary firm reddish-brown tumour which may be painful on pressure and with heat or cold. A clitoral leiomyoma with a leiomyoma of the oesophagus has recently been reported [12].

Lymphocytoma cutis, also a rare lesion in this area, presents as glistening brownish-red nodules, occasionally extending to the urethra and vagina [6].

Endometriosis [1, 2] occasionally occurs on the vulva or in the vagina as a direct implantation. The condition may be becoming more common [3] because of the increased frequency of gynaecological procedures. The lesions are often preceded by uterine curettage or sometimes occur in episiotomy scars after delivery [9]. They present as firm bluish nodules which become tender or bleed during menstruation. The histology is diagnostic.

REFERENCES

1–3 As cited on p. 2201.
4 BLAIR C. (1970) *Br J Dermatol* **83**, 409.
5 GIFFORD R.R.M. & BIRCH H.W. (1973) *Am J Obstet Gynecol* **117**, 187.
6 MATRAS A. (1964) *Hautarzt* **15**, 657.
7 NIELSON N.C. (1973) *Acta Obstet Gynecol Scand* **52**, 387.
8 ONUIGBO W.I.B. (1976) *Arch Dermatol* **112**, 1405.
9 PAULL T. & TEDESCHI L. (1972) *Obstet Gynecol* **40**, 28.
10 SADLER W.P. & DOCHERTY M.B. (1951) *Am J Obstet Gynecol* **61**, 1047.
11 SCHREIBER M.M. (1963) *Arch Dermatol* **88**, 320.
12 STENCHEVER M.A., *et al* (1973) *J Reprod Med* **10**, 75.
13 THOMAS J., *et al* (1979) *Arch Dermatol* **115**, 95.

INFECTIONS OF THE VULVA

Normal flora [1–3, 8]. The skin of the perineal area has a higher pH, temperature and degree of humidity than skin elsewhere and this harbours large numbers of transient and resident organisms, mainly micrococci, diphtheroids and lactobacilli. Only coagulase positive staphylococci are usually considered pathogenic but were found in as many as 67% of normal females [4]. α haemolytic streptococci were present in 44% of the same series; however, only the β haemolytic strain, notably of Lancefield groups A and C, are pathogenic. Gram-negative bacteria (39%) are usually transient but

may sometimes be pathogenic. Health spa whirlpools appear to encourage the growth of these organisms [10].

Candida albicans is a normal inhabitant of the site. Its pathogenicity is discussed below.

Colonization in infancy [8]. Though the subject of much study, the method, extent and pattern of neonatal colonization is not accurately defined and may initially be fortuitous. The significance of the flora in relation to infection in this area is dealt with in Chapter 7.

The effect of diabetes. In well-controlled subjects the flora does not differ materially from that of the normal, but infections, especially candidiasis and erythrasma, are more common, perhaps because of the high skin sugar in diabetic subjects [8].

Vaginal flora. Lactobacilli are probably the more common organisms, particularly on the labial mucosa [8]. However, vaginal swabs from pre-operative women were sterile in about half the cases [7]. A mixed flora, including coliforms, streptococci and *Bacteroides* species, were found in the remainder, more frequently in the first half of the cycle. The frequency of isolation of *Candida albicans* varies with different groups and is probably a matter of selection. It is more frequent in pregnancy. Its significance is also a matter of controversy. In the pregnant woman it may well denote infection [5] but in the non-pregnant woman the significance is still a matter of opinion [6, 9].

REFERENCES

1–3 As cited on p. 2201.
4 ALY R., *et al* (1979) *Br J Dermatol* **101**, 445.
5 CARROLL C.J., *et al* (1973) *J Obstet Gynaecol Br Commonw* **80**, 258.
6 HURLEY R., *et al* (1974) *Symp Society of Applied Bacteriology, No 3* Eds. Skinner, S.A. & Carr J.G. London, Academic Press.
7 NEARY M.P., *et al* (1973) *Lancet* **ii**, 1291.
8 *NOBLE W.C. & SOMERVILLE D.A. (1974) *Microbiology of Human Skin. Vol. 2. Major Problems in Dermatology.* Ed. Rook A.J. London, Saunders.
9 ORIEL J.D., *et al* (1972) *Br Med J* **iv**, 761.
10 SAUSKER W.F., *et al* (1978) *JAMA* **239**, 2362.

Malacoplakia of the vulva [4]. An unusual granulomatous response to infection—usually *Escherchia coli* but sometimes *Pseudomonas* [3] or *Staphylococcus aureus* [5]—has been reported in the vagina, on the vulva [1] and on the perianal skin [3]. More commonly it involves the urinary or gastro-intestinal tract mucosa. The 'soft' plaques may present as an indurated ulcer. Diagnosis is made by searching for and finding Michaelis–Guttmann bodies in the close-packed histiocytes of the infiltrate.

REFERENCES

1 ARUL K.J. & EMMERSON R.W. (1977) *Clin Exp Dermatol* **2**, 131.
2 KHAN A.R. (1979) *J Ind Med Assoc* **72**, 254.
3 LECLERC J.L. & BERNER L. (1972) *Union Med Can* **101**, 471.
4 LEWIN K.J., *et al* (1976) *J Clin Pathol* **29**, 354.
5 PRICE H.M., *et al* (1973) *Hum Pathol* **4**, 381.

VENEREAL AND 'PARAVENEREAL' CONDITIONS

Venereal conditions. For convenience the main forms of venereal disease as a cause of vulvovaginitis will be considered together. The reader is referred to the fuller descriptions of the individual disease given elsewhere.

Syphilis and gonorrhoea must always be thought of in women presenting with vulvovaginitis, particularly as the presentation is not as obvious as in the male.

Gonorrhoea [p. 753]. The incidence is increasing, particularly among younger females. Under poor hygienic conditions, infants may become infected via towels etc. or during birth. In the female the signs of infection may be few or absent. Gonococcal vulvitis is rare but may occur with a mixed discharge. Inflammation involves the urethra and the para-urethral and Bartholin glands, and the rectum and cervix may be involved. The rare soft gonorrhoeal ulcer can occur without urethritis [11]. Several workers [5, 14] stressed the need to take cervical, urethral and rectal swabs if the disease is not to be missed. Repeated cultures may be necessary.

Syphilis (p. 845). The typical primary chancre is now seldom seen in women. The posterior commissure or urethral opening are usually affected, but it may occur anywhere from the cervix to the labia majora. Extensive oedema or induration may simulate cellulitis. The lesion must be distinguished from other causes of ulceration (p. 847).

Condylomata lata are seen in the vulval and anal areas in the secondary stage. The lesions of endemic syphilis resemble condylomata [17], and are also a feature of congenital syphilis. Primary vulval involvement in yaws is rare, but ulcers and crusted nodules may occur on the vulva in the secondary state (p. 871).

Chancroid (p. 764). This is still a relatively rare disease in Britain but is much more common in tropical regions. An initial ulcerating papule is followed by similar lesions in adjacent and opposing sites. The regional glands enlarge and may suppurate. Pain, when present, distinguishes the primary lesion from a chancre. Other venereal diseases may coexist and confuse the clinical picture [8].

Granuloma inguinale (granuloma venereum) (p. 775). This disease of tropical countries is a rare disease of immigrants. The lesions occur in any part of the genitocrural area, vagina or cervix. The bleb or nodule breaks down to form an ulcer with a rolled edge and crazy-paving appearance [2]. Secondary infection is common and may lead to constitutional upset [16]. Dissemination can occur. A post-infective thickening of the involved area is not entirely explained by lymphoedema [7]. The diagnosis is made by finding Donovan bodies in smears from biopsy material or the biopsy specimen.

Mycobacterial infections [10] (Chapter 22). Tuberculosis of the genital tract is rare. The figure of 3–10% of microscopic tuberculosis of the cervix in patients with pelvic infections [1] seems high for the U.K. The primary tuberculous chancre is now extremely rare, with most lesions deriving from foci elsewhere. Exogenous infection may be conveyed by sputum or sexual intercourse. The vulva was involved in three of 26 cases of genital tuberculosis in South Africa [12]. Unilateral Bartholin gland infection has been reported [13]. Haematogenous spread may involve the vulva. Infection of the endometrium and genital tract may cause a tuberculous vulvovaginitis.

Nodules, ulcers with ragged edges or fungating masses are seen in this infection. Suppuration and scarring of the regional lymph glands may occur, followed by lymphoedema of the limb [4]. Smears, histology and culture confirm the diagnosis.

Other foci of a primary source of the tuberculous infection must always be sought, and a full course of antituberculous therapy should be given when there is any doubt of the cause.

Leprosy. Vulval lesions are not common [6, 9]. The pubic hair may be lost [10].

Condylomata acuminata. These affect the mucocutaneous surfaces and form extensive, vegetating masses that may occlude the vaginal orifice and perianal area, especially in pregnancy or in the presence of a vaginal discharge or coincident venereal infection, which should be treated first. Electrocoagulation may be needed if the infection is voluminous and intravaginal. Secondary syphilis, especially in pregnancy, may cause extensive mucous patches, condylomatous masses and erythematopapular or psoriasiform lesions, which must be distinguished.

Lymphogranuloma venereum [3] (p. 7101). This is rare in women. It is due to a chlamydia of a specific serotype. The initial ulcer, papule or herpetiform lesion occurs in the region of the labia clitoris fourchette or in the vagina when pelvic lymphadenopathy is accompanied by a moderate or severe degree of constitutional upset. The subsequent picture of ulceration, scarring, stricture elephantiasis and eventually esthiomène (p. 2219) completes the sequence of events. The Frei test is positive.

Chlamydia of different serotypes have now been recognized as the frequent cause of cervicitis and Bartholinitis in women, both post- and non-gonococcal urethritis in men and conjunctivitis in neonates [15].

REFERENCES

1-3 As cited on p. 2201.

4 ASHWORTH F.L. (1974) *Br Med J* **iv**, 167

5 BHATTACHARYYA M.N. & JEPHCOTT A.E. (1974) *Br J Vener Dis* **50**, 109.

6 BONAR B.E. & RABSON A.S. (1957) *Obstet Gynecol* **9**, 33.

7 DOUGLAS C.P. (1962) *J Obstet Gynaecol Br Commonw* **69**, 871.

8 Editorial (1982) *Lancet* **ii**, 747.

9 GRABSTOLD D.H. & SWAN L. (1952) *JAMA* **149**, 1287.

10 KLOSTERMANN G.F. (1972) In *Handbuch der Speziellen Pathologischen Anatomis und Histologie Weibliche Geschelentsorgave*. Berlin, Spruyer.

11 LANDERGREN G. (1973) *Acta Derm Venereol (Stockh)* **43**, 496.

12 MOORE D. (1954) *S Af Med J* **28**, 666.

13 SCHAEFER G. (1959) *Clin Obstet Gynecol* **2**, 530.

14 SCHROETER A.L. & REYNOLDS G. (1972) *J Infect Dis* **125**, 499.

15 TAYLOR-ROBINSON D. & THOMAS B.J. (1980) *J Clin Pathol* **33**, 205.

16 WILCOCKS C. & MANSON-BAHR P. (1972) *Manson's Tropical Diseases*. 17th ed. London, Balliere, Tindall, Section 7, p. 645.

17 WILCOX R.R. (1964) *Textbook of Venereal Diseases and Treponematoses*. 2nd ed. London, Heinemann, ch. 15.

VULVOVAGINITIS

Inflammation of the female external genitalia may result from infective and irritant causes. It is not always possible to separate these. A vaginal discharge can on occasion give rise to vulval irritation,

and treatment for this may cause a contact dermatitis. Secondary infection of any vulval rash is common owing to the proximity of faeces and urine and the irresistible desire to scratch. The moisture and warmth engendered by inflammation is conducive to further soreness, irritant dermatitis and scratching. Lichenification is frequent and may obscure the original cause of the irritation.

Vaginal discharge. This is a common complaint and is normally unassociated with other symptoms. Five conditions comprise 95% of all vaginal discharges or infections.

Mucorrhoea and epithelial discharge. Between 5% and 10% of women complaining of vaginal discharge do not have infection. They have an excess physiological secretion of mucous and vaginal epithelial debris. The discharge is not irritative, but is odourless and of a thick grey-white pasty consistency. Vaginal pH is normal.

'Non-specific vaginitis' [13]. This is the commonest form of vaginitis. The patient complains of excessive grey thin discharge associated with a 'fishy' malodour which is especially strong immediately after intercourse. Vulval irritation is slight or absent in this group, and symptoms are so few that many women regard their condition as part of the spectrum of normality.

Controversy has surrounded the aetiology but it is now generally agreed that the disorder is almost invariably associated with infection by the small aerobic Gram-negative rod known as *Gardnerella vaginalis*, after its discoverer [8]. It would appear that this organism alone is incapable of causing infection, and non-specific vaginitis is now regarded as a complex interrelationship between *Gardnerella* and anaerobic species of bacteria [12].

Characteristically the vaginal pH is greater than 5 and the fishy odour of the discharge can be accentuated by the addition of an alkali such as 10% KOH (the Whiff test). Treatment with metronidazole (200 mg t.i.d. for 7 days) is effective if the consort is also treated at the same time.

Cervicitis. Nearly one-third of women complaining of vaginal discharge do not suffer from vaginal infection. They suffer from a mucopurulent, occasionally blood-stained, discharge from infected endocervical mucosa.

The four pathogens most commonly involved are *Neisseria gonorrhoeae*, *Chlamydia trachomatis*, *Trichomonas vaginalis* and *Herpes simplex*.

The discharge from chronic cervicitis is not normally irritating to the vulval skin. Patients complaints tend to relate either to the discharge itself or to deep pelvic pain and dyspareunia.

Trichomoniasis [1–3, 6, 7]. Infection with *T. vaginalis* is a frequent cause of vaginitis and vultitis. It is a common inhabitant of the female genital tract, and the problems of pathogenicity are similar to those of *Candida* and depend on a favourable environment for its growth. Infections are rare in children and after the menopause. They are more common in the poorer social groups.

Trichomonal vaginitis causes a frothy malodorous greyish-green watery discharge and a bright-red or petechiae-studded vaginal mucosa. Though the itching is generally less severe than with candida infection, secondary vulvitis occurs from irritation by the discharge [7] which may extend out to the genitocrural area. Erythema and swelling of the vestibule and labia minora are often present.

The diagnosis is made by examination of a fresh *warm* specimen examined on a *warm* slide or by culture of the discharge. The distress and anxiety caused by this mild but persistent condition has often led to an erroneous diagnosis of 'neurodermatitis' and the dermatologist should be careful to exclude this infection before making this diagnosis. Coexistent candida infection should also be excluded.

As the male may harbour the infection and occasionally show signs of it, both partners should receive treatment. Metronidazole (200 mg t.d.s. for 7 days) is usually successful, but other regimes have their advocates. Relapse is due either to re-infection or to failure to take the tablets. Nimorazole may be more effective if there is a coexistent urinary infection [5].

Candidal vulvovaginitis [1–3, 7]. *Candida albicans* may be present in the vagina of 25% of asymptomatic women as commensal. Changes in host factors are probably responsible for transition to pathogenicity and are generally not directly associated with sexual contact. Factors related to cell-mediated immunity are doubtless important but as yet are ill understood. Pregnancy, diabetes, possibly oral antibiotics, the contraceptive pill, immunosuppressive drugs and local tissue damage, e.g. as a secondary invader in incontinence rashes and intertrigo, may all favour precipitation of infection. In general, if microscopy reveals the yeast-like (bunch of grapes) form of organisms, then the commensal state is most likely whilst the pseudohyphal (mycelial) form is most often associated with pathogenicity.

Candida infection accounted for one-third of 478

consecutive cases of discharge and pruritus [9]. The vaginitis may be difficult to diagnose clinically unless the skin is involved. The discharge may be slight, the vagina is reddened and the white curd-like plaques of thrush may be present. The degree of pruritus varies but may be considerable. Candida may, rarely, be the cause of urethral syndrome and cystitis.

The erythema may extend only to the inner aspects of the labia and vestibule, but when it spreads to the genitocrural region it classically presents as well-demarcated sheets with a lightly scaling or vesicopustular edge beyond which are grouped or isolated superficial pustulettes which rupture rapidly, leaving a slight scaly periphery. In such cases microscopy affords an immediate diagnosis. However, all specimens should be cultured, especially those from the vagina.

In the obese middle-aged patient late-onset diabetes should be considered and appropriate tests carried out (Fig. 59.21).

Candidiasis may coexist with other infections, notably gonorrhoea and trichomonal infection (see

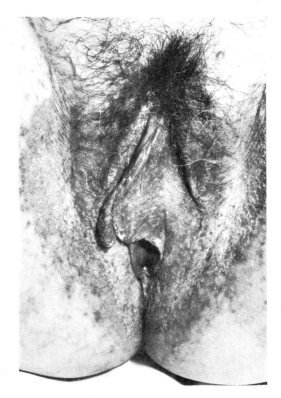

FIG. 59.21. Candidal vulvovaginitis in an undetected 'latent' diabetic woman aged 47 (Stoke Mandeville Hospital).

above). Alternatively, it may supervene as a secondary invasion on other genital dermatoses, especially if predisposing factors are present.

Torulopsis glabrata is very occasionally the cause of a vaginal mycotic infection.

Treatment. The newer imidazole group of drugs (clotrimazole, miconazole and econazole) are now regarded as more reliable than the polyene antibiotics nystatin and amphotericin [10]. Skin and vaginal therapy must be combined; treatment of the consort is almost mandatory since 10% were involved in one series [11]. In refractory cases oral ketoconazole (200 mg b.i.d. for 5 days) is helpful in clearing rectal carriage [4], especially when combined with local therapy.

Other causes of vaginal discharge are less common and are listed in Table 59.1.

TABLE 59.1. Non-infective causes of vaginal discharge

Atrophic vaginitis	Excessive douching
Vaginal ulceration	Contraceptive irritation
Vaginal fistulae	Retained foreign body
Tumours	

REFERENCES

1–3 As cited on p. 2201.
4 BALSDON M.J., et al (1982) *Curr Ther Res* **31**, 511.
5 BURSLEM R.W. (1973) *Prescribers J* **13**, 14.
6 CATTERALL R.D. (1972) *Med Clin North Am* **56**, 1203.
7 FLEURY F.J. (1981) *Clin Obstet Gynecol* **24**, 407.
8 GARDNER H.L. (1980) *Am J Obstet Gynecol* **137**, 385.
9 GRAY L.A. & BARNES M.L. (1975) *Am J Obstet Gynecol* **92**, 125.
10 ODDS F.C. (1977) *Proc R Soc Med* **70** (Suppl. 4), 24.
11 ORIEL J.D., et al (1972) *Br Med J* **iv**, 761.
12 SPEIGEL C.A., et al (1980) *N Engl J Med* **303**, 601.
13 VONTVER L.A. & ESCHENBACH D.A. (1981) *Clin Obstet Gynecol* **24**, 439.

Seminal vulvitis. This is a rare condition characterized by vulva oedema, erythema and pruritus following shortly after intercourse [4]. The pruritus is usually confined to the vulva area but disseminated urticaria may supervene [9]. Most of the patients are atopic and have developed reaginic antibodies to all human seminal plasma [9]. Other antigens may be transmitted through seminal plasma, and a case is recorded of anaphylaxis in a walnut-sensitive lady following intercourse after her husband had consumed walnuts [7].

Salivary vulvitis [5]. A relatively common cause of vulval itching is the increasingly common practice of oro-genital contact. This may present as vulvitis

in the absence of vaginitis. The clinical appearance is non-specific with generalized erythema of the labia, the introitus and the clitoral and periclitoral tissues.

At other times a vaginal discharge is associated with the vulvitis, and unusual pathogens such as *Haemophilus* may be isolated in culture.

In the first group the likely causation is irritation by digestive enzymes in salivary fluid, whilst the infective group involves the transmission of oral pathogens which can often also be recovered from the mouth of the consort.

Miscellaneous causes of vulvovaginitis [1–3]. Infestation with *Enterobius vermicularis* (threadworm) may cause irritation and a secondary vulvovaginitis, especially in children. Occasionally the worm is found in the vagina itself [8]. Scabies may involve the female genitalia and like pediculosis can lead to secondary infection from scratching. Vulval ulceration may occur in infants with amoebic dysentery [3] and filariasis may cause vulval oedema. Schistosomiasis is considered below. Chronic plasma cell vulvitis [6], or a condition closely resembling plasma cell balanitis, has been described. Oedematous red irregular plaques resemble Bowen's disease or erythroplasia but are distinguished by biopsy.

REFERENCES

1–3 As cited on p. 2201.
4 CHANG T. (1976) *Am J Obstet Gynecol* **126**, 442.
5 DAVIES B.A. (1971) *Obstet Gynecol* **37**, 238.
6 GARNIER G. (1957) *Br J Dermatol* **69**, 77.
7 HADDAD Z.H. (1978) *Perspect Allergy* **1**, 2.
8 KACKER T.P. (1973) *Br J Vener Dis* **49**, 314.
9 MATHIAS C.G.T., et al (1980) *Arch Dermatol* **116**, 209.

Vulvovaginitis in children [1]. The vaginal mucosa of the child is an excellent bacterial culture medium. It lacks protective factors such as oestrogen stimulation, glycogen and Doderlein lactobacilli and has a neutral pH. The tissues are thin and easily damaged, the vagina is close to the anus and above all perineal hygiene is frequently poor. The majority of cases in which a specific cause of infection will not be discovered respond well purely to measures designed to improve personal cleanliness [2]. Non-specific irritants such as bubble bath solutions may occasionally be responsible, as may pinworm infestation and foreign bodies. Candida does not infect the vagina of the prepubertal child, although it may induce vulvitis. Gonorrhoea will infect the prepubertal vagina and is becoming a more common cause of vulvovaginitis, especially in more underprivileged parts of North America. Sexual abuse with or without specific vaginal infection accounted for 11% of 54 children with genital problems seen in a recent survey [2].

REFERENCES

1 ALTCHEK A. (1981) *Pediatr Clin North Am* **28**, 397.
2 PARADISE J.E., *et al* (1982) *Pediatrics* **70**, 193.

Corynebacteria [11]. Infection with *C. diphtheriae* occurs rarely as a primary genital infection of children [1]; cases in adults have been reported in past decades. Where diphtheria is still endemic, they may be more common. The typical greyish pseudo-membrane is characteristic. Vaginal adhesions may be prevented by local applications to separate the surfaces [3].

Erythrasma (p. 759). Erythrasma, which is caused by *C. minutissimum*, and is rarely seen in the U.K. before puberty, may be extensive in tropical areas and in the Negro, especially if diabetic. It was also found in the groin of 18% of mentally subnormal patients [14]. Milder forms are often overlooked or unnoticed by the patient. It is confirmed by its coral-red fluorescence under Wood's light. It responds to oral erythromycin and to topical sodium fusidate, Whitfield's ointment, clotrimazole [6] or miconazole. However, recurrences are common. The vigorous use of an antibacterial soap is suggested [3].

Trichomycosis (p. 761). This is caused by various bacteria and may be confused with pediculosis. Careful examination, Wood's light fluorescence and microscopy should enable embarrassing mistakes to be avoided.

Staphylococcal and streptococcal infections. Primary infection with coagulase-positive staphylococci causes impetigo, folliculitis or boils. More chronic forms of pyoderma (lupoid sycosis) are occasionally seen and are exceedingly difficult to treat; combined long-term corticosteroid–antibiotic therapy has been fairly successful in personal cases. Secondary infection occurs in any itchy skin disorder, notably scabies pediculosis and atopic dermatitis.

An exotoxin associated with phage Group 1 staphylococci has been implicated in the production of profound collapse, fever and morbilliform rash seen in a condition known as toxic shock syndrome [17] (p. 738). Whilst the syndrome appears most commonly in menstruating women who use tampons, the association is not exclusive and the exotoxin has not as yet been confirmed [8].

Bartholinitis. Abscesses of Bartholin's gland [10] may be due to pyococcal organisms or to the gonococcus, especially if bilateral [2]. Recent work [7] has shown that *Chlamydia trachomatis* can be involved in the infection, either alone or in association with gonococcus. In another study [10] only 21 of 109 cases were due to the staphylococcus while 50 were due to *E. coli* and 46 to *Strep. faecalis*. The abscess is due to distal blocking of the duct. The patient presents with fever, malaise and a tender swelling arising posterior to the origin of the labium minus. Attacks often follow intercourse and recurrent mild attacks may occur until fibrosis supervenes.

Acute streptococcal infections are rare but erysipelas or cellulitis may follow surgical procedures [12] or destructive and scarring diseases. Persistent lymphoedema usually follows repeated attacks, probably because of progressive damage to an already defective lymphatic system.

Synergistic bacterial gangrene. This severe and rapidly extending disease is due to the synergistic effect of a micro-aerophilic streptococcus and *Staph aureus*. It may follow a pre-existing infection or small injury or without any obvious preceding event. The patient rapidly develops constitutional signs of toxaemia and is severely ill. A bullous or necrotic central zone is surrounded by oedema and erythema. Extension is often rapid.

Necrotizing fasciitis is probably a variant in which the superficial fascia is also destroyed [13]. Most patients are diabetic and the mortality rate is high despite antibiotics and surgery (p. 752). Wide excision, appropriate antibiotics and perhaps hyperbaric oxygen offer the only hope of survival.

Gram-negative and anaerobic organisms. The role of the Gram-negative enterococci in infections of the vulva and vagina remains doubtful [4, 5]. It is unlikely that they are normally pathogenic though they may play a part in the urethral syndrome of dysuria without significant bacteriuria. Anaerobic organisms are often found in the normal vagina. The most common isolates include pepto streptococci, peptococci and *Bacteroides* species.

Women with vaginitis have been reported to have high concentrations of anaerobic organisms [9]. Recent work [15] has shown that in women with *Gardnerella* associated non-specific vaginitis peptococci and *Bacteroides* species were isolated more frequently and in higher concentrations than in normal controls. Perhaps the time has come to cease the use of the term non-specific vaginitis.

Fusobacteria in combination with *Borrelia vincen-*

tii have been associated with erosive vulvitis in the older literature, but this is now rare. The organism can be found in very ill patients with necrotic vaginal tissue or retained secretions [1].

Pseudomonas aeroginosa is not a cause of vulvo-vaginitis [1] but has caused blue staining of napkins in infants [16].

REFERENCES

1–3 As cited on p. 2201.
4 BAILEY R.R., *et al* (1973) *Lancet* ii, 275.
5 CATTELL W.R., *et al* (1974) *Br Med J* iv, 136.
6 CLAYTON Y.M. & CONNOR B.L. (1973) *Br J Dermatol* 89, 297.
7 DAVIES J.A., *et al* (1978) *Br J Vener Dis* 54, 409.
8 DAVIS J.P., *et al* (1980) *N Engl J Med* 303, 1429.
9 LEVISON M.E., *et al* (1979) *Am J Obstet Gynecol* 133, 139.
10 MAYER H.G.K. (1972) *J Gynecol Obstet Biol Reprod (Paris)* 1, 71.
11 NOBLE W.C. & SOMERVILLE D.A. (1974) *Microbiology of Human Skin*. London, Saunders.
12 NORBURN L.M. & COLE R.B. (1960) *J Obstet Gynaecol Br Commonw* 67, 279.
13 REA W.J. & WYRICK W.J. (1970) *Ann Surg* 172, 957.
14 SOMERVILLE D.A., *et al* (1970) *Br J Dermatol* 82, 355.
15 SPIEGEL C.A., *et al* (1980) *N Eng J Med* 303, 601.
16 THEARLE M.J., *et al* (1973) *Lancet* ii, 499.
17 TODD J., *et al* (1980) *Lancet* ii, 1116.

Fungi. Dermatophyte infections of the genital area are uncommon in women. When they are present, other sites are also infected. It may be diagnosed easily. Erythrasma is distinguished by its brown colour and lack of a scaling edge.

Rare but well-documented cases of deep mycoses involving the genital area are recorded by Ridley [3].

In extensive cases pityriasis versicolor can involve the genital region. In the Negro infant the napkin area may be specifically involved, with marked hypopigmentation.

Viruses [1–3]. Three groups of viruses are important causes of infection in the genital area—the pox and papova viruses and the herpes virus. Other viruses seldom give rise to distinctive pictures, though the vulva may be involved in hand, foot and mouth disease.

The pox viruses. Accidental infection of the vulva following smallpox vaccination, once common, is now rarely encountered.

Molluscum contagiosum is becoming very common. Vulval lesions are often seen in childhood and are innocently acquired. In the adult transmission during sexual intercourse tends to produce pubic lesions more often than infection of the external genitalia. Solitary inflamed lesions are often mistaken for boils and the eczematous reaction which may surround lesions can be deceptive. The condition is more fully described on p. 697.

The papova virus. Human papilloma viruses (HPV) have still not been propagated in tissue culture. This makes investigation difficult, but DNA hybridization techniques and restriction enzyme analysis have made it clear that multiple strains of HPV exist [11]. Analysis of viral DNA extracted from anogenital warts has to contain genome sequences related to HPV1 and HPV2. In addition another distinct species of DNA has been found in some anogenital warts and designated HPV6 [18].

The incubation period is between 2 and 3 months [36]. It is now generally accepted that nearly all cases are sexually transmitted. Heterosexual transmission seems clearer than the situation pertaining among male homosexuals where anal warts are many times commoner than penile warts. No satisfactory explanation of this observation is available [37]. The incidence of genital warts has been increasing for several years.

The soft frond-like papilliferous lesions require no description. When numerous they become confluent with a velvety surface. In severe cases they may cover the inner surfaces of the labia and extend far into the vagina. Even the bladder and ureter can be involved. Extension to the perineum and perianal area is common and they may then spread to the rectum. The genitocrural fold is often involved but the thighs are not. In pregnancy, and if an associated vaginal infection is present, condylomata become more profuse.

The only important differential diagnoses are those of syphilitic condylomata, which are flat, broad topped and sparse, and carcinoma, which is harder and usually more localized. However, the so-called 'malignant condyloma' and the Buschke–Lowenstein giant condyloma must always be suspected in cases that do not rapidly respond to appropriate treatment. Close supervision and repeated biopsies may be necessary.

All patients should be investigated for other diseases and any concomitant discharge treated appropriately [29].

Condylomata accuminata on the cervix [33] can also be proliferative and show cytological changes of dyskeratosis and koilocytosis [31]. Similar cytological changes can be found from lesions which are flat and white when viewed on colposcopy. These are now known as flat condylomata, or more correctly as non-condylomatous cervical wart virus infection [30]. It has been concluded that this group of virus-induced lesions can give rise to suspicious smears.

The biological importance of this finding has yet to be evaluated. It seems likely that this virus infection is oncogenic. Recent work [39] has found histological evidence of HPV infection in 91% of 80 women with invasive or pre-invasive cervical neoplasia as compared with only 12·5% of controls. It has long been recognized that early sexual activity, promiscuity and low socio-economic status are major risk determinants in cervical cancer [17, 40, 44, 45]. It has also been shown that there is a threefold increase in cancer of the penis in the husbands of cervical cancer patients [42]. It may well be that HPV infection is the transmissable agent responsible, or tumour promoter, and that HVH II acts as the initiator in cervical neoplasia [22].

Treatment is still based on podophyllin [29]. This is applied in strengths from 10% to 25%, and the patients are instructed to wash it off 8–24 h later. This will need to be repeated at regular intervals and cannot easily be carried out by the patient herself (though a few are very adept with mirrors). Podophyllin should not, however, be used in pregnancy [10] or applied to cervical lesions because of its potential carcinogenicity [21]. Diathermy, electrocautery or liquid nitrogen, using a cryoprobe, are also helpful in difficult cases.

Condylomata may regress after delivery [36] but their management in pregnancy poses a problem—particularly if they are florid near the date of delivery. Diathermy destruction of sections of such florid lesions under general anaesthesia may be attempted.

Prepubertal genital warts. There seems little doubt that this condition is becoming more common [20]. Some workers [43] emphasize an increase in the incidence of sexual abuse of children as a prime cause and this has certainly been in accord with the author's experience.

A more balanced view [46] is that genital warts in childhood can be transmitted either directly at birth, or through close contact of either a sexual or non-sexual nature. However, even in this series two out of four cases showed evidence of sexual molestation.

Transmission of warts to newborns via an infected birth canal can give rise to laryngeal papillomatosis which is very difficult to treat [12] and this has led to suggestions that all affected mothers should be subjected to Caesarian section [19].

The Herpes virus [3, 7, 26, 27]. Both herpes simplex and zoster–varicella affect the vulva. Cytomegalovirus does not. The herpes virus hominis (HVH) type II is mainly concerned in genital infections. The question of antigenic differences [26] is dealt with elsewhere (p. 685). HVH II infection is usually acquired in early adult life. The virus may then lie dormant or give rise to recurrent infections. As HVH I infections are also common, The patient may carry two types of antibody. Neither protects against the other.

Genital herpes [31] due to HVH II is now the commonest cause of genital ulceration [7] and was until recently the most important sexually transmitted disease [16]. Its prevalence is higher than any other of this group of diseases and in 1978 it was estimated to infect nearly 30 per 100,000 population in the U.K. [4].

Many primary and recurrent infections are asymptomatic [38] and recurrences occur in perhaps only one-third of those infected [26].

The primary infection is usually more severe or widespread than subsequent infections. A zosteriform or segmental distribution is not unusual and invites confusion with zoster. The incubation period varies from 2 to 7 days. The grouped vesicles on an inflamed base erode rapidly; deeper ulceration may occur [38]. The vagina, urethra and anal canal may also be involved. Dysuria and retention of urine may occur. The regional glands are enlarged and tender. Cervicitis is common if looked for [23]. Although systemic effects usually subside in a week, ulceration may persist for 2–6 weeks [6].

Recurrences may occur without coitus and be precipitated by trauma, fever, local infection, menstruation or stress. Each individual may have her own pattern, e.g. premenstrual attacks. Prodromal itching and tingling are soon recognized as heralding an attack. These attacks tend to be relatively mild, lasting only 7–10 days, and usually become less frequent with time [16]. It is important to appreciate that this disease is infective even when the patient is asymptomatic and that viral shedding has been found in asymptomatic women up to 6 months after a clinical attack of genital herpes [5].

Familial benign chronic pemphigus has been precipitated by HVH infections. Neurological signs and symptoms have been reported rarely in both primary and recurrent attacks [32]. The diagnosis is usually obvious, though primary attacks may closely resemble zoster or vaccinia. The latter is excluded if giant cells are found in smears but differentiation from zoster requires viral culture. Primary or secondary syphilis may coexist. Aphthosis, Behçet's syndrome and secondarily infected chancroid may pose difficulties in some cases.

The newborn [35] must be protected from contact with active HVH in the mother at the time of delivery, usually by Caesarian section. The whole subject of HVH in pregnancy is well reviewed by Ridley [3].

Treatment. Idoxuridine 40% in dimethyl sulphoxide [25, 26] has been widely used. It is not commercially available in this strength and is probably not as effective as in Type I infections.

Intravenous Acyclovir in a dose of 5 mg/kg every 8 h by slow infusion has been shown to be a safe and effective treatment for the primary attack [34] but does not prevent recurrences.

A 5% Acyclovir ointment has been shown to speed healing and to reduce the duration of viral shedding in both primary and recurrent disease [13]. Oral Acyclovir is now available and doses of 200 mg taken five times daily for 5 days are recommended by the manufacturers for both primary infection and recurrences.

No definite guidelines have yet been issued on the clinical criteria for use of this valuable drug. Resistant mutant strains have now developed [8] and it is advisable to restrict its use at present to life-saving situations.

As an alternative bland applications, wet dressings or 1% aqueous gentian violet are of help. Topical steroids should not be used.

Herpes virus and vulval carcinoma [44]. There is now increasing evidence indicating a close relationship between HVH II and cervical neoplasia in women [14]. Carcinoma *in situ* of the vulval skin, which may be related to Bowenoid papulosis (p. 2226), appears to be increasing in frequency and appearing in a younger age group. The malignant potential of this type of lesion has yet to be established [41]. However, HVH II-induced antigens have now been identified in vulval carcinoma *insitu* [28] and more recently even in one frankly malignant vulval carcinoma [9]. The situation is not yet clear but a connection between virus and malignant change seems likely.

Varicella–Zoster. Varicella only affects the vulva in a random fashion. It may occur in infants by transplacental infection. Zoster may mimic acute primary herpes but is strictly unilateral and segmental and is often preceded by pain. Scattered viraemic vesicles may present elsewhere, especially in immunodeficient patients (p. 683).

Motor involvement leading to bladder and faecal dysfunction is well recognized [15]. When the lesions are sparse, the diagnosis may be difficult. However, a second attack of zoster is ususual [24].

5% Idoxuridine in dimethyl sulphoxide applied very frequently for the first 3–4 days may hasten resolution but must be begun early. Acyclovir is the only reliably effective treatment currently available.

REFERENCES

1–3 As cited on p. 2201.
4 Academic Department (Genito-Urinary Medicine, Middlesex Hospital), Communicable Surveillance Centre (1979) *Br Med J* ii, 1375.
5 ADAM E., *et al* (1979) *Obstet Gynecol* **54**, 171.
6 ALCHECK A. (1981) *Pediatr Clin North Am* **28**, (2), 397.
7 ANSTEY M.S. (1973) *Am J Obstet Gynecol* **117**, 711.
8 BURNS W.H., *et al* (1982) *Lancet* i, 421.
9 CABRAL G.A., *et al* (1982) *Am J Obstet Gynecol* **143**, 611.
10 CHAMBERLAIN M.J., *et al* (1972) *Br Med J* iii, 391.
11 COGGIN J. & ZUR HANSEN H. (1979) *Cancer Res* **39**, 545.
12 COOK T.A., *et al* (1973) *Ann Otol Rhinol Laryngol* **82**, 649.
13 COREY L., *et al* (1982) *Am J Med (Acyclovir Symp.)* **73**, (IA), 326.
14 DREESMAN G.R., *et al* (1980) *Nature* **283**, 591.
15 FUGELSO P.D. (1973) *Br J Dermatol* **89**, 285.
16 GARDNER H.L. (1979) *Am J Obstet Gynecol* **135**, 553.
17 GARDNER J.W. & LYON J.L. (1977) *Gynecol Oncol* **5**, 68.
18 GISSMAN L. & ZUR HAUSEN H. (1979) *Cancer* **25**, 605.
19 GOLDMAN L. (1977) *Arch Dermatol* **113**, 1295.
20 GOLDMAN L., *et al* (1976) *Arch Dermatol* **112**, 1329.
21 GUESON E.J., *et al* (1971) *J Reprod Med* **6**, 159.
22 ZUR HAUSEN H. (1982) *Lancet* ii, 1370.
23 HUTFIELD D.C. (1968) *Br J Vener Dis* **44**, 241.
24 JUEL-JENSEN B.E. (1973) *Br Med J* i, 406.
25 JUEL-JENSEN B.E. (1973) *Br J Hosp Med* **10**, 402.
26 JUEL-JENSEN B.E. & McCALLUM F.O. (1972) *Herpes Simplex, Varicella and Zoster.* London, Heinemann.
27 KAPLAN A.S. (1973) *The Herpes Viruses.* New York, Academic Press.
28 KAUFMANN R.H., *et al* (1981) *N Engl J Med* **305**, 483.
29 KINGHORN G.R. (1978) *Br J Dermatol* **98**, 405.
30 LAVERTY C.R., *et al* (1978) *Pathology* **10**, 373.
31 Leading Article (1980) *Br Med J* i, 1335.
32 Leading Article (1973) *Lancet* ii, 1426.
33 MEISEL S.A., *et al* (1977) *Acta Cytol (Baltimore)* **21**, 379.
34 MINDEL A., *et al* (1982) *Lancet* i, 697.
35 NAHMIAS A.J., *et al* (1970) *Adv Paediatr* **17**, 185.
36 ORIEL J.D. (1971) *Br J Vener Dis* **47**, 1.
37 ORIEL J.D. (1981) *Sex Transm Dis* **8** (Suppl. 4), 326.
38 POSTE G., *et al* (1972) *Obstet Gynecol* **40**, 871.
39 REID R., *et al* (1982) *Cancer* **50**, 377.
40 ROTKIN I.D. (1973) *Cancer Res* **33**, 1353.
41 SCHWARTZ P.E. & NAFTOLIN F. (1981) *N Engl J Med* **305**, 517.
42 SMITH P.G., *et al* (1980) *Lancet* ii, 417.
43 STORRS F. (1977) *Arch Dermatol* **113**, 1294.

44 Symp American Cancer Association (1973) *Cancer Res* **33**, 1345.

45 THOMAS D.B. (1973) *Am J Epidemiol* **98**, 10.

46 DE YONG A.R., *et al* (1982) *Am J Dis Child* **136**, 704.

Chlamydiae and Mycoplasmas [4]. *Chlamydiae* are Gram-negative organisms with many of the features of bacteria but differ in that they are obligatory intracellular parasites [7].

Different serotypes (D–K) of *Chlamydiae* have been found causing cervicitis in the consorts of men with non-specific and post-gonococcal urethritis. The most characteristic picture is a lymphocytic follicular cervicitis [5] most commonly found in the mothers of babies with chlamydial ophthalmia neonatorum [4]. *Chlamydiae* do not cause vaginitis but may cause salpingitis and lead to infertility [7].

Specific serotypes of *C. trachomatitis* are responsible for the disease lymphogranuloma venereum.

Lymphogranuloma venereum (p. 710). Though usually found in tropical areas a number of cases nevertheless occur in the U.K., particularly in men [8]. Transmission is by sexual intercourse or via an alimentary reservoir. The incubation period varies from a few days to a few weeks. The initial papulovesicle, which may quickly ulcerate, occurs at the fourchette or vagina. It is often unnoticed. Lymphadenopathy, often with constitutional upset, follows this in a week or more. This may be unilateral and involve the pelvic and perirectal rather than the inguinal glands. These may become fluctuant and discharge, producing ulceration, fistulae and scarring (esthiomene). Strictures and elephantiasis complete the sequence of events. Carcinoma may ultimately supervene.

Rectal lesions present as proctocolitis followed by rectal stricture, and can be confused with Crohn's disease.

The Frei rest is useful in diagnosis but may give false negative reactions.

Treatment is by full doses of sulphonamides or tetracyclines, often in prolonged or repeated courses.

The Mycoplasmas [6]. *Mycoplasma hominis* and *Urea plasma urealyticum* (T-mycoplasmas) can frequently be isolated from the genital tract. *M. hominis* may have some role in *Gardnerella* vaginitis, and both organisms may be responsible for pelvic inflammatory disease and for post-abortion and post-partum fevers.

REFERENCES

1–3 As cited on p. 2201.

4 DUNLOP E.M.C. (1983) *Br J Hosp Med* **29**, 6.

5 HARE M.J., *et al* (1981) *Br J Obstet Gynaecol* **88**, 174.

6 TAYLOR-ROBINSON D. & MCCORMACK W.M. (1980) *N Engl J Med* **302**, 1003.

7 TAYLOR-ROBINSON D. & THOMAS B.J. (1980) *J Clin Pathol* **33**, 205.

8 WILLCOX R.R. (1974) In *Recent Advances in Sexually Transmitted Diseases*. Eds. Morton R.S. & Harris J.R.W. Edinburgh. Churchill Livingstone, No. 1, ch. 16.

THE INVESTIGATION OF VULVOVAGINITIS [1, 5]

The complexity of factors involved in vulvovaginitis has been indicated in the previous section. Its frequent lack of clear definition, the limitations felt by many dermatologists in regard to gynaecological examination procedures and the frequent high level of anxiety of the patient create an unfavourable milieu in which to work. Moreover, the significance of many of the results obtained from the laboratory remain unknown. In short, the successful investigation requires a little expertise and a lot of time.

A thorough history is essential. The patient should be asked about her initial symptoms and the circumstances under which these occurred, e.g. the relation to menstruation, prior illness, change of contraceptive method, use of deodorants, foreign sojourn, etc. Medication—particularly self-medication—may not be fully disclosed by the referring doctor or admitted by the patient. However, 48% of households contain some topical skin preparation [4] and local anaesthetic ointments are freely available. The family history, especially of diabetes and tuberculosis, should not be neglected. The presence of any urinary or intestinal symptoms should be noted. Tactful enquiries should be made about the presence of any symptoms in the sexual partner and, when necessary and after examination, about family or marital stresses and even sexual technique. Though often irrelevant, these may be a pertinent cause of chronicity or relapse or may increase the perception of pruritus.

The whole skin should be examined in a good light, with special attention to the mucosae, axillae and submammary areas. A rash on one hand is usually a telltale sign of sensitivity to an applied medicament. Examination of the anogenital region demands particularly good lighting and a comfortable but firm couch or bed, especially in the obese. The vagina and cervix should always be examined in adults, if necessary with a vaginal speculum. Proctoscopy may be called for in some cases. The examination of children and young adolescents calls for particular gentleness and care. In some cases a general anaesthetic may be needed but special techniques can be developed [1].

Scrapings from the vaginal wall provide material for hormonal cytology and microbiology; a cervical scrape can be carried out at the same time and will relieve the undisclosed fears of many patients. Smears for *T. vaginalis* must be examined fresh on a warm slide. After cleansing with normal saline, light scrapings from the inner aspects of the labium minus allow a similar assessment of the hormonal state in children and virgins [5]. The use of toluidine blue 1% to detect areas of malignancy [2] is not specific enough to have been accepted for general use in the U.K.

The amine-like fishy odour of the vaginal discharge in *Gardnerella* vaginitis is very characteristic and is accentuated by the addition of 10% potassium hydroxide to vaginal secretions on a glass slide. The vaginal pH is high (5·0–5·5) and a wet mount of vaginal smear in saline will identify 'clue cells'. These are vaginal epithelial cells with granular cytoplasmic appearance and indistinct cellular outlines. This indistinct border is caused by the attachment of the small Gram-negative rods to the cell [3].

Bacteriological specimens must be taken in the correct manner, e.g. moist or transferred to transport medium, and from the appropriate site, e.g. high vaginal, vulval and perhaps perianal and nasal 'in the presence of an infective condition of whatever sort it is wise to assume that others may coexist ...' [5]. It is often valuable to examine the sexual partner and to include penile and perianal swabs where appropriate (especially for staphylococci, yeasts and *Trichomonas*).

A biopsy may be called for at the time or at a later date. The site should be chosen with care.

The urine will have been tested routinely on the first visit but laboratory examination may be necessary to determine infection and a glucose tolerance test if diabetes is suspected. Standard serological tests are called for in all cases of suspected venereal or 'paravenereal' disease, and a full patch test battery is required whenever contact dermatitis is suspected. The routine testing of all cases of vulvovaginitis of unclear origin may, indeed, be rewarding.

The reader is referred to major texts, e.g. ref. 5, for a review of other more specialized procedures of investigation.

General management [6]. During the period of investigation and diagnostic assessment some immediate treatment will be required. The more severe cases require rest and sedation; a few may need admission. All topical irritants and sensitizers should be removed and cotton, rather than nylon, panties worn. Aqueous cream can be used for cleaning, but in the acute phase cool 'sitz' baths or wet dressings will give most comfort. All other topical treatment should be bland but specific agents directed against a likely cause of infection can obviously be used, while the results of culture are awaited. Otherwise, zinc or calamine creams or a hydroxyquinolone–hydrocortisone cream are soothing and do no harm.

REFERENCES

1 Caproro V.J. & Caproro E.J. (1971) *Gynecol Prat* **22**, 169.
2 Collins C.G., et al (1966) *Am J Obstet Gynecol* **28**, 158.
3 Fleury F.J. (1981) *Clin Obst Gynecol* **24**, 407.
4 Office of Health Economics (1973) *Skin Disorders*.
5 *Ridley C.M. (1976) *The Vulva*. London, Saunders.
6 Wilkinson D.S. (1977) *Nursing and Management of Skin Diseases*. 4th ed. London, Faber & Faber.

GRANULOMATOUS LESIONS [2, 3]

Many of these have already been mentioned. All are uncommon in this country but are much more frequent in tropical regions. Here the initial lesion may not by itself produce a granulomatous picture, which develops by neglect and secondary infection and is perhaps accentuated by anaemia and malnutrition. According to Janovski and Douglas [2] granulomas may be the end result of superinfections and abscess formation arising from trivial infections. [2]

Tuberculosis, which is rare in this site, forms areas of granulation tissue, especially at the fourchette, or scrofuloderma from involvement of the inguinal glands. Leprosy tends to avoid the warmer body areas and earlier accounts of vulval involvement are open to doubt. Tertiary syphilis of nodular gummatous form was reported on the vulva some decades ago but may occur where the disease is still prevalent. Crohn's disease (p. 2174) is more likely to involve the perineum but labial lesions have been described [4, 9, 10]. Many protozoal and metazoal diseases can result in granulomatous lesions, often because of secondary infection. Amoebiasis (p. 1013) of the vulva is more likely in babies with severe amoebic dysentery. In the adult cervical lesions are more common [6]. Cutaneous leishmaniasis occasionally affects the vulva and may occur even in the U.K., as in one well-documented case [15]. Diagnosis may be difficult if the lesion is of lupoid type (p. 1020). *Schistosoma* (p. 1005), especially *S. haematobium*, may cause a chronic warty granulomatous reaction in the genital area. Apparently the warty growths may be indistinguishable from condyloma accuminata [11]. The bladder, urethra, vagina and cervix may also be involved. Rectal mucosal snips, examination of urine and vaginal discharge and biopsy should confirm the diagnosis. Genital tract cytology is useful in vaginal infections [5].

Untreated or secondarily infected granuloma inguinale (p. 775) may give rise to a mixed picture of inflammation lymphoedema fistula formation and fibrosis. Fistulae and scarring are also the end result of lymphogranuloma venereum, which may be difficult to differentiate.

Hidradenitis (acne conglobata) commonly affects the perigenital areas, though it is more common in the male. It is fully described elsewhere. The diagnosis is not usually difficult, especially if the axillae are also involved. However, Crohn's disease, deep fungal infection and lymphogranuloma venereum must be excluded. The deep mycoses may themselves cause granulomas and sinus or fistula formation. Pilonidal sinuses have been recorded on the vulva and clitoris [1, 12].

Fat necrosis resulting from corticosteroid injection may cause a painful swelling and the possibility of artefactual granuloma production, when the features are bizarre, recurrent and unusual in behaviour, should finally be remembered. Sclerosing lipogranuloma [7] probably falls into this group. Verruciform xanthoma is a condition first described in the mouth [13] but is now shown to occur on genitalia of both sexes [8, 13, 14]. It is rare and characterized by verrucous epithelial proliferation and xanthoma cells confined to the papillary dermis.

REFERENCES

1–3 As cited on p. 2201.
4 ANSELL I.D. & HOGBIN B. (1973) *J Obstet Gynaecol Br Commw* **80**, 376.
5 BERRY A. (1971) *Acta Cytol* **15**, 482.
6 COHEN C. (1973) *J Obstet Gynaecol Br Commw* **80**, 476.
7 KEMPSON R.L. & SHERMAN A.I. (1968) *Am J Obstet Gynecol* **114**, 271.
8 KRAEMER B.B., *et al* (1981) *Arch Dermatol* **117**, 516.
9 LAUGHIER M.P., *et al* (1971) *Bull Soc Fr Dermatol Syphiligr* **78**, 98.
10 McCALLUM D.I. & KINMONT P.D.C. (1968) *Br J Dermatol* **80**, 1.
11 McKEE P.H., *et al* (1983) *Clin Exp Dermatol* **8**, 189.
12 RADMAN H.M. & BHAGAVAN B.S. (1972) *Am J Obstet Gynecol* **114**, 271.
13 SANTA CRUZ D.J. & MARTIN S.A. (1979) *Am J Clin Pathol* **71**, 224.
14 SHAFER W.B. (1971) *Oral Surg* **311**, 784.
15 SYMMERS W. ST C. (1960) *Lancet* i, 127.

VULVAL DISEASES OF INFANCY [1–3]

These are seldom confined to the vulva but usually involve part or all of the napkin area.

Napkin erythema. Minor degrees are commonplace and the dermatologist, in the U.K. at least, will see only those cases that are severe, unusual or persistent. Though it may appear at any age, especially if the child fails to become continent, napkin erythema is a disease of the first few months of life. The erythema, affecting the area in contact with the napkins and generally sparing the flexures, is characteristic and needs no description. Superficial erosions and even ulceration occasionally occur. The acute phase gives place to a duller scaly rash which may have outlying satellites. When these are micropustular, candidiasis must be suspected.

Some infants appear to be more prone than others to develop napkin erythema, even when the same standards of care and hygiene apply. Infrequent changings, chafing and friction in association with occlusive pants, inadequate rinsing, fabric softeners and excessively strong concentrations of cleansers or antiseptics may contribute to irritancy.

The role of urea-splitting ammonia-producing organisms in napkin rash remains in doubt. Infants with rash do not produce increased amounts of urinary ammonia, and the application of highly ammoniacal urine to intact skin does not induce rash. The fact that prior injury to skin combined with ammoniacal urine under occlusion can induce erythema would tend to support those who ascribe a secondary irritant role to ammonia in the production of nappy rash [9].

Secondary bacterial infection may occur at any stage. The significance of candidal infection has been disputed. Earlier workers found candida in the skin of less than half the affected infants [8]. The problem may arise from trying to consider napkin erythema as a homogenous disease group. It is perhaps best considered as a disorder seen at different times during the course of its natural evolution.

In its early stages it is characterized by chafing and contact erythema. At this stage the dermatologist is rarely involved except perhaps as a parent. Some infants may then progress to an intense erythema with a sharp border and satellite pustules. There is a high return of candida in scrapings from satellite pustules and the faeces from this group, but recovery rates from the area of intense erythema are lower [12].

In infants with intense erythema only, the rate of recovery of candida will be low and conform with findings of earlier observers but the rate of rectal carriage remains high when compared with a control group of atopic infants. It has been shown that *Candida albicans* can activate the alternative pathway of complement and produce severe inflammation which may then suppress further growth of the organism and account for the relative scarcity of organisms within the group [12].

Papular forms. Papular forms of napkin rash which may show central ulceration (Jacquet) are entirely separate from the erythematous form. They are less commonly seen and are generally a manifestation of parental neglect. Long hours of contact with urine and faeces under occlusion with poor general hygiene characterizes this disorder and it may well be that the concept of ammonia in the production of nappy rash lies within this unfortunate group [7].

A particular form, the so-called 'gluteal granuloma' [13], has been described and appears at least in part to be associated with prolonged use of strong steroids. However, a number of cases have now been described in incontinent adults in whom no steroids were used [10].

Treatment. In the papular, necrotic form education, supervision and hygiene are usually sufficient to cure the problem. These infants tend not to relapse or suffer problems with over-sensitive skins.

The erythematous forms do best if they are freed from wearing napkins and, more especially, occlusive pants. Napkins should be washed and rinsed thoroughly; fabric softeners should not be used. The early chafing rashes respond well to zinc creams and even silicone-based barriers. Zinc and castor oil cream alone often suffices in mild lesions. In the type of cases seen by a dermatologist dermatitic changes have usually prevailed and hydrocortisone in association with either a polyene antibiotic or an imidiazole is indicated. Soaps should be avoided and aqueous cream B.P. used for washing the area. Relapse is common but risk of relapse can be minimized by elimination of gastrointestinal candida.

Napkin psoriasis (p. 252). Occasionally an eruption in the napkin area presents as a bright-red glazed well-demarcated sheet of erythema reminiscent of psoriasis. Secondary lesions may be widely scattered and profuse, often with marked scaling. Candida may be found. The appearance is alarming to the mother but the infant seems little worried by the extensive eruption. There is usually a very satisfactory response to simple topical measures but psoriasis may develop in later life [11].

Infantile seborrhoeic dermatitis. This unsatisfactory term (Chapter 7) is applied to a dry scaly parakeratotic eruption involving the folds. Vesiculation does not occur. Secondary infection is common. The cause is unknown and it is probably not the same condition as that called by this name in the adult. The generalized form constitutes Leiner's disease (p. 249).

Dermatophyte infections of the napkin area have been described [6] and are occasionally seen in clinical practice. Their apparent rarity may well reflect the infrequency with which they are sought.

Contact dermatitis. The effect of napkin-washing materials and antiseptic rinses as a primary cause of rashes in the napkin area has been discussed above. These can certainly cause an irritant dermatitis, especially if the general hygiene is poor and the napkin is left unchanged on skin already damaged by ammoniacal breakdown of urine or irritation by loose stools.

A peculiar, apparently idiosyncratic, glazed yellowish-red scaling confined to the area of a paper napkin liner treated with a very weak solution of quaternary ammonium antiseptic has been observed by us in four patients [5]. It resolved rapidly within 48 h when these were left off and did not recur subsequently. The mechanism is unknown. The necrotic reaction to quaternary ammonium agents [14] is now seldom seen but may occur unexpectedly and under unusual circumstances [4]. Other causes of contact dermatitis are rare in the infant.

Other conditions. Acrodermatitis enteropathica is characterized by the general condition of the infant, loss of hair and other typical features. Letterer–Siwe disease (p. 1702) should be considered when yellow-brown papules occur with purpura in the napkin region and elsewhere. The diagnosis is confirmed histologically. Haemangiomas of the vulva and napkin area frequently ulcerate and give rise to parental concern, but they heal satisfactorily with the application of a protective antibacterial ointment.

REFERENCES

1–3 As cited on p. 2201.
4 August P.J. (1975) *Br Med J* i, 70.
5 Bandmann H.J. & Wilkinson D.S. (1977) Unpublished data.

6 CAVANAGH R.M. & GREESON J.D. (1982) *Arch Dermatol* 118, 446.
7 COOKE T.V. (1921) *Arch Dermatol Syphilol* 14, 539.
8 DIXON P.N., *et al* (1969) *Br Med J* ii, 23.
9 LEYDEN J.J., *et al* (1977) *Arch Dermatol* 113, 1676.
10 MAEKAWA Y., *et al* (1978) *Arch Dermatol* 114, 382.
11 NEVILLE E.A. & FINN O.R. (1975) *Br J Dermatol* 92, 279.
12 REBORA A. & LEYDEN J.J. (1981) *Br J Dermatol* 105, 551.
13 TAPPEINER J. & PFLEGER L. (1971) *Hautarzt* 22, 283.
14 TILSLEY D.I. & WILKINSON D.S. (1965) *Trans St John's Hosp Dermatol Soc* 51, 49.

VULVAL PRURITUS

Vulval pruritus occurs consistently with some dermatoses and, with others, to an extent that varies with the individual patient. Any itching of a dermatosis involving the vulva may appear disproportionate, especially in anxious or depressed patients. Scabies, pediculosis, mycotic infections and contact dermatitis are important causes.

Less commonly, pruritus is a presenting symptom of lichen sclerosus et atrophicus, leukoplakia or carcinoma. Cystitis, proctitis, cervicitis and vaginitis of any type cause itching of variable degree. Anal pruritus, whatever its cause, not infrequently spreads to the vulva. Vulvovaginal candidiasis is a very common cause of pruritus, and trichomonal infections to a lesser extent. Fox–Fordyce disease is accompanied by particularly severe itching.

Infestation with *Enterobis (Oxyuris) vermicularis*, was found to be the cause in only 14 of 912 adult women [8].

In 161 patients with pruritus, vulvitis or fungal infections were responsible in 78 and an atrophic or leukoplakic condition in 83 [5]. Paradoxically, dermatologists probably see more cases in which local causes are less obvious.

Vulval neoplasms may also present with pruritus and the symptoms should never be dismissed lightly. An increase of pruritus in patients with lichen sclerosus et atrophicus (see below) may herald the onset of 'leukoplakia' or a premalignant change.

It has been said [3] that 10% of all gynaecological patients present with pruritus. Local and general causes must first be excluded. Diabetes may present in this way and the urine should be tested in all cases. In older patients a glucose tolerance test may be required to detect a mild, late-onset diabetes.

Pruritus vulvae is confined to the vulva or perianal area and does not involve the vagina. However, it may be intense enough to disturb sleep and to affect seriously the mental equilibrium of the patient. In those of a particularly anxious temperament, or when a 'depressive equivalent' is involved, slight degrees of inflammation or infection may give rise to disproportionate itching. The imprecise term 'pruritus vulvae' has been retained to describe those patients in whom there is a complaint of chronic itching without organic cause.

It is important to recognize, however, that short-lived vulval pruritus is not uncommon and is easily induced by friction, chafing, sweating or the vulval engorgement of pregnancy. This is almost physiological. In this group may also be found cases of early candidal vulvitis with infection and symptoms without physical signs.

PSYCHOSOMATIC VULVOVAGINITIS

About 2% of women who present with complaints of vaginal or vulval discomfort defy even the most diligent search for recognizable genital pathology [2]. These patients have usually seen many doctors and been treated with a multitude of medicaments. Their complaints may vary from persistent itching through a spectrum of types of pain which is often localized and described variously as burning, shooting or gnawing. Dyspareunia is virtually the rule among the group and it may well be that avoidance of intercourse is the reward gained for their very genuine discomfort. It is perhaps to preserve this defence against intercourse that these patients will absolutely resist any suggestion that their symptoms might be psychological in origin, although emotional lability, dependent personality and sexual guilt feelings can often be unmasked on relatively superficial questioning.

The pattern of psychosomatic vulvovaginitis appears to be changing over recent years. Until recently the common complaint appeared to be itching without organic cause. This is now much less common [9] and in a recent survey of 900 patients in a combined dermatology–gynaecology clinic no such patient was seen [10].

Complaints of vulval pain are apparently becoming much more common, at least in the U.S.A. and Britain [4, 6]. The term vulvodynia (and even pudendagra) has been used to describe this disorder [10]. The pain is usually described as burning in nature and many patients will indicate the precise locality of the persistently painful area. These patients are often relatively young and may be severely disabled by their symptoms. They are unable to wear tight trousers and even simple activities such as sitting and walking may become impossible.

All manner therapeutic means have been used to

try and alleviate these patients and all to little avail. Even phenol nerve blocks and excision of the painful zones have been attempted [6] but the pain just migrates to an adjacent site. Most observers regard vulvodynia as a modern variant of psychosomatic vulvovaginitis [4].

There are many similarities to other obscure syndromes such as the chronic perianal pain syndrome [7] (p. 2178) and the burning scrotum syndrome described in dysmorphophobic males [1]. Referral for expert psychiatric care is perhaps the only approach that can offer any real hope of full recovery.

TABLE 59.2. Hallmarks of psychosomatic vulvovaginitis [2]

Persistent symptoms of longstanding duration
Lack of demonstrable pathology
Sexual inactivity as a direct result of symptoms
Unsuccessful consultations with many doctors
'Allergy' to many common vaginal medicaments
Reluctance to accept a psychosomatic causation
Emotional lability and dependence

Lichenification of the vulva (syn. Lichen simplex; localized neurodermatitis). Thickening and hypertrophy of the vulva skin are frequently seen as a result of prolonged rubbing rather than scratching. The initial stimulus to itch may be an underlying seborrhoeic dermatitis, intertrigo, tinea or psoriasis, but in most cases the underlying cause is no longer evident and may have been some transient vulvitis or vaginal discharge. Perhaps even more trivial factors such as chafing or sweating may be sufficient to provoke the initial itching sensation. In predisposed individuals the itch–rub cycle supervenes, producing the characteristic picture of lichenification (p. 410).

It is important to appreciate that any itching disease of the vulva can become secondarily lichenified; after treatment all cases must be reviewed in case an under lying 'leukoplakia'. Paget's or Bowen's disease has been revealed.

Treatment. Treatment is identical with management of lichenification elsewhere on the body. The patient should be informed of the need to break the rubbing habit. The cutaneous nerves in involved areas appear to work on a hair trigger mechanism and strenuous efforts should be made to assist the patient by reducing their activation.

In the early stages topical antibiotics may be prescribed if secondary infection is present. Thereafter strong topical steroids injected either locally or in-

tralesionally are usually needed to provide the prolonged relief from itching necessary to break the rubbing reflex.

Application of strong local steroids should not be prolonged for over 1 month because of risks of local atrophy. Such a length of application is usually unnecessary, however. Soaps and cleansing agents other than aqueous cream should be forbidden.

In irritable or extensive cases Grenz ray therapy (p. 2606) in addition to local steroids may be needed to provide the required antipruritic effect. If therapy fails or is only partially effective, a biopsy of the involved area should always be indicated.

REFERENCES

1 COTTERILL J.A. (1981) *Br J Dermatol* **104**, 611.
2 DODSON M.G. & FRIEDRICH E.G. (1978) *Obstet Gynecol* **51** (Suppl. 1), 23.
3 JEFFCOATE T.N.A. (1967) *Principles of Gynaecology.* 3rd ed. Lonson, Butterworths, Ch. 35.
4 LYNCH P.J. (1983) Personal communication.
5 MAIOTTI G.F. (1964) *Riv Ital Ginecol* **47**, 261.
6 MONAGHAN J. (1983) Personal communication.
7 NEILL M.E. & SWASH M. (1982) *J R Soc Med* **75**, 96.
8 OUMPIANISKI R. & SZESKIN Y. (1964) *Hautarzt* **66**, 50.
9 RIDLEY C.M. (1980) *Practitioner* **224**, 481.
10 TOVELL H.M.M. & YOUNG A.W. (1978) *Clin Obstet Gynecol* **21**, 955.

VULVAL AND VAGINAL BULLAE AND ULCERS

Genital ulceration is frequently complicated by secondary infection. Papules and vesicles erode easily on the mucosal surface, and lesions which are not normally ulcerating present as such. Vulval and vaginal ulcers can be divided conveniently into acute, chronic and recurrent types.

Acute genital ulceration. The patient presents with an ulcer or discharge and, sometimes, pain and vulval oedema. Or the ulceration is seen in the course of an acute illness.

Venereal ulcers. These must always be considered first: syphilis (p. 845); chancroid (p. 764); gonorrhoea (p. 753); lymphogranuloma venereum (p. 710); granuloma inguinale (p. 775).

The differential features are discussed elsewhere. The diagnosis is confirmed by the results of specific bacteriological and serological investigations, which should always be carried out to exclude a double infection. Reiter's syndrome has been associated with ulcerative vulvitis [7].

Non-venereal infective ulcers

Tuberculosis (Chapter 22) (typhoid, pneumonia and brucellosis). Ulceration occurs rarely in these and other severe acute illnesses. In diphtheria genital ulcers are seen in children with pharyngeal or nasal infection. The child is ill and the ulcer is characterized by a topical adherent greyish membrane, which often extends over much of the swollen excoriated mucosal surface.

Anaerobic streptococci, *Ps aeruginosa* and fusospirillary organisms alone or as a superinfection cause rapidly spreading burrowing ulcers or phagedaena and gangrene in the debilitated or ill patient. Herpes simplex, herpes zoster, vaccinia and variola are discussed elsewhere.

Hand, foot and mouth disease. Small rapidly eroding vesicles occasionally occur on the vulva of infants (perhaps more frequently than is reported).

Acute non-infective ulcers

Erythema multiforme (p. 1086). This occurs in the form of the Stevens–Johnson syndrome and affects the vulva, often severely.

Artefacts. These are rare on the vulva but may be associated with foreign bodies or trauma from sexual injury or malpractice [1, 18] or with attempts to induce abortions [3]. Frank artefacts may deceive the doctor [15].

We have also seen ulceration follow the use of strong quaternary ammonium solutions used on a speculum.

Chronic genital ulceration. Any chronic ulcer of the genital mucosa must be considered malignant unless proved otherwise. Ulceration occurs particularly on atrophic mucosa (p. 2221) or a patch of leukoplakia (p. 2226). Chronic infective ulcers occur in pyoderma, actinomycosis (p. 982) and other deep mycoses. The late stages of lymphogranuloma venereum cause ulceration and scarring. Vulval ulceration due to the bite of the recluse spider *Loxosceles reclusa* has been reported in certain parts of the U.S.A. [12].

The outdated term *esthiomene* was given to chronic ulcerating, vegetating and lymphoedematous lesions of the vulva and perigenital area. Several of the bullous diseases affect the vulva, but only pemphigus vulgaris [9] and vegetans have a predilection for this area. The flaccid bullae rupture easily to produce erosions. Biopsy (with immunofluorescence studies) will confirm the diagnosis. Juvenile pemphigoid affected the genital area in 36 out of 38 cases [8]. The ruptured vesicles and fissured plaques of benign familial chronic pemphigus may

easily be misdiagnosed. Attacks may follow friction, infection, irritants and herpes simplex infections [10]. Polydysplastic epidermolysis bullosa affects the mucous membranes more frequently than other types. The mouth and conjunctivae are likely to be involved.

Benign mucosal pemphigoid may lead to ulceration and stenosis of the vulva and vagina. Urinary obstruction may be a feature [5, 11]. Erosive lichen planus will be recognizable by its lace-work patterning and oral lesions. Association of erosions of vulva, vagina and gingival mucosa has been reported [14].

Superficial fissures and ulcers occur in lichen sclerosus and may lead also to adhesions and urinary obstructions [6].

Recurrent genital ulceration.[2] A multitude of names, often eponymous, disguise a few entities that can be distinguished clinically. The aetiology of most of them remains unknown; many theories are advocated but few are proven. In this uncertain situation imagination holds rein and 'vitamin deficiency', 'allergy', 'endocrine imbalance' and 'stress', often put forward to satisfy an anxious patient, may be uncritically accepted by her medical attendant. The following patterns can be accepted.

Recurrent erythema multiforme (p. 1086). The genital area is seldom affected in the usual peripheral type but may be involved when oral lesions are predominant.

Bullous fixed drug eruptions. These are less common (or less commonly recognized) on the vulva than on the penis. With the decline in the use of phenolphthalein, sulphonamides and barbiturates, they are becoming rare in any case, at least in the U.K.

Recurrent herpes simplex. This has been discussed earlier. Erosions, rather than ulcers, occur.

Aphthosis, mucosal or with extramucosal manifestations. This common but ill-understood entity of unknown cause, may comprise some or all cases of (a) Sutton's ulcer and (b) Lipschutz's ulcer.

Behçet's syndrome. This, for the present, can be kept apart from aphthosis because of its other manifestations and differing prognosis (Fig. 59.22).

Aphthosis. When aphthae occur in the vulva, the concomitant oral manifestations are usually severe. It is important to differentiate between these ulcers and a recurrent herpetic infection [17]. Premen-

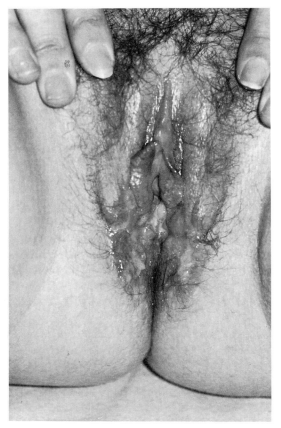

FIG. 59.22. Behçet's disease (Bishop Auckland General Hospital).

strual exacerbations are common and may be the determining feature of attacks. The cause remains unknown. Infection or hypersensitivity reactions to infectious agents, e.g. *Strep. viridans*, have been invoked, but the hypotheses are not borne out by therapy. The role of folic acid deficiency is also uncertain and appropriate treatment by iron and folic acid in combination is not universally successful. There is considerable evidence from patients who suffer from aphthae which relates attacks at sites of minor trauma to periods of stress. This reaction to trauma might be equivalent to the 'prick' reaction obtained to a degree that varies with activity of the disease in patients with Behçet's syndrome. Some patients may, indeed, develop this syndrome later [3].

The genital lesions are multiple, painful, superficial and yellowish with a red areola. They affect the labia particularly and heal quickly. They may be accompanied by vulvitis.

At present only symptomatic treatment is available. Topical corticosteroids, or possibly local tetracyclines, seem to help some patients and will at least console them for the lack of any really effective therapy. Some patients unaccountably respond to a variety of unproven or experimental forms of treatment, suggesting a high degree of placebo response.

Sutton's ulcer (periadenitis mucosae necrotica recurrens). This ulcer is solitary, painful and recurring, and is more common in the mouth [13]. It may be a variant of aphthosis or Behçet's syndrome but normally occurs alone without any associated symptoms. Intralesional triamcinolone has been the most effective form of treatment in personal cases.

Ulcus vulvae acutum (Lipschutz's ulcer). Lipschutz described three types of ulcer but only one of these is now regarded as being a separate entity [4]. The others fall into the pattern of Behçet's syndrome or aphthosis [4]. There remains a form of ulceration, single or sparse, and sometimes associated with infection such as typhoid or paratyphoid fever [16]. It is self-limiting and resolves without treatment. *B. crassus* is no longer regarded as a pathogen in these cases.

Adolescent girls are affected in more than half the cases reported. The lesion is often acute in onset and may be accompanied by fever. Sparse lesions are surrounded by a reddish areola and have a dirty firmly adherent membrane that separates in a few days (Fig. 59.23). The lymphatic glands are usually

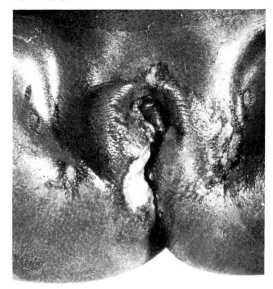

FIG. 59.23. Ulcus vulvae acutum in a girl aged 2 yr (Makerere College Medical School).

enlarged and tests for infectious mononucleosis may be positive.

REFERENCES

1–3 As cited on p. 2201.
4 BERLIN C. (1965) *Acta Derm Venereol (Stockh)* **45**, 221.
5 BOYCE D.C. & VALPREY J.M. (1971) *Obstet Gynecol* **38**, 440.
6 DAMANSKI M., *et al* (1969) *Br Med J* ii, 385.
7 DAUNT S.O.N., *et al* (1982) *Br J Vener Dis* **58**, 405.
8 GRANT P.W. (1968) *Trans Rep St John's Hosp Dermatol Soc* **54**, 128.
9 KAUFMAN R.H., *et al* (1969) *Obstet Gynecol* **33**, 264.
10 LEPPARD B., *et al* (1973) *Br J Dermatol* **88**, 609.
11 McCALLUM D.I. (1969) *Br Med J* ii, 637.
12 MAGRINA J.F. & MASTERSON B.J. (1981) *Am J Obstet Gynecol* **140**, 341.
13 MONTELEONE L. (1967) *Oral Surg Med Pathol* **23**, 586.
14 PELISSE M., *et al* (1982) *Ann Dermatol Vénéréol* **109**, 797.
15 REICH L.H. & WEHR T. (1973) *Obstet Gynecol* **41**, 239.
16 VAN JOOST T. (1971) *Ned Tijdschr Geneeskol* **115**, 1080.
17 WEATHERS D.R. & GRIFFITHS J.W. (1970) *J Am Dent Assoc* **81**, 81.
18 WILSON K.F.G. (1966) *NZ J Obstet Gynaecol* **6**, 191.

THE VULVAL DYSTROPHIES [1–3]

The term vulva dystrophy is applied by gynaecologists to describe a group of diseases presenting as white lesions of the vulva. There has in the past been much confusion over terminology between dermatologists and gynaecologists and it was hoped that the setting up of a Committee on Terminology of the International Society for the Study of Vulvar Disease (ISSVD) might help clear many of the problems and terminology and classification. The recommendations of the Committee [14] suggested classification of vulval dystrophies based on microscopic features as follows [21]:

(1) Hyperplastic dystrophy to include such formerly used terms as leukoplakia, neurodermatitis, lichen simplex, chronicus, leukokeratosis, leukoplakic vulvitis and hyperplastic vulvitis;
(2) lichen sclerosus to include kraurosis vulvae;
(3) mixed dystrophy which is essentially lichen sclerous with areas of epithelial hyperplasia with or without atypia.

There are many problems associated with this form of classification. Some relate to the omission of certain diseases such as lichen planus, and others to the untidiness associated with tagging on some disorders such as extramammary Paget's disease as apparent afterthoughts.

The two major objections relate firstly to the use of the term 'dystrophy', which has been traditionally reserved for describing musculo-skeletal disorders, and secondly to the confusion engendered from its reference to a mixed group of inflammatory, reactive, benign and premalignant hyperplastic epithelial disorders [5].

The classification of ISSVD however, has, finally freed us from the use of such terms as senile atrophy and primary vulval atrophy. These terms presumably relate in major part to the physiological effects of aging and do not represent recognizable disease processes.

A classification using a mixture of clinical and histological criteriae has been proposed [15] which should prove acceptable at least to dermatologists and pathologists (Table 59.3).

TABLE 59.3. Reactive and neoplastic disorders of the vulval epithelium*

(1) Benign dermatoses
(I) Lichenification
(II) Psoriasis
(III) Lichen planus
(VI) Seborrhoeic dermatitis
(V) Eczematous dermatitis (chronic)
(2) Vulvar epithelial hyperplasia
(I) Without atypia
(II) With atypia (leukoplakia)
(3) Lichen sclerosus
(4) Lichen sclerosus with foci of epithelial hyperplasia
(I) Without atypia
(II) With atypia
(5) Squamous cell carcinoma *in situ*
(6) Paget's disease of the vulva

* Adapted from ref. 15.

Benign dermatoses of the vulva

Lichenification (lichen simplex chronicus) (see p. 410). The hyperkeratosis is usually ill defined, merging into normal skin. Pigmentation is common. On the external labia the diagnosis is not difficult. On the mucosal surface the affected area may be localized, thickened and greyish-white in colour, or it may be more diffuse with large areas of thick infiltration merging with obvious lichenification of the adjacent skin. Leukoplakia is dead white and more localized.

Psoriasis. The silvery scaling of patches on the outer aspect of the labia is readily recognized. Psoriasis here is normally of the smooth glazed flexural type.

Lichen planus (p. 1676). The bluish-white papules or delicate lace-like striae are not easily confused with the more opaque lesions of leukoplakia, but in the rare absence of lesions elsewhere a solitary patch of lichen planus, especially if it is itchy, may occasionally cause difficulty and necessitate a biopsy. The vestibule and inner surfaces of the labia minora are most frequently affected (Fig. 59.24). In long-standing and ulcerative lichen planus there may be some risk of malignancy [18].

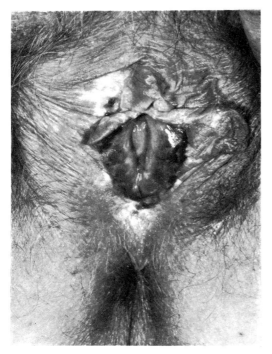

FIG. 59.24. Lichen planus. Reticulate lesions can be seen, though in places the resemblance to leukoplakia is close. (St John's Hospital.)

Seborrhoeic dermatitis (p. 375). The flexures are usually involved. A combination of erythema, scaling and even crusting may spread over the labia majora.

Eczematous dermatitis (p. 373). This relates to irritant and allergic eczema of the vulva.

Vulval epithelial hyperplasia (without and with atypia (leukoplakia)). This seems a ponderous term to have imposed upon the profession. Its necessity appears to stem from the fact that many feel unable to accept that leukoplakia means anything more than literally 'white patch'. If it could be accepted that the term leukoplakia represents a combined clinical and histological diagnosis of vulval epithelial hyperplasia with cellular atypia, most of the dermatologist's difficulties will have been resolved and all the above classification will prove unnecessary. We shall continue to use the term leukoplakia as such in the present text.

Vulval hyperplasia without atypia. This can be limited to such conditions as seborrhoeic warts and epithelial naevi which could involve any area of the skin and appear on the vulva largely by chance.

Vulval epithelial hyperplasia with atypia (leukoplakia) (see also p. 2108)). This is a diagnosis which cannot be made without histological confirmation since its clinical appearance can be imitated by such diseases as lichenification, epithelial naevi and lichen planus. The situation is complicated by the fact that a varying degree of lichenification may be superimposed. In the presence of a confusing biopsy it is perfectly legitimate to use a strong local steroid to clear the lichenification and then re-biopsy the area. Clinically the condition appears as single or scattered plaques of thickened white skin with rather ill-defined edges extending onto or involving the mucosa. Histologically it consists of an irregular hyperplastic epithelium with varying degrees of cellular atypicality or loss of polarity. Occasionally there may be no obvious atypia in the early stages but examination through the block, careful follow-up and re-biopsy, sometimes after clearing superimposed lichenification with steroids, may then show evidence of increased mitotic activity throughout the epidermal layers, which is the earliest sign of atypia.

Thereafter there appears to be a progression from slightly atypical hyperplasia to conditions which approximate to intra-epithelial carcinoma. It has been shown that more than 55% of cases of carcinoma of the vulva were associated with leukoplakic change elsewhere on the genitalia [20].

The white patches of this disease may appear *de novo*, or as a complication of lichen sclerosus. The factors responsible are unknown; syphilis is not one of them. Suspicion is growing that infectious viral agents may be in part responsible [5, 12].

Clinical features and course. Leukoplakia—used in the above context—is usually accompanied by, and may be preceded by, itching which is sometimes severe. This often indicates its development in the course of lichen sclerosus. Pain and soreness also occur, particularly when it becomes fissured.

It presents as one or more well-demarcated thickened dead-white or greyish-white patches which have been likened to white paint that has hardened and cracked. Any part of the vulva except the vestibule and urethral orifice may be affected, but especially the clitoris, the labia minora and the inner aspects of the labia majora. Fissuring, cracking and ulceration are regarded as poor prognostic signs. When it is widespread, leukoplakia causes stenosis of the introitus of the vagina (but not of the urethral meatus).

Leukoplakia is a dynamic process, waxing and waning inexplicably. Different areas in the same patient characteristically vary in extent and appearance within short periods of time, especially in the presence of vulvitis or secondary lichenification (Fig. 59.25).

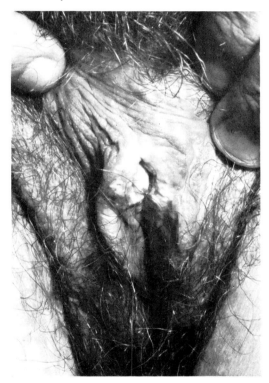

FIG. 59.25. Leukoplakia and lichenification. The latter cleared with corticosteroids; the area on the right labium remained and was confirmed histologically as leukoplakia. (Stoke Mandeville Hospital.)

The course is unpredictable. In some cases the spread is rapid and extensive. In others patches remain inactive for years with little visible change.

Treatment. Excision–biopsy is usually indicated in order to assess the histological picture. However, electrocoagulation or cryotherapy are successful in dealing with lesions that are not frankly neoplastic. If doubt exists, local excision with a margin can be carried out. Local vulvectomy may be necessary if multiple lesions are present but should be undertaken only after careful clinical and histological study and with the fullest consideration of the patient in mind.

Lichen sclerosus [3, 18, 19]. This condition is fully discussed on p. 1368.

Diagnostic features in the genital area. Lichen sclerosus is essentially a disease of women though it occurs on the penis more commonly than is recognized (p. 2190) [6]. It appears to be less common in coloured races, though it has been reported in them [4, 7]. The anogenital area was involved in 190 of 200 women affected [18], the vulva alone in 61, and the vulva and perianal area (the figure-of-eight distribution) in 126. The inguinal area was affected in only 25. The average age at presentation ranges from 45 to 54 yr but it may occur in quite young

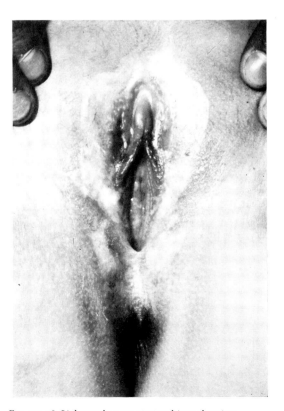

FIG. 59.26. Lichen sclerosus et atrophicus showing ivory-white sheets involving the vulva and perineum (Addenbrooke's Hospital).

children [4, 7]. The presenting symptom is usually pruritus, sometimes soreness and occasionally dyspareunia which may be marked. Vaginitis may precede or accompany any stage of the condition.

The typical appearances of lichen sclerosus as it affects the skin are modified in the anogenital region. The ivory-coloured papules with follicular plugging and hyperkeratosis are most likely to be seen at the edge of perianal lesions and only rarely occur on the vulva. Lesions are present elsewhere on the body in about a fifth of the patients. In 41 patients the skin and the vulva were both affected in 26, the vulva alone in 10 and the skin alone in 5 [4]. As the disease progresses sheets of ivory-white (Fig. 59.26) or light violaceous atrophic skin show the characteristic cigarette-paper atrophy (Fig. 59.27). At times individual papules are absent [16, 18] or there is marked hyperkeratosis or a diffuse irregular scaling. Occasionally the skin feels thick and waxy owing to oedema; when this is marked thick-walled bullae, which are often quite large, may form.

On the mucous surfaces the changes are less distinctive. The labia minora and clitoris are affected early, but a general atrophy with marked narrowing of the introitus may follow. The mucosal surface

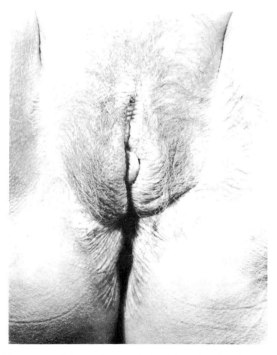

FIG. 59.27. Lichen sclerosus et atrophicus showing the 'cigarette-paper' atrophy extending to the perianal area (St John's Hospital).

is pale and may show flecks of haemorrhage telangiectasia or bulla formation. Fissures, erosions and lichenification may appear in the course of the disease. A statistically significant association with morphoea and a less certain association with vitiligo was demonstrated in 380 cases [18].

The observation that a significant increase of organ-specific autoantibodies [10] can be found in these patients has led to the finding of an increased incidence in general of autoimmune disease of one such group. However, the only specific disease to show a significant association with lichen sclerosus was pernicious anaemia [11]. In males with lichen sclerosus a similar general increase in autoimmune disease was noted [17], but no particular condition was specifically associated.

It has recently been shown that elastic fibres are absent from the superficial dermis in this disease. It is possible that an elastase-type protease is responsible for this degradation of elastic tissue [9].

Histopathology (Fig. 59.28). Hyperkeratosis, follicular plugging with atrophy of the epidermis and epidermal appendages associated with an oedematous-looking degeneration of the collagen in the papillary and superficial dermis, delineated on its deeper aspect by a monomorphic lymphcytic infiltrate, are the hallmarks of lichen sclerosus.

Small areas of epidermal hypertrophy which may represent lichenification or leukoplakia may develop. These areas should be kept under close observation and biopsied regularly [18].

Course and complications. The course is irregularly progressive with periods of relative inactivity. Infection, lichenification, erosion and fissuring occur frequently. Contact dermatitis may complicate treatment.

About two-thirds of the lesions in children remit at puberty leaving little residual change [8, 18]. However, in the other third some degree of stenosis and atrophy persists and leukoplakia may supervene. There is unfortunately no way of differentiating these two groups.

Leukoplakia, often presaged by more intense or persistent itching, eventually occurs in about half the cases [13, 18], though at any one time it is found in substantially less. A carcinoma supervenes in a proportion of these; exactly how many is hard to determine. A figure of 1 in 6 [16] appears to be too high; that of 4·4% in 290 patients [18] is perhaps the minimum for patients under regular observation. The carcinoma always occurs in pre-existing leukoplakia. The labia minora and clitoris are particularly affected. Dysuria and urinary infections may follow meatal stenosis.

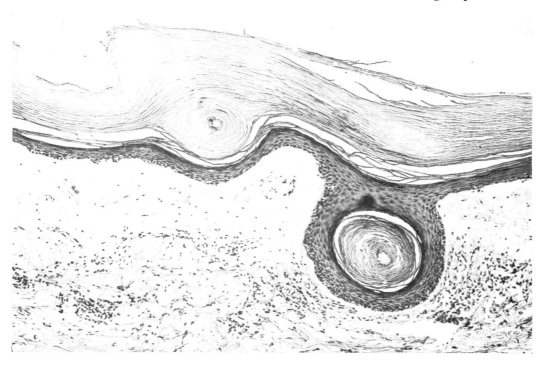

FIG. 59.28. Lichen sclerosus et atrophicus. Hyperkeratosis and follicular plugging. The infiltrate is separated from the atrophic epidermis by a clear area. H&E × 100) (Professor E. Wilson Jones.)

Treatment. There is no specific therapy and no method is known by which this atrophic condition can be halted or slowed down. As the danger to the patient lies in the development of leukoplakia and carcinoma, regular observation by an experienced clinician offers the best safeguard for prognosis. Repeated biopsies of suspicious areas may be needed. The first indication of malignancy will usually be the development of hyperplasia and leukoplakia, the treatment of which is discussed below. Vulvectomy should not be undertaken without very careful consideration, but ablation of areas of early premalignancy may be necessary and can be repeated over a period of many years.

Hydrocortisone cream or even simple emollients and bland agents [19] are of considerable help in overcoming some of the distressing symptoms of the condition and may be used regularly to advantage. The stronger fluorinated corticosteroids may be used under careful supervision. However, local injections of triamcinolone or cryotherapy may be helpful for localized areas.

Differential diagnosis of white vulval patches [1]. A number of conditions of different aetiology and sig-

nificance give rise to white patches or plaques in the vulval region.

Leucoderma (vitiligo). There should be no difficulty in distinguishing this from the other conditions discussed. The genital region is often involved early in the process.

Infections. Candidal infection causes whitish or yellowish-white curd-like patches, typical of 'thrush'. These are readily removed and the associated erosions, superficial ulcers and vaginal discharge distinguish them from other white vulval lesions.

Bowen's disease and Paget's disease (pp. 2227 and 2228). These produce raised velvety or indurated lesions that may at times be confused with leukoplakia. In case of doubt, a biopsy must be performed.

REFERENCES

1–3 As cited on p. 2201.
4 BARCLAY D.L., *et al* (1966) *Obstet Gynecol* 27, 637.
5 CABRAL G.A. (1982) *Am J Obstet Gynecol* 143, 611.

6 CHALMERS R.J.G., *et al* (1982) *Br J Dermatol* **107**, (Suppl **22**), 29.

7 CHERNOSKY M.E., *et al* (1957) *Arch Dermatol* **75**, 647.

8 CLARK J.A. & MULLER S.A. (1967) *Arch Dermatol* **95**, 476.

9 GODEAU G., *et al* (1982) *J Invest Dermatol* **78**, 270.

10 GOOLAMALI S.K., *et al* (1974) *Br Med J* **iv**, 78.

11 HARRINGTON C.I. & DUNSMORE I.R. (1981) *Br J Dermatol* **104**, 563.

12 KAUFMAN R.H., *et al* (1981) *N Engl J Med* **305**, 483.

13 NIKOLAU S.G. & BOLUS L. (1966) *Dermatologica* **132**, 27.

14 Report of the Committee on Terminology (1976) *Obstet Gynecol* **47**, 122.

15 SANCHEZ N.P. & MIHM M.C. (1982) *J Am Acad Dermatol* **6**, 378.

16 SURMOUND D. (1964) *Arch Dermatol* **90**, 143.

17 THOMAS R.H.M., *et al* (1983) *Br J Dermatol* **109**, 661.

18 WALLACE H.J. (1971) *Trans St John's Hosp Dermatol Soc* **57**, 9.

19 WALLACE H.J. & WHIMSTER I.W. (1951) *Br J Dermatol* **63**, 241.

20 WAY S. (1982) *Malignant Disease of the Vulva*. Edinburgh, Churchill Livingstone.

21 YOUNG A.W. & TOVELL H.M.M. (1978) *Clin Obstet Gynecol* **21**, 1023.

BOWENOID PAPULOSIS

Over recent years a number of papers have appeared [3, 6, 7] reporting papular, pigmented, occasionally skin-coloured or de-pigmented lesions [9] in the groins and on the genitalia of young individuals of both sexes. When the female is involved lesions are frequently associated with pregnancy [9].

The clinical appearance of these lesions can vary widely [1]. They have been described variously as verrucous, lichenoid, dry, brown, pigmented or even whitish papules or plaques. The diagnosis is confirmed by biopsy.

These clinically banal asymptomatic lesions have a histological picture which is difficult to distinguish from Bowen's disease (carcinoma *in situ*) [10]. Cellular uniformity, occasional apparent synchronization of mitoses and absence of pilosebaceous involvement are features peculiar to Bowenoid papulosis [9]. Vesicular changes in epidermal cell chromatin have led to comparison with viral balloon cell changes [8] and lesions have been frequently associated with both herpes simplex virus type II [4] and condylomata accuminata [5, 10].

As yet the prognosis is unknown. Major surgery is regarded as contraindicated since so far no cases of invasive squamous carcinoma have been described [10]. Some cases undergo spontaneous regression [2]. Electrodissection or cryotherapy appear to be the treatments of choice, although recurrence has been recorded and long-term follow-up is required to determine the eventual outcome.

REFERENCES

1 BENDER M.E., *et al* (1980) *JAMA* **243**, 145.

2 BERGER B.W. & HORI Y. (1978) *Arch Dermatol* **114**, 1698.

3 BHAWAN J. (1980) *Gynecol Oncol* **10**, 201.

4 CABRAL G.A. (1982) *Am J Obstet Gynecol* **143**, 611.

5 KAUFMAN R.H., *et al* (1981) *N Engl J Med* **305**, 483.

6 KIMURA S., *et al* (1978) *Dermatologica* **157**, 229.

7 LLOYD K.M. (1970) *Arch Dermatol* **101**, 48.

8 SEDEL D., *et al* (1982) *Ann Dermatol Vénéréol* **109**, 811.

9 ULBRIGHT T.M., *et al* (1982) *Cancer* **50**, 2910.

10 WADE T.R., *et al* (1979) *Arch Dermatol* **115**, 306.

PREMALIGNANT AND MALIGNANT LESIONS OF THE VULVA

RONA M. MACKIE

Premalignant vulvar lesions. In a recent study of risk factors associated with vulva malignancy, multiparity, obesity and diabetes emerged as being significantly more common in patients than controls. A striking finding from this study [3] was the fact that 10% of those with vulva malignancy had a past history of viral papillomas. This observation, together with the recent work of Coleman [8] identifying human papilloma virus type 6 (HPV6) in a significant proportion of cases of carcinoma of the cervix, has stimulated interest in the carcinogenic potential of the human papillopma virus. HPV6 is the strain associated with genital warts, and the accumulating evidence suggests that patients with gross and persistent vulva warts may be at future risk of vulva carcinoma.

It is impossible to state definitely how many patients suffering from vulva epithelial hyperplasia with atypia (Leukoplakia) will progress to frank malignancy; one estimate is 10% [18]. Conversely, between 57% and 69% [27] of all squamous cell carcinomas of vulvae show evidence elsewhere on the vulva of hyperplasia and atypia. Progression of true Bowen's disease to vulval carcinoma is probably less frequent despite its sometimes alarming histological appearance [28].

The true incidence of malignancy developing subsequent to lichen sclerosus et atrophicus is not well established. Wallace's classic work [30] suggested that around 5% of patients progress to vulva carcinoma and that those at greatest risk are patients with pruritic ulcerated lesions. Malignancy has not been reported developing after prepubertal lichen sclerosus et atrophicus.

Patients with Fanconi's anaemia, one of the chromosome instability syndromes, appear to be prone to both perineal and vulva cancers [13].

There is evidence from the West Indies [11, 26] that lymphogranuloma venereum and granuloma inguinale increased the likelihood of vulva carcinoma. The patients are younger than those with no evidence of the two diseases, more than half of them show evidence of Bowen's diseases of the vulva and there is a likelihood that the tumour will behave in a virulent fashion. There is some evidence that condyloma acuminatum and herpes virus type 2 infections may be implicated in Bowen's disease and squamous cell carcinoma of the anogenital area [7, 12, 14, 28, 29].

Bowen's disease of the vulva [2, 4, 6, 16, 24]

Clinical features. Bowen's disease of the vulva differs entirely from Bowenoid papulosis (p. 2226), being best regarded as an analogue of erythroplasia. It is characterized by intractable severe itching. In many cases there are multiple lesions which are flat, red or pigmented, velvety or granular plaques with well-demarcated and irregular, occasionally hyperpigmented, margins [1].

A history of bleeding or a palpable mass suggest invasive changes when examination shows induration, ulceration or a verrucous nodular contour. The anterior vulva and especially the labia minora are the main areas involved in contrast with the recto-vaginal area in the post-lymphogranulomatous Jamaican patient [26]. In all patients lymphatic spread is to the inguinal nodes and thence to the iliac nodes.

Diagnosis. It may be difficult to distinguish simple lichenification clinically from epithelial hyperplasia with atypia, 'leukoplakia', Bowen's disease and extramammary Paget's disease.

Any case which does not respond rapidly and completely to the application or intralesional injection of strong steroids must be biopsied. Any indurated, eroded or ulcerated plaque, nodule or warty lesion, especially in the elderly, is more likely to be a squamous cell carcinoma than anything else.

Treatment. Bowen's disease is best treated by complete vulvectomy and multiple sections to exclude invasive malignancy. This may be an unacceptable procedure to relatively young women, and 5-fluorouracil, which is an effective local treatment [33], or cryotherapy may be considered.

Vulvar malignancy. The American statistical service SEER [3] states that in North America there are 1,900 cases annually of vulvar carcinoma. Of these, 82% are squamous cell carcinoma, 5% basal cell carcinoma, 5% adenocarcinoma, 6% melanoma and 1% sarcoma. British statistics report that it is the fourth most common tumour of the female genital tract and comprises 10% of all genital tumours. Sixty per cent occurred in women over 60 yr of age and over 88% were post-menopausal at the onset of the illness. It may develop either *de novo* or from pre-existing areas of 'leukoplakia' or Bowen's disease.

About one-third of patients die within 3 yr of diagnosis despite vigorous therapy [31], and so the prognosis is much less favourable than it should be for so accessible a site. Earlier diagnosis can greatly improve the prognosis. A recent survey of cases of early micro-invasive carcinoma revealed 100% survival after follow-up for 1–24 yr [15].

Clinical features. Any persistent nodule or plaque on the vulva in an older female should be biopsied to exclude vulvar carcinoma. The lesion most commonly presents as an ulcerated nodule, and pre-existing Bowen's disease or leukoplakia will raise clinical suspicion.

Treatment [20, 31]. Until recently radical surgery, frequently complete vulvectomy, offered the only hope of long-term survival. With earlier presentation and new methods of treatment this approach has been somewhat modified and both laser surgery, using the CO_2 laser, and cryotherapy are now considered safe and useful methods of managing patients with early disease, particularly younger patients. Five year survival figures are not yet available to allow accurate assessment of the efficacy of these newer forms of therapy.

Malignant melanoma [5, 10, 32]. American figures indicate that 2% of all melanomas in women occur on the vulva [3]. These lesions are frequently not diagnosed until the tumour volume is considerable and may therefore tend to carry a poor prognosis. The usual clinical presentation is that of a black or brown ulcerating fungated mass.

Basal cell carcinoma. Basal cell carcinoma is rare on the vulva and usually presents as an itchy tumour of long duration. Local excision is associated with a 20% recurrence rate and there is a significant association with other primary malignancies [22]. Secondary tumours and lymphomas are occasionally seen.

Other rarer vulvar tumours. There are recent reports of dermatofibrosarcoma protuberans [25] and benign and malignant mixed tumours of the skin occurring on the vulva [21]. A ductal adenocarcinoma of the vulvar sweat glands has also been reported [23].

Carcinoma of Bartholin's gland [17] should be suspected when there is a persistent cystic or tender and indurated vulval mass [9]. It can easily be mistaken for an inflammatory process and it is wise to biopsy all Bartholin gland enlargements. The lesion is an adenocarcinoma and should be treated by radical vulvectomy.

Vulvar Paget's disease. Extramammary Paget's disease is fully discusssed on p. 2438. However, the vulva is the commonest site for this condition.

The lesion is a moist red oozing plaque which gives rise to the symptoms of burning and pruritus. The great majority are associated with underlying adenocarcinoma of the sweat glands, but cervical [19] and rectal carcinoma may also give rise to this condition.

Complete excision of the lesion and removal of the underlying malignancy is the appropriate therapy.

REFERENCES

1 ABELL M.R. & GOSLING J.R.G. (1961) *Cancer (NY)* **14**, 318.
2 BENDER M.E., *et al* (1980) *JAMA* **243**, 145.
3 BERG E. & LAMP E. (1981) *Cancer* **48**, 432.
4 BERGER B.W. & HORI Y. (1978) *Arch Dermatol* **114**, 1698.
5 BERMAN M.L., *et al* (1981) *Am J Obstet Gynecol* **139**, 963.
6 BHAWAN J. (1980) *Gynecol Oncol* **10**, 201.
7 CABRAL G.A. (1982) *Am J Obstet Gynecol* **143**, 161.
8 COLEMAN D.V., *et al* (1982) *Diagn Gynecol Obstet* **4**, 303.
9 DODSON M.G., *et al* (1970) *Obstet Gynecol* **35**, 578.
10 EDINGTON P.T. & MONAGHAN J. (1980) *Br J Obstet Gynaecol* **87**, 422.
11 HAY S.M. & COLE F.M. (1970) *Am J Obstet Gynecol* **108**, 479.
12 KAUFMAN R.H., *et al* (1981) *N Engl J Med* **305**, 483.
13 KENNEDY A.W. & HART W.R. (1982) *Cancer* **50**, 81.
14 KIMURA S., *et al* (1978) *Dermatologica* **157**, 229.
15 KUNSCHNER, A., *et al* (1978) *Am J Obstet Gynecol* **132**, 599.
16 LLOYD K.M. (1970) *Arch Dermatol* **101**, 48.
17 LURMAN K. (1974) *Zentralbl Gynakol* **96**, 1044.
18 MCADAMS A.J. JR & KISTNER R.W. (1958) *Cancer* **11**, 740.
19 MCKEE P.H. & HERTOGS K.T. (1980) *Br J Dermatol* **103**, 443.
20 MORLEY G.W. (1981) *Cancer* **48**, 341.
21 ORDONEZ N.G., *et al* (1980) *Cancer* **48**, 181.
22 PALLADINO V.S., *et al* (1969) *Cancer* **24**, 460.
23 RICH P.M., *et al* (1981) *Cancer* **47**, 1352.
24 SEDEL D., *et al* (1982) *Ann Dermatol Vénéréol* **109**, 811.
25 SOLTAN M.H. (1981) *Br J Obstet Gynaecol* **88**, 203.
26 STOCKHAUSEN B.Y. (1968) *West Indian Med J* **17**, 103.
27 TAUSSIC F.J. (1940) *Am J Obstet Gynecol* **40**, 764.
28 ULBRIGHT T.M., *et al* (1982) *Cancer* **50**, 2910.
29 WADE T.R., *et al* (1979) *Arch Dermatol* **115**, 306.
30 WALLACE H.J. (1971) *Trans St John's Hosp Dermatol Soc* **57**, 9.
31 WAY S. (1982) *Malignant Diseases of the Vulva* Edinburgh, Churchill Livingstone.
32 WILKINSON T.S. & PALETTA F.S. (1979) *Ann Surg* **35**, 301.
33 WOODRUFF J.D., *et al* (1973) *Am J Obstet Gynecol* **115**, 677.

CHAPTER 60

The Skin and the Nervous System

W. J. CUNLIFFE & J. A. SAVIN

ANATOMY AND PHYSIOLOGY OF THE CUTANEOUS NERVES

In the past decade there have been considerable gains in our knowledge of the structure and functions of the human skin. For example, it is now possible percutaneously to insert a microelectrode into peripheral nerves and to record single fibre activity from both afferent and efferent axons in a conscious volunteer [18].

Such studies have indicated that man differs very little from other mammals, the main differences reflecting the peculiar anatomy of human skin and the evolution of its special sensory mechanisms. Animal studies therefore remain important and contribute vital information [3, 15, 16, 23, 24].

THE AFFERENT NERVE SUPPLY TO THE SKIN AND THE ANATOMY OF SENSE ORGANS

Cutaneous and subcutaneous sense organs are innervated by myelinated (A) and non-myelinated (C) nerve fibres whose cell bodies are located in either the posterior (dorsal) root ganglia or the sensory ganglia of appropriate cranial nerves. These fibres link the sense organs to the central nervous system and it is through them that information is transmitted to the spinal cord and brain. The myelinated fibres in human cutaneous nerves may be divided into $A\alpha$ and $A\delta$ categories on the basis of their conduction velocities. Non-myelinated fibres conduct impulses more slowly [4, 11]. Different sense organs are innervated by axons with different ranges of conduction velocities: sensitive mechanoreceptors are innervated by $A\alpha$ (and possibly $A\delta$) fibres, and nociceptors by both $A\delta$ and non-myelinated fibres [27]; the latter also innervate receptors responding to warmth [17].

Using a variety of techniques such as producing a measured stimulus and biopsying the stimulated site it is now clear that specific sense organs occur in the skin and subcutaneous tissue. The sense organs may be classified into three types: encapsulated receptors, non-encapsulated receptors and non-corpuscular receptors.

Encapsulated cutaneous receptors. In these receptors, usually found in the dermis or subcutaneous tissue, there is a non-nervous capsule that completely invests the nerve-endings. Such receptors are commonly found in glabrous skin. The *Meissner corpuscle* is found in the papillary ridges of the dermis. The single myelinated axon forms flattened sheets of nervous tissue in the form of a coil interleaved with flattened lamina cells [5]. Fine bundles of collagen pass from the corpuscle to the tonofibrils of the overlying keratinocytes, providing a mechanical linkage that transmits displacement of the skin surface to the Meissner corpuscle [1]. The *Krause end-bulb*, uncommonly found in man, is also innervated by a single large axon whose terminal may be a simple expansion surrounded by a small number of lamellae. The *Pacinian corpuscle* which is 0·5–2 mm long is innervated by a single myelinated axon whose terminal extends into the corpuscle as a non-myelinated central core. The central core is surrounded by lamellae which filter mechanical deformations so that only the high frequency components affect the transducer elements in the central core [22, 25]. The *Ruffini ending* has a thin capsule and is innervated by a single large myelinated axon that forms a brush-like inner spindle after losing its myelin sheath [7]. The nerve terminal is intimately associated with collagen fibrilsthat pass longitudinally through the sense organs.

Non-encapsulated corpuscular receptors. The *Merkel cell-neurite complex* [22] consists of a group of Merkel cells at the base of the epidermis in both hairy and glabrous skin. Monoclonal antibodies have recently helped in the better understanding of the functions and origins of this complex. The complex is usually innervated by a single large myelinated ($A\alpha$) axon which splits up into a number of branches each terminating in a flattened expansion enclosed by a single cell [16].

Non-corpuscular receptors. These are of two main kinds. *Hair follicle receptors* surround the hair follicle and are usually innervated by myelinated axons of varying diameters. Other non-corpuscular receptors have been found to be associated with the epidermis. Their role is unclear and they are innervated by non-myelinated fibres [6].

Functional specificity of sense·organs. All types of cutaneous and subcutaneous sense organs have a high degree of functional specificity. However, it is also clear that no cutaneous receptor has absolute specificity and that given a large enough stimulus it will respond in a way other than that to which it is accustomed [15]. A particular problem arises with the response of cutaneous receptors, especially mechanoreceptors, to thermal stimuli, partly because all biological reactions, physical and chemical, are affected by temperature. The mechanoreceptors may change their activity in a way that is typical of other receptors classed as thermoreceptors, and they have been dubbed 'spurious thermoreceptors'.

In functional terms the sensory organs may be classified as mechanoreceptors sensitive to displacement, nociceptors sensitive to damaging or potentially damaging stimuli and thermoreceptors sensitive to temperature changes.

Mechanoreceptors. Cutaneous mechanoreceptors are sensitive to mechanical displacement of the skin and functionally are of two sorts. Dynamic displacements stimulate rapidly adapting receptors whereas a maintained displacement stimulates the slowly adapting receptors.

Meissner's corpuscles and Pacinian corpuscles are rapidly acting mechanoreceptors. The Merkel cell–neurite complex and Ruffini endings are slow to adapt. Meissner's corpuscles and the Merkel cell–neurite complex corpuscles have distinct receptive fields in contrast with the Pacinian corpuscles and Ruffini endings whose fields are indistinct.

Hair follicle units are rapidly adapting mechanoreceptive units responding to movement of the hairs.

Nociceptors. These respond to damaging or potentially damaging stimuli, such as mechanical (cutting, pinching, pricking), chemical (insect bites, experimental application of various substances) and thermal (intense heat or cold). Some nociceptors may respond to mechanical stimuli with little or no

response to thermal or chemical stimuli, whereas others respond to both mechanical and thermal stimuli [3].

Thermoreceptors. There are two kinds of thermoreceptors: those which respond to warming and those which respond to cooling. *Warmth receptors* are probably innervated by non-myelinated axons and are active at constant skin temperatures of 33–35 °C, firing regularly and with an increasing rate as the temperature rises to 45 °C. Cold receptors in humans respond to static temperatures over a range from about 15 to 35 °C.

The skin can appreciate a whole range of sensations and these include light or deep touch and pressure, temperature variation, pain of many types and itch of varied intensity. With the exception of centrally generated sensations (e.g. those from a phantom limb and those produced by drugs) such sensations are interpretations by the brain of information arising in the cutaneous sense organs [18].

Stimulation of single cutaneous axons innervating mechanoreceptors produces the following sensations. Stimulation of the rapidly acting units produce sensations of tapping, Pacinian corpuscle unit stimulation produces vibration or tickle and stimulation of some slowly reacting units pressure. The frequency of the afferent impulses in stimulated axons determines the characteristics of the sensation, e.g. increasing the rate of stimulation of the slowly adapting units results in an increasing sensation of pressure. Attempts to activate single axons innervating nociceptors produced, on the whole, sensations of a painful character [18].

Cutaneous hyperalgesia (increased sensitivity of the skin to pain). This is often present after skin damage or during inflammation [21]. Cutaneous nociceptors may be more easily triggered by heat damage to their receptive fields [9] when they become much more sensitive to mechanical and thermal stimuli and respond to stimuli that were previously ineffective.

The hyperalgesia of inflammation is probably produced by pain-producing mediators from damaged tissue. Such mediators include histamine, serotonin, bradykinin, prostaglandins and leukotrienes. It is a common observation that pain spreads and several possibilities may explain this phenomenon. An axon reflex may be involved [19] or the mechanism may be a central one involving facilitation between neurones in the spinal cord [12]. Substance P, a kinin-like polypeptide, is present in some fine-diameter afferent nerve fibres and may be an important factor in cutaneous hyperalgesia as well as the erythralgia that accompanies it [14]. A central mechanism for cutaneous hyperalgesia resulting from local skin damage seems less likely but cannot be excluded.

Spinal pathways [2]. From neurological experience it is known that the sensation of fine discriminative touch and vibration, together with the sense of position of muscles and joints, is carried by fibres entering the dorsal root which pass into the dorsal columns of the spinal cord to terminate in the gracile and cuneate nuclei in the medulla oblongata. The cruder and less discriminative component of touch, together with temperature sensation, ascends in fibres in the lateral column of the spinal cord, forming the spinothalamic tract. These incoming fibres in the sensory nerve root, mediating primitive sensation, immediately relay to second-order neurones in the substantia gelatinosa of the spinal cord before crossing to the opposite side. Those fibres carrying pain and temperature cross immediately in the same spinal segment, whereas those transmitting touch ascend one or two segments before crossing and joining the opposite spinothalamic tract. It is this separation of fibres entering the spinal cord that is responsible for the dissociated sensory loss encountered in patients with focal spinal cord lesions such as syringomyelia.

The essential basis of this division of incoming fibres is an evolutionary and phylogenetic one. The pain and temperature pathway belongs to an older system in premammals; this unmyelinated system served all the somaesthetic requirements of such an animal. To the older system was added the more efficient myelinated system, also in the lateral column. In mammals a third system of even larger fibres—the dorsal column—appeared in order to provide the abundant accurate afferent information specifically devoted to proprioceptive and manipulative sensations, as well as to fine touch. These tracts are all well developed in the higher mammals.

Autonomic nerves and the skin [13]. The autonomic nervous system is embryologically and phylogenetically a specialized part of the peripheral nervous system which is essentially motor in function. Like the somatic sensory system and the pigmentary system, it arises from a specialized part of the embryonic ectoderm situated between the neural plate and the somatic ectoderm (the neural crest).

In many lower animals the autonomic effector system controls the dispersion of pigment, the circulation of blood through the skin (a respiratory function in the frog) and the flow of blood in the somatic muscles. However, this neural homeostatic function is by no means confined to the body surface and muscles. Together with its specialized endocrine tissue the adrenal medulla (which reinforces the activities of the sympathetic system), the autonomic nerves exert a stabilizing influence and, in times of stress, a stimulating action on both the cardiovascular and the respiratory system. By increasing the cardiac rate and blood pressure the autonomic nervous system controls many of the mechanical aspects of the internal environment and so is of considerable importance to the well-being of the organisms, both at rest and under stress.

The autonomic nervous system is divided into two physiologically distinct components, the sympathetic and the parasympathetic, which to a large extent act in mutual antagonism. The postganglionic fibres of the sympathetic system release noradrenaline, i.e. they are adrenergic, and those of the parasympathetic system release acetylcholine, i.e. they are cholinergic. In man there is one exception: the sweat glands, although having sympathetic drive, have acetylcholine as a postganglionic mediator. In mammals, these systems have become—at least in part—anatomically distinct, and many internal organs have a dual innervation. For example the heart is accelerated by a sympathetic nerve and slowed by a parasympathetic nerve, the cardiac depressor branch of the vagus.

In the skin the sympathetic system plays a major role in that it controls vascular tone, and pilomotor and sudomotor activity. The part played by cholinergic fibres in vasodilatation is controversial. Some researchers, denying the existence of anatomically distinct parasympathetic fibres, have nevertheless assigned a role to so-called sympathetic cholinergic fibres or to 'antidromic', i.e. dorsal root, vasodilator fibres. Others have suggested a role for vasodilator polypeptides known to be secreted by the sweat glands [13].

In general the sympathetic system comes into action at times of stress, although it is now known that there are always a few volleys of sympathetic impulses travelling to the skin, particularly in the extremities. At all times it is concerned with temperature regulation. The α fibres of the system are concerned particularly with the maintenance of blood pressure and the prevention of heat loss by the skin, whereas β function is concerned with the perfusion of muscle, cardiac acceleration and bronchial dilatation.

The fibres of the sympathetic nervous system travel to the skin with the peripheral cutaneous nerve trunks and filaments. These autonomic nerve fibres are postganglionic, emanating from cells in the sympathetic ganglia alongside the spinal cord. The parasympathetic nerve supply to the skin is more controversial and complex. Certainly, active vasodilator fibres are present in some areas of the skin, but the results of experiments are often difficult to interpret because the passive vasodilatation that results from loss of sympathetic tone may closely resemble active vasodilatation due to parasympathetic action.

The parasympathetic nerves are undoubtedly of considerable importance in the pathogenesis of several rare syndromes in which there is aberrant regeneration of parasympathetic fibres into previously damaged sympathetic channels [8]. Certain regional variations in the distribution and function of autonomic nerves are encountered. The circulation within distal parts of the limbs, the nose and the ears is characterized by the existence of many highly specialized arteriovenous anastomoses (glomus bodies), which are innervated by both sympathetic and parasympathetic fibres. These glomera are therefore subject to fine tonal control by the antagonistic fibres, sympathetic impulses provoking vasoconstriction and parasympathetic stimulation increasing the amount of blood flowing through the glomus bodies.

The large surface area of the skin of the trunk represents a considerable vascular pool and the vascular tone of this region is intimately concerned with the control of blood pressure via the carotid sinus reflex. Sudomotor activity of the trunk and proximal parts of the limbs is responsible for the loss of heat by evaporation. However, this function of maintaining a constant body temperature is subservient to the more important one of conserving the systemic blood pressure.

The triple response. This is the well-known physiological triphasic response which follows stroking pressure on the skin and is the result of the coordinated interaction of cellular, vascular and neural factors.

After firm stroking, a transient blanch, which lasts only momentarily, is followed by the first phase, which begins with active vascular dilatation precisely confined to the line of pressure. After only 30 s this well-marginated erythematous line becomes anoxaemic. It is known with certainty that this initial phase of vasodilatation is the result of liberation of histamine from the mast cells that are found in the dermis. The second phase is characterized by the appearance of a peripheral, bright red flare due to arteriolar dilatation. This may extend for several centimetres on either side of the now distinctly cyanotic initial line. This bright halo, called the axon flare, is due to an axon reflex mediated through the peripheral nerve filaments. The final phase is the appearance of a linear weal along the line of pressure.

Apart from mechanical stimulation, the triple response can be elicited by a wide variety of physical and chemical agents. Freezing with carbon dioxide snow, a localized thermal injury, certain polypeptides (e.g. kinins) and insect bites all induce this characteristic sequence of events.

In some patients with atopic or contact dermatitis, and in subjects with erythroderma, whatever its cause, firm stroking will produce not a triple response but a white appearance at the point of pressure, termed white dermographism. It is debated whether this white reaction is due to vasoconstriction or to local oedema blanching the blood vessels [26]. The demonstration of white dermographism may be of some help in suggesting the possibility that a patient may be atopic. The axon reflex is likewise absent when the terminal cutaneous filaments of the sensory nerves in the skin have undergone degeneration. This is encountered in the later stages of any peripheral nerve injury and is found in anaesthetic areas in tuberculoid leprosy. Conversely, the axon flare is often enhanced in skin which has undergone sympathetic denervation, because of the absence of vasoconstrictor tone. The autonomic axon reflex is a combined sudomotor and pilomotor response dependent on intact autonomic fibres in the skin. Mechanical, chemical, thermal, electrical and pharmacological stimuli may act on the afferent limb of the axon reflex causing a sudomotor (acetylcholine-mediated) response around the periphery of the traumatized zone. Thus, intradermal injection of 1×10^{-5} acetylcholine causes localized sweating and pilomotion around the injection site. A higher dilution causes only a direct pharmacological effect upon the sweat glands with sweating within the area of injection.

Cutaneous disorders with combined peripheral sensory and autonomic nerve damage show loss of both the sensory response and the autonomic triple response (e.g. tuberculoid leprosy). In naevus anaemicus there is loss of triple response. The reason for this naevus is sustained adrenergic vasoconstriction; it thus represents a physiopharmacological abnormality rather than an anatomical naevus [10].

REFERENCES

1 ANDRES K. H. & VON DURING M. (1973) In *Handbook of Sensory Physiology* Vol. II. *Somatosensory System.* Ed. Iggo A. New York, Springer.

2 Bishop G. H. (1960) In *Cutaneous Innervation*. Ed. Montagna W. Oxford, Pergamon.

3 Burgess P. R. & Perl E. R. (1973) In *Handbook of Sensory Physiology*. Vol. II. *Somatosensory System*. Ed. Iggo A. New York, Springer.

4 Burke D. R. A., *et al.* (1975) *J Neurol Neurosurg Psychiatry* 38, 855.

5 Cauna N. (1966) In *Touch, Heat and Pain* (Ciba Foundation Symposium). Eds. de Reuck A. V. S. & Knight J. London, Churchill.

6 Cauna N. (1973) *J Anat* 115, 277.

7 Chambers M. R., *et al.* (1972) *Q J Exp Physiol* 57, 417.

8 Cunliffe W. J. (1967) *Br J Dermatol* 79, 519.

9 Fitzgerald M. & Lynn B. (1977) *J Physiol* 265, 549.

10 Greaves M. W., *et al.* (1970) *Arch Dermatol* 102, 172.

11 Hallin R. G. & Torebjork H. E. (1973) *Exp Brain Res* 16, 309.

12 Hardy J. D., Wolff H. G. & Goodell H. (1952) *Pain Sensations and Reactions*. Baltimore, Williams & Wilkins.

13 Herxheimer A. (1960) In *Cutaneous Innervation*. Ed. Montagna W. Oxford, Pergamon.

14 Hokfelt T., *et al.* (1976) *Brain Res* 100, 235.

15 Iggo A. (1977) *Br Med Bull* 33, 97.

16 Iggo A. & Muir A. R. (1969) *J Physiol* 200, 763.

17 Konietzy F. & Hensel H. (1975) *Pflügers Arch* 359, 265.

18 Konietzy F., *et al.* (1981) *Exp Brain Res* 42, 219.

19 Lewis T. (1942) *Pain*. New York, MacMillan.

20 Loewenstein W. R. & Mendelson M. (1965) *J Physiol* 177, 377.

21 Lynn B. (1977) *Br Med Bull* 33, 103.

22 Merkel F. (1875) *Arch Mikrosk Anat (und Entwicklungsmech)* 11, 636.

23 Ochoa J. & Torebjork E. (1983) *J Physiol* 342, 633.

24 Ozeki M. & Sato M. (1965) *J Physiol* 180, 186.

25 Pinkus F. (1904) *Arch Mikrosk Anat (und Entwicklungsmech)* 65, 121.

26 Ramsay C. (1969) *Br J Dermatol* 81, 37.

27 Vallbo A. B., *et al.* (1979) *Physiol Revs* 59, 919.

CUTANEOUS LESIONS IN ORGANIC DISEASE OF THE CENTRAL AND PERIPHERAL NERVOUS SYSTEM

Organic brain disease may be associated with cutaneous bullae [4]. Bullous eruptions have been described in epidemic encephalitis [3] and as a sequel to prefrontal leucotomy [7]. The seborrhoeic facies of chronic encephalitic Parkinsonism is well documented although the mechanism is unknown [2].

Syringomyelia [1, 5, 6]. This is a chronic disorder characterized by the presence of long cavities, surrounded by gliosis, in the central part of the spinal cord, frequently extending up into the medulla (syringobulbia). The principal clinical features are areas of cutaneous analgesia and thermoanaesthesia, often with preservation of the appreciation of light touch and postural sensibility but with muscular wasting and trophic changes, especially in the upper limbs. Symptoms of corticospinal tract degeneration in the lower limbs are common. Loss of sweating or excessive sweating may occur, usually over the face and upper limbs. Sweating may be spontaneous or may be excited reflexly when the patient takes hot or highly seasoned food. Trophic changes in the skin include cyanosis, hyperkeratosis and thickening of the subcutaneous tissues, leading to a swelling of the fingers. The analgesia often renders the patient exceptionally liable to minor injuries which heal slowly; gangrene rarely occurs.

Also seen occasionally is a combination of progressive pain loss, perforating ulcers, loss of soft tissue, and resorption of the phalanges with muscular atrophy (Morvan's syndrome). However, such changes may also occur in leprosy and the hereditary sensory neuropathy.

REFERENCES

1 Barnett H. J. M., Foster J. B. & Hudgson P. (1973). In *Syringomyelia* (Major Problems in Neurology Series) Ed. Walton J. N. London.

2 Haxthausen H. (1932) *Acta Derm Venereol (Stockh)* 13, 408.

3 McLardy T. (1950). *J Neurol Neurosurg Psychiatry* 13, 106.

4 Robertson E. E. (1953) *Br Med J* i, 291.

5 Thrush D. G. & Foster J. B. (1973) *J Neurol Sci* 20, 381.

6 Walton J. N. (1981) *Brain's Diseases of the Nervous System*, Oxford, Oxford University Press.

7 Ziegler L. H. & Osgood C. W. (1945) *Arch Neurol Psychiat Chicago* 53, 262.

SPINA BIFIDA [1–5]

The various forms of spina bifida are due to incomplete closure of the vertebral canal, which is usually associated with a similar anomaly of the spinal cord or, when less severe, with other less striking intraspinal abnormalities.

Aetiology. In the early embryo the nervous system is represented by the neural groove, the lateral folds of which unite dorsally to form the neural tube. An arrest in this process of development leads to defective closure of the neural tube, associated with a similar defect in the closure of the bony vertebral canal. Several varieties of spina bifida are described, differing with respect to the nature and severity of the spinal defect. In the severe form a sac protrudes through the vertebral opening and yields an impulse on crying and coughing. In the least severe cases there is no protrusion but a defect in the lamina may be palpable as a depression which is sometimes covered by a dimple or tuft of hair (spina bifida occulta).

Clinical features. Spina bifida occulta may not give rise to any symptoms and may be an accidental discovery in the course of a routine examination. In such cases a careful history often shows that symptoms were present at an early age, though improvement may have occurred to be followed by a relapse in early adult life due to disproportionate growth between the vertebral column and spinal cord. This results in undue tension upon the lower end of the cord and cauda equina. The neurological symptoms are those of a chronic lesion of the cauda equina; frequently one function is more conspicuously affected than others.

The patient was often slow in learning to walk and walked clumsily at first. Sensation may be impaired over the cutaneous areas innervated by the lowest sacral segments, leading to the characteristic saddle-shaped area of analgesia over the buttocks and posterior surface of the thighs. Trophic changes are conspicuous in some cases, and are rarely altogether lacking. In milder cases the feet are usually cold and cyanosed, and cutaneous injuries are slow to heal and tend to ulcerate, not only on the feet but also in the analgesic skin of the buttocks and thighs.

The severest neurological abnormality is that of a flaccid paraparesis with sphincter paralysis; diagnosis here is easy. Radiography shows defective fusion of the laminae in the affected region, usually the first sacral and fifth lumbar. Myelography may be necessary. Estimation of α-fetoprotein in the amniotic fluid or in the maternal serum may successfully identify a fetus with a severe malformation of the central nervous system such as spina bifida cystica or anencephaly.

Treatment. This is usually in the domain of the paediatrician and the neurologist but the dermatologist may be asked for advice on the trophic ulcers (see p. 2238).

REFERENCES

1 ALLAN L. D., *et al* (1973) *Lancet* ii, 522.
2 BROCK D. J. H., *et al* (1974) *Lancet* i, 767.
3 CAMPBELL S., *et al* (1975) *Lancet* i, 1065.
4 JAMES C. C. M. & LARSMAN L. P. (1967) *Lancet* ii, 1277.
5 SPILLANE J. D. (1975) *An Atlas of Clinical Neurology.* London, Oxford University Press.

TABES DORSALIS [1–3]

The principal symptoms of tabes are readily interpreted as a result of degeneration of the afferent fibres of the dorsal roots. Pain and paraesthesiae are attributable to irritation of the degenerating sensory fibres. Sensory loss, i.e. analgesia and impairment of postural sensibility and vibration sense, is due to interruption of the corresponding sensory fibres.

Usually sensory symptoms, especially pain, precede ataxia by months or years. Pain is the most characteristic early symptom and usually takes the form of so-called lightning pains. Paraesthesiae are not uncommon, especially in the lower limbs. Painful sensibility is also impaired early, the deep tissues becoming insensitive to pain before the skin. Cutaneous sensibility to light touch, heat and cold is usually unimpaired at first, but finally there may be a diffuse loss of all forms of sensibility extending over the whole of the body.

The commonest trophic change in the skin is the perforating ulcer, usually seen beneath the pad of the great toe or at other pressure points on the sole. The first stage is an epidermal thickening resembling a corn, and, either spontaneously or as a result of attempts to cut it away, an indolent ulcer develops. Sometimes a sinus extends deeply as far as the underlying bone and bony disorganization and deformity may then result. Symptomatic herpes zoster may occur, as in other conditions affecting spinal dorsal roots.

REFERENCES

1 BROWN W. J. (1971) *J Infect Dis* 124, 428.
2 SPILLANE J. D. (1975) *An Atlas of Clinical Neurology.* London, Oxford University Press.
3 WALTON J. N. (1981) *Brain's Diseases of the Nervous System.* Oxford, Oxford University Press.

INJURIES OF THE SPINAL CORD [1–3]

The spinal cord may be injured directly by penetrating wounds, such as stabs or gun-shot wounds, in which case it may be penetrated by a missile or by fragments of bone. More frequently in civil life the spinal cord suffers indirectly as a result of injuries to the vertebral column, either fractures, dislocations, or fracture-dislocations. The commonest sites of spinal injury in civil life are the lower cervical region and the thoracolumbar junction.

Seborrhoea and seborrhoeic dermatitis have been reported in quadriplegia patients. The face and scalp are affected and the onset usually occurs in the first month after injury. Dryness of the skin—particularly noticeable on the soles—is the effect of anhidrosis. Chronic decubitus ulceration can be a problem: local osteomyelitis can rarely lead to secondary amyloidosis. Excellent nursing, prevention of pressure and attention to the general health of the patient are essential. The recent development of new patient aids, such as net beds and flotation pads, helps considerably to reduce the pressure. The management of the ulcer itself is as described for other cutaneous ulcers (Chapter 32).

REFERENCES

1 COMARR A.E. (1958) *J Indian Med Assoc* **5**, 2274.
2 KURTZKE J. F. (1975) *Exp. Neurol* **48**, 163.
3 REED W. B., *et al* (1961) *Arch Derm.* **83**, 379.

PERIPHERAL NEUROPATHIES— SENSORY NEUROPATHIES [1–7]

Peripheral neuropathies may in functional terms be motor, sensory or mixed but it is only those with a predominantly or exclusively sensory component which interest the dermatologist since such a patient usually has recurrent acral skin ulcers and a history of repeated injuries that may progress to substantial deformity before the correct diagnosis is made.

Such patients may complain of their extremities feeling 'numb', 'lifeless' or 'dead', or of a vague discomfort specified as 'burning', 'aching' or 'tenderness'. Some neuropathies also affect the autonomic nervous system and in addition to postural hypotension, blurred vision and sphincter problems the patients may notice areas of hypohidrosis. Sometimes it is difficult to be certain whether a patient has autonomic damage or not, and objective measurement of sweating may clearly demonstrate areas of reduction.

Sensory neuropathies are either acquired or congenital. The onset of an acquired peripheral neuropathy is usually obvious to the adult patient who can perceive the change and verbalize his or her problem. Diseases associated with the acquired neuropathies include diabetes mellitus, carcinoma, nutritional deficiencies, alcoholism and the action of cytotoxic drugs, chloroquine, indomethacin, isoniazid, metronidazole and nitrofurantoin.

Some of the congenital sensory neuropathies, of which there are several subgroups, may be genetically determined; they may be manifest at birth or develop in childhood or later.

Hereditary sensory neuropathy (syn. Thévénard syndrome; familial acro-osteolysis; ulceromutilating acropathy). This is a rare familial disorder characterized by the appearance in childhood or early adult life of analgesia of the lower limbs with neurotrophic sequelae and often associated with nerve deafness.

TABLE 60.1. The differential diagnosis of hereditary sensory neuropathy

	Congenital indifference to pain	Congenital sensory neuropathy	Thévénard syndrome	Neuritic amyloidosis	Peripheral polyneuropathy
Aetiology	?Focal cortical agenesis	?Agenesis of sensory ganglion cells	Sensory ganglion cell degeneration	?Amyloid involvement of vasa nervorum	Diabetes, carcinoma, nutritional deficiencies, alcohol, drugs, heavy metals, idiopathic (15%)
Inheritance	Not familial	Not familial	Familial	Familial	Not familial
Age of onset	Congenital	Congenital	15–30 yr	20–40 yr	Any age
Clinical features					
Neurological					
Cornea	Analgesia	Analgesia	Normal	Normal	Normal
Hearing	Normal	Normal	Often deafness	Often deafness	Normal
Pain	Analgesia	Analgesia	Analgesia	Analgesia	Analgesia
Tactile, thermal sensation	Normal	Anaesthesia	Anaesthesia	Anaesthesia	Anaesthesia
Motor function	Normal	Normal	Normal	Impaired	Impaired
Tendon reflexes	Normal	Absent	Absent	Absent	Absent
Sympathetic function	Normal	Normal	Often impaired	Often impaired	Often impaired
Cutaneous					
Axon reflex	Present	Absent	Absent	—	Rarely absent
Trophic ulcers	Rare	Often	Often	Often	Rare
Myelinated fibres	Present	Absent	—	—	Usually present
Osseous					
Fractures	Rare	—	Occasionally	—	Rare
Neuropathic joints	Often	Often	Often	—	Rare
Osteolysis	Often	—	Often	—	Rare

The inheritance is of autosomal recessive type but sporadic cases occur. The cause is unknown, but the basis is a hereditary degeneration of certain of the craniospinal ganglia. The sensory neurones that connect centrally with the spinothalamic tract are particularly affected.

Clinical features. The age of onset is commonly between 15 and 30 yr. The sensory loss is first noted in the lower limbs, and pain and temperature sensations are predominantly affected. Half the patients develop a painless ulcer, especially on the plantar aspect of the large toe, and bilateral foot ulceration is common. Osteoporosis with osteolysis and shortening of the foot is characteristic; in a few cases spontaneous amputation of a digit, without any associated trophic ulceration, has been reported. Trophic lesions have eventually appeared on the fingers in about half the reported cases.

Differential diagnosis. The differential diagnosis from syringomyelia, Morvan's syndrome, leprosy, neuritic amyloidosis and other sensory syndromes is given in Table 60.1.

REFERENCES

1 Bogaert L. van (1953) *Acta Neurol Psychiat Belg* **53**, 90.
2 Card I. & Calnan C. D. (1976) *Clin Exp Dermatol* **1**, 91.
3 Moschella S. L. & Wire G. E. (1966) *Arch Dermatol* **94**, 449.
4 Murray T. J. (1973) *Brain* **96**, 387.
5 Ohta M. et al (1973) *Arch Neurol* **29**, 23.
6 Stanley R. J., et al (1975) *Arch Dermatol* **111**, 760.
7 Thévénard A. (1942) *Rev Neurol (Paris)* **74**, 193.

Congenital pain asymbolia [1]. This is a very rare sensory disorder resulting from a defect in pain perception probably due to a lesion in the region of the parietal lobe; acquired pain asymbolia sometimes results from a tumour in this region.

In both congenital indifference to pain and congenital pain asymbolia, symptoms usually present during early childhood. Trophic ulcers may appear on the heels and pressure-bearing areas of the foot.

An acute abdominal crisis, such as appendicitis, is unaccompanied by pain; fractures of the limbs may first present with deformity or a limp because of the absence of pain sensation.

REFERENCE

1 Winkelmann R. K., et al (1962) *Arch Dermatol* **85**, 325.

Congenital indifference to pain [1, 2]. In some individuals the threshold to pain may be raised; in others the subjective threshold may be within normal limits and yet there may be a high tolerance, so that the subject is indifferent to stimulation which a normal person would regard as painful. In this type of generalized analgesia, sensations apart from pain are normal and all the nerve-endings and sensory fibres connecting to the spinal pathways are apparently normal and functioning.

There are several reports of chromosomal changes in patients with congenital analgesia. The cause is unknown.

REFERENCES

1 Becak W., et al (1964) *Acta Genet Statist Med* **14**, 133.
2 Thrush D. C. (1973) *Brain* **96**, 369.

Congenital sensory radicalopathy and neuropathy [1–3]. This is a very rare disease in which the peripheral nerve endings and myelinated fibres mediating the sensation of pain and often other modalities are absent from the skin.

Aetiology. The cause of this disorder is uncertain, but the sensory spinal ganglia either degenerate or fail to develop during fetal life. A genetically determined defect in differentiation and migration of neural crest elements in early embryogenesis is postulated.

Clinical features. All sensations of pain, temperature and touch are disturbed, although there may be islands of normal sensitivity. There are also variations in the degree of loss of each modality. The cornea is anaesthetic and all the deep reflexes are absent, but motor function is normal. Because of the lack of peripheral nerves in the skin the axon reflex component of the triple response does not appear. The sensory defect may not be noticed for some time but affected children are liable to develop multiple abrasions and burns when they begin to crawl. Painless damage to an ankle joint with resulting deformity of the foot may be a presenting feature.

Diagnosis. The differential diagnosis from other congenital analgesias is shown in Table 60.1. Confusion with epidermolysis bullosa occurs because the lesions occur on traumatized areas. Repeated infections in children may raise the possibility of a congenital agammaglobulinaemia, and the large gaping wounds of Ehlers–Danlos syndrome may cause diagnostic difficulties.

Treatment. These children require careful handling, and the padding of areas liable to trauma may be helpful. When they grow older, explanation, education and protection from injury are important.

REFERENCES

1 BOURLOND A. & WINKELMANN R. K. (1966) *Arch Neurol* 14, 223.
2 OHTA M., *et al* (1973) *Arch Neurol* 29, 23.
3 PERSON J. R. & ROGERS R. S. (1977) *Arch Dermatol* 113, 954.

Post-herpetic syndrome. Zoster is a viral infection of the dorsal root ganglia resulting in degeneration of the sensory nerve; in severe cases regeneration may be incomplete. Unfortunately, post-zoster symptoms are common in elderly patients. One investigation [1] has shown that the duration of the pain increases with the severity of the rash as well as with the age of the patient. A common dysaesthesia is pain which may be spontaneous or provoked by changes in temperature. This 'post-herpetic neuralgia' is sometimes extreme in severity, interfering with sleep and the patient's well-being sufficiently to cause suicidal tendencies. Some patients notice itching in the affected area at night, whilst others complain of a tingling sensation. When the facial skin is affected, the tingling may be provoked by exposure to sunshine and is accompanied by vasodilatation. In mild and moderate cases commonplace analgesics help but in severe cases analgesics are almost useless [4] and interruption of the pain fibres may be required. In spinal zoster, division of the affected dorsal root or tractotomy affords relief. In trigeminal zoster, alcohol injection of the ganglion or sensory root is unreliable. There is evidence that a combination of oral amitriptyline and perphenazine is of most help. Carbamazepine (Tegretol), 200 mg three or four times a day, can be most useful, however. Therapy may have to be continued for many months. There is evidence both for and against the use of local injections of triamcinolone with or without procaine. An expensive form of treatment is prolonged self-administered electrical stimulation from a portable apparatus [3]; such therapy helps about one-third of patients but its mechanism is uncertain.

Many patients with recurrent herpes simplex notice a prodrome of itching but less often herpes simplex is preceded or accompanied by a more diffuse neuralgia-like pain [2].

REFERENCES

1 BAMFORD J. A. C. & BUNDY C. A. P. (1968) *Med J Aus* i, 524.
2 LAYZER R. B. & CONANT M. A. (1974) *Arch Neurol* 31, 233.
3 NATHAN P. W. & WALL P. D. (1974) *Br Med J* iii, 645.
4 WALTON J. N. (1981) *Brain's Diseases of the Nervous System.* Oxford, Oxford University Press.

Trigeminal trophic syndrome [1–7]. Trophic ulceration, commonly beginning in the ala nasi, follows minor trauma to anaesthetic skin within the trigeminal area.

Aetiology. Neurotrophic changes in the trigeminal area follow disease, injury or operation, which destroys fibres conveying pain and temperature sensations. Thus, in leprous trigeminal neuritis erosion of the ala nasi may be found. Facial anaesthesia from interference with sensory function in the brain stem is encountered with occlusion of the posterior inferior cerebellar artery, and syringobulbia may also result in cutaneous ulceration. The ulceration may follow herpes zoster or destruction of the sensory fibres in the Gasserian ganglion with alcohol in an attempt to relieve intractable facial pain. Such patients suffer a permanent total anaesthesia over the affected area of the face, cornea and nasal mucous membranes.

Trauma is an important contributory factor in the production of neurotrophic ulceration. Pronounced paraesthesiae may cause the patient to touch the anaesthetic skin. Sensations include burning, itching, crawling and tickling, and the nose and face may be constantly traumatized by rubbing, picking and scratching. In elderly patients a compulsion for picking may be present. Bleeding may be troublesome enough to produce an iron-deficiency anaemia.

Clinical features. A small crusted area appears, followed by a crescentic ulcer which may extend to destroy the nasal cartilage and slowly spreads towards the cheek and upper lip. The upper lip may be drawn up by a band of scarring, and bleeding may be troublesome. Characteristically the tip of the nose is spared. In rare instances the forehead, scalp and malar region show trophic ulceration. This form of ulceration is particularly intractable and, although painless, often causes considerable distress. The clinical similarity to basal cell epithelioma may be striking, since neurotrophic ulcers show little inflammatory reaction. The pattern of ulceration may be sufficiently bizarre to suggest dermatitis artefacta. Similar ulceration of the ala nasi without anaesthesia has been reported in individuals with chronic postencephalitic Parkinsonism.

Treatment. Therapy should aim at preventing trauma and controlling secondary infection that occasionally complicates the ulceration. A plastic prosthesis is useful as protection. If necessary oral iron supplements should be given.

REFERENCES

1 ECKER A. & PARL A. (1965) *J Neurol Neorosurg Psychiatry* **28**, 65.
2 FREEMAN A. G. (1966) *Br J Dermatol* **78**, 322.
3 HOWELL J. B. (1962) *Arch Dermatol* **86**, 442.
4 KARNOSH L. J. & SHERB R. S. (1940) *JAMA* **115**, 2144.
5 KREBS A. & KUSKE H. (1963) *Schweiz Med Wochenschr* **93**, 1687.
6 ROSENBERG S. J. & STOBAY J. (1931) *Arch Dermatol Syphil* **39**, 825.
7 SAVITSKI M. & ELPERN S. P. (1948) *Arch Neurol Psychiat Chicago* **60**, 388.
8 SPILLANE J. D. & WELLS C. E. C. (1959) *Brain* **82**, 391.

NEUROTROPHIC ULCER [1–4]

SYN. ANAESTHETIC ULCER, PERFORATING ULCER

This is a form of chronic ulceration that develops in anaesthetic skin. It is characteristically painless, persistent and non-inflammatory and appears on areas subject to trauma or pressure.

Aetiology. The essential factors are loss of pain sensation and trauma. Other influences such as interference with the triple response, with autonomic function and with presumed neurotrophic impulses may be of importance.

Some of the neurological disorders responsible for trophic ulceration have already been described and include syringomyelia, spina bifida, tabes dorsalis, spinal cord injuries, hereditary sensory neuropathy, neuropathies, congenital pain asymbolia and congenital indifference to pain.

In one series of 47 patients diabetes complicated by peripheral neuropathy was the most frequent cause of neurotrophic ulcers of the foot. Neurotrophic ulcers on the feet are seen particularly on the pressure-bearing areas, under the heads of the metatarsals and on the heel, from friction and abrasion of badly fitting shoes and from ill-advised treatment of corns. Neurotrophic ulcer of the tongue following lingual nerve block has been described [2].

Clinical features. The denervated skin often shows hyperkeratosis, usually diffuse but occasionally localized in the form of callosities, and is anhidrotic. All injuries heal slowly. The neurotrophic ulcer often begins as a hyperkeratotic and fissured area which becomes infected. A sinus may then develop. Within the ulcer, necrotic material is seen and when the underlying bone is affected small sequestra may be present. The location of the neurotrophic ulcer is determined by trauma, the local topography and the nature of the underlying neurological disorder. Osteoporosis is frequently associated with sensory impairment. On the foot a sinogram may be required to show communication of the sinus with a joint or a subplantar fascial abscess.

Although usually painless, deep sensation may remain intact and referred pain can be present in an anaesthetic ulcer.

Treatment. This is often unsatisfactory, but, particularly in younger patients considerable benefits can be obtained. Efforts should be made to relieve pressure, to control infection and to ensure if possible the return of normal sensation. Education about and protection from unfelt trauma is essential and the provision of individually made shoes can be of considerable help, as can occlusive dressings provided that the ulcer is clean. When the association of ischaemia is present, improvement of the circulation will sometimes initiate healing in elderly patients.

REFERENCES

1 KELLY P. J. & COVENTRY M. B. (1958) *JAMA* **168**, 388.
2 MATIS C. S. (1969) *Oral Surg* **28**, 172.
3 PRICE J. (1965) *Gerontol Clin* **7**, 115.
4 ZAMUDIO L. (1963) *Dermatol Rev Mex* **7**, 3.

OTHER CUTANEOUS MANIFESTATIONS OF PERIPHERAL NERVE ORIGIN

Section or severe contusion of a peripheral nerve has been held responsible for a variety of cutaneous changes. Injury to the lateral femoral cutaneous nerve during appendicectomy [3] was followed 6 days later by the development of bullae on the outer aspect of the right lower leg with subsequent ulceration and scarring. Bullae of the fingertips and nail dystrophy may occur in the carpal tunnel syndrome [1]. Nail dystrophy and other trophic changes are also sometimes caused by a cervical rib [2].

REFERENCES

1 PFISTER P.R. (1954) *Hautarzt* **5**, 440.

2 RUBIN L. C. & CIPOLLARO A. C. (1949) *Arch Dermatol Syphil* **39**, 430.
3 WAGNER W. (1957) *Dermatol Wochenschr* **136**, 971.

CUTANEOUS LESIONS IN DISEASES OF THE AUTONOMIC NERVOUS SYSTEM

The effects of the sympathetic system [3]. When the sympathetic supply of the skin is interrupted, erythema results because of loss of vasoconstrictor impulses reaching the blood vessels. There is passive vasodilatation and the denervated area is anhidrotic. The skin may be noticeably dry with scaliness and fine fissures. The affected area heals only slowly following minor trauma, and some patients complain that the skin is hyperaesthetic. It has been shown that following sympathetic ganglionectomy there can be dissociation of sudomotor and pilomotor activity [1]. In the denervated areas there is no loss of cutaneous sensation and the phenomenon may be due to the regeneration of postganglionic cholinergic fibres. In general, the areas of vasodilatation correspond to the areas of anhidrosis, suggesting a close correspondence of sudomotor and vasoconstrictor fibres [4]. Measurement of sweating and vasomotor response can help to determine the extent of autonomic denervation in such disorders as autonomic neuropathy [2].

When sympathetic denervation is combined with loss of somatic sensation, as for instance in peripheral nerve injury or severe peripheral neuropathy, neurotrophic ulcers may be encountered. These result from local minor trauma and are characteristically painless and slow to heal.

Post-traumatic sympathetic dystrophy is a complex syndrome not infrequently encountered following injury to sympathetic fibres. It usually affects a limb and is characterized by one or several of the following features: (1) prolonged pain (causalgia), (2) vasomotor disturbances including post-traumatic oedema, (3) trophic changes in the skin, and (4) trophic bone changes (Sudeck atrophy).

REFERENCES

1 BROWN G. E. & ADSON A. W. (1929) *Arch Neurol Psychiatry* **22**, 322.
2 HOPKINS A., et al (1974) *Lancet* **i**, 769.
3 MUNRO P. A. G. (1959) *Sympathectomy; An Anatomical and Physiological Study with Clinical Applications.* Oxford, Oxford University Press.
4 SILVER A., et al (1963) *J Invest Dermatol* **40**, 243.

Horner's syndrome [1, 3]. This is a disorder characterized by ptosis, myosis and sometimes eno-phthalmos, anhidrosis and vasodilatation of the affected side of the face, resulting from unilateral paralysis of the sympathetic fibres of the face.

Aetiology. The fibres responsible for the sympathetic nerve supply to the skin of the face travel from the hypothalamus via the spinal cord to relay at the level of the first and second thoracic segments in the lateral column of the spinal grey matter. The preganglionic fibres emerge from the cord in the anterior rami of the first and second thoracic spinal nerves and pass up the cervical sympathetic chain to relay in the superior cervical ganglion. From here postganglionic fibres pass to supply the eye and the skin of a small central area of the face via the internal carotid sympathetic plexus. Other fibres pass along the external carotid artery and its branches to innervate the greater part of the facial skin with vasomotor and sudomotor fibres.

This long and vulnerable pathway can be irritated or interrupted centrally in the spinal cord by vascular disease, syringomyelia, multiple sclerosis or intraspinal tumours. The more peripheral fibres may be damaged by aortic aneurysm, cervical lymphadenopathy, wounds in the neck, cervical surgery, regional anaesthetic procedures or tumours or cannulation of neck vessels [2–6]. In all these cases, whether of central or peripheral causation, Horner's syndrome is usually complete and unilateral. An internal carotid aneurysm or fracture of the base of the skull interrupts only those fibres passing into the orbit, leaving those mediating sweating to the greater part of the face intact. Conversely, lesions affecting the external carotid fibres will leave intact pupillary function whilst interfering with the vascular control and sweating of the face.

Clinical features. An initial irritative phase is described, but rarely seen, in which there is transient unilateral hyperhidrosis and vasoconstriction. The well-known paralytic phase is characterized by ptosis with narrowing of the palpebral fissure, constriction of the pupil, absence of sweating on the affected side of the face and passive vasodilatation. Cases of bilateral Horner's syndrome are rarely encountered.

Treatment. Treatment should be directed to the cause. Unfortunately, this is rarely amenable to therapy. Occasionally, as when following prolonged exaggerated intra-operative lateral flexion of the neck, full recovery is possible [4].

REFERENCES

1 CRAIG J. D. & FULLER R. C. (1948) *Br Med J* **i**, 1182.
2 DAVIS P. & WATSON D. (1982) *Anaesthesia* **37**, 587.

3 GERBER H. & MAAR K. (1977) *Anaesthesist* **26**, 357.
4 JAFFE T. B. & McLESKY C. H. (1982) *Anesthesiology*, **56**, 49.
5 ROWLAND PAYNE C. M. E. (1981) *J.R. Soc Med* **74**, 814.
6 SKAREDOFF M. N. & DATTA S. (1981) *Can Anaesth Soc J* **28**, 82.

Causalgia [1–4]. Causalgia is a sensory disorder usually characterized by a persistent burning sensation, which may be associated with disability and other neurological symptoms. It follows injury to a peripheral nerve containing sensory fibres, but damage to the sympathetic nervous system is also essential. Sometimes oedema, muscular atrophy and osteoporosis are associated.

Aetiology. The disorder follows damage to a peripheral nerve, either by incomplete division or by involvement in scar tissue. The pathogenesis is uncertain but is variously attributed to (a) a breakdown in insulation that causes a 'short-circuit' between postganglionic sympathetic fibres and the sensory nerve travelling from the skin, (b) direct injury to sensory nerves or (c) ischaemia or hyperaemia. Causalgia most commonly follows injury of the median or sciatic nerve or arises in the divided fibres in an amputation stump when the pain is referred distally into the phantom limb. It has also been reported with cervical spondylosis [5].

Clinical features. The upper limb is more frequently affected than the lower. Causalgia may follow penetrating wounds, operations or fractures. The pain begins at the time of injury in about 50% of cases. It is hot and burning in character and is confined to the territory of distribution of the affected nerve. Although continuous it is aggravated by emotional upset and changes in skin temperature. Burning pain is a prominent feature but no longer an essential element in the diagnosis and application of the term causalgia. The burning pain is the most common symptom but is only a part of a spectrum of post-traumatic disabilities. The patient uses the affected extremity less and, after a period of time, this results in muscle atrophy, trophic changes in the skin and demineralization of the bones. Aside from the pain and disuse, other signs of sympathetic dysfunction such as flushing, redness, alterations in temperature, sweating and oedema are seen.

Treatment. Only when the focus of therapy is the sympathetic nervous system is treatment successful. Many patients obtain symptomatic relief from interruption of the sympathetic fibres. This may be achieved by surgical ganglionectomy, local anaesthetic blocking of the paravertebral ganglia by direct infiltration or pharmacological interruption with adrenergic blocking agents. Transcutaneous nerve stimulation may be of help to 40% of patients. Oral guanethidine sulphate may also help [5]. Physiotherapy is essential to improve mobility. In some instances direct infiltration of local anaesthetic into the affected nerve provides relief. In resistant cases spinal cordotomy should be considered and, in rare instances, prefrontal lobotomy may be justified although the response may not be satisfactory.

REFERENCES

1 CASTEN D. F. & BETCHER A. M. (1955) *Surg Gynecol Obstet* **100**, 97.
2 McNEILL R. A. (1963) *Br Med J* ii, 536.
3 O'CONNER F. M. (1958) *Arch Dermatol* **78**, 314.
4 SPEBAR M. J., *et al* (1981) *Am J Surg* **142**, 744.
5 TABIRA T., *et al* (1983) *Arch Neurol* **40**, 430.

Gustatory hyperhidrosis (see p. 1889). The autonomic nervous system has a propensity for regrowth [3]. All postganglionic sympathetic fibres are adrenergic except for the sudorific fibres which are cholinergic. Damage to adjacent preganglionic parasympathetic (cholinergic) fibres and postganglionic sympathetic (cholinergic) fibres may result in parasympathetic fibres regrowing into the sympathetic fibre nerves and thereby directly controlling sweat gland function. In the neck, for example following damage to the sympathetic cervical trunk and vagus (parasympathetic) at the time of thryroidectomy or following trauma, this re-innervation may result in gustatory hyperhidrosis even after eating bland foods [2]. Similarly such an event may occur on the cheeks or chin following surgery to the parotid or submandibular gland, the so-called auriculotemporal syndrome or Frey syndrome [1].

Fortunately topical preparations such as saturated aluminium chloride hexahydrate preparations can often control these symptoms well but may themselves produce an irritant dermatitis.

REFERENCES

1 BLOOR K. (1958) *Br Med J* ii, 1295.
2 CUNLIFFE W. J. & JOHNSON C. E. (1967) *Br J Dermatol* **79**, 519.
3 MURRAY J. G. & THOMPSON J. W. (1957) *J Physiol* **135**, 133.

FAMILIAL DYSAUTONOMIA
SYN. RILEY–DAY SYNDROME [2–5]

This is a rare, viscerocutaneous disease in which there is a combined defect of autonomic, motor and sensory function. Its cause is unknown but it is seen more frequently in Jews and often has a recessive inheritance.

The patient has a characteristic facial appearance. The eyes are almond shaped with a mongoloid slant, the ears large and low set, and the chin pointed. A diagnosis is sometimes made in infancy because the child cries without producing tears; normal babies usually commence lachrymation at the age of 6 weeks.

Blotchy erythema of the face is usual and hyperhidrosis, particularly on the trunk, is common. There is often acrocyanosis of the extremities.

Recurrent vasomotor attacks are common as are acute respiratory distress, abdominal distension and a marked opisthotonic posture, followed by a period of pallor and unresponsiveness.

Corneal analgesia is common and may lead to ulceration. Multiple skin abrasions and ulceration are often seen and the deep reflexes are diminished or absent. Painless arthropathy of the knees is recorded [1].

Treatment. There is no satisfactory treatment. The use of cholinergic blocking agents, atropine or propantheline, would seem logical, and where pulmonary infection is a problem antibiotics should be used to control the infective process.

REFERENCES

1 BRUNT P.W (1967) *Br Med J* iv, 277.
2 DANCIS J. & SMITH A.A. (1966) *New. Engl. J. Med.* **274**, 207.
3 FELLNER M.J. (1964) *Archs Derm.* **89**, 190.
4 GOLSTEIN-NIEVIAZHSKI C. & WALLIS K. (1966) *Adv. Ped.* **206**, 188.
5 RILEY C.M., et al (1949) *Pediatrics, Springfield*, **3**, 468.

SOME DISORDERS AFFECTING THE FACIAL VESSELS

An uncommon group of disorders of uncertain aetiology affect the face. They probably result from an abnormal and paroxysmal discharge of nerve impulses via the autonomic nervous system.

Ciliary neuralgia or 'cluster headaches' [2]. A unilateral and periorbital headache is accompanied by lachrymation with conjunctival injection, nasal congestion and unilateral flushing of the face. The attacks are paroxysmal and sometimes Horner's syndrome is found on the affected side. Ergotamine often proves effective in treating these attacks.

Hypertensive diencephalic syndrome [3]. This paroxysmal disorder is characterized by excessive sweating and blotching of the skin of the face and neck, with salivation, tachycardia and sustained hypertension. These cases require careful assessment and screening for a possible phaeochromocytoma. The Riley–Day syndrome, if occurring in an adult, might also produce such a constellation of symptoms.

Sphenopalatine syndrome [1]. In this disorder there is chronic and intermittent oedema of the face associated with lachrymation on the affected side. In addition, unilateral rhinitis and paroxysms of swelling alternating with erythema affecting the side of the bridge of the nose are sometimes seen.

REFERENCES

1 FEGELER F. (1953) *Hautarzt* **4**, 315.
2 HARRIS W. (1926) *Neuritis and Neuralgia.* London, Oxford University Press.
3 PAGE J. (1935) *Am J Med Sci* **190**, 9.

FLUSHING REACTIONS

The well-known phenomena of blushing and flushing [10, 11] are dependent on transient vasodilatation and are caused by emotional, autonomic or endocrine influences or by the direct action of vasoactive chemicals on dermal blood vessels. Blushing characteristically affects the face, upper chest and epigastric areas and rarely involves other areas such as the buttocks. Frequently no sharp distinction is possible between blushing and flushing, but many distinguish blushing by its emotional provocation and equate flushing with events which are less stress related.

Many aspects of the physiology and pathology of flushing are incompletely understood. Studies are required to clarify the physiology of the autonomic nervous system in the skin with particular attention to the substances acting as chemomediators [9].

Flushing reactions are most frequently seen on the face since the cutaneous vessels are most numerous at this site. In addition neural control of vascular smooth muscle is probably qualitatively different on the face; active control of facial blood vessels is vasodilator rather than vasoconstrictor

TABLE 60.2. Anatomical classification of flushing reactions

Cortex	Emotional (blushing)
Hypothalamus	Oral thermal induced Menopausal
Vasomotor centre (medulla)	Ethanol induced?
Sympathetic nerves	Auriculotemporal syndrome Gustatory flushing
Vascular smooth muscle	Nicotinic acid induced Carcinoid Nitroglycerin induced

TABLE 60 3. Causes of flushing

Widespread
Physiological
    Emotional: anger, guilt
    Menopausal
Drugs: amyl nitrite, bromocriptine, dipyridamole, histamine, hydrallazine, L-dopa, nicotinic acid, reserpine, theophylline, thyrotrophin-releasing hormone and urographic contrast media
Pathological
    Carcinoid tumour: intestinal, bronchial
    Phaeochromocytoma (adrenaline-producing type)
Zollinger–Ellison syndrome
Hereditary angio-oedema

Localized
Physiological
    Triple response, reflex
Pathological
    Urticarial
    Facial
        Rosacea, 'fever flush'
        Auriculotemporal syndrome
        Sphenopalatine syndrome
        Ciliary neuralgia
        Riley–Day syndrome
    Acral
        Erythromelalgia
        Post-Raynaud's attacks

[3]. Table 60.2 provides an anatomical classification of flushing reactions.

A convenient clinical classification of blushing and flushing is shown in Table 60.3.

Emotional flushing [2, 5, 6, 8]. The dermatologist may be confronted with patients who complain about chronic blushing. These patients are often timid and inhibited in social contacts and situations. They dare not express their feelings for fear of disapproval from others, and so they bottle up their emotions and begin to feel inferior. In social situations these patients react with autonomic vasomotor responses, including facial erythema [1].

Based upon their social fear, which expresses itself in symptomatic erythema, a second form of fear often develops, namely the fear of becoming red (erythrophobia), generating a second conditioning process in which the erythrophobia becomes an emotional response. Thus blushing exacerbates the anxiety in a secondary way since the symptom itself embarrasses the patient.

A lack of ability to express emotions is the basic problem, and therapy has to be directed towards learning to experience, to accept and to express the inhibited emotions such as anger, discontent, aggression, friendliness or affection towards other people. Instead of escaping from the situation by not expressing emotions, the patient is trained to behave more frankly in the face of rising fear and thus to overcome it. This method is called assertive training [4]. It has been tentatively proposed that an adrenergic neuro-effector mechanism in the superficial facial veins may be involved [7].

REFERENCES

1 BAR L. A. J. & KUYPENS B. R. M. (1973) *Br J Dermatol* **88**, 591.
2 CALNE D., *et al* (1974) *Br Med J* iv, 442.
3 GONZALEZ G., *et al* (1975) *J Neurosurg* **42**, 696.
4 JAFFE B. M. (1973) *J Clin Invest* **52**, 398.
5 JERNTORP P., *et al* (1980) *Diabetologia* **19**, 286.
6 McDOWELL F., *et al* (1970) *Ann Intern Med* **72**, 29.
7 MELLANDER S., *et al* (1982) *Acta Physiol Scand* **114**, 393.
8 MULLEY G. P. (1978) *J R Coll Physicians Lond* **12**, 359.
9 RYAN T. J. (1973) *The Physiology and Pathophysiology of the Skin*. Ed. Jarrett A. New York, Academic Press, Vol. 2.
10 WILKIN J. K. (1980) *Arch Dermatol* **116**, 598.
11 WILKIN J. K. (1981) *Ann Intern Med*, **95**, 468.

Menopausal and postmenopausal flushing [5]. Hot flushes are the commonest menopausal symptom, affecting at least 70% of women [7, 8] and causing considerable distress. The flushes may last for only a few weeks—but they may persist for years. Hot flushes rarely occur in men.

A hot flush is a vascular phenomenon which is difficult to study, both because of the rapidity of the circulatory response and because women who claim they flush frequently may not always do so in the laboratory. Nevertheless, an appreciable rise in blood flow in the hand coincides with the onset of symptoms [6], the increased flow being sustained over 3 or 4 min and then falling to control levels 6–7 min after symptoms have abated. Forearm blood flow and the pulse rate rise simultaneously but to a lesser extent and for a shorter time, falling to control levels while hand flow is still raised. The blood pressure remains unchanged during the flush. The pattern of circulatory response during the flush (which indicates a substantial increase in blood flow in the skin), the sensation of increased heat, the sweating and the fact that women often feel warmer after the menopause than before (even if they do not experience hot flushes) suggest a disturbance of thermoregulation at this time, although the aetiology is unknown.

Gonadotrophins have been implicated in the genesis of the flush. Their concentration is raised in menopausal women, and oral oestrogens both alleviate menopausal flushing and induce a fall in gonadotrophin concentrations. However, there is no correlation between the severity of the flushes and gonadotrophin concentrations in individual women or between the alleviation of symptoms by oestrogens and the extent of the reduction they induce in gonadotrophin levels. Flushes may continue unabated in menopausal women [1] and may even be induced in premenopausal women [3] after the administration of a gonadotrophin releasing hormone agonist.

Treatment, then, remains empirical. Oestrogens—natural or synthetic—reduce the severity and frequency of attacks in most women. They also improve the associated chronic sleep disturbances [4]. Their precise mode of action is unknown. The addition of a progestogen, given for part of the month to ensure regular withdrawal bleeding and so limiting endometrial hyperplasia, may be associated with unacceptable side effects. Women intolerant of oestrogens, or in whom they are contraindicated, may be helped by compounds which influence vascular responsiveness. Clonidine—an alpha agonist—may reduce the severity of the hot flushes [2]. A beta blocker such as propranolol may also help and may be given in conjunction with the clonidine.

In both men and women, therefore, a reduction in sex steroids consequent on gonadal failure may herald the onset of the vasomotor dysfunction characterized by the climacteric hot flush. Is the signal for the initiation of these flushes a fall in the dominant sex steroid for the gonad in question? Or might it be lack of another, as yet unidentified, compound common to both ovary and testis and in whose absence activity of the hypothalamic centres regulating temperature is disturbed?

REFERENCES

1 CASPER R. F. & YEN S. S. C. (1981) *J Clin Endocrinol Metab* **53**, 1056.
2 CLAYDEN J. R., *et al* (1974) *Br Med J* i, 409.
3 DeFAZIO J., *et al* (1983) *J Clin Endocrinol Metab* **56**, 445.
4 ERIK Y., *et al* (1981) *JAMA* **245**, 1741.
5 GINSBURG J. (1983) *Br Med J* **287**, 242.
6 GINSBURG J., *et al* (1981) *Br J Obstet Gynaecol* **88**, 925.
7 McKINLAY S. M. & JEFFREYS M. (1974) *Br J Preventive Soc Med* **28**, 108.
8 THOMPSON B., *et al.* (1973) *J Biosoc Sci* **5**, 71.

Alcohol-induced flushing. This is common especially in the Chinese and Japanese [6–9]. Certain subjects develop facial flushing from one particular brand of gin, vodka or lager. This abnormal response has been associated with genetically determined differences in alcohol and aldehyde dehydrogenase isoenzymes [2, 3] and is therefore probably due to individual differences in alcohol metabolism. A dominant inheritance has been suggested [4, 7]. The symptoms appear only after blood alcohol exceeds a certain threshold level ($20 \text{ mg}/10^{-2}$) [9]. In patients who are socially incapacitated a combination of H_1 (chlorpheniramine) and H_2 (cimetidine) antagonists helps by reducing the rate of alcohol absorption [9]. However, studies on alcohol-induced flushing using fermented alcoholic beverages such as sherry or beer can be criticized on the grounds that these may also contain vasoactive substances such as tyramine or histamine [10]. Drinking alcohol after exposure to several industrial chemicals produces an 'aldehyde syndrome' with severe flushing and sometimes urticaria and itching. Such chemicals include trichloroethylene, N-butyraldoxine and dimethylformamide. Some diabetics on chlorpropamide or tolbutamide [1, 5] develop facial flushing following modest alcohol intake. This phenomenon may be a dominantly inherited trait [1]; it is mimicked by an enkephalin analogue with an opiate-like activity and is blocked by naloxone [5]. Flushing aggravated by alcohol is seen also with Antabuse and metronidazole [5]. Allergic contact dermatitis from tetramethylthiuram sulphide used in rubber, in certain soaps and as an agricultural fungicide flares up following the ingestion of alcohol.

REFERENCES

1 BARNETT A. H., *et al* (1981) *Br Med J* ii, 939.
2 GOEDDE H. W., *et al* (1980) *Enzyme* **25**, 281.
3 HARADA S., *et al* (1981) *Lancet* ii, 982.
4 JERNTORP P., *et al* (1980) *Diabetologia* **19**, 286.
5 LESLIE R. D. G., *et al* (1979) *Lancet* i, 997.
6 MULLEY G. P. (1978) *J R Coll Physicians Lond* **12**, 359.
7 SCHWITTERS S. Y., *et al* (1982) *Behav Genet* **12**, No. 3.
8 de SILVA N. E. *et al* (1981) *Lancet* i, 128.
9 TAN O. T., *et al* (1982) *Br J Dermatol* **107**, 647.

10 WILKIN J.K. (1983) *Recent Advances in Dermatology* Eds. Rook A.J. & Maibach H.I. Edinburgh, Churchill Livingstone, Vol. 6.

Glutamate-induced flushing. Monosodium glutamate in large doses causes a transient increase in an acetyl-like substance which is responsible for the 'Chinese restaurant syndrome' [2]. Atropine suppresses the flush. As with alcohol the reaction may reflect an inherited sensitivity [3]. Since the reaction may be associated with a delayed onset (12 h or more) of asthma, testing for such flushing should be performed in hospital [1].

REFERENCES

1 ALLEN D.H. & BAKER G.J. (1981) *N Engl J Med* **305**, 1154.
2 GHADIMI H., *et al* (1971) *Biochem Med* **5**, 447.
3 REIF-LEHRER L. (1976) *Fed Proc* **35**, 2205.

Nitrite- and Metabisulphite- induced flushing [1, 2]. Sodium nitrite is common in cured meat products such as frankfurters and salami, and sulphites added as preservatives; both chemicals may uncommonly induce flushing, headache and asthma.

REFERENCES

1 HENDERSON W.R. & RASKIN N.H. (1972) *Lancet* **ii**, 1162.
2 STEVENSON D.D. & SIMON R.R. (1981) *J Allergy Clin Immunol* **68**, 26.

Capsaicin and flushing [1-3]. Red peppers, which contain capsaicin, may induce flushing. This could be due to a direct stimulation of the cutaneous blood vessels or involve substance P through mechanisms (possibly central) which are controversial.

REFERENCES

1 CARPENTER S.F. & LYNN B. (1981) *Br J Pharmacol* **73**, 755.
2 HÄGERMARK O. (1981) *J Invest Dermatol* **77**, 250.
3 THERIAULT E., *et al* (1979) *Brain Res* **170**, 209.

Drug-induced flushing. Most vasodilator drugs such as trinitrin may cause flushing [4]. Nicotinic-acid-induced flushing is probably mediated by prostaglandins [5] and can be blocked by indomethacin and aspirin. Bromocriptine, adenosine, 3'-5'-monophosphate, tamoxifen, thyrotrophin-releasing hormone, cyproterone acetate and cyclosporin have also all been recorded as producing flushing [1-3].

REFERENCES

1 CALNE D.B., *et al* (1974) *Br Med J* **iv**, 442.
2 LEVENE R.A., *et al* (1968) *Clin Pharmacol Ther* **9**, 168.
3 McFARLAND K.F., *et al* (1982) *Arch Intern Med* **142**, 132.
4 WILKIN J.K. (1983) *Recent Advances in Dermatology*. Eds. Rook A.J. & Maibach H.I. Edinburgh, Churchill Livingstone, Vol. 6.
5 WILKIN J.K., *et al* (1982) *Clin Pharmacol Ther* **31**, 478.

Histamine flushing. Histamine flushes can be provoked by therapeutic agents and histamine-releasing drugs. Large amounts of histamine are found in sherry and red wine, less in white wine, beer and port, and none in whisky and cognac, which are distilled [1]. A variety of circumstances produces flushing in patients with mast-cell disease (see p. 1719).

Similarly, extensive urticaria pigmentosa, particularly in children, may be associated with flushing attacks. The erythematous areas are variable in size and sometimes itch. Histamine release is induced by extensive friction to large areas. Associated symptoms include headache (histamine cephalgia), and the urinary excretion of histamine may be increased. Both H_1 and H_2 blockers may modify histamine flushing induced by alcohol.

REFERENCE

1 WILKIN J.K. (1983) *Recent Advances in Dermatology* Eds. Rook A.J. & Maibach H.I Edinburgh, Churchill Livingstone, Vol. 6.

Carcinoid flushing [7-9, 11]. Carcinoid tumours are uncommon, with a prevalence of 1.5 in 10^5. The tumours arise from glandular enterochromaffin cells, some of which show amine precursor uptake and decarboxylation (APUD) [10]. APUD cells are neuro-endocrine cells in that they synthesize and release biogenic amines and low molecular weight polypeptide hormones [10]. Culture of human carcinoid cells has confirmed the ability of the tumour to synthesize, store and release both serotonin and histamine [5].

The common mediators of the carcinoid syndrome produced by the APUD cells are serotonin (diarrhoea and bronchospasm), kallikrein (flushing and bronchospasm) and histamine (occasional flushing) [3, 7, 9]. Calcitonin, ACTH-'MSH' and insulin have also been noted, and unconfirmed reports of glucagon, vasoactive intestinal polypeptides, substance P, catecholamines and prostaglandins exist [12].

Flushing occurs in 94% of patients and is now recognized to be mediated commonly by bradykinin formed after the release of lysosomal kallikrein. This

TABLE 60.4. Types of flushing

	Menopausal	Alcohol-induced	Carcinoid	Phaeochromocytoma	Histamine-induced
Pathogenesis	?Oestrogen lack Menopause Oöphorectomy	'Aldehyde syndrome' Chloropropamide Antabuse Contact dermatitis from TMTS.	?Kinins Tumour of foregut. hindgut, lung, ovary, pancreas	Catecholamine production by tumour of adrenal medulla, accessory adrenal tissue, glomus jugulare	Histaminaemia Urticaria pigmentosa Systemic mast-cell disease Wine (histamine content)
Provocative factors	Spontaneous	Alcohol	Alcohol Overbreathing Noradrenaline	Spontaneous	Certain wines Codeine
Distribution	Head, neck, chest	Head, neck, chest	Face, neck, trunk, arms, legs	Face, neck, chest, trunk	Face, neck, chest, limbs
Duration	5–15 min	15–30 min	15 min to 4 hr	15 min to 4 hr	15 min to 2 hr
Associated features	Hyperhidrosis Tremulous Depression	Urticaria Pruritus	Diarrhoea Abdominal pain Asthma	Hyperhidrosis Piloerection Hypertension	Headache
Investigations Urine	Pituitary gonadotrophin increase		5-HIAA +	VMA +	Histamine +
Treatment	Oestrogens	Avoidance of chemicals or drug exposure	Surgical	Surgical	Antihistamines

release can be provoked by alcohol, emotion, certain foods and catecholamines. Four patterns of flushing have been identified [8].

> Type I lasts less than 5 min and is a diffuse facial and thoracic erythema.
> Type II lasts 15–30 min and presents as a cyanotic flush of the upper face and thorax on a background of telangiectasia.
> Type III lasts from hours to days. It is a disabling erythema affecting the whole body.
> Type IV is transient, producing a well-demarcated 'geographic' flush with red and white areas on the neck.

Other cutaneous carcinoid manifestations include pseudopellagra [4, 13] and (pseudo) scleroderma [6]. This is usually confined to the legs. There have also been isolated reports of scarring abdominal blisters [2], atrophic scarring plaques [2], generalized pruritus, pyoderma gangrenosum, dermatomyositis and leonine facies [7, 14].

The prognosis is related not to the usual histological criteria of malignancy but to the origin of the tumour. Most patients with the carcinoid syndrome will have a midgut lesion with hepatic metastases. Five-year survival for foregut carcinoids is 87%,

midgut 54% (with the exception of appendiceal tumours which have a 99% 5-yr survival) and hindgut 83% [7]. Unusual origins of the tumour include the testis [1].

The pharmacological manipulation of tumour secretions forms the basis of therapy. Table 60.4 illustrates the drugs available and the symptoms affected. Surgery in thoracic foregut carcinoids may be curative. Enucleation of hepatic metastases has a useful role to play in bringing the patient under pharmacological control. Chemotherapy with 5-fluorouracil and streptozotocin may be indicated where tumour enlargement is rapid, symptoms are disabling and surgery is not feasible. The response is transient; death may be due to cardiac failure, secondary to cusp fibrosis, or to the metabolic sequelae of prolonged diarrhoea and flushing.

REFERENCES

1 BATES R. J., *et al* (1981) *J Urol* **126**, 55.
2 BEAN S. F. & FUSARO R. M. (1968) *Arch Dermatol* **98**, 268.
3 CALVERT H., *et al* (1963) *Postgrad Med J* **39**, 547.
4 CASTIELLO R. J. & LYNCH P. J. (1972) *Arch Dermatol* **105**, 574.
5 DEBONS-GUILLEMIN M.-C., *et al* (1982) *Cancer Res* **42**, 1513.

6 FRIES J. F., *et al* (1973) *Arch Intern Med* **131**, 550.

7 GODWIN J. D. (1975) *Cancer* **36**, 560.

8 GRAHAME-SMITH D. G. (1977) *Top Gastroenterol* **5**, 294.

9 KESSELER M. E. (1981) *Clin Exp Dermatol* **6**, 447.

10 METZ S. A. & LEVINE R. J. (1977) *Clin Endocrinol Metab* **6**, 719.

11 MULLEY G. P. (1978) *J R Coll Physicians Lond* **12**, 359.

12 SMITH A. G. & GREAVES M. W. (1974) *Br J Dermatol* **90**, 547.

13 THORSON A., *et al* (1954) *Am Heart J* **47**, 161.

14 WEISS L. & Ingram M. (1961) *Cancer* **14**, 161.

Adrenaline-secreting phaeochromocytoma. In rare instances an adrenal phaechromocytoma produces adrenaline rather than noradrenaline and the clinical manifestations include paroxysmal hypertension with fainting attacks and marked flushing.

Zollinger–Ellison syndrome. A syndrome in which a non-β-cell pancreatic tumour produces peptic ulceration from excessive gastrin secretion [4]. A proportion of cases occur in patients with other endocrine tumours—endocrine polyadenomatosis. Episodes of severe flushing and diarrhoea may be the presenting feature and may persist for 10–15 yr without their nature being detected [3]. The flushing may be due to a vasoactive intestinal polypeptide [1] or increased prostaglandin production [2].

REFERENCES

1 FAHRENKRUG J. (1980) *Clin Gastroenterol* **9**, 633.

2 JAFFE B. M., *et al* (1977) *N Engl J Med* **297**, 817.

3 MURRAY J. S., *et al* (1961) *N Engl J Med* **264**, 436.

4 ROBERTSON J. K., *et al* (1962) *Q J Med* **31**, 103.

ITCHING

Definitions

Itching is the expression in consciousness of the cutaneous sensations that tend to evoke the motor response of scratching or rubbing. The apparent purpose of this reflex action—the scratch reflex—is the removal of noxious agents from the body surface.

Pruritus and itching are synonymous but when used as a diagnostic term pruritus signifies that itching is the primary and presenting complaint unaccompanied by any visible causative lesion of the skin.

Itchy skin is the term applied when the threshold to pruritogenic stimuli is lowered. Itchy skin may surround the area to which an itch stimulus has been applied and may persist when spontaneous itching has ceased.

General considerations [4]. Pruritus is the outstanding sensory feature of many skin diseases. The motor response it evokes, if not controlled, leads to further damage often with perpetuation and intensification of the unpleasant symptom (the scratch–itch cycle). The perception of pruritus may lead to emotional changes so that the entire experience is apt to be a complex one. The severity of pruritus, as of pain, depends upon the intensity of the peripheral stimulus, the integrity of the nervous pathways and the state of awareness of the sensory cortex. Like pain, when intense, pruritus tends to dominate the sensory cortex at the expense of other sensations.

Inherent in the problem of pruritus is its subjective and elusive nature, difficult to quantify for accurate investigation. The tendency to itch varies from person to person and this is borne out by everyday experience of the variability of pruritus in such common dermatoses as pityriasis rosea and psoriasis. However, the presence or absence of itch, and its severity, are of diagnostic value in many dermatoses. Since itching is subjective the physician is dependent on what the patient tells him, aided by the presence or absence of signs of scratching and rubbing such as excoriations, broken hairs and polished or bevelled nails.

The pharmacology of itching [10]. The presumption is that peripheral chemomediators are first liberated by a wide variety of stimuli and that these complex substances acting on the plexus of fine free nerve-endings at the dermo-epidermal junction elicit the distinctive cutaneous sensation of itching. Many pharmacologically active chemicals are known to be capable of this [7], and of these histamine has received most attention. It is distributed widely throughout the human body and causes itching when introduced exogenously or released in the skin; elevated levels have been recorded in pruritic disorders such as atopic eczema [9] and aquagenic pruritus [6]. Both H_1 and H_2 receptors are found in human skin, but H_2 receptors seem to play little or no part in histamine pruritus [3]. Exogenous proteolytic enzymes, such as those in cowhage (mucunain), can cause severe itching, but the role of these enzymes in skin diseases has not yet been evaluated. Prostaglandins are known to be present in increased amounts in inflamed skin [5]. Pretreatment with prostaglandin E significantly lowers the threshold of human skin to itching evoked by histamine and papain [8]. Prostaglandins may thus potentiate pruritus in inflammatory skin disease, possibly by a non-specific effect on nerve endings.

A role for the naturally occurring opioids, the

endorphins and encephalins, as central mediators of the itch sensation has been postulated on the basis of work with naloxone, a pure opiate antagonist. Pretreatment with naloxone diminishes or abolishes histamine-provoked itch [2] and the itching induced by butorphanol, a morphine-like analgesic which does not influence plasma histamine levels [1].

REFERENCES

1 BERNSTEIN J. E. & GRINZI R. A. (1981) *J Am Acad Dermatol* **5**, 227.
2 BERNSTEIN J. E., *et al* (1982) *J Invest Dermatol* **78**, 82.
3 DAVIES M. G. & GREAVES M. W. (1981) *Br J Dermatol* **104**, 601.
4 *GILCHRIST B. A. (1982) *Arch Intern Med* **142**, 101.
5 GREAVES M. W., *et al* (1971) *Br Med J* ii, 258.
6 GREAVES M. W., *et al* (1981) *Br Med J* **282**, 2008.
7 KEELE C. A. & ARMSTRONG D. (1964) *Substances Producing Pain and Itch*. London, Arnold.
8 LOVELL C. R., *et al* (1976) *Br J Dermatol* **94**, 273.
9 RING J., *et al* (1979) *Br J Dermatol* **100**, 521.
10 *WINKELMANN R. K. (1982) *Med Clin North Am* **66**, 1119.

The physiology of itching [6]. Although extensively studied, the physiology of itching is not well understood and many questions remain to be answered. Among these is the relationship between itch and pain, both of which play important and complementary roles in evolutionary survival. Pain is the response to an intense or penetrating stimulus and will lead to withdrawal from it. A noxious stimulus of lower intensity, perhaps operating over a long period and affecting only the superficial layers of the skin, may lead to itching and an attempt to remove the stimulus by scratching.

A wide variety of such stimuli, electrical, mechanical and chemical, can act on peripheral nerve filaments to elicit itching. It is generally agreed that itch spots on the skin have no strict anatomical counterpart, being related to a greater accessibility or a lower threshold of the free nerve-endings possibly of a specific population of polymodal nociceptors in the area [7]. Impulses carrying the sensation of itch pass along the sensory spinal nerves to the spinothalamic tract and thence to the thalamus and sensory cortex. These pathways are shared by the sensation of pain, and in analgesic skin, e.g. in leprosy or congenital analgesia, no itching can usually be elicited, although there is conflicting evidence on this point [3]. However, most researchers now regard itching as a distinct sensory modality rather than as a subthreshold pain sensation. The evidence for this concept may be summarized as follows.

1. Itching can be elicited experimentally only by a stimulus in the deeper epidermis or in the region of the dermo-epidermal junction. An identical stimulus at a deeper level induces only pain.
2. Removal of the epidermis and the subepidermal nerve network abolishes itch although cutaneous pain can still be evoked.
3. Immersion of the skin in water at 40–41 °C quickly abolished itch but intensifies burning pain.
4. Both itch and pain can be experienced simultaneously.
5. Opiates and opiate antagonists have opposite effects on pain and itch.

The central projections of the itch pathway have yet to be defined fully. An itch–scratch centre in the floor of the fourth ventricle has been suggested on the basis of the results of selective brain extirpation and of injections of chemicals into the cisterna magna of experimental animals [4], the itch caused by brain tumours infiltrating that area [1], and the curious side effect of facial itching after spinal opiate anaesthesia [2, 5].

REFERENCES

1 ANDREEV V. C. & PETKOV I. (1975) *Br J Dermatol* **92**, 675.
2 BONNARDOT J. P., *et al* (1982) *Nouv Presse Med.* **11**, 673.
3 DASH M. S. & DESPANDE S. S. (1975) In *The Somatosensory System*, Ed. Kornhuber H. H. Stuttgart, Thieme, p. 94.
4 KOENIGSTEIN H. (1948) *Arch Dermatol* **57**, 828.
5 SCOTT P. V. & FISCHER H. B. J. (1982) *Postgrad Med J* **58**, 531.
6 STÜTTGEN G. (1981) *Münch Med Wochenschr* **123**, 987.
7 TUCKETT R. P. (1982) *J Invest Dermatol* **79**, 368.

Psychological aspects [4]. The literature concerning the importance of the psychological component of itching is complex and often confusing [5]. The threshold for itching varies greatly from person to person [1] and this threshold can be modified by psychological factors. Tense, irritable or anxious patients complain of itching far more frequently than placid emotionally integrated subjects. Moreover it is often observed that in the same person apparently unchanged cutaneous lesions itch more at times of tension, frustration or boredom. The association has been shown experimentally by subjecting patients to stress-provoking situations [2].

A reliable electrical method for causing a short-term itch has been used in conjunction with an estimate of recent life experiences as a measure of psychological stress [3]. Those with high stress had unaltered thresholds for itch but their above average ability to discriminate between weak and strong stimuli was taken to be part of a generalized guarding response pattern. A past history of skin disease was associated with a low itch threshold, and efficiency in detecting itch increased with experience but fell with boredom.

REFERENCES

1 Björnberg A., *et al* (1979) *Acta Derm Venereol (Stockh)* **59**, 49.
2 Cormia F. E. (1952) *J Invest Dermatol* **19**, 21.
3 Edwards A. E., *et al* (1976) *Arch Dermatol* **112**, 339.
4 Rechenberger I. (1981) *Münch Med Wochenschr* **123**, 1005.　　　　,
5 Whitlock F. A. (1976) In *Psychophysiological Aspects of Skin Disease*. London, W. B. Saunders, p. 110.

Scratching [4]. In certain animals there is a spinal reflex pathway for scratching but in man scratching demands the integrity of at least some part of the brain [9]. Scratch reflex responses and their conditioning have seldom been studied in man, but such responses are more easily induced in lichen simplex patients than in controls [6]. The length of the scratch stroke in any area approximates to the distance of two-point discrimination for touch [2]. About one person in five is conscious that scratching an itchy area may produce a sensation of itching elsewhere, this is known as 'referred itch' [3].

Scratch movements have now been assessed in a variety of ways [5, 7, 10]. The pattern of scratching is similar whatever the cause of the itch and during sleep relates to the physiology of individual sleep stages, being especially frequent in stages 1 and 2 of orthodox sleep [8]. In very itchy patients, bouts of scratching may occupy up to 10% of the night. The gate-control theory of pain perception, in which a simultaneous large fibre input is held to slow or abolish the passage of impulses from smaller unmyelinated fibres at spinal cord level, has been extended to itch to provide a neurological basis for the relief supplied by scratching.

REFERENCES

1 Aoki T., *et al* (1980) *Acta Derm Venereol* (Suppl) (Stockh) **92**, 33.
2 Cornbleet T. (1953) *J Invest Dermatol* **20**, 105.
3 Evans P. R. (1976) *Br Med J* ii, 839.
4 Hünecke P. & Bosse K. (1981) *Münch Med Wochenschr* **123**, 992.
5 Koyabashi E., *et al* (1979) *Jpn J Med Electron* **17**, 756.
6 Robertson I. M., *et al* (1975) *Br J Dermatol* **92**, 407.

7 Savin J. A., *et al* (1973) *Lancet* ii, 296.
8 Savin J. A., *et al* (1975) *Br J Dermatol* **93**, 297.
9 Sinclair D. C. (1973) In *The Physiology and Pathology of the Skin*. Ed. Jarrett A. London, Academic Press, Vol. 2.
10 Summerfield J. A. & Welch M. E. (1980) *Br J Dermatol* **102**, 275.

Clinical causes of itching

Localized pruritus. Certain parts of the body have a predilection for certain disease processes which may thus present as localized pruritus. Anogenital pruritus is considered in detail elsewhere (see p. 0000). Some important causes of pruritus in a variety of sites are given in Table 60.5. Certain dermatoses which are normally widespread may, in some instances, show particular localization, e.g. scabies localizing under a wrist-watch, and sweat retention giving rise to prickly heat under a waistband. Systemic disease is usually associated with a widespread pruritus but occasionally the symptom may be localized, e.g. the itching of the lower face and neck which may herald an attack of asthma and which is thought to be referred itch from inflamed bronchi [3]. Solar pruritus may be localized to the elbows [1, 2].

TABLE 60.5. Important causes of localized pruritus

Scalp	Eczema—especially seborrhoeic and contact, neurodermatitis, psoriasis
Eyelids	Airborne irritants or allergens; allergic reactions to make-up and nail varnish
Nose	Hayfever, intestinal worms in children
Fingers	Eczema, scabies, fowl mite infestation
Legs	Gravitational and discoid eczema, asteatosis

REFERENCES

1 Heyl T. (1983) *Arch Dermatol* **119**, 115.
2 Kestenbaum T. & Kalivas J. (1979) *Arch Dermatol* **115**, 1368.
3 Orr A. W. (1979) *J R Coll Gen Pract* **29**, 287.

Generalized pruritus

External causes. No sharp distinction can be drawn between pathological itching and what may be regarded as physiological itching in everyday life, in which slight rubbing or minor thermal changes produce itching which is scarcely noticeable. Some important itch-provoking factors include the following.

Climatic. It is certain that pruritus can result from desiccation of the stratum corneum, where the water content acts as a plasticizer. If this falls with the lowered ambient humidity of cold weather or excessive central heating the stratum corneum becomes brittle and allows minor irritants such as soap to penetrate, causing mild inflammation and itching. With increasing age the skin becomes dry and this type of itching is common. Occupational outbreaks of itchy eruptions due to warm dry air have been resolved by raising the relative humidity [8]. Cholinergic pruritus may be associated with excessive sweating. High humidity can also cause pruritus secondary to sweat retention in some individuals.

Particulate matter. Foreign bodies such as hairs, coarse glass fibres or cactus spines produce a pruritic sensation, often with a burning or tingling character. Skin scrapings treated with 20% caustic potash and examined under the polarising microscope effectively disclose the presence of glass fibres and cactus spines. Industrial exposure to powdered alumina [3] and fibreglass [9] may cause epidemics of itching.

Detergents. A pruritic dermatosis, sometimes with minimal signs, with itching particularly in the evening and at night was traced to optical brighteners used in certain washing powders in Scandinavia [5]. Dish-washing fluids used for bathing have caused generalized pruritus [7].

Aquagenic pruritus [1]. This relatively common condition is distinct from aquagenic urticaria, cholinergic urticaria and the temperature-induced pruritus of polycythaemia. Patients are otherwise well, have elevated blood histamine levels and usually respond to antihistamines. If the condition is not recognized, sufferers are liable to be labelled neurotic.

Insects and infestations. Infestation, particularly scabies, produces marked itching which is especially noticeable at night. Insect bites are pruritic and the itching often lasts for several days after the visible inflammation has subsided. Although stings are characteristically painful, during the phase of resolution itching may be noted.

Familial pruritus. The sudden appearance of pruritus in several members of a household may be caused by scabies or other mites, e.g. chicken mites, by mange from domestic pets [4] or by caterpillar hairs [2]. Such itching has been recorded [6] following contamination of clothing by fibreglass from curtains in a washing machine.

REFERENCES

1 GREAVES M. W., *et al* (1981) *Br Med J* **282**, 2008.
2 HENWOOD B. P. & MACDONALD D. M. (1983) *Clin Exp Dermatol* **8**, 77.
3 JOHANNESSEN H. (1980) *Contact Dermatitis* **6**, 42.
4 KIEFFER M., *et al* (1979) *Vgeskr Laeger* **141**, 3363.
5 OSMUNDSEN P. E. (1969) *Br J Dermatol* **81**, 799.
6 PEACHEY R. D. G. (1967) *Br Med J* ii, 221.
7 RICHARDS W., *et al* (1977) *Ann Allergy* **39**, 284.
8 RYCROFT R. J. G. (1981) *Br J Dermatol* **105** (Suppl. 21), 29.
9 VERBECK S. J. A., *et al* (1981) *Contact Dermatitis* **7**, 354.

Itching caused by skin disease. A wide variety of dermatoses are pruritic, and some of the common ones are listed in Table 60.6. As has been mentioned, pruritus is a variable symptom in many. Individual skin diseases are dealt with in the relevant chapter and will not be discussed further here. Generalized pruritus can precede some skin diseases such as pemphigoid [6].

TABLE 60.6. Some skin diseases causing itching

Severe	Moderate
Scabies, mite infestations	Psoriasis
Pediculosis, insect bites, etc.	Seborrhoeic eczema
Contact and atopic eczema	Pityriasis rosea
Urticaria and dermiographism	Sunburn
Prickly heat	Fungal disease
Lichen planus	Asteatotic skin
Dermatitis herpetiformis	Urticaria pigmentosa
Toxic eruptions	

Systemic causes of pruritus A probable relationship between generalized pruritus and systemic disease was detected in 17 of 34 patients who were sufficiently itchy to need admission for investigation and treatment [43]. Another survey of 32 adult patients found that in 13 the pruritus cleared after 2 yr and in only seven was an underlying systemic disease present [8]. It has been estimated that the prevalence of significant systemic disease in patients attending dermatologists with pruritus may be as low as 10% [39]. The list of posssible systemic causes, however, is a large one (Table 60.7).

Infectious disease. Infectious diseases, with the exception of varicella and rubella, are rarely accompanied by pruritus. However, trichinosis is frequently associated with generalized pruritus at the stage of muscle invasion by the parasite. Onchocerciasis (p. 990) may cause intense pruritus and the rupture of an echinococcal cyst into the circulation is accompanied by pruritus as well as by acute toxic symptoms. Itching is an occasional symptom of schistosomiasis. Severe generalized pruritus has been associated with localized fungal infections [1].

Metabolic disease. Pruritus is sometimes the presenting symptom of diabetes mellitus [38]. In one series [29] of 500 cases of diabetes, 16 had

TABLE 60.7. Some internal disorders causing itching

Endocrine and metabolic
    Diabetes mellitus, diabetes insipidus, myxoedema, hyperthyroidism, hypoparathyroidism
Hepatic
    Intrahepatic and extrahepatic biliary obstruction
Renal
    Chronic renal insufficiency
Blood disease and reticulosis
    Iron deficiency, polycythaemia, lymphatic leukaemia, Hodgkin's disease, mycosis fungoides, lymphosarcoma, mast cell disease
Internal malignancy
    Carcinomatosis
Tropical and intestinal parasites
    Infestation with hookworm, round worm
    Onchocerciasis, filariasis
Autoimmune
    Systemic lupus erythematosus, 'sicca syndrome'
Neurological
    Tabes, general paralysis of the insane, multiple sclerosis, brain tumours
Psychoneurosis
    Anxiety, obsessional neurosis
Pregnancy
Allergic
    Subclinical urticaria
Drugs
    Cocaine, morphine, chloroquine

generalized pruritus and 17 others localized pruritus, principally of the vulva. There is no correlation between the severity of the disease and the pruritus, although control of the diabetes usually relieves the symptoms. Pruritus is a rare accompaniment of diabetes insipidus.

Pruritus may occur in up to 8% of patients with hyperthyroidism [5]. The generalized pruritus of hypothyroidism in most cases is related to the dry scaly skin: administration of thyroxine relieves the symptom. Severe generalized itching occurring half an hour after meals has been recorded in the dumping syndrome [31]; treatment with pectin was successful.

Pregnancy. Up to 2% of pregnant women itch without an obvious dermatological cause [56]. This itching usually develops in the third trimester and is relieved on delivery. Most of these patients have minor abnormalities of liver function [23], and the presence of mild jaundice may be associated with the birth of premature babies of low birth weight [33]. The cholestasis is probably oestrogenically determined and patients may subsequently develop pruritus or jaundice with oral contraceptives.

Hepatic disease. Pruritus in liver disease is a symptom of biliary obstruction: its presence in jaundice therefore implies that this is obstructive in type.

Although pruritus has been recorded in sickle cell anaemia, in general it does not occur with the jaundice of haemolytic anaemia and only infrequently in infective hepatitis.

Generalized pruritus frequently precedes all other symptoms in primary biliary cirrhosis; later a papular or prurigo-like eruption may appear, sometimes with hyperpigmentation. Later still jaundice and xanthomas become a feature of the disease. Pruritus is one of the early symptoms of the intrahepatic biliary obstruction induced by chlorpromazine, testosterone and other drugs.

It has been widely accepted that in obstructive liver disease pruritus is related to the retention of bile salts, and, in support of this, pruritus can be evoked by their application to the base of cantharidin-induced blisters [36]. However, this theory has not been supported by recent studies in which no correlation existed between serum and skin levels of bile acids and pruritus or scratching [7, 11, 23, 24]. Nor does it explain the relief of itching with unaltered bile acid levels by phenobarbitone [25] and with raised bile acids by androgens [2]. Cholestyramine, which is helpful in cholestatic pruritus, will also promote the excretion of other organic anions, and this may explain its action in uraemic pruritus in which bile salts do not seem to be implicated. Cholestyramine is unpalatable and may aggravate steatorrhoea and fat-soluble vitamin deficiency. For this reason other treatments such as hydroxyethyl rutosides [32], phototherapy [30] and plasma perfusion [14] have been tried with some success.

Renal disease. Itching is common among patients with chronic renal failure. In a study of 237 patients undergoing maintenance dialysis 37% were found to be suffering from troublesome itching, and a further 41% had experienced this symptom in the past [27]. Itching was often most marked during or just after dialysis. As a rule itching does not accompany acute renal failure and this has cast doubt upon the role of urea itself as the cause of the symptom.

Some patients with hyperparathyroidism secondary to renal failure improve dramatically after subtotal parathyroidectomy [37] and the itching can be made to return by intravenous calcium injections. However, only a minority of uraemic patients are likely to respond to this operation and the improvement may only last a few months [25].

Other factors have also been incriminated including the dry skin of many uraemic patients [58], a proliferation of mast cells in the skin [15] and high serum concentrations of magnesium [28]. The wide variety of suggested treatments reflects a lack of precise knowledge of the nature of the pruritogenic substances. Restriction of protein intake [10], intravenous heparin [57], lignocaine [53], and oral cholestyramine, have been helpful in some cases. UV light [26,47] is probably the current treatment of choice, with the use of activated charcoal orally being a safe and cheap alternative [42].

Internal malignancy. Pruritus is an important but uncommon manifestation of carcinomatosis [46] and may occur when primary tumours invade the skin [54]. However, the prevalence of pruritus in Hodgkin's disease is much higher, perhaps about 30% [9]. It may be the first symptom, preceding the appearance of papules and melanosis. Severe itching may indicate a poor prognosis [18] and usually increases as the disease progresses. The mechanism is unknown but cimetidine may help some patients [4]. Pruritus is an uncommon presentation of chronic leukaemia but is more often encountered in the lymphatic than in the granulocytic form. Itching due to myelomatosis [17] and paraproteinaemia [59] has also been reported.

Polycythaemia. Fifty-one of 72 patients with polycythaemia reported periods with pruritus [20]. The triggering factor was usually a sudden fall in skin temperature, e.g. after a hot bath. The itching had a characteristic pricking quality and lasted for up to 60 min. Aspirin proved helpful and some patients noted improvement after treatment with phlebotomy or chemotherapy. However, treated polycythaemia may be associated with severe iron deficiency, and the pruritus of six such patients responded to iron therapy [45]. Cholystyramine [16], pizotifen [19] and cimetidine [50] have also been reported to be helpful.

Iron deficiency [49]. When a total of 23,189 men and 19,902 women were screened for iron deficiency, 0.7% of the men were judged to be iron depleted: of these 13.6% reported frequent itching; this was significantly higher than the 5.3% of itchy non-iron-deficient men. The findings were similar, though less striking, for non-iron-deficient women [52]. Iron therapy relieved the pruritus of 59 itchy patients with iron deficiency [55]. Some of these patients were not anaemic but 12 of the 13 men with the combination of a low serum iron, anaemia and pruritus developed or already had underlying neoplasia.

Neurological disease. Pruritus is surprisingly rare among the paraesthesiae of neurological disease. In some cases it is encountered in the pre-eruptive phase of herpes zoster, and a segmental pruritus may be an occasional feature of tabes dorsalis. Paroxysmal unilateral pruritus has been recorded with central nervous system lesions [35]. The activation of artificial synapses between axons lying in areas of partial demyelation may be responsible for the paroxysms of itching affecting patients with multiple sclerosis [22,40].

Thirteen of 77 patients with brain tumours described itching and in six of these, all with tumours infiltrating the floor of the fourth ventricle, the itching was ferocious and persistent but localized to the nostrils [3].

Neuropsychiatric disease [44]. All forms of pruritus, whatever the cause, may be intensified by emotional stress. Pruritus of psychogenic origin is not uncommon and its features are listed in Table 60.8. Itching as a type of tactile hallucinosis has been recorded [34].

TABLE 60.8. Characteristics of psychogenic pruritus

  1 No other cause found
  2 Either widespread or localized to a significant 'symbolic' region
  3 Intensity parallels the emotional state
  4 Rarely prevents sleep unless ano-genital
  5 Tendency to lichenify, thus presenting as lichen simplex
  6 Signs of scratching less than alleged severity suggests
  7 Deep excoriations or bizarre self-induced lesions sometimes seen and suggest psychosis
  8 Patient's symptoms often bizarre, exaggerated
  9 Frequently associated with psychoneurotic traits: coexistent multiple anomalous and exaggerated minor symptoms; suggestible; disinclination rather than incapacity to work; compensation neurosis
 10 Relieved by sedation or antipruritic drugs rather than local applications, but paradoxical exacerbations from sedatives sometimes seen

Iatrogenic pruritus. Pruritus may be a side effect of a variety of drugs including opium alkaloids, central nervous system stimulants, antidepressants and belladonna alkaloids [12]. Itching has followed the administration of hetastarch [41], niacinamide [13,57], cimetidine [51] and chloroquine [48] especially in Africans. It may be an unpleasant side effect of PUVA therapy.

REFERENCES

  1 ALTERAS I. & GRÜNWALD M. (1981) *Mykosen* **24**, 107.
  2 ALVA J. & IBER F.L. (1965) *Am J Med Sci* **250**, 60.
  3 ANDREEV V.C. & PETROV I. (1975) *Br J Dermatol* **92**, 675.
  4 AYMARD J.P. (1980) *Br Med J* **280**, 151.
  5 BARNES H.M., *et al* (1974) *Trans St John's Hosp Dermatol Soc* **60**, 59.
  6 BARRIERE H., *et al* (1981) *Ann Dermatol Vénéréol* **108**, 445.

7 BARTHOLOMEW T.C., *et al* (1982) *Clin Sci* **63**, 65.
8 BEARE J.M. (1976) *Clin Exp Dermatol* **1**, 343.
9 BLUFARB S.M. (1959) In *Cutaneous Manifestations of Malignant Lymphomas*. Springfield, Thomas, p. 534.
10 BOULTON-JONES J.M., *et al* (1974) *Lancet* i, 335.
11 BRAEUNINGER W., *et al* (1981) *Arch Dermatol Res* **270**, 445.
12 BRUINSMA W. (1973) In *A Guide to Drug Eruptions*. Amsterdam, Excerpta Medica, p. 76.
13 BURES F.A. (1980) *J Am Acad Dermatol* **3**, 530.
14 CAREY W.D., *et al* (1981) *Am J Gastroenterol* **76**, 330.
15 CAWLEY E.P. (1975) *Arch Dermatol* **111**, 1663.
16 CHANARIN I. & SZUR L. (1975) *Br J Haematol* **29**, 669.
17 ERSKINE J.G., *et al* (1977) *Br Med J* i, 687.
18 FEINER A.S., *et al* (1978) *JAMA* **240**, 2738.
19 FITZSIMMONS E.J., *et al* (1981) *Br Med J* **283**, 279.
20 FJELLNER B. & HÄGERMARK O. (1979) *Acta Derm Venereol (Stockh)* **59**, 505.
21 FREEDMAN M.R., *et al* (1981) *Am J Med* **70**, 1011.
22 FUKADA T., *et al* (1981) *Rinsho Shinkeigaku* **21**, 296.
23 GAGNAIRE J.C., *et al* (1975) *Nouv Press Med* **4**, 1105.
24 GHENT C.N. & BLOOMER J.R. (1979) *Yale J Biol Med* **52**, 77.
25 GHENT C.N., *et al* (1978) *J Pediatr* **93**, 127.
26 GILCHREST B.A., *et al* (1977) *N Engl J Med* **297**, 136.
27 GILCHREST B.A., *et al* (1982) *Arch Dermatol* **118**, 154.
28 GRAF, *et al* (1979) *Br Med J* ii, 1478.
29 GREENWOOD A.M. (1927) *JAMA* **89**, 774.
30 HANID M.A. & LEVI A.J. (1980) *Lancet* ii, 530.
31 HARRIES A.D., *et al* (1982) *Br J Dermatol* **107**, 707.
32 HISHON S., *et al* (1981) *Br J Dermatol* **105**, 457.
33 JOHNSON M.B. & BASKETT T.F. (1979) *Am J Obstet Gynecol* **133**, 299.
34 KALAMKARYAN, *et al* (1978) *Vestn Dermatol Venerol* **8**, 90.
35 KING C.A., *et al* (1983) *Ann Intern Med* **97**, 222.
36 KIRBY J., *et al* (1974) *Br Med J* iv, 693.
37 KLEEMAN C.R., *et al* (1968) *Trans Assoc Physicians* **81**, 203.
38 KNICK B. (1981) *Münch Med Wochenschr* **123**, 1197.
39 LYELL A. (1972) *Scott Med J* **17**, 334.
40 OSTERMAN P.O. (1976) *Br J Dermatol* **96**, 555.
41 PARKER N.E., *et al* (1982) *Br Med J* **284**, 1405.
42 PEDERSON J.A., *et al* (1980) *Ann Intern Med* **93**, 446.
43 RAJKA G. (1966) *Acta Derm Venereol (Stockh)* **46**, 190.
44 RECHENBERGER I. (1981) *Münch Med Wochenschr* **123**, 1005.
45 SALEM H.H., *et al* (1982) *Br Med J* **285**, 91.
46 SCHOENFIELD Y. (1977) *Dermatologica* **155**, 122.
47 SCHULTZ B.C. & ROENIGK H.H. (1980) *JAMA* **243**, 1836.
48 SPENCER H.C., *et al* (1982) *Br Med J* **285**, 1703.
49 STAUBLI M. (1981) *Schweiz Med Wochenschr* **111**, 723.
50 STAUBLI M., *et al* (1981) *Schweiz Med Wochenschr* **111**, 1394.
51 TAILLANDIER J., *et al* (1981) *Nouv Press Med* **10**, 258.
52 TAKKUNEN H. (1978) *JAMA* **239**, 1394.
53 TAPIA L., *et al* (1971) *N Engl J Med* **296**, 261.
54 TWYCROSS R.G. (1981) *Lancet* ii, 696.
55 VICKERS C.F.H. (1973) *Br J Dermatol* **89** (Suppl **9**) 10.
56 WINTON G.B. & LEWIS C.W. (1982) *J Am Acad Dermatol* **6**, 977.
57 YATZIDIS H., *et al* (1972) *JAMA* **222**, 1183.
58 YOUNG A.W., *et al* (1973) *NY State J Med* **73**, 2670.
59 ZELICOVICI Z., *et al* (1977) *Br Med J* ii, 1154.

Clinical features

Characteristics of the itch. Since itching is subjective, the patient's complaint and his reactions to his discomfort need careful analysis and interpretation. The following characteristics of the itch should be considered.

Itch severity. For practical purposes, pruritus that interferes with sleep should be regarded as severe. A patient may consciously exaggerate or unconsciously minimize his symptoms. Anxiety increases the emotional response to itching.

Itch quality. Patients differ in their ability to describe symptoms accurately—an itch may be described as tormenting or compelling as in scabies.

Time of occurrence. At night parasympathetic activity is predominant and with vasodilatation many itchy disorders tend to become worse. Nocturnal itching is characteristic of scabies. Pruritus ani in children, when due to threadworms, often wakens the child in the early hours of the morning. Night itching tending to waken the patient is usually of organic cause (Table 60.5).

Periodicity. Some patients, such as those with atopic eczema, are liable to bouts of itching which begin in a circumscribed area and with rubbing and scratching can extend to larger and larger areas of the skin surface which itch with an ever increasing severity. The scratching becomes compulsive and after several minutes the patient may develop complete psychic and somatic exhaustion.

Response to temperature changes. A change in temperature from going into a warm room, undressing or sitting close to a fire tends to aggravate itching of cutaneous origin. Itching after a bath is characteristic of, but not diagnostic of, polycythaemia, as it also occurs in aquagenic pruritus and in dermographism as a result of friction from the towel.

Localization. The causes of localized pruritus are covered on p. 2248.

Seasonal Variation. Winter pruritus with asteatosis tends to recur in the autumn, with complete freedom for weeks or months during the summer.

The effects of scratching. The physical signs seen in patients suffering from pruritus result from self-inflicted damage to the skin, and can follow scratching, rubbing, pressing, pinching or kneading, all of which give temporary relief of the itching. Severe pruritus is only relieved by severe self-trauma, which replaces itching by soreness, stinging or pain. Pruritus of central origin is poorly relieved by scratching.

Lacerative injuries are characteristic of scratching and are usually produced by the free margins of the nails, whereas abrasion is more often the result of rubbing and follows trauma inflicted by the nail plate, the soft tissues of the finger tips or the backs of the fingers. Scratching and rubbing may modify the physical signs of an itchy skin disorder e.g. in eczema the tops of papules may be removed to leave multiple small bleeding points.

The immediate effect of pure abrasive injury is the appearance of the triple response which is frequently seen in patients awaiting examination, and this urticarial element is especially important in symptomatic dermographism. Ecchymoses may follow severe rubbing but their presence should lead one to suspect an underlying haemorrhagic disease. The repeated rubbing of a localized area provokes a reactive hyperaemia. Later persistent erection of the hair follicles is seen to be followed by a finely papular lichenifaction. Fractured hair or local alopecia is visible evidence of rubbing. If rubbing continues, confluent plaques of lichenification are seen and in some subjects an eczematous inflammation appears with associated hyperpigmentation or depigmentation. In some patients with pruritic dermatoses haemorrhagic crusts are evidence of scratching or picking. Such lesions may become infected.

As a result of long-continued scratching the nail plates become highly polished and the free margin of the nail bevelled. This bevelled nail sign is helpful in assessing the severity of the pruritus because a patient may deny scratching if he is damaging the skin only whilst asleep.

Psychological reactions. No matter what the cause of the itch is, among factors which tend to influence the psychological response are the following.

1. The ability to relieve the itching by rubbing.
2. The integrity of the sensory end-organs, the conductive pathways and the perceptive centres.
3. Attention and distraction.
4. Previous experience.
5. Current emotional state.

Itching and rubbing may in some individuals be associated with pleasurable emotions (orgasme cutané) but when severe or recurrent, or prolonged and intractable, the personality of the subject may be affected. Some common reactions may be mentioned:

1. Resignation with a brave 'carry-on' attitude—a 'martyr complex'.
2. A depressive state with withdrawal and suicidal tendencies.
3. A secondary anxiety state with apprehension, anxiety, irritability and an inability to 'stand it any longer'.

Combinations of these different responses are sometimes seen but the pattern tends to become fixed in a person with chronic pruritus.

Diagnostic evaluation
History. The diagnostic analysis of pruritus requires a detailed and searching medical history. The location and extent of the itching are important: when limited to one area local causes may be responsible (p. 2248), whereas a widespread and symmetrical pruritus suggests an internal cause. Pruritus affecting only the exposed skin strongly suggests an exogenous cause, as does the simultaneous involvement of family or occupational contacts.

The characteristics of the itch itself should be explored along the lines given on p. 2252. The patient should be specifically questioned about tropical residence as certain tropical infestations such as intestinal ascariasis and onchocerciasis may have marked pruritus.

Questioning should also cover occupational exposure to pruritogenic agents such as fibreglass, cheese mites and red fowl mite and domestic exposure to external parasites such as canine scabies or *Cheyletiella parasitovorax* from a domestic cat or dog.

Clinical examination. In the well-groomed individual, parasitosis may present with minimal signs. A meticulous search may reveal scabetic lesions—a single burrow under a ring, a papule on the nipple in a female or an excoriated penile papule in a male. Any one of these may be the only sign of scabies. An excoriated burrow can easily be missed unless the likely areas are examined with a hand lens. More obvious signs may be present if the patient avoids bathing for a week. Alternatively a therapeutic trial with a scabicide will aid the diagnosis. Scabies is no respecter of persons and the diagnosis should be considered in any patient, whatever the social background, with pruritus which is troublesome at night. Likewise, excoriations in the nuchal region and over the shoulders may be the only sign of pediculosis. Body lice are easily missed unless the seams of the underclothing are closely examined.

The presence of puncture marks on the arm suggests that the subject may be a drug addict. Slight conjunctival icterus draws attention to liver disease as a cause of pruritus, and in this case other stigmata such as spider naevi may be found. In some cases scratch marks with ecchymoses and purpura raise the suspicion of a blood disease, and dryness of the skin with pruritus should suggest possible myxoedema or Hodgkin's disease. Visceral carcinoma should be suspected in elderly patients with bullous eruptions and pruritus; indeed persistent pruritus in any elderly patient should always arouse suspicion of 'occult' carcinoma.

In unexplained generalized pruritus a general physical examination is essential and is directed towards the internal disorders listed in Table 60.6. The diagnoses of psychogenic pruritus and senile pruritus should always be made with reluctance because not infrequently a systemic disease will ultimately declare itself.

Investigative procedures. When the diagnosis is not clear after taking the history and performing a clinical examination (including rectal and gynaecological examinations), certain basic screening tests are employed (Table 60.9). They often quickly

TABLE 60.9. Basic screening tests

Complete blood count, erythrocyte sedimentation rate
Liver function tests
Thyroid function tests
Urea, uric acid, acid phosphatase
Chest X-ray
Urine for albumin, glucose, cells
Stools for blood, worms, ova

indicate the type of disease present and suggest which of the many complex investigations are likely to be helpful in the diagnosis. Sometimes more detailed tests are indicated (Table 60.10).

The treatment of pruritus [1, 2, 10].
Ideally treatment should not start until the diagnosis is established; however, this may be impossible. The primary aim must be to eliminate the causative disease, whether this is a noxious chemical or a physical agent, an external parasite, overt or occult skin disease or a systemic disorder. In practice, however, the patients require treatment whilst investigations are in progress.

Local measures. Provocative influences such as friction from rough clothing, overheating and vasodilators including alcohol and hot drinks are best avoided. Short clipped nails and gloves help to reduce the skin damage from scratching. Likewise occlusive bandaging is valuable in breaking the itch-

TABLE 60.10. Further investigative procedures

Skin diseases
    Scrape for acari, glass fibres, cactus spines
    Scrape and culture for fungus
    Skin biopsy
Endocrine and metabolic disease
    Serum calcium
Liver disease
    Liver biopsy, mitochondrial antibodies
Renal disease
    Pyelogram, renal biopsy
Blood disease and reticulosis
    Serum iron, vitamin B_{12}, folate
    Marrow, lymph node biopsy
    Skeletal X-ray
    Abdominal lymphangiography
Internal malignancy
    Barium enema
    Barium meal and follow-through
    Bronchoscopy
    Liver scan
    Skeletal X-ray, laparotomy
Tropical and intestinal parasites
    Skin snip, blood and stool examination
Autoimmune disease
    Protein electrophoresis, antinuclear factor
    Rheumatoid factor, mitochondrial antibodies
Neurological disease
    Cerebrospinal fluid examination
Psychoneurotic disease
    Psychiatric assessment

scratch cycle in which repeated self-trauma is a perpetuating factor.

The local application of an evaporating shake-lotion such as calamine lotion is soothing to a non-exuding surface although it may make the skin too dry if used for more than a few days. Menthol ($\frac{1}{4}$–1%) in calamine lotion provokes a feeling of surface chilling. Topical antihistamines are the cause of contact sensitization and their use is to be condemned. Local anaesthetics, particularly those containing benzocaine and amethocaine, suffer the same disadvantage. Local corticosteroid ointments along with emulsifying baths, the avoidance of soap and the regular use of emollients also help if the skin is dry. Crotamiton ointment has a useful antipruritic action apart from its effect in scabies. Antibiotics may be needed together with antiseptic baths if secondary infection is present.

Systemic treatment. Trials of systemic antipruritic agents should fulfil certain strict criteria [3], but few have overcome the problems presented by the quantification of the subjective symptom of itching, the placebo effect and the separation of sedative from antipruritic actions [8]. For these reasons nocturnal scratching has recently been used as a measure of itching. In one study [9] both trimeprazine and trimipramine caused a modest reduction in overall scratching, but this was achieved by a reduction in the time spent awake and in stage I of orthodox sleep (when scratching occurs especially frequently) rather than by a specific antipruritic action. Nevertheless, oral antihistamine drugs are often prescribed as palliative treatment, and their sedative effects are of value [6]. Trimeprazine and hydroxyzine are often recommended but many antihistamines are available and the physician should become familiar with the dosage and side effects of a few rather than be master of none. Antihistamines may produce drowsiness but by adjusting the dosage this can be controlled. Usually babies and young children can tolerate proportionately larger doses than adults before feeling drowsy. The newer non-sedative antihistamines seem to have little effect on pruritus.

The H_2 antagonist cimetidine has been used in the treatment of a variety of itchy disorders with unconvincing results [7]. Using a linear itch scale as an index of pruritus in atopic eczema, cimetidine did not confer any therapeutic advantage when added to an H_1 antagonist [4]. The value of opiate antagonists, such as naloxone, and of transcutaneous nerve stimulation [5] has yet to be established. Very occasionally in the most severe cases the use of systemic steroids may be justifiable.

REFERENCES

1 AULEPP H. (1981) *Münch Med Wochenschr* **123**, 999.
2 CAMP R. (1982) *Clin Exp Dermatol* **7**, 557.
3 CORMIA F.E. & DOUGHERTY J.W. (1959) *Arch Dermatol* **79**, 172.
4 DAVIES M.G. & GREAVES M.W. (1981) *Br J Dermatol* **104**, 601.
5 FJELLNER B. & HÄGERMARK O. (1978) *Acta Derm Venereol (Stockh)* **58**, 131.
6 KRAUSE L. & SHUSTER S. (1983) *Br J Dermatol* **109** (Suppl. **24**), 30.
7 ROBERTS D.L. (1980) *Br Med J* **280**, 405.
8 SAVIN J.A. (1980) *Br J Dermatol* **102**, 113.
9 SAVIN J.A., et al (1979) *Arch Dermatol* **115**, 313.
10 *WINKELMANN R.K. (1982) *Med Clin North Am* **66**, 1119.

CHAPTER 61

Psychocutaneous Disorders

ARTHUR ROOK, J.A. SAVIN & D.S. WILKINSON

EMOTIONAL FACTORS IN DISEASES OF THE SKIN [2, 8]

An important area of overlap lies between psychiatry and other clinical disciplines. Many studies confirm that patients with unrecognized psychiatric morbidity often present to medical and surgical clinics [5], and dermatology is no exception to this rule. Indeed the skin has gained the reputation of responding more readily to emotional influences than any other organ of the body. Dermatology outpatients have a higher prevalence of psychiatric disorders than the general population, and dermatology in-patients have a higher prevalence than general medical in-patients [4]. It has been estimated that the effective management of at least one-third of patients attending skin departments depends to some extent at least upon the recognition of emotional factors [7], and yet, despite extensive research devoted to these problems, our knowledge of the psychodynamic and peripheral mechanisms involved is still rudimentary. The literature, though large, remains confusing.

The unfortunate popularity of the term 'psychosomatic dermatoses', often applied to the large numbers of skin conditions in which the emotions are apparently in some way concerned, has tended to obscure the fact that in only a very few, such as dermatitis artefacta, do these emotional factors play a primary and pathogenic role. Similarly, attempts to correlate specific personality profiles with specific skin diseases [9] have been of doubtful value since adequately controlled conditions are difficult to obtain [8].

The relationships between the mind and the skin are more complex than this. This chapter is concerned with delineating the interaction between two broad spectra of conditions. The first ranges from natural anxiety over disfiguring skin lesions, through disproportionate worry over minor blemishes to disturbances of body image which lead patients to become obsessed with their skin in the absence of any abnormality. The second covers the ways in which emotional reactions or psychiatric disease may trigger or exacerbate skin disease. For a further discussion the reader is referred to the recent review by Cotterill [2].

Perhaps the lines of research which are likely to prove most fruitful in this field will be those based not on standard psychological techniques but on the recent advances in biochemistry which are currently shedding new light on the mechanisms involved in anxiety, depression and itching [3]. Thus, the amines involved in the tryptophan and tyrosine metabolic pathways may be involved in depression. Agents such as pimozide are now being shown to have specific biochemical effects [6] and studies of binding sites in the brain of agents such as the benzodiazepines may lead to the discovery of endogenous agents of a similar chemical nature to these anxiolytics [1]. Similarly, advances in our understanding of the opioid receptors, the enkephalins and endorphins and their antagonists may well have far-reaching consequences in opening up a new approach to itch and its perception.

REFERENCES

1 BRAESTRUP C., et al. (1980) Proc Natl Acad Sci 77, 2288.
2 COTTERILL J.A. (1983) In Recent Advances in Dermatology, No. 6. Eds. Rook A.J. and Maibach H.I. Edinburgh, Churchill Livingstone, p. 189.
3 ECCLESTON D. (1982) Br J Hosp Med 27, 627.
4 HUGHES J.E., et al (1983). Br J Psychiat 143, 51.
5 LLOYD G. (1983) Br Med J 287, 539.
6 MUNRO A. (1983) Semin Dermatol. 2, 197.
7 SNEDDON J. & SNEDDON I.B. (1983) Clin Exp Derm 8, 65.
8 WHITLOCK F.A. (1976) Psychophysiological Aspects of Skin Disease. London, W.B. Saunders.
9 WITTKOWER E. & RUSSELL B. (1953) Emotional Factors in Skin Disease. London, Cassell.

Emotional reactions to skin disease. Disfiguring skin lesions may profoundly influence the emotional development of the child, though this is considerably affected by the attitude of the parents and, later, of schoolmates and teachers. The dermatologist's main function at this stage is to explain, to reassure as far as he can and, often, to protect the child from ill-advised interference, e.g. in the unnecessary early treatment of cavernous naevi.

With the approach of puberty, a disfiguring skin disease becomes an increasing anxiety to many children and may handicap them in developing easy relationships with the opposite sex. Some children become increasingly introspective and solitary, while others become aggressive and uncooperative. The dermatologist should interpret such behaviour with equanimity and sympathy.

However, it is impossible to generalize about the effect of such lesions; the number of variable factors is too great. With sensible and affectionate parents and intelligent teachers, children with disfiguring skin lesions will often adjust extremely well, form satisfactory sexual relationships and establish themselves in successful careers. They are blessed with the reverse of dysmorphophobia. However, until the outcome is assured, the dermatologist should not lose touch with the child or the parents.

The psychological importance of the skin [7]. Some cutaneous stimulation is probably a basic need. Newborn mammals need the stimulus of licking and stroking, and caressing favours emotional development. As an organ of touch, temperature and pain sensation and as an erogenous organ, the skin has great psychological significance at all ages. It is an organ of emotional expression and a site for the discharge of anxiety. Psychopathologically, the skin can be used for the expression of hysterical exhibitionism, for the satisfaction of masochistic impulses, and for displaced libidinal discharge. Intense physical stress may override emotional expressions, as in concentration camps or times of war, but the emotional content may recur later in a severe form [8].

The body image [3, 5]. The concept of the body as seen by the patient is of course quite different from that seen by the dermatologist unless he has the gift of being able to integrate, even temporarily, with the person who seeks his help. Our perception of the normal body image bears little relation to that of the anxious and disturbed patient whose vision of himself and his relationship with the environment may be distorted by anxiety, depression or loss of sleep due to itching [4]. In women, the face figures largely in the body image and minor skin affections of this area are a common cause of 'dermatological non-disease' (p. 2259).

Dysmorphophobia is the term given [5, 6] to a patient's excessive preoccupation with a minor complaint that he believes, without reason, to be conspicuous to others. It is a disorder of the body image and may present initially to plastic surgeons [1] and carry a poor prognosis [2]. Attempts to correlate dysmorphophobia with a particular personality type have not given consistent results [5].

REFERENCES

1 ANDREASON N. & BARDACH J. (1977) *Am J Psychiat* **134**, 673.
2 CONOLLY F.H. & GIPSON M. (1978) *Br J Psychiat*. **132**, 568.
3 COTTERILL J.A. (1983) *Dermatol Top Gen Prac* **2**, 1.
4 GADOW S. (1980) *J Med Philos* **5**, 172.
5 *HARDY G.E. (1983) *Semin Dermatol* **2**, 207.
6 HAY C.G. (1970) *Br J Psychiat* **116**, 399.
7 MUSAPH H. (1977) In *Handbook of Sexology*. Eds. Money J. & Musaph H. Amsterdam, Excerpta Medica.
8 SHARON J. (1970) *Br J Dermatol* **83**, 536.

CLASSIFICATION OF SKIN DISEASES DETERMINED OR INFLUENCED BY EMOTIONAL FACTORS

No satisfactory classification can yet be devised. The psychodynamic mechanisms involved remain largely unknown and individual variability is too complex to be assigned to compartments. The following clinical grouping may serve as a general guide, although an alternative classification [1] has much merit.

Dermatoses primarily emotional in origin
   Dermatitis artefacta
   Trichotillomania
   Cutaneous hypochondriasis; dysmorphophobia
   Delusional parasitosis
   Vulvodynia and the perineal syndrome
   Psychogenic purpura

Dermatoses aggravated or perpetuated by self-inflicted trauma
   Lichen simplex
   Acne excoriée
   Prurigo
   Auto-erythrocyte sensitization

Dermatoses due to accentuated physiological responses
   Hyperhidrosis
   Blushing

Phobic states
   Syphilophobia
   Erythrophobia
   Acarophobia, etc.

Dermatoses in which emotional precipitating or perpetuating factors may be important
Vesicular eczema of palms and soles
Atopic dermatitis in the adult
Seborrhoeic dermatitis

In a number of other common diseases the role of emotional precipitating factors is uncertain. Different views are held by different dermatologists. Proof is more elusive than opinion. Such conditions include psoriasis, where stress is believed by some to be an important provoking factor [3], some cases of generalized or localized pruritus [2], alopecia areata, aphthosis, rosacea and, perhaps, some cases of urticaria.

REFERENCES

1 MEDANSKY R.S. & HANDLER R.M. (1981) *J Am Acad Dermatol* **5**, 125.
2 MUSAPH H. (1983) *Semin Dermatol*, **2**, 217.
3 SEVILLE R.H. (1983) *Semin Dermatol* **2**, 23.

DERMATOLOGICAL NON-DISEASE

The term 'non-disease' has been introduced [5] to describe a positive concept of disease in the absence of diagnosable symptoms and signs. Although the original cases were of an endocrine nature, attention has been drawn in recent years to the dermatological aspects of non-disease [3, 6] and to the potentially fatal nature of the condition [1, 2].

Incidence. Although this is unknown, the condition is by no means uncommon though not always diagnosed. Cotterill [2] saw about 50 patients a year, compared with only one with delusions of parasitosis and 10 with dermatitis artefacta. It is more often met in private practice, and teachers and nurses appear to be unduly well represented. Marital disharmony is common [2].

Clinical features. The patients, usually female, present with a dermatological complaint, often described in strongly emotive terms, but with no significant objective disease. Three body areas are particularly involved—the face, the scalp and the perineum (the only area in which males predominate).

Face. A description of burning rather than itching is common and should alert the dermatologist to a psychosomatic cause. Imagined or greatly magnified complaints of redness or facial hair are other modes of presentation, and the patients are prone to mirror-gazing. Although many of these unhappy women suffer from dysmorphophobia [4], depression is common. One out of nine committed suicide and there was a serious risk of this in two more [1].

Scalp. Complaints of excessive hair loss account for most cases, though itching and burning may be the presenting symptoms. Depression and marital difficulties may be present among the women, but schizophrenia should be borne in mind in young men who resist all logical and reasoned arguments about their normality.

Perineal and genital regions. Pain (especially at the tip of the penis) and perineal, scrotal or vulval soreness or discomfort are common. There is no response to topical therapy. The 'perineal syndrome' and vulvodynia (Chapter 59) probably also fall into this group. Personal or social stress or anxiety may be abundantly evident.

Other areas. Glossodynia and the 'burning mouth syndrome' have been attributed to many causes. Contact dermatitis to dentures, *Candida* infection, diabetes, and folic acid and vitamin deficiencies must be excluded. However, in our experience, as in Cotterill's [2], it is rare to find an organic cause. Although it cannot be assumed that these patients necessarily fall into the group of dermatological non-disease, we believe that depression, as well as cancer phobia, plays a part in many patients. Other manifestations include excessive axillary sweating or an unusual pattern of persistent itching or burning of the skin without obvious cause.

The general behaviour of the patient before, during and after the consultation may provide valuable clues to the correct diagnosis [2].

Treatment. The management of these patients takes up a disproportionate amount of time and requires patience and expertise. Antidepressants are of less value than expected, even when depression is evident [1]. Pimozide has not been helpful [1]. Even the placebo response cannot be relied on. A good rapport, sympathy and continued contact are essential. However, the danger of suicide, especially in females with facial symptoms, is real and every effort—though often unavailing—should be made to persuade those in whom this risk seems real to see a psychiatrist.

REFERENCES

1 *COTTERILL J.A. (1981) *Br J Dermatol* **104**, 611.
2 COTTERILL J.A. (1983) *Semin Dermatol* **2**, 204.

3 ECKERT J. (1975) *Acta Derm Venereol (Stockh)* **55**, 147.
4 HAY G.G. (1970) *Br J Psychol* **116**, 399.
5 MEADOR C.K. (1965) *N Engl J Med* **272**, 82.
6 SNEDDON I.B. (1979) *Acta Derm Venereol (Stockh)* **59**, (Suppl. **85**), 177.

MONOSYMPTOMATIC HYPOCHONDRIACAL PSYCHOSIS (MHP)

This disorder has been clearly defined only in recent years [4–6, 10]. Many psychiatric patients exhibit features of undue hypochondriasis, and these must be recognized and referred to psychiatrists. Among such will be those with schizophrenia or severe depression. However, there is a small group of patients with fixed delusional states, not amenable to logical argument, in whom there is no other discernible psychiatric disorder and who appear normal in all other respects. Many of them will have the milder 'neurotic' form of the disease—dysmorphophobia [1, 2]—in which there is a disturbance of the body image, but others show an 'encapsulated' psychotic form in which the fixed delusion may be severe enough to lead to suicide. Munro [5] has defined the syndrome as 'a disorder characterized by a single delusional system, relatively distinct from the remainder of the personality. The delusion may be accompanied by illusional misconceptions, or, at times, possibly by ill-defined hallucinations.' The patients tend to be lonely and self-occupied and may have had long-standing personality problems. The delusion dominates the patient's life. He becomes 'distressed, unhappy and ashamed' [6] and makes those around him equally so. He goes from specialist to specialist in search of relief—and belief—but offers illogical reasons for refusing treatment.

Dermatologists will meet this condition most often in the form of parasitophobia, which made up three-fifths of Munro's series of 50 patients collected over 8 yr [7].

Treatment was notably unsuccessful until the advent of pimozide [9], which gave an 'excellent' response in 32 of 50 patients [6]. However, it may have to be continued in a low dose indefinitely, and the patients have a poor record of compliance. Insomnia, depression and extrapyramidal side effects may require adjuvant corrective therapy. Further studies have confirmed the value of this drug [3, 8].

REFERENCES

1 HARDY G.E. (1982) *Br J Psychol* **141**, 181.
2 HAY G.G. (1970) *Br J Psychol* **116**, 399.
3 KRASS M.E. (1981) *Can Med Assoc J* **124**, 968.
4 MUNRO A. (1980) *Br J Hosp Med* **24**, 34.
5 MUNRO A. (1982) *Delusional Hypochondriasis*, Monograph Series No. 5. Toronto, Clarke Institute of Psychology.
6 MUNRO A. (1983) *Semin Dermatol* **2**, 189.
7 MUNRO A. & CHMARA J. (1982) *Can J Psychol* **27**, 374.
8 REILLY T.M., et al. (1978) *Br J Dermatol* **98**, 457.
9 RIDING J. & MUNRO A. (1975) *Acta Psychiat Scand* **52**, 23.
10 SKOTT A. (1978) *Delusions of Infestations. Rep Psychol Res Centre.* Göteborg, University of Göteborg.

DELUSIONS OF PARASITOSIS [4, 10]

Definition. The patient with delusions of parasitosis remains convinced that his skin is infested by parasites despite all evidence to the contrary. This delusional state differs from a fear of becoming infested: terms such as parasitophobia and acarophobia do not mean the same thing and are best avoided [5].

Aetiology. The term 'monosymptomatic hypochondriacal psychosis' covers patients with a single fixed hypochondriacal delusion sustained over a considerable period but not secondary to another psychiatric illness [6]. Most patients with delusions of parasitosis fit into this category with their delusions occurring either against the background of an otherwise normal personality or perhaps more often showing an acceptable degree of eccentricity with a tendency towards social isolation. Patients referred direct to psychiatrists are more likely to have an underlying depression or schizophrenia than those seen initially by dermatologists [2]. A few patients have organic diseases as a cause of their delusions; pellagra, vitamin B_{12} deficiency, cerebrovascular disease and severe renal disease have been recorded [1, 4, 7]. The delusions may sometimes follow a real infestation even though this has been adequately treated.

Incidence. The condition is uncommon but less so than the number of reports suggests. At one skin hospital 25 cases were seen over a period of 10 yr [11]. It has been estimated that the average dermatologist may see only three or four cases in a lifetime. Women are more commonly affected than men, with the ratio rising to three to one over the age of 50 [4].

Clinical features [3, 4]. Patients with delusions of parasitosis characteristically seek numerous opinions, often complaining about the incompetence of their medical advisers, who are treated with hostility and suspicion. Symptoms include sensations of pruritus, burning, crawling and biting; skin lesions, which are not always present, vary from tiny excoriations to gouged out pits and ulcers which are the result of efforts to dig out the 'parasites'. Many patients offer for examination specimens kept in a small container such as a matchbox. These are usually found to be fragments of skin or hair, but may include living organisms such as ants or flies. With little encouragement the patients will described in detail the appearance of the 'parasites' living in the skin and their life cycles, habits and excesses. Extreme measures may have been taken to cleanse the skin and to disinfest or even destroy clothing and furniture. Cleansing departments and pest control firms may have been called into the home. Sometimes the delusions are shared by others, the commonest pairing being husband and wife; group outbreaks may occur with the imagined parasites infesting factories or kitchens, but these are usually short-lived in contrast with the grimly held delusions of individual patients.

Diagnosis. The diagnosis is usually obvious but a full clinical examination is needed to exclude true infestation, e.g. with scabies. The specimen 'parasites' should always be examined microscopically. An assessment of nutritional status is essential, and organic psychoses of nutritional, cerebrovascular or other origin must be excluded.

Treatment. The management of these patients is always difficult as they are totally convinced of the existence of their 'parasites', becoming angry if their doctors do not believe them. Psychiatric explanations are indignantly rejected, and offers of psychiatric help are often refused and followed by failure to re-attend. Considerable tact is needed to enlist the patient's grudging cooperation, but a direct confrontation over the existence of the parasites and collusion with delusional beliefs are best avoided [3]. A reasonable approach may be to suggest to the patient that he will be offered medication known to have helped others with the same problem [8].

The prognosis in this condition was formerly poor, but pimozide, a neuroleptic drug used mainly to treat schizophrenic patients showing severe apathy, is now the treatment of choice [5] and has been successful in many patients. It is best given as a single morning dose of between 2 and 12 mg daily, and will usually have to be taken indefinitely. Successful treatment with monoamine oxidase inhibitors has also been recorded [9]. It is often reasonable for the dermatologist to prescribe pimozide, but patients with an obvious underlying mental illness should be referred for psychiatric treatment.

REFERENCES

1 ALESHIRE I. (1954) *JAMA* **115**, 15.
2 Editorial (1977) *Br Med J* i, 790.
3 GOULD W.M. & GRAGG T.M. (1976) *Arch Dermatol* **112**, 1745.
4 LYELL A. (1983) *Br J Dermatol* **108**, 485.
5 MUNRO A. (1978) *Arch Dermatol* **114**, 940.
6 MUNRO A. (1980) *Br J Hosp Med* **24**, 34.
7 POPE F.M. (1970) *Practitioner* **204**, 421.
8 REILLY T.M., *et al* (1978) *Br J Dermatol* **98**, 457.
9 ROBERTS J. & ROBERTS R. (1977) *Br Med J* i, 1219.
10 SKOTT A. (1978) *Reports from the Psychiatric Research Centre*, No. 13. Göteberg, St. Jöngen Hospital, University of Göteberg.
11 TULLETT G.L. (1965) *Br J Dermatol* **77**, 448.

SYPHILOPHOBIA

This may be seen in young or middle-aged people who are usually suffering from feelings of sexual guilt. It is surprisingly absent from those who have had the disease and are again at risk. Affected patients may be badly disturbed by this symptom and cannot always be reassured by negative blood tests, the results of which should always be shown to them. If the attitude persists, despite a full and sympathetic discussion and elucidation of their difficulties, early schizophrenia should be considered.

BLUSHING AND ERYTHROPHOBIA

Although blushing itself is normal under certain circumstances, blushing which is grossly excessive in both frequency and extent is sometimes seen in women. It may be the cause of considerable embarrassment and give rise to erythrophobia, a compulsive state related to fear of blushing [1]. Occasionally erythrophobia may represent a hysterical conversion symptom. These patients frequently suffer from emotional difficulties and inhibitions which can be treated only by experts in psychiatry.

Rarely, frequent flushing is a manifestation of hyperthyroidism. The distinctive flushing of the carcinoid syndrome must always be excluded.

REFERENCE

1 PARKES WEBER F. (1947) *Rare Diseases*, 2nd ed. London, Staples, p. 61.

SOLATICS

This term has been suggested [1] for the phenomenon in which a patient has a delusional belief that all her lesions are due to sunlight, sometimes to such an extent that she will venture out only on mooonlit nights.

REFERENCE

1 BERNHARD J.D. & PARRISH J.A. (1982) *Cutis* **29**, 253.

SIMULATED DISEASE
SYN. CONTRIVED DISEASE

This term encompasses patients who, having no real disease, attempt to deceive their doctors by simulating symptoms and signs. The condition is difficult to diagnose, and many patients undergo protracted investigations in the fear of missing an organic disease. They are expert at the deception and manipulation of their doctors [3]. Their symptoms are complex, and their reactions to drugs are bizarre [4]. Simulated disease comes into its own, of course, in times of war when the prospect of a period of invalidity is extremely appealing. However, it may also occur in civil life when emotional pressures become too great or when much is to be gained by litigation.

Simulated disease encompasses many bodily systems. Munchausen's syndrome [1] is one well-known example. Factitious pyrexia, bruising, bleeding or drug-induced colour changes in the skin [5] are others. In this chapter we shall deal only with dermatitis artefacta [2].

REFERENCES

1 ASHER R. (1951) *Lancet* **i**, 339.
2 LYELL A. (1976) *Clin Exp Dermatol* **1**, 109.
3 NAISH J.M. (1979) *Lancet* **ii**, 139.
4 SNEDDON I.B. (1983) *J R Coll Physicians London* **17**, 199.
5 SNEDDON I.B. (1983) *Semin Dermatol* **2**, 177.

ARTEFACTS
SYN. DERMATITIS ARTEFACTA; FACTITIAL DERMATITIS

Definition. Cutaneous artefacts are lesions solely produced or perpetuated by the patient's own actions. They form part of a broad spectrum of artefactual disease which can affect any organ and present to any discipline [7]. It is difficult to define the borderline between such artefacts and the excoriations and other types of damage which can be inflicted upon pruritic disorders, especially by emotionally disturbed patients. The difference is largely one of degree: the artefact is wholly self-inflicted or, if it has been superimposed upon some other process, no longer bears any causal relationship to it.

Patients usually deny any role in producing such artefactual lesions, and in this respect they differ from those with neurotic excoriations [5], a condition which will be considered separately below.

Aetiology. Dermatologists are seldom involved in the management of the very severe self-mutilations, e.g. autocastration, which are usually reported in association with schizophrenia [9], or in the management of the commoner pattern of self-mutilation, superficial slashing of the skin, usually of the extremities, which is classically seen in young women with borderline personality disorders [9] and often a history of anorexia or drug and alcohol abuse [10].

Most artefacts seen in dermatological practice are less obvious and less straightforward. Deliberate self-mutilation by malingerers for direct material gain was formerly common amongst reluctant soldiers and beggars, but the grosser forms are seldom seen now in the developed countries. However, the healing of wounds or eczema may be furtively discouraged when insurance claims are involved or when domestic or social difficulties make hospital a welcome haven.

Malingering apart, women, usually adolescents or young adults and often with some superficial medical knowledge, present with artefacts more commonly than men. One series [11] included 38 females and 5 males, and another [2] included 44 females and 6 males. These patients are often of an inward-looking self-centred disposition with emotional immaturity and restricted interests [3], and against this background a wide variety of recent events may precipitate the artefactual lesions.

Clinical features. Self-inflicted lesions vary widely in their morphology and distribution, and may be difficult to recognize. They will necessarily be in sites readily accessible to the patient's hands and in girls are usually on the face, hands or arms. The individual lesions are often bizarre with irregularly rectilinear outlines and geographical patterning (Figs. 61.1–61.4) not conforming to any spontaneous pathological process. The patient will usually deny that she is producing the lesions and it is often impossible to decide whether or not she is indeed unconscious of her actions.

The changes seen depend on the methods used to injure the skin. These include deep excoriations with the finger nail or a sharp instrument, scarification with a knife or a fragment of glass, the application of caustic chemicals, especially disinfectants, and burning, sometimes with a cigarette.

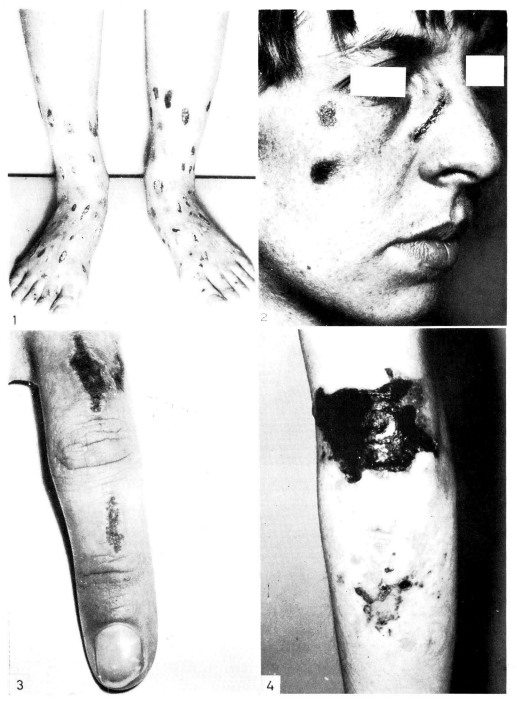

FIGS 61.1–61.4. Artefacts. The lesions are irregularly rectilinear or bizarre in configuration. (FIG. 61.1: Stoke Mandeville Hospital. FIGS 61.2, 61.3 and 61.4: Addenbrooke's Hospital.)

Elastic bands around limbs are used to produce oedema, ulcers and even bone lesions. Hair is plucked or cut. Patients may display extraordinary ingenuity and cunning.

Prognosis. The prognosis seems to be best in young patients who use the artefact to draw attention to a particular problem and who recover when this is solved [11]. Often, however, the artefact is but one incident in a long history of psychiatric illness.

Diagnosis. Lyell [7] cites the 'hollow' history as a helpful diagnostic pointer: the patient does not allow the dermatologist to obtain a clear impression in his mind of the way the lesions form. Suspicion is also aroused by the 'unnatural' configuration of the lesions, and careful observation, including the secure application of occlusive dressings and constant supervision, may be necessary to confirm the diagnosis. This diagnosis should be made with reluctance in a stable and mature person.

Sometimes it may be hard to distinguish artefacts from natural disease: suction blisters have simulated pemphigoid [1], and the lesions of porphyria cutanea tarda on the hands and arms may look like artefacts, as may the bizarre forms of skin necrosis occasionally seen in polyarteritis nodosa.

Treatment. Treatment which is left to the patient to carry out is completely unavailing and the lesions persist or extend. Each patient must be assessed individually. The patient must be interviewed alone. Sometimes the emotional situation which motivated the infliction of the lesions involves her relationship with her parents, in whose presence she will not talk freely. Direct confrontation should be avoided, but usually it is possible to infer that her activities are known but are regarded with understanding and sympathy [4, 6]. The problem may be superficial and easily resolved by modification of the life situation, but at times expert psychiatric treatment will be required [8]. However, the mere suggestion of such a referral may lead to an explosive reaction by the patient and her relatives.

REFERENCES

1 DUFTON P., *et al* (1981) *Clin Exp Dermatol* **6**, 163.
2 FABISCH W. (1980) *Br J Dermatol* **102**, 29.
3 FABISCH W. (1981) *Int J Dermatol* **20**, 427.
4 FRAS I. (1978) *Psychosomatics* **19**, 119.
5 *FRUENSGAARD K., *et al* (1978) *Int J Dermatol* **17**, 761.
6 LYELL A. (1976) *Clin Exp Dermatol* **1**, 109.
7 LYELL A. (1979) *J Am Acad Dermatol* **1**, 391.
8 NOVAK M. (1978) *Cutis* **21**, 713.
9 SCHAFFER C.B., *et al* (1982) *J Nerv Ment Dis* **170**, 468.
10 SIMPSON M.A. (1976) *Br J Hosp Med* **16**, 430.
11 SNEDDON I. & SNEDDON J (1975) *Br Med. J* iii, 527.

NEUROTIC EXCORIATIONS [3]
SYN. ACNE URTICATA; ACNE EXCORIÉE; SUBACUTE PRURIGO

This relatively common condition differs from other artefactual conditions as sufferers readily admit to an uncontrollable urge to gouge and pick at their skin. Women are more commonly affected than men [4]. In one series the average age at presentation was 44 yr, and the average age for the onset of the disease was 10 yr less [2]. The patients commonly seem to be under stress and may be depressed [1]; the most frequent character traits are hypersensitivity and lack of self-confidence [2].

Itching may or may not be present, and a 'primary' lesion is seldom seen, though biopsies may show spongiosis and mononuclear infiltration of the follicular wall and oedema and infiltration by mononuclear cells and eosinophils of the adjoining dermis [5]. The excoriations are usually less than 1 cm in diameter and covered with sanguineous crusts having erythematous edges. Healing leaves a pale scar with a hyperpigmented border. Lesions in all stages can be seen at any one time, and are usually maximal on the extensor aspects of the arms, the face, the neck and the shoulders. Treatment along psychiatric lines is often unsuccessful, though antidepressives may be tried.

REFERENCES

1 FISHER B.K. & PEARCE K.I. (1974) *Cutis* **14**, 251.
2 FRUENSGAARD K. & HJORTSHØOI A. (1982) *Int J Dermatol* **21**, 148.
3 *FRUENSGAARD K., et al (178) *Int J Dermatol* **17**, 761.
4 NIELSEN H., et al (1980) *Psychother Psychosom* **34**, 52.
5 UEHARA M. & OFUJI S. (1976) *Dermatologica* **153**, 45.

FACTITIOUS CHEILITIS [3]
LE TIC DES LÈVRES [1]

A persistent and often gross crusting and scaling of the lips and sometimes the nose [2] follows continued picking, biting or licking in emotionally immature or disturbed patients of both sexes [2, 3]. This condition must be differentiated from cheilitis glandulosa in which an emotional background has also been suggested [4]. The crusts are said to be easily removable with soft paraffin [2].

REFERENCES

1 CARTEAUD A. (1967) *Presse Méd* **75**, 2763.
2 SAVAGE J. (1978) *Br J Dermatol* **99**, 573.
3 THOMAS J.R. III, *et al* (1983) *J Am Acad. Dermatol* **8**, 368.
4 WOODBURNE A.R. & PHILPOTT O.S. (1950) *Arch Dermatol* **62**, 820.

PSYCHOGENIC PURPURA

The deliberate infliction of bruises is a minor form of dermatitis artefacta; the simulation of haemorrhagic states is more serious and more difficult to detect. Auto-erythyrocyte sensitization is described separately as its mechanisms may be more complex.

AUTO-ERYTHROCYTE SENSITIZATION (PAINFUL BRUISING SYNDROME) [2, 7]

In this rare but very characteristic condition (see also p. 1120), which is almost confined to women, exquisitely tender bruises arise after minimal trauma or emotional stress. The onset often follows accidental or surgical trauma. Bleeding from internal organs, abdominal pains and neurological symptoms may occur. Psychiatric symptoms were present in 21 of 30 cases reported [3]. Severe emotional disturbances are a constant feature and it has been claimed that a characteristic psychological profile can be found in affected patients [1, 4, 6]. Typical ecchymoses can be reproduced by the intradermal injection of the patient's own erythrocytes and by phosphatidyl-L-serine.

The psychopathology of the syndrome and its relationship to stigmatization have been interestingly discussed [8].

In 'psychogenic purpura' [5, 6] bruises are produced by patients with the same emotional background, but they are not accompanied by the same degree of tenderness and the intradermal injection of erythrocytes gives a negative reaction. The condition is probably not uncommon as a form of artefact.

REFERENCES

1 AGLE D.P., *et al* (1967) *Psychosom Med* **29**, 491.
2 GARDNER F.H. & DIAMOND L.K. (1955) *Blood* **10**, 675.
3 HERSLE K. & MOBACKEN H. (1969) *Br J Dermatol* **81**, 574.
4 McDUFFIE F.C. & McGUIRE F.L. (1965) *Ann Intern Med* **63**, 255.
5 OGSTON D., *et al* (1971) *Br Med J* i, 30.
6 RATNOFF O.D. (1980) *Semin Hematol* **17**, 192.
7 SHARP A.A. (1966) *Br J Dermatol* **78**, 593.
8 WHITLOCK F.A. (1976) *Psychophysiological Aspects of Skin Diseases*. London, W.B. Saunders.

MISCELLANEOUS CONDITIONS [2]

It is appropriate to mention briefly in this chapter certain curious aspects of deception that are relevant to psychocutaneous disease.

Psychic possession. Alleged outbreaks of industrial dermatitis were instigated by one worker in others (female) with non-industrial dermatolological problems [4]. No industrial cause was found. The phenomenon was likened to the outbreaks of psychic possession common in Europe in the Middle Ages. We suspect that similar situations are probably not uncommon, particularly in factories which employ mainly women.

The 'witchcraft' syndrome. Here an aretefact is produced on others by an aggrieved or emotionally disturbed person. One striking example involved the daughter of a hairdressing salon owner who caused a contact urticaria in numerous clients by touching them with a rubifacient [1].

Habituation to occlusive dressings [3]. An unusual addiction to medicaments long after they ceased to be necessary involved elderly lonely male patients who demanded the reapplication of occlusive bandages for many years after their skin had returned to normal. It was suggested that not only was work avoided but that the subjects found solace in the social contact of attending the 'leg clinic', i.e. group therapy taken to its extreme.

Psychogenic pruritus (see Chapter 60). Subliminal itching is a normal mechanism of everyday activity and occurs constantly. Stronger and consciously recognized bouts of itching may occur in response to an emotional conflict. A psychiatrist's view of the psychosexual and defence mechanisms involved in pruritus with no obvious cause has been well presented recently [5]. Where a careful examination and history suggest that such mechanisms may be operating, referral to a psychiatrist may be of great help.

REFERENCES

1 BANDMANN H.-J. & WAHL B. (1982) *Contact Dermatol* **8**, 145.
2 COTTERILL J.A. (1983) *Semin Dermatol* **2**, 223.
3 LIDDELL K. & COTTERILL J.A. (1973) *Lancet* i, 1485.
4 McGUIRE A. (1978) *Lancet* i, 376.
5 MUSAPH H. (1983) *Semin Dermatol* **2**, 217.

THE TREATMENT OF
PSYCHOCUTANEOUS DISORDERS [8, 9]

'Disease' is a perception of ill-health rather than a physical entity. The same degree of physical affection will be translated into different 'diseases' by different patients. In most patients psoriasis does not itch; in a few it is extremely pruritic. The disease is the same; the perception and interpretation differ. It is necessary to understand the language in which the disease is expressed. Once translated, the key is provided for an understanding of the patient's particular concern and for a valid means of therapeutic communication.

When a rapid cure is possible, there is no great problem in management. A patient's persistence with treatment and faith in the outcome should not be difficult to ensure. However, when a disease is of unknown origin and unpredictable duration, it is likely to become magnified in the patient's mind and to assume undue proportions in his thoughts. In diseases of the skin, as in other spheres of life, the unknown is feared. The spots of acne are magnified in any mirror. The patient and the dermatologist see two different images. It is the patient's that must be treated.

Psychiatry is not an exact science. Some degree of anxiety or depression will be present in a quarter to a third of the patients seen by a dermatologist. This may be unrelated to their skin disease but more often plays some part in the malady or occasionally is the reason for its presentation. When the anxiety is reasonable and openly expressed—fear of cancer, ignorance of prognosis, anxiety about scarring and so on—it is sufficient to reassure the patient with a clear explanation in terms he will understand. Where anxiety is obviously present but at first denied, its nature must be elicited by patient questioning. Those whose conflicts are fully repressed, but whose skin lesions, often factitious in type, leave no doubt about the cause, present the most difficult problem.

All patients with skin disease respond to a receptive and sympathetic approach. Visible illness has a particularly disturbing emotional effect. Itching intensifies this. The physician must have patience, sympathy and insight into human behaviour and must inspire confidence to encourage the patient to talk freely. Advice should be given sparingly and without expecting it to be taken. He must know when a psychological situation is out of his depth and must recognize organic mental disease and endogenous depression as such and seek psychiatric help.

The therapeutic effect of the physician's personality is often underrated. The stronger this is, the less are drugs necessary. Even the act of touching a patient with a skin disease relieves the anxiety of those who have marked feelings of guilt and ostracism—the 'leper complex'. When it is necessary to draw out the patient's emotional difficulties the 'listening ear' is as important as the 'seeing eye'. Tones of voice, hesitancy, a temporary stammer or an unguarded or ambiguous remark (the 'Freudian slip') may provide the key to an important emotional difficulty. Initial explanations given by a patient are often 'cover stories' and are not intended to be believed.

In rosaceous patients a suffusion of the eyes often marks the truth of a probing suggestion. Pruritus or urticaria may likewise become intensified or a patient may rub a patch of lichen simplex vigorously during the consultation.

When a fuller assessment of the social and domestic situation is required, the services of a trained medical social worker are called for [3]. She will extract valuable information about family relationships and stresses and will indicate where these can be helped or eased. Of 1,159 new cases seen by one dermatologist [3] 188 were referred to the social worker; 19 of these were sent on to a psychiatrist.

The first aim in management must be to determine whether any significant emotional situation is present, then whether the reaction is one of anxiety, depression or hysteria, and then how the environmental stresses can be reduced or the patient's frustration, guilt or aggression eased or rechannelled. Hidden fears can often be remedied once they are expressed; anxiety about a child, spouse or parent may lie behind an apparent rudeness or discourtesy. Fatigue alone may provide a 'stressful situation', and adjustment of household burdens, insistence on holidays or proper periods of rest and the provision of 'emotional bunkers', when the situation cannot be avoided, are matters of commonsense and an experience of what is feasible. Feelings of guilt, 'dirtiness' and inadequacy, frequently components of a depressive state, are more difficult to dispel and may require expert help. Obsessional behaviour and phobias are also usually beyond the reach of superficial psychotherapy.

The English language is weak in words expressing emotional disturbances that are not themselves emotive. To ask a patient whether he has 'any worries' is to invite a denial which is often misleading. It is more fruitful to ask if he is tired, worried or depressed. The manner of the reply matters more than the phrasing.

Ancillary aids. The help of relatives must often be enlisted, though their concern is not always disinterested if they are themselves part of the emotional situation. The parents of children with hair pulling or adolescents with acné excoriée or artefacts must be approached tactfully. It is not they who have raised the cry for help but they are often the cause of it. They may feel their honour impugned and their pride at stake.

The medical social worker has been mentioned. She has at her disposal numerous other voluntary bodies and local government agencies who can assist in various ways. She is herself able to undertake a great deal of careful casework and 'gentle psychotherapy'.

Employers, school teachers and rehabilitation officers can give further information or material help in particular situations. To some patients a priest's aid is invaluable.

Drugs [9]. There has been a healthy reaction in recent years against the over-use of drugs in the management of patients with psychoneurotic disorders and patients themselves may refuse to take them. However, short-term therapy with anxiolytics or sedatives may be as helpful to anxious itching patients as analgesics are to those in pain. Sleep deprivation is common and restoration of a normal pattern is an adequate reason for giving hypnotics. Those anxious to avoid giving or receiving such therapy will have to resort, with an easy conscience, to antihistamines with sedative side effects. Some patients will respond well to placebos, but others will develop adverse reactions even to these. Apart from the commonly used diazepoxides, haloperidol, trifluoperazine, promazine, chlorpromazine and chloral can at times be of value. The role of pimozide has already been discussed.

Among antidepressive drugs, imipramine and amitryptyline are of value in lightening the patient's mood and creating a sense of well-being.

The recent recognition of the role of opioid receptors in the elicitation of pain and itch opens new doors to therapeutic advances.

Other measures. Abreactive techniques have been used with some success in elucidating symptoms and relieving tension, but are now seldom employed. Hypnosis, which has always had its adherents and detractors, is now more readily accepted in orthodox medicine. Its potential value in dermatology has not yet been properly studied but is probably limited. However, relaxation techniques, some of which approximate to light autohypnotic states, may be of great value to the stressed or agitated patient, particularly those with adult atopic dermatitis. In recent years interest has grown in biofeedback techniques for reducing tension [2, 5]. These have been claimed to be effective in treating stress-related dysidrotic eczema [7].

Behavioural therapy may be useful in patients with compulsive scratching [1]. Mothers of children with atopic dermatitis should be encouraged to reward failure to scratch.

Group therapy [4] is probably valuable for certain patients but demands too much time and organization to have been generally used in dermatology in the U.K.

There is a small but important group of patients who 'do not want to get better' [10]. They are skilled at deceiving their doctors, their spouses and their friends. They suffer from 'too-good husbands' or 'too-kind doctors' and they are extremely adept at manipulating their simulated disease. Many have a histrionic personality. Dr. Joan Sneddon's illuminating account [10] should be read in full. Once recognized, certain principles of management should be followed [6]; even then, the prognosis is not good [11]. The patient has too much to lose by recovering.

Two general points must be made. The patient may present with a dermatosis that represents only one facet of a complex psychocutaneous situation. It serves its function in expressing an emotional disturbance. If 'cured' too quickly, without attention being paid to the underlying emotional problem, the patient may develop other less accessible ills.

Finally, psychiatrists themselves are of different persuasions. Their views on aetiology and their approach to treatment differ considerably. It is well for dermatologists to discuss these with the psychiatrist to whom he refers his cases lest the patient loses confidence by being given different explanations and advice.

REFERENCES

1 BAR L.H.J. & KUYPERS B.R.M. (1973) *Br J Dermatol* **88**, 591.
2 BROWN B. (1977) *Stress and the Art of Biofeedback*. New York, Harper & Row.
3 COLES R.B. (1959) *Almoner* ii, 466.
4 COLES R.B. (1965) *Med Wld* 1, 128.
5 GREEN E.E., et al (1973) *Ann NY Acad Sci* **233**, 157.
6 KENDALL R.E. (1972) *Medicine* **30**, 1780.
7 KOLDYS K.W. & MEYER R.P. (1979) *Cutis* **24**, 219.
8 LYELL A. (1976) *Clin Exp Dermatol* 1, 109.
9 MEDANSKY R.S. & HANDLER R.M. (1981) *J Am Acad Dermatol* **5**, 125.
10 SNEDDON J. (1983) *Semin Dermatol* 2, 183.
11 SNEDDON I. & SNEDDON J. (1975) *Br Med J* 3, 527.

SKIN DISEASE IN MENTAL DEFECTIVES

Mental deficiency is not a disease in its own right but a condition resulting from a variety of causes, some inborn and others acquired. As a rough guide, some 3% of the population are mentally defective, with an I.Q. of below 70, but the terms idiot, imbecile and moron are now obsolete in the professional sense. The class of higher-grade defectives shades into that of the duller members of the ordinary population [18].

The number of syndromes in which cutaneous lesions and mental deficiency may be associated is large, and many of then have been delineated only during the last few years. Although many of these genetic or developmental conditions are rare, when put together they constitute a formidable part of present-day paediatrics [11]. In addition, there are a number of other skin abnormalities which seem to affect mental defectives in particular.

However, the available statistics must be interpreted with caution as they relate to patients in special institutions to which admission is largely determined by social factors. The proportion of defectives of the lowest grade, and of those of any grade with associated severe physical difficulties, is likely to be higher in such institutions than in the defective population as a whole. In addition, institutional life itself may influence the prevalence of skin disease by allowing the rapid spread of infections, and other conditions may be favoured by unsuspected nutritional deficiencies.

The skin abnormalities of mental defectives fall into three broad groups.

Cutaneous lesions specifically associated with syndromes of genetic or developmental origin. Many of the numerous associations of this type are dealt with in detail elsewhere. Sometimes the nature of the defect is understood at biochemical level (Table 61.1) and sometimes chromosomal abnormalities have been demonstrated (Table 61.2), but in the majority of cases the mechanism of both the cutaneous changes and the mental impairment remains obscure (Table 61.3). The severity of the mental defect and of the cutaneous involvement may run more or less in parallel as in epiloia, but in most of these conditions there is no such relationship and the prevalence and severity of the mental impairment are highly variable.

Non-specific cutaneous lesions showing an increased prevalence in mental defectives
Moniliform hamartoma (see p. 174). Beaded strands of papules, mainly on the forehead and temples,

TABLE 61.1. Some metabolic disorders which may be associated with mental defect and skin changes

Anginosuccinic amino aciduria	Trichorrhexis nodosa
Cretinism	Coarse dry skin and hair
Gangliosidosis (type 1) [19]	Extensive Mongolian spots
Hartnup disease	Photosensitivity
Homocystinuria	Fine hair, livedo reticularis
Hunter's syndrome [12]	Ivory white papules
Lesch–Nyhan syndrome	Self-mutilation
Lipoid proteinosis	Skin nodules and plaques

TABLE 61.2. Some conditions in which chromosomal abnormalities may be associated with mental defect and skin changes

Down's syndrome	See p. 114
Familial X/Y translocation [10]	Ichthyosis
Partial trisomy 2P	Facial hypertrichosis
Patau syndrome (trisomy 13)	Scalp defect, haemangiomas
Ring chromosome 14 [16]	Depigmented spots, café-au-lait patches
Trisomy 18	Nail hypoplasia, lymphoedema
Wolf–Hirschorn syndrome (4P deletion)	Pre-auricular skin tags, scalp defects, flame naevi
XYY syndrome	Acne

develop at puberty in some mental defectives, and more often in Negroids than in Caucasoids.

Atypical keratosis pilaris. A symmetrical eruption of erythematous follicular papules extending from the base of the neck to the lumbar region was found in 10 mental defectives between the ages of 16 and 30 [5]. Similar changes were seen in two imbecile girls [14].

Abnormal hair patterns [3, 14]. The frequency of abnormal patterns of hair growth has been emphasized and is confirmed by our experience. Fusion of the eyebrows and a low frontal hair-line are often seen; the latter is characteristic of true microcephalics but occurs in other defectives. Hypertrichosis of the trunk or limbs is not unusual. The significance of the abnormal patterns is unknown and further surveys are required.

Atopic dermatitis. Only one patient with atopic dermatitis was found among over 200 defective children examined [14]. Others have noticed a low

TABLE 61.3. Some other conditions in which mental defect may be associated with skin abnormalities.

Abnormalities of keratin structures

Alopecia/retardation syndromes [1]	Alopecia
Anhidrotic ectodermal dysplasia	See p. 130
Coffin–siris syndrome [4]	Nail hypoplasia, scalp hypotrichosis
Ibids syndrome [8]	Ichthyosis, brittle hair
Laubenthal's syndrome	Ichthyosis
Menke's syndrome	Twisted hair
Monilethrix	Beaded hairs
Netherton's disease	Bamboo hair
Onchotrichodysplasia with neutropenia [6]	Nail and hair abnormalities
Richner–Hanhart's syndrome [2]	Palmo-plantar keratosis
Rud's syndrome	Ichthyosis
Sjögren–Larsson syndrome [7]	Ichthyosiform erythroderma

Others

Albinism	See p. 1583
Apert's syndrome	Acne
Ataxia telangiectasia	See p. 1094
Basal cell naevus syndrome	See p. 2414
Cockayne's syndrome	See p. 148
Dystrophia myotonica	
De Sanctis–Cacchione syndrome	Xeroderma pigmentosum
Fanconi's anaemia	Hyperpigmentation
Focal dermal hypoplasia	See p. 154
Hallermann–Streiff syndrome	Atrophic skin
Incontinentia pigmenti	See p. 1559
Leprechaunism	Facial hypertrichosis
Marfan's syndrome	See p. 1844
Moynahan's syndrome	multiple lentigines
Naevus sebaceous syndrome	See p. 174
Neurofibromatosis	See p. 119
Papillon–Léage syndrome	Partial alopecia
Poikiloderma congenitale	See p. 150
Rubinstein–Taybi syndrome [17]	Giant keloids, haemangiomas
Russell–Silver dwarfism	Café-au-lait patches
Spina bifida	See p. 223
Sturge–Weber syndrome	See p. 196
Treacher–Collins syndrome	Dermal sinuses
Werner's syndrome	See p. 1816
Wyburn–Mason syndrome	Facial angiomas

prevalence of eczema [3], but atopic dermatitis is frequent in patients with Down's syndrome.

Traumatic keratoses and hypertrichosis [13]. Many mental defectives develop the habit of biting or chewing the forearm, hand or fingers when excited or angry. Repeated biting at the same site induces thickening, hyperpigmentation and hypertrichosis. More rarely there may be atrophic scarring, particularly on the hands. Keratoses in unusual sites may result from the repeated adoption of the same posture.

Traumatic alopecia. This is the result of a hair-pulling tic, and is also not uncommon. The patch selected for plucking is usually in the frontoparietal region, but may be anywhere on the scalp and even in the pubic region [14]. Multiple self-mutilations including traumatic alopecia are seen in children with familial sensory neuropathy (p. 2235).

Crusted scabies. The crusted form of scabies [9] (p. 1065) is particularly frequent in low-grade defectives.

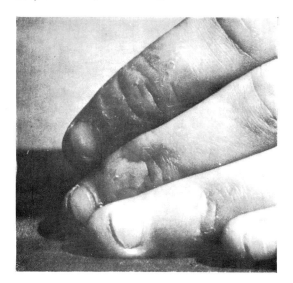

FIG. 61.5. Keratoses induced by biting the fingers ('gnaw-warts') in a mentally defective boy (Addenbrooke's Hospital).

Bacterial infections [14]. Pyogenic infections accounted for 34% of patients referred from an institution for a dermatologist's opinion. The high incidence suggests a low resistance to pyogenic organisms but the part played by the unhygienic habits of the patients is difficult to evaluate. Folliculitis of the thighs occurred in children and adolescents of both sexes, predominantly in the males. Chronic suppurative hidradenitis was seen exclusively in adolescent boys. Erythrasma has a high prevalence [15].

Mycoses. Trichophyton infections are often common and refractory in colonies of mental defectives. It is possible that enzyme induction by other drugs administered reduces the efficacy of griseofulvin.

Intertrigo and perlèche. Genito-crural intertrigo is common in incontinent patients, especially those who are bed-ridden. Perlèche, frequently complicated by fissuring and secondary infection, is seen in a large proportion of patients who dribble constantly.

Primary irritant dermatitis. The failure to take reasonable care in the use of disinfectants and cleansing agents is responsible for a relatively high incidence of primary irritant dermatitis in those patients who are encouraged to carry out simple domestic duties. Allergic contact dermatitis is said to be uncommon [3], perhaps because exposure to potential sensitizing agents is limited.

Drug reactions. The higher incidence of epilepsy in mental defectives accounts for the relative frequency of reactions to drugs.

Non-specific cutaneous lesions the prevalence and cause of which are not proved to differ significantly from those of the general population. There is no reliable evidence that the other common dermatoses are either more or less frequent in mental defectives than in normal individuals [9]. Doubt has recently been cast upon the widely accepted association between epilepsy and acne.

REFERENCES

1 BARAITSER M., *et al* (1983) *J Med Genet*, **20**, 64.
2 BOHNERT A., *et al* (1982) *J Invest Dermatol*, **79**, 68.
3 BUTTERWORTH T. & WILSON M. (1938) *Arch Dermatol Syphil* **38**, 203.
4 CAREY J.C. & HALL B.D. (1978) *Am J Dis Child* **132**, 667.
5 COOMBS F.P. & BUTTERWORTH T. (1950) *Arch Dermatol* **62**, 305.
6 HERNANDEZ A., *et al* (1979) *Clin Genet* **15**, 147.
7 JAGELL S. & LINDEN S. (1982) *Clin Genet* **21**, 243.
8 JORIZZO J.C., *et al* (1982) *Br J Dermatol* **106**, 705.
9 KIDD C.B. & MEENAN J.C. (1961) *Br J Dermatol* **73**, 134.
10 METAXOTOU C., *et al* (1983) *Clin Genet* **24**, 380.
11 OUNSTED C. (1978) In *Developmental Defects and Syndromes*. Ed. Salmon M.A., Aylesbury, H.M. & M., p. ix.
12 PRYSTOWSKY S.D., *et al* (1977) *Arch Dermatol* **113**, 602.
13 RESSMANN A.C. & BUTTERWORTH T. (1952) *Arch Dermatol Syphil* **65**, 458.
14 ROOK A.J. (1950–1953) Unpublished observations at Hensol Castle Hospital for Mental Defectives, Glamorgan.
15 SAVIN J.A., *et al* (1970) *J Med Microbiol* **3**, 352.
16 SCHMIDT R., *et al* (1981) *J Med Genet* **18**, 304.
17 SELMANOWITZ V.J. & STILLER M.J. (1981) *Arch Dermatol* **117**, 504.
18 SIM M. (1981) *Guide to Psychiatry*. Edinburgh, Churchill Livingstone, p. 439.
19 WEISBLUTH M., *et al* (1981) *Br J Dermatol* **104**, 195.

CHAPTER 62

Metabolic and Nutritional Disorders

R.J. PYE, M. BLACK & K. WEISMANN

THE PORPHYRIAS*

R.J. PYE

Definition. The porphyrias are a rare group of disorders characterized by the production of excessive quantities of porphyrins or their precursors; they result from abnormalities in the control of the porphyrin–haem pathway. Each type results from a specific partial enzyme deficiency in the pathway. However, the relationship between this deficiency and substrate overproduction is poorly understood [4].

Porphyrin-haem biosynthesis [8, 12, 13]. Porphyrins and metalloporphyrins are found throughout nature and have numerous functions, but perhaps the most important is the control of biological oxidation and oxygen transport. The haem–porphyrin biosynthetic pathway has now been almost completely elucidated and a simplified scheme of the steps involved is shown in Fig. 62.1. Haem, a tetrapyrrole protoporphyrin chelated with iron, is the end product of this pathway and when bound to other protein moieties forms the cytochrome enzymes and of course haemoglobin.

The pathway starts with the formation of δ-aminolaevulinic acid (ALA) from glycine and succinyl-CoA. This takes place within the mitochondria and is catalysed by the enzyme δ-aminolaevulinic acid synthase (ALA synthase). This is the rate-controlling enzyme of the pathway which is under negative feed-back from haem [6, 7]. After its formation ALA diffuses from the mitochondria into the cytoplasm, and then two molecules combine to form the monopyrrole porphobilinogen (PBG). This is catalysed by the enzyme porphobilinogen synthase (PBG synthase), previously called d-aminolaevulinic acid

dehydrase which is rich in sulphhydryl groups and therefore sensitive to heavy metals. Next four units of PBG are assembled head to tail by the cytoplasmic enzyme PBG deaminase to form an intermediate compound hydroxymethylbilane. Uroporphyrinogen III synthase then closes the ring of the hydroxymethylbilane to form uroporphyrinogen III [1]. It is now thought that these two enzymes act independently of each other with hydroxymethylbilane acting as the substrate of the uroporphyrinogen III synthase reaction. The majority of the PBG is converted to uroporphyrinogen III. It is important to remember that it is only the type III isomers that act as precursors for haem synthesis and that in nature no type I haems have been found. Uroporphyrinogen III is then decarboxylated to coproporphyrinogen III by the enzyme uroporphyrinogen decarboxylase. Coproporphyrinogen re-enters the mitochondrion where it is converted to protoporphyrinogen IX by the enzyme coproporphyrinogen oxidase. Protoporphyrinogen IX is then oxidized to protoporphyrin IX by protoporphyrinogen oxidase. The final step in this pathway is the chelation, by the enzyme ferrochelatase (haem synthetase), of protoporphyrin IX with iron to form the end product haem.

Regulation of haem synthesis [8]. Factors influencing every enzymatic step in haem biosynthesis have been described but the primary regulation is via the level of ALA synthase which acts as the rate-limiting enzyme of the pathway in both liver and erythroid red cells [6, 11].

In the liver ALA synthase is efficiently regulated by feed-back repression. Whilst the precise mechanism is unclear it is suggested that haem reacts with an aporepressor substance to form a repressor, which impedes synthesis of the messenger RNA and blocks the structural gene coding for synthesis of ALA synthase. There is some experimental work to support this hypothesis [15, 17, 18] and the short biological half-life of ALA synthase would make it suited to this type of regulation [15, 17].

*The author wishes to thank Professor G.H. Elder, Department of Medical Biochemistry, Welsh National School of Medicine, Cardiff, for his helpful comments and criticisms.

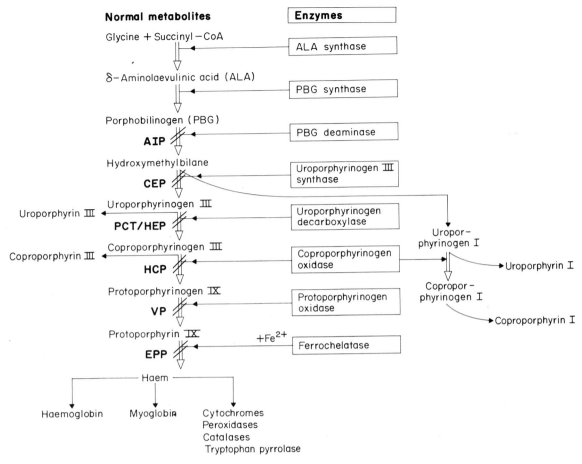

FIG. 62.1. Simplified scheme for the biosynthesis of haem.

A variety of factors are known to influence the induction of ALA synthase in the liver and of particular relevance to hepatic porphyrias are the effects of steroid hormones, iron and carbohydrate. Intermediate metabolites of bile salts and gonadal and adrenocortical hormones induce ALA synthase[5]; however, this induction is dependent on the presence of cortisol. Iron induces ALA synthase[16] but probably of more importance in porphyria, especially porphyria cutanea tarda, is the postulated inhibition of uroporphyrinogen decarboxylase[10]. The induction of ALA synthase is blocked by large intakes of carbohydrate and enhanced by fasting[2, 9]. Although the mechanism for these phenomena is not understood, this glucose effect may explain the reciprocal relationship between carbohydrate intake and porphyrin precursor excretion seen in the hereditary hepatic porphyrias.

A number of lipophilic drugs and chemicals can induce ALA synthase; however, their primary effect appears to be the induction of apoprotein of cytochrome P450, which functions as the terminal oxidase in drug metabolism. This enzyme comprises a haem group and an apoprotein. It is not known how synthesis of these moieties is coordinated but the apoprotein appears to be the rate-limiting component[3, 14], and it is thought that new cytochrome P450 formation depletes the pool of haem and so leads to derepression of ALA synthase[3].

In the erythroid cell, although ALA synthase is the rate-limiting enzyme for haem synthesis its feed-back regulation is uncertain. Hypoxia and erythropoietin, whilst having no effect on hepatic ALA synthase, do increase ALA synthase activity in erythroid tissue. Drugs which induce hepatic ALA synthase have no effect on erythroid cells.

REFERENCES

1 BATTERSBY A.R., *et al* (1980) *Nature* **285**, 17.
2 BOCK K.W., *et al* (1973) *Biochem Pharmacol* **22**, 1557.
3 CORREIA M.A. & MEYER U.A. (1975) *Proc Natl Acad Sci USA* **72**, 400.
4 ELDER G.H. (1983) *Br J Dermatol* **108**, 729.
5 GRANICK S. (1966) *J Biol Chem* **241**, 1359.
6 GRANICK S. & SASSA S. (1971) In *Metabolic Regulations*. Ed. Vogel H.J. New York, Academic Press, p. 77.
7 HARBER L.C. & BICKERS D.R. (1975) In *Year Book of Dermatology*. Eds Malkinson F.O. & Pearson R.W. Year Book Medical Publishers, Chicago, p. 9.
8 KAPPAS A., *et al* (1983) In *Metabolic Basis of Inherited Disease*. Ed. Stanbury J.B., *et al*. New York, McGraw-Hill, p. 1301.
9 KIM H.J. & KIKUCHI G. (1974) *Arch Biochem Biophys* **164**, 293.
10 KUSHNER J.P., *et al* (1975) *J Clin Invest* **56**, 661.
11 LEVERE R.D., *et al* (1967) *Proc Natl Acad Sci USA* **58**, 985.
12 MEYER U.A. & SCHMID R. (1978) In *Metabolic Basis of Inherited Disease*. Eds Stanbury J.B., *et al*. New York, McGraw-Hill, p. 1166.
13 MOORE M.R. (1980) *Clin Haematol* **9**, 227.
14 RAJAMANIKAN C., *et al* (1975) *J Biol Chem* **250**, 2305.
15 SASSA S. & GRANICK S. (1970) *Proc Natl Acad Sci USA* **67**, 517.
16 STEIN J.A., *et al* (1970) *J Biol Chem* **245**, 2213.
17 STRAND L.J., *et al* (1972) *J Biol Chem* **247**, 2820.
18 TYRELL D.L.J. & MARKS G.S. (1972) *Biochem Pharmacol* **21**, 2077.

Mechanism of photosensitivity in porphyria. Photosensitivity of skin is seen in all the porphyrias except in the acute intermittent form. This response of sunlight-exposed skin in patients with porphyria is most marked at around 400 nm with a lesser response at 500–600 nm [6]. This action spectrum responds closely to the absorption spectrum of porphyrins [6] and it seems likely that it is these substances in the skin which produce the photosensitivity. Experimental work to support this idea has been provided by Meyer-Betz who injected himself with haematoporphyrin intravenously and subsequently became very photosensitive [7]. This experiment has been repeated by other workers [9].

Despite the recognized relationship between porphyrins and photosensitivity, the pathogenesis of this reaction is incompletely understood. It is thought that when porphyrins absorb radiation in the 400 nm band there is transient excitation of the molecule to the unstable triplet state. In this state, reaction with molecular oxygen gives rise to free radicals and singlet oxygen [2]. This may cause injury to intracellular membranes such as lysosomes by lipid peroxidation and so release proteases and other inflammatory mediators [1, 8]. This hypothesis is supported by the findings that oxygen is essential for the reaction [1] and that β-carotene, a known quencher of singlet oxygen and free radicals, offers some photoprotection to patients with porphyria [3, 4].

Recently it has been shown in an experimental animal model that if porphyrins are injected prior to exposure to 405 nm light, complement is consumed. This suggests that complement activation may play a role in the production of skin lesions in some porphyrias [5].

Classification of porphyria. No classification of this group of conditions is entirely satisfactory. It is conventional to classify them, on the basis of the major site of abnormal porphyrin synthesis, into two broad groups, hepatic and erythropoietic. More sensitive techniques for the measurement of porphyrins

TABLE 62.1. Classification of porphyria

Erythropoietic		
Congenital erythropoietic porphyria (Gunther's disease)	(CEP)	Uroporphyrinogen III synthase ↓
Erythyropoietic coproporphyria	(ECP)	—
Hepatic		
Acute intermittent porphyria	(AIP)	PBG deaminase ↓
Variegate porphyria	(VP)	Protoporphyrinogen oxidase ↓
Chester porphyria		PBG deaminase ↓ Protoporphyrinogen oxidase
Porphyria cutanea tarda	(PCT)	Uroporphyrinogen decarboxylase
Sporadic		Liver ↓ other tissues **N**
Familial		Liver ↓ other tissues ↓
Hereditary coproporphyria	(HCP)	Coproporphyrinogen oxidase ↓
Erythrohepatic		
Erythrohepatic protoporphyria (erythropoietic protoporphyria)	(EPP)	Ferrochelatase ↓
Hepatoerythropoietic porphyria	(HEP)	Uroporphyrinogen decarboxylase ↓↓

TABLE 62.2 Clinical features and possible types of porphyria

ACUTE ATTACKS—	abdominal and neurological signs and symptoms
	Acute intermittent porphyria
	Hereditary coproporphyria
	Variegate porphyria
	Chester porphyria
CUTANEOUS SIGNS—	skin fragility, bullae, hypertrichosis, pigmentation changes and scarring
Invariably	Hepatoerythropoietic porphyria
	Congenital erythropoietic porphyria
often	Variegate porphyria
	Porphyria cutanea tarda
	Hereditary coproporphyria
—	dermal photosensitivity with pain and swelling
	Erythrohepatic protoporphyria (erythropoietic protoporphyria)

and the enzymes of haem biosynthesis suggest that it is often a 'whole body' disease.

An alternative classification based on deficient enzyme activity might appear more precise but enzyme deficiency alone does not necessarily lead to substrate overproduction and porphyria. Enzyme activity may be altered by drugs or lead poisoning and cause abnormal porphyrin metabolism rather than porphyria.

Grouping according to the clinical features of the diseases is too imprecise to be of real value for classification, but it is perhaps of most value to the clinician since it may prompt him to make the diagnosis of porphyria and to investigate the patient appropriately.

Since there is no single satisfactory classification Table 62.1 shows the porphyrias conventionally classified but with an erythrohepatic group added and the probable enzyme deficiency shown. Table 62.2 shows the clinical features and possible types of porphyria.

REFERENCES

1 ALISON A.C., *et al* (1966) *Nature* **209**, 874.
2 BODANESS R.S. & CHAN P.C. (1977) *J Biol Chem* **252**, 8554.
3 FOOTE C.S. & DENNY R.W. (1968) *J Am Chem Soc* **90**, 6233.
4 FUJIMORI E. & TAVLA N. (1966) *Photochem Photobiol* **5**, 877.
5 LIM H.W. & GIGLI I. (1981) *J Invest Dermatol* **76**, 4.
6 MAGNUS I.A., *et al* (1959) *Lancet* **i**, 912.
7 MEYER-BETZ F. (1913) *Dtsch Arch Klin Med* **112**, 476.
8 SLATER T.A. & RILEY P.A. (1966) *Nature* **209**, 151.
9 ZALAR G.L., *et al* (1977) *Archs Dermatol* **113**, 1392.

ERYTHROPOIETIC PORPHYRIAS

Congenital erythropoietic porphyria (CEP) (Gunther's disease, haematoporphyria congenital).

This is a very rare genetic syndrome in which there is severe mutilating photosensitivity, haemolytic anaemia with splenomegaly and a defect of haem synthesis.

Aetiology. The disorder is inherited as an autosomal recessive character and there is frequent consanguinity. Patients with early onset of this condition appear to be homozygous for a structural gene mutation that decreases uroporphytinogen III synthase in all tissues and leads to the overproduction of type I porphyrin isomers [7, 10]. Enzyme studies have not shown quantitative differences between the early and late onset type of CEP [2].

A patient has recently been described with the clinical features of CEP with normal uroporphyrinogen III synthase but partial deficiency of uroporphyrinogen decarboxylase [6].

A number of mammals appear to develop a disorder which has remarkable similarity to human CEP [1, 3, 11] and bovine CEP may provide an ideal animal model for the human disease. Other abnormalities in porphyrin metabolism have been reported in animals but do not appear to have exact human equivalents [12] and as yet hepatic porphyria has not been reported in animals.

Histology. The changes are similar to those described under variegate porphyria and essentially show subepidermal blister formation with little underlying dermal inflammation.

Clinical features. Soon after birth pink staining of nappies may be noted. The photosensitivity is almost immediate and so severe that infants may scream when put in sunlight or if given phototherapy. Erythema, swelling and blistering follow on exposed sites and may lead to ulcerations which heal slowly with scarring. Repeated episodes of blistering may result in mutilation of ears, nose and

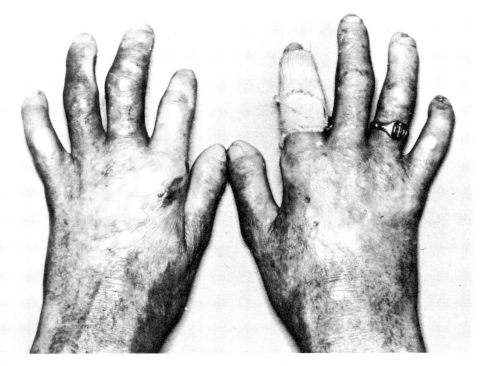

Fig. 62.2. Congenital erythropoietic porphyria—severe scarring and mutilating deformities of the hands. (Royal Hallamshire Hospital.)

fingers. The onset may be delayed until adult life [5, 8] when clinically it may mimic porphyria cutanea tarda. Hypertrichosis occurs in areas of mild involvement and tends to be fine lanugo hair over the limbs with coarser hair on the face. Scarring alopecia may occur in severely affected areas and hyperpigmentation and hypopigmentation are also common features. It is said that the 'werewolf' folklore may have been based on patients with congenital porphyria [4].

Patients may have photophobia and develop ectropion following scarring or even a keratoconjunctivitis leading to blindness. The teeth may be brown and fluoresce reddish pink under Wood's light.

There is usually haemolytic anaemia with splenomegaly. The erythrocytes have a shortened average half-life and it is unclear whether the porphyrins predispose to haemolysis or photohaemolysis in superficial dermal vessels or whether there is some other underlying erythrocyte abnormality.

Investigation. Urine is discoloured pink by uroporphyrin I. Coproporphyrin I is also found in the urine and is excreted in the faeces in large amounts. Fluorescence microscopy shows a stable red fluoresc-

ence, particularly of bone marrow normoblasts but also of circulating erythrocytes. These cells contain high concentrations of uroporphyrin I and somewhat lower levels of coproporphyrin I. There are wide day to day variations of levels of uroporphyrins and coproporphyrins in plasma, erythrocytes, urine and faeces, and this appears largely to be related to the activity of the patient's bone marrow.

Differential diagnosis. The fully developed clinical picture is characteristic and presents no diagnostic difficulties. Early or less severely affected cases in children must be differentiated from erythrohepatic protoporphyria and hepatoerythropoietic porphyria, and in the adult from porphyria cutanea tarda. This can be achieved by accurate porphyrin studies.

Treatment. Treatment is unsatisfactory and largely symptomatic. Sunlight must be avoided. Reflectant sun screens may be of value but are still often difficult for the patient to use. β-Carotene, as widely used in erythrohepatic protoporphyria, does not seem to be of value. Transfusions and even splenectomy may be needed to control the anaemia [9].

REFERENCES

1 CLARE N.T. & STEVEN E.H. (1944) *Nature* 153, 252.
2 DEYBACH J.C., *et al* (1981) *J Lab Clin Med* 97, 551.
3 GIDDENS W.E., *et al* (1975) *Am J Pathol* 80, 367.
4 ILLIS L. (1964) *Proc R Soc Med* 57, 23.
5 KRAMER S., *et al* (1965) *Br J Haematol* 11, 666.
6 KUSHNER J.P., *et al* (1982) *Blood* 59, 725.
7 NORDMANN Y. & DEYBACH J.C. (1982) *Semin Liver Dis* 2, 154.
8 PAIN R.W., *et al* (1975) *Br Med J* iii, 621.
9 POH-FITZPATRICK M.B. (1977) *Semin Hematol* 14, 211.
10 ROMEO G. & LEVIN E.Y. (1969) *Proc Natl Acad Sci USA* 63, 856.
11 WATSON C.J., *et al* (1959) *Arch Intern Med* 103, 436.
12 WITH T.K. (1980) *Clin Haematol* 9, 345.

Erythropoietic Coproporphyria (ECP). This is the rarest of all porphyrias and to date only three cases have been reported [1, 2]. The clinical picture is like erythrohepatic protoporphyria with photosensitivity in childhood. Biochemically a significant increase in coproporphyrins and protoporphyrins has been found in erythrocytes in all the cases.

REFERENCES

1 HEILMEYER H.P., *et al* (1963) *Dtsch Med Wochenschr* 88, 2449.
2 TOPI G., *et al* (1977) *Ann Dermatol Vénéréol* 104, 68.

HEPATIC PORPHYRIAS

Acute Intermittent Porphyria (AIP) (Swedish genetic porphyria, and pyrroloporphyria). This is an uncommon genetically determined disorder, characterized by an overproduction of porphyrin precursors ALA and PBG by the liver. It may be latent for long periods. However, intermittent acute attacks occur, often precipitated by drugs such as barbiturates, and consist of abdominal pain, vomiting and neuropsychiatric illness. Photosensitivity is not a feature of the disorder.

Aetiology. AIP is inherited by an autosomal dominant gene [22]. Most patients with this condition live in Sweden and it has been estimated that the prevalence in Lapland is one per 1,000 [23]. The prevalence in other parts of Europe including the U.K. is one to 3 per 100,000 [24]. PBG deaminase (uroporphyrinogen I synthase) activity is decreased to approximately 50% in the liver and all other extra-hepatic tissues studied [14, 20]. The structural gene for this enzyme has been assigned to a single locus on chromosome 11 [13]. The extent of the reduction in levels of enzyme and the dominant inheritance suggest that patients are heterozygous with a normal gene allelic to one or more mutant genes not expressing the enzyme [1].

Patients with AIP are vulnerable to acute attacks that are often induced by drugs such as anticonvulsants, barbiturate and non-barbiturate sedatives, sulphonamides, griseofulvin and oestrogens [7, 15, 21] (see Table 62.3). These drugs probably act as inducers of the haem pathway (see p. 2271). Attacks may follow a febrile illness, alcohol or fasting (e.g. weight-reducing diets) and may either be related to the menstrual cycle or occur in preg-

TABLE 62.3 Drugs* in AIP, VP and HCP [7,15,21]

Unsafe	Probably safe
Barbiturate	Chloral hydrate
Methyprylone	Pethidine
Glutethimide	Morphine
Meprobamate	Aspirin
Chlordiazepoxide	Phenothiazines
Hydantoins	Diazepam
Succinimides	Bromide
Sodium valproate	Nitrous oxide
Pentazocine	Ether
Halothane	Propranolol
Methyldopa	Atropine
Sulphonylureas	Penicillins
Ergot preparations	Streptomycin
Danazol	Gentamicin
Synthetic progestogens and oestrogens	Cephalosporins
Sulphonamides	
Erythromycin	
Dapsone	
Griseofulvin	

* This is an abbreviated list and more details may be found in the references cited.

nancy. It has been shown that these patients may indeed have a defect in steroid hormone metabolism [10].

Histopathology [17]. All the symptoms of the disease probably result from foci of demyelination at different levels in the somatic and autonomic nervous system. In fatal cases axonal degeneration of the peripheral nerves is found and hepatic changes, commonly centrilobular necrosis, are often noted.

Clinical features. A classical triad of abdominal pain, dark urine and neuropsychiatric symptoms, particularly when associated with multiple laparotomy scars from previous abdominal surgery, should present no diagnostic difficulties to the physician. However, the symptoms and signs may be very variable and subtle. Autonomic neuropathy commonly results in intermittent attacks of abdominal pain associated with nausea, vomiting and bowel disturbance. Patients may also develop tachycardia, postural hypotension, hypertension, sweating and urinary retention or incontinence.

Peripheral neuropathy may be a major feature and again the severity is variable. In some patients it may take the form of mild pain and weakness but in others it may lead to flaccid paralysis, bulbar palsy and death from respiratory failure. Supraoptic nuclei lesions may lead to inappropriate antidiuretic hormone (ADH) secretion and hyponatraemia during attacks [16, 19].

Cutaneous lesions are absent in AIP since it is mainly PBG and ALA that accumulate and these porphyrin precursors are not photosensitizers.

Investigation. The deficiency in PBG deaminase results in elevated levels of ALA and PBG in the urine both during and between attacks.

A quick, simple semi-quantitative test (the Watson–Schwartz test) for the presence of excess PBG during an attack is to mix with equal volumes of Ehrlich's aldehyde reagent and if a pink colour develops then either excess PBG or urobilinogen is present. The PBG–Ehrlich aldehyde complex is insoluble in butane and therefore if this is added, after neutralization with saturated sodium acetate, and shaken the pink colour will remain in the lower portion of the test tube. Recent modifications have increased the sensitivity of this test [11] and quantitative tests are now available but are time consuming. Erythrocyte PBG deaminase can also be measured but it is of no value in assessing the clinical state of patients and is reserved for screening families of patients known to have the disease [14]. The faecal porphyrins are usually normal.

Differential diagnosis. The major problem is differentiating from surgical and medical causes of an acute abdomen and from organic neurological or psychiatric disease [18, 21, 23], including hysteria [9]. Lead poisoning may also have clinical, biochemical and pathological features in common with AIP [6].

AIP differs from variegate porphyria and hereditary coproporphyria both clinically and biochemically; in these, skin lesions are always absent, faecal porphyrins are essentially normal and porphobilinogen is present in the urine in the quiescent phase as well as during the acute attack.

Paroxysmal nocturnal haemoglobinuria (Marchiafava–Micheli syndrome) closely mimics AIP. In attacks the urine ranges in colour from pale red to pale brown. Abdominal and lumbar pain may occur and the attacks may be precipitated by infection or the administration of drugs. Characteristically the urine passed during the night or on waking is red.

Treatment [4]. Since the management of an acute attack is largely supportive it is important that if possible these attacks are prevented. Patients should carry cards warning of the risks that follow treatment with barbiturates, sulphonamides or sex hormones. Skilled nursing is essential for the acute attack and these patients are best managed in an intensive care unit. Pain may be a very distressing symptom and be controlled only with morphine or pethidine. Chlorpromazine may be used to potentiate these analgesics and also alleviate the psychological symptoms. Maintenance of fluid and electrolyte balance is important and may be complicated by the hyponatraemia and hypervolaemia resulting from inappropriate ADH secretion. Patients with muscle weakness and paralysis may develop respiratory failure and require intermittent long-term positive pressure ventilation. The management of convulsions in these patients is extremely difficult since most anticonvulsants are contra-indicated. It has been suggested that bromide is the drug of choice [3], although diazepam may be useful and safe.

More specific treatments have been tried. Carbohydrate [5] and haematin loading [2, 8] have been used to reduce the activity of the rate-limiting enzyme ALA synthase—the latter treatment is reported to have specific benefit in the porphyric neuropathy [12]. The unpredictability of the acute attack has made assessment of these regimes difficult.

REFERENCES

1 ANDERSON P.M., *et al* (1981) *J Clin Invest* **68**, 1.
2 BONKOWSKY H.L., *et al* (1971) *Proc Natl Acad Sci USA* **68**, 2725.

3 BONKOWSKY H.L., *et al* (1980) *Neurology* **30**, 588.
4 *BRODIE M.J. & GOLDBERG A. (1980) *Clin Haematol* **9**, 253.
5 BRODIE M.J., *et al* (1977) *Clin Sci Mol Med* **53**, 365.
6 DAGG J., *et al* (1965) *Q J Med* **34**, 163.
7 *DE MATTEIS F., *et al* (1967) *Pharmacol Rev* **19**, 523.
8 DHAR G.J., *et al* (1978) *Ann Intern Med* **83**, 20.
9 EILENBERG M.D. & SCOBIE B.A. (1960) *Br Med J* **i**, 858.
10 KAPPAS A., *et al* (1972) *Fed Proc* **31**, 1293.
11 LAMON J., *et al* (1974) *Clin Chem* **20**, 1438.
12 McCOLL K.E.L., *et al* (1979) *Lancet* **i**, 133.
13 MEISLER M., *et al* (1980) *Biochem Biophys Res Commun* **95**, 170.
14 MEYER U.A., *et al* (1972) *N Eng J Med* **286**, 1277.
15 *MOORE M.R. (1980) *Int J Biochem* **12**, 1089.
16 PERLROTH M.G., *et al* (1966) *Am J Med* **41**, 149.
17 RIDLEY A. (1969) *Q J Med* **38**, 307.
18 *STEIN J.A. & TSCHUDY D.P. (1970) *Medicine (Baltimore)* **49**, 1.
19 STEIN J.A., *et al* (1972) *Am J Med* **53**, 784.
20 STRAND L.J., *et al* (1970) *Proc Natl Acad Sci USA* **67**, 1315.
21 *TSCHUDY D.P., *et al* (1975) *Ann Intern Med* **83**, 851.
22 WALDENSTRÖM J. (1956) *Acta Genet (Basel)* **6**, 122.
23 WALDENSTRÖM J. (1957) *Am J Med* **22**, 758.
24 YEUNG LAIWAH A.A.C. (1983) *Q J Med* **52**, 92.

Variegate porphyria (VP) (South African genetic porphyria, mixed porphyria, 'Royal malady', protocoproporphyria). This is a genetic disorder with acute porphyric attacks that closely mimic AIP. In addition patients are light sensitive and show fragility of the skin.

Aetiology. Many cases have been reported from South Africa. These have been traced back 13 generations to 1688 and are all descendants of a single Dutch family [5]. The disorder is inherited as a dominant character without sex linkage, although the acute porphyric attacks are commoner in women and the skin manifestation in women may be more apparent during pregnancy. Familial cases have been reported in many parts of the world. The absence of a family history is common in VP, but biochemical tests always show the condition to be inherited as an autosomal dominant.

The site of the defect is still controversial. Initial reports suggested that ferrochelatase activity is reduced [1] but this has not been confirmed and it now seems likely that the primary defect is a deficiency of protoporphyrinogen oxidase [2, 6]. Enzyme activity is reduced to 50% of normal in all tissues except mature erythrocytes since the enzyme is located in the mitochondria. Homozygote variants have been reported [13] and unlike the heterozygotes the skin lesions appear in early childhood.

Histopathology. The blisters are subepidermal, there is little inflammatory cell response in the dermis and the changes closely resemble those of porphyria cutanea tarda. The vessels in the capillary dermis show some deposition of material positive to periodic acid–Schiff reagent (PAS) [11]. On electron microscopy there is reduplication of the basal lamina and perivascular deposition of fine fibrillar material. These changes are not as marked as in erythrohepatic protoporphyria.

Clinical features [3, 9, 12, 14, 15]. Patients present either with cutaneous manifestations following sunlight exposure and minor trauma or as an acute medical emergency with symptoms of acute porphyria. The photosensitivity is not usually present until adult life and the skin lesions are strikingly similar to those of porphyria cutanea tarda. Following exposure to sunlight, vesicles sometimes with obvious haemorrhagic crusted lesions may be seen on the face, neck and the dorsa of the hands. The hands and fingers are also the main sites of post-traumatic blistering. These areas heal with tissue paper scarring and milia. More thickened scars appear on the face and cheeks together with

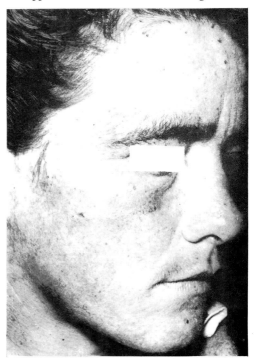

FIG. 62.3. Porphyria variegata in a young woman. Hypertrichosis and scarring contribute to a prematurely aged appearance. (Addenbrooke's Hospital.)

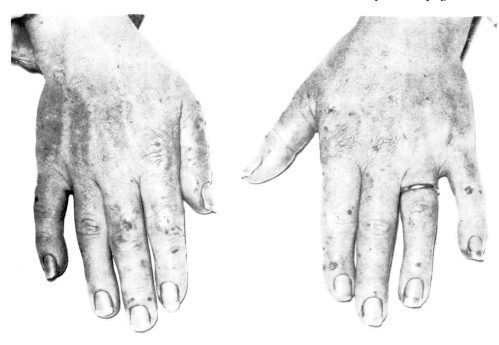

FIG. 62.4. Porphyria variegata—the hands of the patient in Fig. 62.3 showing bullae and scarring. (Addenbrooke's Hospital.)

hypertrichosis and both hypopigmentation and hyperpigmentation. The patients often look older than their years with a weatherbeaten face and excessive furrowing of the forehead. More diffuse thickening of the skin, so-called pseudoscleroderma, has also been reported.

During acute attacks the symptom complex is identical with that of AIP and the patient may present with either a confusional state, hysteria or abdominal pain and peripheral neuritis. Patients with VP, like those with AIP, are vulnerable to the precipitation of these acute attacks by drugs (see Table 62.3).

Investigations. The typical chemical findings in patients with VP are a marked increase in the excretion of protoporphyrin and to a lesser extent coproporphyrin in the faeces both during and between attacks. A quick screening test for these porphyrins is to mix faeces with equal parts of amyl alcohol, glacial acetic acid and ether. If the porphyrins are present pink fluorescence is seen under Wood's light examination. A relatively insoluble porphyrin–peptide complex (X-porphyrin) has been found in the faeces of patients with VP [10, 17]. It was initially thought to be specific but its diagnostic usefulness has now been questioned [8, 9], since it is also found in smaller quantities in patients with AIP and porphyria cutanea tarda.

A fluorescence marker, with a maximum emission at 626 nm, has been described in the plasma of patients with typical VP. This test may prove to be a useful diagnostic marker for the disease [16].

During an acute attack PBG and ALA are elevated but unlike in AIP the levels usually return to normal between attacks. Urinary coproporphyrin is moderately elevated and is higher than urinary uroporphyrin in asymptomatic patients [7].

The coexistence of VP and porphyria cutanea tarda has been described [4]. The biochemical picture in these patients is of porphyria cutanea tarda superimposed on quiescent VP. No clear inheritance pattern for this 'dual' porphyria has emerged.

Differential diagnosis. The signs and symptoms of an acute attack in patients with VP are very similar to those for AIP but usually there are either cutaneous manifestations or a family history of skin fragility. The elevated levels of faecal protoporphyrin and coproporphyrin should confirm the diagnosis.

The cutaneous signs of VP may mimic porphyria cutanea tarda, but in VP the urinary coproporphyrin is more elevated than the uroporphyrin and the majority of patients have markedly elevated faecal porphyrins. The reverse is true for patients with porphyria cutanea tarda. In addition PBG is often increased in VP but never in porphyria cutanea tarda.

Treatment. The management of patients with an acute attack of VP is identical with that discussed under AIP—the drugs to be avoided are the same; carbohydrate and haematin loading have been used [18]. The treatment of the cutaneous lesions is similar to that for porphyria cutanea tarda, namely avoidance of sun and the use of sun-reflectant barrier creams.

It is important that relatives of known porphyrics should be screened and advised accordingly.

REFERENCES

1 Becker D.M., et al (1977) *Br J Haematol* **36**, 171.
2 Brenner D.A. & Bloomer J.R. (1980) *N Engl J Med* **302**, 765.
3 Corey T.C., et al (1980) *J Am Acad Dermatol* **2**, 36.
4 Day R.S. (1982) *N Engl J Med* **307**, 36.
5 Dean G. & Barnes H.D. (1955) *Br Med J* ii, 89.
6 Deybach J.C., et al (1981) *Hum Genet* **58**, 425.
7 Eales L., et al (1966) *S Afr Med J* **40**, 63.
8 Eales L., et al (1975) *Ann NY Acad Sci* **244**, 441.
9 *Eales L., et al (1980) *Int J Biochem* **12**, 837.
10 Elder G.H., et al (1974) *Enzyme* **17**, 29.
11 Epstein J.H., et al (1973) *Arch Dermatol* **107**, 689.
12 Fromke V.L., et al (1978) *Am J Med* **65**, 80.
13 Kordav V., et al (1984) *Lancet* i, 851.
14 *Kramer S. (1980) *Clin Haematol* **9**, 303.
15 *Mustajoki P. (1978) *Ann Intern Med* **89**, 238.
16 Poh-Fitzpatrick M.B. (1980) *Arch Dermatol* **116**, 543.
17 Rimington C., et al (1968) *Clin Sci* **35**, 211.
18 Watson C.J. (1975) *N Engl J Med* **293**, 605.

Chester Porphyria [1, 2]. A large kindred in Chester, England, has recently been described with a previously unrecognised form of acute porphyria. Patients presented with neuro-visceral dysfunction but none experienced photosensitivity. The excretion pattern of haem precursors varied between individuals; some had a pattern typical of AIP, others had a pattern of VP and some were intermediate. Enzyme studies in peripheral blood cells showed a dual deficiency, with reduced activity of both porphobilinogen deaminase, as seen in AIP, and protoporphyrinogen oxidase as seen in VP. The genetic basis for this type of acute porphyria and its relation to other porphyrias are not yet clear.

REFERENCES

1 Quadiri M.R., et al (1985) *Br. Med J* **292**, 455.
2 McColl K.E.L., et al (1985) *Lancet* ii, 796.

Porphyria Cutanea Tarda (PCT) (symptomatic cutaneous porphyria or acquired porphyria). This is a group of disorders characterized by decreased uroporphyrinogen decarboxylase activity in the liver. This defect may either be inherited by an autosomal dominant gene, occur sporadically or be induced by toxic chemicals. Patients are photosensitive but do not have acute attacks of porphyria.

Aetiology. Although it seems certain that the fundamental biochemical abnormality in all patients with PCT is decreased uroporphyrinogen decarboxylase activity in the liver [20], the disorder can be subdivided by measuring this enzyme in extra-hepatic tissues, especially the erythrocytes [45]. In the familial group, the extra-hepatic enzyme activity is reduced to about 50%. The condition is transmitted by an autosomal dominant gene and as might be expected there is often a family history of PCT [2, 16]. The other group is characterized by normal extra-hepatic enzyme activity and because of the lack of family history is referred to as sporadic PCT. Excessive ingestion of ethanol [23], the therapeutic use of oestrogens [6, 32] and hepatic siderosis [18] appear to be important precipitating factors in these patients although the underlying mechanisms are not understood. In addition sporadic PCT may be induced by exposure to toxic chemicals. In Turkey, one major epidemic of PCT was traced to the fungicide hexachlorobenzene used as a dressing for seed wheat [10, 39]—some workers refer to this condition as porphyria turcica [11]. In experimental animals hexachlorobenzene has been shown to inhibit uroporphyrinogen decarboxylase in the liver but not the red cells [15, 33]. Other chlorinated hydrocarbons, tetrachlorodibenzo-p-dioxin [34, 36] and pentachlorophenol [21] may also induce PCT in man. However, it has been suggested that it is the contaminants, dibenzo-p-dioxin and dibenzofurans, which induce the porphyria [21].

Histopathology. The bullae are subepidermal with minimal inflammatory cell infiltration of the dermis and some deposition of PAS-positive material in the vessels of the capillary dermis [7]. Direct immunofluorescence may show IgG in and around blood vessels and less frequently at the dermo-epidermal junction [17]. Biopsy from the sclerodermatous plaques may be indistinguishable from other forms of scleroderma.

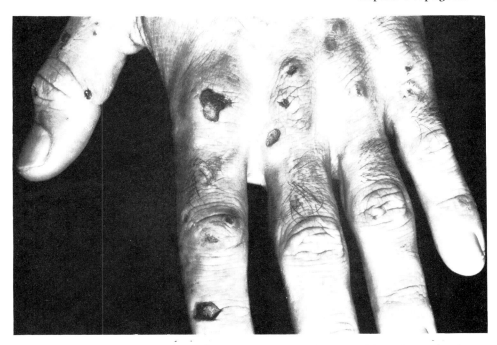

FIG. 62.5. Symptomatic porphyria cutanea tarda—haemorrhagic bullae and scarring of the back of the hand. (St John's Hospital.)

The liver almost invariably shows siderosis [18] and sometimes there are the histological changes of cirrhosis [44].

Clinical features. The clinical presentation closely parallels that of the purely cutaneous phase of variegate porphyria. The diffuse thickening of the skin (pseudoscleroderma) is probably more common in PCT and may be so striking as to suggest the diagnosis of scleroderma. Familial PCT presents at any age, including childhood, whilst sporadic PCT is normally delayed until adulthood (the fourth and fifth decades). Children however, were, affected in the Turkish epidemic and the condition differed in that melanosis and hypertrichosis were marked and led to the description of 'monkey face' [5].

PCT may occur with benign [43] or malignant hepatoma [27, 42], hepatitis [4] and systemic lupus erythematosus [8] and has been reported in patients with chronic renal failure receiving intermittent dialysis [35]. Patients with PCT appear to have an increased risk of developing malignant hepatoma [28].

Investigations. In the urine the main features are the elevated uroporphyrins and a moderate increase in coproporphyrins and 7-, 6- and 5-carboxylate por-

phyrins. The mixture of series 1 and 3 isomers in the urine of patients with PCT is usually distinctive [14, 40] (uroporphyrin is predominantly isomer I, 7- and 6-carboxylate porphyrins are largely III and coproporphyrin and 5-carboxylate porphyrin are approximately equal I:II).

The faeces contain the less soluble coproporphyrin and isocoproporphyrin, together with protoporphyrin [14]. The uroporphyrins and 7-carboxylate porphyrin are present but in much lower concentrations.

A simple screening test is to examine the urine for coral pink fluorescence using a Wood's lamp. The sensitivity of the test can be increased either by first acidifying the urine or by adding talc since this adsorbs the porphyrin and allows the fluorescence to be seen more clearly. However, this test may be negative, especially if the skin lesions are resolving when the patient is seen.

Differential diagnosis. Patients with epidermolysis bullosa acquisita, Hutchinson's summer prurigo (hydroa aestivale), drug-induced photosensitivity, chronic renal failure and frusemide therapy may all have bullae and increased skin fragility similar to that seen in PCT. However, the absence of hypertrichosis, hyperpigmentation and hypertrophic scarring and demonstration of normal porphyrin metabolism should establish the true diagnosis. VP on occasions may present very real diagnostic difficulties. Usually the pattern of porphyrin excretion is diagnostic but VP may coexist with PCT [12] (see also Variegate porphyria).

Treatment. Although general measures such as elimination of alcohol from the diet and avoidance of the use of oestrogens and of iron supplements can induce remissions this may take months and therefore more active therapy is usually required [37].

An effective therapy is regular venesection and at present this remains the treatment of choice [19, 25, 26, 31, 37]. At intervals of 2–4 weeks 500 ml of blood are removed, usually on six to ten occasions. The criteria for stopping are improvement in symptoms, return of porphyrin excretion towards normal and a fall in serum iron or haemoglobin [37]. The mechanism is not clearly understood but this treatment depletes the excessive hepatic iron stores. It is known that biochemical and clinical exacerbations can be induced by the administration of iron [31] and iron has been shown to inhibit uroporphyrinogen decarboxylase [30]—although not all investigators agree with the latter finding [46].

Low dose chloroquine or hydroxychloroquine have been used effectively in the treatment of PCT [24, 29, 38]. One large series showed that 125 mg of chloroquine given twice weekly induced clinical and biochemical remissions which lasted 4 yr or more in nearly three-quarters of the patients [29]. Great care must be taken since higher doses of these antimalarials may produce exacerbation of symptoms, hepatotoxicity and even acute illness [9].

A number of other treatments have been used; however, their value has yet to be established. These include plasma exchange [22], iron chelating agents [13], metabolic alkanization [3], oral cholestyramine [41], vitamin E [1] and penicillamine therapy [23].

REFERENCES

1 AYRES S. & MITHAN R. (1978) *Cutis* **22**, 50.
2 BENEDETTO A.V., *et al* (1978) *N Engl J Med* **298**, 358.
3 BOURKE E., *et al* (1966) *Lancet* i, 1394.
4 BURNETT J.W., *et al* (1977) *Br J Dermatol* **97**, 353.
5 CAM C. & NIGOGOSYAN G. (1963) *JAMA* **183**, 88.
6 COPEMAN P.W.M., *et al* (1966) *Br Med J* i, 461.
7 CORMANE R.H., *et al* (1971) *Br J Dermatol* **85**, 531.
8 CRAM D.L. , *et al* (1973) *Arch Dermatol* **108**, 779.
9 CRIPPS D.J. & CURTIS A.C. (1962) *Arch Dermatol* **86**, 575.
10 CRIPPS D.J., *et al* (1980) *Arch Dermatol* **116**, 46.

11 CRIPPS D.J., *et al* (1982) In *XVI Congr Int Dermatol*, Ed. Mascaro J.M., *et al.* p. 43. Garsi, Madrid.
12 DAY R.S., *et al* (1982) *N Engl J Med* **307**, 36.
13 DONALD G.F., *et al* (1970) *Br J Dermatol* **82**, 70.
14 ELDER G.H. (1977) *Semin Hematol* **14**, 227.
15 ELDER G.H., *et al* (1976) *Clin Sci Mol Med* **51**, 71.
16 ELDER G.H., *et al* (1980) *Clin Sci* **58**, 477.
17 EPSTEIN J.H., *et al* (1973) *Arch Dermatol* **107**, 689.
18 FELSHER B.F. & KUSHNER J.P. (1977) *Semin Hematol* **14**, 243.
19 FELSHER B.F., *et al* (1973) *JAMA* **226**, 663.
20 FELSHER B.F., *et al* (1982) *N Engl J Med* **306**, 766.
21 GOLDSTEIN J.A., *et al* (1977) *Biochem Pharmacol* **26**, 1549.
22 GROSSMAN M.E., *et al* (1979) *Am J Med* **67**, 277.
23 HINES J.D. (1980) *Semin Hematol* **17**, 113.
24 HUNTER G.A. & DONALD G.F. (1970) *Br J Dermatol* **83**, 702.
25 IPPEN H. (1961) *Dtsch Med Wochenschr* **86**, 127.
26 IPPEN H. (1976) *Semin Haematol* **14**, 253.
27 KECZKES K. & BARKER D.J. (1976) *Arch Dermatol* **112**, 78.
28 KORDAČ V. (1972) *Neoplasma* **19**, 135.
29 KORDAČ V., *et al* (1977) *N Engl J Med* **296**, 949.
30 KUSHNER J.P., *et al* (1975) *J Clin Invest* **56**, 661.
31 LUNDVALL O. (1971) *Acta Med Scand* **189**, 51.
32 MALINA L. & CHLUMSKY J. (1975) *Br J Dermatol* **92**, 707.
33 OCHNER R.K. & SCHMID R. (1961) *Nature* **189**, 499.
34 PAZDEROVA-VEJLUPKOVÁ J., *et al* (1981) *Arch Environ Health* **36**, 5.
35 POH-FITZPATRICK M.B., *et al* (1978) *N Engl J Med* **299**, 292.
36 POLAND A.P. & GLOVER E. (1973) *Science* **179**, 476.
37 RAMSAY C.A., *et al* (1974) *QJ Med* **43**, 1.
38 SALTZER E.I., *et al* (1968) *Arch Dermatol* **98**, 496.
39 SCHMID R. (1960) *N Engl J Med* **263**, 397.
40 SMITH S.G. (1977) *Biochem Soc Trans* **5**, 1472.
41 STATHERS G.M. (1966) *Lancet* ii, 780.
42 THOMPSON R.P.H., *et al* (1970) *Gastroenterology* **59**, 779.
43 TIO T.H., *et al* (1957) *Clin Sci Mol Med* **16**, 517.
44 TURNBULL A., *et al* (1973) *QJ Med* **42**, 341.
45 DE VERNEUIL H., *et al* (1978) *Hum Genet* **42**, 145.
46 WOODS J.S., *et al* (1981) *Biochem Biophys Res Commun* **103**, 264.

Hereditary coproporphyria (HCP) [1–3]. This rare inherited disorder is characterized by systemic attacks similar to those seen in AIP or VP but with the cutaneous signs of PCT.

Aetiology. HCP has a world-wide distribution and is transmitted by an autosomal dominant gene. There appears to be a partial deficiency of coproporphyrinogen oxidase activity in patients with the condition [4, 6, 9]. Recently this enzyme has been assigned to chromosome 9 [8]. Measurement of the levels of coproporphyrinogen oxidase have led to the identification of homozygotes [7, 11]. One patient showed a structural abnormality of the enzyme and modified kinetic properties but no detectable levels of normal enzyme. The patient showed marked excretion of harderoporphyrin—an intermediate product of conversion of coproporphyrin to protoporphyrin [11].

Clinical features. Patients may develop acute attacks as in VP and AIP [2], and are vulnerable to the same drugs (Table 62.3). However, the cutaneous signs are less prominent than those seen in VP and usually occur in conjunction with these acute attacks or jaundice [5, 10]. Homozygotes show photosensitivity and haemolytic anaemia in early childhood [11].

Investigations. There is a marked increase in faecal excretion of coproporphyrin, mostly isomer III. Urinary coproporphyrin, PBG and ALA may be normal or mildly elevated in remission but rise sharply during attacks.

Treatment. This is as for VP.

REFERENCES

1 EERGER H. & GOLDBERG A. (1955) *Br Med J* ii, 85.
2 BRODIE M.J., *et al* (1977) *Q J Med* 46, 229.
3 DOBRINER K. (1936) *Proc Soc Exp Biol Med* 35, 175.
4 ELDER G.H., *et al* (1976) *Lancet* ii, 1217
5 GOLDBERG A., *et al* (1967) *Lancet* i, 632.
6 GRANDCHAMP B. & NORDMANN Y. (1977) *Biochem Biophys Res Commun* 74, 1089.
7 GRANDCHAMP B., *et al* (1977) *Lancet* ii, 1348.
8 GRANDCHAMP B., *et al* (1983) *Hum Genet* 64, 180.
9 HAWK J.L.M., *et al* (1978) *J R Soc Med* 71, 775.
10 HUNTER J.A.A., *et al* (1971) *Br J Dermatol* 84, 301.
11 NORDMANN Y. *et al* (1983) *J Clin Invest* 72, 1139.

ERYTHROHEPATIC PORPHYRIAS

Erythrohepatic protoporphyria (EPP) (erythropoietic protoporphyria [12] and protoporphyria). This genetically determined variety of porphyria is characterized by a wide range of photocutaneous changes, occasional liver disease and by an excess of protoporphyrin in erythrocytes and faeces.

Aetiology. It was not clearly defined until 1961 [12] and appears to be inherited by an autosomal dominant gene with variable penetration [3, 11]. However, it has been suggested that two separate genes may operate [17]. Relatives of patients with the disease may show similar biochemical abnormalities but no photosensitivity.

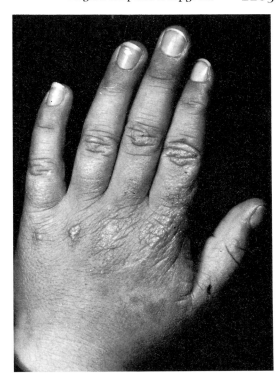

FIG. 62.6. Erythropoietic protoporphyria (reproduced from *Semin Dermatol* 1, 207 (1982) with permission of W. Frain-Bell).

Ferrochelatase activity is reduced to 10–25% in all tissue examined [4, 5, 16]. In an autosomal dominant condition the structural gene mutation should lead to an enzyme reduction of 50% and it is unclear why the activity is so low in EPP.

Histology. The changes are similar to those described under variegate porphyria with a large excess of PAS-positive material in and around the subpapillary capillaries.

Clinical features [12, 13]. The clinical presentation of the photocutaneous lesions may be quite bizarre. The patient may complain of burning and tingling, rather than itching, within a few minutes of exposure to sunlight; oedematous urticaria-like plaques and eczematous areas may appear. In some cases curious linear crusted and pitted areas appear, particularly over the cheeks, nose and dorsa of the hands. The vesicular and crusted lesions show, histologically, marked hyaline deposition around blood vessels and constitute the light-sensitive type of lipoid proteinosis [7].

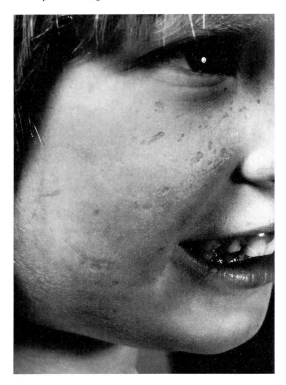

FIG. 62.7. Erythropoietic protoporphyria (reproduced from *Semin Dermatol* 1, 201 (1982) with permission of W Frain-Bell).

In remission, diagnostic clues include pock-like scarring of the nose and cheeks and the distinctive history of burning shortly after exposure to light.

Symptoms develop for the first time in childhood and frequently improve after the age of 10–11. Since the activating wavelengths are 400 nm and to a lesser extent 500–600 nm (the yellow-green spectrum) patients may exhibit symptoms following exposure to sunshine through window glass.

Liver disease may be very mild with marginally raised transaminases and minimal histological changes of liver biopsy. However, hepatic cirrhosis culminating in death has been reported [2, 8, 10]. The incidence of cholelithiasis is high in patients with EPP and the stones consist largely of protoporphyrins.

Differential diagnosis. There is no pigmentation, fragility or hypertrichosis as seen in variegate porphyria. Differentiation from polymorphic light eruption, hydroa vacciniforme, Hutchinson's summer prurigo (hydroa aestivale) and actinic urticaria are often made only by examination of the peripheral blood for protoporphyrins. The disease is missed if only the urinary porphyrins are examined and faecal polyphyrins are also frequently normal [9].

Investigations. Examination of the patients' red cells under lamps emitting 400 nm radiation shows transient red flourescence lasting 5–30 s [15]. Bone marrow normoblasts may show flourescence when the peripheral cells are negative. This screening test together with marked elevation of the red cell protoporphyrin levels are essential diagnostic features.

Faecal protoporphyrin may be elevated, but this increase is an inconsistent finding [9]. There is no increase in urinary excretion of porphyrins, especially uroporphyrin, except in terminal liver failure.

Treatment. Avoidance of sunlight is very important. Where this is not possible the use of a reflectant sunscreen may be helpful, especially where the photosensitivity is relatively mild or in a temperate climate. β-Carotene may offer some photoprotection [6, 14, 18]. A dose of 50–200 mg daily may be required to maintain a serum level of 500 µg/100 ml. Tolerance to sunlight may develop as the summer proceeds and there is a clinical impression that the photosensitivity diminishes as patients age.

Cholestyramine has also been used in three patients with favourable effects and possible reversal of hepatic disease[1].

However, there is still no satisfactory treatment for the severe EPP-associated liver disease except possible liver transplantation.

REFERENCES

1 Bloomer J.R. (1982) *Semin Liver Dis* 2, 143.
2 Bloomer J.R., *et al* (1975) *Am J Med* 58, 869.
3 Bloomer J.R., *et al* (1976) *Lancet* ii, 226.
4 Bonkowsky H.L., *et al* (1975) *J Clin Invest* 56, 1139.
5 Bottomley S.S., *et al* (1975) *J Lab Clin Med* 86, 126.
6 Corbett M.F., *et al* (1977) *Br J Dermatol* 97, 655.
7 Cripps D.J. (1964) *Proc R Soc Med* 57, 1095.
8 Cripps D.J. (1977) *J. Pediatrics* 91, 744.
9 De Leo V.A., *et al* (1976) *AM J Med* 60, 8.
10 Donaldson E.M., *et al* (1971) *Br J Dermatol* 84, 14.
11 Haeger-Aronsen B. & Krook G. (1966) *Acta Med Scand* 179 (Suppl. 445), 48.
12 Magnus I.A., *et al* (1961) *Lancet* ii, 447.
13 Magnus I.A., *et al* (1980) *Clin Haematol* 9, 273.
14 Mathews-Roth M.M., *et al* (1974) *JAMA* 228, 1004.
15 Rimington C. & Cripps D.J. (1965) *Lancet* i, 624.
16 Sassa S., *et al* (1982) *J Clin Invest* 69, 809.
17 Went L.N., *et al* (1972) In *Proc XIV Int. Congr. Dermatol.* Eds Flarer F. & Serri S. Amsterdam, Excerpta Medica, p. 401.
18 Zaynoun S.T., *et al* (1977) *Br J Dermatol* 97, 663.

TABLE 62.4. Major biochemical abnormalities in porphyria

	Erythrocyte	Plasma		Urine	Faeces
Congenital erythropoietic porphyria	UP I++ CP I+	UP I++ CP I+		UP I++ CP I+	CP I++ UP I+
Erythropoietic coproporphyria	CP++ PP++	—		—	—
Acute intermittent porphyria	N	PBG++ ALA++		PBG++ } in an acute ALA+ } attack	N
Variegate porphyria	N	Fluorescence marker	CP+	PBG++ } in an acute ALA+ } attack	PP++ CP+ } Porphyrin X++
Porphyria cutanea tarda	N	UP+		UP++ (I>III) CP+	CP+ (iso CP++) PP±
Hereditary coproporphyria	N	CP+	CP++	PBG++ } in an acute ALA+ } attack	CP++ (III)
Erythrohepatic protoporphyria	PP++	PP+	N	(CP+ in terminal liver failure)	PP±
Hepatoerythropoietic porphyria	PP+	UP+		UP++ CP+	CP+ iso CP++

ALA, δ-aminolaevulinic acid; CP, coproporphyrin fraction; N, normal; PBG, porphobilinogen; PP, protoporphyrin fraction; UP, uroporphyrin fraction; +, increased; ++, greatly increased; ±, sometimes elevated; —, not known.

Hepatoerythropoietic porphyria (HEP). Eight cases to date have been described [1, 3, 4, 6–8] and have the clinical features of congenital erythropoietic porphyria with biochemical abnormalities similar to those of porphyria cutanea tarda [5].

Aetiology. Uroporphyrinogen decarboxylase activity in erythrocytes is reduced to 7% in patients with the condition [2]. A family study has shown an unaffected brother to have 50% enzyme activity, suggesting that patients with HEP may be homozygous for the gene causing familial porphyria cutanea tarda [2]. The identification and investigation of more patients and their families may lead to a reclassification of HEP as hepatoerythropoietic porphyria cutanea tarda [5].

Clinical features. Dark urine is passed from birth. Marked photosensitivity is an early manifestation usually present in the first year of life. The blistering leads to scarring and mutilation, hyperpigmentation, hypertrichosis and sclerodermatous scarring. Haemolytic anaemia associated with splenomegaly has been noted, but the liver on biopsy is structurally normal.

Investigation. There is a marked increased excretion of urinary uroporphyrin and 7-carboxylate porphyrins with the same isomer distribution as in porphyria cutanea tarda. Increased levels of erythrocyte protoporphyrin have been found and in the faeces excretion of coproporphyrin and iso-coproporphyrin are increased.

Differential diagnosis. Detailed porphyrin and enzyme studies are needed to separate HEP from both congenital erythropoietic porphyria and porphyria cutanea tarda.

Treatment. Sun avoidance is clearly the most important measure but reflectant sunscreens and β-carotene might be of value, although as yet untested.

REFERENCES

1 CZARNECKI D.B. (1980) *Arch Dermatol* 116, 307.
2 ELDER H.H., et al (1981) *Lancet* i, 916.
3 ERICKSEN L. & ERICKSEN N (1974) *Scand J Clin Lab Invest* 33, 323.
4 GUNTHER W.W. (1967) *Aust J Dermatol* 9, 23.
5 HERRERO C., et al (1982) In *Proc. XVI Congr. Int. Dermatol.* Eds Mascaro J.M., et al. p. 29. Garsi, Madrid.
6 PIÑOL AQUADÉ J., et al (1969) *Br J Dermatol* 81, 270.
7 PIÑOL AQUADÉ J., et al (1975) *Ann Dermatol Syphiligr* 102, 129.
8 SIMON N., et al (1977) *Br J Dermatol* 96, 663.

XANTHOMAS AND ABNORMALITIES OF LIPID METABOLISM AND STORAGE*

R. J PYE

The classification of hyperlipidaemia is based on clinical assessment, levels of fasting plasma lipids, and the electrophoretic pattern of the plasma lipoproteins, and is divided into six types [1–3] (Table 62.5). It must stressed that these patterns of hyperlipoproteinaemia can be caused by several different genetic diseases and the genetic diseases can produce more than one pattern. Some of the primary hyperlipidaemias have a genetic basis, but most are either polygenic or poorly defined.

Secondary hyperlipidaemia occurs in otherwise normolipidaemic individuals in association with certain acquired systemic diseases. In practice the abnormal lipoprotein pattern may not be diagnostic. For example the hyperlipidaemia of uncontrolled diabetes mellitus and that of lipoprotein lipase deficiency may appear identical—this may be because of similarities in underlying mechanisms. However, there are others, e.g. the hyperlipidaemias associated with biliary obstruction and monoclonal gammopathy, which have unique patterns.

In addition a number of systemic disorders may modify primary hyperlipidaemia, e.g. diabetes mellitus and familial hypertriglyceridaemia.

LIPID METABOLISM [4–7]

Exogenous transport in chylomicrons. Absorbed dietary lipids and cholesterol are packaged with intestinal beta apolipoprotein (apo B 48), a number of A apolipoproteins and a surface layer of phospholipid to form chylomicrons [CM] (See p. 2287). In the circulation chylomicrons (which carry dietary fat and cholesterol) acquire further apolipoproteins, mainly C and E. The apolipoprotein C II present on these particles reacts with lipoprotein lipase on the capillary endothelium; this leads to the rapid hydrolysis of the core triglyceride and entry of the resultant fatty acids into peripheral tissues. Chylomicrons and very low density lipoproteins (VLDL) share this common catabolic pathway and produce chylomicron 'remnants'. The chylomicron remnant re-enters the circulation and is taken up by the liver via specific apo E receptors and metabolized. This transport system is efficient and as a result dietary cholesterol remains in the plasma for only a few minutes.

Endogenous transport from the liver. Triglycerides are produced continuously in large amounts by the liver and must therefore be excreted to prevent steatosis. VLDL convey these lipids and consist of a distinctive apolipoprotein B (apo B 100) and also apolipoprotein C II and E. They are degraded by a similar pathway to chylomicrons. However, the 'remnants' are not taken up by the liver but are modified in a poorly defined process with the loss of triglycerides to form low density lipoproteins (LDL) via the formation of the intermediate density lipoproteins (IDL) consisting of cholesteryl esters, apo B and apo E.

LDL consist mainly of a cholesterol and cholesteryl esters core and apolipoprotein B and E (most of the plasma cholesterol is in LDL). These lipoproteins bind to LDL with receptors which recognize apo E and apo B 100 and enter the liver and extrahepatic tissues where they are metabolized providing cholesterol for membrane and steroid hormone synthesis. LDL are metabolized slowly by this and other pathways over a matter of days. The uptake of LDL regulates both the circulating levels of lipoprotein and the synthesis of cholesterol. The number of receptors and rate of cholesterol synthesis are regulated by the cholesterol concentration of the cell. Cells also take up LDL via other unregulated processes, e.g. the scavenger pathway in macrophages. These are of greater importance when the level of LDL is increased.

High density lipoproteins and reverse cholesterol transport. Cholesteryl esters compose the core of high density lipoproteins (HDL) with a phospholipid layer and the apolipoproteins A (I and II), E and C. The cholesteryl esters are derived from the esterification of cholesterol from lipoproteins and cells with a fatty acyl residue from lecithin (phosphatidyl choline) by the liver enzyme lecithin cholesterol acyltransferase (LCAT). The conversion of polar cholesterol to non-polar cholesteryl esters creates a gradient which allows cholesterol to be continually transferred to HDL. The esters found on the surface of HDLs are transferred by aopolipoprotein D to VLDL and eventually to LDL. These lipoproteins and remnant particles are then taken up by the liver which can hydrolyse the cholesteryl esters and excrete them in bile. Thus HDL may play an important role in the prevention of accumulation of cholesterol in the body, but high concentrations of HDL can produce mild hypercholestolaemia.

*The author wishes to thank Dr Carol Seymour, Consultant and Lecturer, Department of Medicine, Cambridge University for her helpful comments and criticisms.

TABLE 62.5. Classification of hyperlipidaemia

Type	Lipid changes Basic	Lipid changes Lipids	Lipoprotein changes	Primary causes	Secondary causes
I	C↑	TG↑↑	CM↑ HDL↓LDL↓VLD↓	Familial lipoprotein lipase deficiency Apo C II deficiency	
IIA	C↑	TG**N**	LDL↑VLDL **N**	Familial hypercholesterolaemia Common 'polygenic' hypercholesterolaemia Multiple-type hyperlipidaemia	Acute intermittent porphyria Hypothyroidism Anorexia nervosa Hepatoma
IIB	C↑	TG↑	LDL↑ VLDL↑ HDL↓	Multiple-type hyperlipidaemia Familial hypercholesterolaemia	Nephrotic syndrome Cushing's syndrome
III	C↑	TG↑	IDL↑ VLDL remnants↑ LDL↓HDL↓ CM (βVLDL)	Familial dysbetalipoproteinaemia	Monoclonal gammopathy
IV	C**N**	TG↑	VLDL↑ LDL **N** HDL↓ CM absent	Multiple-type hyperlipidaemia Familial hypertriglyceridaemia Sporadic hypertriglyceridaemia	Uraemia Monoclonal gammopathy Alcoholism Lipodystrophies
V	C↑	TG↑↑	VLDL↑ CM↑ HDL↓ LDL↓	Familial type V hyperlipoproteinaemia Familial hypertriglyceridaemia Familial lipoprotein lipase deficiency	Diabetes mellitus

C, cholesterol; CM, chylomicrons; HDL, high density lipoproteins; IDL, intermediate density lipoproteins; LDL, low density lipoproteins; N, normal; TG, triglycerides; VLDL, very low density lipoproteins, ↑, increased levels; ↑↑, markedly increased levels.

TABLE 62.6. Apolipoproteins

Class	Origin	Function (where known)
A I	Intestine, liver	LCAT activator
A II	Intestine, liver	?
B 100	Liver	Neutral lipid transport
B 48	Intestine, liver	?
C I	Liver	LCAT activator
C II	Liver	LPL activator
C III	Liver	?
E	Liver	Receptor mediated lipoprotein remnant (CM remnant) catabolism

LCAT, lecithin cholesterol acyltransferase; LPL, lipoprotein lipase.

Apolipoproteins. These are lipid-free protein components of plasma lipoproteins. They form amphipathic helical structures which allow the formation of stable structures with polar phospholipids at the surface of the plasma lipoproteins and so solubilize lipids for transport (Table 62.6).

REFERENCES

1 BEAUMONT J.L., *et al* (1970) *Bull WHO* **43**, 891.
2 FREDERICKSON D.S., *et al* (1967) *N Engl J Med* **276**, 34, 94, 148, 215, 273.
3 HAVEL R.J. (1977) *Anna Rev Med* **28**, 195.
4 HAVEL R.J. (1982) *Med Clin North Am* **66**, 319.
5 HAVEL R.J., *et al* (1980) In *Metabolic Control and Disease.* Eds Bondy P.K. & Rosenberg L.E. Philadelphia, Saunders, p. 393.
6 HERBERT P.N., *et al* (1983) In *Metabolic Basis of Inherited Disease.* Eds Stanbury J.B., *et al* New York, McGraw-Hill, p. 589.
7 JACKSON R.L., *et al* (1976) *Physiol Rev* **56**, 259.

XANTHOMA

Xanthomas are an uncommon presentation of disorders of lipid metabolism and may be associated with increased risk of arteriosclerotic vascular disease and occasionally with pancreatitis. However, it is the skin manifestations that will bring the patient to the dermatology clinics and therefore these are dealt with separately.

Eruptive xanthomas. Eruptive xanthomas may occur suddenly at any site but are most commonly seen on the buttocks, shoulders and extensor surfaces of the extremities. The oral mucosa and face are sometimes affected. They appear as pinhead or larger yellow papules with a reddish base; they may be fleeting in nature and occur in crops. Occasionally these papules may coalesce and overlie a tuberous xanthoma and are then sometimes called tubero-eruptive xanthomas.

These xanthomas usually signify hypertriglyceridaemia and a high concentration of chylomicrons or VLDL and are therefore associated with type I, III, IV and V hyperlipoproteinaemias. They may also be seen in secondary hyperlipidaemia, usually in association with insulin-dependent diabetes.

Plane xanthomas. These appear as yellow or orange macules or slightly palpable plaques. They involve almost any site, but when plane xanthomas occur in palmar creases (xanthoma palmaris) they are very likely to be associated with either type III hyperlipoproteinaemia or homozygous familial hypercholesterolaemia. Plane xanthomas may also be

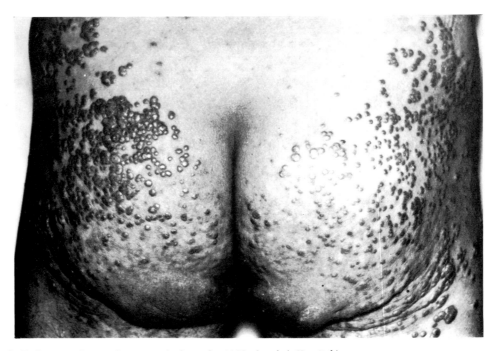

FIG. 62.8. Profuse eruptive xanthomas on the buttocks. (Addenbrooke's Hospital.)

seen in the secondary hyperlipidaemias associated with biliary obstruction and, rarely, monoclonal gammopathy.

Xanthelasma palpebrarum. These usually appear as bilateral and symmetrical soft velvety papules and plaques arranged on the eyelids. The upper eyelid and the region around the inner canthus are the most common sites of involvement. They usually represent a localized cutaneous phenomenon but they may signify a systemic hyperlipidaemia and are then associated with elevation of LDL in type II hyperlipoproteinaemia (such as familial hypercholesterolaemia) or type III hyperlipoproteinaemia. Generalized plane xanthomas may be seen in normolipaemic patients (see later).

Tuberous xanthomas. These lesions vary in size and shape from small papules 0·5 cm in diameter to lobulated tumours 2·5 cm or more across. These are firm and yellow or orange in colour, often with an erythematous halo. Usually they are painless but the larger lesions may be tender on direct pressure. They develop slowly and are seen on the extensor aspect of the limbs, particularly over knees and elbows. These xanthomas are usually seen with hypercholesterolaemia and increased levels of LDL in

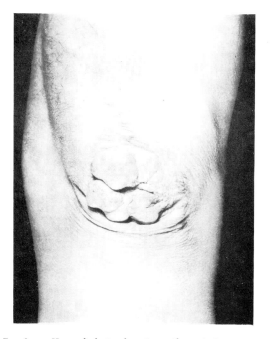

FIG. 62.9. Hypercholesterolaemic xanthomatosis. Tuberous xanthomas of the elbow. (Addenbrooke's Hospital.)

type II (e.g. familial hypercholesterolaemia) and type III hyperlipolipidaemia (e.g. familial dysbetalipoproteinaemia) and in secondary hyperlipidaemia with hypothyroidism, biliary disease and monoclonal gammopathy.

Tendinous xanthomas. These appear as slowly enlarging subcutaneous nodules attached to tendons, ligaments, fascia and periosteum. Usually they are symptomless and the overlying skin appears normal. Although any tendon may be involved, the most frequent are those on the dorsal aspect of the fingers and the Achilles tendons. The subperiosteal lesions tend to involve bony prominences such as the malleoli and elbows but do not appear to calcify.

They appear in association with severe hypercholesterolaemia and elevated levels of LDL found in type II hyperlipoproteinaemia (e.g. familial hypercholesterolaemia). Tendinous xanthomas are also seen in secondary hyperlipidaemias associated with biliary obstruction or primary biliary cirrhosis.

Generalized plane xanthomas. These plane xanthomas cover large areas of the face, neck and thorax and also involve flexures and palms. Many patients with these diffuse plane xanthomas develop a monoclonal gammopathy [6, 9–11] associated with either myeloma, macroglobulinaemia or lymphoma and normal lipid levels [1, 2].

Lipid metabolism may be disturbed and approximately 50% of patients with IgA myeloma have hypolipidaemia with low cholesterol and LDL [8]. Less commonly, endogenous hypertriglyceridaemia may be present [3] and the lipoproteins may be in the density range of VLDL, LDL [5] or intermediate forms [3] and chylomicrons [4]. It is not known how these monoclonal antibodies produce the lipid abnormalities but at least some combine with the lipoproteins [7].

Pathology of xanthomas. Histology of skin biopsies may show the presence of intracellular sudanophilic material in abnormal quantities, particularly around capillaries. Differential staining of this material often shows a characteristic reaction for cholesterol and polariscopic examination of frozen sections may show doubly refractile (anisotropic) droplets.

Treatment of xanthomas. Most of the xanthomas respond well to dietary control and details are given in the following sections. However, occasionally they may need to be removed surgically, although they will recur unless dietary and other measures are also taken. If it is an isolated finding, xanthelasma palpebrarum may be destroyed with cautery or trichloroacetic acid or excised, but they do tend to recur over a period of years.

REFERENCES

1 ALTMANN J. & WINKELMANN R.K. (1962) *Arch Dermatol* **85**, 633.
2 BAZEX A., *et al* (1965) *Ann Dermatol Syphiligr* **92**, 39.
3 COHEN L., *et al* (1966) *Am J Med* **40**, 299.
4 GLUECK H.I., *et al* (1972) *J Lab Clin Med* **79**, 731.
5 MARIEN K.J.C. & SMEENK G. (1975) *Br J Dermatol* **93**, 407.
6 PAGÉ M., *et al* (1974) *N Engl J Med* **291**, 475.
7 RIESEN W., *et al* (1972) *Vox Sang* **22**, 420.
8 SEITANIDIS B.A., *et al* (1970) *Am J Med* **29**, 93.
9 SLACK J. & BORRIE P. (1971) In *Modern Trends in Dermatology*. Ed. Borrie P. London, Butterworth, p. 194.
10 TAYLOR J.S., *et al* (1978) *Arch Dermatol* **144**, 425.
11 WILSON D.E., *et al* (1975) *Am J Med* **59**, 721.

GENETIC PRIMARY HYPERLIPIDAEMIA

Familial lipoprotein lipase deficiency [9] (fat-induced lipoproteinaemia, Bürger-Grütz type [2]). It is a rare disorder probably inherited by an autosomal recessive gene [5] and is due to the lack of lipoprotein lipase [6] which clears chylomicron lipoproteins from the circulation. Vertical transmission has not been documented.

Clinical features. The disease is manifest in childhood and usually presents with recurrent attacks of abdominal pain or acute relapsing pancreatitis and eruptive xanthomas. Hepatosplenomegaly and retinopathy (lipaemia retinalis) are usual findings. The major threat to life in these patients appears to be pancreatitis, and there is no increased risk of arteriosclerotic vascular disease.

Investigation. Lipaemic plasma in young individuals after a 12-h fast should suggest the diagnosis and if the sample is left in the refrigerator (at 4 °C) overnight a creamy layer collects at the top of the tube whilst the infranatant remains relatively clear. The triglyceride level is markedly elevated with only a moderate increase in cholesterol and the level of LDL is normal. A type I pattern on lipoprotein electrophoresis supports the diagnosis but less commonly type V may be found and then measurement of the lipoprotein lipase level [7] on apo C II may be necessary to establish the diagnosis [7].

Treatment. Restriction of dietary fat to 20–30 g per day usually results in loss of the symptoms and signs of the hyperlipidaemia. Medium-chain triglycerides are not normally incorporated in chylomicrons and therefore may be given in unrestricted amounts.

Familial apolipoprotein C II deficiency [9]. This is a very rare autosomal recessive disease [4] in which there is an absence of apolipoprotein C II [1], an essential cofactor for lipoprotein lipase. This results in a functional lipoprotein lipase deficiency and a rise in both chylomicrons and VLDL.

Clinical features. These might be expected to be the same as lipoprotein lipase deficiency but patients usually present in adulthood and do not show hepatosplenomegaly or eruptive xanthomas. Pancreatitis, however, remains a major threat to life.

Investigation. Plasma triglyceride levels are markedly elevated. By strict criteria the lipoprotein electrophoretic pattern is type V, but many patients have an intermediate pattern between I and V [8]. Deficiency of apo C II can be measured by electrophoresis of the very low density apolipoprotein.

Treatment. This is either by fat restriction as in lipoprotein lipase deficient patients or by replacement of the apo C II by transfusion with normal plasma—synthetic apo C II may become more widely available for treatment in the near future [3].

REFERENCES

1 BRECKENRIDGE, *et al* (1978) *N Eng J Med* **298**, 1265.
2 BÜRGER M. & GRÜTZ O (1932) *Arch Dermatol Syphil* **166**, 542.
3 CATAPANO A.L., *et al* (1979) *Biochem Biophys Res Commun* **89**, 951.
4 COX D.W., *et al* (1978) *N Engl J Med* **299**, 1421.
5 FREDRICKSON D.S. & LEVY R.I. (1972) In *Metabolic Basis of Inherited Disease*. Eds Stanbury J.B., *et al.* New York, McGraw-Hill, p. 545.
6 HAVEL R.J. & GORDON R.S. (1960) *J Clin Invest* **39**, 1777.
7 KRAUSS R.M., *et al* (1974) *J Clin Invest* **54**, 1107.
8 MILLER N.E., *et al* (1981) *Eur J Clin Invest* **11**, 69.
9 NIKKILA E.A. (1983) In *Metabolic Basis of Inherited Disease*. Eds Stanbury J.B., *et al.* New York, McGraw-Hill, p. 622.

Familial hypercholesterolaemia [6] (essential familial hypercholesterolaemia). This common autosomal dominant disorder affecting approximately 1:500 of the European and American population. It is characterized by an increase inthe levels of LDL and is the commonest cause of tendinous xanthomas.

Aetiology. The primary defect is a reduction in LDL receptors. Cultured fibroblasts have shown three mutant alleles at the LDL receptor locus. The most common results in a non-functional gene product, the next most frequent in a defective gene product and the rarest produces a receptor that binds LDL normally but fails to transport them into the cells [1, 5].

Homozygotes have two of these mutant alleles and therefore are almost completely unable to clear LDL from the plasma. Heterozygotes have one normal allele and can remove about half the plasma LDL.

Clinical features. Heterozygotes usually present in the third to fourth decades with premature onset of coronary artery disease. Tendinous xanthomas are very common and the incidence increases with the age of the patient. Xanthelasma, tuberous xanthomas and corneal arcus are also seen [3]. The very rare homozygotes usually present in the first year of life with plane xanthomas often at the site of trauma and on the palms. Tendinous and tuberous xanthomas, xanthelasma and corneal arcus are all commonly present. Coronary artery disease is manifest before the age of 20, and in addition cholesterol deposits may give rise to supravalvar aortic stenosis [8].

Prognosis. This depends on the severity of the defect. Homozygotes usually die from heart disease by the age of 20 yr, whilst most of the heterozygotes have had a myocardial infarction by the age of 60.

Investigation. Plasma cholesterol is elevated with a normal triglyceride level. Lipoprotein electrophoresis shows a type IIA pattern. Most patients with type IIA, however, do not have familial hypercholesterolaemia but common 'polygenic' hypercholesterolaemia (see below). The presence of tendinous xanthomas and family members with elevated plasma cholesterol help to establish the diagnosis.

A few patients with familial hypercholesterolaemia have type IIB pattern with raised triglyceride levels. The presence of tendinous xanthomas and family studies should help to separate these patients from 'multiple-type' hyperlipidaemia. A few centres can assay LDL receptors directly in both heterozygous and homozygous patients [6].

Treatment. The treatment of familial hypercholesterolaemia is applicable to any patient with types IIA or IIB hyperlipoproteinaemia. The aim is to reduce the level of LDL to within the normal range. In the heterozygotes the diet should be low in cholesterol and saturated fats and high in polyunsaturated fats [4]. Cholestyramine, a non-absorbable anion exchange resin, may lower the cholesterol by up to 25% [7]. Nicotinic acid may help block cholesterol synthesis and can be used either alone or in conjunction with cholestyramine [9]. Ileal bypass may help in the patients unable to tolerate cholestyramine [2].

Probucol is a moderately effective LDL-reducing drug. It enhances faecal excretion of bile salts and reduces cholesterol synthesis. It may cause a slight increase in triglyceride synthesis and thus has an adverse effect on the levels of HDL. It is of value in the treatment of patients with type IIA hyperlipoproteinaemia but not type IIB because of the effect on triglycerides.

Homozygotes are relatively unresponsive to any of the treatments mentioned and portocaval shunt is currently under trial [10]. Plasma exchange may help but treatment needs to be repeated at least monthly [11].

REFERENCES

1 BROWN M.S. & GOLDSTEIN J.L. (1974) *Science* **185**, 61.
2 BUCHWALD H., *et al* (1974) *Ann Surg* **180**, 384.
3 BULKLEY, B.H. *et al* (1975) *Arch Pathol* **99**, 293.
4 CONNOR W.E. & CONNOR S.L. (1982) *Med Clin North Am* **66**, 485.
5 GOLDSTEIN J.L. & BROWN M.S. (1982) *Med Clin North Am* **66**, 335.
6 GOLDSTEIN J.L. & BROWN M.S. (1983) In *Metabolic Basis of Inherited Disease.* Eds Stanbury J.B., *et al.* New York, McGraw-Hill, p. 672.
7 GRUNDY S.M. (1972) *Arch Intern Med* **130**, 638.
8 KHACHADURIAN A.K. & UTHMAN S.M. (1973) *Nutr Metab* **15**, 132.
9 LEVY R.I., *et al* (1973) *Ann Intern Med* **79**, 51.
10 STARZL T.E., *et al* (1978) *Arch Surg* **113**, 71.
11 THOMPSON G.R., *et al* (1980) *Br Heart J* **46**, 680.

Familial dysbetalipoproteinaemia (familial type III hyperlipidaemia). This is a rare inherited disorder in which plasma triglyceride and cholesterol are elevated because of remnants of chylomicrons and VLDL (beta VLDL [1]).

Aetiology. The defect involves a polymorphic genetic locus for apoprotein E III (apo E III) [6, 7]. Apo E III, a component of remnant lipoprotein derived from chylomicrons and VLDL, is essential for uptake of these remnants by the liver. All patients with this disorder are homozygotes for E^d allele (d,deficient). Heterozygotes are common in the population (1:100) but most individuals can compensate for the abnormal apo E III and it is only those who cannot do so that express the disease. Expression of the disease therefore depends on other genetic or metabolic factors such as the inheritance of multiple-type hyperlipidaemia, familial hypercholesterolaemia, insulin-dependent diabetes, hypothyroidism and obesity [2].

Clinical features [4]. Onset of symptoms is delayed to the second and third decade. Xanthomas are a common presentation and typically patients have tuberous, tubero-eruptive and plane xanthomas involving the palmar and digital creases (xanthoma palmaris) [5]. Xanthelasma may also occur. Premature severe coronary and peripheral vascular disease occurs and patients may in addition have hypoythyroidism, obesity or diabetes mellitus.

Investigation. Plasma cholesterol and triglyceride levels are elevated to almost the same degree. Lipoprotein electrophoresis shows type III pattern with a broad beta band. The IDL fraction, obtained by ultracentrifugation, shows a high cholesterol content, but these changes are not diagnostic. The demonstration of the E^d on iso-electric focusing of the LDL is diagnostic for familial dysbetalipoproteinaemia [2].

Treatment. Treatment of any other metabolic disease such as obesity, diabetes mellitus or hypothyroidism will lower lipid levels. Clofibrate is usually necessary and results in sustained dramatic improvement in plasma lipids; nicotinic acid has a similar effect but is rarely used [3].

REFERENCES

1 BROWN M.S., *et al* (1983) In *Metabolic Basis of Inherited Disease.* Eds Stanbury J.B., *et al.* New York, McGraw-Hill, p. 655.
2 HAVEL R.J. (1982) *Med Clin North Am* 66, 441.
3 LEVY R.I., *et al* (1972) *Ann Intern Med* 77, 267.
4 MORGANROTH J., *et al* (1975) *Ann Intern Med* 82, 158.
5 POLANO M.K. (1974) *Dermatologica* 149, 1.
6 UTERMANN G., *et al* (1975) *FEBS Lett* 56, 352.
7 UTERMANN G., *et al* (1977) *Nature* 269, 604.

Familial hypertriglyceridaemia (endogenous hypertriglyceridaemia). This is a common autosomal dominant disorder with delayed penetrance characterized by increased VLDL and normal levels of LDL [3]. The pathogenesis of the condition is not understood. Obesity and diabetes mellitus are not a primary part of familial hypertriglyceridaemia but they probably exacerbate the condition by increasing VLDL production [2].

Clinical features. The disease is not expressed until early adulthood. Typically patients are obese, with glucose intolerance, hypertension and hyperuricaemia [1, 5]. Severe exacerbations can be precipitated either by ingestion of oestrogen-containing oral contraceptives [5], poorly controlled diabetes [1, 5] or excessive alcohol intake [6], and under these circumstances chylomicrons appear in the plasma and the patient develops' mixed hyperlipidaemia'. During such an exacerbation, patients occasionally develop eruptive xanthomas but xanthomas are not normally a characteristic feature of the condition.

Investigation. A moderate increase in plasma triglyceride, normal cholesterol and type IV pattern on lipoprotein electrophoresis should suggest the diagnosis, although these findings are found in other genetic and acquired hyperlipidaemias [2, 4]. Occasionally patients may have severe triglyceridaemia with increased levels of chylomicrons and VLDL and a type V lipoprotein [4, 5]. There are no other specific tests for familial hypertriglyceridaemia but study of the adult members of the family should show 50% of them to have hypertriglyceridaemia.

Treatment. Patients' weight, diabetes mellitus and thyroid disease if present should all be treated appropriately. Alcohol and the oral contraceptives should be avoided, and the diet should be low in saturated fats. Clofibrate may be necessary if these measures fail and appears to be effective in controlling the hyperlipidaemia.

REFERENCES

1 BIERMAN E.L. & PORTE D. (1968) *Ann Intern Med* 68, 926.
2 FREDRICKSON D.S., *et al* (1978) In *Metabolic Basis of Inherited Disease.* Eds Stanbury J.B., *et al.* New York, McGraw-Hill, p. 641.
3 GLUECK C.J., *et al* (1973) *Metabolism* 22, 1287.
4 GOLDSTEIN J.L., *et al* (1973) *J Clin Invest* 52, 1544.
5 HAVEL R.J. (1969) *Adv Intern Med* 15, 117.
6 MENDELSON J.H. & MELLO N.K. (1973) *Science* 180, 1372.

Familial type V hyperlipidaemia [1]. Within some families there are individuals who in late adult life show`mixed hyperlipidaemia without obvious precipitating agents. These patients present with eruptive xanthomas, abdominal pain and occasionally pancreatitis. The condition may be exacerbated by alcohol, obesity, excess calorie intake and oestrogens. The treatment is essentially as for familial hypertriglyceridaemia.

REFERENCES

1 FREDERICKSON D.S., *et al* (1978) In *Metabolic Basis of Inherited Disease.* Eds Stanbury J.B., *et al.* New York, McGraw-Hill, p. 643.

Familial multiple (lipoprotein type) hyperlipidaemia (familial combined hyperlipidaemia). This is a common disorder probably inherited as an autosomal dominant trait, in which patients show variable plasma lipids and lipoprotein patterns. Family studies show relatives to have either hypercholesterolaemia (type IIA), hypertriglyceridaemia (type IV) or both hyperlipidaemias (type IIB) [1–3]. Its importance is the association with ischaemic heart disease. The condition is not associated with xanthomas.

REFERENCES

1 GOLDSTEIN J.L., *et al* (1973) *J Clin Invest* **52**, 1544.
2 NIKKILÄ. E.A. & ARÖ A. (1973) *Lancet* i, 954.
3 ROSE H.G., *et al* (1973) *Am J Med* **54**, 148.

PRIMARY HYPERLIPIDAEMIA WITH POSSIBLE GENETIC AETIOLOGY

Most patients seen with a hyperlipidaemia cannot easily be placed into a category of the single gene mutation primary hyperlipoproteinaemias. This may in part be due to the lack of diagnostic markers for the disorders, but in most instances it seems likely that the hyperlipidaemia is due to a complex mix of genetic and environmental factors (i.e. polygenic influence).

Common 'polygenic' hypercholesterolaemia [1]. The majority of patients found to have hypercholesterolaemia have this syndrome, usually with type IIA lipoprotein pattern. There are no tendinous xanthomas and no hyperlipidaemias in the patient's family.

REFERENCES

1 HAVEL R.J., *et al* (1980) In *Metabolic Control and Disease.* Eds Bondy P.K. & Rosenberg L.E. Philadelphia, Saunders, p. 445.

Sporadic hypertriglyceridaemia [2]. (common 'polygenic' hypertriglyceridaemia). This is a heterogeneous group of patients who have an elevated plasma triglyceride with or without increased levels of chylomicrons. They differ from familial hypertriglyceridaemia and familial multiple-type hyperlipidaemia in that the first degree relatives are unaffected [1].

REFERENCES

1 GOLDSTEIN R.J., *et al* (1973) *J Clin Invest* **52**, 1544.
2 HAVEL R.J., *et al* (1980) In *Metabolic Control and Disease.* Eds Bondy P.K. & Rosenberg L.E. Philadelphia, Saunders, p. 442.

SECONDARY HYPERLIPIDAEMIA [1]

There are a variety of disorders that may produce or exacerbate a pre-existing hyperlipidaemia (Table 62.7) and of these diabetes mellitus, alcoholism and ingestion of oestrogens are the most commonly encountered.

REFERENCE

1 HAVEL R.L., *et al* (1980) In *Metabolic Control and Disease.* Eds Bondy P.K. & Rosenberg L.E. Philadelphia, Saunders, p. 446.

LIPID STORAGE DISEASES

The first two very rare lipid storage diseases are important in spite of their rarity because these disorders characteristically present with xanthomas. Tangier disease is included but the skin involvement is usually minor.

TABLE 62.7. Secondary hyperlipidaemia

	Cholesterol↑	Cholesterol↑ LDL↑	Triglyceride↑ VLDL↑	Triglycerides↑ HDL↑
Common	Primary Biliary cirrhosis Biliary cirrhosis	Nephrotic syndrome (IIA/ IIB) Hypothyroidism (IIA)	Chronic renal failure (IV) Diabetes mellitus (IV) (less commonly V) Alcoholism (IV)	Oral contraceptives
Rare		Hepatoma (IIA) Acute intermittent porphyria (IIA) Cushing's syndrome (IIB) Anorexia Nervosa (IIA)	Monodonal gammopathy (IV) Lipodystrophy (all forms) (IV)	

Cerebrotendinous xanthomatosis (cholestanolosis). This rare autosomal recessive condition is characterized by widespread tissue deposition of cholestanol and cholesterol resulting in progressive neurological defects and premature death from arteriosclerosis [1].

Aetiology. The primary biochemical defect appears to be in bile acid synthesis. The resulting deficiency of bile acids probably leads to an increased cholesterol and cholestanol synthesis by the liver [2, 5].

Clinical features. Sterol deposits are found throughout the body. Tendon xanthomas, especially over the Achilles tendon, are characteristic of the disorder and clinically are similar to those seen in hyperlipolipidaemias. Xanthelasma and tuberous xanthomas may also be present. Mental retardation and progressive spasticity develop. These neurological signs develop from extensive myelin destruction within the cerebellum and brain stem. Patients also develop juvenile cataracts and are at risk from premature arteriovascular disease [4].

Investigation. Cholestanol levels are elevated in plasma, bile and xanthomas. Plasma cholesterol tends to be low or normal. Correction of bile acid deficiency with chenodeoxycholic acid produces a reduction in plasma cholestanol levels and improvement in the neurological signs [3, 4].

REFERENCES

1 MENKES J., *et al* (1968) *Arch Neurol* **19**, 47.
2 SALEN G. (1971) *Ann Intern Med* **75**, 843.
3 SALEN G., *et al* (1975) *Biochem Med* **14**, 57.
4 SALEN G., *et al* (1983) In *Metabolic Basis of Inherited Disease*. Eds Stanbury J.B., *et al*. New York, McGraw-Hill, p. 713.
5 SETOGUCHI T., *et al* (1974) *J Clin Invest* **531**, 1395.

Sitosterolaemia and xanthomatosis. This very rare condition inherited as an autosomal recessive trait is characterized by xanthomas in childhood and accumulation of plant sterols within the tissues [1, 2].

Aetiology. The biochemical defect has not been established but it has been suggested that absorption of plant sterols campesterol, stigmasterol and sitosterol is increased.

Clinical features. Tendinous xanthomas particularly over the Achilles tendon and extensor tendons of the hand have been present in all cases to date and usually appear in early childhood. Less commonly tuberous xanthomas and xanthelasma may be present. Haemolysis with an enlarged spleen and premature arteriovascular disease has been noted in some patients.

Investigation. The diagnosis is made by the demonstration of increased amounts of these plant sterols by gas–liquid chromatography of plasma or xanthomas. These patients also have hypercholesterolaemia.

REFERENCES

1 BHATTACHARYYA A.K. & CONNOR W.E. (1974) *J Clin Invest* **53**, 1033.
2 SALEN G., *et al* (1983) in *Metabolic Basis of Inherited Disease*. Eds Stanbury J.B., *et al*. New York, McGraw-Hill, p. 713.

Tangier disease (HDL deficiency, α-lipoprotein deficiency disease). This is a very rare autosomal recessive disorder characterized by a deficiency or absence of normal HDL in the plasma [5, 6].

Aetiology. The primary biochemical defect is not known but there may be an abnormality in control of HDL synthesis or catabolism; as a result HDL are markedly reduced and of abnormal composition (apolipoproteins A I and C are present in only trace amounts [1, 2, 6]). This reduction in HDL results in the production of abnormal chylomicron remnants and the accumulation of cholesteryl esters.

Clinical features. Twenty-six patients have been reported to date [6]. Orange–yellow tonsils and adenoids are characteristic but hepatosplenomegaly and peripheral neuropathy are common features. Cholesteryl esters are found in the skin within foamy histiocytes [3, 4, 7]. Slit-lamp examination of the eye shows corneal infiltration in most patients as they age.

Investigation. The combination of a very low level of cholesterol and elevated plasma triglyceride is almost diagnostic. Lipoprotein electrophoresis shows no protein with α motility and ultracentrifugation shows HDL to be absent or present in only trace amounts.

REFERENCES

1 ASSMAN G., *et al* (1977) *J Clin Invest* **59**, 565.
2 ASSMAN G., *et al* (1977) *J Clin Invest* **60**, 242.
3 BALE P.M., *et al* (1971) *J Clin Pathol* **24**, 609.
4 FERRANS V.L. & FREDERICKSON D.S. (1975) *Am J Pathol* **78**, 101.
5 FREDERICKSON D.S., *et al* (1961) *Ann Intern Med* **55**, 1016.

6 HERBERT P.N., *et al* (1983) In *Metabolic Basis of Inherited Disease*. Eds Stanbury J.B., *et al*. New York, McGraw-Hill, p. 607.
7 WALDORF D.S., *et al* (1967) *Arch Dermatol* **95**, 161.

XANTHOMAS IN LYMPHOEDEMA

Xanthomas in association with lymphoedema are reported [1–5]. Lymph stasis with intraluminar and periluminar retention of lipoproteins and ingestion by local histiocytes seems a likely explanation. Scattered firm yellowish papules are seen within lymphoedematous area. Chylous exudation may be spontaneous or follow abrasion. Histologically the epidermis shows irregular acanthosis and hyperkeratosis. Intralymphatic and perilymphatic collections of foam cells are characteristic. Alleviation of the lymph stasis by surgery or pressure bandaging is sometimes effective.

REFERENCES

1 CAIRNS R.J. (1963) *Br J Dermatol* **75**, 123.
2 COBURN J.G. (1963) *Br J Dermatol* **75**, 128.
3 HUNTER J.A.A, *et al* (1970) *Trans St Johns Hosp Dermatol Soc* **56**, 143.
4 POLANO M.K. & PRINS F.J. (1965) *Hautarzt*, **16**, 86.
5 WOOLING K.R., *et al* (1970) *JAMA* **211**, 1372.

XANTHOMA CELLS IN INFLAMMATORY AND NEOPLASTIC DISEASE

Cholesterol deposition is not infrequent in inflammatory disorders, where it appears to result from the liberation of lipids in the tissues. These lipids are ingested by histiocytes producing the characteristic foam cell seen in histological sections. In some instances there may be an abnormal production of cholesterol *in situ*. Diffuse xanthoma may appear in previously inflamed skin [1, 3]. Similar secondary xanthomatous infiltration is also seen in certain localized inflammatory and neoplastic disorders. The diseases in which xanthoma cells may be encountered are listed below.

1. Inflammatory disease
   Histiocytoma
   Juvenile xanthogranuloma
2. Neoplastic disease
   Multicentric reticulohistiocytosis
   Eosinophilic granulomas [2]
   Letterer–Siwe disease, Hand–Schüller–Christian disease
   Mycosis fungoides

REFERENCES

1 JAMES M.P. & WARIN A.P. (1978) *Clin Exp Dermatol* **3**, 307.
2 PINKUS H. (1951) *Med Clin North Am* **35**, 463.
3 WALKER A.E. & SNEDDON I.B. (1968) *Br J Dermatol* **80**, 580.

MUCINOSES

M.M. BLACK

Mucins are jelly-like materials concerned with the hydration of the ground substances and probably play a part in the extravascular exchange of metabolites. Acid mucopolysaccharides, such as hyaluronic acid and heparin, stain with toluidine blue, the coloration depending on the number and nature of the acid groups. PAS stains heparin but not hyaluronic acid. In general acid mucopolysaccharides stain much brighter in frozen fixed tissue.

Neutral mucopolysaccharides are glycoproteins in which the hexosamine sugar polymer is incorporated in a protein chain. Hale and alcian blue stains are negative but PAS stain is positive. The mucins in the skin and their histochemistry have been well reviewed [4].

Mucinous infiltration of the skin is found in many widely differing disorders, some affecting the skin only, others related to systemic disease [3].

Classification
1. Metabolic
   Diffuse myxoedema
   Pretibial myxoedema (p. 2346)
   Lichen myxoedematosus
2. Collagen vascular disease
   Lupus erythematosus
   Dermatomyositis
3. Secondary (catabolic) mucinoses
   Degeneration in tumours
   Fibroma, lipoma, myxosarcoma, liposarcoma, some basal cell carcinomas
4. Localized
   Follicular mucinosis (idiopathic; reticulotic)
   Papular [1]
   Reticulo-erythematous mucinosis syndrome
   Atrophic papulosis (Degos) [2]
   Focal
   'Synovial' cyst

REFERENCES

1 ABULAFIA J. & PIERINI L.E. (1961) *Arch Argent Dermatol* **11**, 1.
2 BLACK M.M. (1971) *Br J Dermatol* **85**, 290.

3 REED R.J., *et al* (1973) *Hum Pathol* **4**, 201.
4 WELLS G.C. (1962) *Trans St Johns Hosp Dermatol Soc* **48**, 35.

LICHEN MYXOEDEMATOSUS
SYN. PAPULAR MUCINOSIS; LICHEN FIBROMUCINODOSIS; SCLEROMYXOEDEMA

Lichen myxoedematosus is a cutaneous myxoedematous state characterized by the formation of numerous lichenoid papules which coalesce together to form generalized plaques, causing extensive thickening and hardening of the skin. It is a rare disorder characterized by proliferation of fibroblasts and excessive deposition of acid mucopolysaccharides in the skin.

Histopathology [7, 8]. Mucinous deposits occur in the middle and deeper layers of the dermis and displace collagen fibres, but do not involve the dermal papillae or accumulate around blood vessels. Histochemically, the mucinous deposits are heterogeneous mixtures of acid mucopolysaccharides which stain positively with alcian blue and toluidine blue. Large stellate and elongated fibroblasts are present within the mucinous stroma. Mucin deposition in the media and adventitia of vessels and in many organs including the myocardium is reported, and the skeletal muscles can be infiltrated with lymphocytes.

Clinical features [9]. Most patients are adults aged 30–50. The clinical manifestations vary, and several types have been described.

1. Generalized lichenoid eruption with discrete papules covering the entire body, but especially the hands, forearms, upper part of the trunk, face and neck.
2. A discrete papular eruption on the trunk and extremities.
3. Localized or generalized over the body.
4. Urticarial plaques and nodular eruptions.

The confluent papular and sclerotic form is called scleromyxoedema [1, 3]—the Arndt–Gottron syndrome—in which diffuse thickening of the skin underlies the papules. The features may be distorted by the exaggeration of the facial ridges and flexion of the fingers may be limited. The involvement of the hands may simulate scleroderma, but the clinical appearance of numerous small papules of more or less uniform size, often in linear patterns on an erythematous and palpably thickened background, is very distinctive.

No endocrine abnormalities have been demonstrated but there are several reports indicating that systemic involvement may occur, for patients with no other evidence of systemic disease may complain of extreme muscular weakness and lassitude.

A paraproteinaemia is commonly found on serum electrophoresis, although total serum protein values are usually normal. This forms a monoclonal-type band that is extremely cationic and is of IgG class [6, 11]. Bone marrow studies may show a mild plasmacytic infiltration. Radiological survey of the skeletal system is normal. In one case the acid mucopolysaccharides in the serum were elevated [10]. It has been shown that serum from patients with lichen myxoedematosus, even after elution of the IgG paraprotein, can stimulate synthesis of DNA and cell proliferation in cultured fibroblasts [4].

Diagnosis. Infiltrates appearing in and around old scars may simulate 'scar sarcoidosis'. Papules on the dorsa of the hands and ears may cause confusion with granuloma annulare. Systemic scleroderma may show many features simulating scleromyxoedema. However, in scleroderma the skin is thickened and bound down, whereas in scleromyxoedema it is thickened but movable over the

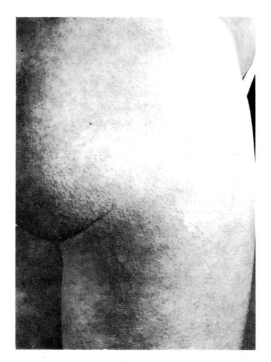

FIG. 62.10. Lichen myxoedematosus. An eruption of small papules on a background of erythematous and diffusely infiltrated skin. (Addenbrooke's Hospital.)

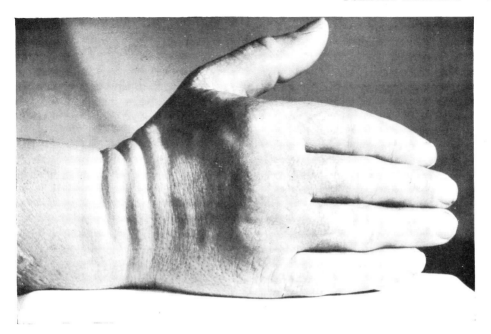

FIG. 62.11. Lichen myxoedematosus. The right hand of the same patient. Note the diffuse infiltration and scattered papules. Movements of fingers and wrists were severely limited. (Addenbrooke's Hospital.)

subcutis. Systemic involvement is minimal in scleromyxoedema and the histological changes are an increase in mucopolysaccharides rather than collagen. Papules are absent in scleroedema and scleroderma, but common in scleromyxoedema.

Prognosis. Prior to the introduction of cyclophosphamide and melphalan the prognosis was usually uniformly poor. Death may result from non-specific complications such as bronchopneumonia, but two patients, both of whom had shown bizarre central nervous symptoms, died of coronary occlusion [10].

Treatment. Treatment with melphalan is probably the treatment of choice, although the therapy may well be toxic. In a recent series long-term low dose melphalan therapy resulted in the gradual resolution of the skin lesions, with noticeable softening of the sclerosis within 3 months [5]. However, the effect of the melphalan on the reversion of the monoclonal protein tended to be variable. Treatment with systemic steroids is ineffective [2], but dermabrasion has helped the papular variety [12].

REFERENCES

1 CROSSLAND P.M. (1953) *Arch Derm Syphil* **67**, 122.
2 DONALD G.F., *et al* (1953) *Aust J Dermatol* **2**, 28.
3 GOTTRON H.A. (1954) *Arch Dermatol Syphil* **199**, 71.
4 HARPER R.A. & RISPLER J. (1978) *Science* **199**, 545.
5 *HARRIS R.B., *et al* (1979) *Arch Dermatol* **115**, 295.
6 LAI A., *et al* (1973) *Br J Dermatol* **88**, 107.
7 McCUISTON C.H. & SCHOCH E.P. (1956) *Arch Dermatol* **74**, 259.
8 MONTGOMERY H. & UNDERWOOD L.J. (1953) *J Invest Dermatol* **20**, 213.
9 *PERRY H.O., *et al* (1960) *Ann Intern Med* **53**, 955.
10 RUDNER E.J., *et al* (1966) *Arch Dermatol* **93**, 3.
11 WRIGHT R.C., *et al* (1976) *Arch Dermatol* **112**, 63.
12 ZEZSCHWITZ K.A.V. (1959) *Arch Klin Exp Dermatol* **208**, 301.

FOLLICULAR MUCINOSIS
SYN. ALOPECIA MUCINOSA

Definition and nomenclature [12]. Follicular mucinosis is an inflammatory disorder characterized clinically by more or less infiltrated plaques with scaling and loss of hair, and histologically by the accumulation of acid mucopolysaccharides in the sebaceous gland and the outer root sheath of the hair follicles.

The condition was first described by Pinkus in 1957 [11] under the name alopecia mucinosa, but alopecia is not always clinically evident, particularly when only vellus follicles are involved.

Aetiology [3, 13]. The cause of follicular mucinosis is unknown. The reported cases fall into three groups. The first and largest group consists of patients with solitary or only a few lesions, clearing spontaneously in 2 months to 2 yr. In a second group are patients in whom the lesions persist or new lesions continue to develop over many years. In the third group are patients in whom the mucinosis is associated with a lymphoma; in such cases histological evidence of the lymphoma is present from the onset, but it may be overlooked until the sections are later re-examined with hindsight.

The cases associated with a lymphoma tend to occur in older patients (age 20–70; average 45) than the benign ones, but there is no absolute distinction in age incidence. The benign forms occur at any age from 2 to 75, with a peak between 20 and 40.

Some authorities regard follicular mucinosis as a non-specific follicular reaction, for similar though perhaps not identical changes have been observed in association with lupus erythematosus [2] and a case is also reported of follicular mucinosis with angiolymphoid hyperplasia [17].

Pathology [3, 5, 14]. The earliest change appears to be oedema of the outer root sheath and sebaceous gland. Cystic spaces form in which mucin accumulates. The entire depth of the follicle may be involved, but the degree of damage to the hair matrix is variable. At a later stage the sebaceous glands may appear to be absent or the whole follicle may be converted into a cystic cavity containing mucin and degenerate root-sheath cells. In the dermis the inflammatory changes are variable in degree, but with a tendency for them to become granulomatous. Electron microscopy studies [6, 10] have shown changes in the keratinocytes of the follicular epithelium. Autoradiographic studies [9] have failed to show increased synthesis of mucopolysaccharides in affected follicles.

Clinical features [3, 7]. In the acute benign form the earliest changes are grouped: skin-coloured papules or plaques of erythema, with some scaling, and with prominent follicles. Each plaque, commonly 2–5 cm in diameter, but sometimes larger, changes little in appearance. Multiple lesions may be present from the onset or may develop within a period of a few weeks. The face, scalp, neck and shoulders are commonly affected. The hairs are shed from the affected follicles, so that alopecia may therefore be the presenting symptoms when the scalp or eyebrow region is involved. Spontaneous recovery usually takes place within a few months but may be delayed for a year or more.

In the chronic form the lesions are often more numerous and more widely distributed and their morphology tends to be more variable. There may be elevated, flat or domed plaques or nodules, some of which may ulcerate. The plaques and nodules are often of soft gelatinous consistency; sometimes, mucin can be squeezed out of affected follicles. Non-infiltrated red scaly plaques, patchy scaling, alopecia and indurated plaques may all be present. In some cases leprosy may be simulated [4, 16]. Exceptionally, follicular papules may be generalized without obvious grouping [1]. Irritation may be troublesome and persistent. Destruction of follicles may give rise to patches of permanent alopecia, which may be studded with horny plugs. This chronic form may persist for many years without any evidence of associated disease.

A coexisting lymphoma is associated with follicular mucinosis in about 15% of cases. Unfortunately there is no single clinical feature which distinguishes such cases from the chronic benign form. Contrary to recent opinion [3] lymphoma-associated follicular mucinosis has now been reported where the lesions occurred on the head and neck [15, 16]. The temporal relationship between the lymphoma and the follicular mucinosis is very variable, and gross manifestations of the lymphoma may have been present for some time before the mucinosis develops. In other cases the first indication of the lymphoma is uncovered by the histological changes in a biopsy.

Diagnosis. The loss of hair in plaques with prominent follicles but minimal inflammatory changes should suggest the diagnosis. Sometimes, mucin can be expressed from the follicles. Eczema, seborrhoeic dermatitis, lichen simplex, pityriasis rosea, traumatic alopecia and tinea capitis can all be closely simulated. Biopsy and serial sectioning of the tissue should confirm the diagnosis.

Treatment. No effective measures are available. Some spontaneously improve and treatments with topical and intralesional steroids have been claimed to be of benefit. Superficial radiotherapy has certainly proved to be of benefit in some of the lymphoma-associated cases [16]. A case of follicular mucinosis responding to dapsone is reported [8].

REFERENCES

1 BAZEX A. *et al* (1962) *Bull Soc Fr Dermatol Syphiligr* **69**, 484.
2 CABRÉ J. & KORTING G.W. (1964) *Dermatol Wochenschr* **149**, 513.
3 *EMMERSON R.W. (1969) *Br J Dermatol* **81**, 395.

4 Fan J., *et al* (1967) *Arch Dermatol* **95**, 354.
5 Haber H. (1961) *Br J Dermatol* **73**, 313.
6 Ishibashi A., *et al* (1974) *J Cutan Pathol* **1**, 126.
7 *Kim R. & Winkelmann R.K. (1962) *Arch Dermatol* **85**, 490.
8 Kubba R.K. & Stewart T.W. (1974) *Br J Dermatol* **91**, 217.
9 Langner A., *et al* (1969) *Acta Derm Venereol (Stockh)* **49**, 76.
10 Orfanos C. & Gahlen W. (1964) *Arch Klin Exp Dermatol* **218**, 435.
11 Pinkus H. (1957) *Arch Dermatol* **76**, 419.
12 Pinkus H. (1976) In *Biology and Disease of Hair*. Eds Toka K., *et al.* Baltimore, University Park Press, p. 287.
13 Plotnick H. & Abrecht M. (1965) *Arch Dermatol* **92**, 137.
14 *Tappeiner J., *et al* (1967) *Arch Klin Exp Dermatol* **227**, 937.
15 Wilkinson J.D., *et al* (1979) *J R Soc Med* **72**, 281.
16 Wilkinson J.D., *et al* (1982) *Clin Exp Dermatol* **7**, 333.
17 Wolff H.H., *et al* (1978) *Arch Dermatol* **114**, 229.

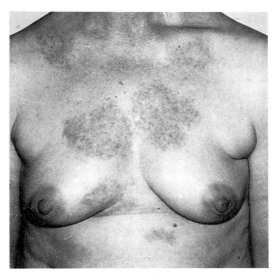

Fig. 62.12. REM syndrome on chest wall (courtesy of Dr S. S. Bleehen, Royal Hallamshire Hospital, Sheffield).

RETICULAR ERYTHEMATOUS MUCINOSIS
SYN. REM SYNDROME: PLAQUE-LIKE CUTANEOUS MUCINOSIS

An entity has been described in which areas of reticular erythema are present on the trunk with a mucinous and round-cell infiltrate in the dermis. This entity is frequently called the REM syndrome.

Aetiology. The aetiology is unknown, but there is some clinical and also experimental evidence that light is a factor in the pathogenesis of this disorder [1].

Pathology. In the papillary and upper reticular dermis there is a perivascular, and occasionally perifollicular, infiltrate largely composed of small mononuclear cells. The epidermis appears normal. There is separation of collagen bundles and fragmentation of elastic fibres. Histochemical stains show an increase in dermal mucin with a profile consistent with hyaluronic acid [1]. Direct immunofluorescence is negative for immunoglobulins, fibrin and complement [1]. Virus-like tubular aggregates have been identified in the cytoplasm of dermal endothelial cells and pericytes [1]. Recent evidence suggests that the lymphocytic cells in the filtrate are not T lymphocytes [2].

Clinical features. Most cases are female [1, 3–5]. Areas of pink reticulate or sheet-like erythema are present on the central part of the chest and back,

particularly over the sternum (Fig. 62.12) and on the upper back. There is usually no pruritus although sometimes the areas become itchy following sun exposure and the erythema may then be more apparent. The areas become infiltrated and then slowly increase in size.

Treatment. Topical steroids are ineffective but fortunately antimalarials are almost invariably effective in controlling the eruption [1, 4, 5].

REFERENCES

1 Bleehen S.S., *et al* (1982) *Br J Dermatol* **106**, 9.
2 Chavaz P., *et al* (1982) *Br J Dermatol* **106**, 741.
3 Quimby S.R. & Perry H.O. (1982) *J Am Acad Dermatol* **6**, 856.
4 Steigleder G.K. & Kanzow G. (1980) *Hautarzt* **31**, 575.
5 Steigleder G.K., *et al* (1974) *Br J Dermatol* **91**, 191.

THE MUCOPOLYSACCHARIDOSES

The mucopolysaccharidoses are genetically determined diseases in which mucopolysaccharides (primarily dermatan sulphate, heparan sulphate and keratan sulphate) are stored in tissues and excreted in large amounts in the urine. The striking alterations in the patient's appearance once led to their being referred to as gargoyles. Research in this field has progressed rapidly and in most of the classic mucopolysaccharidoses it is now possible to delineate the molecular defect in enzyme activity that is the primary product of the abnormal gene and

TABLE 62.8. Clinical and laboratory features of the mucopolysaccharidoses (after Nyhan [11])

MPS	Syndrome	Inheritance	Mental retardation	Eye	First manifestation	Hepato-splenomegaly	Bony defect	Compound stored, excreted	Enzyme defect
I_H	Hurler	Autosomal recessive	+	Corneal clouding	Coarse facial features, motor weakness, mental retardation, hernia	+	+	Dermatan sulphate, heparan sulphate	α-L-Iduronidase
I_S	Scheie	Autosomal recessive	−	Corneal clouding	Coarse features	−	+	Dermatan sulphate, heparan sulphate	α-L-Iduronidase
II	Hunter	X-linked recessive	+	Cornea clear	Weakness, coarse features, mental retardation, aggressive behaviour	+	+	Dermatan sulphate, heparan sulphate	L-Iduronosulphate sulphatase
III_A	Sanfilippo type A	Autosomal recessive	+	Cornea clear	Hyperkinetic behaviour	+	+	Heparan sulphate	Heparan sulphate sulphamidase
III_B	Sanfilippo type B	Autosomal recessive	+	Cornea clear	Hyperkinetic behaviour, mental retardation	+	+	Heparan sulphate	α-N-acetylglucos-aminidase
IV_A	Morquio	Autosomal recessive	+	Corneal clouding	Bony deformities	−	+	Keratan sulphate	N-acetylgalactos-amine-6-sulphatase
IV_B	Morquio-like	Autosomal recessive	+	Corneal clouding	Bony deformities	+	+	Keratan sulphate, heparan sulphate	N-acetylglucos-amine-6-sulphatase
VI	Maroteaux-Lamy	Autosomal recessive	−	Corneal opacities	Growth retardation	+	+	Dermatan sulphate	N-acetylgalactos-amine-4-sulphatase (arylsulphatase B)
VII	β-Glucuronidase deficiency	Autosomal recessive	+	±Corneal clouding	Coarse features	+	+	Dermatan sulphate, heparan sulphate, chondroitin-4,6-sulphate	β-Glucuronidase

fundamental cause of all the manifestations of these diseases. Table 62.8 summarizes the clinical and biochemical features of the mucopolysaccharidoses [11].

HURLER'S SYNDROME; HUNTER'S SYNDROME

These are rare disorders of mucopolysaccharide metabolism characterized by a peculiar facies, dwarfism, widespread skeletal defects, mental deficiency, hepatosplenomegaly and clouding of the cornea.

Aetiology. There are two distinct modes of inheritance:

1. Hurler type, which is severe and inherited as an autosomal recessive trait, in which the molecular defect is the enzyme α-L-iduronidase.
2. Hunter type, which is milder and carried in the X chromosome, in which the molecular defect is the enzyme L-iduronosulphate sulphatase.

There is gross disturbance of mucopolysaccharide metabolism with malformation of cartilage, tendon, periosteum, meninges, cornea and heart valves. The synthesis of acid mucopolysaccharides has been demonstrated in tissue culture [9, 10].

Histopathology [13]. The cutaneous findings are distinctive [6, 12]. In the epidermis, the occasional Malpighian cell develops a pale distended cytoplasm which may displace the nucleus to one side. Vacuolated cells are prominent in sweat glands [2] and, to a lesser extent, in the external root sheaths of hair follicles. Large vacuolated cells (gargoyle cells) are prominent just below the epidermis. In biopsies of scleroderma-like skin, fragmentation and hyalinization of collagen and increased tissue mucin have been demonstrated. Sometimes pooling of metachromatic material between the collagen bundles of the lower reticular dermis is especially marked [5].

Ultrastructurally, the presence of membrane-limited cytoplasmic vacuoles containing fibrillogranular material in dermal connective tissue and Schwann cells has been demonstrated in all varieties of the mucopolysaccharidoses syndrome [5].

Clinical features: Affected children are usually normal at birth and during the first or second year an increasingly grotesque appearance develops. However, corneal haziness may be detected during the first 6 months, when the earliest radiological changes may already be present [3]. Affected infants are dwarfed.

The head is large and scaphocephalic with a prominent sagittal ridge crossing the forehead. The nose is saddle shaped. The lips are large and the tongue protrudes through the open mouth over small, deformed, widely spaced teeth. There is chronic nasal discharge. A stout neck, lumbar kyphosis and protuberant abdomen add to the grotesque appearance. Joint movement is severely limited. Liver and spleen are grossly enlarged and multiple herniae are usual.

Skin changes are not always present but can be distinctive. Ivory-white nodules or ridges occupy symmetrical areas between the angles of the scapulae and posterior axillary lines [1, 4]. The individual nodules range from 1 to 10 mm in size and are a characteristic sign in Hurler's disease [7]. In some cases they have also been present on the upper arms, forearms, pectoral regions and outer thighs. Thickening of the skin of the digits may simulate acrosclerosis [6]. The whole body tends to be abnormally hairy, but after puberty pubic and axillary hair may fail to develop.

Clouding of the cornea is a constant finding which may progress to severe visual loss. Formes frustes have been described with only corneal cloudiness, slight clawing of the hands and a positive urine test [12]. However, in the X-linked (Hunter) type the cornea is normal.

Mental retardation and deafness may be mild or severe. A wide variety of other abnormalities affecting many organs has been reported. The expectation of life is poor, many cases dying of cardiac failure before the age of 20, but some survive to middle age.

Diagnosis: When the Hurler sundrome or another mucopolysaccharidosis is first suspected clinically, the diagnosis can be confirmed by a variety of simple urine spot tests such as that using filter paper impregnated with azure A. The mucopolsaccharide being excreted can be exactly typed with the use of column chromatography.

Differential diagnosis: Differentiating features are listed in Table 62.8.

Treatment: None is available. In one study [8] plasma infusions were given in an attempt to supply the specific corrective factor, but this did not lead to any observable ultrastructural changes after treatment. Bone marrow transplantation is still experimental.

REFERENCES

1 ANDERSON B. & TORDBERG O. (1952) *Acta Paediatr Scand* **41**, 161.
2 BELCHER R.W. (1973) *Arch Pathol* **96**. 339.
3 BURKE E.C. (1962) *Proc Staff Meet Mayo Clin* **37**, 241.
4 COLE H.N. *et al* (1952) *Arch Dermatol Syph* **66**, 371.
5 FREEMAN R.G. (1977) *J. Cutan Pathol* **4**, 318.
6 HAMBRICK G.W., JR. & SHEIE H.G. (1962) *Arch Dermatol* **85**, 455.
7 LARREGUE M., *et al* (1976) *Ann Dermatol Vénéréol* **105**, 57.
8 LASSER A., *et al* (1975) *Arch Pathol* **99**, 173.
9 LEVIN S. (1960) *Am J Dis Child* **99**, 445.
10 MATALON R. & DORFMAN A. (1966) *Proc Natl Acad Sci USA* **56**, 1310.
11 NYHAN W.L. (1980) *Clin Symp* **32**, 25.
12 SHEIE H.G., *et al* (1962) *Am J Ophthalmol* **53**, 753.
13 WALLACE B.J., *et al* (1966) *Arch Pathol* **82**, 462.

THE MUCOLIPIDOSES

The term mucolipidoses refers to a number of Hurler-like syndromes in which there is no accompanying mucopolysacchariduria but in which both polysaccharides and sphingomyelin and related lipids are stored. Dense cytoplasmic inclusions arise in cultured fibroblasts [1, 2].

REFERENCES

1 LEGUM C.P., *et al* (1976) In *Advances in Pediatrics*. Ed. Schulman J. Chicago, Year Book Medical Publishers, Vol. 22, p. 305.
2 MCKUSICK V.A., *et al* (1978) In *The Metabolic Basis of Inherited Disease*. Eds J.B. Stanbury, *et al*. New York, McGraw-Hill, p. 1282.

LEROY'S SYNDROME

This is a rare lipomucopolysaccharide disorder showing skin thickening and bone changes. The X-ray appearances mimic Hurler's disease. No corneal opacities are seen and fibroblast cultures show nuclear inclusions.

REFERENCE

LEROY J.G. & DE MARS R.I. (1967) *Science* **157**, 804.

MORQUIO'S DISEASE

This rare genetic mucopolysaccharide disorder shows general telangiectasia with a loose, wrinkled, yet thickened skin [2]. Gross osteochondrodystrophy is usual. Both qualitative and quantitative analyses of urinary mucopolysaccharides are necessary to distinguish this from Hurler's disease [1,3].

REFERENCES

1 BITTER T., *et al* (1966) *J Bone Joint Surg* **48**, 637.
2 GREAVES M.W. & INMAN P.M. (1969) *Br J Dermatol* **81**, 29.
3 ROBINS M.M., *et al* (1963) *J Pediatr* **62**, 881.

AMYLOID AND THE AMYLOIDOSES OF THE SKIN [2–4]

M. M. BLACK

Amyloid is a proteinaceous substance that is deposited in the tissues in a wide variety of conditions. A number of stimuli can induce its formation and it occurs in association with many diseases.

Amyloid has certain characteristic physicochemical properties: tinctorial properties (Congophilia and green birefringence under polarized light); its distinctive fibrillar ultrastructure; a cross-β pattern on X-ray diffraction.

The β structure of the fibrils probably accounts for the low solubility and resistance to proteolytic digestion of amyloid. A further minor constituent of all types of amyloid, with a characteristic pentagonal ultrastructure, is the doughnut, rod or 'P-component' (protein AP) which may aggregate to form the short rods also seen on electron microscopy. Protein AP has recently been isolated as a normal serum $\alpha 1$ glycoprotein with calcium-dependent binding properties [5] and is a constituent of elastic fibres [1].

REFERENCES

1 BREATHNACH S.M., *et al* (1981) *Br J Dermatol* **105**, 115.
2 COHEN A.S. (1981) *Int J Dermatol* **20**, 515.
3 GLENNER G.G. (1980) *N Engl J Med* **302**, 1283.
4 GLENNER G.G. (1980) *N Engl J Med* **302**, 1333.
5 PEPYS M.B., *et al* (1977) *Lancet* i, 1029.

Staining reactions [1, 2]. These are not entirely specific apart from Congophilia and green birefringence under polarized light [2]. Heparatin sulphate is probably responsible for the metachromasia with various stains and the fluorescence with thioflavine T. The mucopolysaccharide, which constitutes 1·5% of amyloid material, is probably oriented on the surface of the complicated protein molecule.

The staining properties depend to some extent upon the duration of fixation in formalin and tend to be far brighter on frozen fixed material.

In cutaneous amyloidosis the deposits of amyloid are often sparse. It is recommended that a battery of stains be included: (PAS); Congo red with demonstration of green birefringence using polarized light; crystal violet metachromasia of amyloid deposits; thioflavine T fluorescence. The dylon stain appears to be a more promising recent addition [3]. Finally, in some cases it may be necessary to resort to electron microscopy to look for the characteristic ultrastructure of the fibrils.

REFERENCES

1 BLACK M.M. (1976) In *Amyloidosis*. Eds Wegelius O. & Pasternak A. London, Academic Press, p. 1079.
2 COOPER J.H. (1976) In *Amyloidosis*. Eds Wegelius O. & Pasternak A. London, Academic Press, p. 61.
3 YANAGIHARA M., *et al* (1979) *Jpn J Dermatol* **89**, 25.

PRIMARY LOCALIZED CUTANEOUS AMYLOIDOSIS [4, 6]

In primary localized cutaneous amyloidosis the main change consists of a deposition of amyloid in previously apparently normal skin, with no evidence that deposits occur in internal organs. Various localized forms of amyloidosis confined to the skin are recognized. There are the more common papular and macular types and the rare tumefactive forms. Both macular and papular lesions can occur in the same patient.

Aetiology. The aetiology of primary localized cutaneous amyloidosis remains unknown. Racial susceptibility to lichen amyloidosus in the population of the Middle East, Asia, China and Central or South America suggests the role of genetic factors [4]. The presence of an abnormal α2-globulin in the sera of some cases of macular amyloidosis has been reported [22] although this has not been the experience of the author [4, 6]. Y-globulins may also be increased in lichen amyloidosus [12]. Multiple myeloma has developed in four patients with lichen amyloidosis [1, 11]. However, despite the exceptionally long duration of the disease in some, a review of the current literature has revealed no instance of systemic deposition of amyloid.

In lichen amyloidosus the close proximity of the amyloid deposits to the lower epidermis strongly suggests that the epidermis plays a role in its pathogenesis [2, 6]. Although it has been claimed that there is a difference between hyalin bodies (filamentous masses) and amyloid [10], further ultrastructural studies [14, 15] showed no difference in thickness among the tubular filaments of filamentous cells, filamentous masses and amyloid filaments. It is claimed that some of the amyloid substance in primary localized cutaneous amyloidosis derives from epidermal cells through filamentous degeneration [14, 15]. Amyloid fibrils also react to anti-human keratin antibody, indicating further an epidermal origin for the fibrils [14, 15]. Lichen amyloidosus has been reported to follow a lichen-planus-like eruption (19). The author has postulated that in lichen amyloidosus, a specific immunological tolerance develops to the presence of degenerating epidermal cells (filamentous masses), so that amyloid may then be deposited in or around these filamentous masses possibly by fibroblasts [2, 4].

Pathology [4, 7]. In both the papular and macular forms of primary localized cutaneous amyloidosis the deposits of amyloid are confined to the papillary dermis. In papular lichen amyloidosus the focal deposits of amyloid are often large enough to expand the dermal papillae and displace the elongated rete ridges laterally. The overlying epidermis shows considerable irregular acanthosis and hyperkeratosis. The amyloid deposits are in close apposition to the basal layer of the epidermis and contain a few melanophages. The blood vessel walls are never directly involved. Near the amyloid deposits there is usually a sparse lympho-histiocytic perivascular infiltrate.

In macular amyloidosis the deposits of amyloid are smaller and tend to be composed of small faceted clumps whose individual components are similar in size to the hyaline bodies found in lichen planus [6]. In some cases the amyloid deposits in the dermal papillae are so sparse that more than one biopsy is necessary to confirm the diagnosis. The epidermis is usually of normal thickness but pigmentary incontinence with melanophages is a notable feature.

The nodular or tumefactive forms of primary localized cutaneous amyloidosis is entirely different from the papular and macular variants because the dermis, subcutis and blood vessel walls are diffusely infiltrated with amyloid. In addition, there may be a perivascular infiltrate of plasma cells [7]. These features are indistinguishable from those associated with systemic amyloidosis when it affects the skin.

Clinical features [4, 6, 7]. Several distinctive clinical forms of primary localized cutaneous amyloidosis have been described (Table 62.9).

The papular form (lichen amyloidosus) is perhaps the best known. It usually presents as a persistent, pruritic papular eruption on the shins (Figs 62.13

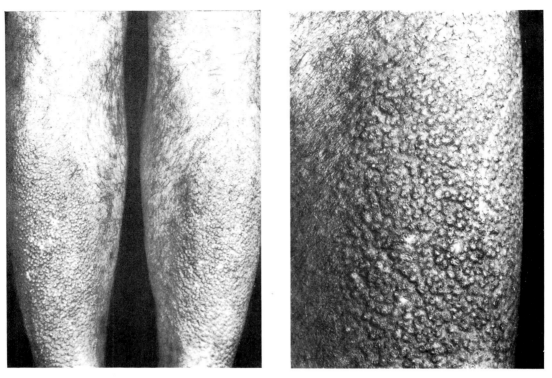

FIG. 62.13. 6 62.14. Lichen amyloidosus (papular form). The distribution of the lesions is characteristic. (St John's Hospital.)

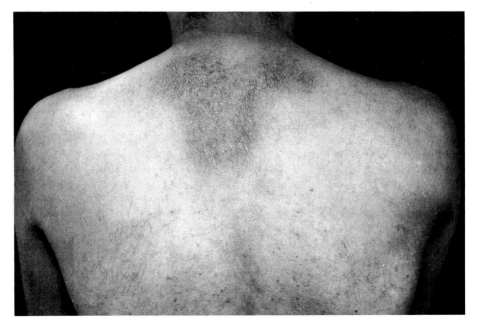

FIG. 62.15. Macular amyloidosis. Interscapular hyperpigmentation in an Asian. (St John's Hospital.)

TABLE 62.9. Clinical classification of primary localized cutaneous amyloidosis

---

(1) Papular or lichen amyloidosus
(2) (a) Macular amyloidosis
    (b) Maculopapular amyloidosis
(3) Nodular or tumefactive
(4) Familial

---

and 62.14) although the extensor aspect of the thighs, forearms and upper arms may also be affected. The individual lesions consist of multiple discrete papules which are scaly and often pigmented. Papules may coalesce into thickened plaques, which may closely simulate hypertrophic lichen planus or lichen simplex chronicus. The condition usually persists for many years with localized pruritus as the prominent symptom. Lichen amyloidosus appears to be more common among the Chinese than among other ethnic groups [17].

Macular amyloidosis [6, 7] is the most subtle of the cutaneous amyloidoses since it can be misdiagnosed as post-inflammatory pigmentation, resolving lichen planus or neurodermatitis. Macular amyloidosis is rare amongst Europeans and North Americans but is much more common among Central and South Americans [13, 21], Middle Easterners [16, 23] and Asians [6]. The lesions may be confined to the interscapular area (Fig. 62.15) but more commonly the lesions are more extensively distributed over the back or chest. Lesions may also occur on the extensor aspect of extremities; macular and papular forms may coexist in the same patient [8]. Periocular pigmentation has also been described [26]. In macular amyloidosis the skin lesions are hyperpigmented, although hypopigmented areas may also occur giving a 'poikilodermatous' appearance. The predominant sign is clusters of small pigmented macules, about 2 or 3 mm in diameter, which may coalesce to produce macular hyperpigmented areas. A reticulate or 'rippled' pattern of pigmentation is a characteristic diagnostic feature in many cases of macular amyloidosis. Micropapules may also occur; thus the maculopapular form is essentially an extension of macular amyloidosis. The lesions tend to be associated with mild to moderate pruritus, but pruritus may be absent in 18% of cases [4]. The condition usually presents in early adult life and persists for many years; both sexes equally affected [4]. Atypical cases occasionally occur presenting with unusual or bizarre patterns of hyperpigmentation [5].

The nodular or tumefactive form is a rare variant of primary localized cutaneous amyloidosis. Most of the reported patients have been females. Single or multiple nodules or plaques may occur on the trunk and limbs. The overlying skin is often atrophic and there may be petechial haemorrhages within the nodules. Most patients have an elevated sedimentation rate and β- and γ-globulin levels. Although amyloid nodules may occur without associated systemic amyloidosis, long-term follow-up is necessary. Progression of nodular amyloidosis to systemic amyloidosis has been reported rarely [7].

Familial forms of primary localized cutaneous amyloidosis are very rare. However, families are described in which the affected members had pigmentation and pruritus [25]. Another family has been described in which the males also had other systemic manifestations [20]. Concurrent nail dystrophy is a further recently described feature [24].

Finally, primary localized cutaneous amyloidosis may show some overlap with collagen vascular diseases. Cases have been described in association with systemic lupus erythematosus [9], systemic sclerosis [3] and primary biliary cirrhosis and scleroderma [4].

Diagnosis. The diagnosis should be strongly suggested clinically in the more typical forms. Cutaneous amyloidosis should always be suspected in a patient presenting with unusual or bizarre forms of hyperpigmentation. The diagnosis should be established histologically and electron microscopy may be necessary [5].

Treatment. No specific treatment is available. Topical steroids under occlusive dressings are certainly helpful in the short term. Dermabrasion can have an extremely long-term beneficial effect on lichen amyloidosus of the shins [27].

REFERENCES

1 ALEXANDER S. (1970) *Bull Soc Fr Dermatol Syphiligr* 77, 707.
2 BLACK M.M. (1971) *Br J Dermatol* 84, 172.
3 BLACK M.M. (1971) *Trans St Johns Hosp Dermatol Soc* 57, 177.
4 *BLACK M.M. (1976) In *Amyloidosis*. Eds. Wegelius O. & Pasternak A. London, Academic Press, p. 479.
5 BLACK M.M. & MAIBACH H.I. (1974) *Br J Dermatol* 90, 461.
6 *BLACK M.M. & WILSON JONES E. (1971) *Br J Dermatol* 84, 199.
7 *BROWNSTEIN M.H. & HELWIG E.B. (1970) *Arch Dermatol* 102, 8.
8 BROWNSTEIN M.H., et al (1973) *Br J Dermatol* 88, 25.
9 DANIELSEN L., et al (1970) *Acta Pathol Microbiol Scand* [A] 78, 335.

10 EBNER H. & GEBHART W. (1975) *Br J Dermatol* **92**, 637.

11 GREAVES M.W. (1963) *Proc R Soc Med* **56**, 791.

12 HABERMANN M.C. & MONTENEGRO M.R. (1980) *Dermatologica* **160**, 240.

13 HUERTA L., CARVAJAL (1976) *Cromograf. Ecuador, S.A.* Guayaquil.

14 KOBAYASHI H. & HASHIMOTO K. (1983) *J Invest Dermatol* **80**, 66.

15 *KUMAKIRI M. & HASHIMOTO K. (1979) *J Invest Dermatol* **73**, 150.

16 KURBAN A.K., *et al* (1971) *Br J Dermatol* **85**, 52.

17 KUTTY M.K., *et al* (1970) *Med J Aust* **i**, 842.

18 MAEDA H., *et al* (1982) *Br J Dermatol* **106**, 345.

19 MASU S., *et al* (1980) *Jpn J Dermatol* **90**, 623.

20 PARTINGTON M.W., *et al* (1981) *Am J Med Genet* **10**, 65.

21 PORTO J.A. (1962) In *Proc. 12th Int. Congr. on Dermatology.* Ed Pillsbury D.M. & Livingood C.S. Amsterdam, Excerpta Medica, p. 783.

22 PORTO J.A., *et al* (1963) *J Invest Dermatol* **40**, 169.

23 SHANON J. & SAGHER F. (1970) *Arch Dermatol* **102**, 195.

24. SHAW M., *et al* (1983) *Clin Exp Dermatol* **8**, 363.

25 VASILY D.B., *et al* (1978) *Arch Dermatol* **114**, 1173.

26 VAN DEN BERG W.H.H.W. & STARINK TH.M. (1983) *Clin Exp Dermatol* **8**, 195.

27 WONG C.K. & LI W.M. (1982) *Arch Dermatol* **118**, 302.

SECONDARY LOCALIZED CUTANEOUS AMYLOIDOSIS

Clinically insignificant microscopic deposits of amyloid material have been described in association with a variety of cutaneous tumours including intradermal naevus, sweat gland tumours, pilomatrixoma, dermatofibroma, seborrhoeic wart, solar keratosis, porokeratosis of Mibelli, Bowen's disease and basal cell carcinoma [1, 4]. A similar phenomenon has been noted following psoralen and long-wave UV radiation (PUVA therapy) [2, 3].

REFERENCES

1 BROWNSTEIN M.H. & HELWIG E.B. (1970) *Arch Dermatol* **102**, 8.

2 GREEN I & COX A.J. (1979) *Arch Dermatol* **115**, 1200.

3 HASHIMOTO K. & KUMAKIRI M. (1979) *J Invest Dermatol* **72**, 70.

4 MacDONALD D.M. & BLACK M.M. (1980) *Br J Dermatol* **103**, 553.

SYSTEMIC AMYLOIDOSIS [3]
SYN. LUBARSH–PICK DISEASE

This is an uncommon disorder of protein metabolism showing various combinations of carpal tunnel syndrome, macroglossia, specific mucocutaneous lesions and visceral (cardiac, renal, hepatic, gastrointestinal) involvement.

Aetiology. Almost certainly the cause of the disease is an underlying plasma cell dyscrasia, although marrow aspiration may not be abnormal.

In primary and myeloma-associated amyloidosis the fibrils are composed of 'protein AL' (amyloid L chain protein) and appear to be a consequence of the plasma cell dyscrasia. Amino acid sequence analysis has demonstrated that protein AL consists of fragments of an immunoglobulin polypeptide light chain, particularly the variable (amino-terminal) region, or of an intact immunoglobulin light chain, or of both [9, 10], and is usually associated with a similar abnormal immunoglobulin light chain in the serum, commonly of λ class. The fibrils of secondary and experimentally induced amyloidosis, by contrast, are composed of a distinctive protein unrelated to any known immunoglobulin and designated 'protein AA' (amyloid A protein) [2]. A precursor of protein AA 'protein SAA', found in small quantities in normal serum and increased in pregnancy, infection and the elderly, appears to be an acute-phase reactant like C-reactive protein.

Almost certainly disturbances in immunoregulatory function may play a fundamental role in the pathogenesis of both primary and secondary amyloidosis [7, 14], with reticulo-endothelial cells governing the final pathway of amyloid fibril formation. Macrophages secrete substances that stimulate B lymphocytes and suppress T lymphocytes, and T lymphocytes normally control the activity and proliferation of macrophages and B lymphocytes. A unifying hypothesis of amyloidogenesis has been proposed [7] in which the initial event in both primary and secondary amyloidosis is macrophage activation associated with T-cell suppression, which is then followed by B-cell proliferation.

In primary and secondary amyloidosis both sexes are affected; the onset is usually in the sixth decade.

Histopathology [3, 5]. In primary and myeloma-associated amyloidosis, deposits of amyloid are usually superficially placed in the papillary dermis as faintly eosinophilic, amorphous, often fissured masses, accounting for the papules seen clinically. Amyloid deposits in the deep reticular dermis and subcutis give rise to the clinical appearance of nodules and tumefactions, and infiltration of blood vessel walls correlates with the clinical finding of purpura. Usually there is little in the way of any inflammatory infiltrate. In areas of alopecia, amyloid deposits may surround and compress pilosebaceous units with resultant atrophy and loss of hair from the shafts. Amyloid may also be deposited in arrector pili muscles and the lamina propria of sweat glands and ducts.

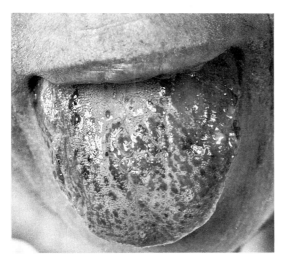

FIG. 62.16. Primary systemic amyloidosis: macroglossia. (St John's Hospital.)

In secondary systemic amyloidosis, small or minute amyloid deposits can be found in small blood vessels and in the subcutis around fat cells—'amyloid rings' [17].

Clinical features [3]. Presenting symptoms may be rather non-specific and include fatigue, weight loss, paraesthesiae, oedema, dyspnoea, light-headedness or syncope secondary to postural hypotension and hoarseness. These features may predate the histological diagnosis by up to 2 yr. The coexistence of the specific symptoms of the carpal tunnel syndrome, macroglossia and cutaneous lesions, however, is classical and should immediately alert the physician to the probable existence of plasma cell dyscrasia-related systemic amyloidosis. Principal initial examination findings usually include macroglossia, mucocutaneous lesions, hepatomegaly and oedema.

The tongue is usually diffusely enlarged and firm, but may also have a number of haemorrhagic papules, nodules, plaques or even bullae on its surface. Macroglossia may be so extensive as to cause dysphagia and reveal permanent tooth indentations along its lateral borders.

Nearly all cases of skin lesions occur in primary or myeloma-associated systemic amyloidosis. The commonest skin lesions are those related to intracutaneous haemorrhage due to infiltration of blood vessel walls by amyloid deposits [5]. Petechiae, purpura and ecchymoses may occur spontaneously or after minor trauma on normal or clinically involved skin especially in the body folds, e.g. eyelids, sides of neck, axillae, umbilicus and oral and anogenital regions. Eyelid purpura after pinching and periorbital purpura after proctoscopy ('post-proctoscopic palpebral purpura'), coughing, and vomiting on the

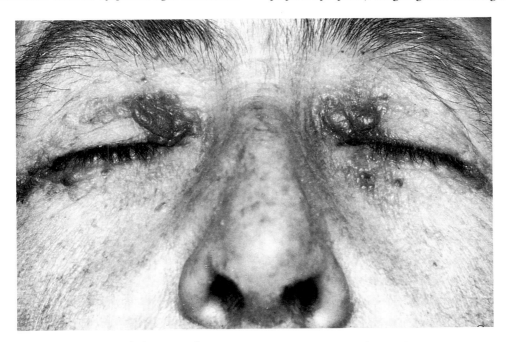

FIG. 62.17. Primary systemic amyloidosis: typical plaques on upper eyelids. (St Thomas' Hospital.)

Valsalva manœuvre are characteristic. Smooth, shiny, waxy papules or plaques, often with a haemorrhagic component, may also be found. Widespread nodules may occur, coalescing to form large tumefactions. Diffuse infiltration of large areas may simulate scleroderma and, on the face, a myxoedema-like appearance. Alopecia may be patchy or widespread and the scalp skin may be thrown into longitudinal folds resembling cutis verticis gyrata. Nail involvement due to infiltration of the nail matrix by amyloid may produce longitudinal striation, crumbling and brittleness [4]. Bullous lesions are rarer but these may resemble porphyria cutanea tarda [11]. The sicca syndrome due to amyloid infiltration of lacrimal and parotid glands has also been recorded [15].

Substantial hepatomegaly occurs in about 50% of cases but spenomegaly in less than 10% [12]. Other predominant findings include oedema, cardiac arrhythmias, orthostatic hypotension, congestive cardiac failure and peripheral neuropathy.

Diagnosis. A strong presumptive clinical diagnosis can be made when a patient presents with the triad of carpal tunnel syndrome, macroglossia and mucocutaneous skin lesions. Biopsy of classical mucocutaneous lesions should be the procedure of first choice. Fine needle biopsies of the subcutaneous fat from clinically normal abdominal skin can yield positive histological results in secondary amyloidosis [16, 17]. Rectal biopsy is positive in over 80% of cases [12]. Carpal tunnel tissue may be diagnostic in up to 90% of cases. About 96% of hepatic and 90% of renal biopsies are positive in primary or myeloma-associated amyloidosis [12]. Percutaneous needle aspiration of the spleen has been reported as a safe procedure of comparable diagnostic accuracy to renal biopsy [13]. Bone marrow aspiration may reveal amyloid in 45% of cases or evidence of plasma cell excess [12].

Immunoelectrophoresis of both serum and concentrated urine is essential if the clinical presentation suggests the presence of a plasma cell dyscrasia, as conventional urine heat tests and simple electrophoresis of serum and urine may not detect small amounts of paraprotein or Bence-Jones protein. Monoclonal proteins are often detected in serum and urine [1, 6, 12]. Nevertheless, there remains a small proportion of patients in which it does not seem possible to find any abnormal proteins.

Skeletal survey may also be useful, as 50% of myeloma cases had radiological abnormalities, compared with only 6% of the primary group [12].

Prognosis. Prognosis in primary systemic and myeloma-associated amyloidosis is poor, the major causes of death being cardiac and renal failure. A mean survival time from diagnosis of 13 months for primary amyloidosis has been reported [1], whereas in myeloma-associated cases the survival time is considerably shorter than this [12]. Occasionally, there are exceptional cases of typical primary systemic amyloidosis that have prolonged survival for many years [8].

Treatment [3]. There are no specific or agreed regimes of treatment; none has produced convincing evidence of success. Theoretical alternatives include the use of melphalan, colchicine, thymosin, dimethyl sulphoxide and renal transplantation.

REFERENCES

1 BARTH W.F., et al (1969) *Am J Med* **47**, 259.
2 BENDITT E.P., et al (1971) *FEBS Lett* **19**, 169.
3 *BREATHNACH S.M. & BLACK M.M. (1979) *Clin Exp Dermatol* **4**, 517.
4 BREATHNACH S.M., et al (1979) *Clin Exp Dermatol* **4**, 495.
5 *BROWNSTEIN M.H. & HELWIG E.B. (1970) *Arch Dermatol* **102**, 20.
6 CATHCART E.S., et al (1972) *Am J Med* **52**, 93.
7 COHEN A.S., et al (1978) *Arthritis Rheum* **21**, 153.
8 CROW K.D. (1977) *Br J Dermatol* **97**, (Suppl. **15**), 58.
9 GLENNER G.G., et al (1971) *Science* **172**, 1150.
10 GLENNER G.G., et al (1973) *Semin Hematol* **10**, 65.
11 HUNTER J.A.A. (1976) *Proc R Soc Med* **69**, 235.
12 KYLE R.A. & BAYRD E.D. (1975) *Medicine* **54**, 271.
13 PASTERNAK A. (1976) In *Amyloidosis*. Eds Wegelius. O. & Pasternak A. London, Academic Press, p. 393.
14 SCHEINBERG M.A. & CATHCART E.S. (1978) *Clin Exp Immunol* **33**, 185.
15 SIMON B.G. & MOUTSOPOULAS H.M. (1979) *Arthritis Rheum* **22**, 932.
16 WESTERMARK P. (1972) *Acta Pathol Microbiol Scand* **80**, 718.
17 WESTERMARK P. & STENKUIST B. (1973) *Arch Intern Med* **132**, 522.

SECONDARY AMYLOIDOSIS [1]

As already mentioned, in secondary amyloidosis the amyloid is composed of amyloid A protein. Secondary amyloidosis commonly involves the kidneys, spleen, alimentary tract and adrenals. A common presentation is that of the nephrotic syndrome. Secondary amyloidosis rarely produces specific skin lesions, although needle aspirates of abdominal wall subcutis may yield positive histological identification of amyloid [9].

Secondary amyloidosis occurs as a complication

of many chronic inflammatory disease in which the immune system is stimulated. Rheumatoid arthritis is perhaps the best known; the approximate frequency of amyloidosis in rheumatoid arthritis is 14–26% [7]. Other important causes include juvenile rheumatoid arthritis, Reiter's syndrome, psoriatic arthritis [8], ankylosing spondylitis, tuberculosis, dermatomyositis, scleroderma, systemic lupus erythematosus and Behçet's syndrome [2]. Important cutaneous diseases associated with secondary amyloidosis include leprosy [6], pustular psoriasis [5], drug abuse and chronic skin suppuration [3].

In secondary amyloidosis the diagnosis should be confirmed by rectal or renal biopsy.

There is no specific treatment, although treatment of the primary disease may arrest progression of the amyloidosis. Renal transplantation is certainly worthy of consideration [4].

REFERENCES

1 *BROWNSTEIN M.H. & HELWIG E.B. (1970) *Arch Dermatol* 102, 1.
2 GLENNER G.G. (1980) *N Engl J Med* 302, 1333.
3 JACOB H., *et al* (1978) *Arch Intern Med* 138, 1150.
4 JONES N.F. & TIGHE J.R. (1976) *Amyloidosis.* Eds Wegelius O. & Pasternak A. London, Academic Press, p. 565.
5 MACKIE R.M. & BURTON J. (1974) *Br J Dermatol* 90, 567.
6 MCADAM K.P.W.J., *et al* (1975) *Lancet* ii, 572.
7 MISSEN G.A.K. & TAYLOR J.D. (1956) *J Pathol Bacteriol* 71, 179.
8 SHARMA S.C., *et al* (1983) *Br J Dermatol* 108, 205.
9 WESTERMARK P. & STENKVIST B. (1971) *Acta Med Scand* 190, 453.

INHERITED SYSTEMIC AMYLOIDOSIS [9]

Several distinct genetic types of amyloidosis are recognized. The kidney, peripheral nerves and spinal ganglia or the heart are predominantly affected [5].

TABLE 62.10. Histological type

Peri-reticulin	Peri-collagen
(1) Nephropathy	(1) Neuropathy
(a) Familial Mediterranean fever [10]	(a) Lower Limb
	(i) Portuguese [1]
	(ii) Japanese [2]
(b) Fever, urticaria, deafness [7]	(b) Upper limb
	(i) Swiss [8]
	(ii) German [6]
(c) Fever, abdominal pain [3]	(c) Lower limb and nephropathy [11]
	(2) Cardiopathy [4]

Table 62.10 allows them to be readily subdivided into nephropathy or neuropathy types.

Familial Mediterranean fever is inherited as a recessive character. Attacks of abdominal pain, fever, joint effusions and renal failure occur from amyloidosis. An erysipelas-like erythema can be seen on the legs. The neuropathy types eventually may cause trophic ulcers on legs or buttocks; some types are dominantly inherited.

No treatment is available for any of these inherited systemic amyloidoses; although colchicine can prevent attacks of familial Mediterranean fever there is no evidence thus far that it can prevent amyloid deposition [9].

REFERENCES

1 ANDRADE C. (1968) *Proc Symp. on Amyloidosis.* Amsterdam, Exerpta Medica, p. 377.
2 ARAKI S., *et al* (1968) *Arch Neurol* 18, 593.
3 BERGMAN F. & WARMENIUS S. (1968) *Am J Med* 45, 601.
4 FREDERICKSON T., *et al* (1962) *Am J Med* 33, 328.
5 GAFNI J., *et al* (1964) *Lancet* i, 71.
6 MAHLOUDJI M., *et al* (1969) *Medicine* 48, 1.
7 MUCKLE T.J. & WELLS M. (1962) *Q J Med* 31, 235.
8 RUCKAVINA J.G., *et al* (1956) *Medicine* 35, 239.
9 *SOHAR E. & GAFNI J. (1976) *Amyloidosis.* Eds Wegelius O. & Pasternak A. London, Academic Press, p. 175.
10 SOHAR E., *et al* (1967) *Am J Med* 43, 227.
11 VAN ALLEN M.W., *et al* (1969) *Neurology* 19, 10.

ANGIOKERATOMA CORPORIS DIFFUSUM

SYN. ANDERSON–FABRY'S DISEASE [17]

M.M. BLACK

This rare hereditary disorder, showing deposition of glycolipid in the smaller blood vessels of the skin and viscera, is characterized by a distinctive cutaneous eruption with vasomotor disturbances, cardiovascular episodes and renal failure.

Aetiology. Angiokeratoma corporis diffusum is a sex-linked disorder of sphingolipid metabolism [15] in which a deficiency of the enzyme ceramide trihexosidase [1] leads to the abnormal deposition of glycolipid throughout the body. Most cases appear in males although there have been some reports in women [11].

Histopathology [6] On light microscopy the skin lesions in angiokeratoma corporis diffusum consist of dilated blood-filled vessels in the upper dermis

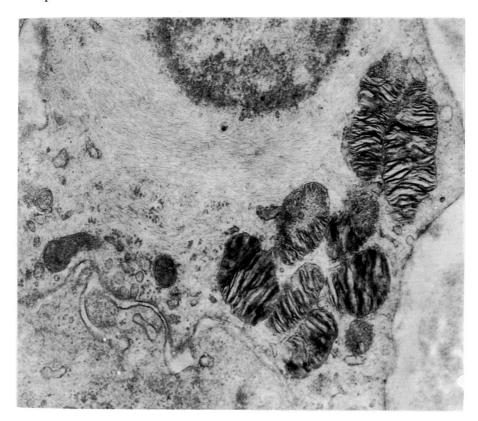

FIG. 62.18. Anderson–Fabry's disease. Electron micrograph showing lamellar bodies in an endothelial cell of a skin capillary (original magnification × 20,000). (Dr S. S. Bleehen.)

lying beneath a thinned epidermis with or without hyperkeratosis. The amount of lipid in the skin is too small to be detected without the use of special fixation and lipid-staining techniques. The characteristic and diagnostic feature of the disease is the presence of vacuolated cells in the walls of capillaries, artérioles and venules. The material, a glycolipid, can be demonstrated in frozen sections in the media and intima of smaller blood vessels in the cutis as a doubly refractile substance by polarized light. The ultrastructural changes are striking and the diagnosis can be made more easily with the electron microscope than the light microscope [14]. Electron-dense cytoplasmic inclusion bodies with a lamellar internal organization, consisting of alternating electron-opaque and light regions with a periodicity of 40–60 Å, are found in endothelial and muscle cells of blood vessels, perithelial and perineural cells, arrectores pilorum muscles and dermal macrophages. It has been suggested that they represent lipid deposits within lysosomes [8, 12]. Inclusion bodies have been reported in the skin of adult patients even in the absence of clinically evident angiectases [3, 18]; they have also been found in 'normal' skin from an infant with the disease [2].

Clinical features [17]. The cutaneous eruption usually first appears shortly before puberty. The initial lesion is a dark red or black telangiectatic macule or papule up to 4 mm across. Overlying hyperkeratosis is not always obvious. The lesions remain unchanged on diascopic pressure. Occasionally, cutaneous lesions may be minimal or even absent. Grouping tends to occur and in mild cases telangiectatic spots may be seen only on the thighs, scrotum or around the umbilicus (periumbilical rosette). In severe cases widespread lesions are present, particularly on the limbs, hips, buttocks, lower trunk and shaft of the penis.

A frequent ophthalmic finding is a symptomless superficial corneal dystrophy which is of diagnostic importance since it can be mimicked only by chloroquine keratopathy [17]. Dilatation and tortuosity

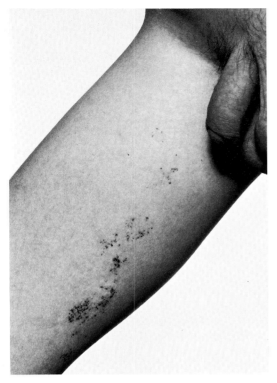

FIG. 62.19. Angiokeratoma corporis diffusum: lesions on the thigh of a 13-year-old boy. (St Thomas' Hospital.)

of the conjunctival and retinal vessels is common and may even be present in childhood. The upper eyelids may be oedematous.

Attacks of pain, often of an excruciating and apparently unique character, occur in 90% of males and in less than 10% of females, usually beginning between the ages of 5 and 15. They occur mainly in the skin of the fingers and toes, but the attacks may be rather episodic in nature. Vasomotor disturbances, which are probably due to involvement of the autonomic nervous system, tend to appear later. The hands may be blue or blanched or there may be flushing of the extremities.

The skin is often dry, lax and hypohidrotic, and mild arthritis of the terminal phalanges is frequent.

Patients with angiokeratoma corporis diffusum are often mildly hypertensive and liable to cerebrovascular attacks, coronary artery disease and renal disease. Albuminuria, haematuria and specific lipophages may be seen in the urine as a result of lipid infiltration of the glomerular vessels.

Varicose veins and stasis oedema are fairly common in these patients.

There is a striking sex difference in the symptomatology. The full syndrome occurs predominantly in men. In women there may be only corneal opacities, retinal vessel tortuosity and urinary signs of renal involvement.

Prognosis. The prognosis is usually grave. Death in the third or fourth decade from vascular accident

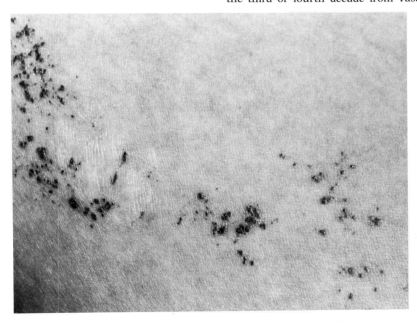

FIG. 62.20. Angiokeratoma corporis diffusum: close-up of the lesions (St Thomas' Hospital).

or uraemia is usual. However, prolonged survival without impairment of renal function is possible [7].

Diagnosis. In many cases a skin biopsy confirms the diagnosis and examination of urinary sediment for birefringent lipid-containing cells provides further evidence. A decreased level of α galactosidase A in plasma, leukocytes and cultured fibroblasts confirms the disorder. In doubtful cases slit-lamp examination of the cornea and renal biopsy should be performed. Careful inspection of the skin may be required to distinguish the lesions from purpura and angioma serpiginosum. It should be remembered that diffuse angiokeratomas have been described with deficiency of the enzymes β-galactosidase [10, 13] and αL fucosidase [5]. The bizarre subjective symptoms may be mistakenly labelled psychogenic neuralgia or erythromelalgia.

Internal vascular episodes, particularly when associated with hypertension and neuritic pains and fever, may cause confusion with polyarteritis nodosa.

Distinction from other types of angiokeratoma— circumscriptum, scrotal (Fordyce type) and Mibelli type—has been reviewed [9].

Treatment. There is no specific treatment but renal transplantation not only corrects the uraemia but also can produce marked improvement in other clinical manifestations of the disease [4].

REFERENCES

1 BRADY R.O., *et al* (1967) *N Engl J Med* **276**, 1163.
2 BREATHNACH S.M., *et al* (1980) *Br J Dermatol* **103**, 81.
3 CLARKE J.T.R., *et al* (1971) *N Engl J Med* **284**, 233.
4 CLEMENT M., *et al* (1982) *J R Soc Med* **75**, 557.
5 EPINETTE W.W., *et al* (1973) *Arch Dermatol* **107**, 754.
6 FROST P., *et al* (1966) *Am J Med* **40**, 618.
7 GOODFELLOW A. & WILLIAMS R.M. (1980) *J R Soc Med* **73**, 373.
8 HASHIMOTO K., *et al* (1976) *Arch Dermatol* **112**, 1416.
9 IMPERIAL R. & HELWIG E.B. (1967) *Arch Dermatol* **95**, 116.
10 ISHIBASHI A., *et al* (1982) In *XVI Int. Congr. on Dermatology, Tokyo.* University of Tokyo Press. p. 43.
11 JOHNSON A.W., *et al* (1966) *Ann Hum Genet* **30**, 25.
12 VAN MULLERN P.J. & RUITER M. (1970) *J Pathol* **101**, 221.
13 NAKAYAMA K., *et al* (1982) In *XVI Int. Congr. on Dermatology, Tokyo.*
14 SCHATZKI P.F., *et al* (1979) *Am J Surg Pathol* **3**, 211.
15 SWEELEY C.C. & KLIONSKY B. (1963) *J Biol Chem* **238**, 3148.
16 VOLK B.W., *et al* (1974) *Neurology* **24**, 991.
17 *WALLACE H.J. (1973) *Br J Dermatol* **88**, 1.
18 *WISE D., *et al* (1962) *Q J Med* **31**, 177.

LIPOID PROTEINOSIS
SYN. URBACH-WIETHE DISEASE [6, 10, 11]; HYALINOSIS CUTIS ET MUCOSAE [9]; LIPOGLYCOPROTEINOSIS [8]

M.M. BLACK

Lipoid proteinosis is a very rare recessively inherited disorder characterized by infiltration of hyaline material into the skin, oral cavity and larynx. It usually presents in infancy with hoarseness.

Aetiology. The nature of the underlying metabolic defect is unknown. However, it has been postulated that lipoid proteinosis may represent a lysosomal storage disease due to single or multiple enzyme defects [2]. More recently, preliminary results strongly suggest that lipoid proteinosis may involve a primary perturbation of collagen metabolism [5]. The sexes are equally affected.

Histopathology [4–7]. The epidermis shows hyperkeratosis and irregular acanthosis. The dermis is considerably thickened, the upper half containing extracellular hyaline material which is at first deposited along the course of capillaries and concentrically around sweat coils. In older lesions broad bands of hyaline material are found in the dermis, tending to be vertically oriented. Lipoid proteinosis must be distinguished from erythropoietic protoporphyria—in the latter condition the hyaline is not so extensively deposited and is never found around sweat coils. Furthermore, in lipoid proteinosis fine droplets of lipid can be demonstrated. The hyaline material stains strongly with periodic acid–Schiff reagent, most probably representing the presence of glycoproteins. Mucosubstances can usually be demonstrated but the histochemical characteristics of the hyaline deposits can vary from site to site and with time [4]. Amyloid stains are usually negative.

Clinical features. Lipoid proteinosis develops early in life and scarring from mild skin inflammation and injury is marked. Hoarseness develops in infancy and becomes prominent within the first few years of life. The mucosae of the pharynx, tongue and lips soon develop firm yellow–white infiltrates. The soft palate, pillars of the tonsils, uvula and undersurface of the tongue show extensive yellow irregular infiltrations. The tonsils are covered with a hard white mass and the larynx is involved to a severe degree, with nodules in the epiglottis and vocal cords. The tongue is enlarged and feels firm on palpation and its range of movement is decreased, so that the patient is usually unable to protrude it beyond the margins of the lips. Occasionally, there is similar involvement of the mucosa of the labia and vagina.

Skin changes frequently become prominent in early life with the development of yellow–brown nodules appearing on the face and lips. Involvement of the scalp leads to loss of hair. Very typical 'beaded' papules are present along the margins of the upper and lower eyelids and there is usually total loss of eyelashes. Nodular lesions on the elbows resemble xanthomas. Deposits may appear in the skin and mucous membranes after trauma. Later the colour of the skin darkens and the lesions become hyperkeratotic or warty. Small nodules are sometimes present on the finger joints, in the axillae and on the knees and scrotum. Dental abnormalities, intracranial calcification and epilepsy are often associated with lipoid proteinosis [6]. Widespread visceral involvement is described [3] and diabetes has been reported [1].

Diagnosis. A combination of hoarseness from early childhood, thickening and stiffening of the tongue and characteristic cutaneous nodules makes the diagnosis relatively easy. In erythropoietic protoporphyria there is solar sensitivity and the scarred areas are confined to exposed skin. In adult life differential diagnosis from lichen myxoedematosus has to be considered. Similarly, myxoedema with hoarseness may produce diagnostic difficulties.

Prognosis. Lipoid proteinosis is progressive until early adult life, but in general the prognosis is good. Involvement of the larynx may lead to respiratory difficulties in childhood, and occasionally tracheotomy is required.

Treatment. Microlaryngoscopy and dissection of the vocal cords can be successful. Apart from dermabrasion no other treatment is known to play any part in influencing the signs and symptoms of this disorder.

REFERENCES

1 BAZEX A. (1939) *Bull Soc Fr Dermatol Syphiligr* **46**, 136.
2 BAUR E.A., *et al* (1981) *J Invest Dermatol* **76**, 119.
3 CAPLAN M. (1967) *Arch Dermatol* **95**, 149.
4 HARPER J.I., *et al* (1983) *Clin Exp Dermatol* **8**, 135.
5 HARPER J.I. *et al* (1985) *Br J Dermatol* **113**, 145.
6 HOFER P.A. (1973) *Acta Derm Venereal (Stockh)* **53** (Suppl. 71), 5.
7 LAYMON C.W. & HILL E.M. (1957) *Arch Dermatol* **75**, 55.
8 LUNDT V. (1949) *Arch Dermatol Syph* **188**, 128.
9 McCUSKER J.J. & CAPLAN R.M. (1962) *Am J Pathol* **40**, 599.
10 ROOK A. (1976) *Br J Dermatol* **94**, 341.
11 URBACH E. & WIETHE C. (1929) *Virchows Arch Pathol Anat Physiol* **273**, 285.

FARBER'S DISEASE [1, 3, 4]
SYN. DISSEMINATED LIPOGRANULOMATOSIS

Farber's disease (disseminated lipogranulomatosis) is a rare and fatal lipid storage disease of infants, probably inherited as an autosomal recessive, although most reports have been of sporadic cases.

Histopathology. In the skin and subcutaneous tissue dense areas of mixed granulomatous infiltrations are found amongst a fibrovascular stroma. Groups of large foamy histiocytes are found towards the centre of the granulomas. At visceral sites (especially the brain) the presence of vacuolated cells is similar to the pathology encountered in other metabolic storage diseases.

Histochemical studies indicate that the deposited material is an acid glycolipid [3] of which ceramide is probably the most important. It has been suggested that estimation of acid ceramidase in cultured fibroblasts or amniotic fluid cells may provide a means of early diagnosis [2]. Ultrastructurally, curvilinear bodies have been found in fibroblasts, histiocytes and endothelial cells; curious banana-like inclusions have been found in Schwann cells [5].

Clinical features. Involvement of the laryngeal joints and the adjoining tissue produces dysphonia, laryngeal stridor, a hoarse cry and noisy respiration. Erythematous papules and nodules appear close to joints and tendons of the hands and feet. The ears, the occipital region and the trunk are other sites of predilection. Gross mental and motor retardation are features of the disease. Cherry-red spots may be noted at the macula [3].

REFERENCES

1 ABUT HAJ S.K., *et al* (1962) *J Pediatr* **61**, 221.
2 DULANEY J.T., *et al* (1976) *J Pediatr* **85**, 59.
3 MOLZ G. (1968) *Virchows Arch [A]* **344**, 86.
4 MOSER H.W., *et al* (1969) *Am J Med* **47**, 869.
5 RAUCH H.J. & AUBÖCH L (1983) *Am J Dermatopathol* **5**, 263.

GAUCHER'S DISEASE

Definition. This is a rare inborn error of metabolism characterized by the accumulation of complex lipid substances in macrophages (Gaucher's cells) within liver, spleen and bones.

Aetiology [2, 4]. The congenital and familial disorder of lipid metabolism is probably transmitted as an autosomal dominant character. The abnormal lipid kerasin accumulates in the cells of the reticulo-endothelial system resulting in enlargement of the spleen, liver and lymph nodes associated with a thrombocytopenia and coagulation defect [1].

Pathology. The classical and distinctive feature of the disease is the presence of numerous characteristic histiocytes (Gaucher's cells) which infiltrate the spleen, liver and bone marrow, lymph nodes and sometimes other organs. Gaucher's cells may be packed into the splenic red pulp and sinuses of lymph nodes. Gaucher's cells are large cells with a small nucleus and a voluminous pale-staining cytoplasm. They differ from other lipid-containing cells because of the delicate striated tissue-paper appearance, best seen in thicker sections (10 μm). Ultrastructurally, Gaucher's cells contain elongated residual bodies containing tubular structures composed of twisted microfibrillar elements [3, 6]. The structures probably represent aggregated glucocerebroside molecules within distended lysosomes. These bodies contain acid phosphatase [8]. In the juvenile neuropathic form, the brain shows loss of neurones and some perivascular accumulation of PAS-positive cells but typical Gaucher's cells are few or absent.

The skin changes consist of diffuse pigmentation which may be due to haemosiderosis or to deposition of melanin [10].

Clinical features

The adult type [7]. This is markedly different from the infantile or juvenile variety, because the adult type of Gaucher's disease shows an insidious onset and thereafter is only slowly progressive, whereas in the infantile variety the onset is relatively acute and death occurs in the first or second year of life. In the adult the initial complaint is usually that of weakness or perhaps of minor bleeding tendencies. Dull pain in the bones is another early feature and patchy pigmentation of the hands and face resembling chloasma may occur early. Deeper pigmentation associated with thickening of the skin and a brownish discoloration of the conjunctivae occur later [4]. Malar flush is a feature in some cases [4]. The skin of the legs may be glossy and small ulcers may appear.

Anaemia is an almost constant finding with a pancytopenia. Generalized osteoporosis of bones due to infiltration by Gaucher's cells leads to gross de-

formity of the skeleton with collapse of thoracic and lumbar vertebrae. Diagnostically the finding of Gauher's cells in sternal marrow is important [5].

The infantile type. This begins during the first 6 months of life and ends fatally before the second year. About 10% of all cases of Gaucher's disease occur in infancy. The symptoms of the acute infantile form are predominantly neurological, and include neck rigidity, increased muscle tone, catatonia and laryngeal spasm. The infant dies of acute respiratory infection complicated by laryngospasm, cyanosis and cachexia. Splenomegaly and hepatomegaly are prominent, but there are no specific skin lesions. Some cases are capable of more prolonged survival and this has been referred to as the juvenile form.

Prognosis. This depends very largely on the age of onset. If the symptoms appear in the first decade of life the prognosis is poor, if in the third or later decades the progress of the disease is much slower.

Treatment. There is no specific treatment. Splenectomy is indicated as a palliative measure to reduce abdominal distension and on occasions to try and relieve anaemia and thrombocytopenia. However, the benefits of splenectomy are rather variable and depend on the extent of marrow destruction by Gaucher's cells [7]. X-ray therapy to the bones may relieve pain. Little can be done for the infantile or juvenile form of Gaucher's disease.

REFERENCES

1 BOKLAN B.F. & SAWITSKY A. (1976) *Arch Intern Med* **136**, 489.
2 *BRADY R.O. (1978) In *Metabolic Basis of Inherited Disease*. Eds Stanbury J.B., *et al.* New York, McGraw-Hill, p. 731.
3 FREDERICKSON D.S. & SLOAN H.R. (1972) In *Metabolic Basis of Inherited Disease*. Eds Stanbury J.B., *et al.* New York, McGraw-Hill, p. 730.
4 GROEN J. (1965) *Isr J Med Sci* **1**, 507.
5 GROEN J. & GARRER A.H. (1948) *Blood* **3**, 1221.
6 HIBBS R.G., *et al* (1970) *Arch Pathol* **89**, 137.
7 MATOTH Y. & FRIED K. (1965) *Isr J Med Sci* **1**, 521.
8 MEDOFF A.S. & BAYRD E.D. (1954) *Ann Intern Med* **40**, 481.
9 PETERS S.P., *et al* (1977) *Medicine* **56**, 425.
10 REICH C., *et al* (1951) *Medicine (Baltimore)* **30**, 1.

NIEMANN–PICK DISEASE

Definition. Niemann–Pick disease is a type of congenital lipidosis bearing a wide spectrum of clinical symptoms. It is usually fatal in early childhood and characterized by emaciation, hepatomegaly and splenomegaly.

Aetiology. Niemann–Pick disease is inherited as an autosomal recessive lack of sphingomyelinase [2]. It is characterized by the accumulation of enormous quantities of sphingomyelin in histiocytes, macrophages and reticulum cells of all organs. The sex incidence is approximately equal [7] and the condition is said to be more common in Jewish infants.

Pathology. There is massive enlargement of the liver, spleen and lymph nodes and infiltrations in lungs and bone marrow. Niemann–Pick cells are readily demonstrated in all organs and recently also in the skin [6]. In the brain and central nervous system a variety of degenerative features similar to those of Tay-Sachs disease have been described. Niemann–Pick cells are usually mononucleate, large, pale and foamy, but accompanied by neither granulomatous nor inflammatory cells. In cryostat sections they stain readily with Sudan stains and contain doubly refractile material. PAS positivity is less marked than with Gaucher's cells. Circulating lymphocytes frequently also show lipid inclusions [5]. Ultrastructurally, the Niemann–Pick cell appears like a histiocyte with cytoplasm containing variably sized lipid cytosomes, many with concentrically arranged whorled features [1].

Clinical features. An apparently normal infant begins to lose weight about the second or third month of life. The abdomen becomes protuberant from massive enlargement of liver and spleen. Lymph nodes are increased in size. The infant becomes progressively more emaciated and apathetic and the face appears mongoloid. Muscle weakness increases and the child is unable to sit or raise the head and all muscle tone is lost. Deafness and blindness are common features. Death takes place usually before the age of 2 yr and often earlier. Exceptionally, older survival has been recorded [4].

The skin involvement in Niemann–Pick disease has been described as waxy induration with transient xanthomas overlying enlarged cervical nodes [3]. Other skin lesions described include suppurative lesions on the face associated with foamy cell infiltration, indurated discoloured patches on the cheeks [6], purpuric lesions, café au lait spots and dark bluish Mongolian spots on skin and oral mucosa [1]. No treatment is known.

REFERENCES

1 BRADY R.O. & KING F.M. (1973) In *Lysosomes and Storage Disease*. Eds Hers H.G. & van Hoof F. New York, Academic Press, p. 439.
2 BRADY R.O., *et al* (1966) *Proc Natl Acad Sci USA* **55**, 366.
3 CROCKER A.C. & FARBER S. (1958) *Medicine* **37**, 1.
4 FORSYTHE W.I., *et al* (1959) *Arch Dis Child* **34**, 406.
5 LAZARUS S.S., *et al* (1967) *Lab Invest* **17**, 155.
6 MARDINI M.K., *et al* (1982) *Am J Dis Child* **136**, 651.
7 MURRAY H.A. & BERNSTEIN T.C. (1946) *Arch Pediatr* **63**, 497.

DISORDERS OF AMINO-ACID METABOLISM

R. J. PYE

The disorders of amino acid metabolism are of growing importance. Patients affected may show mental retardation, abnormalities of skin and hair and interference with general body growth. These disorders are the result of inherited defects of enzymes which mediate the metabolism or transport of amino acids.

THE HYPERPHENYLALANINAEMIA SYNDROMES

Phenylketonuria (PKU) (hyperphenylalaninaemia type I: Folling's disease; phenylpyruvic oligophrenia). This is a rare hereditary disease in which a deficiency of the enzyme phenylalanine hydroxylase leads to an accumulation of phenylalanine in the blood and to the excretion of phenylpyruvic and phenylacetic acids in the urine.

Aetiology [1, 13]. This disorder is inherited as an autosomal recessive character. It accounts for from 0·04 to 1·0% of residents in institutions for the mentally handicapped. Its frequency in the general population has been estimated at four per 100,000. The near complete deficiency of phenylalanine dehydroxylase impairs the conversion of phenylalanine into tyrosine, leading to the accumulation and excretion of abnormal compounds. Heterozygotes have a high fasting serum phenylalanine level and some 'dilution' of hair colour.

The metabolic block in the conversion of phenylalanine to tyrosine leads to the accumulation of phenylalanine, phenylpyruvic acid and related metabolites. The oxidation rate in the brain is probably diminished but, although degenerative changes have been described in the cortex and basal ganglia and in the liver, they are inconstant [3]. The reduction of melanin formation in the hair is probably due to the inhibition of tyrosine–tyrosinase reaction by phenylalanine, since the hair will darken if large amounts of tyrosine are fed [11]. About 1 g of phenylpyruvic acid is excreted daily in the urine.

Clinical features [10]. Affected infants are of average height and weight at birth, but thereafter show wide variation in the ages at which the developmental stages are passed. These patients almost invariably have fair skin and hair (due to the impairment of melanin synthesis), although in the darker races the resultant skin pigmentation may be darker than the average Caucasoid. There is nearly always mental retardation and most of these patients will eventually require special care. Often extrapyramidal manifestations, such as athetosis and exaggerated tendon reflexes, may be found. The electroencephalogram is abnormal in 80%.

The fair and sensitive skin very readily develops eczema. This may be of the atopic variety or of less distinctive type. Although clinical light sensitivity has been reported, the ability to tan and the erythema response to UV radiation are normal [8]. The incidence of pyogenic infections is increased. Scleroderma-like lesions with involvement of the muscles are described [7].

There is some evidence that in mothers with PKU phenylalanine crosses the placental barrier and may cause epilepsy or mental deficiency in the offspring [5, 6]. This diagnosis should therefore be considered in fair-skinned light-sensitive individuals, especially in mothers of mentally retarded children.

Diagnosis. Although the urine may contain phenylpyruvic acid at birth, in some instances the urine test may be negative in the first months of life. The blood phenylalanine, however, is raised from an early date, and therefore it is recommended that screening is performed on blood samples [9, 14].

The most widely used method of screening is the Guthrie test [4]. A method is described for differentiating the hyperphenylalaninaemias based on the response to phenylalanine content in the diet [2]. Some patients with hyperphenylalaninaemia do not have PKU (see also hyperphenylalaninaemia types II to V).

Treatment [10, 12, 13]. It is of prime importance that the diagnosis is made early so that a low phenylalanine diet can be instituted as soon as possible, in order to avoid cerebral damage produced by high blood phenylalanine levels. Unfortunately, the response to dietary treatment is variable despite early and careful control and the effectiveness of treatment varies with individual patients. The amount of phenylalanine supplied in the diet should be low enough to prevent its accumulation in the blood, but high enough to allow proper protein synthesis and growth. Repeated monitoring of the phenylalanine levels is required during treatment.

REFERENCES

1 *Beesman S.P. (1964) *J Pediatr* **64**, 828.
2 Blaskovics M.E., et al (1974) *Arch Dis Child* **49**, 835.
3 Delay J. & Pichot P. (1947) *Sem Hop Paris* **23**, 1749.
4 Guthrie R. & Susi A. (1963) *Pediatrics* **32**, 338.
5 Howell R.R. & Stevenson R.E. (1971) *Soc Biol* **18**, 519.
6 Hsia D. Y-Y. (1970) *Prog Med Genet* **7**, 29.
7 Jablonska S., et al (1967) *Arch Dermatol* **95**, 443.
8 Massel C.W. & Brunsting L.A. (1959) *Arch Dermatol* **79**, 458.
9 MRC Working Party PKU (1968) *Br Med J* iv, 7.
10 Rosenberg L.E. & Scriver C.R. (1980) In *Metabolic Control and Disease*. Eds Bondy P.K. & Rosenberg L.E. Philadelphia, Saunders, p. 709.
11 Snyderman S.E., et al (1955) *Fed Proc* **14**, 450.
12 Sutherland B.S., et al (1966) *Am J Dis Child* **114**, 505.
13 Tourian A. & Sidbury J.B. (1983) In *Metabolic Basis of Inherited Disease*. Ed. Stanbury J.B., et al New York, McGraw-Hill, p. 270.
14 World Health Organisation (1968) *Tech Rep Ser* **401**.

Hyperphenylalaninaemia types II and III. Not all infants with hyperphenylalanaemia have PKU and types II and III represent a continuum from those difficult to separate from typical PKU to those mildly affected. There is a general correlation between phenylalanine hydroxylase activity and blood levels of phenylalanine [1]. Accurate classification usually requires phenylalanine loading [2, 3]. Treatment needs to be modified according to the severity of the enzyme deficiency.

REFERENCES

1 Bartholome K., et al (1975) *Pediatrics* **45**, 83.
2 Guttler F. (1980) *Acta Paediatr. Scand* (Suppl.) **280**, 3.
3 Williamson M., et al (1980) *Pediatrics* **60**, 815.

Hyperphenylalaninaemia types IV and V. Types IV and V are due to deficiencies in the coenzymes dihydropteridine reductase [3] and dihydrobiopterin synthetase [1, 4] respectively. These infants represent only 1·3% of all patients with hyperphenylalaninaemia but need accurate diagnosis since their treatment is very different from that of typical PKU [2, 5].

REFERENCES

1 BARTHOLOME K., *et al* (1977) *Pediatrics* **59**, 757.
2 CURTIUS H-CH., *et al* (1979) *Clin Chim Acta* **93**, 251.
3 KAUFMAN S., *et al* (1975) *N Engl J Med* **293**, 785.
4 LEEMING R.J. (1976) *Lancet* i, 99.
5 SMITH I. (1974) *Arch Dis Child* **49**, 245.

TYROSINAEMIA II [4]
(RICHNER–HANHART SYNDROME)

This is a rare disorder inherited as an autosomal recessive trait and probably due to a deficiency of hepatic tyrosine aminotransferase, the rate-limiting enzyme for tyrosine catabolism [3]. The deficiency leads to tyrosinaemia, tyrosinuria and an increase in the urinary tyrosine metabolites. Mild corneal erosions and dendritic ulcers develop within the first few months of life and may lead to corneal scarring [2]. Ulceration also has occurred on corneal transplants [1]. Painful erosion may develop on palms and soles, especially the tips of digits and thenar and hypothenar eminences. Later these areas become hyperkeratotic [3]. Hyperkeratosis of the tongue has been reported [6]. Mental retardation is common in these patients but not invariable.

Patients respond to a low tyrosine and low phenylalanine diet [5].

REFERENCES

1 BARDELLI A.M., *et al* (1977) *Ophthalmologica* **175**, 5.
2 BIENFANG D.C., *et al* (1976) *Arch Ophthalmol* **94**, 1133.
3 GOLDSMITH L.A., *et al* (1979) *J Invest Dermatol* **73**, 530.
4 GOLDSMITH L.A. (1983) In *Metabolic Basis of Inherited Disease*. Eds Stanbury J.B., *et al.* New York, McGraw-Hill, p. 288.
5 HILL A., *et al* (1970) *J Am Diet Assoc* **56**, 308.
6 LARREGNE M., *et al* (1979) *Ann Dermatol Vénéréol* **106**, 53.

ALKAPTONURIA [3, 4]

This is a rare metabolic disease with deposition of oxidized homogentisic acid pigment throughout the body, particularly in the fibrous and cartilaginous tissues. The disorder is characterized by dark urine, distinctive cutaneous pigmentation (ochronosis) and arthritis.

Aetiology. It is inherited as a Mendelian recessive character. The biochemical defect is homogentisic acid oxidase deficiency, and this leads to an accumulation of homogentisic acid.

Ochronosis is the deposition of a melanin-like brownish-black pigment in the connective tissues and cartilage; this pigment is derived from polymerized homogentisic acid.

The enzyme homogentisic acid oxidase contains an essential SH group which is inhibited by certain chemicals. These include various drugs such as phenol, resorcin, mepacrine and perhaps other antimalarials which cause acquired ochronosis. An exogenous ochronosis can occur from hydroquinone-containing skin bleaching creams [1].

Histopathology. There is deposition of black pigment in the cartilage, fibrous tissue, tendons and atheromatous areas. The intervertebral discs, larynx, tracheal rings and articular cartilages are jet-black as if 'dipped in Indian ink'. Differentiation of the ochronotic pigment from melanin is difficult, and indeed stains do not consistently differentiate between the two pigments.

Clinical features [2, 6]. The patient with the hereditary type is symptom-free until adult life. The only manifestations in childhood are discoloration of the urine and 'spotting or staining' of the napkins or clothing. The constant sequence of events is first alkaptonuria, then ochronosis and lastly ochronotic arthropathy. The cutaneous manifestations appear only in the fourth decade. One of the earliest signs is thickening of the ear cartilage, associated with blue–black or grey–blue discoloration. The pinna feels noticeably thickened and flexible and in later stages there may be gross calcification. The cerumen is often brown or jet-black. Scleral pigmentation is noted as early as the third decade; it appears as brown or grey deposits midway between the corneal margin and the inner canthus. The skin of the eyelids and forehead is also pigmented and the tarsal plates often appear blue on trans-illumination. All the tendons are similarly discoloured; the dark discoloration over the extensor tendons of the knuckles is best seen when the patient makes a fist. Widespread dusky cutaneous pigmentation may be noted, but this feature is particularly marked over the cheeks, forehead, axillae and genital regions. The buccal mucosa and larynx are also affected and the nails are sometimes discoloured distinctly brown. Ochronotic changes affecting the ear drum and ossicles may produce deafness, and prostatic concretions and black renal calculi, as well as calcific aortic disease, have been recorded.

The urine is brown only when alkaline. When of normal colour it darkens on exposure to air or within seconds of adding an alkaline solution.

Patients sometimes observe that both their sweat and urine discolour clothing.

Ochronotic arthropathy follows a fairly consistent clinical pattern. There is low-back pain with stiffness early in the fourth decade; during the next 10 years the knees becomes involved and, later, the shoulders and hips. The friable articular cartilages lead to prolapsed intervertebral discs or a ruptured nucleus pulposus with accompanying acute pain. Spondylosis spreads to the thoracic spine, the patients then assuming a stoop posture losing perhaps 6 in. in height. Limitation of expansion of the chest provokes dyspnoea. Osteoarthritic changes very frequently coexist and the spinal X-ray appearances are diagnostic. In spite of their marked disability many patients reach old age.

Diagnosis. The diagnosis rests on the demonstration of homogentisic acid in the urine by its reducing ability, by specific enzyme tests [5] or by gas–liquid chromatography.

Differential diagnosis. An incorrect diagnosis of glycosuria or diabetes is sometimes made if the urine is tested with Fehling's solution. The pigmentation of acquired ochronosis from exogenous foreign chemicals or drugs is identical, but unaccompanied by homogentisic acid in the urine or by arthropathy. The overall clinical picture and the localization of pigment distinguish the disease from other pigmented disorders. These include Addison's disease, haemochromatosis, argyria, chronic photosensitivity pigmentation, cutaneous porphyria and pellagra. The ferric chloride test gives inconstant results; other phenolic compounds give similar colour reactions and therefore when the test is positive the urine should be examined chromatographically.

Treatment. Low protein diet limiting the amount of phenylalanine and tyrosine is not practicable as a long-term measure. The arthropathy is best treated by analgesics and physical therapy.

REFERENCES

1 FINDLAY G.H., *et al* (1975) *Br J Dermatol* **93**, 613.
2 LAYMON C.W. (1953) *Arch Dermatol Syphil* **67**, 553.
3 McKENZIE A.W., *et al*)1957) *Br Med J* **ii**, 794.
4 O'BRIEN W.M., *et al* (1963) *Am J Med* **34**, 813.
5 SEEGMILLER J.E., *et al* (1961) *J Biol Chem* **236**, 774.
6 WOOLEY P.B. (1952) *Br Med J* **ii**, 760.

HOMOCYSTINURIAS [3, 5, 8]

Homocystinurias are a group of rare, inborn errors of amino acid metabolism.

Aetiology. Initially homocystinuria was thought to be due to deficiency of cystathionine beta-synthase but it is now apparent that homocystine accumulation may also result from acquired or inherited blocks in the methyltetrahydrofolate–homocysteine methyltransferase reaction [2, 6, 9, 11].

Clinical features. Cystathionine beta-synthase deficiency is inherited as an autosomal recessive trait. The newborn infant may be quite normal clinically, but lens dislocation, mental deficiency, growth disorder and cutaneous signs develop slowly over the next few years. Other clinical features include epilepsy, genu valgum and growth changes resembling Marfan's syndrome. Some children develop spontaneous venous and arterial thrombosis from increased platelet stickiness [7].

The hair is fine and sparse and the malar area flushed. In some cases hair examination shows no fluorescence with acridine orange, indicating abnormality of disulphide bonds [4]. The cystine content is normal.

Livedo reticularis of the legs and tissue-paper scars on the hands may be present [4].

Diagnosis. Marfan's syndrome, a hereditary mesodermal dysplasia (see p. 1844), exhibits visceral manifestations without mental deficiency. The hair is normal and homocystine absent from the urine.

Treatment. Diets restricting methionine and supplemented with cystine have been used with encouraging results when started early in life [10]. Large doses of vitamin B_6 (pyridoxine), 200–500 mg daily, produce complete reversal of the biochemical abnormality in some cases [1].

REFERENCES

1 BARBER G.W. & SPAETH G.L. (1967) *Lancet* **i**, 337.
2 BRENTON D.P., *et al* (1965) *J Pediatr* **67**, 58.
3 BRENTON D.P., *et al* (1966) *Q J Med* **35**, 325.
4 CAREY M.C., *et al* (1967) *M J Med* **45**, 7.
5 CARSON N.A.J., *et al* (1963) *Arch Dis Child* **38**, 425.
6 CARSON N.A.J., *et al* (1965) *J Pediatr* **66**, 565.
7 McDONALD L., *et al* (1964) *Lancet* **i**, 745.
8 *McKUSICK V.A. (1972) *Heritable Disorders of Connective Tissue.* 4th ed. St Louis, Mosby, p. 224.
9 *MUDD S.H. & LEVY H.L. (1983) In *Metabolic Basis of Inherited Disease.* Eds Stanbury J.B., *et al.* New York, McGraw-Hill, p. 522.
10 *PERRY T.L. (1971) In *Inherited Disorders of Sulphur*

Metabolism. Eds Carson N.A. & Raine D.N. London, Livingstone, p. 245.

11 ROSENBERG L.E. & SCRIVER C.R. (1980) In *Metabolic Control and Disease*. Eds Bondy P.K. & Rosenberg L.E. Philadelphia, Saunders, p. 662.

HARTNUP DISEASE [3]

This rare hereditary recessive metabolic disorder of amino acid metabolism is characterized by a pellagrous eruption, a temporary and intermittent cerebellar ataxia, and a characteristic renal amino aciduria with excessive indicanuria [1].

Aetiology. The defect is believed to be due to a failure of the transport of tryptophan both from the intestine and from the glomerular filtrate [6, 7]. The defect may be an absence of a specific carrier protein [4]. The failure of absorption of tryptophan results in a deficiency in the synthesis of nicotinamide causing a pellagra-like syndrome.

Clinical features. The onset is usually in childhood between 3 and 9 yr, but the first signs are occasionally encountered in infancy. The cutaneous signs precede the neurological manifestations. The rash is dry, scaly and well marginated, affecting the light-exposed areas, notably the forehead, cheeks, periorbital regions, the uncovered areas of the arms and the dorsa of the hands. After exposure to sunlight the skin reddens and may exude.

Stomatitis, glossitis and diarrhoea have been reported.

Cerebellar ataxia is the predominating neurological feature. Other signs include nystagmus and diplopia, with perhaps tremor of the hands and tongue. Less commonly, there are associated psychic disturbances such as depression, delusions, hallucinations and some mental retardation. Exacerbations are most frequently seen in the spring or early summer [2], cutaneous manifestations being accompanied by transient ataxia. Rarely the attacks are provoked by febrile illness.

Intravenous tryptophan is metabolized normally and the serum amino acids are normal.

The urine contains increased amounts of amino acids of the monoamine monocarboxylic group [5]. Proline and hydroxyproline excretion is normal. There is marked indicanuria.

Differential diagnosis. The eruption in mild cases closely simulates infantile atopic eczema, seborrhoeic eczema and pityriasis alba; in Hartnup disease the covered areas are usually spared.

Florid cases closely mimic nutritional pellagra.

The congenital poikilodermas, particularly the light-sensitive hereditary disorders such as Cockayne's syndrome (p. 148), may present diagnostic difficulties.

Prognosis. Symptoms become milder with increasing age.

Treatment. Nicotinamide should be given in high doses; it controls both the eruption and the cerebral disturbance [2]. Exposure to sunshine should be avoided as much as possible and sun-deflectant creams used.

REFERENCES

1 BARON D.N., *et al* (1956) *Lancet* ii, 421.
2 HALVORSEN K. & HALVORSEN S. (1963) *Pediatrics* 31, 29.
3 *JEPSON J.B. (1978) In *The Metabolic Basis of Inherited Disease*. Eds Stanbury J.B., *et al.* 2nd ed. New York, McGraw-Hill, p. 1568.
4 MATTHEWS D.M. (1971) *Br Med J* iii, 659.
5 MILNE M.D. (1964) *Br Med J* i, 327.
6 *MILNE M.D., *et al* (1960) *Q J Med* 29, 407.
7 SCRIVER C.R. (1965) *N Engl J Med* 273, 530.

GOUT

This heterogeneous group of disorders of purine metabolism is characterized by hyperuricaemia, recurrent attacks of acute arthritis with the deposition of urates in the articular cartilage, urate deposits in the skin (tophi) and renal disease.

Aetiology. Primary gout has long been recognized as a familial disorder with up to 40% of patients having a positive family history [2, 11]. In the majority of patients inheritance appears to be under polygenic control, although some studies suggest a dominant genetic factor. There are two very rare specific enzyme deficiencies associated with gout which have X-linked inheritance. These are partial deficiency of hypoxanthine-guanine phosphoribosyl transferase (HGPRT) and increased activity of phosphoribosylpyrophosphate (PRPP) synthetase. Most patients with primary gout appear to have underexcretion of uric acid [7] but the metabolic abnormalities are poorly understood. Less than 10% of patients with primary gout have an increase in the rate of purine biosynthesis [5]. A number of defects have been suggested but only partial deficiency of HGPRT and increased PRPP synthetase activity are of importance [10].

Secondary gout may result from decreased excretion of uric acid. The most important cause of this is diuretic therapy but it may also occur in a number of disease states, especially renal disease. Increased uric acid production is commonly secondary to increased turnover of nucleic acid in conditions such as polycythaemia rubra vera, lymphoma and myeloma and in patients with leukaemia receiving active chemotherapy.

Histopathology. Sodium urate crystals may be found in joint fluid. The crystals can be identified by microscopic examination and their ability to polarize light strongly. In the dermis and medulla of the kidney the urate crystals provoke a giant-cell reaction [8].

Clinical features. Hyperuricaemia appears at about the age of puberty in males and later in females, often after the menopause. Patients remain asymptomatic until the fourth and sixth decades when the first attack of acute gouty arthritis occurs. Recurrent self-limiting attacks usually follow after a so-called intercritical period of 6 months to 2 yr. Initially, single joints and classically the great toe are involved, but later the condition may become polyarticular and then usually involves the joints of the lower extremities. Later in the disease a chronic tophus state develops with deposits in the cartilage, synovial membranes, tendons, soft tissues and elsewhere. The classical localization for tophi is in the helix and antihelix of the ear.

Acute uric acid nephropathy results from precipitation of uric acid crystals in the collecting ducts of the kidney and is most commonly seen in patients with leukaemia undergoing aggressive chemotherapy. Renal stones develop in up to a quarter of patients [3] and renal colic may be the presenting manifestation of gout. Chronic renal urate nephropathy is a common manifestation [1, 9] and contributes significantly to the morbidity and mortality of gout [9].

Differential diagnosis. Pseudogout [6] (calcium pyrophosphate deposition disease) shows close similarities with gout—acute attacks, familial incidence and later chronic arthropathy, pseudotophi and precipitation by surgical operations and diuretics. The serum uric acid is normal, calcium pyrophosphate is found in synovial fluid and X-rays show articular calcification [4].

Multicentric reticulohistiocytosis (see p. 1709) frequently shows papules and nodules on the ears and fingers with an associated arthropathy.

Rheumatoid arthritis with necrobiotic nodules is usually sufficiently characteristic to avoid confusion with gout. Psoriatic arthropathy may cause diagnostic difficulties (see p. 1511).

Treatment. Acute attacks are treated by rest of the affected joint and with either cochicine or indomethacin. The newer non-steroidal anti-inflammatory agents may be used but experience is still limited. Prophylaxis may be with colchicine, indomethacin or the xanthine oxidase inhibitor allopurinol. Treatment must be tailored to the needs of individual patients and for further details the reader is referred to Kelley [5].

REFERENCES

1 BARLOW K.A. & BEILIN L.J. (1968) *Q J Med* **37**, 79.
2 GRAHAME R. & SCOTT J.T. (1970) *Ann Rheum Dis* **29**, 461.
3 GUTMAN A.B. & YU T-F. (1968) *Am J Med* **45**, 756.
4 HOWELL D.S. (1981) In *Textbook of Rheumatology.* Eds Kelley W.N., *et al.* Philadelphia, Saunders.
5 KELLEY W.N. (1981) In *Textbook of Rheumatology.* Eds Kelley W.N., *et al.* Philadelphia, Saunders.
6 McCARTY D.J., *et al* (1962) *Ann Intern Med* **56**, 711.
7 SNAITH M.L. & SCOTT J.T. (1971) *Ann Rheum Dis* **30**, 285.
8 SOKOLOFF L. (1957) *Metabolism* **6**, 230.
9 TALBOTT J.H. & TERPLAN K.L. (1960) *Medicine* **39**, 405.
10 WYNGAARDEN J.B. & KELLEY W.N. (1976) *Gout and Hyperuricaemia.* New York, Grune and Stratton.
11 YU T.-F. (1974) *Am J Med* **56**, 676.

LESCH-NYHAN SYNDROME [3]

This syndrome is probably determined by a sex-linked recessive gene [1]. The underlying metabolic defect is a lack of hypoxanthine-guanine phosphoribosyl transferase (HGPRT). Blood uric acid levels are high and, although there are no reports of gouty arthritis, renal function is impaired by deposits of urates [4, 5]. Physical and mental development is retarded. Spastic tetraplegia and athetosis are apparent in early childhood. The child grossly mutilates his face and hands, and partial destruction of the lower lip by biting is a characteristic finding. It is not understood what induces the urge to self-mutilation.

Patients with partial deficiency of HGPRT may develop gouty arthritis and/or uric acid calculi without the neurological and behavioural features [2] (see p. 2319).

REFERENCES

1 HOEFNAGEL D., *et al* (1965) *N Engl J Med* **273**, 130.
2 KELLEY W.N., *et al* (1969) *Ann Intern Med* **70**, 155.
3 LESCH M. & NYHAN W.L. (1964) *Am J Med* **36**, 561.
4 NYHAN W.L., *et al* (1965) *J Pediatr* **67**, 257.
5 REED W.B. & FISH C.H. (1966) *Arch Dermatol* **94**, 194.

NUTRITION AND THE SKIN

K. WEISMANN

Lack of essential nutrients may be due to insufficient intake of food, malabsorption, vomiting or increased passage time of food due to diarrhoea and fistulas. Furthermore, certain drugs may interfere with the utilization of the food elements. Mostly the cutaneous changes are variable, reflecting combined deficiencies, so when there is an apparently isolated deficiency an underlying genetic or enzymatic defect should be ruled out. An increased metabolic requirement of nutrients may occur during periods of sudden weight gain. This may lead to relative deficiencies as seen in anabolic patients receiving long-term parenteral nutrition, who become severely deficient in zinc.

MALABSORPTION

Malabsorption is a condition characterized by a decreased intestinal uptake of nutrients associated with an increased faecal excretion of fat (steatorrhoea). The patient suffers from various degrees of lack of proteins, minerals, trace elements, fat-soluble vitamins, carbohydrates and water. Various causes of malabsorption are listed in Table 62.11.

TABLE 62.11. Various causes of malabsorption

Chelating substances in the gut
    Phytates

Insufficient digestive enzyme activity
    Pancreatic diseases (pancreatitis, mucoviscidosis)

Defective micelle formation
    Obstructive jaundice, liver cirrhosis

Contaminated small bowel syndrome (i.e. presence of an abnormal bacterial flora in the small bowel)
    Pernicious anaemia, total gastric resection (lack of hydrochloric acid production)
    Stagnant loop syndrome (strictures, surgical blind loops, scleroderma, diabetic enteropathy)
    Colonic reflux (intestinal fistula, extensive small bowel resection)
    Agammaglobulinaemia

Defective enzyme activity or carrier function in the intestinal mucosa
    Disaccharidase deficiency
    Coeliac disease
    Acrodermatitis enteropathica
    Hartnup disease

Loss of absorption capacity
    Intestinal resection and bypass operation
    Crohn's disease

Interference with intestinal lymphatics
    Lymphangiectasis
    Tuberculous mesenteric adenitis
    Hodgkin's disease

Inadequate transport mechanisms in the blood
Abetalipoproteinaemia

Miscellaneous
    Polyarteritis nodosa
    Lupus erythematosus
    Amyloidosis
    Mastocytosis
    Diabetes mellitus
    Zollinger–Ellison syndrome
    Protein-losing enteropathy
    Hyperthyroidism
    Hypothyroidism
    Cronkhite–Canada syndrome
    Dermatogenic enteropathy

Non-specific cutaneous effects [3, 4]. Non-specific symptoms may be observed in patients who have lost weight due to malabsorption or malignant disease. The skin changes reflect systemic illness rather than specific disease.

Itching and acquired ichthyosis. Itch is mostly caused by dry skin. Elderly patients are especially prone to develop dry skin which easily becomes eczematized. Patients with cancer, chronic liver and kidney diseases and lymphoma may develop an itchy atrophic ichthyosis [1]. Hypoferraemia may cause itch which disappears promptly after initiation of iron therapy [2].

Melanosis. Malabsorption with malnutrition may cause symmetrical melanin hyperpigmentation of the skin. The melanocyte stimulating hormone (MSH) is seldom increased. Apart from hyperpigmentation the skin may change its colour to pallor due to anaemia, wasting and skin atrophy associated with severe malnutrition.

Skin appendages. Brittle nails and hair loss are frequent findings in poorly nourished patients. In some cases lack of zinc, iron and vitamins is the main cause, but in the majority of patients the aetiology is probably multifactorial, and the exact cause remains unknown.

Specific cutaneous effects [3, 4]. Certain vitamin deficiencies may be observed in malabsorption. Lack of fat-soluble vitamins in particular may cause skin changes. The patient may show follicular hyperkeratosis (lack of vitamin A), ecchymoses and haematuria (lack of vitamin K) and cheilitis, glossitis, neuritis and dermatitis (lack of vitamin B complex). Zinc deficiency with specific skin changes may be seen.

Investigations. Patients presenting with skin changes suggestive of malabsorption should have their serum calcium, zinc, folate and albumin levels determined. The faecal fat excretion should be investigated and furthermore X-ray examination of the small intestine should be undertaken.

REFERENCES

1 SHUSTER S. (1967) The gut and the skin. In *Proc 3rd Symp on Advanced Medicine.* London, Pitman Medical.
2 VICKERS C.F.H. (1974) Nutrition and the skin. In *Proc 10th Symp. on Advanced Medicine.* London, Pitman Medical.
3 *WELLS G.C. (1962) Br Med J* ii, 937.
4 *WORMSLEY K.G. (1964) The Skin and Gut in Disease.* London, Pitman Medical.

SOME SPECIAL SYNDROMES WITH MALABSORPTION

Cronkhite–Canada syndrome [2] (see p. 1558)

Whipple's disease. This is a rare disease of uncertain aetiology involving the gastrointestinal tract, skin, joints, heart and lymph nodes [5]. There is diffuse hyperpigmentation of the skin, and leg nodules or erythema nodosum may occur [1]. The involvement of the heart includes inflammatory changes of the pericardium, myocardium and endocardium which may lead to valvular insufficiency.

Dermatitis herpetiformis (see p. 1651). The enteropathy is present in at least two-thirds of all patients and usually responds to a gluten-free diet. Some patients may be managed on a gluten-free diet alone [3, 4]. A dietary regimen enables most patients to reduce their requirement for dapsone [4].

REFERENCES

1 BIENVENU P., et al (1976) *Ann Cardiol Angelol,* (Paris) 25, 207.
2 CRONKHITE L.W. & CANADA W.J. (1955) *N Engl J Med* 252, 1011.
3 HARRINGTON C.I. & REID N.W. (1977) *Br Med J* i, 872.
4 LJUNGHALL K. & TJERNLUND U. (1983) *Acta Derm Venereol* (Stockh) 63, 129.
5 McALLISTER H.A. & FENOGLIO J.J. (1975) *Circulation* 52, 152.

MUCOVISCIDOSIS [2]
FIBROCYSTIC DISEASE; CYSTIC FIBROSIS OF THE PANCREAS

Mucoviscidosis is an inherited syndrome comprising three major symptoms: chronic lung disease, exocrine pancreatic insufficency and an abnormal high sodium concentration of the sweat.

Aetiology. The mode of genetic transmission is autosomal recessive. The basic metabolic defect is unknown. The mucous secretion has an increased viscosity resulting in obstruction of the small bronchial branches, the excretory ducts of the pancreas and the bile ducts of the liver. This eventually leads to respiratory disease, pancreatic insufficiency and hepatic failure. The high sweat sodium concentration is due to an unexplained lowered reabsorption of sodium in the sweat glands [4] (see p. 1886).

Histopathology. The exocrine sweat glands and pancreas show unidentified electron-dense bodies and there are fewer than normal secretory vacuoles in the 'dark cells' of the sweat coils [3].

Clinical features. The main presenting features are chronic pulmonary disease, exocrine pancreatic insufficiency with malabsorption, retarded growth and hepatic disease. Skin changes in the form of acrodermatitis enteropathica-like lesions due to essential fatty acid and zinc deficiency have been seen [1].

Diagnosis. The diagnosis is established by finding a high sweat sodium concentration, absence of pancreatic enzymes in the duodenum, chronic respiratory disease, retarded growth and a family history of the disease.

Treatment. Respiratory infection is controlled by proper prolonged antibiotic therapy according to bacterial cultures. Pancreatic insufficiency is treated by pancreatic enzyme preparations orally and a diet low in fat. The liver disease and the sweat abnormality are not amenable to treatment at present.

REFERENCES

1 HANSEN R.C., *et al* (1983) *Arch Dermatol* 119, 51.
2 *HERBAUT M., *et al* (1965) *La Mucoviscidose*. Paris, Masson.
3 MUNGER B.L., *et al* (1961) *J Pediatr* 59, 497.
4 Report of the Committee for a Study for Evaluation of Testing for Cystic Fibrosis (1976) *J Pediatr* 88, 711.

VITAMINS

Vitamins are biologically active organic compounds which are indispensable for the normal functions of the body. They have no direct function as an energy source or as building material for the tissues, but in most cases act as co-enzymes in various enzyme systems.

VITAMIN A

Vitamin A is a cyclic polyene alcohol. The main dietary sources are liver, eggs and butter. β-Carotene occurs in fruits, carrots and green vegetables and is absorbed and converted to vitamin A in the body. The recommended daily allowance is 5,000 i.u. (equivalent to 6,000–12,000 i.u. β-carotene). The normal blood level is approximately 1·5 μmol/l [3].

Vitamin A is essential for the reproductive system, bone formation, vision and epithelial tissues [1]. *In vitro* studies on human keratinocytes have shown that vitamin A affects their growth and differentiation [2]. In human volunteers 150,000 i.u. of vitamin A produced demonstrable retardation of keratinocyte maturation [4]. Skin disorders with abnormal keratinization such as ichthyosis, pityriasis rubra pilaris and Darier's disease have been treated with high doses of oral vitamin A [6]. There is a risk of intoxication by such treatment and stereoisomers of retinoic acid are now widely used instead [1].

REFERENCES

1 *BOLLAG W. (1983) *Lancet* i, 860.
2 CHOPRA P.P. & FLAXMAN B.A. (1975) *J Invest Dermatol* 64, 19.
3 *KUTSKY R.J. (1973) *Handbook of Vitamins and Hormones*. New York, Reinhold.
4 PINKUS H. & HUNTER R. (1964) *J Invest Dermatol* 42, 131.
5 STÜTTGEN G. (1975) *Acta Derm Venereol (Stockh)* (Suppl) 74, 174.
6 THOMAS J.R., *et al*, (1982) *Arch Dermatol* 118, 891.

VITAMIN A DEFICIENCY

Vitamin A deficiency is seldom seen in the Western world today. It is observed mainly in diseases with malabsorption and often associated with deficiency of other fat-soluble vitamins. Classical manifestations of vitamin A deficiency include xerophthalmia, follicular hyperkeratosis, dryness and scaling of the skin [1]. The diagnosis may be confirmed by the finding of a low vitamin A level in blood and a positive response to vitamin A supplementation.

Zinc deficiency may lead to vitamin A deficiency in the tissues as zinc acts on the retinol binding protein which is the transport protein for vitamin A and indispensable for mobilization of the vitamin from liver stores. Furthermore, zinc acts on the oxidation–reduction interconversion of vitamin A (alcohol dehydrogenase is a zinc metalloenzyme) and lack may trigger off symptoms related to vitamin A deficiency [3]. Night blindness in alcoholics may be due to a combined lack of vitamin A and zinc, and cases of vitamin A refractory night blindness should be given a therapeutic trial with oral zinc [2].

REFERENCES

1 FRAZIER C.N. & HU C.K. (1931) *Arch Intern Med* 48, 507.
2 SOLOMONS N.W. & RUSSEL R.M. (1980) *Am J Clin Nutr* 33, 2031.
3 WEISMANN K., *et al* (1979) *Acta Med Scand* 205, 361.

VITAMIN A INTOXICATION

Aetiology. Chronic hypervitaminosis A may be observed in young children persistently overdosed with vitamin preparations. Most reported adult cases have ingested more than 100,000 i.u. daily for several months. There is probably a risk of toxic effects if more than 50,000 i.u. daily are ingested for long periods [1].

Clinical features. There is lethargy, anorexia and loss of weight and diffuse alopecia. The skin becomes pruritic, rough and dry with desquamation. The lips are dry and cracked. Follicular keratosis, patchy erythema and purpura may occur [2]. In young children painful swellings of the limbs due to bone changes are conspicuous.

Diagnosis. Vitamin A intoxication is diagnosed by clinical findings associated with an increased vitamin A level in the blood. Radiological bone changes are found in young children and in some adults.

Treatment. No treatment is needed except immediate discontinuation of the vitamin supply.

Carotenoderma. A high intake of carrots may induce carotenoderma due to excess carotenes in the sweat. The condition is characterized by orange discoloration of the stratum corneum especially on palms, soles and in areas where sebaceous glands predominate. The condition is quite harmless and subsides gradually when the dietary habits are regulated. It often occurs in pregnancy as a 'pica'.

REFERENCES

1 RAASCHOU-NIELSEN W. (1961) *Dermatologica* **123**, 293.
2 SOLER-BECHARA I. & SOSCIA J.L. (1963) *Arch Intern Med* **112**, 462.

VITAMIN D [1]

Vitamin D is a group of antirachitic steroid derivatives with similar biochemical activity. Vitamin D_2, calciferol, is synthesized from its inactive provitamin ergosterol in plants by the action of UV irradiation. Vitamin D_3, which is present in cod liver oil, butter, eggs and liver, is synthesized from 7-dehydrocholesterol (cholecalciferol), which is present in abundance in the skin, by the action of UV irradiation. It is stored in the liver as hydroxycholecalciferol. In the kidney hydroxylation takes place, and the biologically active 1,25-dihydroxycholecalciferol is formed [2]. 1α-Hydroxyvitamin D_3 is a synthetic highly potent vitamin D analogue used in the management of hypoparathyroidism, vitamin-D-resistant rickets and osteomalacia. Vitamin D regulates calcium and phosphorus absorption and deposition and influences the level of serum alkaline phosphatase. The skin is of unique importance in the synthesis, storage and release of vitamin D into the circulation [2]. Lack of vitamin D in children results in rickets (rachitis) and tetany; in adults osteomalacia develops. In children limited exposure to sunshine may play an aetiological role. The daily need for calciferol is about 400 i.u. Intoxication (long-continued administration of more than 100,000 i.u. daily) causes anorexia, vomiting, headache, diarrhoea, hypercalcaemia and hypercalciuria with osteoporosis, resembling the action of parathyroid hormone. Treatment consists of withdrawal of vitamin D, a low calcium diet and corticosteroids. Recent work has brought some evidence that vitamin D plays an important role in epidermopoiesis but the mode of action remains unknown [2].

REFERENCES

1 FRASER D.R. (1974) *Metabolism and Function of Vitamin D.* London, Biochemical Society.
2 PAVLOVITCH J.H. & DELESCLUSE C (1983) *Int J Dermatol* **22**, 98.

VITAMIN E
TOCOPHEROL

Tocopherols are present in oils of vegetables, seeds and nuts. α-Tocopherol is the most potent compound. Whether the vitamin is essential to man is still a matter of debate, although in rats, guinea pigs and rabbits a true vitamin effect has been demonstrated. Various dermatological diseases and conditions have been claimed to respond to vitamin E [1, 2]. So far, no true benefit has been definitely documented. An inhibitory effect on hyaluronidase and a protective effect on cellular membranes and on vitamin A oxidation have been suggested, but the clinical relevance is still doubtful. Deficiency symptoms in man are not known.

REFERENCES

1 AYRES S. & MIHAN R. (1982) *J Am Acad Dermatol* **7**, 521.
2 POLLACK S.V. (1983) *J Dermatol Surg Oncol* **8**, 667.

VITAMIN B COMPLEX

The vitamins of the B complex are of great clinical significance. Isolated deficiencies of certain B vitamins are probably uncommon; mostly combined deficiencies of several vitamins belonging to the group are involved, often occurring together with an insufficient supply of protein and other nutrients. The group includes

Aneurin (thiamine) (vitamin B_1)
Riboflavine (vitamin B_2)
Pyridoxine (vitamin B_6)
Niacin (nicotinic acid)
Cyanocobalamin (vitamin B_{12})
Folic acid
Pantothenic acid
Biotin (vitamin H)

ANEURIN
VITAMIN B_1; THIAMINE

Aneurin is present in yeast, cereals, liver, meat, eggs and vegetables. It functions as cocarboxylase in carbohydrate metabolism and numerous other enzyme systems. It is involved in growth processes and in the function of the nervous system. Deficiency results in accumulation of pyruvic and lactic acids. Dietary deficiency may be a consequence of polished rice as the staple food or insufficient nutrition associated with chronic alcoholism. Furthermore, avitaminosis B_1 may be associated with pregnancy, lactation, diabetes mellitus, ulcerative colitis, coeliac disease, achlorhydria and myxoedema [1].

Clinical features [1, 3]. The classical form is beriberi, characterized by anorexia, weakness, constipation, symmetrical progressive polyneuritis, cardiac insufficiency with oedema and wasting of musculature. The diagnosis is based on the history and a low urinary aneurin excretion following an injection of 1·0 mg aneurin. Excretion of less than 50 µg usually indicates a deficiency.

Treatment. Aneurin 2–3 mg is given three times daily in mild cases. With severe cardiac and gastrointestinal involvement, or severe polyneuritis and muscular paresis, 20 mg twice daily given parenterally is indicated.

REFERENCES

1 *KUTSKY R.J. (1973) *Handbook of Vitamins and Hormones.* New York, Reinhold.
2 PLATT B.S. (1958) *Fed Proc* **17**, 8.
3 WILLIAM R.R. (1961) *Towards the Conquest of Beriberi.* Cambridge, Harvard University Press.

RIBOFLAVINE
VITAMIN B_2; LACTOFLAVINE

Riboflavine is a *d*-ribitol isoalloxazine derivative widely distributed in plants and animal tissues. Important sources are milk and those of vitamin B_1 [2]. It plays a part in intracellular redox reactions. The human requirement is 1–2 mg daily.

Clinical features. Deficiency becomes clinically manifest after several months of deprivation due to chronic illness and malnutrition, especially in old women who suffer from achlorhydria and in malnourished children with malabsorption. Ariboflavinosis may occur in alcoholic liver cirrhosis and the association with other deficiencies, such as pellagra, is frequent. Clinically [2] there is photophobia due to conjunctivitis, sometimes with corneal vascularization, angular stomatitis (perlèche) and sore lips, tongue and mouth. The tongue is purplish-red and smooth. A scaly seborrhoeic dermatitis-like eruption may be seen around the nose, eyes, ears and genital area (oro-oculo-genital syndrome). Similar findings, including the photophobia, are characteristic of zinc deficiency (see p. 2336). This association is to be expected since the content of the two essential nutrients in foodstuffs is correlated [1, 3].

Treatment. Treatment consists of 5–15 mg riboflavine two to three times daily for 2 weeks and correction of dietary errors.

REFERENCES

1 EGGLETON W.G.E. (1940) *Chin J Physiol* **15**, 33.
2 *GOLDSMITH G.A. (1964) In *Nutrition.* Eds Beaton G.H. & McHenry E.W. New York, Academic Press, Vol. 2.
3 WEISMANN K. (1980) *Zinc Deficiency and Effects of Systemic Zinc Therapy.* Copenhagen, FADL's, forlag p. 46.

PYRIDOXINE
VITAMINE B_6; PYRIDOXAL

Pyridoxine is a pyridine derivative, participating as a co-enzyme in transaminase and decarboxylase reactions and in the metabolism of cystein, tryptophan and essential fatty acids. It is present in many foods including yeast, eggs and various grains. Although much is known about experimental deficiency in many species the manifestations in man are not well defined. Convulsions, anaemia and acrodynia may develop in infants [1]. Dermatitis has occurred and is attributed to a disturbed metabolism of unsaturated fatty acids. Pyridoxine deficiency may follow therapy with isoniazid, hydralazine and penicillamine [2]. The recommended daily allowance is about 2 mg.

REFERENCES

1 HUNT A.D., *et al* (1945) *Pediatrics* **13**, 140.
2 CAPPS J.C., *et al* (1968) *Am J Clin Nutr* **21**, 715.

VITAMIN B$_{12}$
CYANOCOBALAMIN, CYCOBEMINE

Vitamin B$_{12}$ is involved in nucleic acid synthesis and erythrocyte production. Deficiency may occur in extreme vegetarians as plants do not contain the vitamin. More frequently it is due to lack of 'intrinsic factor' in pernicious anaemia. Hyperpigmentation especially in dark-skinned races may occur (see p. 1571).

FOLIC ACID

Folic acid is a compound consisting of pteridine, *p*-aminobenzoic acid and glutamic acid. It is present in liver, meat, green leaves and milk. In the organism folic acid is converted to folinic acid which is the biologically active form. The conversion demands the presence of vitamin C. Folinic acid is needed for the transport of C$_1$ fragments and plays a role in growth and erythrocyte production. The need is not known exactly but is estimated to be about 0·4 mg daily.

Although no constant cutaneous changes are related to folate deficiency, greyish-brown pigmentation on light-exposed parts has been described [2]. Cheilitis, glossitis and mucosal erosions are common. Pigmentation similar to that of vitamin B$_{12}$ deficiency has been described in pregnancy and lactation associated with folate deficiency. Spotty pigmentation of palms and soles and pigmented palmar creases have been found, which cleared with substitution therapy [1]. Folate deficiency is estimated by serum and erythrocyte folate levels. Subclinical deficiency may be present in extensive skin disease [3].

REFERENCES

1 BAUMSCHLAG N. & METZ J. (1969) *Br Med J* ii, 737.
2 GOUGH K.R., *et al* (1963) *Q J Med* **32**, 243.
3 KNOWLES I.P., *et al* (1963) *Lancet* i, 1138.

BIOTIN
VITAMIN H

Biotin is a water-soluble sulphur-containing heterocyclic carboxylic acid involved in bacterial metabolism and possibly functioning as a co-enzyme in decarboxylation and other enzymatic processes. Deficiency can be induced by feeding raw egg-white containing avidin which binds biotin and makes it poorly absorbable [4]. Short-bowel syndrome in association with parenteral nutrition may cause biotin deficiency [2]. Symptoms include alopecia, conjunctivitis, eczema around nose and mouth, hyperaesthesia, paraesthesia, depression and muscle pain [1]. A multivitamin preparation supplying 60 µg of biotin daily cures an adult patient within 3 weeks. Possibly there is a zinc-biotin interaction, as reported in the rat. Biotin seems to possess some antiseborrhoeic actions and has been used in high doses for therapy of Leiner's disease in infants [3] (see p. 249). Biotin-responsive carboxylase deficiency associated with subnormal plasma and urinary biotin levels has been reported [5, 6]. The genetic disorder involves a disturbed biotin metabolism and causes decreased activity of biotin-containing carboxylases. Treatment consists of oral administration of 10 mg biotin daily.

REFERENCES

1 McCLAIN C.I., *et al* (1982) *JAMA* **247**, 3116.
2 MOCK D.M., *et al* (1981) *N Engl J Med* **304**, 820.
3 NISENSON A. (1957) *J Pediat* **51**, 537.
4 *ROTH K.S. (1981) *Am J Clin Nutr* **34**, 1967.
5 THOENE J.G., *et al* (1981). *N Engl J Med* **304**, 817.
6 THOENE J.G., *et al* (1983) *N Engl J Med* **308**, 639.

NIACIN
NICOTINIC ACID; VITAMIN B$_7$

Niacin is an essential component of two co-enzymes, co-enzyme I (NAD) and co-enzyme II (NADP), which either donate or accept hydrogen in a wide range of biochemical reactions. Tryptophan, an essential amino acid, can be transformed to niacin which is converted to the amide in the body.

PELLAGRA [4]

Aetiology. Pellagra is caused by a cellular deficiency of niacin, resulting from an inadequate dietary supply of niacin and tryptophan. In Western Europe and North America pellagra today is only rarely encountered, mostly in subjects living on an unbalanced diet, such as chronic alcoholics and patients with gastrointestinal diseases and severe psychiatric disturbances such as anorexia nervosa. Rare causes are functioning carcinoid tumours (see p. 2244) and Hartnup disease (see p. 2319). Antituberculous therapy with isonicotinic acid hydra-

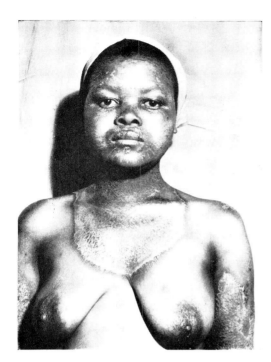

FIG. 62.21. Pellagra. Erythema, scaling and hypermelanosis on light-exposed skin. (Dr Theodore Gillman.)

zide, which competes biochemically with niacin owing to a close structural resemblance, may provoke pellagra [2].

Clinical features. The classical triad is dermatitis, diarrhoea and dementia, not invariably appearing in this order. Redness and superficial scaling appear on areas exposed to sunlight, heat, friction or pressure. The changes resemble sunburn and subside leaving a dusky, brown-red coloration. The tanning occurs more slowly than typically in sunburn [2] and exacerbation follows re-exposure to sunlight. On the face a symmetrical 'butterfly' eruption is frequently observed and there is often a characteristic well-marginated eruption on the front of the neck (Casal's necklace). Asymmetrical lesions may appear at sites of old injury or stasis [1]. Gastro-intestinal symptoms include pain, diarrhoea and achlorhydria in 50% of cases. In mild instances the mental disturbance may pass unnoticed, patients perhaps being slightly depressed or apathetic. Sometimes there is frank disorientation, restlessness and severe symptoms from the central nervous system [3]. Peripheral neuritis and myelitis are occasionally encountered.

Differential diagnosis. Drug eruptions, various forms of porphyria, photodermatitis and actinic reticuloid may cause diagnostic difficulty. A possible concomitant zinc deficiency should be ruled out. The so-called pellagrous vulvitis, vaginitis and scrotal dermatitis may be attributed to accompanying ariboflavinosis and other deficiencies of the vitamin B group.

Treatment. In severe cases intravenous niacin is required in doses of 50–100 mg once or twice daily. Orally, divided doses of niacin amide in a total dose of 0·5 g daily should be given. The amide is to be preferred since it does not precipitate flushing, itching and burning as is seen following ingestion of niacin in large doses. An improvement in the condition is to be expected within a day or two. A

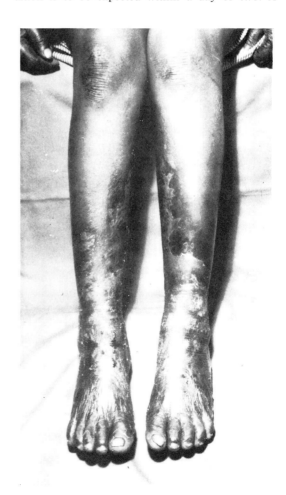

FIG. 62.22. Pellagra. Scaling and hypermelanosis of the lower legs and feet. (Dr Theodore Gillman.)

protein-rich diet and other vitamins of the B group should be administered.

REFERENCES

1 BEAN W.R., *et al* (1944) *Arch Dermatol Syphil* **49**, 335.
2 FINDLAY G.H. (1965) *Br J Dermatol* **77**, 666.
3 RISUM G. (1971) *Ugeskr Laeger* **133**, 935.
4 *STRATIGOS J.D. & KATSAMBAS A. (1977) *Br J Dermatol* **96**, 99.

KWASHIORKOR

Kwashiorkor is a nutritional syndrome with characteristic cutaneous changes due to severe protein malnutrition. In children there is retardation of skeletal and mental development, muscular wasting, fatty infiltration of the liver and oedema.

Aetiology. Protein malnutrition is one of the commonest and most widespread nutritional disorders in the developing countries and is responsible for kwashiorkor. The majority of cases are found in those countries where the diet consists of corn, rice or beans.

Kwashiorkor is more common in children than in adults and is a major paediatric problem in certain parts of the world. The onset in infancy is during the weaning and post-weaning period. In Europe and North America occasional cases are seen in patients suffering from malabsorption or an inadequate protein diet [4] and milder forms are probably not uncommon, particularly in the elderly.

Kwashiorkor refers to the 'deposed child' who is no longer suckled. It is a pluro-deficiency syndrome. The cause is related to lack of essential amino acids, vitamins and trace elements. Zinc deficiency in particular may be involved. The skin manifestations, hair changes and failure to thrive may mimic those seen in acrodermatitis enteropathica. Serum zinc is low, but this may be attributable at least in part to hypoalbuminaemia. Hospitalized children may show persistent hypozincaemia after clinical cure has occurred, indicating a need for zinc supplementation together with vitamins and a protein-rich nutrition [2, 3].

Clinical features [1, 5]. The symptoms of kwashiorkor usually first develop between the age of 6 months and 5 yr; the most important feature in the child is a failure to thrive. As well as inhibition of growth and mental development, oedema and muscle wasting are encountered.

The skin lesions are at first erythematous and later purple and reddish-brown in colour with

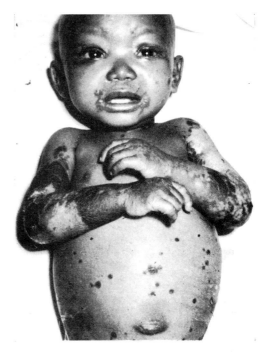

FIG. 62.23. Kwashiorkor. Note the 'flaky paint' lesions, the cheilosis and the pot-belly. (Dr Theodore Gillman.)

marked exfoliation. In milder cases a lacquered 'flaky paint' or 'cracked skin' is present.

The hair is dry and lustreless and may become light red–brown in colour. It may be prematurely grey or show a 'pepper and salt' appearance and become sparse, fine and brittle.

The skin often shows dyschromia with hypopigmentation, perhaps the result of phenylalanine deficiency, and patchy post-inflammatory hyperpigmentation. In florid cases pigmentary changes are particularly striking.

Mucosal lesions such as cheilosis, xerophthalmia and vulvovaginitis are found.

Mental disturbances are variable and may appear either as apathy or irritability. The child does not smile; when it does it is a sign of recovery.

Oedema is the result of hypoalbuminaemia. It affects the α- and β-globulins which are low, whilst an increase in λ-globulin is usual.

Hypoglycaemia with hypothermia, coma and severe bacterial or parasitic disease are rare, but often fatal, complications [6].

Mild cases of kwashiorkor appearing in the elderly show as a 'cracked skin' appearance on the front of the legs and lower abdomen. They have been reported under the title of geriatric nutritional eczema.

Prognosis. The short-term prognosis of mild cases which are given full dietary treatment is good but the mortality is high in severe and relapsing cases.

Diagnosis. Diagnostic difficulties occur in mild cases. The dietary history, 'cracked skin' and oedema, particularly when associated with pigmentary changes, should lead to the suspicion of protein deficiency.

The features distinguishing kwashiokor from pellagra are shown in Table 62.12.

TABLE 62.12. Some features distinguishing kwashiorkor from pellagra

Kwashiorkor	Pellagra
Children more than adults	Adults more than children
Dermatitis with systemic signs of apathy and oedema	Dermatitis precedes gastrointestinal and neuropsychiatric symptoms
Eruption generalized, pale ill-defined 'crackled skin'	Exposed areas only, red, thickened, well-defined; later dry, branny scales
Hair light, 'pepper and salt' appearance, thin	Normal
Nails sometimes soft and thin	Normal
High mortality if untreated	Low mortality

Prevention and treatment. The effective prevention of kwashiorkor depends on increasing the supply of animal proteins, and on education and social welfare in poor areas.

In an established case a complete and balanced diet should be given as soon as possible. Skimmed milk is the most useful treatment presumably through its amino acid content. Appropriate measures should be taken to correct any electrolyte disturbance.

REFERENCES

1 GILLMAN T. (1965) In *Comparative Physiology and Pathology of the Skin.* Eds Rook A. & Walton G.S. Oxford, Blackwell, p. 275.
2 GOLDEN B.E. & GOLDEN M.H.N. (1981) *Am J Clin Nutr* **34**, 892.
3 HAMBIDGE K.M. & WALRAVENS P.A. (1976) In *Trace Elements in Human Health and Disease.* Eds Prasad A.S. & Oberleas D. New York, Academic Press, Vol. I, p. 21.
4 HENINGTON V.M., *et al* (1958) *Arch Dermatol* **78**, 157.
5 *TROWELL H.C., et al* (1954) *Kwashiorkor.* London, Arnold.
6 WHARTON B. (1970) *Lancet* **i**, 171.

VITAMIN C [1]
ASCORBIC ACID

Vitamin C, ascorbic acid, is a relatively strong organic acid, chemically related to the carbohydrates. Only the L-form is biologically active. Ascorbic acid is a strong reducing agent, easily oxidized to dehydroascorbic acid, with which it constitutes a reversible redox system.

Vitamin C plays a central role in collagen and ground substance formation [2], in the metabolism of aromatic amino acids (phenylalanine, tyrosine), in the reduction of folic acid to folinic acid (see p. 2326), and in a broad range of biochemical redox reactions, including the preservation of sulphur-containing enzymes in a reduced form.

It occurs in cabbage, potatoes, green vegetables, and elsewhere. The recommended daily dose is 30–80 mg. A daily intake of 10 mg prevents scurvy.

REFERENCES

1 DICKMAN S.R. (1981) *Perspect Biol Med* **24**, 382.
2 *KUTSKY R.J. (1973) *Handbook of Vitamins and Hormones.* New York, Reinhold.

VITAMIN C DEFICIENCY
SCURVY; SCORBUTUS; HYPOVITAMINOSIS C

In the deficiency state collagen and ground substance synthesis are depressed which leads to a multiplicity of symptoms from bones, muscles, blood, mucous membranes and skin.

Aetiology. Lack of vitamin C is still a serious problem in many parts of the world where access to fruit and vegetables is limited and general malnutrition prevails. Most cases in Europe are a consequence of food faddism, ignorance or alcoholism [4, 5]. Danish beer no longer contains vitamin C as an antioxidant which may cause scurvy in alcoholics [3]. Malnourished children with scurvy (Barlow's disease) are still a paediatric problem as reported from Australia [2] and America [5]. In elderly patients with chronic gastrointestinal disturbances subclinical scurvy may be observed [1].

Clinical features. The initial skin change is follicular keratosis with coiled hairs on the upper arms, back, buttocks and lower extremities. Later perifollicular haemorrhage with blood pigment discoloration especially on the legs (Fig. 62.24), swollen bleeding gums, stomatitis and epistaxis occur. Large skin haemorrhages may be seen. Anaemia is usually present, and the patient appears resentful and mentally depressed. In the infant, dental

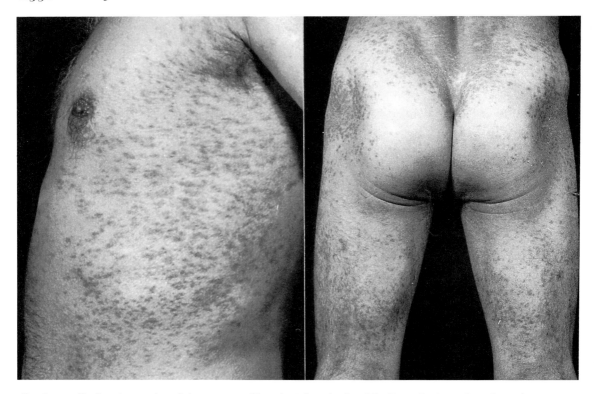

Fig. 62.24. Confluent purpuric rash in a 52-year-old scorbutic beer drinker. (The Finsen Institute, Copenhagen.)

development is impaired and oral changes may be severe. Tender subperiostal haematomas may develop and dominate the picture. Chronic hypovitaminosis C with 'woody' oedema and discoloration of the legs as the presenting feature has been described [6]. Subnormal serum levels of vitamin C are present (normal range about 17–94 µmol/l) but the significance of low values without clinical symptoms is not clear [3].

Treatment. The scorbutic patient should be treated with 300–1000 mg vitamin C daily given by mouth in addition to a protein-rich food. The response is dramatic. It is advisable to continue the therapy for several weeks to ensure repletion of the emptied body stores.

REFERENCES

1 BOOTH J.B. & TODD G.B. (1972) *Geriatrics* **27**, 130.
2 HENDERSON-SMART D.J. (1972) *Med J Aust* **i**, 876.
3 JORGENSEN J., *et al* (1983) *Ugeskr Laeger* **145**, 1525.
4 LEUNG F.W. & GUZE P.A. (1981) *Ann Emerg Med* **10**, 652.
5 Reports of Committee of Nutrition (1962) *Pediatrics* **29**, 646.
6 WALKER A. (1968) *Br J Dermatol* **80**, 625.

ECTOPIC CALCIUM DEPOSITION (CALCIFICATION) AND HETEROTOPIC BONE FORMATION (OSSIFICATION) OF THE SKIN [2]

K. WEISMANN

Calcification is the result of deposition of calcium and phosphate in organic matrices of the tissues. The process occurs in a wide range of different conditions. The mineral phase may be arranged in the manner seen in normal bone formation—ossification. If the deposition is not organized the condition is termed calcification. The organic matrix consists largely of collagen or elastic tissue. All organic matrices of calcified or ossified tissues contain protein-bound phosphorus. In pathological ectopic calcification the matrix is altered and contains acid proteins. In pseudoxanthoma elasticum γ-carboxyglutamic acid, an amino acid present in calcium-binding proteins, has been found in high concentrations in the dermis [1, 2].

The solid phase is made up of hydroxyapatite and amorphous calcium phosphate. Once formed the focus increases in size by growth and may result in disorganized masses of pasta-like material.

TABLE 62.13. Various forms of aberrant calcium deposition (calcification) in the skin

A. DYSTROPHIC CALCIFICATION
    1. Calcification usually associated with localized injury
      Congenital
        fibrodysplasia ossificans
      Traumatic
        foreign-body, haematoma, fat-cell necrosis
      Inflammatory
        acne, varicose veins, tuberculous granuloma, postoperative inflammation in scars
      Degenerative
        infarcts (arterial, venous), venous stasis, parasitic cysts (e.g. echinococcal cysts)
      Neoplastic
      Benign: sebaceous cysts, lipomas, angiomas, calcifying epithelioma of Malherbe
      Malignant: some liposarcomas

    2. Calcification associated with widespread tissue injury
      Dermatomyositis
      Generalized scleroderma (Thibierge–Weissenbach or CREST syndrome)
      Systemic lupus erythematosus
      Acrodermatitis atrophicans
      Pseudoxanthoma elasticum
      Ehlers–Danlos syndrome

B. IDIOPATHIC CALCIFICATION
    Calcinosis universalis; calcinosis circumscripta
    Solitary nodular calcification of the skin ('cutaneous calculus')
    Pinnal calcification
    Tumoral calcinosis

C. METASTATIC CALCIFICATION
    1. Hypercalcaemic
      Hyperparathyroidism
      Sarcoidosis
      Vitamin D excess
      Milk–alkali syndrome
      Destructive bone disease
        Metastatic carcinoma, reticulosis, multiple myeloma, leukaemia, Paget's disease
    2. Normocalcaemic
      Chronic renal failure
      Pseudohypoparathyroidism

Aberrant calcium deposition in the skin may be divided into three main groups: that associated with localized or widespread tissue changes or damage (dystrophic calcification); that unassociated with tissue damage or demonstrable metabolic disorder (idiopathic calcification); and that associated with an abnormal calcium and phosphorus metabolism (metastatic calcification) (Table 62.13).

REFERENCES

1 FOLEY I. & GORDON S. (1979) *Clin Res* **27**, 298A.
2 *GLIMCHER M. (1976) In *Handbook of Physiology*. Eds Greep R.O. & Astwood E.B. Washington, American Physiological Society, Vol. 7, p. 25.

DYSTROPHIC CALCIFICATION [2]

The calcinosis is confined to the dermis or subcutaneous tissue and related to local connective tissue or fat-cell damage. The calcification appears a variable time after the injury: in dermatomyositis after a few years; in generalized scleroderma usually after 10 or more years' duration of the disease.

An accumulation of calcium salts on dermal collagen fibres of pig skin was observed in scars following electrical injury [1]. Deposition of calcium salts in high concentration on a damaged skin surface may induce dermal calcification, as observed following electroencephalography in children [3]. The skin was abraded prior to application of an electrode paste containing calcium chloride. Lesions developed shortly after electroencephalography and disappeared in 2–6 months without therapy. An intact stratum corneum is protective. Soft tissue calcification may be seen in systemic lupus erythematosus [4]. No abnormalities of calcium metabolism can be detected in these cases.

REFERENCES

1 KARLSMARK T., *et al* (1983) *Nature* **301**, 75.
2 KENDRICK J.I., *et al* (1966) *Postgrad Med* **39**, 165.
3 WILEY H.E. & EAGLSTEIN W.E. (1979) *JAMA* **242**, 455.
4 QUISMORIO F.P., *et al* (1975) *Arch Dermatol* **84**, 191.

CALCINOSIS UNIVERSALIS

The deposition of calcium in the dermis, subcutis and muscles is unrelated to any recognizable tissue injury or aberrant metabolic disorder. Many cases reported in the literature under the diagnosis were probably suffering from undetected polymyositis or scleroderma [4] but there remain a number of instances in which no underlying disease is demonstrable.

Aetiology. The cause is unknown. Children, mostly girls, are affected. Some patients absorb calcium in excessive amounts [1] and show decreased urinary calcium excretion.

Histopathology. Initially calcium particles gather around fat cells and deposits are later seen within the cells. Electron microscopy of early lesions has shown apatite crystals lying parallel to the collagen fibres [2].

Clinical features. Nodules or plaques 0·5–5 cm in size are symmetrically distributed over the extremities and, less commonly, the trunk. The lesions may become tender and ulcerate, discharging chalk-like creamy material consisting mainly of calcium phosphate with a small amount of calcium carbonate. After ulceration, a slowly healing sinus remains. Fingertip lesions are often painful, while in other sites there may be limitation of movement due to stiffening of the skin. The disease is eventually fatal.

X-ray examination is valuable for localizing the deeper deposits. Biochemical investigations are normal.

Treatment. Surgical removal of painful deposits may give temporary relief. In some instances corticosteroids may be considered although the response is variable. Cellulose phosphate combined with a low calcium diet should be considered as therapy [3].

REFERENCES

1 AVIOLI L.V., *et al* (1965) *J Clin Invest* **44**, 128.
2 CORNELIUS C.E., *et al* (1968) *Arch Dermatol* **98**, 219.
3 MARKS J. (1970) *Br J Dermatol* **82**, 1.
4 WHEELER C.E., *et al* (1952) *Ann Intern Med* **36**, 1050.

CALCINOSIS CIRCUMSCRIPTA

There may be only a few calcium deposits in the skin. Most cases of calcinosis circumscripta are found in generalized scleroderma or dermatomyositis [5] but rarely it may occur as an idiopathic disorder [1]. Idiopathic calcinosis of the scrotum [3] and penis [2] have been described. Dystrophic calcification in the penis has been reported following trauma, Peyronie's disease and cytostatic therapy. A single case of cheloidal calcification has been reported [4].

REFERENCES

1 EPSTEIN E. (1936) *Arch Dermatol Syphil* **34**, 367.
2 HUTCHINSON I.F., *et al* (1980) *Br J Dermatol* **102**, 341.
3 MOSS R.L. & SHEWMAKE S.W. (1981) *Int J Dermatol* **20**, 134.
4 REDMOND W.J. & BAKER S.R. (1983) *Arch Dermatol* **119**, 270.
5 WHEELER C.E., *et al* (1952) *Ann Intern Med* **36**, 1050.

METASTATIC CALCIFICATION

In metastatic calcification calcinosis occurs in the skin, subcutaneous tissue, muscles and internal organs.

Aetiology. In all cases there is an increase in the serum levels of calcium or phosphate. Hypercalcaemia may be due to hyperparathyroidism, vitamin D intoxication [3], milk-alkali syndrome [2] or destructive bone disease with excessive osteoclastic activity. Metastatic carcinoma, multiple myeloma, leukaemia and Paget's disease of bone may all be associated with metastatic calcification.

Normocalcaemic cases are usually due to raised serum phosphate which is frequently the result of chronic renal insufficiency with phosphate retention [1].

Clinical features. The cutaneous manifestations are similar to those of calcinosis universalis. Additional clinical features reflect the primary disease.

Therapy. Only in hypervitaminosis D and the milk–alkali syndrome can improvement be expected by regulation of dietary habits and withdrawal of vitamin D and milk intake. In cases of renal insufficiency restriction of dietary phosphate and oral administration of an aluminium hydroxide gel may be useful.

REFERENCES

1 KOLTON B. & PEDERSON J. (1974) *Arch Dermatol* 110, 256.
2 WERMER P., *et al* (1953) *Am J Med* 14, 108.
3 WILSON C.W., *et al* (1953) *Am J Med* 14, 116.

TUMORAL CALCINOSIS [1–3]

Tumoral calcinosis occurs most commonly in the native population of Africa, particularly among younger age groups. Clinically the lesions present as swellings around the large joints (hip, elbow, ankle and scapula), but there is no actual involvement of the joint. Extrusion of calcified material, which has been likened to a suspension of procaine–penicillin, may take place. Histologically there is initiallly collagen necrobiosis which results in cyst formation and a foreign body response. The calcification is first granular; later dense deposits are seen [1]. The aetiology is unknown, but it is probably a form of dystrophic calcification caused by mechanical injury.

REFERENCES

1 McKEE P.H., *et al* (1982) *Br J Dermatol* 107, 669.
2 PALMER P.E.S. (1966) *Br J Radiol* 39, 518.
3 WHITING D.A., *et al* (1970) *Arch Dermatol* 102, 465.

PINNAL CALCIFICATION [1]

Calcified ear cartilage has been observed in several conditions such as Addison's disease, ochronosis, acromegaly [2], diabetes mellitus, hyperthyroidism [3], systemic chondromalacia (von Meyenburg disease), familial cold hypersensitivity and frostbite.

REFERENCES

1 McKUSICK V.A. & GOODMAN R.M. (1962) *JAMA* 179, 230.
2 NATHANSON L. & LOSNER S. (1947) *Radiology* 48, 66.
3 SCHERRER F.W. (1932) *Ann Otol Rhinol Laryngol* 41, 867.

CUTANEOUS OSSIFICATION (OSTEOMATOSIS)

Cutaneous calcification with bone formation has been noted in suprapubic prostatectomy scars and in otherwise normal postoperative scars [1]. It may also occur in collagen vascular disease (lupus erythematosus, scleroderma and dermatomyositis) [2, 3]. Cutaneous ossification without any known causative factor (also known as osteomatosis cutis, primary osteoma cutis or osteosis cutis) is rather uncommon in children [1].

REFERENCES

1 LIM M.O., *et al* (1981) *Arch Dermatol* 117, 797.
2 MACLEAN G.D., *et al* (1966) *Arch Dermatol* 94, 168.
3 ROTH S.I., *et al* (1968) *Arch Pathol Lab Med* 76, 44.

IRON METABOLISM [1]

The total iron content of adult man is 4–5 g, 60–70% of which is blood haemoglobin iron. Small amounts of ferritin iron are present in the erythrocytes, in plasma and in leukocytes [1]. The ferritin levels vary with the iron status of the individual and with certain diseases. The body has a limited ability to excrete iron and homeostasis is therefore regulated mainly by adjusting the iron absorption. Iron compounds need to be reduced to the ferrous form (Fe^{2+}) to be absorbed. Ascorbic acid which can reduce and chelate iron enhances iron absorption.

The mechanism of iron absorption is not completely understood. Recent evidence points to an iron transport system involving the binding of iron to the plasma membrane of mucosal cells and the interaction of transferrin in plasma with these sites.

Total iron in faeces lies between 6 and 16 mg/day depending on the amount ingested. Most of it is unabsorbed food iron. Iron is stored in the liver, spleen and bone marrow as ferritin and haemosiderin. It is released readily from these sites according to the body needs.

REFERENCES

1 UNDERWOOD E.J. (1977) *Trace Elements in Human and Animal Nutrition*. New York, Academic Press, p. 13.

IRON DEFICIENCY

General symptoms include fatigue, palpitation on exertion, sore tongue with atrophic filiform papillae, perleche, dysphagia and koilonychia (see p. 2067) [3].

Generalized itch may be present [4]. Hair loss with or without morphological changes of the hair shaft may be observed [1, 3]. In infants and children anorexia, retarded growth and decreased resistance to infections are outstanding features. The recommended daily allowance is 10 mg in infants, 10–15 mg in children, 18 mg in young males and females and 10 mg in both sexes above 20 yr of age [2]. Pregnant women should receive supplemental iron as the increased need for iron can hardly be met by ordinary diets.

The diagnosis of iron deficiency is based on low serum iron levels, clinical symptoms and improvement following iron therapy.

REFERENCES

1 BLANKENSHIP M.L. (1971) *Cutis* 7, 467.
2 Food and Nutrition Board (1974) *Recommended Dietary Allowances*. Washington, National Academy of Sciences.
3 HARD S. (1963) *Acta derm Venereol (Stockh)* 43, 652.
4 VICKERS C.F.H. (1977) *JAMA* 238, 129.

IRON INTOXICATION

Daily ingestion of 50–75 mg iron has been reported as safe [1, 2], and even higher intakes in some individuals turn out to be harmless. Chronic iron intoxication has been reported among Bantus consuming beer which is brewed in iron utensils. The iron is in a soluble form and may supply a net uptake of 2–3 mg iron daily [3]. Iron-contaminated cereals do not induce siderosis because iron is present in a less available form.

REFERENCES

1 CARLTON R.W., *et al* (1973) *Clin Haematol* 2, 383.
2 FINCH C.A. & MONSEN E.R. (1972) *JAMA* 219, 1462.
3 MONSEN E.R. (1971) *J Nutr Educ* 2, 383.

HAEMOCHROMATOSIS [1]
BRONZE DIABETES

Haemochromatosis is a syndrome characterized by the triad of hyperpigmentation, diabetes mellitus and cirrhosis of the liver, associated with increased iron deposition in the internal organs. Hypogonadism is frequently present. The sex ratio is one woman to 10 men. Onset of symptoms is gradual, usually between 40 and 60 yr.

Aetiology. Haemochromatosis can be found in the following conditions: idiopathic or primary haemochromatosis; chronic iron intoxication (e.g. Bantu haemochromatosis); chronic liver disease and iron overload (alcoholic haemochromatosis); hepatic haemosiderosis in anaemic patients with an ineffective erythropoiesis; and congenital transferrin deficiency. The cause of primary haemochromatosis is basically unknown, but a defective control of iron absorption is involved. The abnormality is inherited as an autosomal recessive trait. Erythrocyte ferritin is increased sixtyfold in idiopathic haemochromatosis which allows a distinction between this disorder and alcoholic liver disease with iron overload [6]. In alcoholic haemochromatosis alcohol consumption, particularly red wine and iron-containing beverages, plays an aetiological role. Whether the acquired form develops particularly in patients heterozygous for the trait is not known.

Histopathology. Liver biopsy in primary haemochromatosis shows marked iron deposits in the parenchymal cells and to a lesser degree in the Kupffer cells. Skin biopsy reveals that hyperpigmentation of the skin is due to melanin [4]. Iron deposits can be identified in the deeper dermis.

Clinical features. The skin discoloration may precede other signs by many years although it may appear late in the course. The skin shows a distinctive grey–brown pigmentation especially on the face, flexural creases and exposed parts. Sometimes the buccal mucosa is involved as in Addison's disease but adrenal insufficiency is not present. The various skin changes were studied in 100 patients [2]. There was almost 100% frequency of hyperpigmentation, 75% had hair loss, (including axillary and pubic hair loss), about 50% had koilonychia and 45% had ichthyosis-like, atrophic dry skin. Less frequent symptoms included palmar erythema, onychia striata, leuconychia and spider angiomas. The findings may be seen in cirrhosis of any cause. Hepatomegaly, diabetes, testicular atrophy, heart disease and weight loss are additional findings. Arthropathy, present in 25–50% of the patients, resembles rheumatoid arthritis, but serology is negative.

Diagnosis. The diagnosis may be suspected in a patient with diabetes mellitus, liver cirrhosis and hyperpigmentation. Other pigmentary disorders should be excluded. A skin biopsy shows increased melanin in the basal cell layer of the epidermis and melanophages in the upper dermis. Liver biopsy is usually diagnostic.

Routine laboratory tests may reveal evidence of chronic hepatic disease or of diabetes mellitus. Total serum iron is increased to the range 180–300 mg/100 ml [1], serum transferrin saturation is above

80% [2] and the transferrin level and the TIBC may be reduced [1]. Serum and erythrocyte ferritin is high, reflecting the iron stores on the body [6].

HLA-typing has revealed an increased frequency of HLA-A$_3$ and B$_{14}$ [5].

Treatment. An iron liver concentration above 100 μmol/g weight is an indication for therapy [3]. Organ damage may be reversed by reducing the excessive iron stores by venesection 500 ml weekly for 1–2 yr. Serum iron and serum transferrin and transferrin saturation remain unchanged until excess iron has been removed. Serum or erythrocyte ferritin should be monitored as a guide to the efficacy of treatment. Family members should have their serum iron estimated and where there is evidence of iron overload prophylactic venesection should be undertaken.

REFERENCES

1 *ANHALT G.J. & DUBIN H.V. (1981) In *Cutaneous Aspects of Internal Disease*. Ed. Callen J.P. London, Yearbook Medical Publishers, p. 525.
2 CHEVRANT-BRETON J., et al (1977) *Arch Dermatol* 113, 161.
3 MILMAN N., et al (1983) *Dan Med Bull* 30, 115.
4 PERDRUP A. & POULSEN H. (1964) *Archs Dermatol* 90, 34.
5 SHEWAN W.G., et al (1976) *Br Med J* i, 280.
6 WEYDEN M.B., et al (1983) *Br Med J* 286, 752.

SULPHUR METABOLISM [2]

Sulphur is a vital element for the normal function of the human body. It is an essential component of the amino acids methionine and cysteine and of chondroitin sulphate which are involved in keratinization and formation of dermal collagen respectively. Dietary thionine and cysteine are the main precursors for the synthesis of sulphur-containing components in the body. In homocystinuria (see p. 2318) there is a metabolic block in the pathway and this leads to tissue-paper scars on the hands and sparse fair hair due to impaired keratin formation. When the supply of sulphur-containing amino acids is inadequate less sulphur is available to nail and hair growth, but the keratin produced seems to be normal [3]. The liver plays a central role in degradation of sulphur-containing amino acids. In chronic liver disease low urinary levels of inorganic sulphate are present [2].

In exfoliative psoriasis with increased epidermopoiesis relative sulphur depletion is found and the urinary excretion of inorganic sulphate is decreased. Hair loss in chronic exfoliative dermatoses may be related to diversion of sulphur-containing amino acids to synthesis of skin protein instead of hair keratin formation [3].

Mucopolysaccharide synthesis in the dermis is influenced by certain hormonal factors. Thyrotrophin has a stimulant action on connective tissue and the pituitary somatrophic hormone stimulates chondroitin sulphate formation. Probably growth hormone is a stimulator of sulphation [1].

REFERENCES

1 ASBOE-HANSEN G. (1969) *Br J Dermatol* 81 (Suppl. 2), 2.
2 *MÅRTENSSON J. (1981) *Studies on Human Sulphur Metabolism*. Linköping University Medical Dissertations, No 119, Linköping.
3 ROE D.A. (1969) *Br J Dermatol* 81 (Suppl. 2), 49.

ZINC METABOLISM

Zinc belongs to the group of essential trace elements which at present comprise zinc, iron, copper, manganese, nickel, cobalt, molybdenum, selenium, chromium, iodine, fluorine, tin, silicon, vanadium and arsenic [15]. High concentrations of zinc are present in shellfish, legumes, nuts, whole grain and green leafy vegetables, whereas fruits usually contain insignificant levels [7]. Wine, beer and spirits contain very low concentrations of zinc. The zinc supply depends largely on the protein content of the food and so protein undernourishment will lead to an insufficient zinc supply. Phytate interferes with zinc absorption and a high fibre content of the food also tends to decrease the bioavailability of the element.

Recommended dietary allowance of zinc [6]. The daily oral intake of zinc should average 3 mg in infants less than 6 months, 5 mg in infants 0·5–1 yr old, 10 mg in children 1–7 yr old and 16 mg from the eleventh year and onwards. Pregnant and lactating women should receive 20–25 mg zinc daily.

Biological functions. Zinc is indispensable to the normal function of all cells, cellular systems, tissues and organs in the human body. The essentiality is related mainly to its function as the metal moiety of important enzymes such as alkaline phosphatase, alcohol dehydrogenase and several different dehydrogenases and digestive enzymes [11]. Zinc also regulates DNA and RNA polymerases, thymidine kinase and ribonuclease.

ZINC DEFICIENCY

Zinc deficiency may be caused by a specific absorptive defect present in acrodermatitis enteropathica or by insufficient nutrition as reported from the Middle East and Turkey. These causes of zinc deficiency are referred to as primary. Zinc deficiency may also be consequent upon diseases of the gastrointestinal tract causing diarrhoea and malabsorption. Such cases are called conditional or secondary zinc deficiency.

Primary zinc deficiency [7]

Acrodermatitis enteropathica. The disease was recognized in 1936 by the Swedish dermatologist Thore Brandt [2]. His findings were corroborated and further investigated by Danbolt and Closs [4] who coined the name of the disease. It is a rare disease believed to be transmitted as an autosomal recessive trait. In Denmark the prevalence is about 1 per 500,000 inhabitants. Adema disease in black-pied cattle seems to represent a true animal parallel of the human disease [18].

Aetiology. Zinc absorption in young patients is very low, about 2–3% compared with 27–65% in normal adults (mean 43%) [19]. The cause of the zinc malabsorption is not known. It explains the low serum zinc values invariably found in the patients. The specific malabsorption can be overcome by an oral zinc supply and seems to improve spontaneously with age [19].

Brandt [2] noticed that mothers' milk was an efficient remedy for the disease, probably because of an enhancing effect on zinc absorption mediated by some zinc binding substances in the milk. The nature and existence of zinc binding ligands are still a matter of controversy [5, 12].

Clinical features. The disease typically starts 4–6 weeks after weaning or earlier if the infant is not weaned. The child turns peevish, withdrawn and photophobic, develops a vesicobullous dermatitis on hands, feet and peri-orificial areas and scalp hair is lost. Diarrhoea is often present. Growth is stunted and there is a decreased resistance to infections. Wound healing is poor.

Prognosis. Without proper management the prognosis is dubious and in the past a lethal outcome within 4–5 yr was the rule. Survival up to adult age without therapy has been described in a few cases [9].

Treatment. Halogenated 8-hydroxyquinolines (e.g. Diodoquin) were formerly used for therapy on a purely empirical basis. Experimental studies on rats have shown that iodochlorohydroxyquinoline, a commonly used antibacterial agent, increases ^{65}Zn

absorption significantly in a dose-dependent way [17]. Zinc sulphate for acrodermatitis enteropathica was first introduced in 1973–1974 [1, 13]. Oral zinc in a dose of 2 mg/kg daily was found to cure all clinical manifestations related to the zinc deficiency within a few weeks. Prolonged therapy at least up to adult age is necessary to prevent recurrence of zinc deficiency.

Endemic nutritional zinc deficiency. Endemic zinc deficiency presenting with dwarfism and hypogonadism as the main symptoms has been reported from rural districts in Iran, Egypt [14] and Turkey [3]. The chronic zinc deficiency is attributed to the diet which consists mainly of unleavened whole grain bread with a high fibre and phytate content which makes zinc more or less unabsorbable. The habit of clay eating and concomitant hookworm infestation play a contributory role in the negative zinc balance. Zinc deficiency has been described in severely malnourished children in Jamaica [8], Egypt and various parts of Africa [10]. The significance of zinc deficiency has not been clearly defined but it certainly plays a role in the growth retardation and skin changes of the children. Acrodermatitis enteropathica has been reported from Africa where it is almost invariably first diagnosed as kwashiorkor [16].

REFERENCES

1 BARNES P.M. & MOYNAHAN E.J. (1973) *Proc Soc Med* **66**, 327.

2 BRANDT T. (1936) *Acta Derm Venereol (Stockh)* **17**, 513.

3 CAVDAR O.S., et al (1977) *Am J Clin Nutr* **30**, 833.

4 DANBOLT N. & CLOSS K. (1942) *Acta Derm Venereol (Stockh)* **23**, 127.

5 EVANS G.W. & JOHNSON P.E. (1980) *Pediatr Res* **14**, 876.

6 Food and Nutrition Board (1980) *Recommended Dietary Allowances*, 8th ed. Washington, National Academy of Sciences.

7 FREELAND J.H. & COUSINS R.J. (1976) *J Am Diet Assoc* **68**, 526.

8 GOLDEN P.E. & GOLDEN M.H.N. (1981) *Am J Clin Nutr* **34**, 892.

9 GRAVES K., et al (1980) *Arch Dermatol* **116**, 562.

10 HAMBRIDGE K.M. & WALRAVENS P.A. (1976) In *Trace Elements in Human Health and Disease*. Eds. Prasad A.S. & Oberleas D. London, Academic Press, p. 23.

11 KIRCHGESSNER M., et al (1976) In *Trace Elements in Human Health and Disease*. Eds Prasad A.S. & Oberleas D. London, Academic Press, p. 189.

12 LÖNNERDAL B., et al (1980) *J Inorg Biochem* **12**, 71.

13 MICHAËLSSON G. (1974) *Acta Derm Venereol (Stockh)* **54**, 377.

14 PRASAD A.S., et al (1963) *Arch Intern Med* **111**, 407.

15 UNDERWOOD E.J. (1977) *Trace Elements in Human and Animal Nutrition.* 4th ed. New York, Academic Press, Chs 1, 8.
16 VERHAGEN A.R. (1976) *Dermatoses in Dark-skinned People III.* Basel, Ciba-Geigy, p. 29.
17 WEISMANN K. (1980) *Zinc Deficiency and Effects of Systemic Zinc Therapy.* Copenhagen, FADL's forlag, p. 28.
18 WEISMANN K. & FLAGSTAD T. (1976) *Acta Derm Venereol* (Stockh) **56**, 151.
19 WEISMANN K., *et al* (1979) *Br J Dermatol* **101**, 573.

Secondary (conditioned) zinc deficiency

Zinc depletion syndrome. Adults who receive 0·2 mg zinc daily, which is 1·3% of the recommended allowance, become clinically zinc deficient within 3 months [3]. Where there is disturbed bowel function the zinc loss is increased, and if combined with a decreased absorption and low dietary zinc intake zinc depletion will develop. The zinc depletion syndrome was originally identified because of the acrodermatitis enteropathica-like skin lesions of patients who received prolonged total parenteral nutrition for inflammatory bowel diseases and chronic diarrhoea. Most of the patients have undergone extensive intestinal resections [1, 7]. The cause of the depletion is often triple: pre-existing latent zinc deficiency, prolonged total parenteral nutrition with a low zinc content and a sudden weight gain provoked by high calorie supply with the parenteral nutrition [13]. In most cases reported the parenteral nutrition was given for 2–3 months before signs of zinc deficiency occurred. The serum zinc level is significantly decreased, often less than 20 µg/100 ml (normal about 70–125 µg/100 ml, equivalent to 11–19 µmol/l).

Zinc depletion has been described in infants on total parenteral nutrition [2, 9, 10]. Premature infants are particularly at risk of developing such a state because they are born with negligible zinc stores and undergo rapid growth within their first months of life. Apart from cutaneous lesions of zinc deficiency they may show gastric retention and paralytic ileus [12] which resolves promptly following zinc therapy. Infants of low birth weight fed on mother's milk or cow's milk poor in zinc may also become zinc deficient [4].

Diseases of liver and pancreas. Chronic zinc deficiency may develop in patients suffering from malabsorption–malnutrition associated with alcohol liver cirrhosis and alcoholic pancreatitis [6, 13]. A defective exocrine pancreatic function and elevated urinary zinc excretion associated with liver cirrhosis [11] add to the negative zinc balance.

Intestinal bypass operation. Conditioned chronic zinc deficiency may develop following bypass surgery for obesity, especially in patients with poor eating habits [13].

Cancer chemotherapy. Cancer chemotherapy for leukaemia in children may provoke acute zinc deficiency [5, 8]. The cause is not clear; probably a disturbed bowel function, interference with metallothionine metabolism or other unknown actions are involved.

REFERENCES

1 ARAKAWA T., *et al* (1976) *Am J Clin Nutr* **29**, 197.
2 ARLETTE J.P., *et al* (1981) *J Am Acad Dermatol* **5**, 37.
3 BAER M.T. & KING J.C. (1978) *Fed Proc* **37**, 253.
4 BLOM I., *et al* (1980) *Br J Dermatol* **104**, 459.
5 CUTLER E.A., *et al* (1977) *N Engl J Med* **297**, 168.
6 ECKER R.I. & SCHROETER A.L. (1978) *Arch Dermatol* **114**, 937.
7 KAY R.G., *et al* (1976) *Ann Surg* **183**, 331.
8 LASSON U., *et al* (1979) *Dtsch Med Wochenschr* **104**, 1283.
9 LATIMER J.S., *et al* (1980) *J Pediatr* **97**, 434.
10 PRINCIPI N., *et al* (1979) *Acta Paediatr Scand* **68**, 129.
11 VALLEE B.L., *et al* (1956) *N Engl J Med* **255**, 403.
12 WEBER T.R., *et al* (1981) *J Pediatr Surg* **16**, 236.
13 *WEISMANN K. (1980) *Zinc Deficiency and Effects of Systemic Zinc Therapy.* Copenhagen, FADL's forlag.

Skin changes related to zinc deficiency [9, 10]. Systemic zinc deficiency causes lesions including alterations in nail and hair growth. The findings are similar whether the cause is primary or secondary. A distinction between the changes of acute and chronic zinc deficiency will be made.

Acute zinc deficiency. General symptoms include septicaemia, photophobia and mental depression. There is an acute eczematous eruption on hands and feet, in the anogenital regions and around the body openings. The volar aspects of the fingers show characteristic flat bullous lesions on the flexural creases (Fig. 62.25). There are various degrees of paronychial inflammation on fingers and toes. Oozing lesions may be seen on the heels of bedridden patients. Some lesions are black and necrotic, and burn-like skin changes may be seen. There is angular stomatitis with perioral lesions sparing the vermilion border.

Chronic zinc deficiency. Chronic zinc deficiency lesions are typically seen on skin areas subject to pressure and minor trauma such as elbows, knees, knuckles and malleolar regions of the ankles. The lesions are sharply demarcated, thickened and of a red–brown colour (Fig. 62.26). Lichenification is present as an important clue to distinguish it from

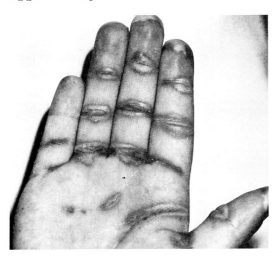

FIG. 62.25. Characteristic bullae on the hands, notably on flexural creases and around nails in a 6-year-old girl suffering from acute zinc deficiency during prolonged total parenteral nutrition.

psoriasis. Seborrhoeic dermatitis-like changes may be seen on the face of adult patients. Pre-existing acne vulgaris tends to flare.

A severe reticulate non-itchy scaly dermatitis on

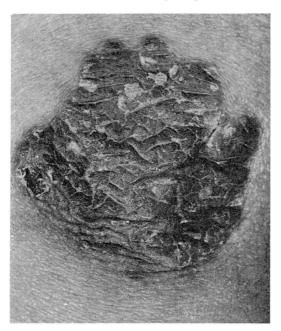

FIG. 62.26. Chronic zinc deficiency lesion on the elbow in acrodermatitis enteropathica. There is a psoriasiform appearance but marked lichenification and only slight scaling of the lesion.

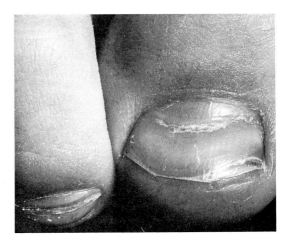

FIG. 62.27. Beau's lines on toe nails progressing after initiation of zinc therapy (the same patient as in Fig. 62.25).

the trunk has been described in chronic zinc deficiency of alcoholics [2, 9, 10]. It remains unresponsive to topical steroid treatment but clears rapidly with oral zinc.

Hair and nail changes [1, 10]. In acute zinc deficiency diffuse thinning of the scalp hair becomes progressive and eventually leads to total alopecia. In chronic zinc deficiency the hair growth is poor and sparse. Structural changes of the hair may be observed with the microscope, e.g. broken spearhead-like endings, transverse striation of the shaft, pseudomonilethrix, longitudinal splits and bayonet hairs. Severe zinc deficiency usually leaves deep transverse depressions (Beau's lines) on the finger nails, which become visible 3–4 weeks after the start of zinc supplementation (Fig. 62.27). White transverse bands may be seen alone or in association with the depressions [3, 8].

Pathology. In acute vesiculobullous acrodermatitis light microscopy reveals pronounced epidermal extracellular oedema with formation of suprabasal cysts and clefts (Fig. 62.28). The horny layer is often separated or lost. Necrosis of the outer epidermis may be seen [5], simulating migratory necrolytic erythema (see p. 2359). In chronic zinc deficiency there is psoriasis-like acanthosis of the epidermis (Fig. 62.29). In the dermis a slight perivascular infiltrate of lymphocytes, neutrophils and a few histiocytes is present.

Electron microscopy of acute lesions shows degenerate basal cells with slender cytoplasmic protrusions and an intact basal lamina with multiple invaginations [11].

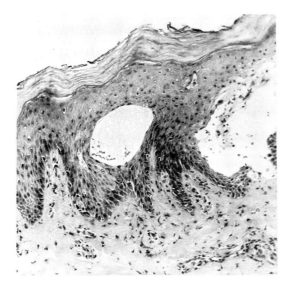

FIG. 62.28. Vesiculobullous dermatitis in acute zinc deficiency (the same patient as in Fig. 62.25). There is extracellular oedema, cysts and clefts low in the epidermis and a degenerate basal cell layer. A mainly neutrophilic perivascular infiltrate is present in the upper dermis.

Diagnosis. Severe zinc deficiency is usually suspected from the clinical findings and the history. The serum zinc and alkaline phosphatase levels are low

[4, 9, 10] but rise promptly during zinc administration. The parallel course of the two parameters can be used for diagnosis and for control of the treatment [6, 9]. It is important always to consider the level of plasma albumin which binds 60–70% of circulating zinc. Severe hypoalbuminaemia therefore is generally associated with low serum zinc values which do not reflect a state of zinc deficiency.

In suspect cases a therapeutic trial with oral or parenteral zinc should be undertaken. If no clinical improvement occurs within 4–5 days and the serum alkaline phosphatase remains unaltered or even decreases despite a rise in serum zinc the patient is not deficient in zinc.

Treatment. In adult patients oral zinc sulphate ($Zn_2SO_4 \cdot 7H_2O$) tablets of 0.2 g are given two to three times daily (about 2 mg zinc/kg). Similar doses on a kilogram basis are given to children. Parenterally 0.2–0.3 mg zinc/kg daily (about 10–20 mg daily in adult patients) is sufficient in severe cases of acute zinc deficiency. For prophylactic purposes total parenteral nutrition should supply no less than 70–80 µg zinc/kg daily. Infants and premature babies on parenteral nutrition should receive a prophylactic dose of 0.1–0.3 mg/kg daily [7].

REFERENCES

1 DUPRÉ A., *et al* (1979) *Acta Derm Venereol* (Stockh) **59**, 177.
2 ECKER R.I. & SCHROETER A.L. (1978) *Arch Dermatol* **114**, 937.
3 FERRANDIZ C., *et al* (1981) *Dermatologica* **163**, 255.
4 JACKSON M.J., *et al* (1982) *Clin Physiol* **2**, 333.
5 OKADA A., *et al* (1976) *Surgery* **80**, 629.
6 ROTHBAUM R.J., *et al* (1982) *Am J Clin Nutr* **35**, 595.
7 SHILS M.E., *et al* (1979) *J Am Acad Dermatol* **241**, 2051.
8 WEISMANN K. (1977) *Acta Derm Venereol* (Stockh) **57**, 88.
9 *WEISMANN K. (1980) In *Recent Advances in Dermatology*. Eds. Rook A. & Savin J. London, Churchill Livingstone, Ch 5.
10 *WEISMANN K. & HØYER H. (1982) *Hautarzt* **33**, 405.
11 WEISMANN K., *et al* (1983) *Acta Derm Venereol* (Stockh) **63**, 143.

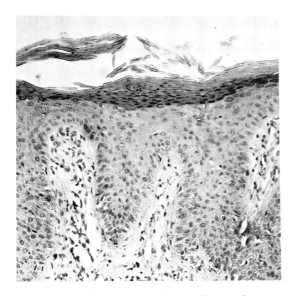

FIG. 62.29. Parakeratosis, irregular acanthosis and moderate spongiosis in the epidermis in chronic zinc deficiency dermatitis of acrodermatitis enteropathica (cf. Fig. 62.26).

SKIN DISORDERS IN DIABETES MELLITUS

Diabetes mellitus [1, 2]. Diabetes mellitus is a heterogenous group of metabolic disorders which have in common an elevated fasting and postprandial blood glucose level and share a variety of multi-system complications, mainly in the blood vessels, eye, kidney, nervous system and integument. Three main types can be distinguished. Type 1, also known as insulin-dependent diabetes mellitus or juvenile-onset diabetes, is characterized by abrupt onset of symptoms, insulinopenia, dependence on insulin injections, proneness to ketoacidosis and lack of ability to produce C-peptide. Type 2, non-insulin-dependent diabetes mellitus or adult-onset diabetes, is characterized by lack of ketoacidosis (except under stressful circumstances), ability to produce C-peptide, a tendency to obesity and improvement following loss of weight. Type 3, secondary diabetes, are miscellaneous types of diabetes which occur as a complication of pancreatic, hormonal or genetic disease or following ingestion of certain drugs or chemical compounds.

REFERENCES

1 National Diabetes Data Group (1979) *Diabetes* **28**, 1039.
2 OYER D.S. (1982) *Arch Dermatol* **118**, 132.

Skin symptoms due to diabetic vascular abnormalities [6, 7]

Diabetic microangiopathy. Both small and large blood vessels are affected in diabetes mellitus. In the diabetic microangiopathy there is a proliferation of endothelial cells and deposits of PAS-positive material in the basement membrane of arterioles, capillaries and venules with resulting decreased luminal area [1]. Basement membrane thickening is a characteristic finding in diabetic and pre-diabetic patients, but it is neither absolute nor pathognomonic for the disease [8]. The diabetic microangiopathy precedes manifest abnormalities of the disease and it is possible that vascular changes are the primary expression of the disease. Microangiopathy is responsible for the retinopathy, nephropathy and possibly also neuropathy and dermopathy associated with the disease.

Erysipelas-like erythema [8]. Well-demarcated red areas occur on the legs or feet of elderly diabetics. Some of the patients have an underlying destructive bone disease caused by a small-vessel insufficiency. It is mostly seen in elderly patients with an average duration of diabetes mellitus of 5 yr. Cardiac decompensation may be involved in some cases.

Wet gangrene of the foot. This is a late manifestation of diabetic microangiopathy. Non-diabetic atherosclerotics tend to develop a dry form which is the result of large-vessel insufficiency.

Diabetic rubeosis [5]. This is a peculiar rosy reddening of the face, sometimes of hands and feet, especially seen in longstanding diabetes. It may be present in mild and latent diabetes. The change has been attributed to a decreased vascular tone or diabetic microangiopathy. Rubeosis may have some practical diagnostic significance, especially in fair-skinned patients.

Diabetic dermopathy. This is the most common dermatosis associated with diabetes mellitus. Microangiopathy and possibly neuropathy are involved [3, 4]. Lesions are predominantly situated on the shin (shin spots), forearms, thighs and over bony prominences. About half of patients show such lesions, more frequently in men than in women. The initial lesion is an oval dull red papule, 0.5–1 cm in diameter. It revolves slowly, producing a superficial scale, eventually leaving an atrophic brownish scar. The colour is due to haemosiderin in histiocytes near the vessels [2]. There are usually multiple lesions, sometimes linear in arrangement. Microscopically, a combination of vascular disease with PAS-positive thickening of the vessel wall and minor collagen changes are found. The presence of shin spots is by no means specific for diabetes. There is no correlation between the presence of the lesions and the duration or severity of the diabetes. In known diabetics the occurrence of dermopathy lesions should initiate an investigation for diabetic microangiopathy and neuropathy [6].

Large-vessel disease [7]. Atherosclerosis is the second form of vascular disease frequently associated with diabetes mellitus. The patient shows intermittent claudication with pallid and cool skin distally on the extremities. The postural test discloses delayed filling of the veins. Common clinical sequelae are myocardial infarction, cerebral thrombosis, nephrosclerosis and ischaemic gangrenous lesions of the legs and feet. Microangiopathy is usually present together with large-vessel involvement, whereas microangiopathy frequently is seen alone.

REFERENCES

1 AJAM Z., *et al* (1982) *Br J Dermatol* **107** (Suppl. **22**) 22.
2 BAUR F.M. & LEVAN N.E. (1970) *Br J Dermatol* **83**, 528.
3 BINKLEY G.W., *et al* (1967) *Cutis* **3**, 955.
4 DANOWSKI T.S., *et al* (1966) *Am J Med Sci* **251**, 570.
5 GITELSON S. & WERTHEIMER-KAPLINSKI N. (1965) *Diabetes* **14**, 201.
6 *HUNTLEY A.C. (1982) *J Am Acad Dermatol* **7**, 427.
7 *KALKOFF K.W. (1982) *Hexagon* **9**, 1.
8 LITHNER F. (1974) *Acta Med Scand* **196**, 333.

Diabetic neuropathy. Elderly patients with an insidious onset of the disease are especially prone to be affected [3]. Commonly, there is a distal symmetrical polyneuropathy with mixed motor and sensory nerve involvement. The motor neuropathy of the foot is characterized by dorsally subluxed digits, distally displaced plantar fat pads, depressed metatarsal heads, hammer toes and pes cavus [1]. At this stage proper foot care is essential to prevent formation of indolent perforating ulcers (mal perforans). A painless and slowly penetrating ulcer of the sole and of other pressure sites is suggestive of diabetic neuropathy. The ulcer is circular and punched out in shape, occurring in the middle of a callosity. An initial subepidermal haemorrhagic bulla may give rise to discoloration of the surroundings [2]. A concomitant loss of temperature and pain sensation and absence of the ankle reflex (an early sign of diabetic neuropathy) show that the ulcer is of neuropathic origin. Sensory abnormalities of the lower extremities include numbness, tingling, aching and burning. Burning feet and restless legs are common complaints which intensify at night while lying down. Autonomic neuropathy may cause decreased or absent sweating of the lower extremities with compensatory increased sweating in other skin areas. Damage to autonomic nerves of the skin in chronic advanced cases is manifested by oedema, erythema and atrophy [1].

REFERENCES

1 *Huntley A.C. (1982) *J Am Acad Dermatol* 7, 427.
2 *Kalkoff K.W. (1982) *Hexagon* 9, 1.
3 Oakley W., *et al* (1956) *Br Med J* ii, 593.

Cutaneous infections in diabetes mellitus. Skin infections due to *Staphylococcus aureus* are more common in diabetics than in normals. The cause is unknown; it cannot be explained on the basis of a higher than normal glucose level in the skin [5]. Before insulin and antibiotics were available infections causing severe furuncles, carbuncles and styes were frequently observed among diabetics. Today, such complications are usually easily dealt with. In malignant external otitis, invasive pseudomonas infection can progress through cellulitis, osteitis to cranial nerve damage and meningitis. A high mortality rate of 53% has been reported [6].

Non-clostridial gas gangrene. This complication develops in the soft tissues near a gangrenous focus. It was diagnosed in 17% of diabetics who were admitted to hospital because of gangrene or ulceration [2]. Pathogens usually involved are *Escherichia coli*, *Klebsiella, Pseudomonas* and *Bacteroides* in various combinations. The outcome is generally good.

Candida albicans infections of the mouth, nail folds, genitals and intertriginous skin areas are more frequent in diabetics than in non-diabetics. Candidiasis may be the presenting feature of the disease, and is frequently seen in diabetics who are not well controlled [3]. The high glucose level of the saliva seems to account for the frequent oral affection [4]. Phimosis is a common complaint of diabetic men, and recurring or chronic candidal infection may be causative. Dermatophyte infections are not more frequent in diabetics than in non-diabetic individuals [1].

REFERENCES

1 Alteras J. & Saryt E. (1979) *Mycopathologica* 67, 157.
2 Bessman A.N. & Wagner W. (1975) *JAMA* 233, 958.
3 *Huntley A.C. (1982) *J Am Acad Dermatol* 7, 427.
4 Knight L. & Fletcher J. (1971) *J Infect Dis* 123, 371.
5 Marples M.J. (1965) *Ecology of the Human Skin*. Springfield, Thomas, p. 117.
6 Zaky D.A., *et al* (1976) *Am J Med* 61, 298.

Various skin disorders associated with diabetes mellitus

Necrobiosis lipoidica (see p. 1691). Necrobiosis lipoidica is frequently associated with diabetes mellitus. In two series of necrobiosis patients 62% [9] and 42% [12], respectively, were found to be diabetics. Among diabetics only 0·3% show necrobiosis [8]. It occurs three times more frequently in women than in men.

Granuloma annulare (see p. 1687). The evidence that granuloma annulare is associated with diabetes mellitus is inconclusive [1]. It is rarely seen in diabetics [6].

Idiopathic bullae [2, 6, 10]. Various forms of diabetic bullae have been described. They occur as spontaneous atraumatic lesions mostly on feet and hands. A typical blister arises on a non-inflamed base and heals without scarring in 2–5 weeks. Histological examination shows intra-epidermal separation and lack of acantholysis.

Pruritus. Pruritus was once considered a typical symptom of diabetes mellitus. The frequency of generalized pruritus in diabetics is unknown. Anogenital pruritus is often caused by candidiasis.

Stiff joints and waxy skin. Waxy tight skin on the back of the hands and joint limitation may be seen in insulin-dependent diabetics [11].

Scleroedema of diabetes mellitus. Scleroedema following bacterial infection of the skin, often due to streptococci, tends to resolve slowly over several months. Whether the postinfectious scleroedema and diabetic scleroedema are identical diseases with a more severe course in diabetes due to altered host response is still a matter of debate [7].

Vitiligo (see p. 1591). Vitiligo occurs more frequently in diabetics. In late-onset diabetes a 4·5% frequency has been reported [4].

Lichen planus (see p. 1665). An increased incidence of abnormal glucose tolerance tests in lichen planus patients has been found in a Danish study [5]. Other studies have failed to link the two diseases.

Haemochromatosis (see p. 2334). The main symptoms are liver disease, hyperpigmentation, joint disease, hypogonadism and eventually diabetes.

Eruptive xanthomas of the skin (see p. 1288). Eruptive xanthomas of the skin may develop in diabetics with hyperlipidaemia. The lesions slowly resolve when the diabetes is properly managed.

Reactive perforating collagenosis (folliculitis). There have been some reports of perforating collagenosis or folliculitis in patients with diabetes and/or renal insufficiency. The cause is attributed to diabetic microangiopathy and mechanical injury due to scratching [3].

REFERENCES

1 ANDERSEN B.L. & VERDICH J. (1979) *Clin Exp Dermatol* **4**, 31.
2 CANTWELL A.R. & MARTZ W. (1967) *Arch Dermatol* **96**, 42.
3 COCHRAN R.J., *et al* (1983) *Cutis* **31**, 55.
4 DAWBER R.P.R. (1971) *Br J Dermatol* **84**, 600.
5 HALEVY S. & FEUERMAN E.J. (1979) *Acta Derm Venerol (Stockh)* **59**, 167.
6 *HUNTLEY A.C. (1982) *J Am Acad Dermatol* **7**, 427.
7 KRAKOWSKI A., *et al* (1973) *Dermatologica* **146**, 193.
8 MULLER S.A. (1966) *Mayo Clin Proc* **41**, 689.
9 MULLER S.A. & WINKELMANN P.K. (1966) *Arch Dermatol* **93**, 272.
10 ROCCA F. & PEREYA E. (1963) *Diabetes* **12**, 220.
11 ROSENBLOOM A.L., *et al* (1981) *N Engl J Med* **305**, 191.
12 SMITH J.G. (1956) *Arch Dermatol* **74**, 280.

CHAPTER 63

The Skin in Systemic Disease

S. O. B. ROBERTS & K. WEISMANN

The systemic associations of skin diseases have been stressed throughout this book. In this chapter many of these associations are listed again, along with some other important conditions. They are grouped so as to be helpful to the general physician or internist. It is hoped that such a presentation will also be useful to the dermatologist who is asked to help in the diagnosis of obscure internal disease. Many further references may be found by turning to the chapter in which the relevant dermatosis is considered in detail. The texts listed below provide much more information than it is possible to give here, and are also a source of additional references.

REFERENCES

1 BRAVERMAN I. M. (1981) *Skin Signs of Systemic Disease.* *2nd ed* Philadelphia, Saunders.
2 JONES J. H. & MASON D. K. (Eds.) (1980) *Oral Manifestations of Systemic Disease.* London, Saunders.
3 SHUSTER S. & MARKS J. (1970) *Systemic Effects of Skin Disease.* London, Heinemann.

ENDOCRINE DISORDERS

Endocrine influences on the skin have been mentioned in many chapters of this book. The effects on pigmentation, hair growth, sebaceous glands and connective tissue have been described in some detail and the cutaneous changes of puberty, pregnancy and the menopause have been related to the underlying endocrine phenomena. Certain specific syndromes of endocrine origin have also been described.

Here we shall consider the cutaneous manifestations of endocrine disorders not covered in other chapters.

Parathyroids. See p. 2332

Diabetes. See p. 2339

PITUITARY SYNDROMES

Acromegaly and gigantism [1, 4]. Excessive secretion of growth hormone (somatotrophin) causes hypertrophy of skin and subcutaneous tissues and periosteal bone growth. This leads to acromegaly in the adult who has stopped growing and, rarely, to gigantism in children who are still capable of linear growth.

Aetiology. The usual cause is a benign adenoma or hyperplasia of the acidophilic cells of the adenohypophysis. The growth hormone effect is very complex. One of its main effects is the ability to increase collagen and mucopolysaccharides in the skin and skeleton. This gives rise to hypertrophy of skin and subcutaneous tissues and bone growth of acral parts of the body. The skin is thickened and furrowed, in extreme cases producing cutis gyrata of the scalp (see p. 2033). Individual viable epidermal cells are larger than normal and epidermal cell turnover is increased [3].

Clinical features. The facial expression of the patient is characteristic. There is prognathism, frontal bossing, widely spaced teeth, a protruding thickened lower lip, oedematous thick eyelids, a large and furrowed tongue, triangular large ears, numerous skin tags, widened skin pores, and wet and oily skin due to hyperhidrosis and increased sebum production. Acne may develop. The elongated fingers are blunt and thickened. In about half the patients skin pigmentation is accentuated, a phenomenon which is believed to be secondary to the effect of melanocyte-stimulating hormone (MSH) or to other unknown hormonal effects. The scalp hair usually turns coarse but in late stages it is often fine, silky and sparse. There is loss of body hair due to a decrease in gonadotrophin production. The nails are flat and wide and grow fast. Additional changes include hirsutism in females, hypothyroidism and diabetes which are present in 10% and eventually develop in 30% of patients. Hypogonadism (amenorrhoea and impotence) is frequent. Visual disturbances and a burning headache are common early complaints. Acanthosis nigricans may occur; it usually regresses following therapy of the pituitary tumour [2]. Pachydermoperiostosis (see p. 157) is an important differential diagnosis. In this disease there is no macroglossia or prognathism and the fingers are characteristically clubbed.

Treatment. Bromocriptine inhibits the pituitary secretion of prolactin and growth hormone [5]. It may be used alone or in conjunction with radiation therapy. The response to radiation alone is slow. Occasionally spontaneous remission may be seen and in some patients the disease burns out despite a continuous elevation of growth hormone levels.

REFERENCES

1 *BRAVERMAN I. M. (1981) *Skin Signs of Systemic Disease.* 2nd ed. Philadelphia, Saunders.
2 BROWN J., *et al* (1966) *JAMA* **198**, 619.
3 HOLT P. J. A. & MARKS R. (1976) *Br Med J* i, 496.
4 *LANG P. G. (1981) In *Cutaneous Aspects of Internal Disease.* Ed. Callen J. P. London, Year Book Medical Publishers, p. 463.
5 WASS J. A., *et al* (1977) *Br Med J* i, 875.

Hypopituitarism (Sheehan's syndrome) [1, 3]. In hypopituitarism all endocrine cell functions of the pituitary gland are involved to a various degree.

Aetiology. Insufficiency of the adenohypophysis is mostly due to a chromophobe adenoma, craniopharyngioma, infection (syphilis, tuberculosis), sarcoidosis or histiocytosis X. During pregnancy oestrogens cause hypertrophy of the pituitary gland. Delivery complicated by excessive bleeding and hypotension may result in pituitary ischaemia and infarction [4]. Severe hypertension may cause deleterious haemorrhage into the gland with subsequent hypofunction.

Clinical features. The various endocrine dysfunctions are typically insidious and less impressive than those seen in the primary glandular disorders.

Pallor of the skin often with a yellow tinge is due to carotenaemia and decreased MSH production [3]. In contrast with anaemia the mucous membranes retain their normal colour. The decreased MSH secretion results in generalized hypopigmentation, most prominently seen in sexual areas. There is an increased sensitivity to sunlight. Loss of terminal hair is observed in all patients, first in the axillae and later, but not invariably, in the pubic area. Decreased gonadotrophin secretion occurs. Fine

wrinkling of the skin simulates advanced age. The face appears expressionless due to diminution of the facial skin folds. The activity of sebaceous and sweat glands is compromised. Onycholysis, longitudinal ridging and brownish discoloration of the nail plate may be seen [2].

Pituitary dwarfism. Pituitary dwarfism is characterized by proportionate retardation of somatic growth in conjunction with normal mental development. The cutaneous changes of old age may develop from the third decade (for differential diagnosis see p. 279).

REFERENCES

1 *DAUGMADAY W. H. (1974) In *Textbook of Endocrinology.* Ed. William R. H. Philadelphia, Saunders, p. 55.
2 DENICHOLA P., *et al* (1974) *Nail Diseases in Internal Medicine.* Springfield, Charles C. Thomas, p. 69.
3 *LANG P. G. (1981) In *Cutaneous Aspects of Internal Disease.* Ed. Callen J. P London, Year Book Medical Publishers, p. 467.
4 MURDOCH R. (1962) *Lancet* i, 1327.

SUPRARENAL SYNDROMES

Hypercorticism (Cushing's syndrome) [1, 4]. Hypercorticism is a systemic metabolic dysfunction caused by an excess production or supply of glucocorticoid hormones or hormonal substances.

Aetiology. Increased endogenous glucocorticoid synthesis is usually caused by suprarenal hyperplasia secondary to pituitary overproduction of ACTH. Up to 80% of patients have pituitary microadenomas, mostly chromophobe [4]. Basophil adenoma as described in Cushing's original report is less frequent [3]. Exogenous or iatrogenic hypercorticism is seen during therapeutic administration of glucocorticoids and nowadays has become the most familiar cause. The hormones, among other effects, impair synthesis of collagen and mucopolysaccharides which leads to atrophy and vascular fragility of the skin.

Clinical features. The cutaneous manifestations are quite similar whether caused by endogenous or iatrogenic hypercorticism. The exception is the effects mediated by androgens in the genuine suprarenal form. The appearance of the patient is characterized by deposits of fat over the clavicles and back of the neck (buffalo hump) and the puffy telangiectatic cheeks (moon face, tomato face). The obese trunk contrasts with the slender wasting limbs. Purplish striae develop over the skin, which becomes fragile. Skin lesions heal poorly. Telangiectasia and osteoporosis and compression fractures of the vertebrae add to the altered physiognomy of the patient. Hirsuitism is seen in the majority of patients. In genuine Cushing's syndrome acne and hirsutism may be pronounced owing to additional overproduction of suprarenal androgens. Associated features in women are clitoral hypertrophy and male-pattern baldness. In iatrogenic hypercorticism, hypertrichosis is limited and usually confined to the cheeks in the form of lanugo hair. Acneform eruptions are common. In contrast with acne vulgaris the lesions are uniform, and comedones and cysts are absent.

About 6–10% of patients with the genuine form have Addisonian-like pigmentation [1] due to associated overproduction of MSH.

Treatment. Radiation therapy of the pituitary gland will cure most children and about 20% of adult patients. Cyproheptadine in high doses (24 mg daily) and bromocriptine inhibit pituitary ACTH release and seem to work in 50% of patients [2]. Bilateral adrenalectomy if performed requires lifelong replacement therapy with glucocorticoids and mineralocorticoids. A substantial number of such patients eventually develop a pituitary tumour and cutaneous hyperpigmentation (Nelson's syndrome), but pretreatment with metyrapone or aminoglutethimide seems to prevent this. Medical adrenalectomy using *o-p*-dichlorophenyl-dichlorethane destroys cortisol-producing adrenal cells but frequently causes gastrointestinal side effects.

REFERENCES

1 *Braverman I. M. (1970) *Skin Signs of Systemic Disease.* Philadelphia, Saunders, p. 366.
2 Doyle D. & O'Donovan D. K. (1977) *N Engl J Med* **296**, 576.
3 Editorial (1977) *Br Med J* i, 1049.
4 *Lang P. G. (1981) In *Cutaneous Aspects of Internal Disease.* Ed. Callen J. P. London, Year Book Medical Publishers, p. 451.

Suprarenal insufficiency (Addison's disease, hypocorticism) [4].

Hypocorticism refers to a metabolic state caused by insufficient secretion or supply of adrenocortical hormones or hormonal compounds, mainly cortisol and mineralocorticoids.

Aetiology. Addison's disease may be due to insufficiency of the suprarenal glands (primary insufficiency) or to hypopituitarism. In primary insufficiency, infections (tuberculosis, histoplasmosis and viral infections), autoimmunity or metastatic malig-nant diseases may be causative. Acute suprarenal insufficiency may develop following abrupt discontinuation of prolonged corticosteroid therapy which suppresses ACTH production. In secondary cases the condition is usually one aspect of the pituitary pan-insufficiency. In idiopathic hypocorticism 98% of patients show circulating antibody to the cortex cells and 40% have other autoimmune related disorders [5].

Clinical features [1, 3]. General symptoms include wasting, fatigue, hypotension, dizziness, anorexia, abdominal pain and amenorrhoea. Uniform hyperpigmentation of the skin is the cardinal symptom. It is most pronounced on light-exposed areas, around scars and on the genitalia and mucous membranes and is often seen under the nails. It is due to pituitary MSH and ACTH excess, and gives a clue to differentiating between suprarenal insufficiency and hypopituitarism. Lesions on mucous membranes often occur as spots or patches. Pigmentation of palmar and finger creases is characteristic, but it should be remembered that this may be normal. Moles and hair become darker [1]. Females lose axillary and pubic hair, and acne improves due to a decrease in suprarenal androgen secretion.

Treatment. Primary suprarenal failure requires glucocorticoid and mineralocorticoid replacement. In secondary cases related to pituitary insufficiency usually only cortisol is required [1].

During stress, such as when undergoing major surgery and in severe systemic infections, the need for cortisol is increased. The hyperpigmentation regresses only slowly during continued replacement therapy. The prognosis of Addison's disease is good, unless it is a part of the mucocutaneous candidiasis–endocrinopathy syndrome [2].

REFERENCES

1 *Braverman I. M. (1970) *Skin Signs of Systemic Disease.* Philadelphia, Saunders, p. 366.
2 Kirkpatrick C. H., *et al* (1971) *Ann Intern Med* **74**, 955.
3 *Lang P. G. (1981) In *Cutaneous Aspects of Internal Disease.* Ed. Callen J. P. London, Year Book Medical Publishers, p. 457.
4 *Nerup J. (1974) *Dan Med Bull* **21**, 201.
5 Nerup J., *et al* (1969) *Clin Exp Immunol* **4**, 355.

THYROID DISEASES

Hyperthyroidism. This is a hypermetabolic state which results from excessive production of thyroid hormones (thyroxine (T_4) and triiodothyronine (T_3)). It may result from diffuse toxic goitre, ectopic thyroid tissue or excess intake of thyroid hormones. Only rarely is there increased production of thyroid-stimulating hormone (TSH) or thyrotropin-releasing hormone (TRH) (secondary hyperthyroidism).

Aetiology. There is increasing evidence that Graves' disease is an autoimmune disorder [1]. There is a high incidence of antithyroid antibodies, circulating long-acting thyroid stimulator (LATS, a 7-S-immunoglobulin), lack of allergic responses to dinitrochlorbenzene (DNCB) [2] and concurrence of other autoimmune diseases [3].

Clinical features. The classical triad of Graves' disease is diffusely enlarged toxic goitre, exophthalmos and dermopathy. Various other cutaneous symptoms may be seen (Table 63.1). Pretibial myxoedema (see

TABLE 63.1.   Cutaneous symptoms in hyperthyroidism [5]

Thickening of epidermis [3]
Soft, velvety and dry skin
Increased skin temperature and perfusion due to increased
     sympathetic activity
Palmar erythema
Flushing of the face
Increased sweating (especially palms and soles)
Fast nail growth; distal onycholysis (Plummer's nail) [6,7]
Diffuse Addisonian hyperpigmentation (spares the buccal
     mucosa)
Diffuse thinning of scalp hair
Pruritus and urticaria (uncommon) [4]
Pretibial myxoedema
Acropachy

below) which is present in 1–10% may precede, occur concomitantly with or follow the thyroid disease and its therapy. Almost all patients with pretibial myxoedema show ophthalmopathy, whereas ophthalmopathy is frequently present alone [5]. Acropachy is seen in less than 1% of patients.

Treatment. Beta-blockers (*e.g.* propranolol) may be used in the initial phase of therapy with the purpose of suppressing the increased sympathetic activity. The hyperthyroid state can be reversed by surgery, radioactive iodine or therapy with antithyroid drugs such as propylthiouracil and carbimazole. All symptoms caused by the excessive thyroid hormone production will remit whereas changes unrelated to the hormone production tend to persist. Ophthal-

mopathy is not influenced by return to euthyroidism and the prognosis in severe cases is doubtful.

REFERENCES

1 BRODY J.L. & GREENBERG S. (1973) *J Clin Endocrinol Metab* **36**, 358.
2 *FREITAS J. E. (1981) *Int J Dermatol* **20**, 207.
3 HOLT P.J.A. & MARKS R. (1977) *J Invest Dermatol* **68**, 299.
4 ISAACS N.J. & ERTEL N.M. (1971) *J Allergy Clin Immunol* **48**, 73.
5 *LANG P.G. (1981) In *Cutaneous Aspects of Internal Disease.* Ed. Callen J.P. London, Year Book Medical Publishers, p. 437.
6 PARDO-CASTELLO V. & PARDO O.A. (1960) *Diseases of the Nails.* Springfield, Charles C. Thomas, p. 106.
7 SAMMAN P.D. (1972) *The Nails in Disease.* London, Heinemann, p. 215.

PRETIBIAL MYXOEDEMA
SYN. LOCALIZED MYXOEDEMA

Localized oedematous and thickened pretibial plaques are seen in patients with hyperthyroidism, although sometimes the lesions are not clinically evident until anti-thyroid treatment has been initiated.

Aetiology. A thyroid-stimulating hormone from the pituitary is implicated and is suggested as being responsible for the deposition of mucin. Most patients with pretibial myxoedema whether thyrotoxic or not have elevated levels of long acting thyroid stimulator (L.A.T.S.) in their serum, but this does not seem to be causally involved [4, 5]. There is however a factor in the serum of pretibial myxoedema patients which in tissue culture causes a 2 to 3 fold increase in hyaluronic acid production by fibroblasts from the pretibial area of patients and normal subjects, but which has no effect on those from the shoulder or prepuce [2]

Histopathology [1]. There is oedema of the corium with mucinous infiltration and separation of the collagen fibres. Extensive deposits are found, particularly in the lower dermis, and the dermis is greatly thickened on account of oedema and mucin infiltration.

Clinical features. In many instances the lesions first appear on the anterolateral aspect of the lower limbs and only later extend to the back of the legs and feet. The nodules are pink or skin-coloured,

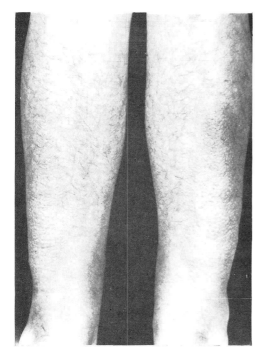

FIG. 63.1 Pretibial myxoedema. Diffuse plaques of non-pitting oedema with prominent follicles (St John's Hospital).

sometimes yellow and waxy, with prominent hair follicles giving a 'peau d'orange' appearance. Localized hypertrichosis over the lesions is often noted.

Three clinical types are recognized:

1. Sharply circumscribed—in which both nodular and tuberous lesions appear on the shins and toes.
2. Diffuse—producing solid non-pitting oedema of the shins and feet.
3. Elephantiasic—in which there are both oedema and nodule formation.

The legs and lower abdomen may be affected [6] and lesions are reported on the arms [3].

Treatment. Corticosteroids applied under occlusive plastic dressings to enhance penetration are useful in the control of pretibial lesions.

REFERENCES

1 ASBOE-HANSEN G. (1965) *Hautarzt*, **16**, 246.
2 CHEUNG H.S., *et al* 1978. *J Invest Dermatol* **71**, 12.
3 COHEN B.D., *et al* (1963) *Arch intern Med* **111**, 641
4 LYNCH P.J., *et al* (1973) *Arch Derm* **107**, 107

5 SCHERMER D.R., *et al* (1970) *Arch Derm.* **102**, 62
6 SUNSERI J. (1943) *Arch Derm Syph* **48**, 70.

Thyroid acropachy [1, 2] Clubbing of the fingers and toes—periosteal new bone formation involving the phalanges and other distal long bones—is frequently associated with past or present hyperthyroidism, exophthalmos and pretibial myxoedema. Acropachy usually appears some time after the other components of the syndrome.

Soft-tissue thickening is an important diagnostic feature. Stiffness is a frequent complaint, and pain and heat, characteristic of hypertrophic pulmonary osteoarthropathy, are absent. Pachydermoperiostosis (p. 157) shows some resemblance to acropachy but other features of the syndrome are absent.

REFERENCES

1 FREEMAN A.G. (1985) *Lancet*, **ii**, 57
2 GIMLETTE T.M.D. (1960) *Lancet*, **i**, 22.

Hypothyroidism (myxoedema) [4]. In hypothyroidism there is a slowed metabolic rate involving all organs. This is caused by a decreased concentration of free thyroid hormone in the blood or blockage of the peripheral hormone effect.

Aetiology. The most common cause is idiopathic hypothyroidism (primary hypothyroidism) in adults, probably triggered off by autoimmune disease. The thyroid gland is atrophic and fibrotic. Congenital hypothyroidism (cretinism), usually due to absence of the thyroid, is rare. Other rare causes include pituitary failure (Sheehan's syndrome) (see p. 2344) and pituitary tumour, a disturbed hormone synthesis (goitrous hypothyroidism) and lack of TSH or TRH production. A high percentage of Hashimoto's thyroiditis patients eventually develop hypothyroidism [3].

Clinical features. There is a close connection between hyperthyroidism, Hashimoto's thyroiditis and idiopathic hypothyroidism. Exophthalmos, pretibial myxoedema and acropachy and associated disorders such as vitiligo may therefore be observed in all conditions. The most prominent manifestation of hypothyroidism is related to dermal accumulation of mucopolysaccharides, in particular chondroitin sulphate and hyaluronic acid, which bind excessive water in the tissue and lead to puffiness of the skin

[6]. The TSH is involved in the pathogenesis of such lesions in primary hypothyroidism [1] but not in cases secondary to pituitary failure.

In the cretinous infant coarseness of features, lethargy, macroglossia, cold dry skin with livedo, umbilical hernia and poor muscle tone are pathognomic. Without treatment physical and mental development is retarded. The scalp hair is coarse, eyebrows tend to confluence, and pubic and axillary commonly fail to develop at puberty.

In juvenile hypothyroidism abnormal physical and mental development is the principal manifestation of the disease. Some children develop hypertrichosis of the upper back and shoulders [8]. In the rare syndrome in which juvenile hypothyroidism is associated with sexual precocity [9], the penis and scrotum enlarge or menstruation and galactorrhoea begin, but axillary and pubic hair does not develop.

In the adult hypothyroid patient, typically a woman of 30–70, the expression of the syndrome is very variable. Cutaneous changes are early and conspicuous features (Table 63.2).

TABLE 63.2.   Cutaneous symptoms of hypothyroidism [4]

Pale, cold, scaly and wrinkled skin [6]
Absence of sweating
Ivory–yellow skin colour
Puffy oedema of hands, face and eyelids
Eczema craquelé [9]
Coarse sparse scalp hair; loss of pubic, axillary and facial
   hair; loss of lateral eyebrows
Brittle and striated nails [7]
Purpura and ecchymoses
Punctate telangiectases on arms and fingertips [2]
Poor wound healing

Diagnosis. Protein-bound iodine, T_4 and T_3 levels are low. In primary hypothyroidism the TSH level is elevated; in pituitary failure it is low or undetectable. The histological changes in the dermis may provide evidence in difficult cases [5]. Recognition of hypothyroidism in the elderly may be difficult. Chronic renal failure with anaemia and Down's syndrome are important differential diagnoses.

Treatment. Therapy is given in the form of L-thyroxin. In patients over 45 yr initially 0·05 mg L-thyroxin is given daily for 1 month, and thereafter 0·1 mg daily for another month. The maintenance dose is usually 0·15 mg daily. When hypothyroidism is caused by pituitary insufficiency additional replacement of other hormones is needed.

REFERENCES

1 ASBOE-HANSEN G. (1960) *Arch Dermatol* **82**, 32.
2 CROTTY C. P. & DICKEN C. H. (1981) *Arch Dermatol* **117**, 158.
3 FREITAS J. E. (1981) *Int J Dermatol* **20**, 207.
4 *LANG P. G. (1981) In *Cutaneous Aspects of Internal Disease* Ed. Callen J.P. London, Year Book Medical Publishers, p. 444.
5 MEANS M. A. & DOBSON R. L. (1963) *JAMA* **186**, 113.
6 MOORE T. J., et al (1976) *Ann Intern Med* **85**, 731.
7 PARDO-CASTELLO V. & PARDO O. A. (1960) *Diseases of the Nails.* Springfield, Charles C. Thomas, p. 215.
8 PERLOFF W. H. (1955) *JAMA* **157**, 651.
9 WARIN R. P. (1973) *Br J Dermatol* **89**, 289.

CUTANEOUS MARKERS OF INTERNAL MALIGNANCY [1,8,31,56]

There are many well-known examples of skin changes associated with internal malignancy apart from cutaneous metastases, Paget's disease of the breast and direct tumour invasion. It is convenient to classify these cutaneous markers in three broad groups:

(1) the genetically determined syndromes with a cutaneous component in which there is also an inherent predisposition to internal neoplasia;

(2) the cutaneous markers of exposure to a carcinogen capable of inducing internal malignancy;

(3) a group of varied cutaneous syndromes which appear to represent reactions to the neoplasm itself—paraneoplasia.

The genetic group [31]

Gardner's syndrome (p. 126) [36]. This is characterized by epidermal cysts, osteomas and fibromatous tumours associated with polyposis coli in which carcinomatous change is a frequent and early finding. Familial cases of simple epidermal cysts are, of course, frequent and apparently have no sinister significance.

Peutz–Jeghers syndrome (p. 1156). There is pigmentation of the lips, oral mucous membranes, perioral region, etc., regularly associated with polyposis of the small intestines and, on rare occasions, with neoplastic change [40].

Palmoplantar keratoderma (Howel-Evans syndrome) (p. 1453). In the two families reported, 70% of cases with tylosis developed oesophageal carcinoma [25]. A single case of carcinoma of the oesophagus occurred in an Indian family with tylosis [61] but this and reports suggesting an excess of tylosis in patients with carcinoma of the oesophagus must be interpreted with caution. Generally tylosis of the diffuse type does not imply a genetic susceptibility to cancer but a distinct form of palmar hyperkeratosis may occur as a reaction to a neoplasm (see below).

Basal cell naevus syndrome (Gorlin's syndrome) (p. 2416). In this disorder medulloblastoma is probably more prevalent than expected and multiple meningiomas have been reported [48].

Werner's syndrome (p. 1816). Sarcomas and other malignancies are frequent in this condition.

Von Hippel–Lindau's syndrome (p. 198). There are associations with hypernephroma and phaeochromocytoma in this condition.

Neurofibromatosis (p. 119). Nephroblastoma, childhood leukaemia, optic nerve gliomas and sarcomatous changes in deep neurofibromas are all important malignant associations while acoustic neuromas are also more common [41, 49].

Mucosal neuromas, medullary thyroid carcinoma and phaeochromocytoma (multiple endocrine neoplasia type 3) [8, 31]. This probably autosomal dominant condition is characterized by the development in early life of multiple mucosal neuromas. They involve the tongue, the lips, which are typically bumpy, and the eyelids, which are thickened. Thus a striking facial appearance is produced and it is associated with a Marfanoid habitus. There is a marked tendency to develop medullary carcinoma as early as the second decade of life, with the production of excess thyrocalcitonin. This in turn may result in parathyroid hyperplasia or adenomas. Phaeochromocytomas also occur in many cases. The corneal nerves may be seen to be hypertrophic and neuromas may involve the gut, leading to gastrointestinal symptoms. Pigmentation and myopathy have been described in this syndrome [14].

There is no doubt that the risk that medullary carcinoma will develop is high in members of such families who show neuromas. Estimation of thyrocalcitonin and screening for thyroid nodules is mandatory and must be repeated at intervals indefinitely. Prophylactic thyroidectomy may be justified. Screening for phaeochromocytoma is also warranted.

Multiple hamartoma syndrome (syn. Cowden disease) [11, 21, 28, 44]. In this rare disorder multiple hamartomatous lesions of ectodermal, endodermal and mesodermal origins are associated with a pre-disposition to malignant tumours of the breast and thyroid. The eponymous family were sufferers from the disease which appears to be of autosomal dominant inheritance. Characteristic cutaneous lesions may develop in childhood but become obvious in adult life. There are lichenoid papules and papillomas distributed on the face around the mouth, nostrils and eyes. Histologically these are revealed as trichilemmomas. The lips may be involved particularly near the angles of the mouth and the ears are often affected. Hyperkeratotic flat-topped papules are found on the dorsal surface of the hands and forearms and translucent punctate keratoses occur on the palms and soles and flexor surfaces of the digits. Equally constant in published cases are numerous papules of the gums and palate giving a cobblestone appearance. Papillomatous lesions of the buccal and faucial regions and of the tongue are also common and are simple fibromas. The genital mucous membrane may be similarly affected in the female. Inconstant superficial features include multiple lipomas and angiomas.

The benign internal anomalies are manifold and variable but goitre and fibrocystic disease of the female breasts are present in most cases and gastrointestinal polyposis, pectus excavatum and adenoid facies are commonly found. Nervous system involvement is particularly varied, with mental retardation, fits, meningiomas of the auditory canals and perhaps neuromas and ganglioneuromas being included.

Frank neoplasia presents frequently as breast carcinoma, sometimes bilateral, and less often as follicular thyroid carcinoma. (Benign thyroid adenomas are also found.) Carcinoma of the caecum has been reported but gut malignancy is less common than might be expected from the presence of multiple polyps.

Sebaceous neoplasia and visceral carcinoma (syn. Torre's syndrome, Torre–Muir syndrome) [31, 32]. The association of multiple sebaceous adenomas (or carcinomas) with visceral neoplasms of early onset usually of the gastrointestinal tract is well established. In several instances multiple primary growths have been reported with surprisingly good survival rates [7]. Unfortunately the cutaneous lesions may be insignificant or may postdate the visceral malignancy. Moreover Lynch and his associates have demonstrated that malignant disease may be equally common among members of these families who have no sebaceous tumours. They therefore prefer to regard this syndrome as a subgroup of the cancer family syndrome characterized simply by a genetically determined (autosomal dominant) predisposition to visceral malignancy. Gut polyposis, malignancies of the duodenal area (ampulla of Vater for example) and multiple keratoacanthomas have also been noted as features in some patients reported as examples of Torre's syndrome [60].

Wiskott–Aldrich syndrome [16] (p. 251). Malignancy usually expressed as lymphoma or leukaemia is extremely common in those few patients who survive to adult life.

Ataxia telangiectasia [16] (p. 1094). There is a high incidence of malignant lesions (14 out of 200 reported cases) in this condition, including reticulum cell sarcoma (five patients), Hodgkin's disease (two patients), lymphosarcoma (two patients) and gastric carcinoma (two patients). Some increased predisposition to malignancy may extend to heterozygous relatives [51].

Chediak–Higashi syndrome [16] (p. 1586). The terminal illness in many of these patients has features strongly suggestive of a lymphoma.

The last three syndromes are all ones in which there is defective immunity. It has been presumed that defective immunosurveillance is responsible for the high incidence of neoplasia, but other mechanisms may also operate.

Exposure to a carcinogen

Arsenical pigmentation (p. 1573), *keratoses* (p. 2429) *or superficial basal cell carcinomas* are associated with an increased tendency to develop internal carcinomas, especially of the bronchus.

Bowen's disease of covered skin (p. 2428). In Bowen's disease of covered skin (i.e. when sunlight can be excluded as a carcinogen) there is a high incidence of internal neoplasia. Between one-third and one-half of the patients will develop an internal malignancy within 5–10 yr of when the skin diagnosis is made.

Nicotine staining of the fingers. This is clear evidence of exposure of the bronchi to a carcinogen.

X-ray damage to the skin of the neck. This should alert the physician to the increased risk of carcinoma of the thyroid.

Multiple basal cell carcinomas over the spine may result from X-ray treatment of ankylosing spondylitis. Such patients show an increased tendency to develop leukaemia.

Vinyl chloride disease. Acrosclerosis-like changes with or without acro-osteolysis and papular skin lesions are inconstant markers of the serious industrial disease of workers involved in polyvinyl chloride manufacture. In some patients with this syndrome angiosarcoma of the liver has been reported [3].

Paraneoplastic dermatoses and other associations

Acanthosis nigricans (p. 1460). When this syndrome develops for the first time in adult life in the absence of obesity, endocrinopathy and ingestion of nicotinic acid [38] and with a negative family history, there is an associated internal neoplasm in virtually all cases [43]. The lesion is usually abdominal (91%) and generally a gastric carcinoma is present (60%). Unfortunately it is rarely curable [33]. Even in childhood, tumour-associated acanthosis nigricans has been reported on several occasions [22]. Generalized pigmentation with hyperkeratosis, both removable by tape stripping, has been reported as a sign of neoplasia in three patients and may be related to acanthosis nigricans [18] as may 'tripe palms' (see below).

Acanthosis palmaris (syn. tripe palms). There have been several recent reports of a distinctive rugose thickening of the palms (sometimes of the soles) associated, apparently causally, with carcinomas of the lung and stomach [10, 27, 55]. Some patients have had coexisting (malignant) acanthosis nigricans [27], but in others this dermatosis has developed independently. Rapid clearance of the palmar thickening after surgical excision of the neoplasm has been described [55]. The condition may also occur, however, in association with exfoliative psoriasis without any neoplasm [10].

Dermatomyositis (p. 1376). When this occurs in adults, the condition is linked with malignancy in perhaps 25% of cases. The neoplasia may be curable so that as soon as the diagnosis is made investigation should be undertaken [54]. Multiple carcinomas have been reported with dermatomyositis [58]. Though childhood dermatomyositis is not normally associated with neoplasm, four cases have been recorded [47].

Digital ischaemia [23]. A report of six cases of atypical Raynaud's syndrome of late onset (bilateral in five cases, progressing to gangrene in four) suggests that this syndrome may be a reliable marker of internal neoplasia. Persistent pain was a marked feature. All these patients had malignancy (of maxillary antrum, kidney, ovary, Hodgkin's disease, double primary—colon and body of uterus—and indeterminate, either ovary or pancreas) and all were dead within 18 months of presenting with ischaemic symptoms. In one of three similar but milder cases reported by Palmer [35] there was lessening of digital pain after removal of a gastric carcinoma, but his other patients with reticulum cell sarcoma and abdominal carcinomatosis had died at the time of writing.

Annular erythemas [53] (p. 1088). Most annular erythemas are not associated with neoplasia. In the erythema gyratum repens or 'woodgrain' type a frequent, but not invariable, association of internal carcinoma does occur however (Fig. 63.2).

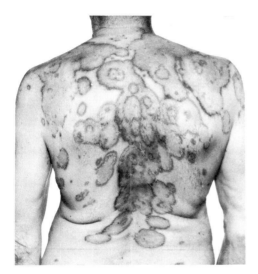

FIG. 63.2 Erythema gyratum repens in a patient with carcinoma of the bronchus (Addenbrooke's Hospital).

The glucagonoma syndrome (syn. necrolytic migratory erythema) (see p. 2359). This distinctive syndrome is almost 100% specific for islet cell carcinoma of the pancreas.

Multicentric reticulohistocytosis (p. 1709). Approximately 25% of patients with the condition appear from the literature to have coexisting neoplasia and in one report four of eight patients had cancer—of breast, cervix and ovary (two) [13]. Whether there is a genetic or paraneoplastic association is unclear.

Paraneoplastic acrokeratosis (syn. Bazex's syndrome) [4, 5, 37]. There are now at least 50 reported cases of this condition, all but one occurring in men [37]. Hyperkeratotic psoriasiform plaques affect the

hands and feet, the digits, the nose and the ears. The facial lesions tend to be less well defined and more eczematous or lupus erythematosus-like. The palms and soles may show diffuse hyperkeratosis and the nails become thickened and friable. Acrokeratosis may suggest Reiter's syndrome. In all reported cases there has been an association with a neoplasm of the pharynx or upper respiratory tract or deposits in nodes of the cervical or submaxillary areas without a proven site of origin. The cutaneous changes may with time spread to involve the limbs more proximally and the trunk. The histological changes are those of a dermatitis with a mixed inflammatory infiltrate and in older lesions marked hyperkeratosis and focal parakeratosis [37]. Immunoglobulin may be demonstrated in the buccal layer.

Acquired ichthyosis. This is an occasional finding during the course of a lymphoma, usually Hodgkin's disease; it is rarely the presenting feature, however. Acquired ichthyosis may occur with other neoplasms [19] and in the malabsorption syndrome. It should not be confused with asteatotic eczema which, of course, is a common feature in elderly patients. Whether pityriasis rotunda should be regarded as a marker of neoplasia is not clear. One report suggests this [29].

Pruritus. Pruritus is a well-recognized symptom of Hodgkin's disease, although only occasionally the presenting one. Alcohol-induced pruritus has also been reported in this condition, though it is much rarer than alcohol-induced pain [9]. Because pruritus is so common in the elderly, it is not unusual to find it in patients with neoplasia, but although a causal relationship has often been claimed it is difficult to find definite proof of this. Severe intractable pruritus or paraesthesiae of the nostrils, a long-recognized symptom, was found in 13 of 77 patients with brain tumours [2].

Bullous eruptions. In general, patients with bullous eruptions are no more likely to have a hidden neoplasm than age-matched controls. Certainly this is so in pemphigoid [17, 50]. Isolated reports of close, apparently causal, associations in pemphigoid [24, 52] and pemphigus of the foliaceous and erythematosus group [34] suggest that there are occasional exceptions to the general rule. Because of this, and because pemphigoid patients, being elderly, must be expected to be cancer prone, some screening investigations should be considered. Reports of dermatitis herpetiformis associated with neoplasia may be significant in view of the suggested increased incidence of neoplasia in patients with coeliac syndrome, but the link here is probably a genetic one. The association between porphyria cutanea tarda and hepatoma is considered elsewhere (p. 2280).

Erythema multiforme and erythema nodosum. Occasional reports of such cases are difficult to evaluate. Some cases of erythema multiforme seem closely linked with radiotherapy, usually for lymphomas. Cases of erythema nodosum may be related to drug therapy rather than the primary condition.

Migratory thrombophlebitis. Although not always associated with neoplasia, many cases do show an underlying neoplasm, carcinoma of the pancreas being the commonest.

Pyoderma gangrenosum. This, with leukaemia, is discussed elsewhere (p. 1148).

Erythroderma (p. 408). Erythroderma may be an expression of mycosis fungoides and Sézary syndrome but if these conditions are excluded there is still a small number of patients with an apparently banal erythroderma in whom an underlying lymphoma or leukaemia will eventually be discovered. The percentage of such cases is not reliably known, but in one large series one in eight patients who had no prior skin disorder eventually turned out to have neoplasia [59].

Leser–Trélat sign [30, 42]. Sudden development of large numbers of seborrhoeic keratoses with associated pruritus is a rare, but apparently reliable, marker of internal malignancy. Multiple seborrhoeic keratoses are such a common feature that this sign should be diagnosed with care. There are many recent reports in which the causal association is far from convincing.

Miscellaneous skin tumours. Eruptive keratoacanthomas have been reported with carcinoma of the fallopian tube and stem cell leukaemia but are not usually sinister [57]. Keratoacanthomas are reported in Torre's syndrome (see above).

Seed keratoses of the palms and soles. These have been both implicated and exonerated as markers of internal malignancy. A very recent report indicates that although they occur on the palms in more than a third (36%) of healthy subjects over 50 yr old, they are significantly more common in patients with carcinoma of the bladder (87%) and bronchus (71%)

[15]. The nature of the association is unknown and their value as a marker is clearly limited.

Multiple eruptive angiomas simulating pyogenic granulomas or Campbell de Morgan spots have been reported as a paraneoplastic phenomenon in four patients with neoplasias as varied as Hodgkin's disease, chronic lymphatic leukaemia, multiple myeloma and probable disseminated melanoma [39].

Flushing. Flushing, later a fixed erythema, suggests a diagnosis of carcinoid usually with extensive metastases which, however, may still be compatible with prolonged survival.

Unilateral lymphoedema. Sudden onset of this symptom over the age of 40 suggests obstruction of the abdominal lymphatics by malignant deposits or a pelvic neoplasm [6].

Clubbing. There are many causes of this sign, of which carcinoma of the bronchus is perhaps the commonest in middle and later life.

Scleroderma-like skin changes. These have been reported without Raynaud's phenomenon in some cases of carcinoid syndrome with metastases [20].

Herpes zoster [45] (p. 680). Herpes zoster occurs more frequently, with greater severity and with a higher incidence of disseminated lesions in patients who have an underlying reticulosis, but the uncomplicated form is common in the elderly and does not demand intensive investigation.

Urticaria. Reports suggesting that urticaria may be linked with neoplasia are difficult to evaluate. When there is also sensitivity to cold and peripheral gangrene the patient may have cryoglobulinaemia, and myelomatosis or lymphoma should be considered.

Acquired hypertrichosis lanuginosa (p. 1959). This excessively rare condition has been reliably linked with carcinoma in most patients [26, 46]. It can also be induced by diazoxide and minoxidil used for treating hypertension. Assuming drugs can be excluded, a search for neoplasm should be undertaken.

Generalized hyperhidrosis (p. 1887). This, too, appears to be a rare, but reliably established, association with a malignant disease.

Conclusions. The response by the physician to the discovery of one of these cutaneous markers of internal neoplasia must depend on the reliability of the marker and on the likely prognosis of the carcinomas he may expect to find. Unfortunately, one of the best markers, acanthosis nigricans, is associated with the poorest prognosis.

Dermatomyositis presents the most important challenge. The number of patients in whom an underlying neoplasm will be found is sufficently high to make a search worthwhile. Moreover in this condition a good history, careful examination and simple investigations such as a chest X-ray, urine analysis and stool examination for occult blood are probably sufficient as a screening procedure [12].

REFERENCES

1 ANDREEV V.C. (1978) *Skin Manifestations of Visceral Cancer*. Basel, Karger.
2 ANDREEV V.C. & PETKOV I. (1975) *Br J Dermatol* 92, 675.
3 Anonymous Leading Article (1974) *Br Med J*, i, 590.
4 BARRIERE H. (1975) *Ann Med Interne (Paris)* 126, 177.
5 BAZEX A. (1979) *Hautarzt* 30, 119.
6 BEAZLEY J.M. & CHANDIOK S. (1976) *Hosp Update* 2, 58.
7 BITRAN J. & PELLETTIERE E.V. (1974) *Cancer* 33, 835.
8 BRAVERMAN I.M. (1981) *Skin Signs of Systemic Disease*. 2nd ed. Philadelphia, Saunders.
9 BRAVIN T.B. (1966) *Br Med J* ii, 437.
10 BREATHNACH S.M. & WELLS G.C. (1980) *Clin Exp Dermatol* 5, 181.
11 BROWNSTEIN M.H., et al (1979) *Br J Dermatol* 100, 667.
12 CALLEN J.P. (1982) *J Am Acad Dermatol* 6, 253.
13 CATTERALL M.D. (1980) *Clin Exp Dermatol* 5, 267.
14 CUNLIFFE W.J., et al (1968) *Lancet* ii, 63.
15 CUZICK J., et al (1984) *Lancet* i, 530.
16 DOLL R. & KINLEN L. (1970) *Br Med J* iv, 420.
17 EBNER H. & SPANGLER E. (1974) *Wien Klin Wochenschr* 16, 449.
18 EWER R.W., et al (1963) *Arch Intern Med* 111, 634.
19 FLINT G.L., et al (1975) *Arch Dermatol* 111, 1446.
20 FRIES J.F., et al (1973) *Arch Intern Med* 131, 550.
21 GENTRY W.C., et al (1975) In *Birth Defects*. Original Article Series, II. New York, National Foundation, p. 137.
22 GRUPPER CH., et al (1974) *Bull Soc Fr. Dermatol Syphiligr* 81, 297.
23 HAWLEY P.R., et al (1967) *Br Med J* iii, 208.
24 HODGE L., et al (1981) *Br J Dermatol* 105, 65.
25 HOWEL-EVANS A.W., et al (1951) *Q J Med* 27, 107.
26 IKEYA T., et al (1978) *Dermatologica* 156, 274.
27 LARREGUE M., et al (1979) *Ann Dermatol Vénéréol (Paris)* 106, 781.
28 LAUGIER P., et al (1979) *Ann Dermatol Vénéréol (Paris)* 106, 453.
29 LEIBOWITZ M.R., et al (1983) *Arch Dermatol* 110, 607.
30 LIDDELL K., et al (1975) *Br J Dermatol* 92, 449.
31 LYNCH H.T. & FUSARD R.M. (Eds.) (1982) *Cancer Associated Genodermatoses*. New York, Van Nostrand Reinhold.
32 LYNCH H.T., et al (1981) *Arch Intern Med* 141, 607.
33 MOLLER H., et al (1978) *Acta Med Scand* 203, 245.
34 NAYSMITH A. & HANCOCK B.W. (1976) *Br J Dermatol* 94, 695.
35 PALMER H.M. (1974) *Br J Dermatol* 91, 476.
36 PALMER T.H. (1982) *Am J Surg* 143, 405.
37 PECORA A.L., et al (1983) *Arch Dermatol* 119, 820.
38 PEDRO S. (1974) *N Engl J Med* 291, 422.
39 PEMBROKE A.C., et al (1978) *Clin Exp Dermatol* 3, 147.
40 PERZIN K.H. & BRIDGE M.F. (1982) *Cancer* 49, 971.
41 RICCARDI V.M. (1981) *N Eng J Med* 305, 1617.
42 RONCHESE F. (1965) *Cancer* 18, 1003.
43 SAFAI B., et al (1979) *Int J Dermatol* 18, 312.
44 SALEM O.S. & STECK W.D. (1983) *J Am Acad Dermatol* 8, 686.
45 SHANBRON E., et al (1960) *Ann Intern Med* 53, 523.
46 SINDHIPHAK W. & VIBHAGOOH A. (1982) *Int J Dermatol* 21, 599.
47 SINGSON B.H., et al (1976) *J Pediatr* 88, 602.
48 SOUTHWICK G.J. & SCHWARTZ R.A. (1979) *Cancer* 44, 2294.
49 STAY E.J. & VAWTER G. (1977) *Cancer* 39, 2550.
50 STONE S.P. & SCHROETER A.L. (1975) *Arch Dermatol* 111, 991.
51 SWIFT M. (1975) *Int J Dermatol* 14, 733.
52 TANAKA T., et al (1983) *Arch Dermatol* 119, 704.
53 VERRET J.L., et al (1979) *Hautarzt* 30, 213.
54 VESTERAGER L., et al (1980) *Clin Exp Dermatol* 5, 31.
55 VOTION V., et al (1982) *Dermatologica* 165, 660.
56 WALDENSTROM J.G. (1978) *Paraneoplasia. Biological Signals in the Diagnosis of Cancer*. New York, Wiley.
57 WEBER G., et al (1970) *Arch Klin Exp Dermatol* 238, 107.
58 WILSON E., et al (1965) *Br Med J* ii, 80.
59 WILSON H.T.H. (1954) *Arch Dermatol Syphil* 69, 577.
60 WORRET W.I., et al (1981) *Hautarzt* 32, 519.
61 YESOUDHAN P., et al (1980) *Br J Dermatol* 102, 597.

THE GASTROINTESTINAL TRACT AND THE SKIN

Skin changes related to under-nutrition, malabsorption and nutritional defects have been discussed in Chapter 62. Here certain gastrointestinal conditions often associated with skin manifestations are mentioned.

Gastrointestinal bleeding [1]. Various cutaneous lesions may be observed in association with bleeding gastrointestinal diseases (Table 63.3).

Regional ileitis (Crohn's disease) [1, 4]. Skin lesions are frequently seen in Crohn's disease [3, 6–8]. Often the cutaneous involvement is an extension of the intestinal disease, presenting as perineal abscesses and fistulas in nearly 20% [8, 9]. Sinus

TABLE 63.3.   Skin lesions associated with gastrointestinal disorders which may present with bleeding

Disease	Gastrointestinal lesion	Skin symptom
Blue rubber-bleb naevus	Haemangiomas	Haemangiomas
Crohn's disease	Inflammatory changes of the intestinal	Acquired epidermolysis bullosa
Ulcerative colitis	wall	Pyoderma gangrenosum
		Necrotizing vasculitis
		Aphthous stomatitis
		Erythema nodosum
		Erythema multiforme
Neurofibromatosis (Von Recklinghausen)	Neurofibromas	Café-au-lait spots
		Atrophic spots
		Neurofibromas
Cronkhite–Canada syndrome	Gastrointestinal polyposis	Diffuse hyperpigmentation, alopecia, nail defects
Gardner's syndrome	Polyposis of colon (cancer)	Lipomas, epidermoid cysts
Peutz-Jeghers syndrome	Polyposis of the small intestine	Hyperpigmentation on lips, circumoral area and fingertips
Cowden disease	Polyposis	Papules, lipomas, angiomas
Osler–Weber–Rendu disease	Telangiectasia	Telangiectasia
Degos' syndrome	Intestinal perforation	White atrophic lesions
Henoch–Schönlein	Vasculitis	Allergic purpura
Pseudoxanthoma elasticum	Involvement of visceral arteries	Yellowish papules and plaques
Ehlers–Danlos syndrome	Fragility of visceral arteries	Hyperelasticity of skin and joints

formation involving the abdominal wall, groins and even submammary folds are nearly as common. In a minority of cases distinctive dermatoses such as erythema multiforme, aphthous stomatitis and cutaneous vasculitis are seen. Erythema nodosum occurs in about 1% of patients, pyoderma gangrenosum less often. Cutaneous vasculitis of the lower legs is perhaps the least common cutaneous manifestation [2, 5]. Nodules of cutaneous vasculitis with livedo and joint pain may be linked with the underlying disease [2, 12]. Epidermolysis bullosa acquisita has been reported repeatedly [10, 11, 13]. The disease clinically resembles other mechano-bullous diseases but is acquired in relation to systemic diseases such as amyloidosis, multiple myeloma, diabetes mellitus and inflammatory bowel disease [10]. Immunological serum factors are present in affected areas, suggesting their involvement in the cutaneous lesion. Anchoring fibrils below the basal lamina are present; thus differentiation from dystrophic epidermolysis bullosa is possible by electron microscopy. Recurrent aphthous stomatitis and glossitis are common. They often follow the course of the bowel disease [1]. Cutaneous Crohn's disease ('metastatic Crohn's disease') with numerous eroded cutaneous granulomas at sites distant from the affected bowel has been reported. There is a granulomatous histology in the dermis and subcutis [6]. A thickened corrugated appearance of the oral

mucosa and lips may be associated with the disease [4].

REFERENCES

1 *Callen J. P. (1981) In *Cutaneous Aspects of Internal Disease*. Ed. Callen J. P. London, Year Book Medical Publishers, p. 511.
2 Chalvardijan A. & Nethercott J. R. (1982) *Cutis* 30, 645.
3 Greenstein A. J., *et al* (1976) *Medicine (Baltimore)* 55, 401.
4 *Johnson W. T. & Narva W. M. (1975) In *The Systemic Manifestations of Inflammatory Bowel Disease*. Eds. Lukasch W. M. & Johnson R. B. Springfield, Thomas, p. 212.
5 Kahn E. L., *et al* (1980) *Dis Colon Rectum* 23, 258.
6 Levine N. & Bangert J. (1982) *Arch Dermatol* 118, 1006.
7 McCallum D. I. & Gray W. M. (1976) *Br J Dermatol* 95, 551.
8 McCallum D. I. & Kinmont P. D. C. (1968) *Br J Dermatol* 80, 1.
9 Mountain J. C. (1970) *Gut* 11, 18.
10 Ray T. L., *et al* (1982) *J Am Acad Dermatol* 6, 242.
11 Roenigh H. H., *et al* (1971) *Arch Dermatol* 103, 1.
12 Solley G. O., *et al* (1975) *Gastroenterology* 69, 235.
13 Tan R. (1977) *Br J Dermatol* 97, 46.

Ulcerative colitis [2, 7]. The cutaneous manifestations of ulcerative colitis and regional enteritis are almost identical, although there are differences in their frequency. In large series of patients skin lesions have been reported in 10% of patients with ulcerative colitis and in 5% of patients with regional ileitis [6]. Non-specific eruptions are seen, including urticaria, angio-oedema, erythema and purpura. Butterfly erythema has been reported mainly in children [8]. Other skin changes may be related to malabsorption. The distinctive cutaneous lesions associated with ulcerative colitis are pyoderma gangrenosum, pyostomatitis vegetans and erythema nodosum.

Pyoderma gangrenosum [5] (see p. 1148). This is characterized by necrotic ulceration surrounded by undermined borders but the morphology is very variable, as are its course and distribution. The pyoderma usually reflects the severity of bowel involvement. Trauma is sometimes a predisposing factor [9]. Papules and pustules are followed by ulcerating and vegetating epithelial proliferation. In some patients there are extensive gangrenous ulcers necessitating total colectomy to control the disease. The lesions may be extremely persistent. Dermatitis herpetiformis-like eruptions may be seen. In pyoderma gangrenosum, gastrointestinal investigation should be carried out as about half of the patients may have or may develop inflammatory bowel disease.

Pyostomatitis vegetans [12]. This is characterized by miliary pustules with epithelial proliferation which form vegetating lesions. The eruption may occur in association with pyoderma gangrenosum or alone.

Nodular vasculitis (see p. 1166). This occurs in up to 10% of patients with ulcerative colitis. There are red indurated nodules mainly on the shin but occasionally elsewhere. An eruption of new elements is accompanied by fever, malaise, joint pain and swelling. The nodules may ulcerate to form persistent pyodermal lesions. Erythema multiforme is rarely associated with ulcerative colitis and regional ileitis [4]. Other causes such as drug reactions should therefore be considered first [3]. The eruption follows the course and severity of bowel inflammation and recurrences are common [2]. Necrotizing leukocytoclastic vasculitis has been reported in both ulcerative colitis and regional enteritis [1, 10, 11].

REFERENCES

1 CALLEN J. P. (1979) *Arch Dermatol* **115**, 226.
2 *CALLEN J. P. (1981) In *Cutaneous Aspects of Internal Disease*. Ed. Callen J. P. London, Year Book Medical Publishers, p. 511.
3 CAMERON A. J., *et al* (1966) *Br Med J* ii, 1174.
4 CHAPMAN R. S., *et al* (1977) *Dermatologica* **154**, 32.
5 GREENBERG S. J., *et al* (1982) *Arch Dermatol* **118**, 498.
6 GREENSTEIN A. J., *et al* (1976) *Medicine (Baltimore)* **55**, 401.
7 *JOHNSON W. T. & NARVA W. N. (1973) In *The Systemic Manifestations of Inflammatory Bowel Disease*. Eds. Lukasch W. B. & Johnson R. B. Springfield, Thomas, p. 212.
8 LAGERCRANTZ R. (1958) *Acta Paediatr Scand* **47**, 675.
9 RUSSELL B. (1950) *Br J Dermatol* **62**, 114.
10 SAMITZ M. H. (1966) *Cutis* **2**, 383.
11 WACKERS F. J., *et al* (1974) *Br Med J* iv, 83.
12 ZEGARELLI E. V. & KUTSCHER A. H. (1962) *Am J Dig Dis* **7**, 281.

Cronkhite–Canada syndrome. The syndrome, which was described in 1955 by Cronkhite and Canada [2], is characterized by concurrent pigmentation, alopecia, nail defects and polyposis of the gastrointestinal tract [3]. The disease is rare and only sporadic cases have been reported. The intestinal lesions occur extensively from oesophagus to anus. The cause remains unknown. Inheritance has been implicated but has never been documented. Possibly the condition is acquired. Most of the approximately 50 patients reported so far were middle aged or elderly, with a male to female incidence ratio of 3:2 [1].

Clinical features. Wasting and chronic diarrhoea are the usual presenting features. There is protein deficiency with hypoalbuminaemia due to protein-losing enteropathy associated with the intestinal polyposis. Hypokalaemia and hypocalcaemia may be present due to persistent diarrhoea and malabsorption. Histological examination of the bowel has revealed enterocolitis with inflammatory pseudopolyposis [1]. Pigmentation of the skin is due to hypermelanosis. It is diffuse with accentuation over the face, neck and extremities. Palms and volar aspects of the fingers are also involved. The scalp hair becomes thin and sparse, initially resembling alopecia areata; later total loss of hair occurs. All fingernails and toenails are dystrophic showing a peculiar triangular residual nail plate. Initially, shedding of the nails may take place. Many of the symptoms and metabolic disturbances may be due to deficiencies associated with altered digestive, motility and secretory functions of the bowel [1]. The course is usually slowly progressive, the outcome dubious. No adequate therapy is at hand [1, 4]. Improvement after hemicolectomy, gastrectomy and a course of ampicillin [3] has been noted.

REFERENCES

1 CHAN H. L., *et al* (1979) *Arch Dermatol* 115, 98.
2 CRONKHITE L. W. & CANADA W. J. (1955) *N Engl J Med* 252, 1011.
3 CUNLIFFE W. J. & ANDERSON J. (1967) *Br Med J* iv, 601.
4 JOHNSON G. K., *et al* (1972) *Gastroenterology* 63, 140.

Dermatogenic malabsorption [1, 2]. Malabsorption may occur in patients suffering from extensive skin diseases. It is to be regarded as a gut complication of erythroderma whether it is due to psoriasis, eczema or pityriasis rubra pilaris, but it can occur with less extensive rashes. Stool examination reveals steatorrhoea of a mild to moderate degree. Though the severity is correlated with the extension of the skin lesions it is unrelated to the total duration of the dermatosis or to the length of the immediate attack. There is regularly malabsorption of folic acid and usually of D-xylose and iron. The fate of zinc has not been investigated. Vitamin B_{12} and calcium absorption may be compromised. Jejunal biopsy is normal and the malabsorption does not respond to a gluten-free diet.

The gut function is restored within a few weeks after the dermatosis has healed. Relapses with recurrent episodes of erythroderma are likely. The mechanism of the enteropathy is unknown. Any patient who has an extensive skin disorder or erythroderma may be expected to suffer from dermatogenic steatorrhoea. Only if the malabsorption fails to clear with successful treatment of the cutaneous disease should further investigation, including jejunal biopsy, be undertaken.

REFERENCES

1 SHUSTER S. & MARKS J. (1965) *Lancet* i, 1367.
2 SHUSTER S. & MARKS J. (1970) *Systemic Effects of Skin Disease*. London, Heinemann.

The bowel bypass syndrome (intestinal bypass arthritis–dermatitis syndrome) [2, 5, 8]. Intestinal bypass surgery for morbid obesity has been used for nearly 25 yr. Since 1971 mainly the end-to-end jejunoileal bypass has been performed [6]. The advisability of such a procedure is still controversial. A variety of serious complications have been reported, such as persistent diarrhoea with water and electrolyte imbalance, hepatic failure, renal stones, gallstones, polyarthritis, zinc deficiency, vitamin A deficiency, dermatitis, bypass enteropathy and emotional disturbances [1, 3, 5]. The bowel bypass syndrome occurs in about 7% of patients [5]. It is characterized by constitutional symptoms such as fever, tenosynovitis and myalgia associated with a non-destructive polyarthritis and recurrent pustular or vasculitis-like lesions on the skin.

Aetiology. The cause seems to be related to bacterial overgrowth in the bypassed bowel segment. Bacterial antigens in the form of peptidoglycans are probably released from the intestinal flora, particularly *Escherichia coli* [2]. Circulating immune complexes can be demonstrated in most patients actively developing skin lesions [5, 7].

Histopathology [5]. Macular, vesicular and pustular lesions show dilated dermal venules and capillaries and perivascular neutrophil granulocytes. In vesicopustular lesions there is a more pronounced accumulation of polymorphs and more extensive dermal oedema leading to dermo-epidermal separation. Epidermal necrosis may be found. The pustular lesions are sterile.

Clinical features. The syndrome has been reported to occur between 1 and 63 months after operation [2]. The characteristic manifestation consists of crops of erythematous papules or vesicopustules. The lesions range in appearance from indurated papules resembling insect bites to necrotic lesions similar to those of gonoccaemia [4, 7]. Erythema nodosum and panniculitis-like lesions may be found [1]. Leukocytoclastic vasculitis is not the rule but has been reported on the lower extremities [7]. The joint involvement is variable and similar to the type of arthritis recognized in regional ileitis and ulcerative colitis. The bypass enteropathy may manifest itself as acute massive abdominal distention resembling intestinal obstruction, but milder and chronic forms have been described.

Treatment. In about half of the patients the illness abates spontaneously [5]. Some patients respond to oral tetracyclines 1–2 g daily. Non-steroidal anti-inflammatory agents can be added for relief of arthritis. Dapsone may be useful in some cases with recurrent episodes [7]. In recalcitrant cases, reconstitution of the bowel may be necessary.

REFERENCES

1 DICKEN C. H. & SEEHAFER J. R. (1979) *Arch Dermatol* 115, 837.
2 *ELY P. H. (1980) *J Am Acad Dermatol* 2, 473.
3 FALDON W. W. (1977) *Hosp Pract* 12, 73.
4 GOLDMAN J. A., *et al* (1979) *Arch Dermatol* 115, 725.
5 *KENNEDY C. (1981) *Br J Dermatol* 105, 425.
6 SCOTT H. W., *et al* (1971) *Ann Surg* 174, 560.
7 *SIMON S., *et al* (1981) *Cutis* 28, 545.
8 STEIN H. B., *et al* (1981) *Arthritis Rheum* 24, 684.

LIVER DISEASE

Hepatobiliary diseases are frequently associated with abnormalities of the skin, nails and hair. Various forms of cirrhosis share similar clinical features, except for biliary cirrhosis. As a general rule, the cutaneous findings are non-specific as they may be present in other diseases and absent in patients even with advanced liver dysfunction. There is no clear correlation between the degree of the skin changes and the severity of liver dysfunction. Importance should be given to the overall picture of the patient rather than to the presence of particular cutaneous symptoms.

Pruritus. Pruritus is the most common skin symptom associated with liver disease. It may precede the onset of jaundice. Often the trunk and extremities are affected, rarely the genitals. Itch may be transient or prolonged, mild or severe. As the disease progresses and liver insufficiency develops the itch may clear. With obstructive liver disease the itch is believed to be due to the presence of bile salts in the skin [3, 5] but other liver products may be involved. In hepatitis B infection [2] itch is often associated with urticaria, maculopapular exanthema and arthralgia. In syphilis cholestatic jaundice may be the cause [4]. There is no indication that release of histamine plays an important role in the pathogenesis of hepatobiliary itch [3]. Accordingly, the therapeutic response to antihistamines is limited. Oral cholestyramine 8–12 g daily and a diet rich in polyunsaturated fatty acids may provide significant relief [1].

REFERENCES

1 ANHALT G. J. & DUBIN H. V. (1981) In *Cutaneous Aspects of Internal Disease*. Ed. Callen J. P. London, Year Book Medical Publishers, p. 536.
2 DUFFY J., *et al* (1976) *Medicine* (Baltimore) **55**, 19.
3 KIRBY J., *et al* (1974) *Br J Dermatol* **91**, (Suppl. 10), 11.
4 SARKANY I. (1973) *Proc R Soc Med* **66**, 237.
5 VARADI D. P. (1974) *Arch Dermatol* **109**, 678.

Urticaria [2]. Urticaria and transitory erythema may occur in the pre-icteric phase of acute viral hepatitis [1]. It is often associated with a *serum sickness-like picture* (generalized malaise, fever and arthralgia) present in 20–30% of patients with hepatitis [2]. Circulating immune complexes are probably involved [3].

REFERENCES

1 KURWA A. & WADDINGTON E. (1968) *Br J Dermatol* **80**, 839.
2 MCELGUNN P. S. J. (1983) *J Am Acad Dermatol* **8**, 539.
3 NEUMANN H. A. M., *et al* (1981) *Br J Dermatol* **104**, 387.

Persistent skin changes in liver disease [1]. Jaundice or icterus is first visible as a yellowish hue of the sclerae and soft palate before it becomes generalized. It is due to hyperbilirubinaemia. Carotenaemia and skin discoloration following mepacrine and busulphan therapy should be excluded.

Telangiectasia. Rapid development of multiple spider angiomas occurs in patients with severe chronic liver disease [2]. The cause is not known; hyperoestrogenaemia may be involved. A spider angioma consists of an abnormal coiled artery which ends up with radiating thin-walled vessels emerging from a central point. With pressure, blanching is produced, and when relieved the thread-like vessels are quickly refilled with blood from the centre.

Diffuse telangiectasia occurs as palmar erythema, which is most pronounced on the thenar and hypothenar regions. It is seen in many other conditions and is not specific for liver disease. Diffusely scattered telangiectatic vessels are referred to as 'paper money skin'. Purpuric lesions especially on the legs may be due to lack of clotting factors or consequent to deficiency of vitamins D, K and C (see chapter 62).

In progressive liver disease with portal obstruction collateral blood flow creates visible coiled varicose veins on the abdominal wall ('caput Medusae').

Hyperpigmentation is regularly seen in the form of diffuse muddy-grey hypermelanosis. There may be a yellowish tinge due to supervening jaundice. Usually pigmentation is more prominent in sun-exposed areas. Localized hyperpigmentation in the perioral and periorbicular areas may resemble chloasma. Males frequently show increased pigmentation of the areola in association with gynaecomastia and testicular atrophy [1]. Spotty hypomelanosis is seen on the back, buttocks and thighs, often in relation to spider angiomas.

Hair and nail changes. The body hair is thinned or lost and males tend to develop a female pubic hair pattern. When there is loss of scalp hair, zinc deficiency should be suspected (see p. 2335). Nail changes are several and frequent in cirrhosis. Typical findings include clubbing, white flat nails, striation and white bands. White nails showing a uniform whitish tinge with an invisible lunula may be seen in chronic conditions other than cirrhosis. White bands may be seen in hypoalbuminaemia [6] and may be associated with Beau's lines caused by zinc deficiency. In hepatolenticular degeneration

(Wilson's disease) the lunules attain a characteristic azure colour [3]. A diagnostic sign, the Kayser–Fleischer ring around the cornea, should be looked for.

Striae distensae. Cutaneous stretch marks occur in both sexes, especially on the lower abdomen, thighs and buttocks. Hormonal imbalance with oestrogen overweight is possibly involved.

Xanthomatosis (see p. 2286). Patients with biliary cirrhosis may show multiple xanthomatous lesions widely distributed over the trunk, face and extremities. Extensive plane xanthomas may develop on hands and fingers [1].

Porphyria cutanea tarda (see p. 2280). Chronic liver disease is involved in the skin changes of porphyria cutanea tarda. The lesions consist of bullae, scarring and hyperpigmentation of sun-exposed skin areas and hypertrichosis of the face.

Lichen planus. Lichen planus lesions have been reported in a number of diseases with abnormal immune function. The occurrence or erosive oral lesions in primary biliary cirrhosis [5] and chronic active hepatitis [9] may be related to a common immunological pathogenesis. Most reported patients have received penicillamine therapy which is believed by some to be the cause of the eruption [7, 11].

Hepato-cutaneous syndrome. In chronic active hepatitis (juvenile cirrhosis, lupoid hepatitis) and in primary biliary cirrhosis reddish firm papules leaving slightly depressed atrophic scars have been reported [8, 10]. The lesions erupt on the trunk and extremities and may show some resemblance to pityriasis lichenoides chronica or lymphomatoid papulosis. Histological examination reveals a capillaritis of the skin. In one of our patients the eruption subsided when he was started on Antabuse. The cause of the skin changes is unknown; some sort of allergic reaction is believed to be involved. In the *Gianotti–Crosti syndrome* (see p. 718) of childhood a papular rash develops associated with hepatitis B infection, usually in an anicteric form. The lesions disappear gradually over 3–6 weeks.

Pseudo-glucagonoma syndrome (see p. 2359). Skin changes consistent with the classical glucagonoma syndrome have been reported in cirrhosis [4].

REFERENCES

1 *ANHALT G. J. & DUBIN H. W. (1981) In *Cutaneous Aspects of Internal Disease*. Ed. Callen J. P. London, Year Book Medical Publishers, p. 530.
2 BEAN W. B. (1958) *Vascular Spiders and Related Lesions of the Skin*. Springfield, Charles C. Thomas.
3 BEARN A. G. & McKUSICK V. A. (1958) *JAMA* 166, 904.
4 DOYLE J. A., et al (1979) *Br J Dermatol* 100, 581.
5 GRAHAM-BROWN R. A. C., et al (1982) *Br J Dermatol* 106, 699.
6 MUEHRCKE R. C. (1956) *Br Med J* i, 1327.
7 POWELL F. C., et al (1982) *Br J Dermatol* 107, 616.
8 RAI G. S., et al (1977) *Br Med J* i, 817.
9 REBORA A., et al (1982) *Acta Derm Venereol (Stockh)* 62, 351.
10 SARKANY I. (1970) *Proc R Soc Med* 63, 819.
11 SEEHAFER J. R., et al (1981) *Arch Dermatol* 117, 140.

PANCREATIC DISEASE

Apart from jaundice, skin changes associated with pancreatic disease are uncommon (if primary diabetes mellitus (see p. 2339) is excluded). Most signs are non-specific, whereas others such as the glucagonoma syndrome are distinct and therefore of diagnostic value [8].

Cutaneous haemorrhage [9]. Within 1–2 days after the onset of acute pancreatitis spread of haemorrhage from the tail of the organ may be clinically manifest as a bruise-like discoloration of the skin of the left flank (Grey–Turner's sign). If the bleeding spreads along the falciform ligament bruising appears around the umbilicus (Cullen's sign). Rupture of the common bile duct, ectopic pregnancy, perforated duodenal ulcer [2], hepatoma [6] and other haemorrhagic diseases may lead to similar cutaneous bruising.

Livedo reticularis [9]. In acute pancreatitis dull red livedo reticularis may occur on the abdominal skin and upper thighs. The sign is non-specific as it may occur in other disease states, especially those with vascular involvement. Urticaria has been described in postpartum pancreatitis.

Nodular fat necrosis (nodular panniculitis) [8]. Systemic nodular fat necrosis is a rare syndrome which may or may not be associated with diseases of the pancreas. Examples are acute and chronic pancreatitis, post-traumatic pancreatitis and pancreatic carcinoma [4]. Most of the reported pancreatic neoplasms were acinous adenocarcinoma, which is rare [2]. A diagnostic tetralogy for acinous adenocarcinoma of the pancreas has been suggested: nodular fat necrosis, fever, eosinophilia in the blood and pain in bones and joints [3]. Subcutaneous fat necrosis associated with acute pancreatitis in a newborn has been reported [1].

Aetiology. Subcutaneous fat necrosis is thought to be produced by released pancreatic lipases and other enzymes which act on the peripheral fat tissue, producing free fatty acids, cholesterol, neutral fats and glycerol.

Clinical features. Synovitis of the small joints in connection with nodular fat necrosis affects 2–3% of patients with pancreatic disease [8]. Either the nodules or the arthralgia may predominate. Nodular lesions are usually 1–3 cm in diameter, tender or symptomless. The areas of predeliction are the trunk and the lower extremities, especially the anterior shins, but lesions may occur anywhere. They persist for 2–3 weeks and usually heal without scar formation, leaving slightly depressed hyperpigmented spots. The joint changes consist of synovitis of small- and medium-sized joints, but more severe changes due to periarticular fat necrosis may occur. Polyserositis may be a part of the syndrome [7].

Histopathology. There are foci of subcutaneous fat necrosis with ghost cells and a surrounding inflammatory infiltrate of neutrophils and eosinophils. At the periphery of the lesion histiocytes, foam cells and foreign body giant cells are seen. Secondary calcification may be observed in necrotic areas.

Diagnosis. In pancreatitis the serum amylase and lipase are increased. Enzyme determination of the urine may be helpful. The pathogenesis of cases not associated with pancreatic disease is not known.

Migratory thrombophlebitis [8]. Multiple superficial and deep venous thromboses may develop in patients with pancreatic cancers. The frequency has been reported to be high, but more recent studies indicate that lung cancer is the most common associated neoplasm in men over 40 [8]. The phlebitis is distributed on trunk, neck and extremities and is usually limited to a short segment of the vein. The cause is unknown but probably related to disordered fibrinolysis.

Haemochromatosis (bronze diabetes) (see p. 2334). Haemochromatosis often involves the pancreas, resulting in diabetes mellitus.

Insulinoma and gastrinoma. The most common islet cell tumours are insulinoma of β-cells and gastrinoma of δ-cells (Zollinger–Ellison syndrome).

The tumours are not associated with specific skin changes but they may occur together with other tumours that secrete ACTH, MSH and serotonin. Severe diarrhoea in the Zollinger–Ellison syndrome and the pancreatic cholera syndrome are life threatening and may cause secondary hypovitaminosis and other nutritional deficiencies giving rise to skin and hair changes [8].

Pancreatic disease of the tropics. Pancreatic disease of the tropics [5] is an acquired inflammatory disorder of the pancreas of unknown aetiology that occurs widely in East Africa, affecting mainly young adult men. It is a frequent cause of malabsorption syndrome. There is widespread cutaneous scaling, hair loss and a unique and occasionally dramatic loss of hair and of skin pigmentation. The patients respond well to pancreatic enzyme replacement. Zinc deficiency may be involved but has not been studied. Recurrent attacks of zinc deficiency may be observed in alcoholics suffering from chronic pancreatitis with malabsorption [10] (see p. 2337).

REFERENCES

1 DAWSON T. A. J. & SLATTERY C. (1979) *Br J Dermatol* **101**, 359.
2 EVANS D. M. (1971) *Br Med J* i, 154.
3 GRACIANSKI P. (1967) *Br J Dermatol* **79**, 278.
4 GRACIANSKI P., et al (1965) *Soc Med Hôp Paris* **116**, 261.
5 KLAUS S. N. (1980) *Int J Dermatol* **19**, 508.
6 MABIN T. A. & GELFAND M. (1974) *Br Med J* i, 493.
7 POLTS D. E., et al (1975) *Am J Med* **58**, 417.
8 *SIBRACK L. A. (1978) *Cutis* **21**, 763.
9 SIGMUND W. J. & SHELLEY W. B. (1954) *N Engl J Med* **251**, 851.
10 WEISMANN K., et al (1978) *Arch Dermatol* **114**, 1509.

Necrolytic migratory erythema (glucagonoma syndrome) [6, 7, 10]. Necrolytic migratory erythema is a peculiar cutaneous reaction with a prolonged fluctuating course characterized by migratory annular erythematous lesions, usually associated with hyperglucagonaemia. The syndrome was first described in 1942 [1], redefined in 1967 [2] and the term coined in 1971 [11]. Originally it was thought to represent a specific cutaneous marker of a pancreatic islet cell tumour, but recent reports dispute this [3–5, 10].

Aetiology. The cause of the skin eruption is not clear. Low serum amino acid levels may be implicated in the dermatitis [3]. The role of the hyperglucagonaemia is uncertain. Cases with no substantial elevation of plasma glucagon and lack of pathological changes of the pancreas have been reported [3, 5].

An aberrant zinc metabolism has been suggested but seems unlikely since most patients have normal serum zinc values.

Clinical features. The typical patient is a woman of 45–65, often seen first because of loss of weight, anaemia, a smooth tongue and a rash which is found especially on the lower abdomen, groins, buttocks and thighs. There is a cyclic pattern in the course of the eruption. First there is a macule, with a central bulla at friction sites. Seven to fourteen days later the central part heals leaving post-inflammatory pigmentation while the erythematous periphery becomes encrusted. There is irregular centrifugal extension of the annular lesions, which coalesce into a geographic serpiginous pattern. Burning and itch accompany the eruption. Most patients in addition complain of painful glossitis and perianal and genital lesions. The clinical spectrum includes anaemia, diarrhoea, wasting, weakness, venous thromboses and psychiatric disturbances. Diabetes without ketoacidosis or abnormal glucose tolerance is present in most patients. With a glucagon-producing tumour an elevated plasma glucagon level in the range 700–7,000 pg/ml (normally 50–150 pg/ml [4]) is found [6]. Half of the patients show low plasma amino acid levels [7]. Other reports corroborate this [3, 9]. In most reported cases with hyperglucagonaemia the cause was a glucagon-secreting islet cell tumour of the pancreas but aberrant glucagon-secreting tumours may be involved. A case of necrolytic migratory erythema with hyperglucagonaemia associated with advanced hepatic cirrhosis but without evidence of pancreatic disease has been reported ('pseudo-glucagonoma syndrome') [4]. In another case chronic pancreatitis was associated with the syndrome [10].

Histopathology [8, 11]. Biopsy should be taken from the edge of early lesions. The characteristic histological feature is a well-demarcated necrolysis ('sudden death') of the outer cell layers in the stratum Malpighii. Later, clefts and separation occur at the site. In the dermis a mild perivascular lymphocytic and histiocytic infiltrate is seen. Older lesions show various degrees of dyskeratosis, acanthosis and a lymphocytic infiltrate in the dermis. The histological changes may mimic those observed in acute zinc deficiency. Here cell degeneration and the formation of clefts and vesicles is situated at the level of the basal cells which may be helpful to distinguish the

two disorders. In the electron microscope there are distinct differences (see p. 2338).

Diagnosis. Pancreatic and hepatic scans and arteriography are helpful in locating a primary pancreatic tumour and its metastases if present. Serum amino acid, glucose and plasma glucagon levels should be determined. In cases with an elevated plasma glucagon level and a clinical and histological picture suggestive of the disease surgical exploration should be performed.

Treatment. Where there is a glucagonoma surgical treatment is indicated. When the tumour is removed a marked improvement of the skin will follow. In cases with hepatic metastases, present in about 50% at the time of diagnosis, streptozocin (a nitrosurea compound used for the ablation of β-cell adenoma) has proved beneficial [6]. Parenteral amino acid infusions may be helpful as an initial form of therapy [3].

REFERENCES

1 BECKER S. W., *et al* (1942) *Arch Dermatol Syphil* **45**, 1069.
2 CHURCH R. E. & CRANE W. A. J. (1967) *Br J Dermatol* **79**, 284.
3 DOLL D. C. (1980) *Arch Dermatol* **116**, 861.
4 DOYLE J. A., *et al* (1979) *Br J Dermatol* **100**, 581.
5 GOODENBERGER D. M., *et al* (1979) *Arch Dermatol* **115**, 1429.
6 *GUILLAUSSEAU P.-J., *et al* (1982) *Gastroenterol Clin Biol* **6**, 1029.
7 MALLINSON C. N., *et al* (1974) *Lancet* **ii**, 1.
8 OHYAMA K., *et al* (1982) *Arch Dermatol* **118**, 679.
9 PEDERSEN N. B., *et al* (1976) *Acta Derm Venereol (Stockh)* **56**, 391.
10 THIVOLET J., *et al* (1974) *Ann Dermatol Syphiligr* **101**, 415.
11 WILKINSON D. S. (1973) *Trans St John's Hosp Dermatol Soc* **59**, 244.

RENAL DISEASE [5]

Skin and the kidneys may be affected by the same pathological process. A list of the more important of these so-called renocutaneous syndromes is given in Table 63.4.

In angiokeratoma corporis diffusum patients commonly show proteinuria and microscopic haematuria, and usually they die of renal failure. In Von Recklinghausen's disease there may be obstruction to urinary flow at bladder level or elsewhere by a neurofibroma. Patients with this condition may also have vascular lesions of the kidneys,

TABLE 63.4. Renocutaneous syndromes

Hereditary syndromes
   Angiokeratoma corporis diffusum
   Neurofibromatosis
   Tuberous sclerosis
   Sickle-cell disease
   Pseudoxanthoma elasticum
   von Hippel–Lindau disease
   Hereditary haemorrhagic telangiectasia

Metabolic disorders
   Primary systemic amyloidosis
   Calcinosis

Collagen disease and vasculitis
   Allergic vasculitis
   Systemic lupus erythematosus
   Polyarteritis nodosa
   Scleroderma
   Wegener's granulomatosis
   Erythema multiforme
   Anaphylactoid purpura
   Drug-induced toxic epidermal necrolysis

of which the most important are those resulting in renal artery thrombosis with hypertension [4, 14]. Renal dysplasia presenting as chronic glomerulonephritis occurs in some and electron microscopy evidence of glomerular abnormalities in all cases of the nail–patella syndrome [3]. In partial lipoatrophy, renal disorders occur with high frequency, and renal failure in children and young adults is common [9]. In familial Mediterranean fever with urticaria (see p. 1108) there is often early death from renal failure due to amyloid. In systemic amyloidosis renal failure tends to be fatal fairly rapidly. A quarter of patients show some cutaneous or mucosal changes helpful in the diagnosis; primary cutaneous amyloidosis has no renal associations. Cutaneous lesions of sarcoid may explain the cause of polyuria and nocturia.

Polycystic disease of the kidney and liver occurred in three out of four cases of the oral–facial–digital syndrome that came to autopsy, and in von Hippel–Lindau's disease 20% of patients ultimately develop hypernephroma.

Renal involvement may occur in many forms of vasculitis and should always be considered in classical Henoch–Schönlein purpura (especially in the adult), in cases usually labelled allergic vasculitis and in arteriolitis with livedo reticularis [7]. It occurs in some cases of erythema multiforme [6] and has been reported in drug-induced toxic epidermal necrolysis [19]. The renal changes in these conditions and in polyarteritis nodosa, systemic lupus

erythematosus and scleroderma are considered elsewhere.

Streptococcal impetigo is an acknowledged cause of acute nephritis and as both nephritis and guttate psoriasis may follow streptococcal tonsillitis it is reasonable to expect such renal and skin pathology occasionally to coexist. Secondary syphilis is a rare cause of the nephrotic syndrome [21]; herpes zoster affecting several dermatomes may sometimes cause neurogenic bladder dysfunction [16].

Signs of renal failure. Cutaneous signs of renal failure are present only in fairly advanced cases and are therefore of little diagnostic value. The most dramatic sign, urea frosting, in which crystalline urea is deposited on the skin, is rarely seen. Many uraemic patients, however, have dry skin, sometimes with fine scaling. The reduction in the size of eccrine sweat glands in uraemia may be important here [20].

A common sign is pallor from the anaemia, but there is also a muddy-brown discoloration of the skin, attributed to the retention of chromogens and deposition of excess melanin perhaps due to the kidney's failure to metabolize or excrete MSH [13]. Increased nail pigmentation, usually confined to the distal half, was found in 9 of 59 patients by Kint *et al* [17]. Purpura due to platelet dysfunction, partly corrected by dialysis, and attributed to an unknown factor in serum is extremely common [27]. Troublesome pruritus occurs in 30–40% of patients in terminal renal failure and minor symptoms in many more [12]. In a majority of patients the itching is relieved by dialysis but that procedure itself may cause pruritus in some subjects. In those who are not improved, secondary hyperparathyroidism must be considered, as parathyroidectomy may be remarkably effective [22]. It probably does not account for all patients whose irritation fails to respond to dialysis. Moreover, many patients with secondary hyperparathyroidism have no pruritus. In intractable cases of itching due to renal failure UV-B radiation is an effective treatment [26] and UV-A (without psoralens) has been reported to work nearly as well [15]. Calcifying panniculitis has now been reported several times in patients with renal failure [25] and has in each case been attributed to the phenomenon of calciphylaxis described by Selye. Calcinosis cutis, presenting as tender woody infiltrated nodular plaques around the axillae, thighs, large joints and perineum, is a rare but well-recognized complication of renal failure. It may be reversed by a low phosphorus diet and aluminium hydroxide gel [18].

Most recent research on the skin in renal failure

has inevitably concentrated on dialysis populations in whom the effects of prolonged partially corrected renal failure may be studied along with side effects of dialysis (haemo or peritoneal) itself. Patients with renal failure may develop gynaecomastia when they undergo dialysis; 10 out of 24 showed this in one series [10]. It may be reversed by a low phosphorus diet and aluminium hydroxide gel [18]. Premature ageing of the skin and solar keratoses have also been described [1], a reason for avoiding over enthusiastic UV-B for pruritus; moreover, perforating folliculitis with keratoses of the Kyrle type has been observed [2, 23] and may be related to hypervitaminosis A [2]. The significance of a cutaneous microangiopathy uncorrected by dialysis but reversible by successful renal transplantation is as yet obscure [11] but the unexplained porphyria-like bullous eruptions in dialysis patients reported some years ago now seem likely to be due to porphyria after all. Recent publications stress the need for more sophisticated porphyrin biochemistry to reveal porphyria cutanea tarda in these patients [8, 24, 28].

REFERENCES

 1 Altmeyer D., *et al* (1982) *Hautarzt* **33**, 303.
 2 Bardach H. F. (1982) *Hautarzt* **33**, 584.
 3 Bennett W. M., *et al* (1973) *Am J Med* **34**, 304.
 4 Bourke E. & Garenby P. B. B. (1971) *Br Med J* iii, 681.
 5 Christianson H. B. & Birchall R. (1964) *South Med J* **57**, 2053.
 6 Comaish J. S. & Kerr D. N. S. (1961) *Br Med J* ii, 84.
 7 Cream J. J., *et al* (1970) *Q J Med* **39**, 461.
 8 Disler P., *et al* (1982) *Am J Med* **72**, 989.
 9 Eisinger A. J., *et al* (1972) *Q J Med* **41**, 343.
10 Freeman R. M., *et al* (1968) *Ann Intern Med* **69**, 67.
11 Gilchrest B. A., *et al* (1980) *Lancet* ii, 1271.
12 Gilchrest B. A., *et al* (1982) *Arch Dermatol* **118**, 154.
13 Gilkes J. J. H., *et al* (1975) *Br Med J* i, 656.
 4 Hamburger J. *et al* (1979) *Nephrology.* Philadelphia, Saunders, Vol. II, Ch. 30.
15 Hinson C., *et al* (1981) *Lancet* i, 215.
16 Izumi A. K. & Edwards J. (1974) *Arch Dermatol* **109**, 692.
17 Kint A., *et al* (1974) *Acta Derm Venereol (Stockh)* **54**, 137.
18 Kolton B. & Pederson J. (1974) *Arch Dermatol* **110**, 256.
19 Krumlovsky F. A., *et al* (1974) *Am J Med* **57**, 817.
20 Landing B. H., *et al* (1970) *Am J Clin Pathol* **54**, 15.
21 Lebon P., *et al* (1975) *Ann Dermatol Syphiligr* **102**, 354.
22 Massry S. G., *et al* (1968) *N Engl J Med* **279**, 697.
23 Noble J. P., *et al* (1979) *Nouv Presse Méd* **8**, 2905.
24 Poh-Fitzpatrick M. B., *et al* (1982) *J Am Acad Dermatol* **7**, 100.
25 Richens G., *et al* (1982) *J Am Acad Dermatol* **6**, 537.
26 Shultz B. C. & Roenigk H. H. (1980) *JAMA* **243**, 1836.
27 Stewart J. H. & Castaldi P. A. (1967) *Q J Med* **36**, 409.
28 Topi G. C., *et al* (1981) *Br J Dermatol* **104**, 579.

CARDIAC DISEASE AND SKIN SYMPTOMS

There are several cardiac diseases in which skin symptoms may be present. A full description and delineation of all such conditions is beyond the scope of this chapter. From a dermatologist's point of view the following disorders may be of interest.

Ischaemic heart disease. Ischaemic heart disease occurring in early life may be linked with progeria, Werner's syndrome, hypercholesterolaemic xanthomatosis (Frederickson type II) and Fabry's disease. Cases of sudden death from myocardial ischaemia have been reported in pseudoxanthoma elasticum.

Bacterial endocarditis [7]. More than half of the patients have a past history of heart disease (rheumatic fever, congenital heart disease, heart valve operation) or parenteral drug addiction. About 75–80% of cases are caused by *Staphylococcus aureus* or streptococcal species, predominantly *Streptococcus viridans*. Cutaneous lesions are probably often related to circulating immune complexes [2]. Osler's nodes are small red papules mainly situated on the distal finger and toe pads. The lesions are often preceded by soreness at the site of the eruption. Faint red macular lesions may develop on the thenar and hypothenar eminences (Janeway lesions). Splinter haemorrhages of the nail fold and conjunctiva may be seen in half of the patients but as such changes are often traumatically induced the sign is of no diagnostic value.

Rheumatic fever. Papular lesions on the extensor surface of the extremities, particularly near the joints, have been described in 2–3% of patients with rheumatic fever. With the same incidence subcutaneous nodules occur around the elbow or knee joints, almost exclusively in patients with rheumatic carditis [9].

Erythema marginatum. Erythema marginatum together with subcutaneous nodules constitute the major cutaneous criteria for guidance in the diagnosis of rheumatic fever. It is a transitory gyrate erythema mainly situated on the trunk and proximal parts of the extremities. It may occur at any time during the course of the disease. Within hours it expands to form figurate lesions with a dull red border which fades in 1–2 days. In itself it is not specific of rheumatic fever as it may be seen in other diseases [3].

Urticaria, erythema nodosum and purpura are noted in about 2% of patients [9].

Sarcoidosis of the heart (see p. 1764). Sarcoidosis may affect the heart causing conduction defects and arrhythmia, especially heart block and ventricular tachycardia. Cutaneous sarcoidosis may or may not be present. Congestive heart failure and sudden death due to ventricular arrythmia or complete block is common.

Cardiac amyloidosis (see p. 2306). In primary amyloidosis this is frequent although seldom the presenting manifestation of the disease. Most commonly there is congestive heart failure, low voltage on the ECG and conduction disturbances. Cardiomegaly is present in about one-third of the patients. A positive skin histology may be useful in suspected cases of cardiac amyloidosis.

Lentiginosis (a mnemonic term is 'leopard syndrome') [5]. In this syndrome there are widespread *l*entigines, *E*CG abnormalities, *o*cular hypertelorism, *p*ulmonary stenosis, *a*bnormal genitals, *r*etardation of growth and *d*eafness. The cardiac involvement includes left-axis deviation on the ECG, ventricular hypertrophy and arrhythmia.

Angiokeratoma corporis diffusum (Fabry's disease) (see p. 2309). Evidence of cardiac involvement is present in the majority of cases. Arrhythmia, an abnormal P–R interval on the ECG and left ventricular hypertrophy are the most common findings. ECG abnormalities may also be found in persons heterozygous for the gene.

Whipple's disease. Pericarditis, myocarditis and endocarditis may be present in conjunction with diffuse melanosis, leg nodules and joint pain which are characteristic of the disease.

Lupus erythematosus (see p. 1282) [4]. It appears that myocarditis, mitral valve thickening, vegetations and fibrinous pericarditis have become less common since the introduction of corticosteroid therapy. Congenital heart block in the newborn may be associated with systemic lupus erythematosus of the mother.

Generalized scleroderma (progressive systemic sclerosis) (see p. 1351). A focal or diffuse myocardial fibrosis may give rise to ECG abnormalities. In addition, cardiac symptoms may develop secondary to pulmonary hypertension (cor pulmonale). There is an increased incidence of pericardial effusion and pericarditis.

Dermatomyositis and polymyositis (see p. 1376). Cardiac involvement is probably more frequent in dermatomyositis and polymyositis than previously believed [6]. The most common changes are conduction abnormalities and various arrhythmias, often causing no symptoms. Cardiomyopathy is a rare complication.

Relapsing polychondritis. The cardiovascular system is affected in a high proportion of cases. Cardiac involvement includes aortic aneurysm, mitral regurgitation, pericarditis and cardiac ischaemia.

Erythroderma. Erythroderma causes a hyperkinetic circulatory state which may lead to cardiac failure in predisposed patients. In patients with exfoliative erythroderma a raised cutaneous blood flow is invariably demonstrable, whereas a significantly raised cardiac output is only present in a minority of cases. Effective local therapy causes improvement of the cardiac function but, before this can be achieved, digitalization may be indicated.

Diffuse neonatal haemangiomatosis [8]. In this rare disorder there are numerous haemangiomas scattered over the body and visceral involvement is common. This may lead to high-output cardiac failure. Hepatic artery ligation has been performed with consequent improvement of the cardiac function.

Cardiac pacemaker. Cutaneous reactions over the site of implanted cardiac pacemakers have been reported [1]. Irritant, toxic or allergic mechanisms may be operative. Rejection of the implanted material is the rule.

REFERENCES

1 ANDERSON K. E. (1979) *Arch Dermatol* **115**, 97.
2 BAYER A. S. (1976) *N Engl J Med* **295**, 1500.
3 BURKE J. B. (1955) *Arch Dis Child* **30**, 359.
4 FRIES J. F. & HOLMAN H. R. (1975) *Major Problems in Internal Diseases.* Vol. 6, *Systemic Lupus Erythematosus: A Clinical Analysis.* Philadelphia, Saunders, p. 30.
5 GORLIN R. J., *et al* (1969) *Am J Dis Child* **117**, 652.
6 GOTTDIENER J. S., *et al* (1978) *Am J Cardiol* **41**, 1141.
7 *GREER K. E. (1981) In *Cutaneous Aspects of Internal Dis-*

ease. Ed. Callen J. P. London, Year Book Medical Publishers, p. 389.
8 KELLER L. & BLUHM J. F. (1979) *Cutis* 23, 295.
9 *LYNCH P. J. (1981) In *Cutaneous Aspects of Internal Disease.* Ed. Callen J. P. London, Year Book Medical Publishers, p. 383.

RESPIRATORY SYSTEM AND SKIN DISEASES

Asthma is associated significantly with atopic dermatitis and ichthyosis of the dominant type. In the carcinoid syndrome attacks of dyspnoea and asthmatic wheezing may occur during flushing periods. Asthma with erythema multiforme and nodular lesions on the trunk and extremities occur in allergic granulomatosis (Chapter 31). In the larva migrans syndrome asthma and bronchitis form part of the syndrome.

In *relapsing polychondritis* (see p. 1856) there may be dyspnoea and inspiratory stridor due to swelling of the respiratory tract, collapse of cartilages of larynx and trachea and nasal obstruction. Cutaneous hallmarks are chronic otitis externa with cellulitis of the pinna. There is a potential risk of obstructive suffocation. Dyspnoea may occur with the lung fibrosis of generalized *scleroderma* and in *dermatomyositis* with interstitial infiltration of the lung bases [7]. Dyspnoea and even asphyxia may occur if the mucous membranes of the respiratory tract are involved in *xanthoma disseminatum*. Involvement of the respiratory tract in *primary amyloidosis* is common but often symptomless. Amyloid infiltrates in the alveolar septa can produce dyspnoea [5].

In *familial dysautonomia* (the Riley–Day syndrome) (see p. 2241) there are acute episodes of bronchopneumonia with profuse mucous secretion causing dyspnoea. Skin changes include multiple excoriations, erythematous mottling during the attack and pallor as it subsides. Progressive emphysema causing cor pulmonale is a severe manifestation in some cases of *generalized cutis laxa* of early life. The vast majority of patients with *cutaneous sarcoid* and erythema nodosum (see p. 1156) probably have enlargement of the hilar glands but exact figures are lacking. Pleural involvement is a frequent manifestation of *systemic lupus erythematosus*. It also occurs with pancreatic disease associated with fat necrosis (see p. 1864) and in the form of recurrent pleural effusion in some cases of the yellow nail syndrome. Pleural effusions, moreover, have been reported in *adenoma sebaceum* [2]. Pulmonary involvement is uncommon, but there may be numerous small cysts which on X-ray can be mistaken for tuberculosis or sarcoidosis [6]. The changes are characteristically found in adult female patients.

In *hereditary haemorrhagic telangiectasia* (see p. 1093) there may be vascular deformities in the lung in the form of arteriovenous shunts. In *Darier's disease* diffuse lower lobe fibrosis and laryngeal involvement has been reported [3]. *Psittacosis*, or ornithosis, may be accompanied by erythema nodosum and erythema multiforme (Bateman's syndrome). Mycoplasma pneumonia is frequently associated with erythema multiforme. The combined finding of lung infiltrates by X-ray, a nonproductive cough and erythema multiforme is suggestive of mycoplasma infection. In *primary pulmonary tuberculosis* the ide reactions of erythema multiforme, erythema nodosum, lichen scrofulosorum, Bazin's disease and papulonecrotic tuberculide occasionally are present. Chest symptoms, X-ray findings suggestive of chronic pulmonary tuberculosis and erythema nodosum suggest *North American blastomycosis*. The erythema multiforme or erythema nodosum of *pulmonary coccidioidomycosis* typically are seen late in the course. Cutaneous granulomas occur in the progressive form. *Pulmonary melioidosis* may run a subacute course and last for one to several weeks. It may be contracted by inhalation causing early pneumonic symptoms or via skin defects. In this case abscess formation precedes the septic stage. In chronic forms urticaria may be seen [8].

Hoarseness from laryngeal or tracheal involvement is an important audible sign of certain systemic diseases with skin involvement [1]. Examples are *pachyonychia congenita*, *Lange's syndrome*, *Farber's disease*, erythema multiforme, sarcoidosis, secondary syphilis, epidemic typhus, lupus erythematosus and dermatomyositis. Voice changes are of major diagnostic value for the recognition of *lipoid proteinosis*, *pemphigus vulgaris*, *relapsing polychondritis* and *hypothyroidism*. In these examples it is important to consider and exclude a possible carcinoma of the larynx as the cause of the voice changes. Lung tumours may cause local destruction of the overlying thoracic tissue and spread to the skin. Sympathetic nerve function may be disturbed due to tumour growth, and this may cause ipsilateral or contralateral segmental hyperhidrosis [4].

REFERENCES

1 BERNHARD J. D. (1983) *Cutis* 31, 189.
2 BROUGHTON R. B. K. (1970) *Br Med J* i, 477.
3 DELLON A. L., *et al* (1975) *Arch Dermatol* 111, 744.
4 McCOY B. P. (1981) *Arch Dermatol* 117, 659.

5 POH S. C., *et al* (1975) *Thorax* **30**, 186.
6 REED W. B., *et al* (1963) *Arch Dermatol* **87**, 715.
7 SCHWARTZ M. I., *et al* (1976) *Medicine (Baltimore)* **55**, 89.
8 STECK W. D. & BYRD R. B. (1969) *Arch Dermatol* **99**, 80.

HAEMATOLOGY

Anaemia. The mucocutaneous signs of hypochromic anaemia—pallor, koilonychia, glossitis—are of little diagnostic value, in view of the ease with which the haemoglobin can be estimated. Any of the syndromes in which cutaneous markers are associated with gastrointestinal bleeding may be associated with iron-deficiency anaemia; perhaps the most important of these is hereditary haemorrhagic telangiectasia. There are no absolute cutaneous markers of pernicious anaemia. The deep red, cobblestone tongue changes are classical but, like the diffuse pigmentation of the skin, are a late feature. Patients with pernicious anaemia have vitiligo 10 times more frequently than normal controls and, conversely, in one series pernicious anaemia occurred in 10·6% of patients with vitiligo. This is 30 times more common than in the general population [4]. Vitiligo of late onset may be especially significant. Sickle cell anaemia may be suggested by leg ulcers which occur in 75% of adult patients with this condition, often in association with haemosiderosis and melanosis of the legs [9]. From time to time iron-deficiency anaemia is causally linked to pruritus in single case reports [12, 13].

In patients with dermatitis herpetiformis anaemia is often due to dapsone-induced haemolysis [1], but malabsorption from gluten enteropathy is likely to be a factor in some cases. In patients with erythroderma, anaemia is a common finding. In one report [10] 28% of patients had a haemoglobin of 12 g or less. In many patients haemodilution seems to be the explanation, but more study of the whole problem is necessary. Much iron may be lost from the skin in psoriasis, and there may be defective absorption of iron in dermatogenic enteropathy, yet in most cases hypoferraemia appears to be a reflection of abnormal handling of iron rather than real body depletion [7]. There is often a true folate deficiency in extensive skin disease and sometimes in more limited skin involvement. Macrocytic anaemia is not usually present but cases do occur.

Leukocytosis. Leukocytosis in the absence of infection is a very common feature in erythroderma (six out of 42 patients had a white cell count of more than 15,000 per cubic millimetre in one series [10]). Leukocytosis also occurs in pustular psoriasis, pustular miliaria and erythema multiforme.

ESR. A raised ESR is common in erythroderma, nearly two-thirds of Shuster's patients having levels above 20 mm in the first hour [10]. In most cases this was associated with a raised gamma globulin.

Leukaemias. These are discussed in Chapter 47

Miscellaneous. Blood dyscrasias are common in dyskeratosis congenita and in Fanconi's anaemia, 85% of cases of which show olive–brown pigmentation. In one reported series of patients diagnosed as having hypereosinophilic syndrome half had either irritable erythematous papules and nodules or urticarial weals [6]. In another report 11 out of 15 patients had skin lesions or pruritus [11]. Livedo and erythromelalgia may both be causally associated with thrombocythaemia and polycythaemia rubra vera. In the latter condition pruritus classically accentuated by bathing is well recognized and may on occasion be caused by iron deficiency [8]. There have been a few reports of concurrent polycythaemia and mastocytosis; the significance of these is not yet clear [5]. Idiopathic cryoglobulinaemia may present as purpura of exposed parts on cooling, as livedo reticularis, cold urticaria or frank gangrene. In symptomatic cryoglobulinaemia there are no skin signs. Cold agglutinins are manifest as Raynaud's syndrome, acrocyanosis or gangrene, usually in elderly patients. Cold haemolysins may give cold urticaria or Raynaud's syndrome. Extensive or multiple strawberry angiomas, especially if rapidly enlarging, may be associated with thrombocytopenia with purpura. Purpura may be simulated by asteatotic eczema with superficial haemorrhage in the fissures of the skin. Some cases of von Willebrand's disease may show albinism, and in the Hermansky–Pudlak syndrome albinism is associated with platelet dysfunction as it is in a similar disorder with the additional feature of pulmonary fibrosis [2, 3].

REFERENCES

1 CREAM J. J. & SCOTT G. L. (1970) *Br J Dermatol* **82**, 333.
2 DAVIES B. H. & TUDDENHAM E. G. D. (1976) *Q J Med* **45**, 219.
3 FRENK E. & LATTION F. (1982) *J Invest Dermatol* **78**, 141.
4 GRUNNET I., *et al* (1970) *Arch Dermatol* **101**, 82.
5 HANDLER G., *et al* (1981) *Clin Exp Dermatol* **6**, 43.
6 KAZMIEROWSKI J. A., *et al* (1978) *Arch Dermatol* **114**, 531.

7 REIZENSTEIN S., *et al* (1968) *Acta Derm Venereol (Stockh)* **48**, 70.
8 SALEM H. H., *et al* (1982) *Br Med J* **285**, 91.
9 SERGEANT G. R., *et al* (1968) *Br Med J* iii, 86.
10 SHUSTER S. & MARKS J. (1970) *The Systemic Effects of Skin Disease.* London, Heinemann.
11 SPRY C. F. J., *et al* (1983) *Q J Med* **52**, 1.
12 TAKKUNEN H. (1978) *JAMA* **239**, 1394.
13 VALSECCHI R. & CAINELLI T. (1983) *Arch Dermatol* **119**, 630.

BONE AND JOINT DISEASES

There are several systemic diseases in which symptoms from bones and joints occur together with skin changes. Arthralgia and/or arthritis is frequent in systemic lupus erythematosus, polyarteritis nodosa, scleroderma, sarcoidosis, serum sickness, allergic purpura (Henoch–Schönlein purpura), intestinal bypass syndrome and Sweet's syndrome [8]. Various infections may show concurrent skin and joint lesions. Examples are yersiniosis, gonococcal arthritis–dermatitis syndrome and hepatitis B infection [6]. The combined reactions from skin and joints usually reflect systemic disease and mostly other organs or organ systems are involved. In arthropathic psoriasis and Reiter's disease a joint disease may dominate the clinical picture. Primary joint diseases such as rheumatoid arthritis (see p. 1386) and rheumatic fever (see p. 1392) may show a broad range of cutaneous reactions.

In secondary and tertiary syphilis osteitis and osteomyelitis may be seen. In the secondary stage of the disease the presenting symptom may be intense bone pain and arthralgia occurring alone or together with cutaneous markers of the disease [2].

Maffuci's syndrome (dyschondroplasia) (see p. 209). This is characterized by bony deformities, pathological fractures, hard cartilaginous subcutaneous nodules and multiple haemangiomas.

Conradi's disease (chondrodysplasia punctata) (see p. 163). The joints are stiff and contracted and usually there are developmental defects of the skeleton. The skin shows congenital ichthyosiform erythroderma with adherent hyperkeratoses, patchy atrophoderma in a linear and blotchy pattern and alopecia [3].

Osteogenesis imperfecta (see p. 1845). There are brittle bones, otosclerosis, blue sclerae and translucent macular atrophic skin with an aged appearance [1].

Ehlers–Danlos syndrome (see p. 1837). This is characterized by thin velvety hyperelastic skin and hyperextensibility of the joints. Osteoarthritis and kyphoscoliosis may eventually develop.

Tuberous sclerosis (see p. 122). Skin symptoms include adenoma sebaceum, fibromas, shagreen patches and dull white hypopigmented lesions. Pseudocysts of the finger phalanges of young children occur commonly; in adult patients thickening of the cortex of ribs, pelvis and phalanges is the typical finding.

Werner's syndrome (see p. 1816). This causes premature greying of hair, osteoporosis and a high frequency of sarcoma. The skin is tense and shining, the joints become fixed and sclerodactyly may be present.

Albright's disease (polyostotic fibrous dysplasia) (see p. 1562). There is a unilateral irregular pattern of hyperpigmented skin patches, with absence of involvement of the axilla which is an important clue to separating it from neurofibromatosis. There is precocious puberty, frequently in females, and fibrous dysphasia of long bones, appearing as cystic lesions on X-ray. There is an increased risk of bone fracture caused by even minor trauma, but the lesions heal rapidly and completely. There are hyperostotic changes of the skull.

Histiocytosis X (eosinophilic granuloma of bone). Skin changes may be seen but are rare [5].

Basal Cell Naevus Syndrone (Gorlin's syndrome) (see p. 2416). Spina bifida, bifid or splayed ribs, scoliosis and kyphosis each occur in about one-third of patients.

There may be developmental bone lesions in *incontinentia pigmenti* and in *Ota's naevus*, in which defects of the posterior cranial fossa have been described. In *relapsing polychondritis* (see p. 1856) migratory arthritis of small and large joints, usually sparing the hands, is an essential feature [4]. The various forms of acro-osteolysis, the epidermal naevus syndrome [7] and Behçet's syndrome are further examples of osteocutaneous syndromes.

REFERENCES

1 BLEGVAD O. & HAXTHAUSEN H. (1921) *Br Med J* ii, 1071.
2 DISMUKES W. E., *et al* (1976) *JAMA* **236**, 2646.
3 HAPPLE R. & KASTNER H. (1979) *Hautarzt* **30**, 590.

4 O'HANLAN M., *et al* (1976) *Arthritis Rheum* **19**, 191.
5 RODMAN O. G. & COOPER P. H. (1980) *Cutis* **26**, 487.
6 SHUMAKER J. B., *et al* (1974) *Arch Intern Med* **133**, 483.
7 SOLOMON L. M. (1968) *Arch Dermatol* **97**, 273.
8 STORER J. S., *et al* (1983) *Int J Dermatol* **22**, 8.

CUTANEOUS MANIFESTATIONS OF IMMUNOLOGICAL DEFICIENCY SYNDROMES

Since the recognition by Bruton of agammaglobulinaemia in 1951, many other forms of congenital and acquired immune deficiencies have been recognized. They are of interest to the dermatologist because they may present with recurrent or chronic mucocutaneous infections, because in some of them eczema is a striking feature, and because in others there are cutaneous markers which may be of considerable diagnostic importance. It is convenient to classify these conditions according to the component of the immune defence system which is defective, and although deficiencies of granulocyte function are often excluded from this group they are considered here alongside deficiencies of antibody formation and defects of the complement system because of the similarity of their clinical presentation. It is now clear that a great many different syndromes exist, but it is still useful to think of them under the following main headings:

Primary defects (may be congenital or appear later) [1–6]
(1) Defects of T-lymphocyte function—defects of delayed hypersensitivity
(2) Defects of antibody formation—B lymphocyte deficiency—broad or narrow, restricted to one class of immunoglobulin
(3) Combinations of (1) and (2)
(4) Defects of the secretory (mucosal) IgA system
(5) Defects of phagocyte function [7]
(6) Defects of the complement system (usually manifest as defective phagocyte function)

Secondary defects [2, 5, 7], i.e. associated with, and caused by, systemic disease, e.g. Hodgkin's disease, leukaemia, renal failure, malnutrition and sarcoidosis. Drugs, other than those used specifically as immunosuppressants, may depress immune function. Some infections such as influenza and leprosy are known to be capable of causing defects of immunity and a viral infection is the explanation for the acquired immune-deficiency syndrome (AIDS) (see p. 719). Secondary defects of immune function in general tend to be broad and often less easy to define than the primary syndromes so that at present classification, except by identifying the causal agent when possible, is difficult.

REFERENCES

1 ASHERSON G. L. & WEBSTER A. D. B. (1980) *Diagnosis and Treatment of Immunodeficiency Diseases.* Oxford, Blackwell Scientific.
2 BERGSMA D. (Ed.) (1975) *Immunodeficiency in Man and Animals.* New York, National Foundation.
3 BERGSMA D. & GOOD R. A. (Eds.) (1968) *Immunologic Deficiency Disease in Man.* New York, National Foundation.
4 ROSEN F. S. (1978) In *Immunological Diseases.* Ed. Samter M. 3rd ed. Boston, Little Brown, Vol. I, Ch. 24.
5 STIEHM E. R. & FULGINITI V. A. (Eds.) (1973) *Immunologic Disorders in Infants and Children.* Philadelphia, Saunders.
6 WEBSTER A. D. B. (Ed.) (1982) *Assessment of Immunocompetence. Clinics in Immunology and Allergy.* Philadelphia, Saunders, Vol. 1, No. 3.
7 WESTON W. L. (1976) *Arch Dermatol* **112**, 1589.

THE DERMATOLOGICAL FEATURES

The dermatological features of primary and secondary immune defects can be grouped under four main headings:

(1) Chronic and recurrent, sometimes atypical, infections of the skin and mucous membranes caused by viruses, bacteria and fungi (*Candida* species mainly)
(2) Eczemas
(3) Independent cutaneous markers
(4) Graft-versus-host reactions

Table 63.5 indicates most of the important conditions and shows the clinical features including the cutaneous ones. The various dermatological points are now considered briefly.

Viral infections [17]
Warts. The wart virus is so ubiquitous, and clinical infections with it are so common, that the significance of warts in a patient with any of the immune defects is always difficult to establish. Warts have been specifically mentioned in Wiskott–Aldrich syndrome, in some types of dysgammaglobulinaemia [11] and in Hodgkin's disease, lymphoma and chronic lymphatic leukaemia [30].

Mollusca contagiosa. This infection has been reported in sarcoidosis, a condition in which T-cell function is often depressed [16].

Herpes simplex. Serious herpes simplex infections are typically associated with the Wiskott–Aldrich

TABLE 63.5. Some syndromes of defective immunity and their cutaneous features

Syndrome	Immunological defect	Genetics	Cutaneous infections					Other cutaneous features	Associated features	Other infections
			Viruses	Pyoderma	BCG complications	Chronic mucocutaneous candidiasis	Eczema			
The granulocytopathies (chronic granulomatous disease(s); Job's syndrome)	Various defects of granulocyte function	Various (X-linked recessive; autosomal recessive)	—	+		+	+ reported in some. + in Job's syndrome			Otitis, pericarditis, liver abscess, etc.
Chediak-Higashi syndrome	Defective granulocytes (large granules)			+				Pigment dilution. Skin + hair		Pneumonias common
C3 defect of complement	Low C3 } Defective granulocyte function	—		+				Urticaria	Klinefelter's syndrome associated	Otitis media. + +
C5 defect of complement	Low C5 }						+ at 10 days	Exanthema before eczema		Systemic infections, +
Bruton's disease (X-linked hypoglobulinaemia)	Gross lack of all immunoglobulins and of antibody responses. T-cell function normal	X-linked recessive	Many vaccinated normally	+ fairly common (rarely pyoderma may be only infection)	+ has been reported		Increased prevalence of atopic eczema			Recurrent bacterial infections common. Pneumonia, meningitis, septicaemia
Severe combined immunodeficiency (several subgroups)	Very low immunoglobulins. T-cell and B-cell responses severely defective	Autosomal recessive and X-linked recessive variants	Vaccinia +	+ (two-thirds of patients)	+. main cause of fatal generalized BCG	+ (three-quarters patients). Some systemic candidiasis too	+. increased prevalence almost from birth in some	Exanthomas common. ? Graft-versus-host reactions	Diarrhoea. Failure to thrive	Sino-pulmonary gastrointestinal infections, septicaemia
Nezelof syndrome	Deficient T-cell responses to all antigens. Immunoglobulins normal. Antibody responses defective	Autosomal recessive	Herpes zoster and varicella +	+		+	—	Diffuse erythema, koilonychia	Diarrhoea, wasting	Systemic infections are common. Viruses, fungi, pneumocystis carinii
DiGeorge syndrome	Absence of T-cell response to all antigens. Immunoglobulins normal but antibody responses show some defects	—		Subcutaneous abscesses		+	—		Absence of parathyroids (tetany). Cardiovascular abnormalities. Diarrhoea	Systemic infections are common. Viruses, fungi, pneumocystis
Immunodeficiency with short-limbed dwarfism	Defective T- and B-cell function	Autosomal recessive	Varicella + +	—	—	—	—		Achondroplasia	Sinopulmonary infections
Cartilage hair hypoplasia	Defective T-cell function	Autosomal recessive	Varicella + +	—				Fine sparse hair, later bald	Achondroplastic dwarfism	
Ataxia telangiectasia	T-cell responses to some antigens defective. Immunoglobulins often show some deficit	Autosomal recessive	Some have been vaccinated safely	—			Reported	Telangiectasia, face and ears, etc. Later scleroderma-like features	Telangiectasia of conjunctiva and other tissues. Cerebellar ataxia. ovarian dysgenesis	Sinopulmonary infections common
Wiskott-Aldrich syndrome	Defective T- and B-cell responses due to defective antigen recognition. Immunological attrition	X-linked recessive	Herpes simplex + + (some fatal) Warts + Herpes zoster + Varicella	+			+ always at some stage	Purpura	Thrombocytopenia. Reticuloses in older survivors	Sinopulmonary infections and otitis common

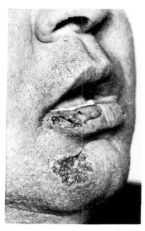

Fig. 63.3. Persistent herpes simplex in renal transplant recipient treated with systemic steroids and azathioprine (Addenbrooke's Hospital).

syndrome. In one series three out of 18 cases had this condition, and in two of them it was fatal [11]. It seems likely that the underlying eczematous condition may be of importance as well as the immune defect.

Varicella/Zoster. Severe or fatal varicella may occur in severe combined immunodeficiency or in immunodeficiency with short-limbed dwarfism [36]. Herpes zoster of prolonged course, sometimes with disseminated lesions, has been reported in the Wiskott–Aldrich syndrome [11] and, of course, in Hodgkin's disease, chronic lymphatic leukaemia and other lymphomas [17, 30] more frequently than in the general population. Patients with granulocyte defects do not seem to have difficulty in handling this virus. Deficient interferon production may be of importance [3].

Vaccinia [15]. Many patients with hypoglobulinaemia X-linked (Bruton's disease) have been successfully vaccinated without complications [22] as have some patients with granulocyte defects. Most cases of simple disseminated vaccinia were not attributable to the well-recognized immune-deficiency diseases. The syndrome of progressive fatal vaccinia, however, was closely linked to severe combined immunodeficiency, the Nezelof syndrome [1] and immunodeficiency with short-limbed dwarfism [36]. It occurred in two siblings with thymic deficiency and dysgammaglobulinaemia and in another child with thymic dysplasia and defective IgM production [9]. If there is any suspicion of an immune deficit, any live vaccine should be withheld. Even in Bruton's disease occasional fatalities may occur.

Measles. This may occur in severe or fatal form in defects of T-cell function sometimes without the development of a rash [36]. Fatalities after immunization with attenuated virus have occurred. In one case associated with dysgammaglobulinaemia the eruption was florid, reticulate, hyperkeratotic and crusted [26].

Bacterial infections
Pyoderma. Pyoderma may be follicular, impetiginous or periungual. In some cases reported, impetiginized eczema appeared to be implicated rather than a primary pyoderma.

Bacterial infection of the skin is characteristic of granulocyte dysfunction. It occurs in two-thirds of cases of chronic granulomatous disease [5] and in Chediak–Higashi syndrome [38]. It is also found in defects of C3 [2] and C5 [36] of the complement system, and it is present in some cases of classical Bruton's disease, rarely as the only infection [20], and in selective IgM deficiency [39]. Pyoderma is more common in severe combined immunodeficiency in which there is a defect of T-cells as well as antibodies. It does *not* appear to be an important feature of the Nezelof syndrome, nor is it a feature of DiGeorge's syndrome (thymic aplasia with hypoparathyroidism) or of ataxia telangiectasia in which deficiency of delayed hypersensitivity is found. Pyoderma is common in the Wiskott–Aldrich syndrome [11]. Here, although the immune deficit does lead to defective delayed-type hypersensitivity, the basic defect is probably a specific inability to appreciate certain carbohydrate bacterial antigens, i.e. a defect of the 'afferent loop of the immune response' [7]. The coexisting eczema is probably also important.

Mycobacterial infections. The commonest mycobacterium with which the immune-deficient infant is likely to be confronted is BCG. The syndrome of fatal generalized BCG infection has occurred in isolated T-cell deficiency [33], in cases of severe combined immunodeficiency [8] and in Bruton's disease but the absence of reports in other syndromes may simply reflect a much smaller number of patients exposed [25].

Septicaemia. Meningococcal septicaemia presenting with purpura may be linked with IgM deficiency [19] and in Bruton's disease ecthyma gangrenosum has been reported in *Pseudomonas* septicaemia [35].

Fungal infections
Candidiasis (chronic mucocutaneous candidiasis, p. 958). Infection of the mouth, the face, scalp, nail

folds, and nail plates with *Candida*, which persists in spite of vigorous topical therapy and which usually relapses even after clearance with systemic amphotericin B, is a reliable indication of defective immunity. It may be found in company with other infections, cutaneous or systemic, in several of the well-known immunodeficiency syndromes but occurs as an isolated finding in patients who are otherwise well. In the latter case it may not be possible, with existing techniques, to demonstrate any clear immune defect. In general, however, it seems that defects of delayed-type hypersensitivity and granulocyte function are the most likely to be associated with this condition (see p. 950). Chronic candidiasis is a prominent feature of DiGeorge's syndrome, and where the defect of delayed hypersensitivity has been reconstituted by thymic grafting the *Candida* infection has cleared with striking rapidity [10]. It is found in severe combined immunodeficiency and again cleared rapidly after grafting [23]. In the syndrome of biotin-dependent carboxylase deficiencies with T- and B-cell defective immunity [12], chronic mucocutaneous cadidiasis has responded to biotin therapy. It is present in some types of chronic granulomatous disease and is a prominent feature in many patients with acquired immune-deficiency syndrome (see p. 719). In those patients who do not fit into any of these categories a variety of different defects of delayed hypersensitivity or defective macrophage function [37] may be found.

Other fungal infections. Although there are occasional reports of patients with chronic mucocutaneous candidiasis who also have extensive and persistent dermatophytosis, ringworm infections are not particularly common in patients with immune defects. This is probably partly related to exposure factors. However, even among adult patients with acquired immune defects, tinea appears to be only an occasional problem. Recurrent *T. rubrum* infections have been reported in a family with defective neutrophil chemotaxis and ichthyosis [29]. Systemic mycoses occur, cryptococcosis being particularly associated with Hodgkin's disease and sarcoidosis [6].

Eczemas. Eczema is invariably present at some stage in the Wiskott–Aldrich syndrome [11, 34] and closely resembles, if it does not actually represent, atopic eczema. It is flexural and may occur early, within the first few weeks of life. In severe combined immunodeficiency it is an occasional feature (two out of 14 patients in one series [18]) and it may be present from birth. In two cases so far described of complement deficiency of the C5 type, severe extensive eczema was present from about 10 days of life in both [27, 28]. Again, the relationship to atopic eczema is interesting. There was a positive family history of atopy in these cases. Some patients with chronic granulomatous disease, including the variant known as Job's syndrome [13], have eczematous eruptions. There appears, too, to be an increased incidence of eczema of the atopic type in patients with the Bruton type of hypogammaglobulinaemia, and perhaps in type I dysgammaglobulinaemia. Eczema was also present in a patient with the so-called immunologic amnesia syndrome described by Kretshner [24] and in a new syndrome of antihistamine responsive immunodeficiency [21]. The significance of these eczematous eruptions is still obscure. Reports indicate that they may be complicated by considerable secondary pyoderma, and that the whole cutaneous condition may clear rapidly if it is possible to restore immunological function by grafting [4].

Independent cutaneous markers

Purpura. Purpura, usually petechial, due to a numerical and functional deficiency of platelets, is classical in the Wiskott–Aldrich syndrome.

Telangiectasia. Telangiectasia starting with changes on the bulbar conjunctivae and spreading to involve the cheeks, the ears, the sides of the neck and the antecubital fossae is a reliable marker of ataxia telangiectasia, in which it is associated with immune defects and cerebellar ataxia starting in infancy [4]. The telangiectases usually follow the neurological change. The immune defect of delayed type hypersensitivity does not normally result in any mucocutaneous infections, although there may be ear infections and purulent nasal discharge.

Pigment dilution. In the Chediak–Higashi syndrome [38], in which there is widespread defect of certain subcellular organelles, the cutaneous marker is dilution of pigment. This presents as albinism in white races and as a curious mottled greyish skin colour with greying of the hair in darkly pigmented people.

Fine sparse hair. This occurs as part of the cartilage hair hypoplasia syndrome in some forms of short-limbed dwarfism with immune defects [36].

Miscellaneous. Pigmented dyskeratotic skin of the neck from birth associated with dystrophic nails, lacrimal duct atresia and oral leucoplakia are all features of the Zinsser–Engman–Cole syndrome in which hypogammaglobulinaemia is present [32].

Urticaria has been described in complement deficiency of the C3 type [2], koilonychia in the Nezelof syndrome [31], and exanthems are reported in several syndromes. Some of these appear to be the initial signs of an eczema; in others they may represent mild degrees of graft–versus–host reaction.

Cutaneous signs of discoid or systemic lupus erythematosus should be included here, as autoimmune disorders are a feature of primary immune defects, e.g. IgA deficiency and some complement system defects [14, 36].

REFERENCES

1 ALLIBONE E. C., *et al* (1964) *Arch Dis Child* **39**, 26.
2 ALPER C. A. (1970) *N Engl J Med* **282**, 349.
3 ARMSTRONG R. W., *et al* (1970) *N Eng J Med* **283**, 1182.
4 ASHERSON G. L. & WEBSTER A. D. B. (1980) *Diagnosis and Treatment of Immunodeficiency Diseases*. Oxford, Blackwell Scientific.
5 BASS L. J., *et al* (1972) *Arch Dermatol* **166**, 68.
6 BELCHER R. W., *et al* (1975) *Arch Dermatol* **111**, 711.
7 BLAESE R. M., *et al* (1968) *Lancet* i, 1056.
8 BOULTON J., *et al* (1963) *Br Med J* i, 1512.
9 CHANDRA R. K., *et al* (1969) *Lancet* i, 687.
10 CLEVELAND W. W., *et al* (1968) *Lancet* ii, 1211.
11 COOPER M. D., *et al* (1968) *Am J Med* **44**, 499.
12 COWAN M. J., *et al* (1979) *Lancet* ii, 115.
13 DAVIS S. D., *et al* (1966) *Lancet* i, 1013.
14 DAY N. K. & GOOD R. A. (1975) In *Immunodeficiency in Man and Animals*. Ed. Bergsma D. New York, National Foundation.
15 FULGINITI V. A., *et al* (1968) In *Immunologic Deficiency Diseases in Man*. Eds. Bergsma D. & Good R. A. New York, National Foundation.
16 GANPULE M. & GARRETTS M. (1971) *Br J Dermatol* **85**, 587.
17 GRIECO M. H. (Ed.) (1980) *Infections in the Abnormal Host*. New York, Yorke Medical.
18 HITZIG W. H. (1968) In *Immunologic Deficiency Diseases in Man*. Eds. Bergsma D. & Good R. A. New York, National Foudation.
19 HOBBS J. R., *et al* (1967) *Br Med J* iv, 583.
20 Hypogammaglobulinaemia in the United Kingdom. Summary report of an M.R.C. Working Party (1969) *Lancet* ii, 163.
21 JUNG L.K.L., *et al* (1983) *Lancet* ii, 185.
22 KEMPE C. H. (1960) Pediatrics **26**, 176.
23 DE KONING J. (1969) *Lancet* i, 1223.
24 KRETSCHNER R., *et al* (1969) *N Engl J Med* **182**, 285.
25 MATSANIOTIS N. & ECONOMOU M. C. (1968) In *Immunologic Deficiency Diseases in Man*. Eds. Bergsma D. & Good R. A. New York, National Foundation.
26 MAWHINNEY H., *et al* (1971) *Br Med J* ii, 380.
27 MILLER M. E. & NILSSON U. R. (1970) *N Engl J Med* **282**, 354.
28 MILLER M. E., *et al* (1968) *Lancet* ii, 60.
29 MILLER M. E., *et al* (1973) *J Lab Clin Med* **82**, 1.
30 MORISON W. L. (1975) *Br J Dermatol* **92**, 625.
31 NEZELOF C., *et al* (1964) *Arch Fr Pédiat* **21**, 897.
32 ORTEGA J. A., *et al* (1972) *Am J Dis Child* **124**, 701.
33 PASSWELL J., *et al* (1976) *Am J Dis Child* **130**, 433.
34 SAURAT J-H., (1985) *Acta Derm Venereol* (Stockh) **114**, 125
35 SPIERS C. F., *et al* (1963) *Lancet* ii, 710.
36 STIEHM E. R. & FULGINITI V. A. (1973) *Immunologic Disorders in Infants and Children*. Philadelphia, Saunders.
37 VALDIMARSSON H., *et al* (1973) *Cell Immunol* **6**, 348.
38 WINDHORST D. B., *et al* (1968) In *Immunologic Deficiency Diseases in Man*. Eds. Bergsma D. & Good R. A. New York, National Foundation.
39 YOCUM M. W., *et al* (1976) *Am J Med* **60**, 486.

CUTANEOUS MANIFESTATIONS OF IMMUNOSUPPRESSIVE THERAPY

Suppression of homograft rejection by the use of corticosteroids, azathioprine and by antilymphocyte globulin is a well-established procedure. Recently cyclosporin A has been used alone or in combination with other drugs in renal, hepatic and cardiac transplantation. Established immunosuppressive drugs are, of course, widely used in other medical situations and cyclosporin is likely to join them. Most of the published series relate to renal transplant patients but similar incidence figures are found, at least with regard to infections, after transplantation of other organs and where these agents are used for other purposes [2].

The cutaneous complications of their use include the changes associated with Cushing's syndrome, atrophy, striae, telangiectasia, hirsutism, acne, etc., some of the changes typical of cytotoxic drugs (mouth ulcers, purpura, hair loss, etc.) and a general susceptibility to infection [20].

Infections. Virus infections are common. The incidence probably depends on the doses of immunosuppressant drugs used. Koranda *et al* [10] reported that 43% of their 200 renal transplant patients had warts; in a personal series 19% of 93 patients were affected. In one very recent series the overall incidence was 31% (about 10 times that in the control population) but warts were much commoner still in those immunosuppressed patients with high sun exposure (58%) [4]. Warts may be widespread, some being very large, and others may show malignant change histologically [10] although this seems rare. Herpes zoster usually follows a quiet course [11]—quite different from the outlook in leukaemia. Atypical examples with erythema and virtually no vesicle formation may be encountered. Again incidence varies from 13% [10], 12·5% [17], 7·5% [18] to nil

[8]. Varicella occurring during immunosuppression is likely to be life-threatening [9, 14] but one personal case with a history of previous childhood varicella survived a mild attack with minimal symptoms. This case indicates the value of prior exposure to this virus in patients requiring immunosuppression. Uncomplicated herpes simplex is common, affecting perhaps 50 or 60% of patients [2], but persistent ulcers of the mouth and perioral skin are well-documented occasional problems, sometimes with secondary bacterial infection. Systemic infections have also been reported [14]. Widespread eruptions of molluscum contagiosum should also be included in the list of cutaneous viral infections [6, 19].

Furunculosis, impetigo and cellulitis are found more often than in the normal population [8, 17] but would be a greater problem if it were not for the frequent use of antibacterial agents for wound and systemic infections. Staphylococcal toxic epidermal necrolysis—a condition normally rare in adults—is a recognized hazard and may be related to a deep-seated staphylococcal infection [17, 18]. Gram-negative septicaemia may present with vasculitis-like dermal nodules in a patient who is, initially, otherwise well. Long-standing leprosy, quiescent after treatment, may relapse dramatically on immunosuppression [1], nor should atypical mycobacterial infection be forgotten [11]. Nocardiasis, a well-recognized pulmonary hazard of immunosuppression, may present with early cutaneous pustules [3].

Candidiasis of the mouth and intertriginous areas of the skin is common [8, 17] but the incidence of infection can probably be lowered by routine oral prophylaxis with amphotericin lozenges to reduce the gut reservoir of this organism. Cutaneous signs of candida septicaemia are not reliable and are, it seems, more likely to be found in leukaemia (see chapter 47). Dermatophyte infections are probably only a little more common on immunosuppression [10, 17], but pityriasis versicolor is undoubtedly very prevalent, with figures of 18% [10], 59% [17] and 70% [18], confirming earlier reports referring to corticosteroid therapy alone.

Most deep fungal infections reported in transplant patients do not show cutaneous lesions but cryptococcosis, reported in seven of 149 patients by Murphy [13], may present with erythema nodosum-like lesions, some showing a striking bruise-like quality. As successful treatment without loss of the kidney may follow prompt diagnosis, early biopsy of such nodules is mandatory. A variety of saprophytic moulds may invade damaged skin in the immunosuppressed patient but the possibility of systemic involvement requires consideration. Phycomycosis of the sinuses may present as facial cellulitis in the immunosuppressed [8] as well as in the diabetic, and Park *et al* [14] have reported a remarkable erysipelas-like case of histoplasmosis after transplantation. Scabies, usually of the Norwegian variety, has been noted several times in immunosuppressed patients [15, 24].

Neoplasms. There is now clear evidence of susceptibility to Kaposi's sarcoma in transplant recipients [16] and reticulum cell sarcoma, which may also involve the skin, appears to be causally related to immunosuppression too [5]. These neoplasms may be reversible if immunosuppression is stopped or reduced [21]. Squamous carcinoma, basal cell carcinoma and keratoacanthoma may all be more common after transplantation [10, 23] and recent work in Glasgow confirms the East Anglian impression that these neoplasms are largely restricted to patients with high levels of sun exposure [4]. The wart virus should not be forgotten as another possible carcinogen in ordinary squamous [10] and verrucous [22] carcinoma.

Miscellaneous. The rapid extension of a long quiescent case of linear porokeratosis of Mibelli was closely related to immunosuppression [12]. Although a widespread eruption of lipid deposits in the skin has now been seen twice in Cambridge [7, 18] it is perhaps surprisingly rare in view of the abnormalities of lipid metabolism commonly found in renal homograft recipients. Gangrene and ischaemic lesions are frequent in such patients in whom arterial disease is almost universal. Livedo reticularis, sometimes with ulceration, may present immediately after surgery or later [18].

REFERENCES

1 ADU D., *et al* (1973) *Br Med J* ii, 280.
2 AXELROD J. L. (1980) In *Infections in the Abnormal Host*, Ed. Grieco M. H. New York, Yorke Medical, Ch. 19.
3 BACH M. C., *et al* (1973) *Lancet* i, 180.
4 BOYLE J., *et al* (1984) *Lancet* i, 702.
5 DEODHAR D. S., *et al* (1969) *N Engl J Med* 280, 1104.
6 GOERZ G. & ILLGNER M. (1972) *Hautarzt* 23, 37.
7 GOLDIN D., *et al* (1975) *Br J Dermatol* 93, (Suppl. 11), 59.
8 HAIM S., *et al* (1973) *Br J Dermatol* 89, 169.
9 HARPER J. R., *et al* (1969) *Br Med J* iii, 637.
10 KORANDA F. C., *et al* (1974) *JAMA* 229, 419.
11 LOMVARDIAS S. & MADGE G. E. (1972) *Arch Dermatol* 106, 875.
12 MACMILLAN A. L. & ROBERTS S. O. B. (1974) *Br J Dermatol* 90, 45.

13 MURPHY J. F. *et al* (1976) *Arch Intern Med* 136, 670.
14 PARK R. K. *et al* (1967) *Arch Dermatol* 95, 345.
15 PATERSON W. D., *et al* (1973) *Br Med J* iv, 211.
16 PENN I. (1979) *Transplantation* 27, 8.
17 PERIS Z. & COHAR F. (1975) *Acta Dermatol Iug* 2, 145.
18 ROBERTS S. O. B. Unpublished observations.
19 ROSTENBERG E. W. & YUSK J. W. (1970) *Arch Dermatol* 101, 439.
20 SAVIN J. A. & NOBLE W. C. (1975) *Br J Dermatol* 93, 115.
21 STARZL T. E. *et al* (1984) *Lancet* i, 583.
22 TURNER J. E. *et al* (1980) *Arch Dermatol* 116, 1074.
23 WALDER B. K., *et al* (1971) *Lancet* ii, 1282.
24 YOUSHECK E. & GLAZER S. D. (1981) *JAMA* 246, 2608.

Graft-versus-host disease [1, 3, 6]. If subjects with defective immunity are given immunologically competent lymphocytes a reaction involving particularly the skin, the gastrointestinal tract and the liver may develop. This is known as graft-versus-host disease. It is frequently seen in patients with aplastic anaemia, leukaemia or immune defects treated by bone marrow grafting and is the major cause of death in these circumstances. It may occasionally follow leukocyte infusions in an immunosuppressed subject [10].

There are two forms of this disease: the acute, occurring between 1 week and 3 months after transplantation, and the chronic form, which appears later [6]. For either form to develop the graft must include immunologically competent cells, the host should possess important (non-HLA) antigens which are lacking in the donor and the host must be incapable of mounting an effective immune reaction against the graft. Although mature T-cells in the graft tissue are thought to be the important initiators of the reaction the mechanisms underlying the full expression of the graft-versus-host process are not fully understood [1]. Humoral antibodies may well have a role and infections, viral and otherwise, are believed to influence the process and certainly they affect the outcome. In one series patients with HLA B18 were three times more likely than others to develop graft-versus-host disease while HLA BW35 appeared to be associated with a lower than average incidence of this complication [9].

Clinical features [3]. The acute form of graft-versus-host disease, typically occurring a few weeks after transplantation, is characterized by fever, an erythematous macular rash often beginning on the face but spreading to the hands, the trunk and the limbs, and diarrhoea and liver dysfunction. The cutaneous signs may settle or evolve into a diffuse maculopapular erythema, with scaling lichenoid papules or bullae. These blisters sometimes resemble toxic epidermal necrolysis of the erythema multiforme type.

Chronic graft-versus-host disease is generally defined as that which follows grafting by a period of at least 3 months [8]. Most patients will have previously shown signs of the acute form but in a minority of approximately 20% there is no such history. This form is very variable but patients show features of several different collagen diseases. The cutaneous eruption is often widespread and papular, and it may closely resemble lichen planus [7, 11]: scaling and hyperpigmentation may appear and later the face and the extremities may show severe systemic sclerosis-like changes with contractures and ulceration. Morphoeic lesions without the classic violaceous peripheral erythema are also found [5, 12]. There may be dystrophic nails and partial alopecia: mouth lesions suggesting lichen planus and oesophagitis occur, while Sjögren syndrome features—dry mouth and eyes—are common. Polymyositis is a recognized part of the syndrome in some cases: hepatic changes are relatively mild but pulmonary function is often impaired as a result of fibrosis.

In the acute form liver function tests are typically abnormal. In the chronic cases eosinophilia, hypergammaglobulinaemia and autoantibody formation are common.

Histology [4, 8]. In the mild acute maculopapular form there is focal or diffuse vacuolation of epidermal basal cells. In severe examples focal or diffuse spongiosis with eosinophilic degeneration of epidermal cells and closely applied lymphocytes are seen; the picture may be similar to that of epidermal necrolysis. With the chronic form the initial changes may resemble those described above but a lichen planus-like lymphocytic invasion of the dermo-epidermal junction with marked basal cell degeneration is also found. Later the collagen bundles of the dermis tend to become hyalinized, coarse and tightly packed with a sparse lymphocytic infiltrate resembling that seen in scleroderma. There may be either thickening or atrophy of the overlying epidermis.

Differential diagnosis. In the acute form drug eruptions and the exanthems of various infections must be considered. Lichen planus and scleroderma developing months after transplantation strongly suggest graft-versus-host disease but such a diagnosis should not be forgotten in any immunosuppressed patient who has received a lymphocyte infusion and who develops any of the clinical syndrome within the range outlined above [10].

Treatment. Mild acute cases with only skin lesions often settle without treatment but more severe acute or chronic cases are commonly fatal, a mortality up to 50–70% being usual without treatment. Because infections appear to play a major role a combination of antibiotic and immunosuppressant therapy was originally used. It now seems that cyclosporin A prophylaxis (rather than treatment) by greatly reducing the severity of the reaction will lead to a much reduced mortality [2]. Alternatively pretreatment of the graft tissue with monoclonal antibodies to remove all mature functioning T-cells may be equally effective. It prevents the development of graft-versus-host disease while still allowing satisfactory engraftment [1].

REFERENCES

1 Anonymous leading article (1984) *Lancet* i, 491.
2 BARRETT A. J., *et al* (1982) *Br Med J* **285**, 162.
3 GLUCKSBERG H., *et al* (1974) *Trqnsplantation* **18**, 295.
4 LERNER K. G., *et al* (1974) *Transplant Proc* **6**, 367.
5 MASTERS R., *et al* (1975) *Arch Dermatol* **111**, 1526.
6 MATSUOKA L. Y. (1981) *J Am Acad Derm* **5**, 595.
7 SAURAT J. H., *et al* (1975) *Br J Dermatol* **92**, 591.
8 SHULMAN H. M., *et al* (1980) *Am J Med* **69**, 204.
9 STORB R., *et al* (1983) *Lancet* ii, 816.
10 TOLBERT B., *et al* (1983) *J Am Acad Dermatol* **9**, 416.
11 TOURAINE R., *et al* (1975) *Br J Dermatol* **92**, 589.
12 VAN VLOTEN W. A., *et al* (1977) *Br J Dermatol* **96**, 337.

CHAPTER 64
Tumours of the Skin

RONA M. MacKIE

INTRODUCTION

Definition. Because tumours are identified most precisely by the pathologist, many definitions of their nature and classifications of their types have been made from the pathologists' point of view. Willis [2] defines a true tumour as '. . . an abnormal mass of tissue, the growth of which exceeds and is uncoordinated with that of the normal tissues, and persists in the same excessive manner after cessation of the stimuli which evoked the change'. This definition excludes reparative proliferations, hyperplasias and malformations. Whilst it is true that these are the result of quite separate pathological processes, it is convenient in a clinical textbook to include certain hyperplasias and malformations among skin tumours. This is justifiable, in that some of these conditions may become truly neoplastic if their natural evolution is permitted.

When all the facts, clinical and pathological, are considered it becomes impossible to draw a line between malformations and tumours. It is sometimes equally difficult to separate completely benign from malignant tumours. In fact tumours, like most other biological processes, vary continuously between the extremes, and elude precise definition and classification. The definition proposed by Willis is used as the basis for this section because it is more generally true than any other so far advanced and has the merit of emphasizing that neoplasms are the result of stimuli which previously have acted on the diseased tissue.

Classification. The most logical method of classifying tumours is on their histogenesis [2]. The tissue of origin can usually be identified on microscopy, but the exact direction of differentiation of tumour cells is often hard to determine. Electron microscopy and histochemical techniques are adding more precise information than can be obtained by ordinary histological examination.

The tumours of the skin have suffered from overclassification. A variety of schemes has been proposed, but there is no uniformity between different countries, and nomenclature varies not only from one nation to another but even within a single country and between dermatologist, pathologist and surgeon. The aim in this chapter is to reduce the number of categories to as few as possible and to require a distinctive clinical pattern of behaviour and microscopical appearance as a justification for each type. The classification conforms closely to that suggested by the W.H.O. International Reference Centre [1].

The fundamental divisions are into epithelial, melanocytic and mesodermal tumours. Tumours of the lymphoreticular system are considered in Chapter 47. Epithelial tumours can be subdivided broadly into those of the epidermis, which differentiate toward keratin formation, and those of the appendages and the germinal layer of the epidermis which differentiate toward glandular structures. Basal cell carcinoma falls more naturally into the second subdivision. Cysts of the skin form a third epidermal category. In the classification of melanocytic, neural and mesenchymal tumours, common ground on most points has been established between clinician and pathologist, and the accepted classification is followed here.

Terminology. The benign tumours have long been named in a way that defies rationalization. Pathologists object to the use of the term naevus and in particular to 'cellular naevus', which many of them consider should be called benign melanoma. Melanocytic naevus has been accepted by some as a compromise and is preferred in this section. The general approach here to the nomenclature of benign tumours is conservative and in line with current clinical usage. It is reasonable to term malignant epithelial tumours carcinomas, and malignant connective-tissue tumours sarcomas, and to qualify the title to indicate the derivation and direction of differentiation of the tumour cells. The various titles which will be used, and their synonyms, will be given in each section of the text.

REFERENCES

1 TEN SELDAM R. E. J., *et al* (1974) *International Histological Classification of Tumours No. 12. Histological Typing of Skin Tumours.* Geneva, W.H.O.
2 WILLIS R. A. (1967) *Pathology of Tumours.* London, Butterworths.

Incidence and epidemiology. Common experience suggests that most people suffer from one or more benign tumours, such as melanocytic naevi, skin tags and seborrhoeic warts. The exact prevalence of benign tumours is unknown, but their frequency is much greater than hospital or private practice statistics would suggest.

Most of the sources of information on the frequency of malignant skin tumours are worthless from an epidemiological point of view because they are based on selected series of cases seen in the clinic, or by pathologists, and cannot be related to the populations from which they are drawn. The best epidemiological approach, and the one used by the surveys of cancer incidence in the U.S.A. ('Ten cities' survey') by the National Cancer Institute [6] is to examine the medical histories of all patients treated in geographically and demographically defined areas during a known period. The results of such surveys [6, 15] allow the problem to be viewed in relation to cancer incidence in other organs, and make clear some of the predisposing factors and environmental causes.

Carcinoma of the skin is most prevalent in countries such as Australia, South Africa and the southern part of the U.S.A., where fair-complexioned people are exposed to sun and wind. Mortality rates are the most readily available data, but are influenced by factors other than the prevalence of the disorder and may reflect the quality of medical care or the readiness of the population to seek attention. Crude mortality rates for malignant melanoma have shown a progressive increase in a number of countries with predominantly European populations between 1950 and 1958, while the rate for other skin malignancies was decreasing [27]. The age-adjusted mortality rate in males is highest in Australia, with South Africa, Ireland, New Zealand and the U.S.A. ranked in descending order [22].

The peculiar susceptibility of people of Irish and Scottish descent to sunlight-induced tumours is well known in Australia and the U.S.A. [7, 23], and has been attributed to the natural selection of a thin poorly pigmented skin, through the effect over many generations of rickets and other disorders, as a biologically desirable characteristic of the countries of origin. This racial characteristic, and the importance of agricultural pursuits, probably account for the high mortality rate in the Irish Republic.

In the U.S.A. the incidence rate of skin cancer in white people of the same age group increases as their place of living becomes closer to the equator, doubling for each 265 miles [3]. The incidence in coloured people shows only a slight increase with added exposure to sunlight. The overall incidence of skin cancer of the exposed skin is 15 times greater in Caucasians than in Negroes in the U.S.A. [6]. The relative immunity of dark-skinned people is found in all countries, and is due to skin colour rather than any other racial characteristic as is shown by the high incidence of skin cancer in the albino Bantu [5]. The most susceptible of the fair-skinned people are those with blue or grey irises, red hair and freckles [7]. A multivariate analysis of a number of factors in Queensland has shown that age and occupation are highly significant in their relation to skin cancer. Other important factors are a sunburn reaction to sunlight, complexion, ancestry and eye colour, in that order [23]. The capacity to tan readily without sunburn protects the skin by dispersing the pigment in the epidermis in a manner similar to the pigment distribution in Negroes [17]. In sunny climates susceptible subjects develop their keratoses and skin cancers a decade or more before those who tan easily and have been exposed to similar conditions. They also develop tumours in greater numbers [7]. In East Africans squamous cell carcinoma commonly occurs in scars, mainly those due to burns [4].

The facts relating skin cancer to occupational environment have been extensively reviewed [8–13, 26]. The prevalence of industrial skin cancer is determined by the potency of the carcinogens and by the thoroughness of the measures used to protect workers from them. The likelihood of an individual developing tumours depends also on the duration of the exposure. An inverse relationship between age at first exposure and the latent period has been noticed with cutting oils and some other industrial carcinogens. As the latent period between exposure and development of tumours may be several decades, exact statistics are difficult to determine, and many of the published figures represent the lowest approximation to the true incidence. In the case of arsenic there is conflicting evidence about its carcinogenicity in industry [14, 19], which is hard to explain, except in terms of the duration and thoroughness of the follow-up. The analysis of death certificates by occupation correlates high rates with known occupational hazards [8], but is, again, a rough approximation only.

It would be a mistake to assume that skin cancer

occurs mainly in people with skin which does not tan easily on sun exposure or that it is rare in a relatively sun-starved country like the U.K. The data of Payne & Chilvers [18] show quite marked geographical variation of incidence in Southern England which can be attributed to the different proportions of farm and other outdoor workers in the regional populations. There is an obvious difference in the prevalence of actinic damage to the skin and of skin cancer between coalminers and farmers or gardeners [2]. In areas like Australia the majority of the white population tan readily, and tumours may occur in such people, although at a somewhat later age than those who do not tan.

Surveys in Texas [15, 16] showed a considerable increase in the prevalence of skin cancer in two decades, and the rates appear to have doubled in Minnesota in the last 10 yr [21], confirming the impressions of dermatologists working in high incidence areas. This may be partly due to the changing age structure of the population, but changing habits of dress and recreation must also be important. It is unlikely that the U.S. government will make sunbathing illegal or that the Australian or South African governments will prohibit fair-complexioned migrants. We must anticipate, therefore, an ever-increasing incidence of skin cancer in such countries unless the popular attitude to sunbathing changes.

Regional and occupational incidence of skin cancer can be influenced by other enviromental factors, such as arsenic in drinking water [1, 25] or as an occupational hazard [20, 24], contact with mineral oils or the products of combustion of coal and exposure to X-rays or radiant heat. These agents will be considered in more detail in the following section.

REFERENCES

1 ARGUELLO R. A., *et al* (1950) *Rev Fac Cien Med Univ nac Córdoba* **8**, 409.

2 ATKINS M., *et al* (1949) *Br J Cancer* **3**, 1.

3 AUERBACH H. (1961) *Public Health Rep* **76**, 345.

4 BURKITT D. P., *et al* (1968) *Br J Cancer* **22**, 1.

5 COHEN L., *et al* (1952) *S Afr Med J* **26**, 932.

6 *DORN H. F. & CUTLER S. J. (1959) *Morbidity from Cancer in the United States*. Public Health Monograph No. 56.

7 HALL A. F. (1950) *Arch Dermatol Syphilol* **61**, 589.

8 HENRY S. A. (1950) *Ann R Coll Surg Engl* **7**, 425.

9 *HUEPER W. C. (1942) *Occupational Tumors and Allied Diseases*, Springfield, Thomas.

10 HUEPER W. C. (1948) *Public Health Rep* (Suppl.) 209.

11 HUEPER W. C. (1954) *AMA Arch Pathol* **58**, 360, 475, 645.

12 HUEPER W. C. (1963) *Nat Cancer Inst Monogr* **10**, 377.

13 KENNAWAY E. L. & KENNAWAY N. M. (1946) *Cancer Res* **4**, 49.

14 LEE A. M. & FRAUMENI J. F. (1969) *J Natl Cancer Inst* **42**, 1045.

15 MACDONALD E. J. (1959) *J Invest Dermatol* **32**, 379.

16 MACDONALD E. J. & BUBENDORF E. (1964) In *Tumors of the Skin*. Eds. Cumley R. W., *et al*. Chicago, Year Book Publishers, p. 23.

17 OLSEN R. L. (1971) *Cutis* **8**, 225.

18 PAYNE P. M. & CHILVERS J. S. W. (1963) *South Metropolitan Cancer Registry* Report for 1960.

19 PINTO S. S. & BENNETT B. M. (1963) *Arch Environ Health* **7**, 583.

20 ROTH F. (1957) *Ger Med Mon* **2**, 172.

21 SCOTTO J., *et al* (1974) *Cancer* **34**, 1333.

22 SEGI M. (1963) *Natl Cancer Inst Monogr* **10**, 245.

23 SILVERSTONE H. & SEARLE J. H. A. (1970) *Br J Cancer* **24**, 235.

24 THIERS H., *et al* (1970) *Ann Dermatol Syphiligr* **94**, 133.

25 TSENG W. P., *et al* (1968) *J Natl Cancer Inst* **40**, 453.

26 WATERHOUSE J. A. H. (1971) *Ann Occup Hyg* **14**, 161.

27 W. H. O. (1960) *Epidemiol Vit Stat Rep* **13**, 426.

AETIOLOGY

Genetic factors. The tendency to develop some types of benign skin tumours may be genetically determined, usually by an autosomal dominant mode of inheritance. The tumours are commonly multiple, symmetrically disposed and in some instances most profuse on the head and upper trunk. Their appearance may be delayed until puberty or later and there may be defects in other tissues. The late onset is not incompatible with genetic influences because the skin, and particularly its appendages, continues to develop until adult life. A degree of histological variation may occur in the tumours of a family, or even of an individual. Included among these tumours are tricho-epithelioma, dermal cylindroma, steatocystoma multiplex, basal cell naevus, neurofibroma, glomangioma and, probably, seborrhoeic keratosis. It is more difficult to make judgement on the genetics of common tumours than on that of rare tumours, and the inheritance of melanocytic tumours and basal cell carcinoma is not clear.

There is some evidence that the susceptibility of the skin to carcinogenic agents may be genetically influenced. The extreme sensitivity of patients with xeroderma pigmentosum (p. 144) is a recessive characteristic, and has been attributed to a defective repair replication of DNA [7–9]. The influence of constitutional factors, for which no genetic basis has yet been shown, is of importance in some conditions. Perhaps the most striking of these is that of the patients with multiple sebaceous adenomas and multiple primary malignant tumours of the viscera (Torre's syndrome, p. 2349). Arsenical cancer of the skin is exclusively squamous cell in some individuals and basal cell in others, while many patients show both types [27]. The variation in response to dose schedules of the same order presumably depends on some constitutional factor. The larger question of why only some members of a group of individuals exposed to a carcinogen develop tumours is still unsolved. An interesting possibility is that the ease of induction of enzymes such as aryl hydrocarbon hydroxylase within the target tissue may determine how sensitive it is to chemical carcinogens [22]. This is discussed further on p. 2385.

Oncogenes and malignancy [6, 10, 31]. A number of human malignancies have recently been found to contain within their nuclear DNA sequences of amino acids which are also found in animal tumours. These sequences or *oncogenes* have the ability to transform cultured murine cells (NIH 3T3 strain) from the benign to the malignant state. The oncogenes do exist in premalignant lesions and as 'proto oncogenes' in normal tissue but appear to become 'de-repressed' in malignant cells. Recent work has demonstrated that at least one oncogene is structurally very similar to platelet-derived growth factor (PDGF). Oncogene activity is also associated with chromosomal translocations.

Environmental causes. Percivall Pott described cancer of the scrotum in chimney sweeps two centuries ago. The immediate cause of this cancer was prolonged soiling of the rugose skin with soot from coal fires. The circumstances which lay behind it were more complex, involving such things as a widespread fear of a recurrence of the Great Fire of 1666, changing styles of domestic architecture, the composition of coal mined in England, the laws and customs governing the care of orphans and foundlings, and the general standards of personal hygiene. It took a hundred years for reformers to overcome powerful interests and to persuade

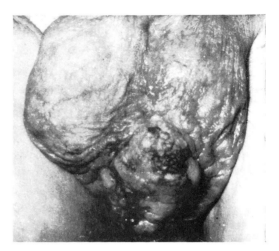

FIG. 64.1. Chimney sweeps' cancer of the scrotum. For many years the patient had ridden a bicycle with his brushes on the cross-bar. (Stoke Mandeville Hospital.)

Parliament to pass laws preventing children being used as sweeps.

A number of other environmental carcinogens acting on the skin have been recognized; the more important are shown in Table 64.1.

Legislation to protect later industrial workers has been less tardy than in the case of chimney sweeps. Preventative measures are not yet completely successful against occupational hazards or those which occur in the practice of medicine. Cases of scrotal cancer due to lubricating and cutting oils [10] still occur, although machines are now generally shielded to prevent splashing and adequate washrooms for bathing are provided by employers [5]. Legislation cannot make workers use protective measures and wash properly. The final responsibility for his cancer rests with the workman. The occurrence of subsequent malignancies in other

TABLE 64.1. Some important skin carcinogens for man [10, 21, 23, 30]

Agent	Average latent period (in years)	Range	Year recognized
Coal tar	20	1–50	1874
Creosote oil	25	15–45	1920
Mineral oil	50	4–75	1870 (shale oil)
			1910 (shale lubricating oil)
Crude paraffin	15	3–35	1930 (petroleum lubricating oil)
Cutting oil	35	5–55	1950
Arsenic	18	3–46	1888 (medicinal)
Sunlight	20–30	15–40	1875
X-rays	21	1–64	1902

organs, as well as the skin, following scrotal cancer [20] suggests that oil may be a carcinogen by inhalation or ingestion. Arsenical skin cancer was described in 1888, and the records of the first case suggest the patient may have died from primary carcinoma of the lung. Arsenic is still used in dermatology [14] and in the treatment of asthma [19] in doses in the hazardous range.

Although chemical agents, especially those derived from coal and mineral oil, are the main industrial danger, the most important environmental cause, as the epidemiological statistics show, is exposure of susceptible people to sunlight. The most damaging part of the spectrum is in the 290–330 nm range (UV B) [1]. This is effectively removed by passage through glass, or through air containing high concentrations of water vapour. Dry sunny climates are therefore the most dangerous. The atmospheric absorption of UV B increases as the angle of incidence of the solar rays decreases, which accounts for the statistical correlation of prevalence to decreasing latitude. It is of practical importance that as much as 50% of UV B may reach the skin as scattered radiation from the sky and by reflection from sand and other surfaces [11, 13, 29]. Protection from the direct rays of the sun is not sufficient to prevent solar damage. The reaction of the skin to different dose rates and different intervals between doses of UV B radiation, e.g. frequent lower dose rates as might be experienced by outdoor workers compared with less frequent higher dose rates from weekend radiation, has not been established in man. Analogy with superficial radiotherapy and with animal experiments [2] suggest that such differences may be important.

The effect of sunlight is cumulative and produces other changes in the skin before malignancy appears. The rugged appearance of the males and the weather-beaten complexion of the females in middle-aged Texans and Australians stand out in comparison with the fresher complexions of their British and Scandinavian counterparts. These changes in the skin texture are due mainly to dermal elastosis, which personal observation suggests may be reversible in the early stage if further sun exposure is avoided. Transposition of skin grafts between exposed and covered areas has given further evidence of reversibility [18].

Exposure to ionizing radiation may occur as an accidental occupational hazard or as the result of medical investigation or treatment. The skin is relatively insensitive to the carcinogenic effect of ionizing radiation compared with tissues such as the thyroid gland. However, doses which leave no evidence of atrophy, such as were used to treat tinea capitis or ankylosing spondylitis, have produced multiple malignancies, usually basal cell carcinoma or fibroepithelioma. The improved apparatus of the last two decades, and the increased knowledge of the hazard of even low doses of irradiation, should make iatrogenic radiation cancer a rare event in the future. Whether this will also be true of occupational exposure depends on the awareness of the danger among workmen and those who supervise them.

Longer-wavelength radiant energy may be carcinogenic. Radiant heat produced the Kangri cancer of Kashmir and occasional cases of cancer on the lower legs of people who huddle too close to coal fires [25]. Grenz rays may also be carcinogenic [3]. Carcinoma may occur in the scars of past pathological processes such as tuberculosis, syphilis, leprosy, burns and other injuries. Although some tumours may be the result of the treatment of the primary disorder with X-rays, UV radiation or other carcinogenic agents, it seems likely that scar tissue is abnormally susceptible. Malignant transformation may occur in venous ulcers of the lower leg. The rare examples of psoriasis becoming malignant are probably due to the use of tar and UV radiation in treatment [26].

Patients often give a history of recent injury to explain a skin tumour. Critical examination of these claims will usually show them to be groundless or, at the least, unable to satisfy the criteria laid down by Ewing [15] for such an association to be valid. This is a point of more than academic interest where the injury has been sustained at work and compensation is claimed. In those writings specifically concerned with the medico-legal aspects [4], the opinion is generally advanced that there is no evidence that injury can cause tumours, although some writers are careful to say that this applies only to normal skin [1]. The findings of both experimental pathologists [24] and clinicians [16] suggest tht injury can localize and promote a skin tumour in skin previously exposed to a carcinogenic stimulus. At least two series of cases claim to meet Ewing's criteria [12, 17]. In most instances the injury has been a small burn or a penetrating injury by a hot fragment. The commonest type of tumour has been basal cell carcinoma. It is likely that there is a much larger number of unreported cases where a valid connection is probable; the figures of Pack & Treves [28] suggest that 1 in 500 skin malignancies follow directly on a burn to the area. The author has experience of three cases of carcinoma of the vermilion of the lip following immediately on a burn, two sections of squamous cell carcinoma with wood splinters embedded under them and a case of squamous cell carcinoma of the upper eyelid following a burn with a fragment from a blast furnace. Fragments of mineral material seen beneath the tumour on microscopic examination confirmed the patient's history in the last of these cases.

REFERENCES

1 *BLUM H. F. (1959) *Carcinogenesis by Ultraviolet Light.* Princeton University Press, Princeton.

2 BLUM H. F. (1969) In *Biologic Effect of Ultraviolet Radiation.* Ed. Urbach F. Oxford, Pergamon, p. 543.

3 BRODKIN R. H. & BLEIBERG J. (1968) *Arch Dermatol* **97**, 307.

4 BRODKIN R. H. & BLEIBERG J. (1970) *Med Trial Tech Q* **17**, 37.

5 BROWN A. J., *et al* (1975) *Report on a Study of Occupational Skin Cancer.* Birmingham, University of Birmingham.

6 CAPON D. J., *et al* (1983) *Nature* **302**, 33.

7 CLEAVER J. E. (1968) *Nature* **218**, 652.

8 CLEAVER J. E. (1970) *J Invest Dermatol* **54**, 181.

9 *CLEAVER J. E. (1974) *Adv Radiat Biol* **4**, 1.

10 CRUIKSHANK C. N. D. & SQUIRE J. R. (1950) *Br J Ind Med* **7**, 1.

11 DER C. J., *et al.* (1982) *Proc Natl Acad Sci USA* **79**, 3637.

12 DIX C. P. (1960) *Plast Reconstr Surg* **26**, 546.

13 DUKE-ELDER SIR STEWART (1972) *System of Ophthalmology.* London, Kimpton, Vol. 14, Part I, p. 701.

14 EHLERS G. (1968) *Z Haut Geschlkrankh* **43**, 763.

15 EWING J. (1935) *Arch Pathol* **19**, 690.

16 EWING M. R. (1971) *Aust NZ J Surg* **41**, 140.

17 GARDINER A. W. (1959) *Lancet* **i**, 760.

18 GERSTEIN W. & FREEMAN R. G. (1963) *J Invest Dermatol* **41**, 445.

19 HARTER J. G. & NOVITCH A. M. (1967) *J Allergy* **40**, 6.

20 HOLMES J. G., *et al* (1970) *Lancet* **ii**, 214.

21 HUEPER W. C. (1963) *Natl Cancer Inst Monogr* **10**, 377.

22 KELLERMAN G., *et al* (1973) *N Engl J Med* **289**, 934.

23 MARTIN H., *et al* (1970) *Cancer* **25**, 61.

24 ORR J. W. (1935) *Br J Exp Pathol* **16**, 121.

25 PETERKIN G. A. G. (1955) *Br Med J* **ii**, 1599.

26 ROOK A. J., *et al* (1956) *Br J Cancer* **10**, 17.

27 SANDERSON K. V. (1963) *Trans Rep St Johns Hosp Dermatol Soc* **49**, 115.

28 TREVES N. & PACK G. T. (1930) *Surg Gynecol Obstet* **51**, 749.

29 *URBACH F., *et al* (1966) In *Advances in Biology of Skin.* Vol. 7. *Carcinogenesis.* Eds. Montagna W. & Dobson R. L. Oxford, Pergamon, p. 195.

30 WATERHOUSE J. A. H. (1971) *Ann Occup Hyg* **14**, 161.

31 WEINBERG R. A. (1981) *Biochim Biophys Acta* **651**, 25.

32 WOODHOUSE D. L. (1960) In *Progress in the Biological Sciences in Relation to Dermatology.* Ed. Rook A. Cambridge, Cambridge University Press, p. 356.

GENERAL PATHOLOGICAL CONSIDERATIONS

Clinicopathological links. Many tumours have a distinctive micro-anatomical structure, which is partly evident in histological preparations and can be more fully displayed by special techniques [10, 12, 13]. Some features of the architecture can be deduced from the external appearance. Many benign tumours have a symmetrical shape, suggesting equal growth about an axis. Malignant tumours frequently have an irregular contour. A papillary surface implies elongation of dermal papillae, either in combination with epidermal proliferation or because an accumulation of cells within the papillae has expanded the epidermis covering them. The clear-cut margin of a circumscribed and expansive tumour like a nodular basal cell carcinoma contrasts with the vague or indeterminate edge of an infiltrating growth such as a morphoeic or terebrant basal cell carcinoma. The terms exophytic and endophytic, used by European dermatologists, correspond roughly to these two patterns of growth.

The first step in diagnosis is to decide whether the tumour is basically epidermal or dermal. The state of the surface can be seen only if adherent keratin and crusts are removed. Firmly attached hyperkeratosis indicates disturbance of maturing prickle cells. Ulceration and erosion may be due to a more deeply situated disorder of epidermal cells, to their replacement by malignant cells from elsewhere or to alterations in the papillary dermis affecting their nutrition. The appearance of the epithelium at the margin of the tumour may indicate whether the growth is arising in or beneath the epidermis. The shape of benign intradermal tumours and cysts is, in general, of little help in their diagnosis, but the stony-hard lobular consistency of trichomatrixoma may be.

The presence of specialized cells in a tumour may be apparent from the surface. The brown colour of melanin is an example and, when present in excess, presupposes functioning melanocytes at some stage of the tumour's evolution. Spreading and fluctuating pigmentation may be more reliable than the histological features as a sign of macular malignant lentigo in some cases (p. 2446). Melanin produced within the dermis and dispersed among the collagen looks blue, owing to the subtractive mixing of colours [3]. Maturing keratinocytes, whether benign or malignant, give an opaque quality to the surface. Cells with little cytoplasm, such as those of basal cell carcinoma or intradermal melanocytic naevus, give a jelly-like translucency to the tumour.

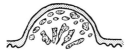

Intradermal melanocytic naevus

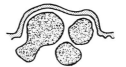

Nodular basal cell carcinoma

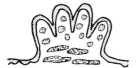

Compound melanocytic naevus

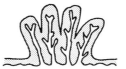

Verrucous seborrhoeic wart

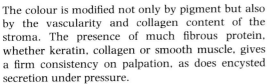

Ulcerated squamous cell carcinoma

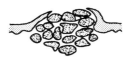

Ulcerated malignant melanoma

FIG. 64.2. Architectural features of some common tumours.

The colour is modified not only by pigment but also by the vascularity and collagen content of the stroma. The presence of much fibrous protein, whether keratin, collagen or smooth muscle, gives a firm consistency on palpation, as does encysted secretion under pressure.

Multiple and symmetrical tumours are generally determined genetically, even if their eruption is delayed until adolescence or later. Many of these are hamartomas composed of two or more elements, which have made an incomplete and distorted attempt to form one of the normal parts of the skin.

Those of ectodermal origin have a distinctive stroma [8].

The natural history of tumours is determined by their architecture and pattern of growth. Hamartomas tend to reach a limiting size and to regain this if partly removed. Kerato-acanthoma enlarges rapidly, not only because of frequent cell division but also because the products of the proliferating squamous cells are retained within the lesion instead of being shed, as might occur with a growth on the surface, or absorbed, because the products are more labile, as in basal cell carcinoma.

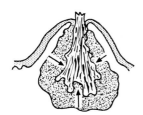

Keratoacanthoma

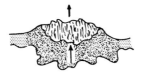

Squamous cell carcinoma

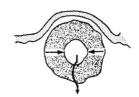

Cystic basal cell carcinoma

FIG. 64.3. Cellular currents which may influence the rate of tumour growth.

The rate of growth and the invasiveness of a tumour may alter fairly abruptly owing to a change either in the character of the tumour cell or in the cellular and humoral response of the host. Some lesions react to external stimuli. Leiomyoma cutis may contract if the skin is chilled. Some cystic sweat gland tumours increase in size when the skin is exposed to heat. Tumours of smooth muscle, peripheral nerve or sweat gland origin may be painful on pressure or with temperature change, or even without stimulation. Pulsations may be found in cutaneous metastasis from hypernephroma, thyroid carcinoma and multiple myeloma, as well as in vascular sarcomas, arterial aneurysms and arterio-venous fistulae [14].

Criteria of malignancy. If by its growth and invasion a tumour destroys the patient, there is no doubt that it is malignant. This is the ultimate criterion of biological malignancy; the occurrence of metastasis or lymphatic spread is an equally valid criterion. Much of the dispute about the benign or malignant nature of basal cell carcinoma [9] would have been avoided if the results of neglected or failed treatment had been considered. Skin tumours are most favourably situated for treatment to frustrate these natural criteria. In practice the pathologist is the judge; a skin tumour is regarded as malignant or not by its appearance under the microscope, and in most cases a definite verdict is possible. The importance of checking histological criteria against clinical evidence is shown in kerato-acanthoma and juvenile melanoma, which were both regarded as malignant tumours by the majority of pathologists until quite recently.

In a small proportion of cases there may be disagreement among expert pathologists on the nature or potentialities of a tumour, or a definite opinion may be impossible. Amelanotic malignant melanoma may be indistinguishable from anaplastic carcinoma or sarcoma, but the outcome is not usually altered for the patient. The distinction between a melanocytic naevus with active junctional proliferation and an early malignant melanoma is much more important and may require great experience and the concensus of several opinions. The stage at which a lesion such as a solar keratosis or Bowen's disease becomes malignant is largely a semantic question, depending on the criteria of malignancy adopted by the individual pathologist as much as on the stage of development of the process. It is a point of more than academic interest, however, when there is the possibility of metastasis. There is no sharp boundary between innocence and malignancy, and there are no infallible criteria. The

higher magnification of electron microscopy has not revealed specific features of malignant cells that cannot be seen by light microscopy [4]. The diagnosis of pre-invasive malignancy is, in general, made on the presence of abnormal cells replacing the epithelium, and it is distinguished from overt malignancy by the confinement of these cells within the natural boundaries of the epithelium. The inflammatory response found immediately beneath such lesions is probably part of an immune defence against invasion by the altered epidermal cells, which are antigenically indistinguishable.

Histological criteria

Cellular changes. The orderly and graduated arrangement of cells which gives the normal structure its distinctive appearance may be disturbed, a phenomenon which can be described as loss of polarity. This may result in incomplete differentiation (anaplasia), delayed maturation in some areas and premature maturation in others. Functions which demand the organization of numbers of cells, such as the formation of a hair shaft, are more easily disturbed than those, like melanin production, which can be performed by a single cell. Metaplasia (differentiation in an abnormal direction) is uncommon in epithelial tumours of the skin, but it is a feature of mucin-secreting hidradenocarcinomas of the anogenital area (extramammary Paget's disease). Mucin secretion is not a major function of the sweat glands from which these tumours arise [7].

Aberrations of cellular function and organization alone are insufficient evidence of malignancy. Changes in cellular dynamics must be looked for. An increased rate of cell multiplication is shown by more than the normal number of mitoses, and a more radical and characteristic alteration is the presence of abnormalities of the cell nuclei. They may be larger and darker, containing more densely packed nucleoprotein arranged in an atypical way; nucleoli may be prominent and some cells may be multinucleated. Bizarre mitotic figures may be seen.

Patterns of growth. The histological diagnosis and grading of malignancy are achieved by correlating the cellular changes with the effect they produce on the normal structure around the tumour. The components of a hamartoma are organized into a deformed copy of a normal part of the skin. The growth rate tends to be that of normal tissue. The cells are polarized in relation to each other and to the stroma. Nuclear abnormalities and excessive mitotic activity are not seen. The cells are more or less mature. This degree of organization is lacking in malignant tumours. A semblance of tumour–stroma polarization takes place at the margin of many basal cell carcinomas (p. 2417), and in the most highly differentiated of these tumours distinction from a hamartoma, e.g. tricho-epithelioma, may be impossible on histological evidence alone. In rare instances a hamartoma may give rise to a malignant tumour, a happening seen most frequently in naevus sebaceus in the skin. The prevalence of basal cell carcinoma in a relatively unselected series of naevus sebaceus has been put at 6·5% [18].

Spread of tumours. Malignant skin tumours behave as if they start in a small focus and spread locally by multiplication of their cells. The mathematics of cell division in tumour growth makes it obvious that many of the cells must die without dividing. Recent studies of cell proliferation in basal cell carcinoma [17] suggested an experimentally determined cell-doubling time of 9 days if all the cells were to continue dividing, a finding out of keeping with the rather slow clinical growth rate. Tumours often show areas of cell maturation or necrosis. The cause of the necrosis is not always ischaemia as it can occur in parts of tumours not too far from an adequate blood supply. Selective necrosis causes some tumours to separate from their point of origin. In general, however, a complete cross-section of a tumour leaves little doubt of the way it began and has since evolved.

The best pathological evidence of malignancy is invasion of neighbouring tissues by atypical cells. Slowly invasive tumours may induce around themselves a well-organized stroma. Local spread by expansion or infiltration leads to destruction of adjacent structures and alteration of the small-vessel network. Extension through the dermis is often impeded by the fibrous reticular layer, so that tumour cells spread in the looser perineural and periadnexal connective tissues, a phenomenon also

seen with some benign tumours such as melanocytic naevi and juvenile melanomas.

Collagenolytic activity has been demonstrated in the cells of squamous cell carcinoma, basal cell carcinoma and malignant melanoma [6, 19]. The dissolution of the fibrous component of the dermis is probably partly effected by histiocytes, and it is likely that the cellular response around many malignant growths is not just tissue resistance to foreign invaders [1, 16]. The importance of the defence reaction has been demonstrated in carcinoma of the breast [5], the reaction being a cell-mediated immune response whose histological expression correlates well with prognosis. There have been extensive studies of the immune response to malignant melanoma (p. 2455) where the cell-mediated response also operates. The same type of reaction is seen around some basal cell carcinomas, whilst others may show a predominantly histiocytic response. The former group usually appear to be well contained, whereas the latter are invariably invasive and may show greater mitotic activity and cellular pleomorphism.

The planes of invasion determine in part the clinical appearance of the lesion and to a large extent the size of the area to be treated, and thus are of importance to the clinician. There are three fundamental directions: outwards (exophytic) leading to a vegetating growth and eventually to destruction of the epidermis and ulceration, laterally, producing a plaque-like lesion, and downwards (endophytic) to produce a tumour. The more malignant tumours grow in all three directions. The importance of the direction of growth as an indicator of the invasiveness of malignant melanoma, and hence of the prognosis, has been amply demonstrated (p. 2448).

Some neoplasms, especially when ulcerated, may stimulate the adjacent epidermis to pseudo-epitheliomatous hyperplasia and cause errors of diagnosis. An amelanotic malignant melanoma may thus

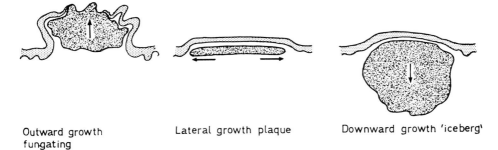

Outward growth fungating   Lateral growth plaque   Downward growth 'iceberg'

FIG. 64.4. The form of tumours produced by different directions of growth.

mimic an anaplastic squamous cell carcinoma. Growing tumours induce their own blood supply by distorting the normal vascular architecture. The degree of hyperaemia partly reflects, and perhaps partly governs [15], the rate of growth. The capillaries within a malignant melanoma may be very profuse, and it is not surprising that haematogenous dissemination of this tumour is so common. Lymphatic dissemination is hard to gauge using microscopy, although it is obvious that the lymph channels are the weak spot in the collagen–ground substance complex of the reticular dermis. Lymphatic and blood stream dissemination occur most commonly in those tumours such as malignant melanoma whose cells have little natural tendency to adhere together. There is, indeed, evidence that the more malignant squamous cells may have lost the capacity to induce a basement membrane substance which normally acts as a bonding material [2]. The presence of actinomyosin-like microfilaments within epidermal cancer cells is indirect evidence that they are actively mobile [11].

Examination of various areas within a single tumour often shows different patterns of growth and cell type. This is an unsuperable obstacle to a neat classification of a heterogeneous group such as basal cell carcinoma and related tumours.

REFERENCES

1 ANDERSON M. R. & GREEN H. N. (1967) *Br J Cancer* **21**, 27.
2 DE MORAGOS J. M., *et al* (1970) *Cancer* **25**, 1404.
3 FINDLAY G. H. (1970) *Br J Dermatol* **83**, 127.
4 HAGUENAU F. (1969) In *The Biological Bases of Medicine.* Eds. Bittar E. E. & Bittar N. New York, Academic Press, p. 433.
5 HAMBLIN I. M. E. (1968) *Br J Cancer* **22**, 383.
6 HASHIMOTO K., *et al* (1973) *Cancer Res* **33**, 2790.
7 HELWIG E. B. & GRAHAM J. H. (1963) *Cancer* **16**, 387.
8 KLIGMAN A. M. & PINKUS H. (1960) *Arch Dermatol* **81**, 922.
9 LEVER W. F. (1948) *Arch Dermatol Syphilol* **57**, 679.
10 *MADSEN A. (1941) *Acta Derm Venereol* (Suppl) (Stockh) **22**, (7).
11 MALECH H. L. & LENTZ T. L. (1974) *J Cell Biol* **60**, 473.
12 OBERSTE-LEHN H. (1954) *Z Haut GeschlKrankh* **16**, 334.
13 SANDERSON K. V. (1961) *Br J Dermatol* **73**, 455.
14 SELMANOWITZ V. J. (1969) *Dermatologica* **138**, 59.
15 TANNOCK I. F. (1968) *Br J Cancer* **22**, 528.
17 WEINSTEIN G. D. & FROST P. (1970) *Cancer Res* **30**, 724.
18 WILSON JONES E. & HEYL T. (1970) *Br J Dermatol* **82**, 99.
19 YAMANISHI Y., *et al* (1973) *Cancer Res* **33**, 2507.

Experimental carcinogenesis. In the last decade advances in different branches of biological research have made the processes of carcinogenesis more comprehensible. They have also shown that cancer is a heterogeneous disease due to a variety of agents working through different mechanisms, and that a simple answer to the cause and nature of cancer is not to be expected [28]. It is possible to touch on only a few aspects of the very extensive literature here, and it is becoming increasingly difficult to cite reviews [6–8, 16, 17, 20, 28] which are sufficiently broad-based to be valuable to clinicians. Perhaps the most interesting aspect of recent work is that which shows the importance of an immune response in the natural history of malignant tumours (p. 2386) and which gives hope that more effective and refined ways of treatment may be at hand.

Chemical agents. Tumours were first reproduced experimentally in 1915 by the application of coal tar to rabbit's skin. Between this event and Pott's description of chimney sweeps' cancer in 1775, arsenic, sunlight, mineral oil, radium and X-rays were all identified as causing skin cancer. Except for arsenic, all these agents, and many others besides, have now been shown to produce tumours in animals. The classical experiments on carcinogenesis were carried out with polycyclic hydrocarbons, mainly on mouse skin, and were at first concerned with the isolation and assay of the chemical agents rather than with the tissue response.

Attempts to correlate chemical structure with carcinogenicity were unconvincing [2] until it was shown that most carcinogens were 'activated' by cellular enzyme systems to produce the ultimate electrophilic carcinogen [22, 23, 30]. The action of such carcinogens is limited to those species and tissues which possess the specific enzyme for the conversion. A clinical example of this is bladder cancer in rubber workers owing to degradation of β-naphthylamine by hydrolysing enzymes in the bladder epithelium. There is a theoretical necessity for activation; the exact site of action, although it may be uncertain, is somewhere within the target cell. To obtain the maximum effect it is desirable that an agent should not react with the extracellular components or cell membranes in its passage from the exterior into the target cell. Carcinogenic potency of chemicals may therefore be a function of the ease with which they can be transported to and across the cell membranes, and the degree to which intracellular mechanisms can uncover their active radicals.

Activation of carcinogenic aromatic hydrocarbons involves the formation of epoxide groups

[30]. A direct effect of carcinogenic hydrocarbons on DNA synthesis has been demonstrated; this is not shared by non-carcinogenic compounds, although both stimulate RNA synthesis [25]. There is no proof, however, of specific qualitative alterations in DNA associated with the action of chemical carcinogens in skin. It may be that they cause an alteration in specific proteins or RNA which results in relatively stable and hereditable changes in genome expression [21]. An even more indirect effect has been suggested, e.g. on the supporting connective tissue in epithelial tumours [24], or on the metabolic activity of cells [34].

Modes of action [19]. The direct effects have been studied in great detail in the case of radiant energy, and the mechanisms of damage and repair that follow UV irradiation are of general significance. The formation of pyrimidine dimers is one of the specific changes induced by UV radiation in the DNA molecule. Free radicals may be the mediators of this reaction, perhaps by forming perhydroxyl radicals through their action on water in the presence of oxygen as has been suggested in the case of ionizing radiation. Whatever the mechanism, the prevalence of such changes was not appreciated until the DNA repair mechanisms were revealed. Strangely, one of these is performed by an enzyme system requiring visible light as a cofactor. Other systems (dark-repair enzymes) have been found which do not require light. Much of the research on these systems, and on irradiation damage and protection, has been carried out either on bacterial nucleoprotein or on cell cultures. In such systems it became apparent that variations in resistance to irradiation effects, for instance, were due mainly to variations in the effectiveness of the repair mechanisms. That the same is true for the human skin was demonstrated when the defect causing xeroderma pigmentosum (p. 144) was discovered.

A most important distinction is made between carcinogens, which initiate the process, and cocarcinogens, which promote neoplasms in tissues already exposed to a carcinogen but which are not carcinogenic on their own. The two-stage hypothesis was developed using polycyclic hydrocarbons as carcinogens and croton oil as the promoting agent in mouse skin. Further work has shown that there are a large number of promoting agents, and that the situation is rather more complex when other agents and systems are used. For instance, hydrocarbons carcinogenic on mouse skin can act as cocarcinogens in rabbits infected with Shope fibroma virus by suppressing immune responsiveness [25]. Thus, initiation and promotion are activities which depend on the biological system in which the agent is acting as well as on the intrinsic character of the agent. It has not been possible to extrapolate these laboratory findings directly to human cancer, but their influence on clinical concepts of cancer is very important. The major carcinogen in the human skin, i.e. sunlight, produces multiple effects on the epidermis and dermis, and is likely to be a promoter as well as an initiator. Cancer becomes a less random and arbitrary event if it is dependent not just on chance somatic mutations but also on a continuing promotion which can be avoided at will. It is obvious from experiments that a cocarcinogen or anticarcinogen can be the deciding factor in whether or not a tumour develops in animals exposed to the same dose of carcinogen [28].

The yield of tumours and their histological type, rate and mode of evolution in response to a particular carcinogen vary greatly between species, and indeed between different strains of mice, rats or rabbits. For instance, the influence of species on skin response is well shown by mice and rats. Mice produce squamous papillomas and carcinomas, while rats, after a longer latent interval, produce basal cell carcinomas as well as a variety of follicular and squamous tumours. Both species may develop sarcomas, but the mutant hairless varieties differ in producing few sarcomas in proportion to epithelial tumours. Many of the older experiments on record can be criticized for lack of attention to the character of the tumours produced by the chemicals. The value of this aspect is shown in the very close similarity found between the behaviour and the microscope appearance of lesions induced in rabbits by hydrocarbons and human kerato-acanthoma. Besides demonstrating that the lesion begins in the hair follicles, the experiments showed a different tumour architecture depending on whether the change began in anagen or telogen follicles [14, 35]. The kerato-acanthoma-like lesions regress spontaneously, and so do many of the papillomas in mice and rats if they are observed for a long enough time.

The influence of the stroma on the behaviour of tumours which have already appeared (as distinct from its effect on their induction) [24] has been shown by the much enhanced invasiveness of basal cell carcinomas of rats when they grow into adjacent sarcomas [29]. In such collision tumours the character of the sarcoma is also altered by the presence of the carcinoma, showing that the interaction works both ways.

The ability of a tissue to become neoplastic seems to be as fundamental a property as the ability to proliferate and repair a damaged area. Many of the more recently described chemical carcinogens act on connective-tissue cells and not on epithelia, presumably because connective-tissue cells respond directly to the molecular and textural nature of foreign material. The production of tumours by embedding cellophane in connective tissue when the sheet is unbroken, but not when it is perforated, suggests that anoxia or accumulation of metabolites may be a factor in carcinogenesis, the proces being analogous to the modification of the biological effects of ionizing radiation by variation of the oxygen tension [16]. This could be significant in tumours which develop in scarred areas in man.

Physical agents. The oncogenic effect of UV radiation has been reproduced in animals [6, 10] and the effective wavelength range seems to be 280–320 nm. A carcinogen of natural origin (cholesterol α-oxide) is formed *in vitro* in UV-irradiated human skin [4], and in increasing quantities in UV-irradiated hairless mice [3]. The connective-tissue changes have also been produced in rat skin [23], and followed from the earliest vascular changes to the final elastosis. The effects of UV and ionizing radiation are considered in Chapter 19.

Viral carcinogenesis [9, 15, 17, 18]. This subject is of importance, not for clinical practice, but for the light it is throwing on mechanisms of carcinogenesis. Viruses causing animal tumours have specific host requirements and some, indeed, need to be introduced to the host in unnatural circumstances. Polyoma virus, for instance, is oncogenic only in large dosage in animals made immunologically incompetent or when given to newborn animals. Experiments with inoculated animals are time consuming and reveal little about basic mechanisms because of the many uncontrollable factors. The use as the host of animal cells in tissue culture allows precise biochemical and genetic comparison of normal and transformed cells, and the application of the methods of immunology and molecular biology is revealing the relationship of the virus to the cell.

The DNA tumour viruses polyoma and SV 40 have been used in cultures with fruitful results. In cell cultures which accept the virus, infected cells may act either as hosts for virus replication or become transformed and behave like tumour cells. In most systems transformation is a very uncommon event in which the viral DNA becomes incorporated in the cell's DNA. The virus can no longer multiply, but the cell produces a virus-specific antigen. Transformation may require similar base sequences between the DNA of the virus and of the susceptible cell; it occurs more easily when there are chromatin breaks, and cell division after virus integration seems to be necessary for stable transformation.

Transformed cells grow more rapidly than normal and establish permanent lines. Their metabolic requirements are less exacting, and contact inhibition and orientation in culture are less likely to occur. The cells may show chromosome abnormalities and will produce tumours when implanted in an animal with which they are compatible. However, the cells lack invasive properties and grow as expansile masses, stimulating an immune response. In some respects, therefore, the behaviour of these transformed cells resembles that of cells in carcinoma-*in-situ*.

The RNA ocogenic viruses differ in many respects from DNA viruses in their mode of action. They can, for instance, transform a cell and multiply within it at the same time. Their requirements for successful growth in tissue culture are more exacting than those of DNA viruses, and their widespread latency in susceptible species has made their investigation difficult. There is experimental evidence suggesting that the genetic information for the formation of type C RNA tumour viruses may be transmitted from parent to progeny in some species [32]. If this virogenic-oncogene hypothesis is valid it follows that activation of the normally repressed gene rather than infection from outside is the common mechanism of production of spontaneous RNA virus tumours. Whether such activation can be promoted by other carcinogenic stimuli and how likely it is to be concerned in human cancer remain to be shown. There is evidence that some human tumours contain RNA sequences homologous with animal neoplasms [31].

The association between viruses and malignant change [27] has recently been strengthened by the identification of the human T-cell leukaemia–lymphoma virus (HTLV-I) which is found in a subset of patients from Japan and the Caribbean with severe rapidly progressive T-cell lymphoma [5, 13, 33]. A further association is with the human papilloma virus (HPV). HPV3, HPV5 and HPV8 are found in association with cutaneous malignancies developing in patients with epidermodysplasia verruciformis, and HPV6 has been identified in cases of vulvar carcinoma.

Immune responses and tumour growth. Many facts indicate that immune responses modify the evolution of some malignant tumours [11]. Antigens have been found on the plasma membrane of many neoplastic cells, and the hypothesis that malignant cells are eliminated when the immune system recognizes them as foreign is supported by the increased incidence of lymphomas in patients with hypogammaglobulinaemia [22], the development of malignancies and dysplastic cells in many tissues following prolonged immunosuppressive treatment [12], the association of autoimmune haemolytic anaemia and lymphoma in man [22] and NZB mice, and the behaviour of malignant cells unwittingly transferred with kidney homografts [36]. This problem has recently been reviewed [26]. However, the great majority of patients and experimental animals that develop malignant tumours have competent responses to other antigens. Certain questions therefore need to be answered. Do all tumours from their initial stages produce antigen? How do early tumours evade rejection by the immune response? Do enlarging tumours paralyse the immune response, or do they enlarge because of an ineffective response? What are the relative roles of circulating antibody and cytotoxic cells, and what determines whether tumour cells disseminate through the bloodstream? The evidence from human tumours is fragmentary. Studies on experimental sarcomas in rats [1] have clarified some of these questions for that particular tumour. A developing sarcoma causes transformation of lymphocytes into immunoblasts in the regional lymph nodes. Growing tumours fix the immunoblasts in the nodes, perhaps by continuously flooding them with antigen, because removal of the primary tumour is followed by a shower of circulating immunoblasts. However, the cells are presumably producing circulating antibody because metastases arise only in animals depleted of the fluid component of lymph. In this system it seems that the tumour initially evades rejection because few immunoblasts reach it in their random passage around the body and because neither cells nor circulating antibody enter the tumour in effective concentrations. The immobilization of effector cells in the regional lymph nodes may be both a result and a cause of the proliferation of the tumour.

The importance of the permeability of the neoplastic process to cells and antibody is made obvious by a study of premalignant conditions of the skin in man. There is invariably a brisk lymphocyte reaction to Bowen's disease, solar keratoses and premalignant melanosis, but little evidence of interaction between lymphocytes and the cells on the epidermal side of the basement membrane. It has still to be determined whether cytotoxic lymphocytes play a part in preventing dermal invasion, but clinical evidence indicates that they may be important in several methods of treatment. It is common experience that comparatively trivial damage by freezing with CO_2 slush will cure many solar kera-

toses. Neither this method nor the more recently introduced sensitization to, and challenge with, DNCB is likely to kill all the aberrant cells, but both increase the permeability of vascular endothelium and the basement membrane region.

Immunotherapy for cancer may therefore require both the enhancement of a specific response and a means of making tumour cells accessible to it at the earliest possible stage.

REFERENCES

1 ALEXANDER P. & HALL J. G. (1970) *Adv Cancer Res* **13**, 1.
2 BADGER G. M. (1954) *Adv Cancer Res* **2**, 73.
3 BLACK H. S. & DOUGLAS D. R. (1973) *Cancer Res* **33**, 2094.
4 BLACK H. S. & LO W.-B. (1971) *Nature* **234**, 306.
5 BLATTNER W. A., et al (1983) *Lancet* **i**, 639.
6 *BLUM H. F. (1959) *Carcinogenesis by Ultraviolet Light*. Princeton, Princeton University Press.
7 BOYLAND E. (Ed.) (1958) *Br Med Bull* **14** (2).
8 BOYLAND E. (Ed.) (1964) *Br Med Bull* **20** (2).
9 DULBECCO R. (1969) *Science* **166**, 962.
10 EPSTEIN J. H. (1966) In *Advances in Biology of Skin*. Vol 7. *Carcinogenesis*. Eds. Montagna W. & Dobson R. L. Oxford, Pergamon, p. 215.
11 *FAIRLEY G. H. (1969) *Br Med J* **ii**, 467.
12 FEINGOLD M. L., et al (1969) *Arch Intern Med* **126**, 66.
13 GALLO R. C., et al (1982) *Proc Natl Acad Sci USA* **79**, 5680.
14 GHADIALLY F. N. (1961) *Cancer* **14**, 801.
15 *GLASER R., et al (1975) *In Vitro* **11**, 151.
16 GRAY L. H., et al (1953) *Br J Radiol* **26**, 638.
17 *GROSS L. (1970) *Oncogenic Viruses* Oxford, Pergamon.
18 HABEL K. (1968) *Cancer Res* **28**, 1825.
19 HADDOW A. (1972) *Adv Cancer Res* **16**, 181.
20 MILLER E. C. & MILLER J. A. (1966) *Pharmacol Rev* **18**, 805.
21 MILLER J. A. (1970) *Cancer Res* **30**, 559.
22 MILLER R. W. (1968) *J Natl Cancer Inst* **40**, 1079.
23 NAKAMURA K. & JOHNSON W. C. (1968) *J Invest Dermatol* **51**, 251.
24 ORR J. W. (1938) *J Pathol Bacteriol* **46**, 495.
25 PAUL D. (1969) *Cancer Res* **29**, 1218.
26 PENN I. (1974) *Cancer* **34**, 1474.
27 RAPP F. & DUFF R. (1974) *Cancer* **34**, 1353.
28 *ROE F. J. C. (1969) In *The Biological Basis of Medicine*. Eds. Bittar E. E. & Bittar N. New York, Academic Press, Vol. 5, p. 487.
29 SANDERSON K. V. (1962) *Nature* **194**, 95.
30 SIMS P. & GROVER P. L. (1974) *Adv Cancer Res* **20**, 165.
31 SPIEGELMAN S., et al (1974) *Cancer* **34**, 1406.
32 TORADO G. J. (1975) *Am J Pathol* **81**, 590.
33 UCHIYAMA T. J., et al (1977) *Blood* **50**, 487.
34 WARBURG O.. (1956) *Science* **123**, 309.
35 WHITELEY H. J. (1957) *Br J Cancer* **11**, 196.
36 WILSON R. E., et al (1968) *N Engl J Med* **278**, 479.

SUPERFICIAL BENIGN EPITHELIAL TUMOURS

There is a heterogeneous collection of conditions, not all of them neoplastic, which could be included under this heading. Some are hyperplasias of specific cause, such as virus warts and mollusca contagiosa; these belong with the virus diseases. Others are placed more appropriately among the naevi, but because of their hamartomatous nature are included in the list that follows.

Verrucous naevus (p. 169)
Naevus comedonicus (p. 172)
Naevus sebaceus (p. 174)
Seborrhoeic keratosis
Stucco keratosis
Skin tag
Acquired digital fibrokeratoma
Intra-epidermal epithelioma (Borst-Jadassohn)
Haber's syndrome
Clear-cell acanthoma
Kerato-acanthoma
Pseudo-epitheliomatous hyperplasia

Seborrhoeic keratosis (syn. seborrhoeic wart, senile wart, basal cell papilloma)

Definition. A benign tumour, frequently pigmented, more common in the elderly and composed of epidermal cells whose maturation is retarded.

Aetiology and incidence. Profuse seborrhoeic keratoses may be a familial trait, with an autosomal dominant mode of inheritance [11]. It has been suggested that the lesion is a naevoid tumour; its occasional association, in the same patient, with the fibroepithelial type of basal cell carcinoma [10] is said to support this concept. A genetically determined predisposition, based perhaps on a mosaic pattern of aberrant response to epidermal chalone [14], would explain those cases where a profuse eruption follows an inflammatory dermatosis [17] or occurs as a manifestation of visceral malignancy [2] or during oestrogen administration [16].

Seborrhoeic keratoses are very common in white races and are often not remarked by the patient, being accepted as a harmless and inevitable consequence of ageing. Males and females are equally affected. The keratoses usually appear in the fifth decade, and thus in women they may more or less coincide with the menopause. Careful examination of patients, however, shows that the flat variety is not uncommon in the fourth decade, and can be seen in the third. There is little tendency to spontaneous disappearance and new lesions may continue to appear for many years. Stucco keratosis (p. 2391) is probably a non-pigmented seborrhoeic wart occurring principally on the limbs.

Seborrhoeic keratosis is uncommon in Negroes and Indians. Multiple tumours of the face found in dark-skinned races, and termed *dermatosis papulosa*

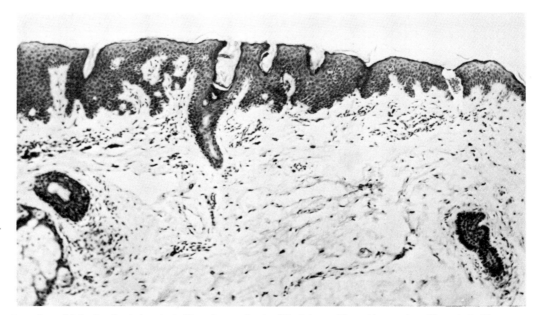

FIG. 64.5. Superficial seborrhoeic keratosis. There is acanthosis of the interpapillary ridges and papillomatosis. The surface is broken by a series of small clefts. (H&E. × 85) (Dr. K. V. Sanderson.)

nigra (see p. 2391), have a similar histology to seborrhoeic keratosis, but appear earlier in life [3].

Pathology [13]. The essential change is an accumulation of immature keratinocytes between the basal layer and the keratinizing surface of the epidermis. Melanocytes usually proliferate among the immature cells and transfer melanin to them. The dermal papillae elongate and branch to nourish the thickened epithelium. Focal keratinization may occur within the mass of immature cells to produce horn cysts, which enlarge, may coalesce and can be carried to the surface by the tide of epidermal cells. If the formation and discharge of horn cysts is considerable, a verrucous surface will be formed. Marked papillomatosis will also cause an irregular 'church steeple' outer border which retains keratin. If, in contrast, the main mass of the lesion is composed of immature cells, the surface will be smooth and rounded, and the melanocyte population and degree of pigmentation will be considerable. The parenchymal cells are rather small and polygonal, possessing tonofibrils and intercellular bridges, and they are arranged in an orderly fashion.

Inflammation is frequent in those seborrhoeic keratoses excised surgically and may be due to bacterial infection in keratin crypts. It produces not only oedema and cellular infiltration of the wart, but also stimulates the parenchyma to mature [12]. As a result the cells become more squamous in type, and mitotic figures may be seen. This appearance has been mistaken for malignant transformation. It has also been named baso-squamous-cell epidermal tumour [6].

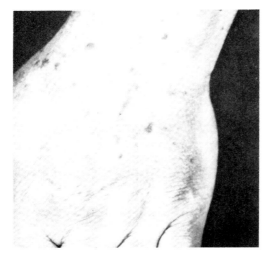

FIG. 64.6. Superficial seborrhoeic keratoses on the back of the hand (Dr. H. J. Wallace, St. John's Hospital).

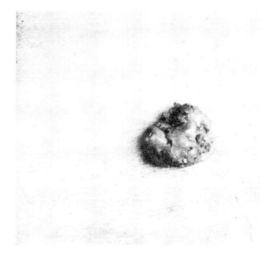

FIG. 64.7. An acanthotic type of seborrhoeic keratosis on the breast. The tumour is dark brown, the surface is lustreless and the follicles contain keratin plugs. (Dr. Forman, St. John's Hospital.)

Malignant transformation in seborrhoeic keratoses has been reported [1, 15], and indeed might be expected to occur in skin exposed to a carcinogen, but considering the frequency of the lesion such change, usually of a squamous cell type, is remarkably rare. A recent report suggesting that malignant change is not uncommon [5] does not give convincing evidence to support its author's view.

Clinical features. Seborrhoeic keratoses occur in any area where there are pilosebaceous follicles, although seborrhoea plays no part in their genesis. They are most frequent on the face and median parts of the upper trunk. The first evidence is slight hyperpigmentation and a fine granular loss of lustre of quite small areas. A hand lens will show the granularity to be caused by a series of fine depressions making an incomplete network around the capillary loops of the papillary dermis. On the hand and face, seborrhoeic keratoses may remain superficial for a long period, or indeed may never become thicker and can be mistaken for melanocytic tumours. It may indeed be difficult to distinguish superficial seborrhoeic warts from senile melanosis (senile lentigo) and from pigmented actinic keratosis. More florid warts may be smooth surfaced, domed and heavily pigmented (acanthotic), but in contrast with melanocytic naevi they are relatively lustreless and usually have plugged follicular orifices punctuating their surface. Indeed, seborrhoeic keratoses usually bear fewer hairs than the skin

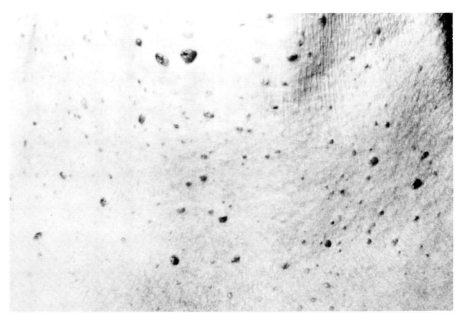

FIG. 64.8. A profuse eruption of seborrhoeic keratoses in a patient with an internal malignant neoplasm (Stoke Mandeville Hospital).

they arise from. The commonest appearance is that of a verrucous plaque stuck on the epidermis, varying from dirty yellow to black in colour and having loosely adherent greasy keratin on the surface. The shape is usually ovoid and multiple lesions may be aligned in the direction of the skin folds. The size varies from 1 mm to several centimetres. The smallest lesions are placed around follicular orifices, particularly on the trunk. On the eyelids and major flexures seborrhoeic warts may be pedunculated and not keratotic (Fig. 64.9). Irritation or infection of a wart causes swelling, sometimes bleeding, oozing and crusting, and a deepening of the colour due to inflammation. An eruption of seborrhoeic keratoses may be precipitated by an inflammatory dermatosis [17]. The keratoses may be very itchy. The lesions may disappear when the dermatosis is cured.

Seborrhoeic keratoses usually increase in number over the years, and some elderly patients have an appreciable proportion of their total skin surface affected. The keratotic surface may be shed or removed artificially from time to time, only to form again. Considering the frequency of seborrhoeic keratoses, malignant change within them is remarkably rare. Indeed, it is likely that there is less chance, in high-incidence regions, of malignancy in an exposed seborrhoeic keratosis than in the adjacent unaffected skin.

Diagnosis. The superficial type of seborrhoeic keratosis has to be distinguished from simple and malignant lentigo (p. 2450) and from actinic keratosis, especially on the face. The patterned fine fissures on the surface are perhaps the most useful sign but it requires a powerful loupe to see them. The pigmented domed variety may closely resemble a melanocytic naevus, but the surface is less lustrous and the follicular orifices are plugged. An inflamed keratosis may be interpreted as a malignant melanoma, but where there is reason to doubt the more serious diagnosis it is best to observe carefully the effect of local antibacterial treatment and protection from injury for a few days; a seborrhoeic keratosis rapidly returns to its normal state. Pigmented basal cell carcinoma is usually rather irregular with a rolled edge, a thin shiny epidermis with telangiectases and a somewhat depressed or ulcerated centre.

Treatment. This is the most satisfying skin tumour to treat. Removal with a small sharp curette leaves a flat surface which becomes covered by normal epidermis in a week. Cautery or diathermy should be used as little as possible to avoid scarring. Satisfactory results can be obtained by freezing briefly, a technique especially suitable for large superficial lesions, or by carefully painting the surface with pure trichloracetic acid and repeating if the full thickness is not removed on the first occasion.

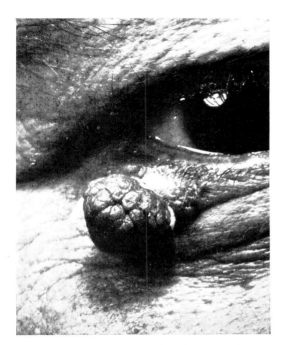

FIG. 64.9. A pedunculated seborrhoeic keratosis. The surface is cerebriform and etched with very fine fissures. (St. John's Hospital.)

Melano-acanthoma. This term has been used for a very rare lesion, originally described by Bloch as 'non-naevoid melano-epithelioma, type I', and has been considered to be a benign combined neoplasm of epidermal keratinocytes and large dendritic melanocytes [8]. The writer doubts whether it is an entity. Some deeply pigmented acanthotic seborrhoeic keratoses contain, dispersed among the parenchymal cells, numerous dendritic melanocytes which are demonstrable by the dopa technique [9]. Normally they transfer melanin to the surrounding immature keratinocytes. However, if irritation or inflammation caused the parenchymal cells to become more mature, the transfer of melanin would be impeded and pigment might be retained in the melanocytes, producing a microscopic appearance similar to that described as melano-acanthoma.

Stucco keratosis [4, 18]. This title has been given to small, rough whitish keratotic plaques which are easily lifted off the skin with a finger nail and come away without causing bleeding. They are situated principally on the extremities, especially the ankle region, and occur in middle-aged or elderly persons. They have the same stuck-on appearance of seborrhoeic warts and a similar microscopic architecture.

Basaloid cells and horn systs are not seen and the histology is more that of a regular spiky papillomatosis, with loose lamellated hyperkeratosis capping the epidermis. If treatment is called for, any superficial destructive measure would do.

REFERENCES

1 CHRISTELER A. & DELACRÉTAZ J. (1966) *Dermatologica* 133, 33.
2 DANTZIG P. I. (1973) *Arch Dermatol* 108, 700.
3 HAIRSTON M. A., et al (1964) *Arch Dermatol* 89, 655.
4 KOCSARD E. & CARTER J. J. (1971) *Aust J Dermatol* 12, 80.
5 KWITTKEN J. (1974) *Mt Sinai J Med (NY)* 41, 792.
6 LUND H. Z. (1957) *Tumors of the Skin. Atlas of Tumor Pathology*, Section 1, Fasc. 2. Armed Forces Institute of Pathology, Washington, DC, p. 48.
7 *MEHREGAN A. H. & PINKUS H. (1964) *Cancer* 17, 609.
8 MISHIMA Y. & PINKUS H. (1960) *Arch Dermatol* 81, 539.
9 MOLOKHIA M. M. & PORTNOY B. (1971) *Br J Dermatol* 85, 254.
10 PINKUS H. (1953) *Arch Dermatol Syphilol* 67, 598.
11 REICHES A. J. (1952) *Arch Dermatol Syphilol* 65, 596.
12 ROWE L. (1957) *J Invest Dermatol* 29, 165.
13 SANDERSON K. V. (1968) *Br J Dermatol* 80, 588.
14 SANDERSON K. V. (1969) *Trans Rep St Johns Hosp Dermatol Soc* 55, 127.
15 TSUJI T., et al (1969) *Jpn J Clin Dermatol* 23, 601.
16 WILKINSON D. S. (1970) *Personal communication*.
17 WILLIAMS M. G. (1956) *Br J Dermatol* 68, 268.
18 WILLOUGHBY C. & SOTER N. A. (1972) *Arch Dermatol* 105, 859.

Dermatosis papulosa nigra

Aetiology [3]. This cumbersome term describes a lesion which is common in Negroes and is probably genetically determined. The incidence rises from about 5% in the first decade to over 40% by the third, and is rather higher in females than males.

Pathology [2, 3]. The lesions, which are naevoid developmental defects of the pilosebaceous follicles, show irregular acanthosis and hyperkeratosis, and somewhat resemble seborrhoeic keratoses.

Clinical features [1, 3, 4]. The individual lesions are black or dark brown flattened or cupuliform papules 1–5 mm in diameter. They are rare under the age of 7, after which they increase steadily in frequency, number and size. They are most numerous in the malar regions and on the forehead. They are rare on the lower parts of the face and the chin, but in a few individuals may be found on the neck, chest and back [2].

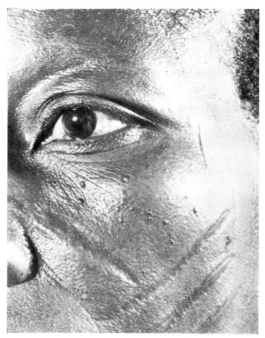

FIG. 64.10 Dermatosis papulosa nigra in a Yoruba woman aged 40 (University College, Ibadan, Nigeria).

Treatment. Treatment is seldom requested. Removal with the diathermy or cautery is practicable.

REFERENCES

1 CASTELLANI A. (1925) *J Trop Med Hyg* **28**, 1.
2 DIASIO F. A. (1933) *Arch Dermatol Syphilol* **27**, 751.
3 HAIRSTON M. A., *et al* (1964) *Arch Dermatol* **99**, 655.
4 MICHAEL J. C. & SEARLE E. R. (1929) *Arch Dermatol Syphilol* **20**, 629.

Skin tags (syn. soft warts, achrochordon)

Definition. A common tumour in the middle-aged and elderly, occurring mainly on the neck and major flexures as a small, soft, pedunculated and often pigmented protrusion.

Incidence and aetiology. The condition is very common, particularly in women at the menopause or later. It may also occur in pregnancy. It is frequently found together with seborrhoeic keratoses.

Pathology. The protruding mass is connected to the skin by a narrow pedicle. The bulk of the lesion is loose fibrous tissue, similar to that of the pars papillaris. The epidermis is thin, and the basal cell layer is flat and often hyperpigmented. Melanocytic proliferation and naevus cells are not usually seen and the majority of such lesions probably come within the seborrhoeic keratosis spectrum. There is, however, an overlap with melanocytic naevi and neurofibromas.

Clinical features. The lesions are always pedunculated and are frequently constricted at their base. They vary in size and are about 2 mm in diameter on average. They are round, soft and inelastic. The colour may be unchanged, but they are frequently hyperpigmented. The most common situation is on the sides of the neck, where they may be mixed with typical small sessile seborrhoeic keratoses. When more profuse they can extend onto the face or down to the back and chest. Similar lesions may be found in and around the axillae and groins.

Diagnosis. The lesions are unmistakable. They are smaller than the average pedunculated melanocytic naevus or the lesions of neurofibromatosis.

Treatment. Menopausal skin tags can be the cause of considerable anguish and may at times be the focal symptom of mental depression. Their treatment is relatively simple. Destruction by fulguration or electrocoagulation can usually be done without local anaesthesia. A convenient way to freeze them is to grip them with haemostat forceps that have been chilled in liquid nitrogen. Liquefied phenol or trichloracetic acid applied on a pointed wooden applicator is effective. New lesions are likely to appear and periodic retouching may be required.

Acquired fibrokeratoma. An uncommon papillary or keratotic outgrowth, usually from the region of a finger joint but in a few cases on the hand, foot or elsewhere, has been described [1, 2]. It affects adults, and males predominate. Trauma is the most likely cause. Microscopically, both dermis and epidermis are relatively normal, elastic fibres being somewhat sparse in most specimens and the epidermis being acanthotic and hyperkeratotic in some. The condition must be distinguished from rudimentary supernumerary digit, which is congenital, or from a cutaneous horn, which lacks the dermal core. Simple excision cures all cases.

Intra-epidermal epithelioma (Borst–Jadassohn). It is a natural consequence of the inelastic coherence of the epidermis that if abnormal cells, either immature keratinocytes or foreign cells, establish focal colonies within it they will form rounded nests in which the cells often have a whorled appearance. The above title given to this phenomenon thus includes a variety of conditions such as Bowen's disease, intra-epidermal hidro-acanthoma, invasion by malignant melanoma, Paget's disease and epidermotropic carcinoma of more distant origin. The greater number of examples are, however, a variant of seborrhoeic keratosis [3], and the nests of immature cells can be induced to mature by irritation of the surface or inflammation in the dermis beneath the lesion. The seborrhoeic keratosis with this focal arrangement of immature epidermal cells is unusual in often being a solitary, deeply pigmented and rather irregular plaque, frequently situated on a limb, and it is quite easy to recognize clinically. There is now no justification for retaining the title, as even the original cases of Borst and Jadassohn were of different pathological conditions [3].

REFERENCES

1 BART R. S., *et al* (1968) *Arch Dermatol* **97**, 120.
2 HARE P. J. & SMITH P. A. J. (1969) *Br J Dermatol* **81**, 667.
3 MEHREGAN A. H. & PINKUS H. (1964) *Cancer* **17**, 609.

Haber's syndrome

Definition. A familial condition characterized by a persistent rosacea-like eruption associated in some cases with keratotic plaques on the trunk and limbs.

Incidence. A family in which five members have been affected was originally described [1]. Another case, with 15 affected relatives, has been described from Japan [2]. The rosacea-like eruption appears in childhood, and the keratotic lesions somewhat later. The mode of inheritance seems to be a simple autosomal dominant.

Pathology. The facial eruption shows perivascular inflammation leading to fibrosis, acanthosis and parakeratosis of the epidermis, distortion of pilosebaceous complexes with dilated follicular orifices, and proliferation of immature glands and basal cell strands. The warty lesions are produced by papillomatosis, acanthosis in the interpapillary ridges and dyskeratosis with areas of pale-staining cells giving a parakeratotic stratum corneum. Mitotic figures are present, but there is no evidence of malignancy.

Clinical features. The cheeks, nose, forehead and chin are permanently flushed. The skin surface shows a combination of erythema and telangiectasia, prominent follicles, comedones, small papules, some of which are scaly, and tiny atrophic pitted areas. There is little fluctuation in the erythema although sunlight may aggravate it. The warty

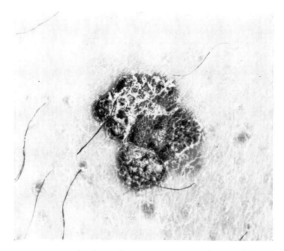

FIG. 64.11. Haber's syndrome. Warty acanthoma of the thigh.

lesions occur mainly on the trunk and thighs. They are scaly or keratotic, flat and non-indurated plaques 1 cm or so in size. Their disposition lacks symmetry and they are not progressive. The combined clinical picture is unmistakable.

Treatment. The facial eruption was controlled in the young patient in the first family and in the Japanese patient by steroid creams locally. The warty lesions responded to radiotherapy. Presumably, simple destructive measures would also be effective.

REFERENCES

1 SANDERSON K. V. & WILSON H.T.H. (1965) *Br J Dermatol* **77**, 10.
2 SEIJI M. & OTAKI N. (1971) *Arch Dermatol* **103**, 452.

Clear-cell acanthoma (syn. Degos' acanthoma, acanthome à cellules claires) [3, 8, 9]

Definition. A scaly plaque or nodule which has a characteristic accumulation of clear glycogen-containing cells in the epidermis when examined under the microscope.

Incidence and aetiology. It is a relatively uncommon condition occurring in adults of middle-age or older. The sexes are equally affected [9]. There is no suggestion that injury, toxic substances or medicaments provoke it. Experimental transmission and virus cultures have failed [4].

Pathology [1, 3, 5]. The epidermis is thickened and papillomatous with sharply outlined areas of light-coloured cells, which contrast with the normal

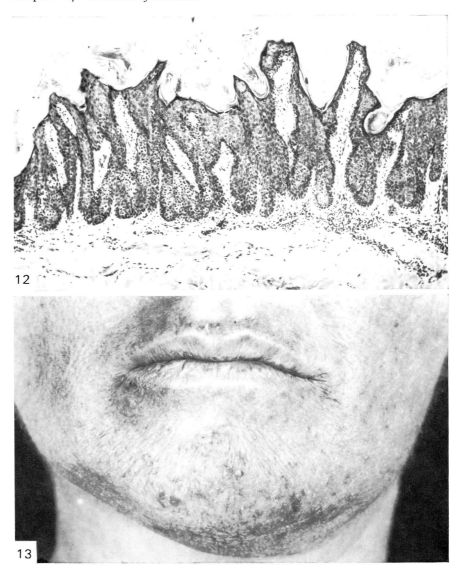

FIG. 64.12. Haber's syndrome. Warty acanthoma with nests and columns of pale cells. Atypical epidermal cells and mitotic figures give a resemblance to Bowen's disease. (By courtesy of the Editor, *Br J Dermatol.*)

FIG. 64.13. Haber's syndrome. Persistent rosacea-like erythema and telangiectasia with follucular papules, scaling and small, depressed scars. (By courtesy of the Editor, *Br J Dermatol.*)

basal cells below and Malpighian cells around them. The cytoplasm of the clear cells contains an abundance of glycogen, which with electron microscopy is seen to displace tonofibrils [6, 7]. The cells do not have the enzymes characteristic of eccrine sweat glands. There is intercellular oedema and an infiltrate often containing many polymorphonuclear leucocytes. The papillary body is oedematous and the superficial capillaries and veins are increased in number. There may be syringomatous sweat gland elements and evidence of sebaceous differentiation beneath the lesion [2].

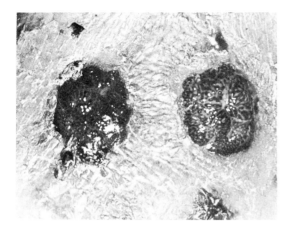

FIG. 64.14. Two adjacent clear-cell acanthomas. The patient had multiple lesions. (Dr. A. R. Kurwa.)

Clinical features [3, 5, 9]. The lesion is usually solitary, but several patients have had more than one. It is a slightly elevated to dome-shaped plaque or nodule with an abrupt margin and a wafer-like scale adherent at the periphery, which leaves a moist or bleeding surface when removed. The colour varies from pink to brown, but is most characteristically red with vascular puncta and blanches on diascopy. It varies from 3 to 20 mm in diameter, and occurs most commonly on the lower limbs. The duration may be of many years, and there are usually no symptoms. The diagnosis can be suspected on the clinical evidence. The lesion may be mistaken for a histiocytoma, seborrhoeic keratosis or pyogenic granuloma, among others. Excision allows it to be diagnosed microscopically. There is no record of it recurring after excision, or of it disappearing spontaneously [3].

REFERENCES

1 BROWNSTEIN M. H., *et al* (1973) *Am J Clin Pathol* **59**, 306.
2 CRAMER H. J. (1971) *Dermatologica* **143**, 265.
3 DEGOS R. & CIVATTE J. (1970) *Br J Dermatol* **83**, 248.
4 DUPERRAT B. & MASCARO J. M. (1965) *Ann Dermatol Syphiligr* **92**, 5.
5 FINE R. M. & CHERNOSKY M. E. (1969) *Arch Dermatol* **100**, 559.
6 FU H. & SISSONS J. H. (1969) *J Invest Dermatol* **52**, 185.
7 HOLLMANN K. H. & CIVATTE J. (1968) *Ann Dermatol Syphilogr* **95**, 139.
8 WELLS G. C. & WILSON JONES E. (1967) *Br J Dermatol* **79**, 249.
9 ZAK F. G. & GIRERD R. J. (1968) *Hautarzt* **19**, 559.

Kerato-acanthoma (syn. molluscum sebaceum)
Definition. A rapidly evolving tumour situated

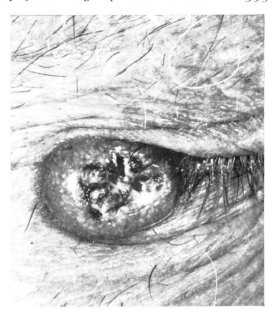

FIG. 64.15. Kerato-acanthoma. Typical crateriform nodule. (St. John's Hospital.)

mainly on the exposed areas of the skin, composed of keratinizing squamous cells originating in pilosebaceous follicles and resolving spontaneously if untreated.

Incidence. It is a common tumour, and in white races tends to occur with about a third of the frequency of squamous-cell carcinoma, despite differences in climate [24]. It is uncommon in dark-skinned races and in the Japanese [21]. Males are affected about three times as often as females. The adjusted age distribution shows that it is frequent in middle life and does not become markedly more frequent in old age, unlike basal and squamous cell carcinomas.

Aetiology. The epidemiological data indicate that incidence is related to sun exposure, and the localization of the tumours mainly on the head and upper limb supports this idea. Contact with tar and mineral oil has also been shown to cause an increased incidence [4, 10, 15], and very similar lesions have been produced in animals by painting with carcinogenic hydrocarbons. In some cases the lesion follows injury to the skin, which suggests that infection may play a part in its origin, a view supported by the occurrence of multiple kerato-acanthoma in skin grafts of patients with the tumour, in the recipient site [22], the donor site [33] or both sites [12]. Final proof of a virus causing it is still lacking. Cases are recorded of kerato-acanthoma associated with carcinoma of the larynx [7], multiple internal malignancy [23], leukaemia [29] and deficient cell-mediated immunity [9].

Pathology. The distinctive features are best seen when the fixed specimen is being cut before processing or in sections under low magnification. The tumour has a symmetrical more or less globular form and is situated in the dermis, usually extending down no deeper than the sweat glands although deep penetration has occasionally been recorded [17]. The epidermis around the tumour is normal or slightly acanthotic, but becomes thinned as it rises over the tumour. A narrow spur of connective tissue separates the epidermis from the proliferating squamous cells, except where the two connect at the mouth of the keratin-filled crypt. The architecture is thus that of a tumour originating in the appendages. Serial sections of an early lesion have shown connection of the masses of squamous cells with the upper part of a hyperplastic follicle [18].

The histological features vary with the stage of evolution. The early lesion is composed of a mass of rapidly multiplying squamous cells. These are large and rather pale with vesicular nuclei, prominent nucleoli and frequent mitoses. Hyperchromatic cells, atypical mitotic figures, individual cell keratinization and other evidence of loss of polarity may be found. The marginal cells invade the surrounding dermis aggressively, while those more centrally placed keratinize to form a branched core of keratin which communicates with the surface. The stroma is vascular and is infiltrated with round cells and histiocytes.

Resolution occurs through maturation of the hyperplastic masses. The accumulating keratin dilates the central pore, the epidermal lips recede from the centre and the lesion opens like a flower bud. When the horn is finally shed, the irregular epithelium beneath it replicates the scalloped outline of the active mass. The cells take on the morphology of epidermis, and a scar is formed which is depressed and may have papillomatous tags at the margin, the remnants of the epidermal lip.

The possibility of malignant change in kerato-acanthoma exists but is difficult to prove [26]. In one case [5] it may have been precipitated by treatment with oral methotrexate for a recurrence. The conjunction of two independent lesions in sun-damaged skin may account for the finding of a basal-cell carcinoma in the scar of kerato-acanthoma in this and other cases.

Experimentally produced lesions differ in their form, depending on whether the hair follicles are in anagen or telogen when the proliferation begins [14, 30]. Virus-like particles have been seen under electron microscopy [34].

Clinical features [2, 19, 24]. The first evidence of kerato-acanthoma is a firm, rounded, flesh-coloured or reddish papule which may resemble molluscum contagiosum or, if keratotic, a virus wart. The patient rarely seeks advice at this stage, and only realizes that the 'pimple' is not commonplace when it enlarges rapidly. In a few weeks it may become 10–20 mm across and palpation often shows it to have a globular shape. There is never a spreading infiltration at the base. The epidermis over the nodule is smooth and shiny; the colour is flesh to red with telangiectases just beneath the surface. The centre contains a horny plug or is covered by a crust which conceals a keratin-filled crater. As the lesion matures the accumulating keratin expands the outermost part making the edge overhang the base somewhat, but the radial symmetry is usually well preserved. The keratin may project like a horn or it may soften and break down. Spontaneous resolution is achieved by the epidermal covering receding towards the base and the horny core being shed. The base is revealed as irregular and puckered and the edge may remain as soft but thickened epidermis, either as a continuous rim or a series of tags. The process of spontaneous healing usually takes about 3 months.

A small proportion of kerato-acanthomas grow to much larger dimensions, 50 mm or more in diameter being not exceptional on the forearm. One lesion on the chest became over 150 mm across [13]. In some cases the maximum size may be reached in a month or two; others may enlarge for many months. After growth ceases, involution may not occur for some months or may occur at part of the periphery whilst growth continues elsewhere. There may be recurrences after curetting or excision, more frequently in lesions on the lips and fingers [26] and when treatment is carried out in the early stages [25]. Recurrence may happen after spontaneous resolution [3].

The most frequently affected area is the central part of the face—the nose, cheeks, eyelids and lips. The dorsum of the hand, the wrist and the forearm are commonly affected, the thigh, chest, shoulder and scalp less so, and the anogenital area uncommonly except in those exposed to occupational hazards. Lesions have occurred in the subungual region [20, 27], in the vermilion of the lips [28] and on the buccal mucosa.

In most cases the tumour presents as a solitary lesion. Multiple or recurrent tumours are more

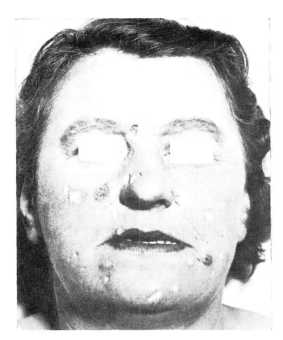

FIG. 64.16. Multiple self-healing epitheliomas. (Dr. R. J. Cairns).

likely to be present in several circumstances. Recurrent lesions occur in the patient who has been exposed to pitch or tar [10] and in rare cases as a familial disorder, although there are reasons for keeping this Ferguson–Smith type as a separate entity (see below). There are a few cases of eruptive kerato-acanthoma recorded. Multiple lesions have occurred with defective cell-mediated immunity and also as part of Torre's syndrome, with multiple internal malignancies [23] and with sebaceous adenomas (p. 2349).

Diagnosis. The main problem is to distinguish kerato-acanthoma from squamous-cell carcinoma. In most cases the more rapid evolution to relatively large size, the regular crateriform shape and keratotic plug, the undamaged surrounding skin and the younger age of onset make a distinction relatively easy for the clinician. Spontaneous healing makes the diagnosis certain. The problem is made more difficult in sunny areas where actinic damage and squamous cell carcinoma are more common, and the most important single point in these areas is the history of rapid growth from previously normal skin. Of a long list of other conditions to be differentiated [1, 2], the most confusing are cutaneous horn and hypertrophic solar keratosis, virus

wart, molluscum contagiosum, pseudo-epitheliomatous hyperplasia and granulomas of various types. Secondary deposits from internal cancer can occasionally mimic kerato-acanthoma.

Treatment. The end result of leaving the tumour to regress is usually a rather unsightly scar. Curettage and coagulation of the base, or excision and suture, produce a much more acceptable result. Excision is desirable if the diagnosis is in doubt, because curetted specimens yield poor sections. A further reason for treating the lesion is that even if the clinician is sure of the benign outcome, the patient may not be convinced and, especially when the growth is on the face, may desire to be relieved of it as soon as possible. Radiotherapy shortens the course and improves the scar, and can be used in patients who refuse surgery. A total of 2,000 rad in two closely spaced doses of adequate penetration can be given.

The application of 5-fluorouracil ointment twice daily may reduce the time taken for natural resolution and diminish the scarring [16]. If there is real doubt about the diagnosis, surgical removal or radiotherapy should be carried out as for squamous cell carcinoma, and the patient followed up.

Familial primary self-healing squamous epithelioma of the skin. This condition is fully described on p. 127. The published descriptions do not always emphasize the clinical differences between the tumours and scars of this condition and kerato-acanthoma; the majority of dermatologists who have seen both agree that they are distinct, although very closely related [6]. The familial incidence is of the autosomal dominant type. The majority of lesions occur on the exposed surfaces, but there is no evidence of exposure to a common carcinogen [11]. The lesions usually first appear in early adult life and continue to erupt at intervals for years—for nearly 50 years in one case [8].

The clinical appearance, course and pathology of individual tumours are so similar to those of kerato-acanthoma that some authors regard it as a variant of that lesion. There are, however, minor differences. The tumours have a rather slower evolution, tend to be more deeply set in the skin and are more variable in their maximum size, and therefore in the scars that result, than is the average solitary kerato-acanthoma. Sometimes, sinus-like scars form with epithelial bridges and undermining of the margin owing to lateral invasion by the tumour columns.

Histologically, the process is often less well circumscribed. Proliferating columns of squamous cells may burrow into the dermis, undermining the epithelium [11] but not always raising it up in the bud-like tumour characteristic of kerato-acanthoma. In sections of early lesions which the writer has examined, the arrangement of epithelial columns suggests an origin from both follicles and eccrine sweat ducts as in the case reported by Witten & Zak [32].

Generalized eruptive kerato-acanthoma [31]. A small number of cases of widely disseminated lesions, some of them typical kerato-acanthoma, has been reported. Both sexes have been affected. The primary lesions are flesh-coloured to red dome-shaped follicular papules 1–3 mm in size and affecting particularly the face, where they may be confluent, the trunk and the roots of the limbs. Itching is a prominent symptom, and ectropion and narrowing of the mouth may be produced by the keratotic facial change. Scattered among the papules are larger more typical kerato-acanthomas, which resolve spontaneously. The palms and soles are spared, but the oral and laryngeal epithelium can be involved.

Histological examination shows the papules to consist of a dilated and plugged follicle duct with acanthotic follicular epidermis around it, the mucosal lesions to be irregular acanthosis and the nodules to be kerato-acanthoma, but with no inflammatory changes.

The nodular lesions heal in a few months. The papules are not influenced by cytotoxic drugs, but one case responded to topical vitamin A [31] and current trials of the synthetic retinoids are encouraging.

REFERENCES

1 *BAER R. L. & KOPF A. W. (1962) *Yearbook of Dermatology*, Chicago, Year Book Publishers, p. 7.
2 *BAPTISTA A. V. B. P. (1964) *Querato-Acantoma*. Coimbra Editoria.
3 BEARE J. M. (1955) *Lancet* i, 182.
4 BRAUN W. & ENAYAT M. (1960) *Berufsdermatosen* 8, 61.
5 BURGE K. M. & WINKELMANN R. K. (1969) *Arch Dermatol* 100, 306.
6 CALNAN C. D. & HABER H. (1956) *J Pathol Bacteriol* 69, 61.
7 CHAPMAN R. S. & FINN D. A. (1974) *Br J Dermatol* 90, 685.
8 CHARTERIS A. A. (1951) *Am J Roentgenol* 65, 459.
9 CLAUDY A. & THIVOLET J. (1975) *Br J Dermatol* 93, 593.
10 COLOMB D., et al (1966) *Rev Lyon Med* 15, 449.
11 CURRIE A. R. & SMITH J. F. (1952) *J Pathol Bacteriol* 64, 827.
12 DIBDEN F. A. & FOWLER M. (1955) *Aust NZ J Surg* 25, 157.
13 DUANY N. P. (1958) *AMA Arch Dermatol* 78, 703.
14 *GHADIALLY F. N. (1961) *Cancer* 14, 801.
15 GHADIALLY F. N., et al (1963) *Cancer* 16, 603.
16 GRUPPER C. (1970) *Dermatologica* 140 (Suppl. 1), 127.
17 HURIEZ C., et al (1957) *Rev Pract* 7, 1.
18 KALKOFF K. W. & MACHER E. (1961) *Hautarzt* 12, 8.
19 KINGMAN J. & CALLEN J. P. (1984) *Arch Dermatol* 120, 736.
20 LAMPE J. C., et al (1964) *J Bone Jt Surg* 46, 1721.
21 MIYAJI T. (1963) *Natl Cancer Inst Monogr* 10, 55.
22 PILLSBURY D. M. & BEERMAN H. (1958) *Am J Med Sci* 236, 614.
23 POLEKSIC S. (1974) *Br J Dermatol* 91, 461.
24 *ROOK A. & CHAMPION R. H. (1963) *Natl Cancer Inst Monogr* 10, 257.
25 ROOK, A. & MOFFATT J. L. (1956) *AMA Arch Dermatol* 74, 525.
26 ROOK A., et al (1967) *Med Cutan Iber Lat Am* 11, 17.
27 SHAPIRO L. & BAREF C. S. (1970) *Cancer* 25, 141.
28 STEVANOVIC D. V. (1960) *Dermatologica* 121, 278.
29 WEBER G., et al (1970) *Arch Klin Exp Dermatol* 238, 107.
30 WHITELEY H. J. (1957) *Br J Cancer* 11, 196.
31 WINKELMANN R. K. & BROWN J. (1968) *Arch Dermatol* 97, 615.
32 WITTEN V. H. & ZAK F. G. (1952) *Cancer* 5, 539.
33 WULSIN J. H. (1958) *Am Surg* 24, 689.
34 ZELICKSON A. S. (1962) *Acta Derm Venereol (Stockh)* 42, 23.

Pseudo-epitheliomatous hyperplasia [2]

Aetiology. Epidermal hyperplasia is an early and essential feature in the healing of any breach of the skin surface. Under ordinary circumstances this is coordinated with the repair of the dermis, and the downgrowths are eventually broken up [1]. When the dermis is diseased, however, a persistent and much more extensive hyperplasia may occur. This is seen, for instance, at the margin of chronic ulcers, as in venous hypertension, over chronic granulomas like lupus vulgaris, tuberculosis verrucosa cutis, insect-bite granulomas and halogen granulomas, and, in a rather unusual form, over a small proportion of histiocytomas (p. 1706). It is also a component of some cases of lupus erythematosus and of lichen planus of the hypertrophic type. It may occur in association with tumours, particularly granular-cell myoblastoma and malignant melanoma.

Pathology. The nature of the primary disorder modifies the picture greatly. In simple ulcers and in-

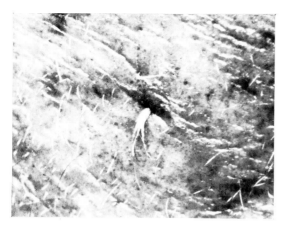

FIG. 64.17. Trichofolliculoma on the forehead of a 22-yr-old man. (Addenbrookes's Hospital).

flammatory lesions, by far the commonest causes, there is disturbance of the upper part of the dermis, often with young fibroblasts and a rather myxomatous connective-tissue stroma replacing the normal dermal collagen. Columns of prickle cells grow down into the dermis in an irregular fashion. In some areas there is maturation of the central parts of the columns to produce horny pearls. The general appearance is that of invasive proliferation of the epithelium. The individual cells, however, do not show the atypical features that suggest malignancy. The columns may be penetrated by inflammatory cells, a feature which is not seen in malignant proliferations. In most instances a weighing of the dermal changes against the epidermal suggests that the former are the cause and not the consequence of the latter.

Clinical features. The appearance will vary with the primary disorder. Granulomas may be covered by a thickened, warty or heaped-up epidermis, perhaps best seen in chromomycosis. In chronic ulcers the margin is heaped-up, often giving the appearance of being rolled, and has an irregular surface. The edge is not usually indurated to the extent that occurs in squamous cell carcinoma. It is characteristic that the hyperplasia will subside as the ulcer is treated and heals. It is wise to remember that an ulcer whose margin has been affected by pseudo-epitheliomatous hyperplasia in the past may eventually be the cause of metastasing squamous cell carcinoma.

REFERENCES

1 GILLMAN T. (1964) In *Progress in the Biological Sciences in Relation to Dermatology*. Eds. Rook A. & Champion R. H. Cambridge, Cambridge University Press. p. 113.
2 WINER L. H. (1940) *Arch Dermatol Syphilol* **42**, 856.

HAIR FOLLICLE TUMOURS [13]

Tumours related to the hair follicle, like those of sweat glands, are of greater variety microscopically than in their clinical features, and it is arguable how meticulously they should be subdivided. In this section a rather simplified classification is used. A more comprehensive subdivision has been advanced [7] which includes dermatosis papulosa nigra, follicular poroma, a tumour of the follicular infundibulum, tricholemmoma (external root sheath tumour), trichogenic adnexal tumour and tricho-adenoma, as well as tricho-epithelioma, basal cell naevus and certain types of basal cell carcinoma. In hair follicle hamartomas the epithelial elements are enveloped by a characteristic thickened fibrous stroma, and a small number of cases where the stromal element constitutes the tumour (perifollicular fibroma) have been reported [38], including one where the lesion was congenital and presumably most unlikely to have been reactive in nature [9]. The following tumours will be described in this section:

> Trichofolliculoma
> Inverted follicular keratosis
> Tricholemmoma
> Tricho-epithelioma
> Multiple eruptive milia
> Pilomatrixoma
> Trichogenic adnexal tumour
> Trichodiscoma

Trichofolliculoma (syn. hair-follicle naevus)
Definition. A tumour composed of multiple malformed hair roots arising from an enlarged follicular canal.

Incidence. The tumours are rare. Though obviously a maldevelopment, the lesions may not appear until middle age.

Pathology [17]. The tumour is situated in the dermis and has at its centre a large sinus joining the epidermis. Numerous well-formed hair roots bud from the sides and base of the sinus. These possess a dermal papilla, a hair matrix and the rudiments of root sheaths. Some may form fine hair shafts, whereas others are only crumbling fragments of keratin. Sebaceous glands are inconspicuous and rudimentary, and pilomotor muscles are usually absent. The stroma is well formed and fibrous.

Clinical features. The lesion is solitary and is most common on the face. There is a central crater or punctum containing keratin surrounded by a firm, somewhat elevated, pearly tumour. If hairs issue from the crater (Fig. 64.17), the diagnosis is obvious [25,30]. If not, it can only be guessed at.

Inverted follicular keratosis (syn. benign intra-epidermal follicular acanthoma [23] porome folliculaire). This tumour, which is not as uncommon as reports might suggest, usually occurs on the face in middle-age as a slightly projecting keratotic plug surrounded by a more or less raised fleshy epithelial collar. The keratin may be fasciculated in a perpendicular direction and more crumbly than in a cutaneous horn or kerato-acanthoma, but firmer than in molluscum contagiosum. Microscopically, there is a mass of immature cells resembling those of a seborrhoeic keratosis, but with eddies of more mature cells. The central cells keratinize and may connect with the surface by canals resembling follicle ducts. It is regarded by some as a benign tumour of the intra-epidermal part of the hair duct [20], and by others as a seborrhoeic keratosis, which usually shows histological evidence of irritation [32]. The latter view is the more plausible. It is cured by simple excision.

Tricholemmoma [14, 16]. This name has been given to a small benign tumour occurring principally on the face of elderly patients. It is characterized microscopically by lobules and plaques of squamoid cells containing glycogen and attached to the epidermis and follicular ducts. There is a vitreous sheath and the marginal tumour cells may be palisaded. This tumour has some features in common with inverted follicular keratosis. It usually occurs as a solitary tumour on the face or neck, and men are more often affected than women. It is seen mainly in the middle-aged or elderly [3]. It is usually diagnosed clinically as basal cell carcinoma.

Tricho-epithelioma (syn. epithelioma adenoides cysticum) [11, 18]
Definition. A tumour differentiating towards hair follicles, usually multiple and often familial.

Incidence and aetiology. This is an uncommon condition. Patients with multiple lesions often have a family history indicating autosomal dominant inheritance, but there is a disproportionate prevalence of females in published pedigrees [31]. This appears

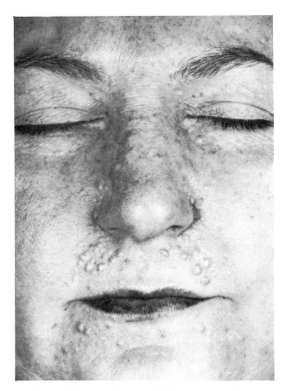

FIG. 64.18. Tricho-epithelioma. Multiple symmetrical tumours of the face. (St. John's Hopsital.)

to be due to a deficit of affected males through lessened expressivity and penetrance of the gene [1]. Tricho-epithelioma and dermal cylindroma may be a single genetic entity [36]. There is no evidence of genetic or clinical overlap between tricho-epithelioma and naevoid basal cell carcinoma [15].

Pathology. The individual tumour cells and their arrangement resemble those of basal cell carcinoma. There are rounded masses enclosed by a well-developed fibrous stroma. The marginal cells tend to be in a palisade, and it is not uncommon to find lace-like strands of cells composed simply of a double palisade. The more central cells of the masses are often fusiform, have a more abundant cytoplasm and may mature to form cystic spaces filled with lamellae of keratin. These can later calcify, or evoke a foreign body reaction. Connection of the tumour islands with hair follicles and the epidermis can often be seen. At times differentiation to rudimentary hair roots is apparent in some areas. Melanin may be deposited in and around the tumour. The general outline of the tumour is symmetrical and the epidermis is intact. Tricho-epithelioma may be found in combination with adnexal hamartomas, for example superficial or nodular hidradenoma, either as separate lesions or separate foci in a single tumour [10, 18, 22]. A combined tumour with a melanocytic naevus can occur [27]. Histologically, there is no sharp boundary between tricho-epithelioma and trichofolliculoma on the one hand, and basal cell carcinoma on the other.

Clinical features. The tumours usually appear at puberty and are small, rounded and rather translucent. The cheeks, eyelids and nasolabial folds are the common sites, but other parts of the face, and exceptionally the upper trunk or arms, may be affected. The disposition is symmetrical. Larger lesions may be yellow or pink, or sometimes bluish from pigmentation, and there may be dilated blood vessels over the surface. Individual tumours reach a limiting size, but the numbers may increase over the years. Continued growth or ulceration raises the suspicion of change to basal cell carcinoma.

Diagnosis. The typical case, with multiple tumours on the face and a family history, presents no problem. Some tumours may mimic milia, others syringoma. The solitary tumour which is not familial may cause difficulty, and is hard to distinguish from a basal cell carcinoma. A darkly pigmented lesion can be mistaken for malignant melanoma.

Treatment. Any suspicion of malignant change calls for adequate excision and histological examination. The only other reason for treatment is to improve the patient's appearance, and is probably best done by a plastic surgeon. Partial destruction is usually followed by regrowth.

Multiple eruptive milia. Several cases have been described [33, 34] in which large numbers of milia-like nodules are present in the skin of the face and upper trunk. They develop in adult life, without any external cause, in contrast with the lesions of chloracne. They are symmetrical, varying from 1 to 5 mm in size, and some are punctuated by a central black comedo which can be expressed. Sections show deformed follicles, from which fine strands of epithelium extend into the surrounding dermis and up to the adjacent epidermis. Horn cysts develop in some of these strands; others have the morphology of the collars of vellus hair follicles with rudimentary sebaceous differentiation. The deformed pilosebaceous complexes are enveloped by a thick connective-tissue sheath. It is possible that 'Haarschiebe tumours' [24, 26] and 'disseminated dermatofibrosis and skin tags with microscopic cyst formation' [35] are related conditions. The familial occurence of milia with tricho-epithelioma and cylindroma affecting males in three consecutive generations has been described [28].

Pilomatrixoma (syn. benign calcifying epithelioma of Malherbe, trichomatrioma)
Definition. A benign tumour composed of cells resembling those of the hair matrix, which undergo 'mummification' and may calcify.

Incidence. It is a relatively uncommon tumour, which may occur at any age from infancy [2]. The majority of the patients are under 20, and females are affected more often than males. It is not hereditary but a number of familial cases are recorded. It may occur in black and oriental races. An association with myotonia atrophica has been reported [5]. The tumour is considered to be a hamartoma of the hair matrix [8].

Pathology [8, 19, 21]. The tumour is situated in the dermis, and is composed of well-circumscribed rounded islands giving a lobulated contour. The outer cells are small, and their rounded nuclei crowded together make this region deeply basophilic. Mitotic figures can usually be seen and may be frequent. The cytoplasm is scanty and the cell margins indistinct, but intercellular connections can be seen. Towards the centre of the mass the cytoplasm becomes more abundant and eosinophilic: the nuclear outline persists, but the chromatin is sparse and clumped in dark granules; then, all the basophilic material disappears, leaving a 'ghost cell'. The ultrastructure and histochemical characteristics of these cells mark them as hair-matrix cells maturing towards cortex or root sheath [12]. The central areas often calcify, and calcium can be demonstrated in the basophilic cells. In older lesions the basophilic cells may be much reduced or disappear entirely. Melanin may be present, and dendritic melanocytes have been found between the tumour cells [6]; the stroma which encapsulates the masses usually contains inflammatory and foreign body giant cells, and occasionally ossifies.

Clinical features. The lesion is usually a solitary deep dermal or subcutaneous tumour 3–30 mm in diameter situated in the head, neck or upper extremity [2]. The skin over the tumour is normal and the lesion has a firm to stony-hard consistency and a lobular shape on palpation. In adult life there may be quite a short history, and there is usually no evidence of a preceding cyst. It may be subject to periodic inflammation, and on occasions presents as a granulomatous swelling [4]. Malignant change has been reported [34, 37].

Diagnosis. The diagnosis can be suspected if a tumour feels hard and lobular. The presence of calcium salts may be apparent on radiographs, but these are deposited in other cysts and tumours of the skin. The microscopical picture is diagnostic.

Trichogenic adnexal tumour. This has been suggested as a generic term for hair matrix neoplasms of the skin which show identifiable differentiation towards hair follicles and in which there is an intimate stromal–epithelial relationship [14]. The diagnosis is made microscopically.

Trichodiscoma. Three cases are described of multiple 1–5 mm diameter domed flesh-coloured papules appearing on the face, trunk and extremities. They tend to remain unchanged for years, and there are histological grounds for regarding them as originating from the Haarscheibe, a richly vasculated dermal pad containing nerve endings closely associated with hair follicles [25].

REFERENCES

1 ANDERSON D. E. & HOWELL J. B. (1976) *Br J Dermatol* **95**, 225.
2 BINGUL O., *et al* (1962) *Pediatrics* **30**, 233.
3 BROWNSTEIN M. H. & SHAPIRO L. (1973) *Arch Dermatol* **107**, 866.
4 BUREAU Y., *et al* (1968) *Bull Soc Fr Dermatol Syphiligr* **75**, 363.
5 CANTWELL A. R. & REED W. B. (1965) *Acta Derm Venereol (Stockh)* **45**, 387.
6 CAZERS J. S., *et al* (1974) *Arch Dermatol* **110**, 773.
7 DUPERRAT B. & MASCARO J. M. (1965) *Ann Dermatol Syphiligr* **92**, 19.
8 FORBIS R. & HELWIG E. B. (1961) *Arch Dermatol* **83**, 606.
9 FREEMAN R. G. & CHERNOSKY M. E. (1969) *Arch Dermatol* **100**, 66.
10 GRAUL E. G. (1953) *Dermatol Wochenschr* **128**, 949.
11 GRAY H. B. & HELWIG E. B. (1963) *Arch Dermatol* **87**, 102.
12 HASHIMOTO K., *et al* (1966) *J Invest Dermatol* **46**, 391.
13 HEADINGTON J. T. (1976) *Am J Pathol* **85**, 480.
14 HEADINGTON J. T. & FRENCH A. J. (1962) *Arch Dermatol* **86**, 430.
15 HOWELL J. B. & ANDERSON D. E. (1976) *Br J Dermatol* **95**, 233.
16 INGRISH F. M. & REED R. J. (1968) *Dermatol Int* **7**, 182.
17 KLIGMAN A. M. & PINKUS H. (1960) *Arch Dermatol* **81**, 922.
18 KNOTH W. & EHLERS G. (1960) *Hautarzt* **11**, 535.
19 McGAVRAN M. H. (1965) *Cancer* **18**, 1445.
20 MEHREGAN A. H. (1964) *Arch Dermatol* **89**, 229.
21 MOEHLENBECK F. W. (1973) *Arch Dermatol* **108**, 532.
22 MULLER-HESS S. & DELACRÉTAZ J. (1973) *Dermatologica* **146**, 170.
23 OSWALD F. H. (1971) *Dermatologica* **142**, 29.
24 PINKUS H. (1966) *Arch Argent Dermatol* **16**, 7.
25 PINKUS H. & SUTTON R. L. (1965) *Arch Dermatol* **81**, 922.
26 PINKUS H., *et al* (1974) *J Invest Dermatol* **63**, 212.
27 RAHBARI H. & MEHREGAN A. (1975) *Cutan Pathol* **2**, 225.
28 RASMUSSEN J. E. (1975) *Arch Dermatol* **111**, 610.
29 ROSENBERG E., *et al* (1968) *Cutis* **4**, 1079.
30 SANDERSON K. V. (1961) *Trans Rep St Johns Hosp Dermatol Soc* **47**, 154.
31 SERRA A., *et al* (1957) *Acta Genet Stat Med* **7**, 207.
32 SIM-DAVIS D., *et al* (1976) *Acta Derm Venereol (Stockh)* **56**, 337.
33 THIES W. & SCHWARZ E. (1961) *Arch Klin Exp Dermatol* **214**, 21.
34 VAN DER WALT J. D. & ROHLOVE B. (1984) *Am J Dermatopathol* **6**, 63.
35 VERBOV J. (1969) *Br J Dermatol* **87**, 69.
36 WELCH J. P., *et al* (1968) *J Med Genet* **5**, 29.
37 WOOD M. G., *et al* (1984) *Arch Dermatol* **120**, 770.
38 ZACKHEIM H. S. & PINKUS H. (1960) *Arch Dermatol* **82**, 913.

Desmoplastic trichoepithelioma [1] (sclerosing epithelial hamartoma [2])

These two terms were introduced almost simultaneously. The Americans, Brownstein & Shapiro [1], chose the term 'desmoplastic trichoepithelioma', while the British group [2] suggested the term 'sclerosing epithelial hamartoma' to describe essentially the same process.

The lesion is a slowly growing locally invasive proliferation of tissue in which elements of hair follicle are predominantly represented. Lesions are found mainly on the face and have a depressed centre and a raised rolled edge in many cases, causing clinical confusion with basal cell carcinoma. To date, more females than males have been reported with the condition.

The three essential pathological features are firstly the presence of numerous keratin-filled cysts, secondly the presence of strands and ribbons of small dark tumour cells and thirdly a dense fibrous stroma surrounding the first two structures. The striking palisading of the basal cell carcinoma is absent. There is, however, a considerable similarity to the sclerosing variant of basal cell carcinoma, but the number of cysts should help to differentiate between the two.

Local excision is reported as being effective in the majority of cases.

REFERENCES

1 BROWNSTEIN M.H. & SHAPIRO L. (1977) *Cancer* 40, 2979.
2 MACDONALD D.M., *et al.* (1977) *Clin Exp Dermatol* 2, 153.

TUMOURS OF SEBACEOUS GLANDS

The following tumours or tumour-like conditions of sebaceous glands are considered here or elsewhere in the book.

Naevus sebaceus (p. 170)
Senile sebaceous hyperplasia (p. 1934)
'Sebaceous' cyst (p. 2404)
Steatocystoma multiplex (p. 2406)
Sebaceous adenoma
Sebaceous carcinoma

Sebaceous adenoma

Definition. A benign tumour composed of incompletely differentiated sebaceous cells of varying degrees of maturity.

Incidence and aetiology. This is a fairly rare tumour. The solitary type may occur in either sex, and most cases have been in elderly patients. There is no evidence that actinic radiation or other recognized carcinogens are to blame. The relationship of 'basal cell carcinoma with sebaceous differentiation' to sebaceous adenoma is undecided (see below).

The multiple type [1, 7, 10] is important as it is associated with multiple visceral malignancy (Torre's syndrome).

Pathology [7, 12]. Terminology may cause confusion, because some workers regard all sebaceous tumours as carcinoma [8] whilst others distinguish between sebaceous adenoma, sebaceous epithelioma and basal cell carcinoma with sebaceous differentiation. The last of these is a diagnosis which has not yet been validated by modern techniques, and there is no good reason for differentiating between degrees of benignity as the first two titles do. A reasonable compromise seems to be to regard as sebaceous adenomas all lesions which show no evidence of malignancy whatever the proportions of immature to maturing cells.

The tumour is multilobular and is situated in the upper dermis. The lobules are well defined, and are composed of small basophilic sebaceous matrix cells peripherally and larger cells containing cytoplasmic fat globules. The proportion of immature, transitional and mature sebaceous cells may vary widely from one area to another. There may also be cystic spaces lined by a thin layer of eosinophilic

material similar to the intraglandular sebaceous ducts [4]. The outline of the tumour is less regular than the normal sebaceous glands, and may be frankly irregular. The lobules often connect to, and may displace, the epidermis above them. Mitotic figures are not frequent.

Clinical features. The tumour is rounded, raised and may be either sessile or somewhat pedunculated. It is usually less than 10 mm in diameter, but older less-differentiated lesions may form plaques or ulcerate. The colour may be fleshy or of a waxy-yellowish hue, and the surface may be verrucose. The common situation is the face or scalp, and it may occur on the eyelid. It usually grows slowly, but a sudden increase in growth rate can occur.

Diagnosis. The colour, when yellowish, may be suggestive, but clinical differentiation from other epithelial tumours, especially basal cell carcinoma, may be impossible. The microscopical diagnosis is more certain when fat can be demonstrated, but sebaceous accumulations in the cytoplasm can usually be distinguished in ordinary sections [8].

Treatment. The best treatment is surgical excision. It may recur if incompletely excised. It is radiosensitive.

Sebaceous carcinoma

Definition. A malignant tumour composed of cells showing differentiation toward sebaceous epithelium.

Incidence. The variable incidence reported for this tumour reflects the differing diagnostic criteria of different workers, and the figure given by Stout [9]—namely 0·2% of skin malignancies—is, in the writer's experience, not too low. It has been reported following radiodermatitis [5], and the writer has seen a tumour in a patient with multiple arsenical skin cancers.

Pathology [11]. The same problem of terminology exists with sebaceous carcinoma as with the adenomas. There is a range of malignant tumours within which some of the lesions called 'basal cell carcinoma with sebaceous differentiation' can quite easily be fitted. It is uncommon for the lesion to be aggressively invasive on the skin, although it frequently is when situated on the eyelid [3].

The essential feature is cytological evidence of sebaceous differentiation, and a diagnosis resting on paraffin-embedded material only must be open to some doubt. The proportion of cells showing fat globules and the degree of cytoplasmic vacuolation are variable. The undifferentiated cells are of moderate size, with round centrally placed nuclei, rather basophilic cytoplasm and tending to group themselves in masses of a multilobular configuration. The differentiating cells tend to be more central. There are, in addition, cytological features of malignancy and evidence of local tissue invasion. Fat droplets may be found in the cells of some squamous and basal cell carcinomas and malignant melanomas. These tumours are differentiated by their own characteristic features. Sebaceous carcinoma is usually rather deeply set in the dermis, and the epidermis is involved only secondarily.

Clinical features. The tumour is solitary, firm, somewhat raised, more or less translucent and covered with normal or slightly verrucose epidermis. The colour may be yellow or orange [5]. The face and scalp are the commonest sites. The evolution may be very slow, and a size of 50 mm or more may be reached after many years without metastasis. Some tumours grow rapidly and invade early, but metastasis is uncommon [2]. In the absence of the yellow colour there is no feature to indicate the diagnosis clinically.

Treatment. Adequate surgical excision should cure the majority of cases.

REFERENCES

1 BAKKER P. M. & TJON A. JOE S. S. (1971) *Dermatologica* **142**, 50.
2 CIVATTE J. (1961) *Épithéliomas et États Pré-épithélio, Mateux Cutanés.* Paris, Masson, p. 281.
3 DOXANAS M. T. & GREEN W. R. (1984) *Arch Ophthalmol* **102**, 245–9.
4 ESSENHIGH D. M., *et al* (1964) *Br J Dermatol* **76**, 330.
5 JUSTI R. A. (1958) *AMA Arch Dermatol* **77**, 195.
6 NIKOLOWSKI N. (1951) *Arch Dermatol Syphilol* **193**, 340.
7 RULON D. B. & HELWIG E. B. (1973) *Cancer* **33**, 82.
8 SALM R. & WRIGHT G. E. (1975) *Beitr Pathol* **115**, 221.
9 STOUT A. P. (1946) *Arch Dermatol Syphilol* **53**, 597.
10 TORRE D. (1968) *Arch Dermatol* **98**, 549.
11 WARREN S. & WARVI W. N. (1943) *Am J Pathol* **19**, 441.
12 ZACKHEIM H. S. (1964) *Arch Dermatol* **89**, 711.

CYSTS OF THE SKIN

Nomenclature. The term sebaceous cyst should be confined, strictly speaking, to one uncommon condition, steatocystoma multiplex, containing oily sebum. Histological examination of all other cysts reveals the lining wall to be keratinous in nature

and the contents to be greasy, cheesy and semisolid with a foul or rancid odour in some cases. Keratinous cysts are divisible into two types, those with a lining identical in its stratification with epidermis and pilosebaceous duct and those with a lining resembling the external root sheath of the follicle. The latter variety is less common, and is often familial, multiple and largely confined to the scalp [7]. Of the many names this type has been given, trichilemmal cyst [11] seems the most apt. If sebaceous cyst is to survive as a diagnosis it would be best to use it as a generic term, in the way that surgeons still do, until the true pathology of these lesions becomes more widely known. The cysts found in Gardner's syndrome are epidermoid in type [5] and are characterized by their appearance in childhood. There is no genetic overlap between trichilemmal cysts, cysts of Gardner's syndrome or steatocystoma multiplex, although all have an autosomal dominant mode of inheritance.

Histogenesis. Steatocystoma multiplex is most likely to be a genetically determined failure of canalization between the sebaceous lobules and the follicular pore. The common epidermoid cyst is the result of squamous metaplasia in a damaged sebaceous gland. Milia may result from either keratinization within the sebaceous anlagen ('collars') of vellus hair follicles or cystic dilatation of an interrupted sweat duct. Trichilemmal cysts may be due to survival of fragmented segments of the hair root during catagen.

The following cysts are described in this section or elsewhere in the book.

Keratinous cyst
  Epidermoid
  Trichilemmal
Dermoid (p. 221)
Milium
Steatocystoma multiplex
Eccrine hidrocystoma (p. 2408)
Apocrine hidrocystoma (p. 2410)
Bartholin's cyst (p. 2203)
Myxoid cyst of the skin (p. 1855)
Branchial cyst (p. 219).

Epidermoid cyst (syn. sebaceous cyst, steatoma, epithelial cyst)
Definition. A cyst containing keratin and its breakdown products, surrounded by an epidermoid wall.

Incidence and aetiology. Epidermoid cysts are common, most frequently affecting young and middle-aged adults. They are rare in childhood. Many are the result of inflammation around a pilosebaceous follicle, and they are frequently seen following the more severe lesions of acne vulgaris. Some may result from deep implantation of a fragment of epidermis by a blunt penetrating injury. Those which occur as a part of Gardner's syndrome and of the naevoid basal cell carcinoma syndrome are probably due to a developmental defect.

Pathology. An epidermoid cyst is unilocular and spherical, unless flattened by firm tissue beneath it. There may be an obvious connection with the surface by a keratin-filled duct, but this is probably less common than surgical texts would suggest. The cyst is situated within the dermis. The lining wall reproduces the layers of the epidermis, although attenuated in large cysts. The keratin is lamellated and birefringent. Cholesterol clefts may be seen. The basal layer may be flattened and surrounded by fibrosis, or may show papillary indentations similar to the epidermis. Some cysts have a chronic inflammatory or foreign body type of reaction around them, at times producing (or caused by) partial disruption of the wall. Occasionally, a hair shaft may be found coiled up within the cyst. These cysts probably result from inflammatory destruction of the sebaceous matrix cells and connective tissue investment of the gland and subsequent re-epithelization of the abscess cavity, or from squamous metaplasia following impaction of a hair shaft within the sebaceous gland.

Clinical features. An epidermoid cyst is situated in the dermis and raises the epidermis to produce a firm elastic dome-shaped protuberance which is mobile over the deeper structures. It is tethered to the epidermis, and there may be a central keratin-filled punctum. The spherical form can be felt where the skin is sufficiently lax. Cysts near the surface, as in the ear lobe or scrotum, are yellowish or white. The size varies from a few millimetres to 50 mm or so. The common sites are the face, neck, shoulders and chest, which are areas favoured by acne vulgaris. Lesions may be solitary but are commonly multiple. They enlarge slowly and may become inflamed and tender from time to time. Suppuration may occur. Cysts that follow acne and have been subject to recurrent inflammation are rather difficult to remove completely. Calcification of the contents of epidermoid cysts cannot usually be detected clinically; when it occurs in multiple cysts of the upper part of the trunk it can give a confusing picture in a radiograph of the chest.

Traumatic inclusion cysts usually occur on the palmar or plantar surfaces, buttock or knee. A history of penetrating injury is not always obtained.

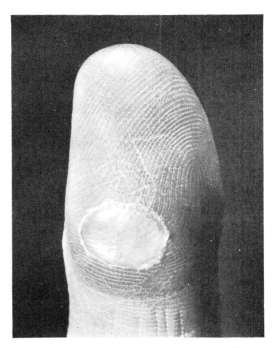

FIG. 64.19. Implantation epidermoid cyst which followed a penetrating injury by a blunt object (St. John's Hospital).

Diagnosis. The uncomplicated cyst can usually be diagnosed with confidence. Other benign and rounded dermal tumours may be mistaken for epidermoid cysts, and inflammatory granulomas such as cutaneous leishmaniasis may mimic an inflamed cyst.

Treatment. A cyst which has not recently been inflamed can be dissected out. An inflamed cyst is better incised, drained and phenolized.

Trichilemmal cyst (syn. sebaceous cyst, pilar cyst)
Definition. A cyst containing keratin and its breakdown products, usually situated on the scalp, multiple and familial, with a wall resembling external hair root sheath [4].

Incidence and aetiology. It is quite a common condition, and accounts for about 5–10% of keratinous cysts seen in surgical pathology services. Women are affected more frequently than men, and it is seen mainly in middle age [2]. It is inherited as an autosomal dominant [6, 7].

Pathology. Trichilemmal cysts differ from epidermoid cysts in the way the lining cells mature. As they move centrally they do not flatten and form a granular layer, and keratinization seems to occur mainly in the region of the cell membrane. The cells appear to disintegrate at the inner margin of the lining. The contents are not brightly birefringent lamellae, but may calcify.

The wall of a trichilemmal cyst may become ruptured and the contents invaded by granulation tissue. The reaction is much less acute than in ruptured epidermoid cysts and produces proliferation rather than destruction of the wall. The proliferation may be progressive and simulate, clinically and histologically, a well-differentiated squamous cell carcinoma [14]. Acceptable cases of clinically proved malignant degeneration in scalp cysts are very rare.

Clinical features. The lesion occurs mainly on the scalp, and is a smooth, mobile, firm and rounded nodule. Larger lesions may be lobular and multiple cysts are commonly found. Tenderness occurs with inflammation, and the surface may break down over a suppurating cyst. The cyst wall may fuse with the epidermis to form a crypt (marsupialized cyst) which can occasionally terminate by discharging its contents and healing spontaneously [6]. In contrast, the contents may protrude above the surface to form a soft cutaneous horn (Fig. 64.19).

Treatment. Uncomplicated cysts shell out of the dermis with remarkable ease. Proliferating cysts need to be excised with a margin because they will recur if tissue is left behind.

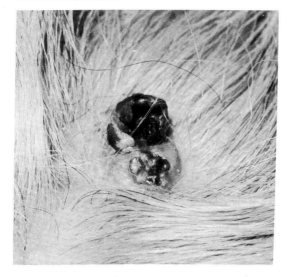

Fig. 64.20. Marsupializing trichilemmal cyst of the scalp. (Royal Marsden Hospital).

Milium
Definition. A small subepidermal keratin cyst.

Incidence and aetiology. Milia are quite common at all ages from infancy onwards. Many arise in undeveloped sebaceous glands. This may occur in young women as an eruptive phenomenon, and is sometimes a sequel to sunbathing. Others may arise in the proximal part of divided sweat ducts. The cause of the duct damage is usually avulsion accompanying an acute subepidermal bulla, particularly in second degree burns, epidermolysis bullosa, porphyria cutanea tarda and bullous lichen planus. They may also follow dermabrasion and occur in areas of chronic corticosteroid-induced atrophy. Destruction of skin appendages by radiotherapy may result in a ring of milium-like lesions at the margin of an area treated with tumour doses. These, unlike other forms, can be expressed easily.

Pathology. The lesion is so easily treated that specimens for histological examination are uncommon. The milia that follow blistering can, in the writer's experience, often be traced to eccrine sweat ducts in serial sections. Those at the margin of an irradiated area are usually situated in the distorted remnant of the pilosebaceous duct. The much commoner milia of the face are found to be situated within the undifferentiated sebaceous collar that encircles many vellus hair follicles. The white milium body is composed of lamellated keratin.

Clinical features. The lesions are white or yellowish, rarely more than 1 or 2 mm in diameter and appear to be immediately beneath the epidermis. They are usually noticed only on the face, and occur in the areas of vellus hair follicles, on the cheeks and eyelids particularly. Those that follow blisters are scattered more or less at random in the affected area.

Diagnosis. Milia can hardly ever be confused with any other lesion.

Treatment. Incision of the epidermis over the milium with a cutting edge needle or sharp-pointed scalpel and squeezing out the contents with two finger nails is usually effective. Recurrence is uncommon. Spontaneous disappearance occurs in many milia in infants.

Steatocystoma multiplex (syn. sebocystomatosis, hereditary epidermal polycystic disease)
Definition. Multiple cysts in the dermis having sebaceous gland lobules in their wall and containing sebum.

Incidence and aetiology. It is a very uncommon condition, which usually begins in adolescence or early adult life [8]. The condition is inherited as an autosomal dominant in many cases [10, 12]. The sexes are affected equally [1].

Pathology. The cyst is situated in the mid-dermis. The wall is thin and composed of keratinizing epithelium. In some sections, lobules of sebaceous glands can be seen to form part of the wall or to empty by ducts into the cyst. The contents are oily, and are composed of the unsplit esters of sebum [9]. They may contain hairs. Hair roots and, occasionally, sweat glands may be found connected with the cyst, and the whole complex is joined to the epidermis by a short strand of undifferentiated cells [3].

Clinical features. There are multiple smooth elastic swellings within the dermis varying in diameter from a few millimetres to 20 mm or more. They usually appear, or become larger, at puberty, and reach a limiting size. The trunk and proximal part of the limbs are most commonly involved, with the presternal region as the site of election. No punctum is usually apparent over the cyst, but there may be widespread comedones [13]. The more superficial lesions may have a yellowish colour. If pricked an oily fluid can be expressed. Some lesions become inflamed, suppurate and heal with scarring.

Treatment. The multiplicity of the lesions makes excision unpractical in most cases. There is no reason, apart from the cosmetic one, for treating them.

REFERENCES

1 AMERLINCK F. (1949) *Arch Belg Dermatol Syphiligr* **5**, 187.
2 HOLMES E. J. (1968) *Cancer* **21**, 234.
3 KLIGMAN A. M. & KIRSCHBAUM J. D. *J Invest Dermatol* **42**, 383.
4 MCGAVRAN M. H. & BINNINGTON B. (1966) *Arch Dermatol* **94**, 499.
5 LEPPARD B. J. & BUSSEY H. J. (1966) *Clin Exp Dermatol* **1**, 75.
6 LEPPARD B. J. & SANDERSON K. V. (1976) *Br J Dermatol* **94**, 379.
7 LEPPARD B. J., *et al* (1977) *Clin Exp Dermatol* **2**, 23.
8 MOUNT L. B. (1937) *Arch Dermatol Syphilol* **36**, 31.
9 NICOLAIDES N. & WELLS G. C. (1957) *J Invest Dermatol* **29**, 423.
10 NOOJIN R. O. & REYNOLDS J. P. (1948) *Arch Dermatol Syphilol* **57**, 1013.
11 PINKUS H. (1969) *Arch Dermatol* **99**, 544.
12 SACHS W. (1938) *Arch Dermatol Syphilol* **38**, 877.
13 SCHIFF B. L. (1958) *Arch Dermatol* **77**, 516.
14 WILSON JONES E. (1966) *Arch Dermatol* **94**, 11.

SWEAT GLAND TUMOURS

It is not yet possible to give a definitive classification of sweat gland tumours, despite much work on the problems of histogenesis [12, 30]. The kinship of a number of tumours to either apocrine or eccrine structures is known with reasonable confidence. The origin of the nodular hidradenomas is still uncertain, and the evidence for attributing an eccrine origin to dermal cylindroma and spiradenoma is, to the writer's view, inadequate. The grouping together of the less mature eccrine duct tumours as eccrine acrospiroma has much to commend it [29]. Eccrine poroma, hidro-acanthoma simplex and dermal duct tumour form a fairly homogeneous family derived from eccrine duct and pore. Eccrine hidradenoma, though closely related, has features suggesting both secretory and ductal differentiation, which makes the title acrospiroma misleading, and is perhaps best kept in a separate category.

Malignant tumours of sweat glands are relatively rare. Their morphology and behaviour are variable, and a malignant counterpart for most of the benign tumours exists. They will not be considered in much detail here.

Syringoma (syn. hidradenomes éruptifs, syringocystadenoma, syringocystoma) [6]
Definition. A benign tumour which is usually multiple and results from malformation of sweat ducts.

Incidence. It is an uncommon tumour, and is more common in females than males. It is most likely to appear at adolescence, and further lesions may develop during adult life. It does not appear to be hereditary.

Pathology [13]. Collections of convoluted and cystic sweat ducts are seen in the upper half of the dermis. Most are lined by a double layer of cells similar to, but flatter than, those which line normal ducts. The lumina contain amorphous debris. A characteristic feature is the tail-like strand of cells projecting from one side of the duct into the stroma, giving a resemblance to a tadpole or comma. The ducts may be enclosed in a fibrous stroma similar to the hair follicle hamartomas, but in most cases it is narrower and less cellular. When the stroma is dense it may be difficult to differentiate from the morphoeic basal cell carcinoma in which, however, well-developed duct structures are not associated with cellular strands.

Clinical features. The individual small dermal papules are skin-coloured, yellowish or mauve, but

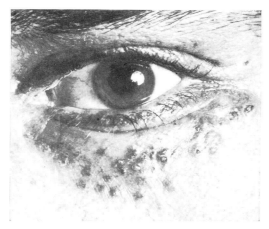

FIG. 64.21. Syringoma (hidrocystoma) of the eyelids. (Dr. I. Muende, St. John's Hospital).

sometimes appearing translucent and cystic. The surface may be rounded or flat-topped and the outline is sometimes angular. Rarely, injury to the surface will allow a drop of clear watery fluid to escape. They vary in size from 1 to 5 mm; the majority are less than 3 mm. In most cases there are multiple tumours, and they tend to have a bilateral symmetry in distribution. The front of the chest, face and neck are the chief areas affected. A few lesions are usually found on the eyelids when the cheeks are involved. The onset may be eruptive in adolescence (hidradenomes éruptifs) in one or more eruptions, and the front of the chest or lower abdomen is the initial site. Each lesion reaches a limiting size, but some patients report minor fluctuations.

Diagnosis. Syringoma is most likely to be confused with tricho-epithelioma on the face. The syringomas tend to be smaller, rather less superficial, more flat-topped and disposed more evenly over the cheeks and eyelids, rather than favouring the nasolabial creases. There is no family history. Lesions on the lids may be mistaken for xanthelasma, but lack the orange colour. Those erupting on the trunk may be mistaken for disseminated granuloma annulare.

Treatment. The main reason for treatment is disfigurement. Careful destruction with diathermy can produce good cosmetic results. Excision of lesions on the lower eyelid can be very pleasing to middle-aged women, but requires a plastic surgeon. Partial removal, by planing for instance, is often followed by regrowth.

Eccrine hidrocystoma

Definition. A tumour, usually situated on the face and often multiple, produced by mature deformed eccrine sweat units whose secretions dilate the ducts.

Incidence and aetiology. It is generally regarded as a rare tumour which occurs mainly in middle-aged women. It was formerly more common in those who had to work exposed to heat, such as cooks. A recent report indicating that the lesion is usually solitary and situated close to the eyelid [35] must be treated with reserve until it can be shown convincingly that the lesions referred to are not apocrine hidrocystomas.

Pathology. The general features are similar to syringoma, but secretory cells are usually found and the stroma tends to be inflammatory rather than fibrosing. The histochemical reactions are eccrine in pattern.

Clinical features. The lesions are largely confined to the cheeks and eyelids; they may seem to be cystic on examination and there is frequently a history of enlargement when the skin is exposed to heat. A recent report of predominantly solitary lesions in a series of 45 cases [35] changes the traditional ideas of this condition. Many of these lesions were bluish in colour and most were in the vicinity of the eyelids, features more typical of apocrine hidrocystoma (p. 2410).

Treatment. Diathermy produces satisfactory results.

Eccrine acrospiroma [21]

Definition. A tumour derived from eccrine sweat-duct epithelium which may be intra-epidermal (hidro-acanthoma simplex), juxta-epidermal (eccrine poroma) or intradermal (dermal duct tumour).

Incidence and aetiology. The members of the group are comparatively uncommon. Eccrine poroma has been the most written about; the sexes are equally affected, and the tumour usually begins in middle age. More than half the reported lesions have been on palms and soles. Some cases of hidro-acanthoma simplex have been included in the Borst–Jadassohn (intra-epidermal epithelioma) category. Cases of dermal duct tumour may be mistaken for eccrine hidradenoma ('myo-epithelioma'). There is no indication that heredity or external agents cause these tumours.

Pathology. The unifying feature of the three conditions is the type of cell that proliferates. It is smaller and more cuboidal than Malpighian cells, and resembles sweat ducts in containing glycogen and an abundance of glycolytic enzymes [34].

In hidro-acanthoma simplex [16, 37] the cells form nests, which may be discrete and rounded, or spread more diffusely within the epidermis. Eccrine poroma is a tumour in which these cells replace the epidermis and usually extend down into the dermis for a short distance; in the dermal tumour, nodular masses of the cells are found in the upper or mid-dermis, more or less separate from the epidermis. Slits or lumina may be found in the cellular masses. Because of its situation, eccrine poroma stimulates the adjacent epidermis to become thickened and hyperkeratotic, especially on palmoplantar skin, and there is usually a vascular fibrous stroma penetrating the under surface of the tumour. Pigmented eccrine poroma has been reported [23]. Malignant change has been observed in hidro-acanthoma simplex [20] and in eccrine poroma [30].

Clinical features. Eccrine poroma is the best documented [11, 18] and most easily recognized variety. The tumour is pink to livid-red in colour and sessile or slightly pedunculated. The diameter may be up to 10 mm or more. The surface may be smooth or somewhat keratotic, there is little tendency to bleeding or oozing and it is not tender. Many lesions have occured on the sole of the foot and have a somewhat flattened contour with a thickened, hyperkeratotic collar of epidermis immediately around them. A similar collar may occur on the palm. Elsewhere on the body the lesion is usually raised and vascular, and it may be ulcerated [17]. It grows slowly, and even after several years the majority of tumours are less than 10 mm in diameter. Thirty-one cases of malignant eccrine poroma are recorded in the literature [23].

Hidro-acanthoma simplex is a verrucous plaque or ring with a hyperkeratotic brownish surface. Ulceration or elevation of the lesion suggests invasive growth. From the few reports available, it appears that the limbs are more likely to be involved than the trunk or head.

Dermal duct tumour may present as a nodular dermal tumour or as a tumour with verrucous changes in the epidermis over it.

Diagnosis. On the palmoplantar aspects it may be mistaken for granula telangiectaticum, but may be distinguished by its slower rate of growth, thicker epidermal covering and lack of bleeding and erosion. Other dermal lesions such as histiocytoma and neurofibroma can cause a similar nodule surrounded by a collarette. There is not the thick accumulated keratin of a virus wart, and the vascular papillae are broader and blunter. The nature of the surface also distinguishes it from amelanotic malignant melanoma, where the epidermis is thin and fragile, and from squamous cell carcinoma. Hidro-acanthoma is most commonly mistaken for seborrhoeic keratosis or superficial basal cell carcinoma.

Treatment. Local excision will cure. Curettage may be sufficient for eccrine poroma [31]. A rather wider margin is necessary for the other two varieties.

Eccrine hidradenoma (syn. clear-cell myoepithioma, solid cystic hidradenoma, clear-cell hidradenoma).

Definition. A tumour of sweat gland origin which is distinguishable microscopically.

Incidence. It is an uncommon tumour, found mainly in adults and more common in women than in men.

Pathology. The tumour may connect with the epidermis, forms lobulated circumscribed masses and is composed of two cell types—polygonal cells, whose glycogen content may give the cytoplasm a clear appearance, and elongated darker and smaller cells, which may occur at the periphery. Cuboidal or columnar cells are seen lining duct-like spaces and clefts. The histochemical reactions and fine structure indicate an eccrine origin [32, 42], with features of both secretory and duct cells. Rarely, the tumour may be malignant.

Clinical features. The tumours are firm dermal nodules 5–30 mm in size, and may be attached to the overlying epidermis which can be either thickened or ulcerated. Growth is slow and there may be a history of serous discharge. The lesions are usually solitary and are most likely to be found on the scalp, face or anterior trunk.

Diagnosis. When the tumour is attached to the epidermis the diagnosis may be suspected on clinical grounds, especially with a history of discharge. Ulcerated lesions may resemble basal cell carcinoma. Dermal nodules are undiagnosable.

Treatment. Surgical excision will cure benign lesions. Malignant eccrine hidradenoma may metastasize.

Syringocystadenoma papilliferum. This is described in the section on naevi (naevus syringocystadenomatosus papilliferus). It frequently occurs in association with naevus sebaceus, although it may not develop until adult life. It may also occur combined with tricho-epithelioma. Composite lesions of this type, where the other element is pilosebaceous, are in favour of an apocrine histogenesis. The glandular structures have the architectural and cytological features of apocrine glands. The electron microscopic and histochemical features, however, are, equivocal, and a larger series needs to be examined before they can be regarded as proving one origin or the other. Fortunately, the name remains neutral.

Hidradenoma papilliferum
Definition. A tumour of the anogenital area of adult females composed of frond-like papillae lined by apocrine epithelium.

Incidence [19]. It is an uncommon tumour, which occurs predominantly in women. In one large series [27] they were exclusively white, and 75% were between the ages of 25 and 40. It occurs four times as commonly on the vulva as in the perianal area.

Pathology. The tumour is well circumscribed and located just below the skin surface. It is usually spherical in shape and enclosed by compressed connective-tissue stroma. The tumour is composed partly of slender fronds of connective tissue lined by one or two layers of epithelial cells, and partly of glandular structures. The epithelial cells have histochemical characteristics in keeping with an apocrine origin [27, 39]. The lesion may receive a pathological diagnosis of adenocarcinoma, but follow-up studies indicate that it is benign.

Clinical features [19]. The patients usually seek advice for a lump in the vulval or perianal area which may be symptomless or, less frequently, may be tender or liable to bleed. The tumour is rounded, freely mobile, often elevated and may feel firm, soft or even cystic. It may range in size from 1 to 40 mm. The commonest site is the labium majus, but it may occur elsewhere on the vulva or perianal area and, less frequently, in other sites.

Occasionally, the epithelial surface will ulcerate and the tumour become everted to form a reddish-brown papillary mass which may be suspected of being malignant [7].

Diagnosis. The tumour is usually mistaken for a cyst, polyp, angioma or haemorrhoid. A prolonged history and a firm spherical form make the last three diagnoses unlikely.

Treatment. Simple excision is curative.

Erosive adenomatosis of the nipple (syn. florid papillomatosis of the nipple ducts, adenoma of the nipple, papillary adenoma of the nipple, subareolar duct papillomatosis).

Definition. A benign tumour of the lactiferous ducts of the nipple which frequently causes erosion of the surface.

Incidence. This is a relatively uncommon tumour, occurring mainly in middle-aged women, but it has been reported in males and at any age [38]. The association with other breast diseases such as intraduct papilloma and chronic cystic disease appears to be fortuitous.

Pathology. There is a subepidermal proliferation of duct and gland-like structures which may spread down to form a circumscribed tumour of the nipple and subjacent tissues. The luminal cells are columnar and are surrounded by flat myoepithelial cells. The epidermis may show acanthosis and hyperkeratosis.

Clinical features. The condition usually starts with a bloodstained or serous discharge and the nipple may look eroded, crusted or eczematous. Symptoms may be worse in the premenstrual phase. Some lesions have been symptomless [33]. A clinical diagnosis of Paget's disease or intraduct papilloma is usually made.

Treatment. Simple excision is all that is needed.

Apocrine hidrocystoma (syn. apocrine cystadenoma) [36]
Definition. A tumour produced by cystic proliferation of apocrine secretory glands.

Incidence. The lesion is not uncommon, but is most often seen in opthalmic or surgical clinics. It occurs in adult life in no particular age group. Males and females are equally affected.

Pathology [28]. Large cystic cavities are found in the dermis if the lesion has been dissected out carefully. Commonly, the cyst is punctured and has collapsed before fixation. The cavities are lined by cuboidal or high-columnar apocrine secretory cells within flattened myoepithelial cells. Papillary projections or solid buds of secretory cells may break the smooth contour of the cyst lining. The secretory cells may contain pigment which is neither melanin nor haemosiderin. The secretions in the cysts may be coagulated and stained using the periodic acid–Schiff (PAS) technique. There is a well-organized fibrous stroma. Electron microscopy confirms the apocrine nature of the secretory epithelium [10].

Clinical features. The lesions are solitary well-defined dome-shaped translucent nodules. The surface is smooth and the colour varies from a skin colour to greyish or blue-black. The pigmentation may affect only part of the cyst. The commonest site is around the eye, particularly lateral to the outer canthus. It has also been reported on the penis [9]. There are no symptoms. The cyst increases slowly in size, and may become 10 mm or more in diameter.

Diagnosis. Basal-cell carcinoma is usually of a firmer consistency, less regular in its surface contour, and has surface telangiectases. The cystic nature of the lesion, which can be shown by transillumination in the larger ones, separates it from blue naevi and malignant melanoma when pigment is present.

Treatment. It is cured by surgical removal.

Nodular apocrine hidradenomas. Under this title are included dermal cylindroma, 'eccrine' spiradenoma and chondroid syringoma. Eccrine spiradenoma and dermal cylindroma are closely related, and perhaps the simplest illustration of this is their occurrence together as different parts of a single tumour [4]—an uncommon, but not rare, phenomenon; the writer has a section of a tumour in which these two elements are combined with chondroid syringoma. More refined evidence of similarity is shown by the presence in both of small undifferentiated basal cells and of four other cell types with varying directions of differentiation electron microscopically, by the presence in both of duct-like spaces, of hyaline droplets within and a hyaline membrane around the tumour islands, and of microdecapitation secretion of some cells [12]. Both tumours can be surrounded by a strongly positive acetyl cholinesterase network. These features suggest that both tumours derive from the coiled part of the sweat glands which are part secretory and part duct. Enzyme studies on cylindroma are indefinite but, in conjunction with some features of the fine structures, they favour apocrine rather than eccrine derivation.

There is some conflict in the published enzyme reactions of eccrine spiradenoma [11, 41] and a recent report suggests that the histochemical and electron microscopic findings show the cells to be basaloid in character [3]. However, there is a body of evidence suggesting an eccrine derivation for spi-

radenoma, which makes judgement on its histogenesis difficult. It is included in the apocrine category here with these reservations in mind.

Chondroid syringoma has a characteristic stroma in which are embedded gland- and duct-like structures and nests or festoons of tumour cells [15, 24]. It is likely that these criteria include tumours of both apocrine and eccrine origin, and possibly some mixed apocrine and hair follicle hamartomas also. Metastasis has been reported [26].

It is of little practical importance to determine whether the nodular hidradenomas are differentiating towards eccrine or apocrine structures. With these tumours, as with basal cell carcinoma, effort expended trying to interpret the maturation potential of immature cells is largely wasted. Using the fine structures of fetal cells as the standard for proving histogenesis is to reintroduce Cohnheim's still unsubstantiated hypothesis in a modern disguise. As sweat gland tumours occur in domestic and other animals [40] a study of their comparative pathology in the classes of mammals might be more valuable in understanding their nature.

Dermal cylindroma (syn. cylindroma, turban tumour, Spiegler's tumour)
Definition. A tumour of sweat gland origin with a characteristic histology and usually manifest as nodules or tumours of the scalp.

Incidence. It is an uncommon tumour, affecting females about twice as frequently as males. It is frequently familial [8]; its inheritance is determined by an autosomal dominant gene. It has been reported to follow X-ray epilation of the scalp [1]. The onset is usually in early adult life, but may be in childhood or adolescence [4].

Pathology. The tumours have a rounded outline and are composed of closely set mosaic-like masses and columns of cells which are invested by a narrow band of hyaline material and separated from one another by thin bands of stroma. The cells are of two types—one large, with a moderate amount of cytoplasm and a vesicular nucleus, and the other small, with little cytoplasm and a compact nucleus. The small cells tend to be peripheral; they also surround duct-like spaces or masses of hyaline material within the tumour lobule.

Clinical features. The tumours are frequently multiple, smooth, firm, pink to red in colour and often somewhat pedunculated. The rate of growth is slow and often seems to cease when a certain size

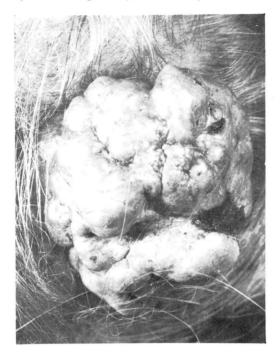

FIG. 64.22. Dermal cylindroma of the scalp (St John's Hospital).

has been reached. Some tumours become 50 mm or more in diameter, but most are smaller. Some tumours are painful. The commonest site is the scalp and adjacent skin. The tumours here may be almost hairless when pedunculated, but the smaller lesions form dermal nodules with little loss of hair over them. Multiple tumours have attracted much attention in the literature, but solitary lesions are not uncommonly seen in surgical pathology services. A proportion of lesions occur on the face and neck away from the scalp margin; in less than 10% of cases are they situated on the trunk and limbs. When the lesions are multiple, new tumours arise over the years. In some patients there may be an admixture with tricho-epithelioma either in separate tumours or sometimes in the same tumour. Malignant change is very rare [25].

Diagnosis. The multiple type on the scalp is most likely to be confused with trichilemmal cyst, which is, however, usually smoother, firmer and more mobile. Small tumours are difficult to diagnose, and must be distinguished from tricho-epithelioma, steatocystoma multiplex or basal cell carcinoma if solitary. Large, pedunculated and lobular tumours are almost unmistakable.

Treatment. Surgery is the treatment of choice. Extensive involvement of the scalp may require wide excision and replacement of the whole area by a graft.

Spiradenoma (syn. eccrine spiradenoma) [22]
Definition. A benign tumour of sweat gland origin which is usually solitary and is distinguished by its microscopical features.

Incidence. It is relatively uncommon, appears mainly in young adults equally in both sexes and is not familial.

Pathology. The tumour is lobular, with two cell types in the islands. Larger paler cells may be grouped around lumina, and smaller darker cells form the periphery. Small tubular structures or cystic spaces may occur. The lobules are surrounded by condensed connective tissue which may encroach on the islands as hyaline droplets. The tumour may also contain lakes of blood. Malignant transformation has been reported [5].

Clinical features. The lesion is usually solitary, may be tender and shows as a firm rounded dermal nodule 3–50 mm in diameter and raising the normal skin over it somewhat. The usual site is on the front of the trunk and proximal limbs.

Diagnosis. Clinical differentiation from other dermal tumours and cysts may be made if the tumour is a firm domed elevation of a dark blue colour.

Treatment. Surgical excision should be complete, as recurrence may occur.

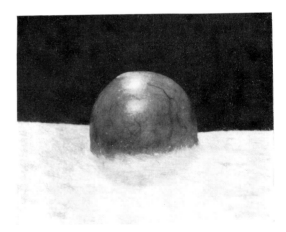

FIG. 64.23. Cystic eccrine spiradenoma (St. John's Hospital).

REFERENCES

1 BLACK M. M. & WILSON JONES E. (1971) *Br J Dermatol* **85**, 70.

2 BOTTLES K., *et al* (1984) *Cancer* **53**, 1579.

3 CASTRO C. & WINKELMANN R. K. (1974) *Arch Dermatol* **109**, 40.

4 CRAIN R. C. & HELWIG E. B. (1961) *Am J Clin Pathol* **35**, 504.

5 DABSKA M. (1971) *Nowotwory* **21**, 37.

6 *DAICKER B. (1964) *Dermatologica* **128**, 417.

7 DEACON A. L. & TAYLOR C. W. (1952) *J Obstet Gynaecol Br Commonw* **59**, 64.

8 DORN H. (1956) *Z Haut GeschlKrankh* **21**, 248.

9 GRINSPAN D., *et al* (1968) *Dermatol Iber Lat Am* **10**, 397.

10 GROSS B. G. (1965) *Arch Dermatol* **92**, 706.

11 *HAENSCH R. (1966) *Dermatol Wochenschr* **152**, 1481.

12 HASHIMOTO K. & LEVER W. F. (1968) *Appendage Tumours of the Skin.* Springfield, Thomas.

13 HASHIMOTO K., *et al* (1966) *J Invest Dermatol* **46**, 347.

14 HASHIMOTO K., *et al* (1967) *Arch Dermatol* **96**, 500.

15 HIRSCH P. & HELWIG E. B. (1961) *Arch Dermatol* **84**, 835.

16 HOLUBAR K. & WOLFF K. (1966) *Cancer* **23**, 626.

17 HUNTER G. A. & DONALD G. F. (1961) *Aust J Dermatol* **6**, 59.

18 *HYMAN A. B. & BROWNSTEIN M. H. (1969) *Dermatologica* **138**, 29.

19 IOANNIDES G. (1966) *Am J Obstet Gynecol* **94**, 849.

20 ISHIKAWA K. (1971) *Arch Dermatol* **104**, 529.

21 JOHNSON B. L. & HELWIG E. B. (1969) *Cancer* **23**, 641.

22 KERSTING D. W. & HELWIG E. B. (1956) *AMA Arch Dermatol* **73**, 199.

23 KRINITZ K. (1967) *Hautarzt* **18**, 504.

24 LENNOX B., *et al* (1952) *J Pathol Bacteriol* **64**, 865.

25 *LUGER A. (1949) *Arch Dermatol Syphilol* **188**, 155.

26 MATZ L. R., *et al* (1969) *Pathology* **1**, 77.

27 MEEKER J. H., *et al* (1962) *Am J Clin Pathol* **37**, 182.

28 MEHREGAN A. H. (1964) *Arch Dermatol* **90**, 274.

29 MEHREGAN A. H. & LEVSON D. N. (1969) *Arch Dermatol* **100**, 303.

30 MISHIMA Y. & MORIOKA S. (1969) *Dermatologica* **138**, 238.

31 MORRIS J., *et al* (1968) *Arch Dermatol* **98**, 162.

32 O'HARA J. M., *et al* (1966) *Cancer* **19**, 1438.

33 PERZIN K. H. & LATTES R. (1972) *Cancer* **29**, 996.

34 SANDERSON K. V. & RYAN E. A. (1963) *Br J Dermatol* **75**, 86.

35 SMITH J. D. & CHERNOSKY M. E. (1973) *Arch Dermatol* **108**, 676.

36 SMITH J. D. & CHERNOSKY M. E. (1974) *Arch Dermatol* **109**, 700.

37 SMITH J. L. S. & COBURN J. G. (1956) *Br J Dermatol* **68**, 400.

38 SMITH N. P. & WILSON JONES E. (1977) *Clin Exp Dermatol* **2**, 79.

39 TAPPEINER J. & WOLFF K. (1968) *Hautarzt* **19**, 101.

40 WEISS E. & FRIZE K. (1974) *Bull WHO* **50**, 79.

41 WINKELMANN R. K. & WOLFF K. (1967) *J Invest Dermatol* **49**, 173.

42 WINKELMANN R. K. & WOLFF K. (1968) *Arch Dermatol* **97**, 651.

Adenoid cystic carcinoma of the skin. This tumour arises principally in salivary glands and less often in lacrimal and ceruminous glands and the mucous glands of the upper respiratory tract. The microscopic appearance is characteristic and the behaviour predictable no matter what the site. The small number of cases arising primarily in the skin has been reviewed [1] and a further case was unusual in having pulmonary metastases [2]. Three of the seven cases have been situated on the scalp. The tumour grows slowly, invades along fascial planes, nerves and into bone, and is rarely excised completely. It is not radiosensitive. Wide excision with meticulous histological control of the margins is recommended [1].

REFERENCES

1 HEADINGTON J. T., *et al* (1978) *Arch Dermatol* **114**, 421.

2 SANDERSON K. V. & BATTEN J. C. (1975) *Proc R Soc Med* **68**, 649.

Hidradenocarcinoma (sweat gland carcinoma)
Definition. A group of malignant epithelial tumours showing evidence of derivation from sweat glands.

Incidence. Hidradenocarcinoma is relatively rare. It occurs with equal frequency in men and women and is more frequent in the second half of life.

Pathology. The tumour is an adenocarcinoma situated within the dermis. It shows cytological features of malignancy, invasion of surrounding tissue and differentiation to acinar or duct-like structures, although much of the tumour may be anaplastic carcinoma. Eccrine and apocrine varieties may be differentiated on histological or histochemical features and by elelctron microscopy. Eccrine carcinoma is the more common and may frequently metastasize [9], first to regional lymph nodes but later becoming widespread [13]. Distant metastases from eccrine carcinoma have invaded the overlying epidermis and established symbiotic foci ('epidermotropism'), a remarkable and interesting phenomenon [10, 12]. Metastatic deposits from other organs, especially from the breast, may be difficult to differentiate [1] and must always be considered before the diagnosis is made. Primary mucinous carcinoma [6, 8] has enzyme histochemical reactivity suggesting eccrine secretory epithelium, mucin histochemistry of sialomucin formation and electron microscopy of a highly differentiated neoplasm with a mode of secretion similar to that observed in the dark (mucinous) cell of the eccrine coil. Adenoid basal cell carcinoma and pseudo-glandular squamous cell carcinoma must be separated; the histological evidence of differentiation into duct structures in these cases is spurious, and the behaviour of the tumours is different, resembling that of basal or squamous cell carcinoma. Apocrine carcinoma may show the characteristics of apocrine secretory epithelium [7]. The special case of extra-mammary Paget's disease is considered on p. 2438.

Clinical features. The tumours, which may be painful [3], are reddish- or violet-coloured nodules arising in the dermis, and tend to be firm or hard and irregularly lobular. They may occur anywhere on the skin surface, including the palm [4], but the scalp and face are affected more often than can be explained on a random distribution [13]. The course may be slow and the history may suggest that the tumour has arisen within a benign lesion of long duration. The primary mucinous variety is usually very indolent, with a predilection for face and scalp, but may metastasize [6]. The diagnosis is unlikely to be made on clinical grounds. The tumour can be mistaken for dermatofibrosarcoma protuberans, cheloid, metastatic carcinoma or a malignant lymphoma of the skin.

Treatment. The tumour should be excised widely. It frequently spreads to regional lymph nodes and there may be metatatic nodules in draining lymphatics, requiring radical surgery.

Microcystic Adnexal Carcinoma (Sclerosing or syringomatous sweat duct carcinoma) [2, 5].

This recently described entity presents as a slow-growing indurated plaque, usually on the central panel of the face. The salient histological features are the presence of cords of cytologically banal keratinocytes with some ductal differentiation set in a very sclerotic stroma. The importance of this tumour is that perineural permeation is common, and for this reason microscopically controlled surgical excision is recommended.

REFERENCES

1 CIVATTE J. (ed.) (1961) *Épitheliomas et États Pré-épithéliomateux Cutanés.* Paris, Masson, p. 281.
2 COOPER P.H., *et al.* (1985) *Am J Surg Path.* **9**, 422.
3 EL-DOMIERA A. A., *et al* (1971) *Ann Surg* **173**, 270.
4 FRENSEN O. (1960) *Hautarzt* **11**, 15.
5 GOLDSTEIN D.J., *et al,* (1982) *Cancer* **50**, 566.
6 HEADINGTON J. H. (1977) *Cancer* **39**, 1055.
7 KIPKIE G. F. & HAUST M. D. (1958) *Arch Dermatol* **78**, 440.
8 MENDOZA S. & HELWIG E. B. (1971) *Arch Dermatol* **103**, 68.
9 MILLER W. L. (1967) *Am J Clin Pathol* **47**, 767.
10 MISHIMA Y. & MORIOKA S. (1969) *Dermatologica* **138**, 238.
11 PANET R. G. & JOHNSON W. C. (1973) *Arch Dermatol* **107**, 94.
12 PINKUS H. & MEHREGAN A. H. (1963) *Arch Dermatol* **88**, 597.
13 TELOH H. A., *et al* (1957) *Arch Dermatol* **76**, 80.

BASAL CELL TUMOURS
NAEVOID BASAL CELL CARCINOMA SYNDROME
PREMALIGNANT FIBRO-EPITHELIAL TUMOUR (PINKUS)
BASAL CELL CARCINOMA

The term basal cell carcinoma is preferred to the various other titles that have been proposed, such as rodent ulcer, rodent cancer, non-Malpighian epithelioma, adnexal carcinoma, etc., for the commonest malignant tumour of the skin. It is the term which is most generally recognized by clinicians and pathologists; its use is justified by the histological resemblance of the tumour cells to those of the epidermal basal layer and the undifferentiated cells of the appendages. The abbreviated title basalioma, much used in Germany, is to be commended and may become accepted in English-speaking countries.

The tumour cells show little evidence of maturation towards either keratin formation or adnexal structures. They are dependent upon connective tissue influences for their growth, and all but the most malignant induce a well-organized stroma around them. They invade and destroy adjacent tissues, but rarely metastasize. The majority of tumours develop without an obvious premalignant change in the skin, although some behave in so indolent a fashion as to suggest that they might themselves be only premalignant.

The two other conditions described in this section have many histological features in common with basal cell carcinoma. They usually behave in a benign way, but many become invasive if left sufficiently long.

Naevoid basal cell carcinoma syndrome (syn. basal cell naevus, Gorlin's syndrome)
Definition. A genetically determined disorder in which multiple skin tumours indistinguishable from basal cell carcinoma may be associated with palmoplantar pits and defects in other tissues such as cysts of the jaws, abnormalities of the ribs and vertebrae, and a variety of less common changes.

Aetiology and incidence. Genetic studies [1, 2] show that the syndrome is a hereditary dysplasia conditioned by an autosomal dominant gene with multiple and variable effects. Chromosome studies have not shown a consistent abnormality and the suggestion has been made that the disorder may be mosaic. The sexes are affected equally. The majority of patients are white-skinned, but cases have been reported in Negroes and Asians [11]. The condition is uncommon.

Pathology [15]. From their earliest stages the skin lesions are indistinguishable from basal cell carcinoma. Small buds grow into the dermis from the underside of the epidermis producing, as they enlarge, a filigree-like pattern resembling premalignant fibro-epithelioma (p. 2416) or more solid islands of cells. The reticular dermis is not usually invaded in the earlier and benign phase. The tumour induces a fibrous stroma as occurs with tricho-epithelioma or nodular basal cell carcinoma, and the lesions may become papular or pedunculated. Deeper penetration, ulceration and invasion can occur, with lymphocytic infiltration. There may be pigment in and around the masses. The presence of calcification and the general architecture can give a resemblance to tricho-epithelioma. The palmo-plantar pits are due to a premature shedding of defective keratin resulting from delay in maturation of the epidermal basal cells [14, 19]. Basal cell carcinoma has developed in palmar pits [12, 17]. The dental cysts may be either keratinous or dentigerous.

Clinical features. The skin manifestations may be present at birth or appear in infancy, but are usually first brought to notice in childhood or adolescence. The distribution of tumours is usually bilateral and symmetrical, but a zosteriform pattern [3], quadrant distribution or localization in a dog-bite scar [7] are recorded. The eyelids, nose, cheeks and forehead are the usual sites, but the neck, trunk and axillae are quite frequently involved. The scalp and limbs are usually spared. There may be few tumours or hundreds.

The individual lesions are smooth-surfaced rounded elevated papules, flesh-coloured or pigmented and varying in size from 1 to 15 mm in diameter. There may be fine telangiectasia and milium-like bodies just below the surface. Tumours of the axillae, neck and eyelids tend to be pedunculated. They increase in size and number up to late adolescence. The majority of lesions behave in a benign fashion. Some may become, or be from their beginning, truly invasive. This is most fre-

quent on the eyelids or nose, and can cause gross destruction. Ulceration is almost always due to invasive change.

A variety of other skin manifestations occur. There may be multiple epidermoid cysts and milia. The palms and soles show diffuse or punctate hyperkeratosis, but the characteristic change is the presence of more or less circular pits, varying in size from pinpoint to several millimetres in diameter. The edges are perpendicular and the base, formed by normal keratin, is about 1 mm below the surface. The base is redder than the surrounding skin. There may be larger irregular areas of ham-coloured erythema in which skin texture is altered. The change in texture is most obvious when the extremities are cold.

The dental cysts are usually multiple, occurring in either jaw or both, and are odontogenic keratocysts [4]. They are the most common stigma of the syndrome; spina bifida occulta, bifid or splayed ribs, scoliosis or kyphosis occur with a third of the frequency of the cysts or the basal cell naevi [1]. Among associated anomalies are broad nasal root and hypertelorism, frontal bossing, syndactyly, shortened metacarpals, defective dentition, cleft palate and hare lip, soft tissue calcification (especially of the falx cerebri), bicornuate uterus, ovarian fibromas, hypogonadism in males, lymphatic mesenteric cysts, dystopia canthorum, cataracts and congenital blindness, agenesis of the corpus callosum, mental deficiency and a variety of neurological disorders [4, 6, 8, 9, 11, 13, 18]. The changes in the eyes, bones and central nervous system may be present in childhood before the naevi appear. Some patients show a renal defect in tubular resorption of phosphate which may be demonstrated by an impaired response to parathormone, suggesting a relationship to Albright's pseudohypoparathyroidism [5, 6]. Other patients show some of the changes of Turner's syndrome, Marfan's syndrome, Weil–Marchesan syndome or Klippel–Feil syndrome [6]. Medulloblastoma has occurred in siblings of patients with the condition [10]. Maxillary antral carcinoma has been reported in one case [16].

Diagnosis. In most cases the skin lesions resemble melanocytic naevi, von Recklinghausen's neurofibromatosis or skin tags rather than basal cell carcinoma, and their true nature may be suspected only because of the associated features or the family history. The pathological diagnosis is usually basal cell carcinoma, with no qualification to suggest a benign behaviour, and this has led to radical treatment and severe cosmetic disability [13].

Treatment. As the tumours may become malignant it is advisable to destroy them early in their evolution, especially those situated on the central part of the face. This can be done with cautery, cryotherapy or diathermy with minimal damage to the normal skin. Radiotherapy should not be used on the 'benign' lesions, and is inferior to surgery for the malignant ones.

REFERENCES

1 ANDERSON D. E., *et al* (1964) *Tumors of the Skin.* Chicago, Year Book Medical Publishers, p. 91.
2 *ANDERSON D. E., *et al* (1967) *Am J Hum Genet* **19**, 12.
3 ANDERSON T. E. & BEST P. V. (1962) *Br J Dermatol* **74**, 439.
4 BERLIN N. I., *et al* (1966) *Ann Intern Med* **64**, 403.
5 BLOCK J. B. & CLENDENNING W. E. (1963) *N Engl J Med* **268**, 1157.
6 CLENDENNING W. E., *et al* (1964) *Arch Dermatol* **90**, 38.
7 DAVIDSON F. (1962) *Br J Dermatol* **74**, 439.
8 GORLIN R. J. & GOLTZ R. W. (1960) *N Engl J Med* **262**, 908.
9 *GORLIN R. J., *et al* (1963) *Acta Derm Venereol (Stockh)* **43**, 39.
10 GORLIN R. J., *et al* (1965) *Cancer* **18**, 89.
11 GRINSPAN D., *et al* (1968) *Dermatol Iber Lat Am* **10**, 255.
12 HOLUBAR K., *et al* (1970) *Arch Dermatol* **101**, 679.
13 HOWELL J. B. & CARO M. R. (1959) *AMA Arch Dermatol* **79**, 67.
14 HOWELL J. B. & MEHREGAN A. H. (1970) *Arch Dermatol* **102**, 586.
15 MASON J. K., *et al* (1965) *Arch Pathol* **79**, 401.
16 MATTEY W. E., *et al* (1976) *J Med Soc NJ* **73**, 971.
17 TAYLOR W. B. & SILKINS J. W. (1970) *Arch Dermatol* **102**, 654.
18 VAN DIJK E. & SANDERINK J. F. H. (1967) *Dermatologica* **134**, 101.
19 ZAZZHEIM H. S., *et al* (1966) *Arch Dermatol* **93**, 317.

Follicular atrophoderma and basal-cell carcinoma (Bazex syndrome). This is another disorder in which multiple basal cell carcinomas are genetically determined. Two families have been reported [1, 2, 3] with a dominant inheritance, but there is insufficient evidence to decide whether it is autosomal or X-linked. Follicular atrophoderma is present at birth or in early childhood, and shows as 'ice-pick marks', enlarged folliclar ostia on the dorsa of hands, elbows, feet and face. The follicular changes are not due to injury or inflammation but there may be facial eczema soon after birth. There may be anhidrosis of the face and head and hypotrichosis. The basal cell carcinomas appear on the face in the second or third decade and resemble cellular naevi [2]. Histologically they are indistinguishable from the tumours of Gorlin's syndrome. The patients do not have skeletal abnormalities, plantar pits or the other features of Gorlin's syndrome.

REFERENCES

1 BAZEX A., *et al* (1966) *Ann Dermatol Syphiligr* **93**, 241.
2 VIKSNINS P. & BERLIN A. (1977) *Arch Dermatol* **113**, 948.
3 PLOSILA M., *et al* (1981) *Clin Exp Derm* **6**, 31.

Premalignant fibro-epithelial tumour
Definition. A premalignant tumour composed of cells resembling those of basal cell carcinoma arranged in a thin honeycomb around a prominent overgrown papillary stroma.

Incidence. The tumour is relatively uncommon. Several examples have arisen in areas treated by radiotherapy for ankylosing spondylitis [1, 5]. The writer has seen one case on the chest of a patient with multiple post-arsenical basal cell carcinomas.

Pathology. The outline is domed and the surface is formed of normal epidermis. The bulk of the tumour is composed of considerably enlarged dermal papillae, more cellular and fibrotic than normal, which are surrounded by strands of small dark cells that extend down from the underside of the epidermis. Small buds of cells may arise from the strands and enlarge to form basal cell carcinoma, replacing part or all of the tumour [2, 4].

Clinical features. The tumour is sessile with a domed surface, firm and flesh-coloured to pink or brown. Most of the recorded lesions have been found on the

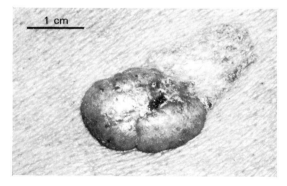

FIG. 64.24. Fibro-epithelioma of Pinkus of the lumbar region, with a superficial basal cell carcinoma in continuity. The patient had been exposed to X-rays 30 yr before when working as a radiographer and also had two basal cell carcinomas of the back. (St. George's Hospital.)

abdomen or loins. There may be seborrhoeic keratoses or basal cell carcinomas, or both, elsewhere [3]. Increase in size, when it occurs, is slow. The tumour is most likely to be diagnosed as a fibroma [4].

Treatment. Local excision is sufficient.

REFERENCES

1 COLOMB D., *et al* (1975) *Sem Hop* **51**, 2655.
2 DEGOS R. & HEWITT J. (1955) *Ann Dermatol Syphiligr* **82**, 124.
3 JAEGER H. & DELACRÉTAZ J. (1956) *Dermatologica* **112**, 364.
4 PINKUS H. & MEHREGAN A.H. (1969) *A Guide to Dermatohistopathology*. London, Butterworths, p. 464.
5 SARKANY I., *et al* (1968) *Br J Dermatol* **80**, 90.

Basal cell carcinoma [26, 50] (syn. basalioma, rodent ulcer)

Definition. A malignant tumour, which rarely metastasizes, composed of cells similar to those in the basal area of the epidermis and its appendages, and requiring a characteristic stroma.

Aetiology and incidence. Basal cell carcinoma may arise in skin damaged by sunlight and ionizing radiation (p. 2379). It may occur in burn scars [19] or vaccination scars [6, 24, 53]. Arsenic salts are also a proven cause [68]. The tumour may on occasion have a familial incidence independent of these causes, and it has been reported in identical twins [46]. Tumours of naevoid basal cell carcino-

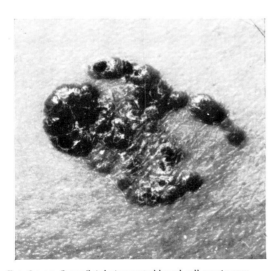

FIG. 64.25. Superficial pigmented basal cell carcinoma. (Stoke Mandeville Hospital.)

mas may become invasive carcinomas if untreated (p. 2414). The effect of developmental influences is shown also in those cases of basal cell carcinoma complicating naevus sebaceus and other adnexal hamartomas. In a considerable proportion of cases no cause can be found [16, 20, 22, 42].

In white races basal cell carcinoma is the commonest malignant tumour of the skin, whether the climate is sunny or not. The prevalence increases greatly with exposure to sunlight. However, the distribution of the lesions on the face does not correlate well with the area of maximum exposure to light; the tumour is common on the eyelids, at the inner canthus and behind the ear, and is uncommon on the back of the hand and forearm. The palm, sole and vermilion of the lips are rarely, if ever, involved. It is obvious that regional factors, perhaps related to the density and type of pilosebaceous follicles, are important in determining the distribution of the tumour. By contrast, the prevalence and distribution of squamous cell carcinoma correlates well with exposure to UV light (p. 2379).

Basal cell carcinoma is rather more frequent in males than females. It is extremely uncommon in dark-skinned races, and less common in Chinese, Japanese and other Mongoloids than in Causasoids [44, 57]. Although it may occur at any age from childhood [51], more than three-quarters of patients are over 40 yr old. It occurs earlier, and multiple tumours are more common, in those with a fair freckled complexion. On the lower leg the incidence in women is three times as great as in men [35]. Basal cell carcinoma appears to arise more frequently, and at a younger age, in patients who are immunosuppressed. These lesions are frequently aggressive [11, 21, 65]. It is occasionally seen adjacent to leg ulcers.

Pathology. The tumour cells resemble those [14, 32, 33, 49] of the basal layer of the epidermis and the matrix cells of the appendages in the relatively small amount of cytoplasm they possess and in their ability to interact with the dermis adjacent to them. Their nuclei are compact, rather darkly staining and closely set. Their cytoplasm stains poorly and the cell margins are rather indistinct. Adjacent cells are connected by bridges. The sparsity of keratin fibrils gives these connections a different appearance from the 'prickles' of the Malpighian layer, but the presence of desmosomes and tonofibrils has been shown electronmicroscopically [71]. The interaction with the dermis (which is one of the principal functions of the normal epidermal basal cell) produces the characteristic marginal palisade of tumour cells and the well-organized stroma

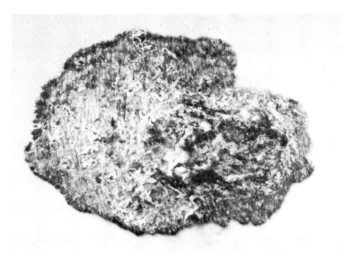

FIG. 64.26. Superficial pigmented basal cell carcinoma (St. John's Hospital).

that surrounds it. The dependence of the tumour on its stroma has been shown by transplantation and cultural experiments [18, 62]. The cells within the palisade usually show little evidence of organization or differentiation. Mitotic figures are not frequent as a rule, and in the cases where they are this is not necessarily an indication of rapid growth. Data on cell kinetics indicate that a considerable proportion of cells in the tumour die fairly rapidly [66]. Bizarre and atypical cells occur commonly in arsenic-induced tumours [41, 64, 68]. In some tumours the cells may become acantholytic [41] and amyloid may be diagnosed [64].

In early lesions the tumour buds can be seen arising from the epidermis [69]. In very small lesions multiple buds have been seen. These very soon become confluent, and the three-dimensional examination of superficial basal cell carcinoma shows a coherent margin of tumour with a reticular pattern of growth along the interpapillary ridges and larger more discrete masses centrally [38, 39, 56]. As the tumour progresses the masses extend into the dermis, and may separate from each other and from their point of origin. Growth in one area may be accompanied by involution of the tumour in nearby areas, leaving an atrophic epidermis. A common site of origin in man, and in the experimental tumours of the rat [70], is the junction between a pilosebaceous duct and the epidermis. From here the tumour may extend along the epidermis and down the duct. It is difficult to prove a purely adnexal origin for basal cell carcinoma, but some lesions behave as though this were so. In all considerations about the origin of the tumour

one must remember that the tumour can either sever its connection with epithelial structures or establish a secondary connection to structures to which it has grown close.

The variability of the natural history of basal cell carcinomas is reflected in its pattern of growth. Most tumours are composed of rounded expansile islands. These throw out small buds that grow in the same way to produce multilobular masses with thin strands or septa of fibrous tissue penetrating them [56]. In some regions a limited capacity to grow around and enclose adjacent connective tissue may be associated with a reticular or cystic pattern of growth. The capacity to invade in thin strands is often accompanied by an excessive, and almost exclusive, fibroblastic response, in contrast with the lymphocytic response around the expansile masses. Invasive strands may spread for long distances along nerve sheaths. Basal cell carcinoma is truly invasive in only a small proportion of cases. In these the tumours show no tendency to grow as rounded masses, have no palisade or organized stroma and penetrate the dermis and deeper structures, destroying them as they go. Such tumours are almost always ulcerated, usually from an early stage. In the less invasive tumour ulceration occurs when the epidermis is replaced by the tumour. An eroded vegetating type of growth is rather uncommon.

Most basal cell carcinomas provoke a round-cell inflammatory reaction of some degree. It increases in extent with ulceration and is often conspicuous in the papillary body, with superficial patterns of growth. Mast cells are often present in numbers among the fibroblasts of the stroma, and Langer-hans cells have been demonstrated within and near the tumour [37]. This infiltrate has recently been correlated with the aggressive nature of the tumour [58].

The diversity of histological patterns of basal cell carcinoma is due in part to features which have no direct bearing on the clinical course of the tumour. Not infrequently, melanocytes proliferate within the tumour. The melanin they produce causes the tumour to be pigmented, and numerous melano-phages collect in the stroma, and sometimes in cys-tic cavities. Mucin is commonly found in the stroma, particularly at the margin of the tumour, and may be encysted within it. Cystic cavities also form when the centrally placed cells undergo nec-rosis. There is no evidence that such cavities repre-sent glandular differentiation. Evidence of true se-baceous or sweat gland differentiation has been seen, but is very rare. Within some tumours there are strands of fusiform cells with more abundant eosinophilic cytoplasm, which may form whorls or keratinizing cysts and which probably represent ru-dimentary differentiation towards hair roots. Citrul-line can be demonstrated as a histochemical con-firmation in such cases [25] but does not help in the sometimes difficult separation from tricho-epi-thelioma. Histochemical and electron microscopy investigations show little evidence of differentiation of the tumour cells [23, 25, 67]. However, *in vitro* culture of tumour cells from nodular tumours pro-duces evidence of keratinization after 30 days, sug-gesting that the cells possess the biochemical mech-anisms for keratinization but that some factor, possibly dermal in origin, inhibits them [17].

Histogenesis. Theories about the nature and origin of the cells of basal cell carcinoma have been put forward at intervals over the last 80 yr or more. The histological variability does not accord with a derivation from any individual epithelial structure, and is now generally considered to stem from the pluripotentiality of immature cells of the epidermis. It is thus capable of maturing towards any of the epithelial structures and its behaviour is governed, as is the normal immature cell, by the connective tissue in its proximity. Thus the stroma dependence, the range of histological patterns and the way these merge with the more organized hamartomas are explained. It has been rightly emphasized that the stroma is an essential part of the neoplastic process [49] and it must also be removed in treatment.

Clinical features [1, 63]. The early tumours are com-monly small, translucent or pearly, raised and rounded areas covered by thin epidermis through which a few dilated superficial vessels show. Tiny flecks of pigment may be seen with a hand lens. Other modes of presentation are as a small pearly erythematous lichenoid papule or plaque, as a ker-atotic and slightly indurated area, or as a small and superficial ulcer resembling an excoriation by a fin-ger nail. It may occasionally be pedunculated and telangiectatic, resembling a pyogenic granuloma [36].

The more advanced tumours have as wide a var-iety of forms as the early lesions and tend to main-tain the same pattern of growth throughout their course. One common type grows slowly as a well-marginated expanding nodule or thickened plaque. The thinned epidermis closely covers the tumour and may periodically scale or erode and crust. In this variety ulceration occurs relatively late, and may re-epithelialize and break down several times before becoming permanent. The surface contour usually becomes more irregular as the lesion grows. The degree of vascularity varies. There may be a few surface telangiectasia over a flesh-coloured mass or the tumour may be pink or red colour. Pigment, when present, is usually unevenly distri-buted through the tumour. Some, or all, of the com-ponent nodules may have cystic centres, which add to the translucent appearance; the cystic parts may be more deeply pigmented than the peripheral parts.

Less commonly, the tumour spreads only super-

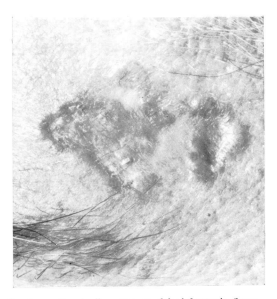

Fig. 64.27. Basal cell carcinoma of the left temple. Some areas are scarred, and the thickened rim is incomplete. (St. John's Hospital.)

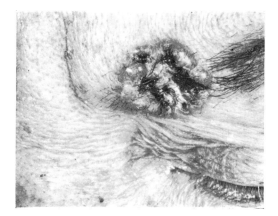

FIG. 64.28. Nodular and ulcerated basal cell carcinoma (St. John's Hospital.)

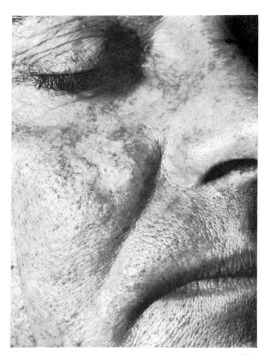

FIG. 64.29. Basal cell carcinoma of morphoeic type (St. John's Hospital.)

ficially. It is bounded by a slightly raised thread-like margin which is irregular in outline and may be deficient at part of the circumference. The epidermis covering the central zone is usually atrophic and may be scaly. This, combined with an increased vascularity, gives a resemblance to Paget's disease of the nipple. There may be a series of thickened papular islands of growth within the margin, and these may be crusted or eroded. Superficial tumours are often pigmented [38].

The atypical rodent ulcer has an indurated edge and base, but no thread-like margin. The edge is usually raised above the normal level but in some areas, particularly in the nasolabial furrows, it may be flush with the surface. The floor of the ulcer is depressed below the skin surface, fleshy in appearance and not very vascular. There is, however, more or less inflammation around the tumour. Such an ulcerated lesion may have begun as a nodule, but more frequently it is crusted or eroded from an early stage of its evolution. If left, the tumour and its following ulcer may spread deeply and cause great destruction, especially around the eye, nose or ear. There may be wide extension in the peri-orbital tissues; the bones of the face, the skull and even the meninges may be invaded, and advanced cases amply justify the title 'ulcus terebrans'.

The morphoeic or sclerodermiform basal cell carcinoma is very uncommon, and is so named because dense fibrosis of the stroma produces a thickened plaque rather than a tumour. The exact margin of the lesion is impossible to define, but palpation reveals a firm skin texture which extends irregularly beyond the visible changes.

The surface is smooth and may be slightly raised above, or sometimes slightly depressed below, the normal level. The colour is yellowish and has been compared with old ivory. Ulceration is uncommon and only very superficial when it does occur. Many patients, and not a few doctors, may take little notice of this type of basal cell carcinoma until its slow extension produces a sizable lesion.

The fibro-epithelial tumour of Pinkus probably belongs within the basal cell carcinoma group (p. 2461).

The majority of basal cell carcinomas arise on the head and neck, with a particular predilection for the upper central part of the face. The morphoeic type occurs almost exclusively on the face. The superficial type, however, is found mainly on the trunk. The palms and soles are rarely affected [38, 40]. Basal cell carcinomas may be multiple. The lesions which arise in patients who have been treated with potassium arsenite are almost invariably multiple, and are most profuse on the trunk. The tumours are usually well-circumscribed plaques or nodules and may number several hundred. The post-irradiation tumours of the scalp [55], and those which occur in sun-damaged skin of the face, may be multiple and show various stages of development. A few cases of genuine basal cell carcinoma have been reported to arise from the epidermis over histiocytomas, but the not uncommon basaloid buds seen in sections of histiocytoma are of doubtful significance [49].

The typical basal cell carcinoma runs a slow progressive course of peripheral extension, which produces the thread-like margin, the nodule with a central depression or the expanding rodent ulcer. Some tumours grow at so slow a rate that they are, for all practical purposes, benign. This is true for many of the superficial lesions and some of the nodular cystic lesions also. There may be spontaneous fluctuation in size, and areas of scarring can be found within many superficial tumours. A patient who has had one basal cell carcinoma treated should always be followed up, not only for local recurrence but also to detect fresh tumours arising elsewhere. There is no recognized premalignant stage of basal cell carcinoma equivalent to solar keratosis or Bowen's disease for squamous cell carcinoma.

Rapid growth is so uncommon as to throw doubt on the accuracy of the patient's history. Invasive rodent ulcers, if neglected, may cause death. This is

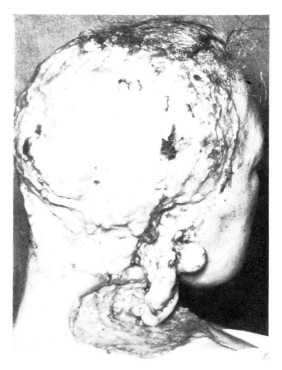

FIG. 64.31. Extensive basal cell carcinoma in a young woman. The hairy scalp and the right ear have been largely destroyed and the neck deeply invaded. The patient died from haemorrhage when an artery was eroded. (Stoke Mandeville Hospital.)

preceded by prolonged mutilation of the face or scalp, with destruction of the nose or eye and exposure of the paranasal sinuses or the skull, dura or brain. A few giant exophytic tumours have occurred on the back [10].

In rare cases the tumour may disseminate [4, 5, 12, 15, 30, 31, 54, 59, 62]. When the ulceration involves the airway, fragments of tumour cells and stroma may be inhaled and become implanted in the lungs. Authentic cases of blood stream metastasis are on record in which, for example, deposits in the viscera or spinal column have caused the presenting symptoms of the terminal illness [9]. Other cases have spread via lymphatics to the regional lymph nodes before disseminating [5, 15, 30].

Diagnosis. The common nodular type of tumour has a distinctive appearance when it is more than a few millimetres in diameter. In the initial stages it may be hard to separate from a melanocytic naevus (especially when pigmented), molluscum contagiosum or senile sebaceous hyperplasia without the

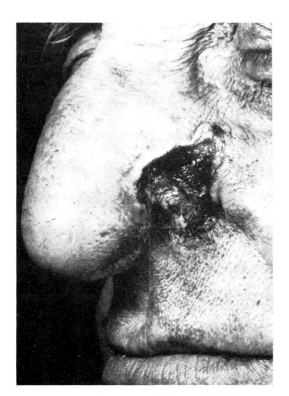

FIG. 64.30. Basal cell carcinoma (rodent ulcer) of the nasolabial sulcus (St. John's Hospital).

aid of a biopsy. Naevi can be distinguished if hairs grow from the surface, and in molluscum contagiosum and sebaceous hyperplasia there is a central keratin-filled pit. Scaling or crusting on the surface can cause confusion with warts, keratoacanthoma, squamous cell carcinoma or molluscum contagiosum. In all cases the debris should be removed, and this is easily done in basal cell carcinoma. The friable relatively avascular tissue beneath is characteristic, and if fragments are removed and smeared on a slide the diagnosis can be confirmed by cytology (p. 79). Darkly pigmented ulcerated tumours are occasionally confused with malignant melanoma. The margin of basal cell carcinoma is usually rolled, telangiectatic and multinodular, and there is no pigmented halo. The colour tends to be more definitely brown, in contrast with the dusky greyish-brown of malignant melanoma.

Perhaps the most difficult problems (though least crucial from the patient's viewpoint) are found with superficial basal cell carcinoma. Casual inspection may suggest that these are patches of eczema, psoriasis or Bowen's disease. When the scale is removed and the edge stretched the thread-like margin will reveal the true diagnosis. Careful inspection will almost always rule out eczema or psoriasis, which the patient's history will have also made unlikely. There are some cases, however, where distinction from Bowen's disease can be made only after biopsy. The consistency of a morphoeic basal cell carcinoma may resemble morphoea; the outline is usually less sharp and the evolution more gradual and relentless. A recently described elastotic nodule on the anterior crus of the antihelix of the ear in sun-damaged skin may resemble a nodular basal cell carcinoma on cursory examination [8].

Treatment. In most carcinomas treatment of an advanced lesion is usually palliative because metastasis makes a cure unlikely. This is not so in basal cell carcinoma, but there is a great risk that treating an insufficiently large area will allow recurrence and deep invasion. There is a 50% recurrence rate after retreatment of tumours treated inadequately in the first instance [43]. A knowledge of the pathological pattern of the particular tumour, and an appreciation of the modes of extension of the tumour in general, are the only real safeguards against inadequate treatment. Those that ulcerate early, particularly when situated in the nasolabial crease, usually behave aggressively. Some send strands of cells along the fine nerves of the skin for a considerable distance beyond the obvious clinical edge of the tumour [45] and are likely to give marginal recurrences after any form of treatment. The

lateral margin of superficial tumours can be difficult to define. The edge of the morphoeic basal cell carcinoma may be hard to find clinically, and the extent of this lesion is often underestimated. The outlook is bad when cartilage, bone or the orbit have been invaded. In the common nodular and plaque forms of the tumour, however, careful inspection with a loupe enables the margin to be determined to within 0.5 mm of the histologically proven border [15].

In experienced hands there is little to chose between the several methods of treatment in common use, and the decision as to which to employ may often be made on the cosmetic result. The patient's best interests are served by the establishment of a combined tumour clinic in which the various specialities are represented.

Radiotherapy. Modern techniques of dividing the dose into a number of small fractions over several weeks have reduced greatly the scarring and likelihood of necrosis which were a frequent sequel to single-dose treatment. Atrophy of some degree is inevitable and tends to become more prominent as time passes. Lack of response, or recurrence within the treated area, is unusual. Radiotherapy is best suited for elderly and timorous patients, particularly with rather extensive lesions, for whom major surgery would be a strain. An analysis of the late results of a large series of patients treated by radiotherapy suggests that surgery is preferable for tumours of the ear, the lower limbs and possibly the eyelids [17], although extensive lesions on the eyelid present the reconstructive surgeon with great problems. Radiotherapy should not be used a second time for recurrences, nor for treating morphoeic lesions which are radioresistant. The technical details are discussed elsewhere (p. 2604).

Surgery. Excision with primary closure, or a sliding or full-thickness graft to make good the defect, produces a good scar in expert hands and enables the pathologist to confirm the completeness of excision; in general, the cosmetic result improves as time passes. With both surgery and radiotherapy, the lateral margin of the growth may be underestimated and marginal recurrence result. This can usually be recognized early and dealt with. Excision has the added hazard of inadequate removal in depth. If this happens the recurrence may not be apparent until deeper structures have become invaded [3]. The pathologist cannot always be certain that every point on the periphery is clear of malignant cells, but he can almost always give a verdict on clearance in depth. Morphoeic basal cell carcinoma requires wide surgical excision with histological confirmation of adequate clearance [34].

Cryosurgery. Freezing with liquid nitrogen has been advocated for basal cell carcinoma as well as for many other accessible tumours. It is claimed to be a quick and relatively tolerable procedure which does not require anaesthesia. Thermometer probes can be inserted beneath the tumour to ensure that the freezing is adequate at its base. The operator can therefore have a good knowledge of the pattern of growth of the tumour. This form of treatment is considered in more detail on p. 2596.

Curettage. The common pattern of growth as circumscribed masses makes this a very suitable method of treatment for many tumours. The tumour tissue is soft and friable, and the stroma is fibrous and resists the curette. After the bulk of the lesion has been enucleated by curettage, the smaller extensions can be scraped with a Meibomian curette. The stroma and surrounding dermis are then charred with diathermy or cautery for a depth of 1 mm and curetted, and the destruction is repeated. Healing is accomplished with remarkably little scarring in most cases. The need for cauterization of the margin has been questioned [52]. The recurrence rate is comparable with those of surgery or radiotherapy [29, 60].

Chemosurgery [45, 48, 61]. This is probably the best technique to employ for the extensively invading tumours, as it uses microscopic control of the completeness of removal at the whole periphery of the tumour and enables strands penetrating along neurovascular bundles to be followed to their extremities. There are only a limited number of centres with the equipment and trained staff to perform the exacting technical work involved (see Chapter 68).

Cytotoxic agents. Small and superficial basal cell carcinomas would seem to be admirably suited for local treatment by cytotoxic drugs. A variety of compounds has been used, including podophyllin, methotrexate, colchicine analogues and 5-fluorouracil. Of these, 5-fluorouracil has been widely used in recent years, although more particularly for keratoses and Bowen's disease. Recurrence rates are considerably greater than with other forms of treatment of basal cell carcinoma [47] and it seems likely that the method will be reserved for domiciliary treatment of bedridden patients with a short life expectation.

A treatment of greater interest is tumour destruction by the induction of a specific immunological response in the area of the skin neoplasia. This is done most easily by contact sensitization to a hapten such as dinitrochlorobenzene and then challenging the affected area with a concentration of the sensitizer just sufficient to produce a response in normal skin [27]. Follow up for 7–10 yr of 24 patients with multiple epitheliomas showed that more than 90% of tumours were eradicated without recurrence [28].

Basisquamous or metatypical basal cell carcinoma [7, 15, 49]. This term is used for tumours which on pathological study appear to have features of both basal and squamous cell carcinoma. The biological significance is that this pathological pattern is associated with a significantly higher incidence of metastatic spread. The pattern in these lesions is of small aggregates of cells lacking classic palisading and embedded in dense and profuse fibrous stroma. The cells are larger with a larger paler nucleus than in the classic basal cell carcinoma and have a more eosinophilic cytoplasm.

There are two groups of basal cell carcinomas which should not be termed metatypical or basiquamous tumours.

(1) Basal cell carcinomas whose more central cells show some evidence of maturation towards stratum corneum in being larger, more eosinophilic and forming whorls or keratin cysts. This appearance is not uncommon, and is possibly evidence of differentiation towards hair follicles. It is, if anything, associated with a low degree of local malignancy and no tendency to metastasize.

(2) In skin damaged by actinic or ionizing radiations multiple malignant lesions may develop close to each other. Thus basal and squamous cell carcinomas of separate origin may collide and even intermingle. The squamous cell component may, however, arise at a rodent ulcer's margin as pseudo-epitheliomatous hyperplasia. In either case the prognosis depends upon an accurate assessment of the danger of the squamous cell proliferation, and it is important to realize that, in those rare cases of collision tumour, the squamous cells have an altered appearance when they grow in basal cell carcinoma. In examples seen by the author the double origin was obvious when sections were cut from different parts of the specimen.

REFERENCES

1 AFZELIUS L., *et al* (1980) *Acta Pathol Microbiol Scand* **88**, 5.
2 ANDERSON F. E., *et al* (1969) *Med J Aust* **ii**, 385.
3 *BAER R. L. & KOPF A. W. (1964) *Year Book of Dermatology*, Chicago, Year Book Medical Publishers, p. 7.
4 BINKLEY G. W. & RAUSCHKOLB R. R. (1962) *Arch Dermatol* **86**, 332.
5 BLEWITT R. W. (1980) *Int J Dermatol* **19**, 144.
6 BURNS D. A. & CALNAN C. D. (1978) *Clin Exp Dermatol* **3**, 443.

7 BURTON J. & CLAY R. D. (1959) *J Clin Pathol* **12**, 73.

8 CARTER V. H., *et al* (1969) *Arch Dermatol* **100**, 282.

9 CRAWFORD H. J. & JOSLIN C. A. F. (1964) *J Pathol Bacteriol* **87**, 437.

10 CURRY M. C., *et al* (1977) *Arch Dermatol* **113**, 316.

11 DELLON A. L. (1978) *Plast Reconstr Surg* **62**, 37.

12 VON DOMARUS H. & STEVENS P. J. (1984) *J Am Acad Dermatol* **10**, 1043.

13 *DUPONT A. & PIERARD J. (1961) In *Epitheliomas et Etats Pre-epitheliomateux Cutanes*. Paris, Masson, p. 223.

14 EPSTEIN E. (1973) *Br J Dermatol* **89**, 37.

15 FARMER E. R. & HELWIG E. B. (1980) *Cancer* **46**, 748.

16 FERGIN P. E., *et al* (1981) *Clin Exp Dermatol* **6**, 111.

17 FLAXMAN B. A. (1972) *Cancer Res* **32**, 462.

18 FLAXMAN B. A. & VAN SCOTT E. J. (1968) *J Natl Cancer Inst* **40**, 441.

19 GAUGHAN L. J., *et al* (1969) *Arch Dermatol* **99**, 594.

20 GOLDBERG H. S. (1980) *Cutis* **25**, 295.

21 GORMLEY D. E. & HIRSCH P. (1978) *Arch Dermatol* **114**, 782.

22 HANSEN P. B. & JENSEN M. S. (1968) *Acta Radiol* **7**, 307.

23 *HASHIMOTO K. & LEVER W. F. (1968) *Appendage Tumors of the Skin*, Springfield, Thomas, p. 115.

24 HENDRICKS W. M. (1980) *Arch Dermatol* **116**, 1304.

25 HOLMES E. J., *et al* (1968) *Cancer* **22**, 663.

26 HOWELL J. B. (1984) *J Am Acad Dermatol* **11**, 98.

27 KLEIN E. (1968) *NY State J Med* **68**, 900.

28 KLEIN E., *et al* (1975) *Transplant Proc* **7**, 297.

29 KNOX J. M., *et al* (1967) *South Med J* **60**, 241.

30 LARSON D. L., *et al* (1980) *South Med J* **73**, 647.

31 LATTES R. & KESSLER R. W. (1951) *Cancer* **4**, 866.

32 LEWIS W. R., *et al* (1973) *J Cutan Pathol* **2**, 284.

33 LILLIS P. J. & CEILLEY R. J. (1979) *Cutis* **23**, 310.

34 LITZOW T. J., *et al* (1968) *Am J Surg* **116**, 499.

35 LYNCH F. W., *et al* (1970) *Cancer* **25**, 83.

36 LYNFIELD Y. L. & GRIER W. (1970) *Cutis* **6**, 898.

37 MACADAM R. F. (1978) *J Pathol* **126**, 149.

38 *MADSEN A. (1941) *Acta Derm Venereol (Stockh)* **22**, Suppl. 7.

39 MADSEN A. (1965) *Acta Pathol Microbiol Scand*, (Suppl. 7).

40 MCEVOY R. & HELM F. (1969) *Z. Haut GeschlKrankh* **44**, 91.

41 MEHREGAN A. H. (1979) *J Cutan Pathol* **6**, 280.

42 MEHTA V. R. (1980) *Indian J Med Sci* **34**, 8.

43 MENN H., *et al* (1971) *Arch Dermatol* **103**, 628.

44 MIKI Y. (1968) *Aust J Dermatol* **9**, 304.

45 *MOHS F. E. (1956) *Chemosurgery in Cancer, Gangrene and Infections*. Springfield, Thomas.

46 OETTLE A. G. (1956) *Arch Dermatol* **74**, 167.

47 PENICHE J. & RUIZ GODOV V. M. (1968) *Dermatologia (Mexico City)* **12**, 137.

48 PHELAN J. T. (1968) *Ann Surg* **168**, 1023.

49 PINKUS H. & MEHREGAN A. H. (1969) *A Guide to Dermatohistopathology*. London, Butterworths, p. 454.

50 *POLLAK S. V., *et al* (1982) *J Am Acad Dermatol* **7**, 569.

51 RAHBART H. & MEHREGAN A. (1982) *Cancer* **49**, 350.

52 REYMANN F. (1973) *Arch Dermatol* **108**, 528.

53 RICH J. D., *et al* (1980) *J Clin Pathol* **33**, 134.

54 RICHTER G. (1957) *Hautarzt* **8**, 215.

55 RIDLEY C. M. & SPITTLE M. F. (1974) *Lancet* **i**, 509.

56 SANDERSON K. V. (1961) *Br J Dermatol* **73**, 455.

57 SHANMUGARANAM K. & LA BROOY E. B. (1963) *Natl Cancer Inst Monogr* **10**, 127.

58 SHERERTZ E. F., *et al* (1982) *Clin Res* **30**, 266 (Abstract).

59 STELL J. S., *et al* (1966) *Arch Dermatol* **93**, 338.

60 SWEET R. D. (1963) *Br J Dermatol* **75**, 137.

61 TROMOVITCH T. A. & STEGEMAN S. J. (1974) *Arch Dermatol* **110**, 231.

62 VAN SCOTT E. J. & REINERTSON R. P. (1961) *J Invest Dermatol* **36**, 109.

63 WADE T. R. & ACKERMAN A. B. (1978) *J Dermatol Surg Oncol* **4**, 23.

64 WEEDON D. & SHAND E. (1979) *Br J Dermatol* **101**, 141.

65 WEIMAR V. W., *et al* (1979) *J Dermatol Surg Oncol* **5**, 609.

66 WEINSTEIN G. D. & FROST P. (1970) *Cancer Res* **30**, 724.

67 WOLFF K. & HOLUBAR K. (1965) *Arch Klin Exp Dermatol* **223**, 483.

68 YEH S., *et al* (1968) *Cancer* **21**, 312.

69 ZACKHEIM H. S. (1963) *J Invest Dermatol* **40**, 283.

70 ZACKHEIM H. S., *et al* (1959) *J Invest Dermatol* **33**, 385.

71 ZELICKSON A. S. (1962) *J Invest Dermatol* **39**, 183.

PREMALIGNANT CONDITIONS

Certain changes in the epidermis are important because they may, if left untreated, go on to become malignant tumours. Some, such as solar keratosis and leukoplakia of mucosal surfaces, may show little evidence of cellular unrest for much of their natural history. Others, like Bowen's disease or erythroplasia of Queyrat, may have the microscopical features of intra-epidermal carcinoma from the beginning, but remain confined by the dermal–epidermal junction. A feature common to all is a chronic inflammatory cell infiltrate in the papillary dermis beneath [34]. The stage at which the lesion becomes a malignant tumour is determined by the breaching, or disappearance, of the basement membrane, and the cancer is of the squamous cell type. Basal cell carcinoma is probably never truly intra-epidermal [27]. Skin damaged by ionizing radiation, radiant heat or exposure to tar and other carcinogenic compounds, and the keratoses that follow ingestion of inorganic arsenic compounds, are also potentially malignant. Occasionally, long-standing scars, sinuses and ulcers may be the site of cancer. Rarely a burn or other injury may be followed almost immediately by a squamous cell carcinoma (p. 2431). The majority of squamous cell carcinomas, in areas where they are frequent, are found to have been preceded by a premalignant lesion.

The malignancy which follows exposure to tar or arsenic is presumably the result of direct action of the chemical on the epithelial cell, whereas that which follows irradiation must, in some cases at least, be due to dermal changes which later act on the epithelium that has grown in to replace that destroyed by the radiation [14]. The effect of UV radiation is to act directly on the epidermis and indirectly through the dermal change which is an almost invariable accompaniment. Bowen's disease has been found to be associated with visceral cancer in a significant proportion of cases [18], and the same has been shown with arsenical keratoses [41] and solar keratoses [18]. An area of Bowenoid change has been found in a perianal wart shown by electron microscopy to be viral [31]. Malignant change has been described in epidermodysplasia verruciformis [36].

Solar keratosis (syn. actinic keratosis, keratosis senilis)
Definition. A dermatosis occurring in sun-exposed fair skin, at or after middle age, and showing itself clinically as areas of adherent hyperkeratosis, the result of changes in the epidermal cells which may later progress to squamous cell carcinoma.

Aetiology and incidence. The process is due to the cumulative effect of radiant energy. The great majority of cases occur in fair-skinned people exposed to sunlight. Similar changes may be induced by ionizing radiation or radiant heat and in workers exposed to pitch and other products of coal distillation.

The geographical prevalence depends upon the amount of UV radiation reaching the earth in the area, the proportion of susceptible individuals in the population, and the time spent in outdoor occupations and recreations. The maximum prevalence is probably found in Queensland, Australia, where the majority of elderly people have one keratosis or more [16].

Pathology [13, 32]. The boundary between unaffected and affected epidermis is a sharp line which slopes upwards and inwards, and there is a similar margin where the appendage ducts perforate the epidermis as funnel-shaped columns of orthokeratosis. The epidermal cells have a paler cytoplasm and mature through an absent or diminished granular layer to form a parakeratotic scale of varying thickness. There is usually some acanthosis, and the more dysplastic lesions show epidermal hypertrophy with hyperkeratosis and parakeratosis. The interpapillary ridges may be reduced in number and broader than normal. The affected zone tends to grow under the normal epidermis and around the ductal epithelium, and may separate from it by a cleft. The basement membrane is intact but basaloid cells may form multiple buds at the junction; the combination of clefting, budding and papillomatosis produces a Darier-like change. Within the epidermis there may be a simple dysplasia or a range of abnormalities up to a picture indistinguishable from Bowen's disease.

The papillary vessels are irregularly increased and there is a round-cell infiltrate beneath the lesion. There is a variable degeneration of dermal collagen and deposition of material staining like elastin in the upper half of the dermis, except for a narrow band at the basement membrane; this change is more or less uniform, unlike the discontinuous keratosis.

Flat keratoses may resemble discoid lupus erythematosus; the distinction is made by the altered epidermal cells, deficient granular layer and parakeratosis, the band-like, rather than perivascular, nature of the inflammatory reaction and the absence of immunoglobulin in the basement membrane region. Occasionally, the appearance may mimic lichen planus [39] or appear pseudo-epitheliomatus [4].

The transition of a keratosis to squamous cell carcinoma is indicated by acanthosis, with irregular proliferation of the lower epidermis to produce buds and branching columns of large eosinophilic squamous cells that penetrate the dermis and do not induce the formation of a basement membrane. However, the proliferation does cause an increase in capillaries in the region.

The occurrence of funnel-shaped columns of normal epidermis, derived from appendage ducts which appear to be trying to cover the diseased epidermis like an umbrella, suggests an effort at biological compensation [32]. This probably explains the rapid recovery after treatment with CO_2 slush. It must be remembered, however, that in keratoses and Bowen's disease sleeves of dysplastic cells growing down appendage ducts may survive damage by freezing or cytotoxic applications [33].

Clinical features [6]. The first evidence of a solar keratosis is usually a collection of telangiectatic capillaries a millimetre or two in diameter. This will pass unnoticed by most patients, and the diagnostic changes appear later as a dry rough adherent and often yellow or dirty brown coloured scale. This can only be picked off with difficulty, and a hyperaemic base with bleeding points is revealed. The scale forms and in time may become thick and horny. The edge of the keratosis is rather sharp. In the majority of cases there are a number of lesions. The

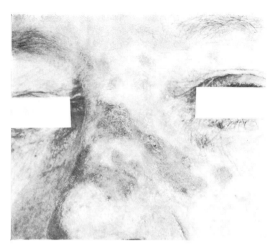

FIG. 64.32. Multiple solar keratoses. Their surface is rough, brownish and opaque on an erythematous base. (St. John's Hospital.)

principal sites are the backs of the hands and forearms and the face. The cheeks, temples and forehead are more commonly affected than the lower face. The sides of the neck are involved in both sexes, but the ears predominantly in men. The vermillion of the lower lip, but not often of the upper, may also show keratosis, with a much higher incidence in men than women. The elastotic degeneration which is almost always seen in patients who have solar keratosis produces a rather coarse, yellowish weather-beaten look to the exposed skin generally.

Solar keratoses are potentially malignant, but do not show the progressive lateral growth which is a feature of some other lesions of this type. It is, indeed, hard to explain the discontinuous nature of the epidermal changes in skin which has had fairly uniform exposure, except as due to clones of disordered cells. The transition to malignancy is suggested by the induration at the base of the keratosis, which must be distinguished from the hard consistency of the horn, and by an increase in the vascularity of the dermis beneath. In the transitional phase the induration and inflammation beneath a keratosis may flutuate independently of external irritants. The latent period is probably at least 10 yr, and the squamous cell carcinoma which develops in a keratosis is almost always very slow growing and has little tendency to metastasize [18]. Malignant change occurs in a minority of keratoses, and patients who observe their lesions closely may report that some will disappear spontaneously. In the earliest stages both solar keratoses and elastotic degeneration may disappear if the patient goes to live in a less sunny environment.

Diagnosis. The flat keratosis is most likely to be mistaken for discoid lupus erythematosus, which is usually bright red in colour and has an easily detachable scale. When the keratosis is pigmented it may resemble a superficial seborrhoeic wart, but it lacks the regular granular texture of this lesion. Bowen's disease on the exposed areas usually has a more irregular contour and a more erythematous base.

Treatment. Superficial lesions are most easily removed by rapid freezing with CO_2 slush or liquid nitrogen on a swab-stick. It is not necessary to produce an obvious blister, and 10–30 s is time enough. Destruction with cautery or diathermy current, preceded by curettage of horny lesions, is equally effective but is rather more likely to leave superficial scarring. Indurated lesions are best excised. Radiotherapy should not be used for solar keratoses.

Where large areas of skin are covered by numerous keratoses, cytotoxic applications such as podophyllin or 5-fluorouracil may be used, the latter preparation as a 1% lotion in propylene glycol or a 5% cream. If it is applied twice daily for 3–4 weeks, most keratoses erode and clinically unsuspected areas may react whilst normal skin is unaffected. These applications may damage the conjunctival epithelium; they take longer to work and produce an unsightly reaction, but they have established a place for themselves in the treatment of the more severely affected skin [23, 40].

In view of the improvement that follows avoidance of sunlight, an effective sunscreen is important in treatment, as well as in prophylaxis [12]. The present fashion for both sexes to have long hair will, if widely adopted, reduce damage to the ears.

Disseminated superficial 'actinic' porokeratosis. This disorder was first recognized in Texas, where a considerable number of cases have been seen [1, 3], and it is not uncommon in Australia [7]. It appears on sun-exposed areas of Caucasoids, becomes more prominent in summer and may improve in winter, and new lesions have been provoked by exposure to a UV sun lamp [2]. The tendency to develop these lesions is inherited as an autosomal dominant [1]. The preponderance of females in reported cases has been attributed to their greater awareness of minor blemishes. The average age at which Texan patients first notice it

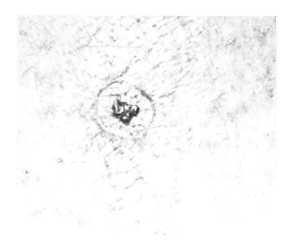

FIG. 64.33. Disseminated superficial actinic porokeratosis on the leg of a 58-yr-old sun-loving woman who had lived all her life in southern England. Most of her lesions had a central scale. (St. George's Hospital.)

is about 40, and its frequency in members of affected families seems to increase linearly with age. It has not been seen before the age of 16 [1]. There are English patients with multiple lesions who have never lived abroad (Fig. 64.33), and the true role of the sun in the aetiology of the condition has recently been questioned.

Pathology [3, 35]. There is no microscope feature which separates this disorder from Mibelli's porokeratosis, and both have been explained as the result of localized clones of abnormal epidermal cells [7], an idea supported by the successsful autotransplantation of the disseminated superficial variety [3]. The distinctive feature of porokeratosis is the cornoid lamella at the margin. This is a narrow column of altered or parakeratotic keratin, seated in a slight depression in the epidermis and directed obliquely inwards in some cases. It may involve the ostia of follicles and sweat ducts. The granular layer of the indented epidermis is usually missing and there may be dyskeratotic cells. The epidermis enclosed by the ridge is usually thinned, the interpapillary ridges and dermal papillae may be flattened, and the basal cells may show liquefaction degeneration. In addition to solar elastosis, decrease in collagen and telangiectasia, the upper dermis may have a non-specific inflammatory infiltrate with vascular proliferation, oedema and fibrosis. Malignant change has not been recorded.

Clinical features [3]. The lesion begins as a 1–3 mm conical papule, brownish-red or brown in colour,

and usually around a follicle containing a keratotic plug. It expands and a sharp slightly raised keratotic ring, a fraction of a millimetre thick, develops and spreads out to a diameter of 10 mm or more. The skin within the ring is somewhat atrophic and mildly reddened or hyperpigmented, but a hypopigmented ring may be seen just inside the ridge. The ridge itself is sometimes darkly pigmented. The central thickening usually disappears, but it may persist with an attached scale, follicular plug or central dell. Sweating is absent within the lesions. Sun exposure may cause them to itch. In sunny areas lesions may be present in very large numbers and may change from a circular to a polycyclic outline. In less sunny climates like Britain patients have fewer lesions, which tend to remain circular (Fig. 64.33). In a few cases, the centre of the area has become considerably inflamed and covered by thick hyperkeratosis, or has even ulcerated and crusted. The disorder affects areas exposed to sunlight, appearing mainly on the distal extremities and arising more frequently on the lower legs in women than men. The malar regions and the cheeks may be affected. It has not been seen on areas habitually covered by clothes, or on the scalp, palms or soles.

Diagnosis and treatment. Porokeratosis is distinguished from other dermatoses by its sharp margin and history of outward expansion. The rim of disseminated superficial actinic porokeratosis is very much smaller than in Mibelli's porokeratosis and never contains a cleft. The onset of Mibelli's porokeratosis is often in childhood, and the lesions are usually solitary or few in number and do not necesssarily affect exposed parts. Where the central keratosis and inflammation are prominent, the disseminated superficial variety may be mistaken for solar keratosis if the marginal ridge is not noticed. Lesions respond satisfactorily to freezing with slush or liquid nitrogen [3, 7].

Cutaneous horn. This is a clinical diagnosis [26]. Horny plugs or outgrowths may be caused by various epidermal changes such as hard naevus, virus wart, molluscum contagiosum, kerato-acanthoma, seborrhoeic keratosis, or marsupialized trichilemmal or epidermoid cyst. In most of these cases the primary diagnosis is suggested by the appearance and clinical course and, in most, the horn has a friable quality. The gradual continuing development from relatively normal-looking skin of a hard keratotic protusion resembling an animal horn in miniature, however, is the result of dysplastic epidermal changes similar to those in a solar keratosis. Histologically, there is usually no atypicality or loss of

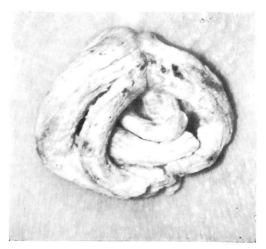

FIG. 64.34. Cutaneous horn of many years' duration over the sternum.

polarity of the epidermal cells but the granular layer is deficient or absent. In long-established lesions there may be budding from the basal layer, signalling transition to a squamous cell carcinoma. Clinical examination shows a hard yellowish-brown excresence, often curved and having circumferential ridges, which is surrounded either by normal-looking epidermis or by a somewhat acanthotic colarette. Recurrent injury may cause the base to be inflamed; a combination of inflammation and induration beneath the horn is suggestive of malignant transformation. The lesions are most common on the exposed areas—particularly the upper part of the face and the ears. They are commonly single, but may be multiple; it is usual to find some more typical solar keratosis or other evidence of solar damage. Nodular actinic keratoses, which are largely confined to the dorsum of the hand and forearm and in which the histology may show an almost pseudo-epitheliomatous picture, occupy a position midway between cutaneous horns and the more usual flat solar keratoses.

Bowen's disease

Definition. A persistent progressive non-elevated red scaly or crusted plaque which is due to an intra-epidermal carcinoma and is potentially malignant.

Aetiology and incidence. If those keratoses with a Bowenoid histology (p. 2425) are considered to belong here, sunlight would be considered an important cause. If, however, these are separately classified, the cause most frequently found is trivalent arsenic compounds. Many of the patients are un-

aware of having been exposed to arsenic, as its presence in a mixture taken medicinally or as an occupational hazard may have been concealed from them or forgotten. The importance of this cause came to light when the association between Bowen's disease and internal cancer [17] was being investigated [18]. Although less than 5% of a large series of patients with Bowen's disease gave a history of arsenic medication, arsenic was found in a statistically significant higher proportion of the patients' skin than in that of the controls [19].

The possible sources of arsenic vary in different localities. In the U.K. the majority of cases with a history of arsenic exposure have been treated for psoriasis with Fowler's solution, or for epilepsy, chorea and other such complaints with a mixture of bromide and arsenic. There is evidence that arsenic was commonly used quite recently by dermatologists in Germany [8]. It is the basis of Gay's solution, a treatment for asthma used in the U.S.A. [20]. It has also been sold as proprietary eczema and psoriasis mixtures and 'blood tonics'. Agricultural workers may be exposed to arsenic salts used as a fungicide, weed killer, sheep dip or pesticide, and frequently take inadequate precautions against accidental ingestion or inhalation. It may be a hazard in smelting and other industrial processes. In some countries, notably parts of Argentina and Taiwan, the water supply has been contaminated [43].

It is the writer's experience that very few patients admit to exposure to arsenic on direct questioning, but detailed enquiry into their occupations and past medical history provides suggestive evidence of exposure in a much higher proportion. In more than half the patients, however, the history does not suggest the cause. Bowen's disease is a comparatively uncommon condition, and occurs equally on exposed and covered areas. It may localize at sites of repeated trauma [41].

Pathology [21, 24]. Atypical squamous cells proliferate through the whole thickness of the epidermis. There is more or less acanthosis, with increase in the length and thickness of the interpapillary ridges, but retention of a distinct dermo–epidermal junction. The atypical cells have hyperchromatic nuclei, often larger than normal, giving a freckled appearance to the epidermis. Giant forms and multinucleate cells are seen, and mitotic figures may be frequent. There is a conspicuous disturbance of epidermal organization, and cells keratinize prematurely and lose their intercellular connections. The surface is formed by a thickened loose parakeratotic scale. The papillary body shows an inflammatory infiltrate which is often quite dense. In some cases the proliferating cells may penetrate the surrounding epidermis, to give a 'Borst–Jadassohn' appearance. The epidermis above the ducts of appendages may be normal, as in solar keratosis, but the Bowen cells often grow down around the ducts like a collar. The condition can become invasive, and when it does it is always squamous cell in type. Arsenical Bowen's disease is said to be characterized by the presence of numerous vacuolated atypical cells [29]. Electron microscope features have been described [30, 38, 46].

Clinical features. The lesions may occur anywhere on the skin surface or on mucosal surfaces. The initial change is a small, red and slightly scaly area which is symptomless and gradually enlarges in a somewhat irregular fashion. The scale is white or yellowish, detached without much difficulty to give a moist, reddened and at times granular surface, but without producing bleeding. The margin is sharp and the lesion slightly raised; the surface is usually flat, but may become hyperkeratotic or crusted. Ulceration is usually a sign of invasive growth, and may be delayed for many years after the appearance of the intra-epidermal change. Persistent superficial ulceration may, however, be the early clinical evidence of Bowen's disease of palmar skin without invasion. There may be several lesions, either widely spread or sometimes close and becoming confluent with extension.

When there is good evidence of chronic arsenicalism, either from the history or because of associated changes such as pigmentation or punctate palmoplantar keratoses, the possible evolution of a

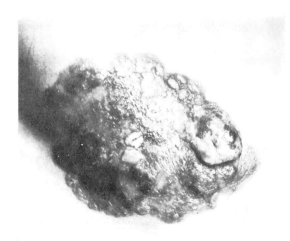

FIG. 64.35. Bowen's disease of the breast in a man
(Radcliffe Infirmary, Oxford.)

visceral malignancy, especially of the lung, should be borne in mind.

Diagnosis. The condition must be distinguished from lichen simplex, psoriasis and other papulo-squamous dermatoses. If the diagnosis is uncertain on the first examination, the lack of improvement when steroids are applied is suggestive of Bowen's disease. The superficial ('Pagetoid') type of basal cell carcinoma can produce a very similar appearance, but can usually be differentiated by the finely elevated, 'thread-like' margin. Bowen's disease and superficial basal cell carcinoma can be seen in the same patient. Distinction from the flat type of solar keratosis may be impossible.

Treatment. Destruction of the epidermis by adequate freezing, cauterization or diathermy coagulation is often effective. Radiotherapy, if used, has to be in full tumour doses and, although a low penetrating quality may be used, it is likely to cause obvious scarring and possibly radionecrosis in large lesions. Local cytotoxic agents such as podophyllin or 5-fluorouracil can be applied to good effect. Recurrences are not infrequent, and may come from extensions of the carcinoma *in situ* around appendage ducts which were not affected by treatment. Surgical excision is the best treatment if the lesion is not too large [18].

Intraepidermal carcinoma of the eyelid margin. This condition, which may resemble a banal warty lesion in its early stages, represented about 6% of all eyelid malignancies in one series [25]. Occupational exposure to oils and grease may be important. The dysplastic changes seen on biopsy may not be sufficiently severe to warn of the dangers of inadequate treatment. One clue is the way the intraepidermal carcinoma invades the deepest ciliary adnexae, causing loss of eyelashes and nodularity of the margin on clinical examination. Squamous cell carcinoma may supervene and complete excision is essential.

Arsenical keratosis
Definition. A corn-like punctate keratosis, more profuse on the extremities and characteristically affecting the palms and soles, which may progress to squamous cell carcinoma.

Incidence. A considerable proportion of any population exposed to chronic aresenic intoxication develops keratoses, the frequency increasing with the degree of intoxication and its duration [43]. There is great individual variation in tolerance, and it is not possible, on present data, to construct a precise dose–response curve.

Pathology. A range of changes may be seen from a benign-looking hyperplasia or dysplasia, the common appearance of the palmoplantar corns, through mild or moderate atypia to frank Bowen's disease [22, 45]. There is no microscopic feature that allows a positive diagnosis of arsenic as the cause. In most lesions there is no elastotic degeneration of the upper dermis.

Clinical features. [15] The keratoses usually begin on the palms or soles as small areas of hyperkeratosis resembling corns. These enlarge, thicken and increase in number. The fingers, backs of the hands and more proximal parts of the extremities may be involved. Induration, inflammation and ulceration occur when the lesion becomes malignant. There may be areas of Bowen's disease in other sites and multiple basal cell carcinomas, mainly of the trunk, may occur in association.

Diagnosis. The palmar lesions have to be differentiated from the various types of punctate keratosis, such as disseminated punctate keratoderma (p. 1455), which usually appears in early life, and Darier's disease and lichen planus, which usually have characteristic lesions elsewhere. Plantar warts differ, in being papillomatous.

Treatment. The multiplicity of the keratoses makes radical treatment impracticable. Where it is necessary, the use of a keratolytic ointment and trimming down of the surface is helpful. The patient should be examined periodically for evidence of malignant change and for signs of visceral malignancy.

Erythroplasia of Queyrat. This condition is described with the genital disorders (p. 2199). The histological appearance and natural history suggests that the lesion is Bowen's disease of the mucosa of the penis. However, the lack of association with visceral malignancy and its prevalence in the uncircumcised only indicate a different, and locally acting, cause [18].

Leukoplakia. This condition is described with diseases of the oral cavity (p. 2108).

Leukokeratosis of the lips (see p. 2125). This disorder is a solar keratosis when it occurs on the vermilion border. The patient almost always gives a history of recurrent sunburn of the lips, and the lower lip is predominantly affected. There is no certainty about the part that smoking plays. Some observers have not found a correlation [28], but others claim that this is the reason for the high incidence in men [44]. The use of lipstick by women may be protective, especially in preventing dehydration. It is common experience that a hot, dry wind potentiates the burning effect of the sun. The lower lip shows persistent dry scaling, a tendency to fissure and atrophic changes beneath and around the keratosis. Removal of the affected area by shaving it off through the superficial dermis often produces a good result.

Post-irradiation keratoses. [9] These may occur in an area of scarring following radiotherapy or excessive fluoroscopy where there is obvious dermal damage. They may also be seen in radiologists, surgeons, dentists and others who have injudiciously exposed their skin to frequent small doses of X-rays and where the dermis is less grossly changed, although such cases are now becoming rare. The epidermal changes are similar to solar keratosis. Histologically, the dermis shows a much more extensive replacement of collagen by scar and elastotic material, obliterative changes in the vessels and, at times, the presence of abnormally large and irregular fibroblasts.

Tar keratoses [10, 11, 37]. Several different types of warts are seen in workers with tar and pitch. There may be small keratotic plaques, not unlike plane warts, or flat seborrhoeic keratoses on the face and hands which have the microscopic features of benign acanthomas. These usually disappear when the exposure ceases. There may also be lesions resembling solar keratoses, which persist and may become malignant. Other lesions with the appearance of kerato-acanthomas may erupt [5]. Their course is usually more prolonged and, particularly on the scrotum, they may become malignant.

Radiant heat may produce changes very similar to those of sunlight (p. 2379).

PUVA therapy and malignancy [42]. It is not yet clear whether or not patients receiving PUVA therapy for severe psoriasis are at increased risk of developing cutaneous malignancy as a result of this therapy *per se*. Series in which patients on PUVA therapy have developed squamous carcinoma and basal cell carcinoma include a high proportion of patients who have in the past received other better established carcinogens as therapeutic agents. These include arsenic and X-irradiation. Careful prospective documentation of all patients on PUVA is needed to establish its true carcinogenic potential either as an initiator or a promoter.

REFERENCES

1 ANDERSON D. E. & CHERNOSKY M. E. (1969) *Arch Dermatol* **99**, 408.
2 CHERNOSKY M. E. & ANDERSON D. E. (1969) *Arch Dermatol* **99**, 401.
3 CHERNOSKY M. E. & FREEMAN R. G. (1967) *Arch Dermatol* **96**, 611.
4 CIVATTE J., *et al* (1973) *Ann Dermatol Syphiligr* **100**, 29.
5 COLOMB D., *et al* (1966) *Rev Lyon Méd* **15**, 449.
6 *DELACRÉTAZ J. (1961) In *Épithéliomas et États Préépithéliomateux Cutanés*. Paris, Masson, p. 41.
7 DONALD G. F. & HUNTER G. A. (1968) *Aust J Dermatol* **9**, 335.
8 EHLERS G. (1968) *Z Haut GeschlKrankh* **43**, 763.
9 EMMERSON R. W. (1975) *Proc R Soc Med* **68**, 345.
10 FISHER R. E. W. (1961) *Proc 13th Int Congr on Occupational Health* p. 250.
11 FISHER R. E. W. (1965) *Trans Assoc Ind Med Off* **15**, 122.
12 FREEMAN R. G. (1968) *Cancer* **21**, 1114.
13 *FREUDENTHAL W. (1926) *Arch Dermatol Syphilol* **152**, 505.
14 GLUCKSMANN A. (1963) *Natl Cancer Inst Monogr* **10**, 509.
15 GOLDMAN A. L. (1973) *Am Rev Respir Dis* **108**, 1205.
16 GORDON D. & SILVERSTONE H. (1969) In *The Biologic Effects of Ultraviolet Radiation*. Ed. Urbach F. Oxford, Pergamon, p. 625.
17 GRAHAM J. H. & HELWIG E. B. (1959) *AMA Arch Dermatol* **80**, 133.
18 GRAHAM J. H. & HELWIG E. B. (1964) In *Tumors of the Skin*. Eds. Cumley R. W., *et al*. Chicago, Year Book Medical Publishers, p. 209.
19 GRAHAM J. H., *et al* (1961) *J Invest Dermatol* **37**, 317.
20 HARTER J. G. & NOVITCH A. M. (1967) *J Allergy* **40**, 6.
21 HELWIG E. B. & GRAHAM J. H. (1964) In *Tumors of the Skin*. Eds. Cumley R. W., *et al*. Chicago, Year Book Medical Publishers, p. 131.
22 HUNDEIKER M. & PETERS J. (1968) *Arch Klin Exp Dermatol* **231**, 355.
23 KLEIN E. (1968) *NY State J Med* **68**, 886.
24 LLOYD K. M. (1970) *Arch Dermatol* **101**, 48.
25 McCALLUM D. I., *et al* (1975) *Br J Dermatol* **93**, 239.
26 MEHREGAN A. H. (1965) *Dermatol Dig* **4**, 45.
27 MEHREGAN A. H. & PINKUS H. (1964) *Cancer* **17**, 609.
28 MOLESWORTH E. H. (1934) *Dermatol Wochenschr* **99**, 945.
29 MONTGOMERY H. & WAISMAN M. (1941) *J Invest Dermatol* **4**, 365.
30 OLSEN R. L., *et al* (1969) *Br J Dermatol* **81**, 676.
31 ORIEL J. D. & WHIMSTER I. W. (1971) *Br J Dermatol* **84**, 71.
32 *PINKUS H. (1958) *Am J Clin Pathol* **29**, 193.
33 *PINKUS H. & MEHREGAN A. H. (1969) *A Guide to Dermohistopathology*. London, Butterworths, p. 408.
34 PINKUS H., *et al* (1963) *J Invest Dermatol* **41**, 247.
35 READ R. J. & LEONE P. (1970) *Arch Dermatol* **101**, 340.
36 RUTTER, M. (1973) *Acta Derm Venerol* (Stockh), **53**, 290.
37 SANDERSON K. V. (1974) *Proc R Soc Med* **67**, 23.
38 SEIJI M. & MIZUNO F. (1969) *Arch Dermatol* **99**, 3.
39 SHAPIRO L. & ACKERMAN A. B. (1966) *Dermatologica* **132**, 386.
40 SINCLAIR M. H. (1969) *Cancer Bull* **21**, 56.
41 SOMMERS S. C. & McMANUS R. G. (1953) *Cancer* **6**, 347.
42 STERN R. S., *et al* (1979) *N Engl J Med* **300**, 809.
43 TSENG W. P., *et al* (1968) *J Natl Cancer Inst* **40**, 453.
44 WYNDER E. L. & BROSS I. J. (1957) *Br Med J* i, 1137.
45 YEH S., *et al* (1968) *Cancer* **21**, 312.
46 YEH S., *et al* (1975) *J Natl Cancer Inst* **53**, 31.

SQUAMOUS CELL CARCINOMA OF THE SKIN
SYN. EPIDERMOID CARCINOMA, SPINOCELLULAR CARCINOMA, SPINALIOMA

Definition. A malignant tumour arising within the epidermis or its appendages whose cells show some degree of maturation towards keratin formation.

Aetiology and incidence. Only a relatively small number of these tumours arise without some previous exogenous cause. Any of the environmental carcinogens (p. 2378), singly or in combination, may be responsible, but sunlight is the commonest. Rare causes are frostbite [8] and radioactive gold jewellery [13]. A few tumours are reported to have occurred at the site of a previous herpes infection [37, 38].

Squamous cell carcinoma is an occasional complication of long-standing chronic granulomas such as venereal granulomas, syphilis, lupus vulgaris and leprosy and lupus erythematosus, chronic ulcers, osteomyelitis sinuses, old burn scars and hidradenitis suppurativa. It may complicate scarring dermatoses such as poikiloderma congenitale, dystrophic epidermolysis bullosa [35] and porokeratosis of Mibelli [20]. It is, of course, necessary to separate pseudo-epitheliomatous hyperplasia from carcinoma in the granulomatous and ulcerative lesions and to give due weight to carcinogens like X-rays and UV radiation which may have been used in treatment before accepting all reported cases as due to the primary disorder. This is especially so in tumours occurring in patients who have been treated for psoriasis.

The prevalence of squamous cell carcinoma varies greatly from one country to another and between people employed in different occupations, depending on the carcinogenic hazards of the environments and the susceptibility of the population. It is a common tumour in those of Celtic descent living in sunny climate such as Queensland [3] or Texas [19]. It is uncommon in dark-skinned people, and in the Bantu many of the tumours follow injury to the leg or foot [4]. There is a high incidence in albino members of the dark-skinned races; there is no evidence of an increased incidence in vitiliginous skin of Negroids [21]. There is possibly a similar innate variation in susceptibility to industrial carcinogens such as tars and oils. The therapeutic application of tar has, in a few cases, been followed after many years by squamous cell carcinoma [25]. A single injury such as a burn from hot metal fragments (p. 2379) or tar [22], a scratch or, in two cases seen by the writer, an embedded splinter of wood may be followed by a tumour—sometimes within a matter of weeks or months. In such cases previous actinic or other damage to the skin may have prepared the way for the carcinoma to start [3]. Radiant heat from coal and peat fires may cause squamous cell carcinoma in women who habitually sit with their legs too close to the fire [23].

Squamous cell carcinoma develops mainly in later life. The age-specific incidence increases steeply after the age of 55–59 [4]. Males are affected almost twice as often as females. Tumours on the lower legs, however, are much more likely to occur in women than men [29]. In highly susceptible subjects like albino Bantus [26] and in patients with xeroderma pigmentosum, the tumours may appear in early adult life or before.

Pathology [17]. Squamous cell carcinoma is a tumour which may arise in any epithelium, and its behaviour in the skin is essentially similar to the behaviour in the respiratory tract and elsewhere. Because of the accessibility of the skin, the precancerous changes that lead to the tumour are more easily observed and followed.

The precancerous conditions—solar keratoses, Bowen's disease and leukoplakia—have already been described (p. 2424). Squamous cell carcinoma begins when the atypical Malpighian cells break through the normal dermal basement membrane and invade the dermis. The exact point at which this change occurs is impossible to define; the basal cells in the precancerous conditions are usually more or less atypical, some degree of acanthosis precedes the actual invasion and the basement membrane is a plastic structure. The distinction is thus architectural rather than cytological, and is based on the presence of descending strands of cells which can no longer be regarded as distorted inter-

papillary ridges. The distinction is further complicated by the phenomenon of pseudo-epitheliomatous hyperplasia, which may occur at an ulcer margin or over certain inflammatory or neoplastic states in the dermis (p. 2398).

The cells of squamous cell carcinoma vary from large well-differentiated polygonal cells with vesicular nuclei, prominent nucleoli and an abundant cytoplasm containing numerous tonofibrils and well-developed intercellular bridges, through to completely anaplastic cells with basophilic cytoplasm which provide no cytological evidence of their origin. Some tumours have large bizarre cells, in others the cells may have a clear almost vacuolated cytoplasm and in yet others the cells may be spindle shaped. Well-differentiated tumours show areas of maturation which form parakeratotic horny pearls and individually keratinized cells, or, by dyskeratosis, produce lacunae and lumina which contain shed rounded degenerating cells. The latter appearance is pseudoglandular, and has been called 'adeno-acanthoma of sweat glands'. The terms adenoid or acantholytic squamous cell carcinoma are to be preferred [15, 24].

Most tumours invade as coherent strands and columns, and reproduce the same pattern in their metastases. Many of them are composed of cells uniform in type and showing only moderate mitotic activity. They excite an inflammatory reaction in the dermis. The capillary pattern is abnormal and the number of vessels considerably increased [32]. Increasing anaplasia is associated with hyperchromatic nuclei, decreasing eosinophilia and tonofibril formation in the cytoplasm, and lessened intercellular adhesions. The cell outlines may be rounded or spindle shaped. Mitotic figures become more frequent and abnormal mitoses can be found. Even in extensively ulcerated tumours the connection with the epidermis is usually maintained, and the origin can be traced to atypical epidermal cells which may enable a distinction to be made from an anaplastic amelanotic melanoma. Its origin from an area of abnormal epidermis distinguishes it from keratoacanthoma, where the architecture suggests a derivation from adnexal ducts. In rare instances squamous cell carcinoma may arise in a keratinous cyst. Many reported instances of this occurrence, however, can now be considered as proliferating trichilemmal cysts.

Local extension of squamous cell carcinoma may occur around nerves, sometimes for considerable distances, and may require extensive surgery [6]. It is unusual for squamous cell carcinoma originating in a solar keratosis of the hand or arm to show evidence of anaplasia or to metastasize until very

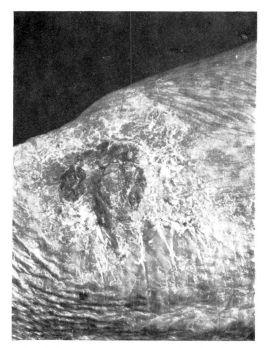

FIG. 64.36. Squamous cell carcinoma of the hand. There are multiple solar keratoses, atrophy and elastosis. (St. John's Hospital.)

well advanced. In a recent Scandinavian series [30] less than 8% of tumours of the upper limb metastasized. Lesions of the vermilion of the lip, and to a lesser extent of the ear, metastasize much earlier even when they are relatively well differentiated. Those elsewhere on the face appear to be less aggressive. Squamous cell carcinoma of the external genitals is also inclined to early invasion and metastasis. Spread is almost always by the lymph vessels.

Various ways of predicting the likelihood of metastasis from the histological features have been suggested. One that has been widely used is Broders' classification based on the proportion of differentiated to atypical tumour cells. From the practical point of view this method needs to be supplemented by the depth of invasion. For tumours of the hand, for instance, metastasis is unlikely when the penetration does not extend deeper than the sweat coils [14]. At the two extrememes of differentiation this criterion does not apply. A very well-differentiated lesion like 'epithelioma cuniculatum' may invade the soft tissues of the foot extensively without metastasis [1], while a completely undifferentiated tumour, of the lip for instance, may disseminate at a very early stage.

Clinical features. Squamous cell carcinoma does not often arise from healthy looking skin. Commonly there are signs of damage from sunlight: elastotic degeneration of the dermis, keratosis, irregular pigmentation and telangiectasia of the skin, or leukokeratosis and fissuring of the lip. The first clinical evidence of malignancy is induration. The area may be plaque-like, verrucous, tumid or ulcerated, but in all cases the lesion feels firm when pressed between the finger and thumb. The limits of the induration are not sharp and usually extend beyond the visible margin of the lesion. The resistance to pressure is much greater than that given by an inflammatory lesion or benign epithelial hyperplasia.

The tissue around the growth is hyperaemic and the edge is an opaque dirty yellowish-red colour. The better-differentiated tumours are usually papillary and are capped by a keratotic crust in the earlier stages. This may be shed later to reveal an ulcer or eroded tumour with an indurated margin and a purulent exuding surface which bleeds rather easily. The outline may be rounded, but is often irregular, and in premalignant lesions the induration and elevation is often asymmetrical at first. On mobile structures like the lip or genitalia the presenting sign may be a fissure or small erosion or ulcer which fails to heal and bleeds recurrently.

The commonest sites for squamous cell carcinoma are those most exposed to the sun. They occur on the backs of the hands and forearms, the upper part of the face and, especially in males, on the lower lip and pinna. Special habits associated with occupation may modify the distribution. Australian fishermen who expose their feet and legs to

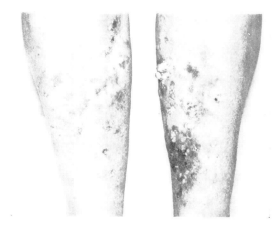

FIG. 64.37. Erythema ab igne complicated by multiple keratoses, and a squamous cell carcinoma on the left shin (St. George's Hospital).

the sun in their boats have a tendency, which is rare in the general male population, to develop lesions on the lower extremities [34]. The susceptiblity of the scrotum in chimney sweeps, mule spinners and capstan-lathe operators is due to the retention of the carcinogen on the skin surface. The high incidence of lesions on the lower leg in the natives of tropical countries is related to the frequency of ulcers and scars. The nail bed is an uncommon site, which may be overlooked until the lesion is large enough to produce radiographic changes in the distal phalanx [9].

The evolution of squamous cell carcinoma is usually faster than that of basal cell carcinoma, but is conspicuously slower than that of kerato-acanthoma which may attain the same size in as many weeks as squamous cell carcinoma does in months or even years. Tumours arising in keratoses on the dorsum of the hand are particularly indolent and late in metastasizing. Some workers [11, 18] have cast doubt on whether they are truly malignant. Early ulceration, and the absence of tumid outgrowth, are usually due to an anaplastic lesion [28], and are more commonly seen on the lip and genital area than elsewhere. Regional nodes may become enlarged, either as a result of infection of the ulcer or from metastases. In the latter case they feel harder, are more irregular and become fixed to the adjacent tissues. Spread by the blood stream is uncommon [36].

There are several uncommon tumours which are so well differentiated that the diagnosis may be in doubt if the unrelenting course is not taken into account. One such has been reported on the sole of the foot under the title 'epithelioma cuniculatum' [1]. There is a bulbous mass with a squashy consistency on the distal part of the sole. Multiple sinuses open on the surface and, when pressed, greasy, rancid and foul-smelling material can be expressed 'like toothpaste from a tube'. It is possible that the appearance of a vegetating pyoderma may at times be due to the same process. In such cases the distinction from pseudo-epitheliomatous hyperplasia (p. 2398) may be very difficult. A few examples of 'giant condyloma acuminatum' have eventually become low-grade squamous cell carcinoma [7, 27].

At the other extreme anaplastic squamous cell carcinoma may arise from skin not showing a premalignant lesion and in a form very difficult to recognize. The lesion is a red papule or nodule, relatively fast growing and looking inflammatory rather than neoplastic. It tends to ulcerate early. It may resemble a kerato-acanthoma, but the central keratin core is usually absent. Induration is present, but may be less marked than in well-differentiated

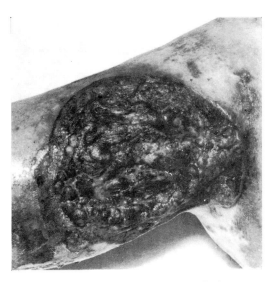

FIG. 64.38. Marjolin's ulcer. An old scar on the lower leg ulcerated and healed with treatment on several occasions. The ulcer eventualy recurred and extended widely and deeply. The patient died of metastatic squamous cell carcinoma. (St. George's Hospital.)

tumours. It can infiltrate deeply and metastasize quite early. It has been designated 'squamous cell carcinoma—*de novo*' [11].

Diagnosis. The indurated well-differentiated tumour arising in skin damaged by sunlight or X-rays presents no problems. The distinction from kerato-acanthoma is usually easy, as the rate of growth and domed appearance of that lesion are characteristic. On occasions, however, a tumour develops like a typical kerato-acanthoma, but proves by its progress to be a squamous cell carcinoma [4]. In such cases the histology of the early stage may not be conclusive one way or the other. The most important clinical distinction is between a poorly differentiated carcinoma arising *de novo* from normal skin, and an inflammatory ulcer or granuloma on the one hand, or an amelanotic melanoma or basal cell carcinoma on the other. The characteristic induration and opaque colour are the most important signs, but any doubt is usually dispelled by biopsy. The only contra-indication for biopsy is the possibility of malignant melanoma. Warty lesions such as viral warts or seborrhoeic keratoses are not indurated, and are frequently multiple.

Treatment. There are three different approaches to the cure of squamous cell carcinoma: local destruction, radiotherapy or surgery. Each method has its advocates. A balanced judgement of the claims is difficult, because most of the reports give inadequate details of the type of case, pathology or precise techniques used and cannot, therefore, be compared. In many countries the majority of these tumours are sent to surgeons or radiotherapists, and the dermatologist is not in a good position to obtain a comprehensive view of the results of treatment. In countries of high prevalence, where it is the practice for dermatologists to do much of the radiotherapy or surgery themselves, a more adequate experience is possible; it is obvious that no one embarks on these specialized treatments without first acquiring the basic training by working with an expert. Details of radiotherapeutic or surgical techniques are considered to be outside the scope of this chapter.

In deciding what is best for the patient the first consideration is complete eradication of the carcinoma, and the next is the final cosmetic and functional result; the cost of treatment to the patient (or to the National Health Service) is a subsidiary, but not insignificant, factor.

A good biopsy—preferably from the centre to the margin of the tumour, down to and including the connective tissue around it—is essential before treatment is planned. As a general rule a very well-differentiated tumour is best treated by surgery or local destruction and a poorly differentiated tumour is best treated by radiotherapy. If the regional nodes are enlarged the patient should be seen by the surgeon before any other treatment is undertaken.

Local destruction. Treatment by curettage and cauterization or diathermy (Chapter 68) is used extensively in areas where actinic cancer is common. It is the method of choice for tumours of the upper limb which are too large for simple excision and primary closure. It can be used for tumours of the head and neck if they are less than 15 mm in diameter and well differentiated; some dermatologists treat large tumours in this way [10]. The results of the local destruction are claimed to be superior to surgery or radiotherapy, giving a 5 yr cure rate of better than 95% in large series [10, 16]. Experience and skill are required in selecting the cases suitable for the treatment and in judging the limits to which the destruction must be taken. For this, as for all forms of treatment for cancer, a knowledge of the dynamic pathology is fundamental.

Cryosurgery [31]. The modern apparatus using liquid nitrogen either to chill a cryoprobe continuously or to spray on a surface allows the local destruction of tissue to quite a considerable and calculable depth. The technique has the advantage of simplicity as it requires no other local anaesthetic and is relatively free of post-operative complications. However, the successful treatment of malignant tumours requires adequate freezing of the tumour and a margin all round it. The lateral clearance can be judged by observation. The clearance in depth depends upon knowledge of the depth of invasion from an adequate biopsy and preferably the use of temperature-recording probes which can be accurately positioned beneath the tumour. The cytotoxic effect of freezing and thawing can be enhanced if the tumour is refrozen once or twice. Collagen, cartilage and bone are less sensitive than cells to injury by freezing, and thus scarring and late effects are greatly reduced.

Radiotherapy. This treatment leaves rather fragile scars on the hand and forearm, and it may be followed by radionecrosis on the trunk. Its main use is, therefore, in tumours of the head and neck. It is particularly indicated for poorly differentiated squamous-cell carcinoma which has not spread to bone or cartilage nor metastasized. It is usually preferred by the very old patients (who form a considerable proportion of the cases), and in them the final cosmetic result and durability of the scar is less critical than in younger patients. The quality of the scar following superficial X-ray therapy depends, to a considerable extent, upon the number of doses into which the total treatment dose is divided and the time taken to complete the treatment. In many centres a total dose of 5,000 rad is given in 10 doses over a period of 2 weeks. Large lesions, especially when situated on the trunk, require more protracted treatment, lasting for up to 6 weeks. Except where the skin to be treated lies over bone or cartilage, it is desirable to use a fairly penetrating ray generated at 100–140 kV with suitable filtration.

In a number of situations, especially where a curved area has to be treated, radium or radioactive cobalt applied as a surface mould gives excellent results. This technique is now being used more frequently, since after-loading of the moulds enables the technicians to be protected from exposure. Interstitial radiation from radium needles, gold grain or iridium wire is a convenient and effective way of treating mobile areas, such as the lip and tongue, or curved surfaces. Electron beam therapy can be used in areas, such as over nasal cartilage, where conventional radiation might result in radionecrosis.

The planning of radiotherapy requires cooperation between the clinicians and the physicist. The advice of the dermatologist and pathologist on the diagnosis is essential, but the choice of the type, quality and dosage of irradiation for squamous cell carcinoma is, in the writer's view, the province of the radiotherapist and physicist.

Surgery. This is the treatment of choice for small tumours when primary closure or a simple sliding graft can make good the defect. The palpable margin of the tumour should be outlined before any local anaesthetic is injected, and at least 3–5 mm clearance allowed beyond it. Surgical removal is quick and the wound heals in 2 weeks. The specimen provides better material for the pathologist than a biopsy, and very much better material than curettings which are always difficult to interpret. Surgery is also the best treatment for lesions which have invaded bone or cartilage or when lymph node metastases have developed, and it is usually employed on cases which have recurred after other treatment has been given or on those tumours which are sclerosing or have ill-defined margins [10]. These cases have the worst outlook, so that any truly representative series of surgical cases is likely to give a lower cure rate than the other methods.

It is not necessary to do prophylactic lymph node clearance in squamous cell carcinoma of the skin. Even in carcinoma of the lip only 10% of patients develop metastases [33], and half of these are found when the patient is first seen. Therefore only 5% of patients would gain any benefit from the procedure, and careful frequent follow-up examinations should detect these cases at an early stage. Surgery is an optional form of treatment for larger lesions which have not spread, and whether or not it is used may depend on the availability of skilled radiotherapy services or dermatologists trained in the method of curettage.

Treatment of lesions at special sites. The dorsum of the hand should not be treated by radiotherapy. Most tumours on this area are brought for treatment when quite small, and curettage or excision gives equally good results.

The lip may be treated by any of the methods. Extensive superficial lesions are suitable for lipshave or curettage and cautery; radiotherapy of a large area leaves considerable scarring, and surgical excision calls for plastic repair. Smaller tumours may be excised by wedge excision, which is a relatively simple operation but leaves the lip shorter and thus changes the shape of the mouth. Equally good results are claimed if an excision is performed around and beneath the tumour and the wound is left to heal by granulation. Some surgeons prefer to use a galvanocautery or diathermy needle rather than a scalpel to cut out the tumour [2]. Poorly differentiated and invasive tumours of the lip should be irradiated unless they invade the mandible, when an extensive surgical removal is required [33]. Lesions at or near the angles of the mouth are better treated with radiotherapy because of the difficulty of plastic reconstruction in this region.

The face can be treated by any of the methods according to the general considerations already mentioned. Tumours of or adjacent to the scalp are better treated surgically if atrophic alopecia of the marginal skin is to be avoided.

The ear is a relatively uncommon area for squamous cell carcinoma. Small tumours not involving cartilage can be treated by any of the techniques. Involvement of cartilage is an indication for surgery, and lesions on the helix can be excised with a wedge of cartilage. If it is important to preserve the symmmetry of the ears, a wedge from the other ear of up to 1 cm in length at the helix can be used as a free graft.

The final results of any of the methods depends on the experience of the person using it, rather than the technique itself. In good hands all the techniques give 5 yr cure rates of about 90% in a wide variety of squamous cell carcinomas at different sites. Almost all tumours arising in solar keratoses of the upper extremity can be cured. Those developing from Bowen's disease or arsenical keratoses are more aggressive and require careful follow up for metastases. The cure rate for lip cancer is about 90%. Squamous cell carcinoma of the ear is rather more aggressive and a somewhat larger proportion of cases metastasize early.

REFERENCES

1 AIRD I., *et al* (1954) *Br J Surg* **42**, 245.
2 ARIEL I. M. (1959) In *Treatment of Cancer and Allied Diseases.* Eds. Pack G. T. & Ariel I. M. London, Pitman, Vol. 3, p. 53.
3 BELISARIO J. C. (1959) *Cancer of the Skin.* London, Butterworths, p. 20.
4 COHEN L., *et al* (1952) *S Afr Med J* **26**, 932.
5 CROSS F. (1967) *Proc R Soc Med* **60**, 1037.
6 DANDY D. J. & MUNRO D. D. (1973) *Br J Dermatol* **89**, 527.
7 DAVIES S. W. (1965) *J Clin Pathol* **18**, 142.
8 DI PIRRO E. & CONWAY H. (1966) *Plast Reconstr Surg* **38**, 541.
9 DRIBAN N. E. & LACOGNATA J. J. (1975) *Dermatologica* **150**, 186.
10 FREEMAN R. G., *et al* (1964) *Cancer* **17**, 535.
11 GRAHAM J. H. & HELWIG E. B. (1963) *Natl Cancer Inst Monogr* **10**, 323.
12 HAY D. M. & COLE F. M. (1970) *Am J Obstet Gynecol* **108**, 479.

13 HOLUBAR K., *et al* (1973) *Hautarzt* **24**, 489.

14 JOHNSON R. E. & ACKERMAN L. V. (1950) *Cancer* **3**, 657.

15 *JOHNSON W. C. & HELWIG E. B. (1966) *Cancer* **19**, 1639.

16 KNOX J. M., *et al* (1967) *South Med J* **60**, 241.

17 *LUND H. Z. (1957) *Tumors of the Skin. Atlas of Tumor Pathology*, Section I, Fasc. *2*. Armed Forces Institute of Pathology, Washington, DC, p. 235.

18 LUND H. Z. (1965) *Arch Dermatol* **92**, 635.

19 MACDONALD E. J. (1959) *J Invest Dermatol* **32**, 379.

20 OBERSTE LEHN H. & MOLL B. (1968) *Hautarzt* **19**, 399.

21 OETTLÉ A. G. (1963) *Natl Cancer Inst Monogr* **10**, 197.

22 PELLERAT J. & COUDERT J. (1948) *Rev Lyon Med* **179**, 442.

23 PETERKIN G. A. G. (1955) *Br Med J* ii, 1599.

24 PINKUS H. & MEHREGAN A. H. (1969) *A Guide to Dermatohistopathology*. London, Butterworths, p. 413.

25 ROOK A. J., *et al* (1956) *Br J Cancer* **10**, 17.

26 SHAPIRO M. L., *et al* (1953) *Br J Cancer* **7**, 45.

27 SOUTH L. M., *et al* (1977) *Clin Oncol* **3**, 107.

28 STOUT A. P. (1946) *Arch Dermatol Syphilol* **53**, 597.

29 SWANBECK G. & HILLSTROM L. (1969) *Acta Derm Venereol (Stockh)* **49**, 427.

30 SWANBECK G. & HILLSTROM L. (1970) *Acta Derm Venereol (Stockh)* **50**, 350.

31 TORRE D. (1976) In *Cancer of the Skin*. Eds. Andrade R., *et al*. Philadelphia, Saunders, p. 1569.

32 URBACH F. (1963) *Natl Cancer Inst Monogr* **10**, 539.

33 WARD G. E. & HENDRICK J. W. (1950) *Surgery* **27**, 321.

34 WARD W. H. (1955) *Aust J Dermatol* **3**, 27.

35 WESCHLER H. L., *et al* (1970) *Arch Dermatol* **102**, 374.

36 WILLIS R. A. (1960) *Pathology of Tumours*. London, Butterworths.

37 WYBURN-MASON R. (1955) *Br Med J* ii, 1106.

38 WYBURN-MASON R. (1957) *Br Med J* ii, 615.

PAGET'S DISEASE OF THE NIPPLE

Definition. A progressive, marginated, scaling or crusting of the nipple and areola due to invasion of the epidermis by characteristic 'foreign' cells, which probably originate in the intraduct carcinoma of the breast which accompanies the condition.

Incidence and aetiology. Paget's disease of the nipple is an uncommon occurrence, considering the frequency of breast cancer. In one series it occurred in less than 3% of breast cancers [10]. It occurs chiefly in women, although cases have been recorded in men [2]. It is rare before the fourth decade and is most frequent in the fifth and sixth. Published cases suggest that the disease is more common in Anglo-Saxon countries [7]. The associated breast carcinoma is of the intraduct variety, and presumably the incidence of this, as of breast cancer as a whole, is reduced by suckling.

Pathology. The epidermis is somewhat thickened at the beginning, with papillomatosis, enlargement of the interpapillary ridges and hyperkeratosis or para-keratosis on the surface. Within the epidermis characteristic Paget cells are dispersed between the prickle cells. They vary in number, and when profuse the Malpighian layers may be disrupted and the surface covered by a crust. There is a chronic inflammatory reaction in the upper dermis. In the later stages the epidermis may be atrophic or eroded.

The Paget cells have a clear abundant cytoplasm and do not establish intercellular bridges with the adjacent prickle cells. Both the cells and their nuclei are rounded; the nuclei are vesicular or hyperchromatic and show the stigmata of malignancy. The cytoplasm is PAS positive and diastase resistant [1], which indicates the presence of neutral polysaccharides and supports the glandular origin of the cells [11]. The cells are disposed singly among the prickle cells or in clusters which, if basal in situation, may mimic a malignant melanoma. The Paget cells may also extend down the ducts of appendages.

The underlying breast carcinoma is not always seen on biopsy, as it may be deeply set. Careful examination of the amputated breast shows an intraduct carcinoma, sometimes of quite small dimensions, situated most usually distally, but sometimes in the terminal ducts, and often appearing to spread between the two layers of epithelial cells of the duct. This is a type of carcinoma *in situ*, and the cells accumulate within and distend the ducts and spread in both directions. A number of ducts are usually involved. At a later stage the carcinoma becomes invasive and behaves like any other breast carcinoma. If there is anything peculiar to the breast tumour of Paget's disease, it is probably that the intraduct phase is more prolonged than in the average breast carcinoma.

Clinical features. The early changes may be minimal, perhaps a small, crusted and intermittently moist area on the nipple giving a brownish stain on the undergarments or night attire, or producing itching, pricking or burning sensations. Less often, there is a serous or blood-stained discharge from the nipple, or a lump may be noticed in the breast. The surface changes persist and gradually spread to produce an eczematous appearance. The nipple, areola and, at a later stage, the skin of the breast are erythematous and moist or crusted. The change is sharply marginated and may spare a segment of the areola. The edge is slightly raised and irregular in outline. If the crusts are removed a red, glazed, moist or vegetating surface is revealed. Itching may be a prominent symptom and excoriations found in

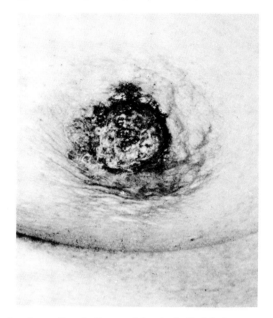

FIG. 64.39. Paget's disease of the nipple (St. John's Hospital.)

the established lesion. Superficial induration gives a 'visiting card' texture on palpation. Some areas may be ulcerated. The change is confined to one nipple. The nipple itself may be retracted, and a subjacent mass or a lump deeper in the breast may be felt. The regional glands should be examined; they are rarely enlarged when a mass cannot be felt, but are so in more than half the cases with a detectable tumour. The rate of spread of the skin changes is slow, and patients often wait a year or more before seeking advice. The change may occasionally involve not only the skin of the breast but also spread on to the chest wall.

Diagnosis. The principal disease to be distinguished is eczema of the nipple. This is frequently bilateral and runs a more fluctuating course, improving in response to local treatment and spreading rapidly when irritated. Eczema lacks the sharp, raised and rounded margin and the superficial induration. In doubtful cases a few days' treatment with a local steroid should provide the answer. Bowen's disease and superficial basal cell carcinoma produce a similar clinical picture. They are both very uncommon on the nipple and can be differentiated histologically. The chief pathological problem is to distinguish the changes from a superficial malignant melanoma, and as the Paget cells may contain pigment [3] this can be difficult. The absence of

melanophages and the presence of neutral mucopolysaccharides in the cells are helpful.

Treatment. Mastectomy should be carried out by a surgeon as for carcinoma of the breast. Radiotherapy may be palliative.

EXTRAMAMMARY PAGET'S DISEASE

Definition. A marginated plaque resembling Paget's disease clinically and histologically, but occurring in the anogenital region or the axilla.

Incidence and aetiology. It is a very uncommon disease. It occurs more frequently in women than in men and starts usually in the fifth decade or after [7]. In a proportion of cases (18 of 56 in one series [6]) an underlying adnexal carcinoma is found. In 20% of cases [12] a primary carcinoma of other organs is found, principally rectum, urethra or cervix uteri, but also more distant organs such as breast, examples of epidermotropic spread or metastasis [12].

Pathology [6]. The changes in the epidermis are essentially similar to Paget's disease. There is perhaps a greater tendency for the Paget cells to accumulate in the basal area, and especially in the interpapillary ridges. The cells stain positively for acid as well as neutral mucopolysaccharides. They may contain melanin granules. Recent studies using antibody against carcinoembryonic antigen (CEA) have demonstrated the presence of this material in most cases [8].

Clinical features. The lesion has many features in common with Paget's disease of the nipple. The margin is sharp, rounded and slightly raised, and encloses an area somewhat erythematous to distinctly red. The surface may be scaly, and here and there small greyish crusts may cover erosions. Itching is a prominent feature and there may be excoriations or lichenification.

The appearance varies somewhat according to the site. The commonest area involved is the vulva, followed by the perianal area (which is more frequently affected in men than women), the scrotum, penis and axilla. The first symptom, especially in vulval lesions, is itching and burning, which may persist for a long time and spread. It is quite frequently regarded as a banal pruritus or dermatitis [4] and eczematization may occur from local applications. The mucosal surfaces of the labia are frequently a rather more vivid red than the skin when both areas are involved, and the change may spread to the thighs or the mons pubis and into the vaginal introitus. There may occasionally be a papillomatous surface. Perianal lesions may extend up into the anal canal. Those of the scrotum spread to the thigh or on to the shaft of the penis. Perhaps the most characteristic features are the relentless progression, despite all local applications, and the sharp margin. Eventually, one area may become thickened and ulcerated as evidence of invasion downwards. Lymph node or distant metastases can occur.

Although most of the cases in which a primary carcinoma is found result from an underlying sweat gland adenocarcinoma, it is necessary to examine the patient for evidence of carcinoma of the cervix, the rectum [5, 14] (especially in perianal lesions) and the breast. The majority of patients with a primary carcinoma develop widespread metastases [6].

Diagnosis. The diagnosis from eczema, intertrigo and pruritus vulvae is made by the inexorable course and the sharp and extending margin. Bowen's disease is usually more raised and verrucous, and superficial basal cell carcinoma has a thread-like margin. It may be difficult to differentiate leukoplakia or Bowen's disease of the mucosal surfaces, but in cases of doubt a biopsy is conclusive.

Treatment. The proper treatment is surgical excision of the area to an adequate depth, which may be a major undertaking in the vulva. The margin may be a little difficult to define when the vagina or anal canal is involved, and microscopic control of the adequacy of this excision at multiple points is necessary.

REFERENCES

1 CAWLEY L. P. (1957) *Am J Clin Pathol* **27**, 559.
2 CRICHLOW R. W. & CZERNOLBILSKY B. (1969) *Cancer* **24**, 1033.
3 CULBERTSON J. D. & HORN R. C. Jr. (1956) *Arch Surg* **72**, 224.
4 DEGOS R., *et al* (1963) *Bull Soc Fr Dermatol Syphiligr* **70**, 2.
5 GUNN A. & FOX H. (1971) *Br J Dermatol* **85**, 476.
6 HELWIG E. B. & GRAHAM J. H. (1964) In *Tumors of the Skin*. Eds. Cumley R. W., *et al*. Chicago, Year Book Medical Publishers, p. 131.
7 *HURIEZ C., *et al* (1961) *Épithéliomas et États Préépithéliomateux Cutanés*. Paris, Masson, p. 121.
8 KARINIEMI A. L., *et al* (1984) *Br J Dermatol* **110**, 203.
9 KAY S. (1966) *Surg Gynecol Obstet* **123**, 5.
10 LUBSCHITZ K. (1944) *Acta Radiol* **25**, 127.
11 NICOLAU S. G. & BALUS L. (1959) *Dermatologica* **119**, 93.
12 PINKUS H. & MEHREGAN A. H. (1969) *A Guide to Dermatohistopathology*. London, Butterworths, p. 470.
13 POTTER B. (1967) *Acta Derm Venereol (Stockh)* **47**, 259.
14 YOELL J. H. & PRICE W. G. (1960) *AMA Arch Dermatol* **82**, 986.

METASTATIC MALIGNANT TUMOURS

Definition. A tumour formed by malignant cells originating from another site, and frequently from another tissue, which are conveyed to the skin by the blood or lymphatic circulation.

Incidence and aetiology. Most malignant tumours can produce cutaneous metastases, but some seem to seed to the skin more frequently than others. Hypernephroma is one of the less common malignancies, yet it accounts for 9% of skin metastases [1]. The skin is involved by metastases in 3–4% of malignant tumours [1, 6]. On occasions, the skin lesion may be the first evidence of internal malignancy. The most frequent primary sites are breast, stomach, lung, uterus, large intestine, kidney, prostate gland, ovary, liver and bone. It is obvious that, in general, the incidence of skin deposits is related to the frequency of the primary cancer in the population. Thus hepatoma is a rare cause in Europeans, but not in Africans or West Indians. The likelihood of a visceral malignancy producing deposits in the skin is increased if the lesion is anaplastic and of long duration. Widespread haematogenous circulation occurs when emboli of malignant cells are discharged into the pulmonary venous circulation, and is most common with primary carcinoma of the lung. Although it is debatable whether direct spread to the skin from a deeper tumour by way of lymph channels should be classed as metastasis, such secondary deposits will be included in this section.

Pathology. Skin deposits from an internal malignancy are recognized by the presence of foreign cells. These may be sufficiently distinctive to enable the primary site to be predicted. In many instances, however, the cells are anaplastic and can only be described as 'carcinoma' or 'sarcoma', or possibly 'an undifferentiated malignancy'. In general the metastatic cells resemble those of the primary growth [9, 11].

The commonest skin tumour to metastasize to the skin is malignant melanoma. The differentiation between primary and secondary melanoma is made by the presence of junctional proliferation in primary lesions.

Carcinomatous deposits in the dermis tend to spread in the lymphatic channels. This produces

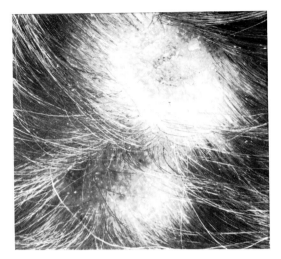

FIG. 64.40. Metastatic carcinoma of the scalp (St. John's Hospital.)

either the 'Indian file' appearance of strands of cells, usually with hyperchromatic nuclei and rather scanty cytoplasm, packing the spaces between the collagen bundles, or bulkier islands and columns of cells dilating the lymphatics whose fine endothelium surrounds the masses. Obstruction of the lymph circulation may produce oedema or, on occasions, gross cystic dilatation of lymphatics [5]. There is usually some degree of capillary engorgement, and in the case of 'Indian file' type of spread there may be fibrosis as well. Hypernephroma produces a marked vascular proliferation, and the acinar arrangement of the clear tumour cells may be a relatively inconspicuous feature [8].

Clinical features Skin metastases are usually late events in the course of internal malignancy and point to a hopeless outcome. Patients survived for an average of 3 months in one series [6]. In hypernephroma there may occasionally be an early solitary skin deposit which can lead to the diagnosis. Treatment of the primary and the deposit may be followed by a considerable period of freedom.

The lesions themselves are usually more vascular than normal skin, and may appear to be inflammatory rather than neoplastic in nature. They are often not noticed until they are 5 mm or more in diameter. The rate of growth is variable. The deposits may be solitary, few or very many, and the configuration varies from nodular to a raised plaque or thickened fibrotic area. There is no consistent pattern associated with any particular primary tumour, but certain trends are seen.

In carcinoma of the breast the skin of the in-volved breast is the region most commonly affected, and the process tends to spread by contiguity. The more rapidly growing deposits take the form of inflammatory plaques with a clear-cut raised margin resembling erysipelas (carcinoma erysipeloides) or of firmer flatter telangiectatic plaques and papules (carcinoma telangiectoides). There may be dilated lymphatics and superficial haemorrhage, giving a vesicular appearance resembling a lymphangioma. Lymph stasis produces dermal oedema which may look like pigskin or orange peel. This may involve a large area (*cancer en cuirasse*). More distant metastases may have a variety of forms; one rather distinctive pattern is produced by a scirrhous dermal reaction which looks like morphoea, and may produce rounded areas of thickening and alopecia on the scalp.

A characteristic clinical picture in lung carcinoma is produced when the tumour discharges large numbers of emboli into the pulmonary venous circulation. A considerable number of nodules appear suddenly in the skin, particularly of the trunk and scalp, and develop more or less rapidly and at much the same rate. They are firm, usually of a reddish colour, symmetrical and, on the chest, tend to follow the direction of the intercostal vessels. On the scalp, at first sight they may suggest dermal cylindroma. A similar appearance has been caused by carcinoma of the prostate [7].

Hypernephroma can produce solitary deposits in the skin which are conspicuously vascular or even pulsatile, tend to be pedunculated and may bear a close resemblance to a granuloma telangiectaticum [10]. The scalp is involved in a high proportion of cases, and the operation scar may also be selectively affected [3].

The situation of lymph-borne metastases depends upon the site of the primary growth and the direction of the efferent lymph vessels. It is not uncommon for a tumour to spread along the planes of operation incisions and produce nodules in the scar. Intra-abdominal malignancy may produce umbilical metastasis [2, 4]. The primary cancer is usually in the stomach or ovary, and is spread by way of the peritoneal cavity. The prognosis is thus grave, but the finding of the deposit may permit microscope confirmation of the diagnosis without laparotomy. The lesions themselves are firm nodules, usually rather deeply set, and are discovered by palpation rather than inspection.

Diagnosis. In the majority of cases the history and general examination will suggest the presence of an internal cancer or give evidence of a treated cancer in the past.

Treatment. Although the presence of skin deposits almost always indicates wide dissemination of the primary tumour, removal of the affected area of skin is justifiable on two counts. There is always the possibility that the metastasis may be solitary, and its removal, combined with or following treatment of the primary, may cure the patient. This is most likely to occur with the lymph-vessel metastases of malignant melanoma which follow excision of the tumour and block dissection of the regional glands. These should always be widely excised. Even if cure is impossible the patient may be saved much discomfort and disfigurement if the skin deposits are removed completely at an early stage.

REFERENCES

1 BEERMAN H. (1957) *Am J Med Sci* **233**, 456.
2 CLEMENTS A. B. (1952) *JAMA* **150**, 556.
3 CONNOR D. H., et al (1963) *Arch Pathol* **76**, 339.
4 DUPERRAT M. B. & DUPERRAT N. (1968) *Bull Soc Fr Dermatol Syphiligr* **75**, 638.
5 FREEMAN C. D. & LYNCH F. W. (1937) *Arch Dermatol Syphilol* **35**, 643.
6 REINGOLD I. M. (1966) *Cancer* **19**, 162.
7 RONCHESE R. (1940) *Arch Dermatol Syphilol* **41**, 639.
8 ROSENTHAL A. L. & LEVER W. F. (1957) *AMA Arch Dermatol* **76**, 96.
9 STECK W. D. & HELWIG E. B. (1965) *Cancer* **18**, 907.
10 TAYLOR H. B. & CONNOR D. (1963) *Arch Pathol* **76**, 339.
11 WILLIS R. A. (1960) *Pathology of Tumours*. London, Butterworths.

TUMOURS OF MELANOCYTES

The tumours which belong to this class are listed below. Melanocytic naevi are described with other naevi in Chapter 6. They are, however, the benign members of a coherent class whose most conspicuous clinical feature (although it may be absent in some tumours) is pigmentation. Malignant melanoma is extremely dangerous, and the differential diagnosis of a pigmented tumour is thus one of the most important problems in dermatology. Not all pigmented tumours contain melanin, and some of those that do are not tumours of melanocytes. The majority of pigmented lesions seen in the clinic can be diagnosed with confidence, but a comparison of clinical and histological diagnoses reveals a higher proportion of mistakes than is made with malignant epithelial tumours, for instance.

In some countries *melanoma* is used as a synonym for malignant melanoma. This may cause misunderstanding, because many pathologists use this term for melanocytic naevi. Other synonyms like melanosarcoma, melanoblastoma, melanocarcinoma, naevocarcinoma, naevoblastoma, malignant naevocytoma and melano-epithelioma cannot be justified on pathological or etymological grounds, and deserve to be forgotten.

Lentigo (p. 180)
Melanocytic naevi (p. 181)
    Common forms
        Junctional
        Compound
        Intradermal
    Special forms
        Oculocutaneous
        Sutton's naevus
        Pigmented hypertrichotic
        Congenital
    Neurocutaneous melanosis (p. 188)
    Spitz naevus
Dermal melanocytosis
    Mongolian spot
    Blue naevus
    Ota's naevus
Melanotic freckle
Precancerous melanosis
Malignant melanoma

When to excise an apparently benign pigmented mole. Advice on when to excise an apparently benign pigmented naevus is often sought. No absolute guidelines can be given but the following recommendations should be of some value.

(1) All small pigmented naevi which are apparently congenital and can easily be locally excised should be considered for excision under local anaesthesia once the child has reached an age where this will not cause significant psychological disturbance. This may result in over-excision of benign congenital naevi but data are not yet available on the true lifetime risk of malignant change (p 2554).

(2) In an adult, any pigmented naevus which is showing signs of growth, of change in colour, whether this be darkening or lightening, or bleeding should be excised without delay and submitted for histological examination.

(3) Any pigmented naevus which acquires signs of irritation or a surrounding inflammatory flare should be excised.

(4) Most acquired naevi appear before the age of 30. Any apparently 'new mole' developing for the first time over the age of 35 should be regarded with suspicion, carefully examined and excised if any of the above signs are present.

(5) The average benign mole, acquired or congenital, is asymptomatic. Any mole in which symp-

toms develop, whether these be itch, pain or just increased sensation, should again be regarded with suspicion. If the mole is in a site where cosmetic considerations are not overwhelming, an excision biopsy is recommended.

(6) Difficult problems arise with regard to acquired benign pigmented moles on certain sites which are continually subjected to trauma. These are usually on the waistband, under shoulder straps and on the beard area where regular shaving occurs. Evidence that continual trauma can convert a benign naevus into a malignant melanoma is extremely slight and is mainly based on the historical account of the predominance of malignant melanoma on the soles of barefoot African negroes. These individuals are now shod in the same way as their counterparts in Europe but still develop malignant melanoma on this site, suggesting that trauma is not in fact the predominant feature. Despite this, concern over trauma and melanoma continues. Advice here is difficult to give on logical grounds, but if the individual is concerned about his or her naevi prophylactic excision is obviously a relatively harmless procedure.

(7) In the past it has been stated that benign moles on the palms, the soles and the genitalia have a higher incidence of malignant change and should therefore be excised as a preventive measure. Once again, the evidence to support this statement is poor, and epidemiological studies of moles on palms and soles suggest that the proportion of moles on these sites which go on to malignant change is probably the same as if not less than that on other body sites. The reason for this belief may well be the fact that the very early clinical signs of acral melanoma on the soles or palms are often subtle and difficult to interpret. Even in a lesion which is relatively well advanced and entering the vertically aggressive stage of growth there may be very little surface change or interruption of the normal skin lines. It is highly likely that in the past lesions of this type were interpreted as benign naevi when in fact they were already malignant melanoma. For these reasons it is suggested that any pigmented lesion on the palm or sole which the individual considers is growing or changing in any way should be excised without delay.

Spitz naevus (juvenile melanoma) [1, 17, 18]
Definition. A benign tumour most common in children, probably melanocytic in origin but differing both clinically and histologically from the common pigmented naevus; the cells may be sufficiently bizarre in type and arrangement to give a specious resemblance to malignant melanoma.

Incidence. The tumour usually occurs in children but may be found in adults [2, 10]; it has been reported to have developed before birth at one extreme or in the seventh decade at the other. The sexes are equally affected and it is seen rarely in Mongoloid or negroid races. It has occurred in identical twins [18]. It is impossible to estimate the prevalence of juvenile melanoma, because most series of surgical pathology specimens will be highly biassed towards the unusual lesion. From one large series [17] it can be said that it is likely to be less than 1% of melanocytic naevi in children. The prevalence declines sharply after puberty.

Pathology [3, 14, 18, 30]. In its general architecture the Spitz naevus resembles a compound naevus. The cells proliferating at the junction are, however, much larger, with an abundant eosinophilic cytoplasm. They may be either spindle shaped and stream into the dermis in interlacing bundles or epithelioid and arranged in clusters with giant and multinucleated cells among them. The giant cells are irregular in outline and like a tadpole in shape. Cleavage artefacts between the cells are due to decreased intercellular cohesion. Mitotic figures may occur but abnormal mitoses are not seen. The deepest cells are often smaller and more mature. The dermal vessels are usually dilated, and the stroma may be oedematous and infiltrated with lymphocytes. The epidermis is often acanthotic and may show spongiosis. The higher levels of the epidermis are not invaded by tumour cells. Melanin is rarely abundant, and may often be absent [14, 18]. Histochemical studies have shown little evidence of phenoloxidase or cholinesterase activity [32], although conflicting views have been reported [18]. Electron microscopy shows the presence of melanosomes [22].

Clinical features. The tumour usually appears in early childhood as a firm, rounded red or reddish-brown nodule. The colour is due to excessive vascularity and much of it can be expressed by pressure to show the true degree of pigmentation.

The lesion grows rapidly at first and may attain a diameter of 1–2 cm. The surface can remain smooth, and the epidermis is often thinned and fragile. It is not uncommon for it to become warty; bleeding and crusting may occur after minor injury [9]. The commonest sites are the face, particularly the cheeks, and the legs, but other areas may be affected. After its initial growth it may remain static for years.

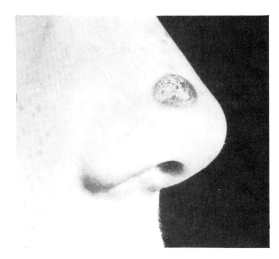

FIG. 64.41. Spitz naevus (St. John's Hospital.)

Diagnosis. Most Spitz naevi are red rather than brown, and are likely to be confused with vascular tumours, granuloma telangiectaticum, histiocytoma, juvenile xanthogranuloma or granulomas such as a lupus vulgaris. When the surface is warty, distinction with epidermal naevus or common wart may be difficult. Pigmented tumours may be indistinguishable from a common pigmented naevus. Clinically, confusion with malignant melanoma only occurs after puberty, and the histological criteria establish the diagnosis in most cases [1, 3]. Microscopic differentiation can be difficult at times, and the pathologist may still make an error. Malignant transformation in a Spitz naevus is a possibility which is not yet well documented.

Treatment. Once the diagnosis has been established it is desirable to excise the lesion. Before puberty a limited excision is adequate. If the pathologist has any doubts about the innocence of a tumour after puberty a more radical removal should be performed.

Organoid neuro-ectodermal neoplasm of the skin [26]. Two cases which had an unusual histological apppearance have been reported under this title. Large cells with large, lobulated or folded nuclei, prominent nucleoli and abundant granular or fibrillar cytoplasm are arranged in pseudo-alveolar fashion in the dermis. Some of the cells are multinucleated, and in general they bear a close resemblance to adult ganglion cells. The nests of cells are surrounded by flattened cells, resembling the lemmoblastic capsule around ganglion cells.

Clinically, the two lesions were firm pink or red

dermal nodules, one on the foot and the other on the lower leg, and occurred in young men. The condition may be an unusual variant of Spitz naevus. The histological picture is very similar to alveolar soft-part sarcoma (p. 2464), but that tumour does not occur in the dermis.

Mongolian spot
Definition. Macular blue-grey pigmentation present at birth on the sacral area in normal infants of mongoloid and some other races.

Incidence [11]. It is present in over 90% of infants of Mongoloid race, and has been found in about 1% of Caucasoid infants in Europe, where the incidence is highest in the Mediterranean region. The incidence in other races lies between these extremes. It has been found in some 80% of East African infants [27].

Pathology. Ribbon-like melanocytes are dispersed between the collagen fibres and around the neurovascular bundles of the dermis. They run parallel to the skin surface and contain very fine granules of melanin. There is no disturbance of the pattern of collagen and elastic fibres. Melanophages are not found. The last two characteristics enable it to be differentiated from blue naevus.

Clinical features. The pigmentation is macular, diffuse and more or less uniform, slatey-blue to grey and usually relatively faint. The patches are usually rounded or oval in shape, up to 10 cm or so in diameter, and usually single but occasionally multiple. The lumbosacral region is the common site, and the buttocks, flanks or even shoulders may be affected in extensive lesions. The pigmentation develops in fetal life, increases in depth for a period after birth and then diminishes. It has usually disappeared by the age of 7, and almost invariably by the age of 13, but has occasionally persisted into adult life.

Blue naevus
Definition. An area of blue or blue-black dermal pigmentation produced by aberrant collections of functioning benign melanocytes.

Incidence and aetiology. Blue naevi are relatively common, and usually go unremarked by the patient. A ratio of 2·5:1 of female to male patients in a recent series [29] probably represents the relative desires of the sexes to have blemishes removed. Blue naevi are due to a defect of development and can be regarded as arrested migration of melanocytes bound for the dermal–epidermal junction. Dermal melanocytes are normal in many other animals, especially in relation to neurovascular bundles. Lesions similar to the cellular blue naevus have been produced experimentally by painting the dorsal pigmented spots on hamsters with carcinogenic hydrocarbons [7, 28].

Pathology. Two forms exist, the rarer being termed 'cellular blue naevus'. In the common variety bipolar and dendritic melanocytes lie singly or in masses in the dermis. They tend to be profuse in the lower dermis and are often concentrated around appendages or in the perivascular and perineural areas. Deeper tissues may be involved [19]. The melanocytes are relatively inconspicuous, containing fine granules of melanin dispersed through their cytoplasm. There are varying numbers of melanophages in which the melanin granules are coarse and more closely clumped. This type of blue naevus is usually neither very extensive nor of sufficient bulk to raise the surface much.

The cellular type is composed of the same elements as the ordinary type, but in addition possesses islands of larger cells arranged in a neuroid ('pigmented neurofibroma') or sarcomatoid fashion [20]. The appearance may raise suspicions of malignant melanoma, but the lack of mitotic activity, vascularity or inflammatory reaction, the regularity of the cells and the absence of junctional proliferation in continuity with the cellular masses enable the distinction to be made. Exceptionally, a blue naevus may be combined with a pigmented cellular naevus [16, 20].

Clinical features. There is a rounded area of dark-blue pigmentation, usually slightly raised and smooth surfaced, less often nodular, and 10 mm or less in diameter. Lesions larger than this are usually of the cellular type. The common situations of the blue naevus are on the extremities, particularly the dorsa of the hands and feet, the buttocks and the face. The onset may be before birth, but eruption in later life is not uncommon [8]. Progressive growth is rare, and change to malignant melanoma very rare [3, 8, 21].

Diagnosis. The condition is characterized by its colour and must be differentiated from other dermal melanoses. The long and unchanging course should set it apart from malignant melanoma, but this diagnosis is not infrequently sent with surgical pathology specimens.

Treatment. When this is demanded, plastic excision should be carried out and should include some subcutaneous fat to ensure complete removal.

Naevus of Ota (syn. naevus fuscocaeruleus ophthalmomaxillaris) [24]; extensive blue patch-like pigmentation [25]; persistent aberrant Mongolian spots [6]; mesodermal melanosis of the face and sclera [5]; ocular and dermal melanocytosis [13])

Definition. A diffuse bluish pigmentation of the skin adjacent to the eye and of the sclera due to the presence of dermal melanocytes.

Incidence. This disorder is not uncommon in the Japanese, but is comparatively rare in Caucasians and Negroes. Unlike the Mongolian spot, it is not usually present at birth, becomes progressively darker in childhood and persists in adult life.

Pathology [23]. The features are the same as those of Mongolian spot.

Clinical features. The pigmentation is somewhat speckled and is composed of deeper bluish and more

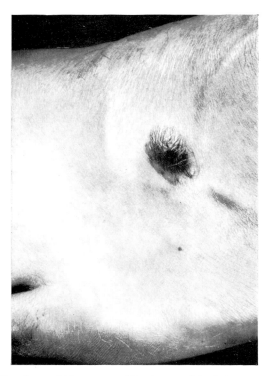

Fig. 64.42. A blue naevus of the dorsum of the foot. Histologically, it was of the 'cellular' type. (Dr. H. J. Wallace, St John's Hospital.)

superficial brownish elements, which do not always coincide. The two colours are perhaps best seen on the eye, where the affected sclera is blue and the conjunctiva brown. The brown pigmentation is patchy and may be patterned in a reticular or geographical way; the blue pigmentation is more diffuse. The areas involved are the eyelids, the bulbar and palpebral conjunctiva and the sclera, and the cheeks, forehead, scalp, alae nasi and ears. The mucosa of the palate and cheeks may also be affected [12]. The distribution is usually restricted to the first and second divisions of the trigeminal nerve, but rarely patches may occur on the trunk [5].

The pigmented spots usually appear in childhood and increase in number and extent to become confluent in some areas. There is one report [31] of the onset following trauma, and in another [13] the ocular pigmentation became much more pronounced after an attack of conjunctivitis. The distribution is usually, but not always, unilateral.

In three cases [5, 12] ballooning of the posterior fossa to produce a step-like deformity of the occiput has been reported. There has also been one case with facial hemiatrophy [4].

In very rare instances malignant melanoma has developed in naevus of Ota [8].

Treatment. Heavy make-up disguises the blemishes. Frequent short applications of CO_2 snow may reduce the depth of pigmentation.

Naevus of Ito [15]. This type of dermal melanocytosis involves the acromioclavicular region and the upper chest and, like Ota's naevus, is largely confined to the Japanese.

REFERENCES

1 ALLEN A. C. (1960) *AMA Arch Dermatol* **82**, 325.
2 ALLEN A. C. (1963) *Ann NY Acad Sci* **100**, 29.
3 *ALLEN A. C. & SPITZ S. (1953) *Cancer* **6**, 1.
4 AUBRY, *et al* (1949) *Algér Méd*, p. 265.
5 CARLETON A. & BIGGS R. (1948) *Br J Dermatol* **60**, 10.
6 COLE H. N., *et al* (1950) *Arch Dermatol Syphilol* **61**, 244.
7 DELLA PORTA G., *et al* (1956) *AMA Arch Pathol* **61**, 305.
8 DORSEY C. S. & MONTGOMERY H. (1954) *J Invest Dermatol* **22**, 225.
9 DUPONT A. & VANDAELE R. (1957) *Arch Belg Dermatol Syphiligr* **13**, 217.
10 *ECHEVARRIA R. & ACKERMAN L. V. (1967) *Cancer* **20**, 175.
11 EL BAHRAWY A. A. (1922) *Arch Dermatol Syphilol* **141**, 171.
12 FINDLAY G. H. (1951) *S Afr J Clin Sci* **2**, 281.
13 FITZPATRICK T. B., *et al* (1956) *Arch Ophthalmol* **56**, 830.
14 GARTMANN H. (1959) *Med Kosmet* **9**, 301.
15 ITO M. (1954) *Tohoku J Exp Med* **60**, 10.
16 KAWAMURA T. (1950) *Arch Dermatol Syphilol* **62**, 395.
17 *KERNEN J. A. & ACKERMAN L. V. (1960) *Cancer* **13**, 612.
18 KOPF A. W. & ANDRADE R. (1966) *Year Book of Dermatology.* Chicago, Year Book Medical Publishers, p. 7.
19 LEOPOLD J. G. & RICHARDS D. B. (1967) *J Pathol Bacteriol* **94**, 247.
20 *LUND H. Z. & KRAUS J. M. (1962) *Melanotic Tumors of the Skin. Atlas of Tumor Pathology*, Section 1, Fasc. 3. Armed Forces Institute of Pathology, Washington, DC.
21 MERKOW L. P., *et al* (1969) *Cancer* **24**, 888.
22 *MISHIMA Y. (1967) In *Ultrastructure of the Normal and Abnormal Skin.* Ed., Zelickson A. S. Philadelphia, Lea & Febiger, p. 388.
23 MISHIMA Y. & MEVORAH B. (1961) *J Invest Dermatol* **36**, 133.
24 OTA M. (1939) *Jpn J Dermatol Urol* **46**, 369.
25 PARISER H. & BEERMAN H. (1949) *Arch Dermatol Syphilol* **59**, 396.
26 PEACE R. J. (1955) *AMA Arch Pathol* **59**, 359.
27 PIERS F. (1946) *E Afr Med J* **23**, 210.
28 RAPPAPORT H., *et al* (1961) *Cancer Res* **21**, 661.
29 *RODRIGUEZ H. A. & ACKERMAN L. V. (1968) *Cancer* **21**, 393.
30 *SPITZ S. (1948) *Am J Pathol* **24**, 591.
31 STUART C. (1955) *Br J Dermatol* **67**, 317.
32 WELLS G. C. & FARTHING G. J. (1966) *Br J Dermatol* **78**, 380.

MALIGNANT MELANOMA [69]

Definition A malignant tumour arising in the skin from epidermal melanocytes, from the junctional component of a cellular naevus or, rarely, within a blue naevus.

Incidence and aetiology [31, 51] The incidence of cutaneous malignant melanoma is rising rapidly in all parts of the world for which adequate data are available. In Norway the incidence doubles every 10 yr and is currently 12 new cases per 10^5 population per year [65]. In Queensland, Australia, the incidence is currently the highest in the world at $39 \cdot 6/10^5$ annually, and here also it has been doubling each decade [39]. In the 'sunbelt' states of North America [84, 90] the incidence has quadrupled in the past 10 yr in Arizona, but the increase has been confined exclusively to the white-skinned population of North European extraction—the so-called 'Anglos'. No increasing incidence is seen in those of Spanish or Mexican descent in either Arizona or New Mexico.

In the UK [97] there is clear evidence of a rising incidence in England and Wales with incidence figures of $2 \cdot 3 \times 10^5$ for males and $4 \cdot 4 \times 10^5$ for females for 1977. In Scotland the incidence for 1979 is $5 \cdot 1 \times 10^5$ [63]. A striking feature of the British data is the fact that the sex incidence is consistently two females to one male. This imbalance is not seen in other parts of the world with a higher incidence, and has been interpreted by Lee and Storer [53] as suggesting the involvement of endocrine cofactors in aetiology which are masked or overwhelmed in areas of higher solar exposure.

These rising incidence figures and the geographic pattern with high figures close to the equator strongly implicate sunlight exposure as an aetiological agent in cutaneous melanoma. The evidence, however, is conflicting, as the typical melanoma patient is a Caucasian female in the fourth or fifth decade with an office job and of high socioeconomic status [54]. This does not describe the individual who has the maximum lifetime sun exposure—an elderly outdoor male worker in the seventh or eighth decade of low socio-economic status. Current evidence suggests that short sharp periods of intense sun exposure resulting in severe sunburn may be important in the development of cutaneous malignant melanoma rather than cumulative lifetime dose [44, 62].

The studies by Lee and Merril [52] showing increased incidence of malignant melanoma on both exposed and non-exposed sites have led them to postulate the existence of 'solar circulating factor', a substance which is activated or generated by melanocytes on exposure to sunlight and which then acts on melanocytes in covered sites. Proof of the existence of such a substance is not forthcoming and a point against its existence is the lack of an increased incidence of ocular melanomas. The alternative explanation of inadequate protection of 'covered sites' by thin layers of cotton clothing in warm climates seems well worthy of consideration.

Racial susceptibility is a further important feature and both Australian and North American studies demonstrate the increased susceptibility of individuals of Celtic or Caledonian descent [36, 50] who tend to be fair skinned and blue eyed. In dark-skinned races the tumour is most frequently seen on the sole of the foot or the nail fold. This may be attributable to trauma or to a metabolic aberration of melanocytes which are not realizing their full melanogenic capacity [70].

It is hard to assess the importance of an injury as the agent provoking a tumour or converting a melanocytic naevus to malignant behaviour. There are a certain number of cases where penetrating or thermal injuries to normal skin have been followed after a short time by a malignant melanoma. With moles the history may be misleading, as early malignant change often makes the epidermis more fragile to trivial injury. Although the general impression is that trauma is of little importance, statistical comparison of the histories of patients with malignant melanoma and basal cell carcinoma shows a highly significant difference in favour of malignant melanoma following trauma. Pregnancy appears to increase the size and number of metastases, but comparison of matched series of pregnant and non-pregnant patients indicates that the eventual outcome is little altered [37]. Familial cases are uncommon, but some striking family histories have been recorded [4, 46, 47].

Malignant melanoma is rare before puberty [1]. Transplacental metastasis to the fetus can occur [13]. Many of the tumours of childhood have begun in large congenital melanocytic naevi [38, 94].

Pathology [2, 3, 10–12, 15–17, 68–71]. The essential feature of primary cutaneous malignant melanoma is the presence of neoplastic melanocytes invading the dermis, but retaining in portions of the section a contact with the basal layer of the epidermis. The neoplastic melanocytes are generally larger than the keratinocytes surrounding them and individual cells have a high nuclear-to-cytoplasmic ratio. The melanocytes may be epithelioid, spindle shaped or form a mixed population. Upward movement of individual melanocytes through the epidermis is observed in a proportion of cases, and a dermal round-cell infiltrate may be present.

Valuable contributions to the clinical significance of pathological features in malignant melanoma have been made by Mishima [76–78] who proposed the existence of two distinct developmental pathways from the neural crest, one via the naevus cell to the naevocytic melanoma and one via the melanocyte to the melanocytic melanoma. Clark, McGovern and co-workers have classified primary malignant melanoma into three distinct histogenetic types—the lentigo maligna melanoma, the superficial spreading melanoma and the nodular melanoma. These variants are based on a study of the epidermis more than three rete ridges lateral to the invasive portion of the tumour.

Mishima's concept of a dual developmental pathway is based on the clinical observation of very different prognoses for the more slowly evolving lentigo maligna melanoma by comparison with nodular and superficial spreading melanoma. Mishima offers clinical evidence to support the dual origin of malignant melanoma. On the one hand he considers that the lentigo-maligna-derived lesion is radiosensitive, does not develop an amelanotic form, occurs later in life and is almost entirely confined to exposed skin sites. The naevocytic malignant melanoma on the other hand is found on both exposed and non-exposed sites, affects a younger age group, may be found in an amelanotic form and is relatively radioresistant.

Further evidence, both histochemical and ultrastructural, is advanced for the dual pathology theory [76]; lentigo-maligna-derived lesions show melanocytes which are intensely dopa positive and dendritic in outline, whereas naevocytic melanoma cells are more rounded in outline, tend to occur in clumps or theques and tend to lose dopa positivity in the deeper parts of the lesion. At the ultrastructural level Mishima demonstrates ellipsoid structures, frequently with a ring-like structure in the melanocytic malignant melanoma, whereas melanosomes within the naevocytic melanoma are cigar shaped and average 850×350 μm in size.

This dual pathway theory for the development of malignant melanoma has caused much interest and has been a catalyst for much valuable work, particularly on the ultrastructure of malignant melanoma. An important argument against such a system is the assumption that all non-lentigo-maligna-derived malignant melanomata arise in association with a pre-existing junctional naevus. This is histologically demonstrable in only a minority of cases, the incidence reported varying widely from 20% to 50%. Even taking the highest figure for this observation, it seems very unlikely that all evidence of a pre-existing naevus is obliterated in 50% of lesions.

The work of Clark and co-workers [15–17], and McGovern and colleagues [68–71] has greatly stimulated ideas on the biological behaviour of evolving malignant melanoma. Clark considers that the majority of primary cutaneous melanomas can be divided into histogenetic types based on a study of the epidermal changes adjacent to the portion of the lesion invading the dermis. The superficial spreading melanoma comprises 60–70% of most reported series, and is characterized by epidermal hyperplasia and associated nests of neoplastic melanocytes at various levels in the epidermis lateral to the invasive area of the tumour. This may at times be so striking that Paget's disease may be simulated. The tumour cell population may be spindle, epithelioid or mixed and in the early stages of dermal invasion a round-cell infiltrate may be present.

The lentigo maligna melanoma which comprises about 10% of reported series occurs in 90% of cases on exposed sites—the face, scalp and backs of the hands. Adjacent to the invasive component of the lesion the epidermal change is that of lentigo maligna which may exist for many centimetres around the lesion. The epidermis is generally thin and atrophic, and the basal layer is replaced by abnormal melanocytes. These are large spindle-shaped cells, frequently heavily melanized. Individual cells vary considerably in size and nuclear cytoplasmic ratio, so that the overall picture is pleomorphic; mitotic figures are relatively infrequent. Neoplastic melanocytes are not commonly observed in the upper portion of the epidermis. Areas of regression within a lentigo maligna melanoma are common and are comprised of circumscribed areas resembling granulation tissue or frank scarring. Lymphoid cells may be observed and at times form a dense boundary at the invading edge of the lesion. Melanin-filled macrophages and melanin lying free in the dermis are frequently seen adjacent to such areas. The papillary dermis around lentigo maligna melanoma shows gross solar elastosis, and McGovern considers this feature an essential part of the histological pattern of lentigo maligna melanoma [69].

In Clarke's classification, malignant melanoma of the nodular type is a lesion with only a vertically invasive component; the epidermis on either side of the invasive component is normal with no abnormal melanocyte activity in either the epidermis or the basal layer. These lesions form around 12% of reported series and are found twice as frequently in males as in females.

Lesions on the soles and palms have in some cases a distinct pathological appearance although the superficial spreading melanoma can also occur on these sites. The so-celled acral lentiginous pattern shows extensive lateral lentiginous change on either side of the invasive nodule with replacement of the basal layer keratinocytes by atypical melanocytes. Within the epidermis there are scattered atypical melanocytes seen at various levels, and downward dermal invasion may initially be very localized. The early changes are subtle and the unwary may be inclined to consider the lesion benign. A further useful diagnostic point is the presence scattered along the dermo–epidermal junction of foci of lymphocytes. Lesions of this type are particularly common in the Japanese population and comprise 40–50% of reported Japanese series of malignant melanomas [92].

In addition to these four clinicopathological variants of malignant melanoma there is a small number of tumours in which a lateral radial growth phase with neoplastic and abnormal melanocytes is observed, but which cannot be classified as either that of the superficial spreading or the lentigo maligna pattern. The frequency with which this pattern, termed malignant melanoma with an unclassified radial growth phase, is observed will vary according to the individual pathologist, but a figure of around 10% of all lesions is commonly reported.

The McGovern classification [68] divides depths of invasion of the tumour into five stages.

Level I.   Intraepidermal only—an *in situ* situation. This level would not be used in a clinical report but is reserved for research studies.

Level II.   Invasion into the upper layers of papillary dermis.

Level III. A filling and distorting of the papillary dermis with tumour cells.

Level IV.   Invasion of the reticular dermis.

Level V.   To subcutaneous tissues.

The significance of the level of invasion of tumour, which is discussed in detail together with other histological features in several specialist publications, is that it has been shown to have clinical prognostic significance as illustrated in Tables 64.2 and 64.3.

The most important histological feature available for prognostic information is the measurement in millimetres of the thickest part of the melanoma, measuring from the granular layer to the deepest underlying easily identified tumour cell (Fig. 64.44). This measurement is termed the Breslow thickness, after the late Alexander Breslow who showed a clear inverse linear correlation between tumour thickness using this measurement and 5 yr survival [10–12]. Thus in his series no patient with a tumour thinner than 0.76 mm died of their tumour during this period but 5 yr survival for those with tumours of 3.5 mm or greater was only 50%. Many groups around the world have confirmed the value of this measurement in predicting survival, and it is a pathological feature which should be made available to all clinicians in charge of the management of patients with melanoma. It is of course essential that absolutely vertical sections are taken through the apparently thickest part of well-fixed tissue if this measurement is to be obtained accurately. Although some published papers have measured

TABLE 64.2 Level of invasion of primary tumour and survival (after Clark *et al* [15])

Level	% survivors of 208 patients 5–7 yr
II	72
III	47
IV	32
V	12

TABLE 64.3. Depth of invasion in millimetres correlated with lymph node metastases and 5 yr survival (after Wanebo *et al* [99])

Depth of invasion (mm)	% with nodal metastases at block dissection	5 yr survival
0.0–0.5	0	100
0.6–1.0	9	100
1.1–1.5	5	89
1.6–2.0	8	82
2.1–3.0	22	58
<3.1	39	55

Breslow thickness retrospectively the validity of these figures must be questioned because of the possible inappropriate selection of blocks for this measurement. Although at first consideration this may seem to be a duplication of the measurement of level of invasion in the Clark and McGovern classifications, this is clearly not the case in lesions where marked elevation above the surrounding skin is present. In fact the two measurements both have prognostic significance and the use of both Clark's levels and Breslow's direct thickness measurement are strongly recommended in any histological protocol for malignant melanoma relationship between lesional thickness, presence of metastases in draining lymph nodes and survival [99].

In both the superficial spreading and nodular varieties of the tumour there may be very little clinical or indeed histological evidence of the presence of melanin pigmentation on conventional haematoxylin and eosin sections. This situation arises more frequently in subungual lesions. The neoplastic cells can be shown to be melanocytes by use of the dopa

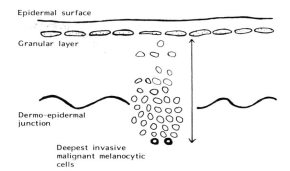

FIG. 64.43. Details of the Breslow thickness measurement (in millimetres). The measurement is read on an eyepiece micrometer, measuring from the granular layer in the epidermis down to the deepest easily identified tumour cell in the dermis.

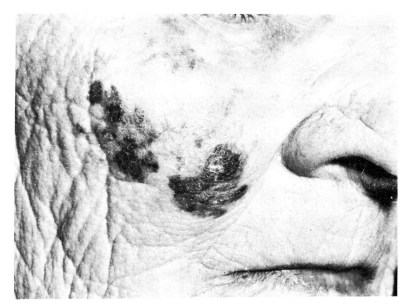

FIG. 64.44. Lentigo maligna melanoma on the cheek of an elderly woman. Fig. 64.45. shows histology from this lesion.

or tyrosinase reaction. Even in an amelanotic or, more correctly, a hypomelanotic lesion this reaction will be positive, proving the presence, within the cells under study, of the enzymatic pathways necessary for melanin synthesis.

Secondary spread of malignant melanoma may take place locally by direct tissue invasion, by lymphatics or by vascular channels.

The commonest pattern of secondary spread of any of the three histogenetic types of malignant melanoma is to the local draining lymph nodes, but bypassing of these nodes and involvement of any organ by blood spread is also observed. Common sites are liver, lung and the central nervous system. A rather more unusual pattern of spread is where the secondary tumour is confined to subcutaneous

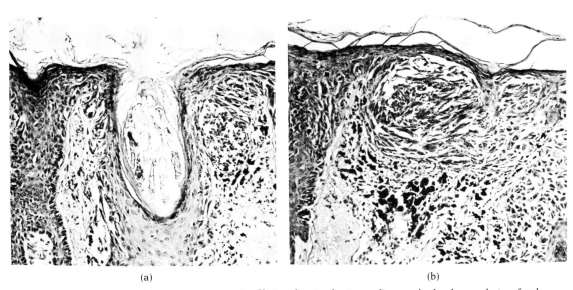

(a)   (b)

FIG. 64.45. Lentigo maligna: (a) area at outer margin of lesion showing lentigo maligna and solar damage but no frank dermal invasion or neoplastic melanocytes; (b) raised central nodule showing invasion of melanocytes into dermis.

tissues and other organs are spared. This pattern may result in a patient with large numbers of subcutaneous nodules in areas distant from the site of the primary tumour. There is some evidence to suggest that such a pattern of spread is more amenable to adjuvant therapy with immune stimulants or cytotoxic agents.

The cellular characteristics of a secondary deposit of malignant melanoma may be strikingly similar to the primary lesion, but this is by no means always the case. A high mitotic rate and abnormal mitotic figures are frequently observed in secondary deposits. The presence of a lymphoid cell infiltrate in secondary deposits is extremely rare.

Clinical features [72, 73]. The first visual indication of any of the four histogenetic types of malignant melanoma is generally one of colour change, either of pigmentation appearing on previously normally pigmented skin or of pigment variation in an antecedent pigmented naevus. Before any visible change, however, the patient may be aware of altered sensation over the lesion, described by many as a mild itch or tingling. Bleeding from a pigmented lesion should certainly arouse suspicion, but this is usually a later clinical alteration than pigment variation or altered sensation.

The change in pigmentation may take the form of increased or decreased melanin pigmentation or be attributable to an increased blood supply to the area. Often all factors are present simultaneously and it is therefore difficult to be dogmatic about the specific changes which should arouse suspicion. In general, however, any previously uniform brown lesion which acquires darker brown irregular areas, central or peripheral, or elevated nodules or an inflammatory border should be viewed with great suspicion.

In addition, however, to these general features which should arouse suspicion of malignant melanoma developing either *de novo* or in association with a pre-existing naevus there are specific clinical features suggestive of the three histogenetic types of malignant melanoma, and these will be described below.

Superficial spreading melanoma [49, 78]. This lesion presents most frequently in a patient in the fourth or fifth decade and the commonest sites are the trunk and leg. It is twice as common on the trunk in males by comparison with females, but three times as common on the leg in females. Other sites which may be involved, but which have a less marked sex difference, are the head, neck and foot. Early presentation is generally that of a slightly ele-

vated and at times hyperkeratotic brown pigmented lesion with a well-defined but irregular margin. Loss of normal skin surface marking can be observed on careful examination, and an area of inflammation may be present at the periphery of the lesion. A lesion of this type may be present for months or even years prior to invasive growth of the tumour, and during this time there may be considerable clinical alteration due to concomitant growth and regression. Notching of the margin of the lesion is a common feature, and partial regression may cause central pigment loss while extension continues peripherally. This pattern of growth may result in a crescentic area of dense blue–black pigmentation with some adjacent inflammatory response and a central area of thin atrophic scar tissue. Elevated nodules and a history of bleeding or serous ooze from the lesion are seen when the lesion changes to the vertically invasive stage of growth. Colour variation in the superficial spreading melanoma is often marked and deep shades of brown and black may be admixed with pink or violet hues.

Acral Lentiginous Melanoma (Palmo-plantar malignant melanoma) This type of melanoma comprises around 10% of all melanomas on white skin, but about 50% of all melanomas in Japan. The lesions are found mainly on the sole of the foot but also on the palm of the hand, and are characterised, as their name would suggest, by a large macular lentiginous pigmented area around an invasive raised tumour. Approximately 50% of all melanomas on the foot come into this category.

Lentigo maligna melanoma. In this histogenetic variant the preceding radial growth phase is the lentigo maligna (Hutchinson's melanotic freckle; melanosis circumscripta precancerosa of Dubreuilh). By comparison with the radial growth phase of the superficial spreading melanoma, this is a much more prolonged period of lateral extension, and many lesions never develop a vertically invasive component. Most occur on the face, commonly on the upper cheek, temple or forehead. Ocular structures may be involved in the process. A small proportion of lentigo maligna melanomas (10% in most series) are observed on extrafacial exposed sites such as the hand or leg. The age of presentation is more advanced than in the case of superficial spreading melanoma and patients are commonly in the sixth or seventh decade. Initially the lentigo maligna is a flat brown stain-like lesion, and this extreme flatness with loss of skin markings is a useful clinical point in the differentiation of the lesion from such lesions as actinic keratoses or seborrhoeic keratoses.

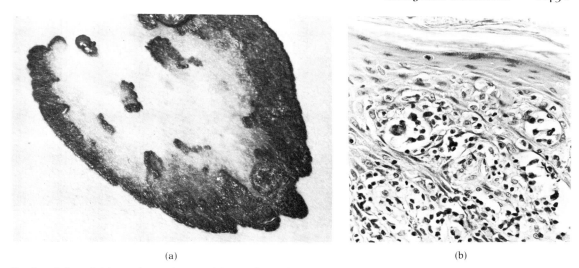

(a)
(b)

FIG. 64.46. Superficial spreading melanoma: (a) central area shows depigmentation representing partial regression, the lateral margin of the tumour is heavily pigmented and some central nodules of tumour persist; (b) upward migration of neoplastic melanocytes through the epidermis.

Associated with this completely smooth surface is a dull non-reflecting quality of the skin surface. As with superficial spreading melonoma, the clinical picture of such a lesion may change strikingly over a period of years and sequential photographs may demonstrate marked migration of the lesion, leaving an area of previous pigmentation as thin atrophic scar tissue. Although the initial colour is generally a fairly uniform mid-brown, this tends to change to a more irregular pattern of dark brown, black and blue hues. Red, pink or violet shades are much less commonly seen in lentigo maligna melanoma than in superficial spreading melanoma.

The change from radially spreading lentigo maligna to vertically invasive lentigo maligna melanoma is indicated by the development of an elevated nodule within the area of pigmentation. The nodule itself is not invariably pigmented. Serous ooze, bleeding and crusting are all associated with nodule formation.

Nodular melanoma. This variety presents most commonly in the fifth or sixth decade and occurs more frequently in males than in females. A male:female incidence ration of 2:1 is commonly reported, and in males increased incidence is mainly seen on the head, neck and trunk.

This tumour carries a poor prognosis which is, at least in part, due to the fact that there is no prodromal radial growth phase, but the lesion would appear to be vertically invasive *ab initio*. A benign pigmented lesion may, however, have been present at the site of development of a nodular melanoma. The lesion presents clinically as an elevated, dome-shaped or even pedunculated structure and the predominant colour is a reddish brown. Melanin pigment may be sparse in these lesions and a raised red central area, with only a peripheral brown ring of melanin, is a common clinical pattern. Ulceration and bleeding from the lesion occurs frequently. This variety of malignant melanoma is misdiagnosed prior to surgery more frequently than either superficial spreading melanoma or lentigo maligna melanoma. The reason for this is probably the rapid growth and relative lack of melanin pigment which may lead to confusion with vascular lesions.

The situation occasionally arises of a secondary malignant melanoma presenting as an isolated non-pigmented subcutaneous nodule with no primary source of the tumour apparent [5]. In such a situation the possibility of an ocular or mucosal primary tumour should be carefully investigated. A further possibility in such a situation is that the primary lesion has undergone spontaneous resolution, and examination of the skin distal to the secondary nodule may reveal a depigmented area suggestive of such a pattern.

Diagnosis. On clinical inspection an uncomplicated pigmented naevus is unlikely to be mistaken for a malignant melanoma. If, however, it becomes inflamed or a granuloma develops within it, suspicion may be aroused. The resulting enlargement is not associated with a change in colour, and examination will show a tender swelling beneath the naevus. Melanocytic naevi erupting in adolescence or adult life are rather more difficult. They have a more regular form than malignant melanoma and, after a brief initial burst of growth, usually become static. A common error is to mistake a dark, inflamed or infected acanthotic seborrhoeic keratosis for a melanoma, especially when it enlarges rapidly or when there is itching and a tendency to bleed or ooze, or even erode and crust. The characteristic 'stuck on' appearance of the seborrhoeic keratosis is a help. When there is uncertainty, the result of applying an antibiotic preparation and protection from injury will usually settle the matter in a few days. A blue naevus is unlikely to be mistaken if a proper history is obtainable; these lesions have almost always been stationary for a considerable time. Pigmented basal cell carcinoma may be ulcerated, but the characteristic translucence, rolled margin and fine telangiectasia are usually sufficient to differentiate it. A small haemangioma which has thrombosed ('capillary aneurysm') [31] or a skin tag which has become strangulated may easily be mistaken for a very early malignant melanoma. The history of the preceding lesion is of help. A haematoma, especially when subungual, should cause no confusion when there is a history of trauma. Spontaneous thrombosis in a plantar wart has been known to trap the élite; paring down the surface will reveal inspissated blood in papillary projections of keratin. A histiocytoma is occasionally sufficiently large and darkly pigmented to mimic a malignant melanoma, but its dermal situation and firm rubbery texture, as well as its yellowish-brown colour, usually permit differentiation. Amelanotic malignant melanoma is difficult to diagnose clinically, and vascular tumours such as pyogenic granuloma are common pitfalls. The use of cytology on imprints, or scrape and smear preparations, has been helpful in the tumours on the feet of Africans.

Black heel (talon noir) (p. 606) may cause some initial concern, but lack of any elevation of the lesion and continuity of the normal skin lines are both reassuring features which should be sought.

Subungual malignant melanoma. A brown tumour beneath the nail plate may be taken for a subungual haematoma. Other modes of presentation in this area are a brown longitudinal band in the nail (which may, however, occur with a pigmented naevus of the nail matrix), a painful spot with a history of enlargement or darkening, longitudinal splitting of the nail, which may not be discoloured, and an oozing and resistant paronychia or nail dystrophy. As the tumour develops the nail is destroyed.

Depigmentation in relation to malignant melanomas [41]. Haloes of depigmentation are occasionally seen around each of the three clinical types of malignant melanoma; as they may also occur around benign pigmented lesions, their presence is not diagnostic of malignant melanoma. The haloes around benign lesions tend, however, to be symmetrical, whereas those around a neoplastic lesion may be highly irregular. Haloes may also appear around benign naevi in a patient with a growing malignant melanoma, and vitiligo is fairly frequently associated with malignant melanoma. The significance of these observations is not yet clear but they would appear to be related to the immunological mechanisms known to be active, particularly in patients with early disease.

Differential diagnosis. The proportion of accurate diagnosis by clinicians varies from 30% to 50% [45]. The dangers of errors of judgment are twofold: the proper treatment of a malignant lesion will be delayed and allow dissemination, or treatment for a malignant melanoma might lead to severe and totally unnecessary cosmetic disability if employed for a benign tumour.

There is a body of opinion that incisional biopsy may lead to premature dissemination [83]. Excisional biopsy and immediate frozen section will differentiate seborrhoeic keratoses, pigmented basal cell carcinoma, granuloma telangiectaticum, thrombosed angioma and thrombosed plantar wart. The pathologist may have difficulty in distinguishing compound or junctional naevi, cellular blue naevi, juvenile melanoma or histiocytomas from malignant melanoma without the assistance of paraffin-embedded sections and special stains, and it is not reasonable for a surgeon to demand an immediate clear-cut answer in all cases.

Malignant melanoma in childhood [95]. The rarity of malignant melanoma before puberty and its comparative commonness in young adults suggest that the tumour may be hormone dependent. Widespread maternal metastases may involve the uterus, placenta and fetus. Such congenital malignant melanomas are rapidly fatal. In exceptional cases congenital tumours may occur in infants with healthy mothers. Of the remaining cases reported in children a quarter have arisen in congenital melanocytic naevi [94]. All the children died. The outlook is rather better for malignant melanoma arising on normal skin, but the tumours behave in more malignant fashion than in adults: the 3 year survival rate in children is almost exactly the same as the 5 year survival rate in adults. Otherwise, there

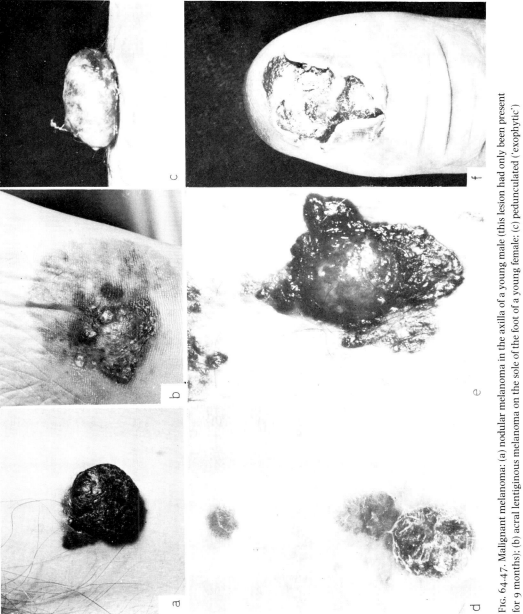

FIG. 64.47. Malignant melanoma: (a) nodular melanoma in the axilla of a young male (this lesion had only been present for 9 months); (b) acral lentiginous melanoma on the sole of the foot of a young female: (c) pedunculated ('exophytic') melanoma (St. John's Hospital); (d) melanoma with satellite metastases (St. John's Hospital); (e) melanoma with satellite metastases (Stoke Mandeville Hospital); (f) melanoma of the nail bed (a pigmented crusted tumour has destroyed the nail plate) (St. John's Hospital).

is nothing to distinguish the behaviour of the tumour in the two age groups.

The association between benign melanocytic naevi and malignant melanoma. At the present time there is considerable interest and controversy over the proportion of malignant melanomas which arise on the basis of a pre-existing acquired naevus. The average figure for all studies from around the world, based on histological evidence of naevus cells adjacent to malignant melanoma cells, is that 25–50% of melanomas arise in association with acquired melanocytic naevi, but in high incidence areas there is preliminary information that this association is even more common. As, however, the young adult has approximately 30 acquired melanocytic naevi on his body, it must be stated firmly that the very great majority of acquired melanocytic naevi are not premalignant and appear not to have premalignant potential under normal circumstances.

The two groups of melanocytic naevi which appear to be associated with a significantly higher risk of malignant transformation are firstly the group of naevi present at birth—congenital naevi—and secondly a recently described group of naevi showing histological features of dysplasia. These lesions may be either familial or sporadic.

In the case of congenital naevi the risk of malignant change has to date mainly been reported in association with the giant bathing trunk or garment type of naevi, and studies from a number of plastic surgery units over the past 20 yr have put the risk of malignant change at between 2% and 28%. The average risk from accumulated studies of this type is around 12%, but this is almost certainly an overestimation due to positive reporting of those lesions which do undergo malignant change and a lack of reporting of lesions which do not. The most useful study to date in this area is that by Lorenzen *et al* [56] who carried out a retrospective study on 150 patients with large congenital naevi followed for 60 yr through the Scandinavian Tumour Registries. From this extremely valuable epidemiological study they suggest that the cumulative lifetime risk of malignant change in such a lesion is around 4%.

More recently, considerable interest has been devoted to the smaller congenital naevi and their possible association with malignant change. In 1973 Mark *et al* [66] clearly defined the histological criteria for separating the small congenital naevus from the acquired naevus. This information was based on family histories and included such features as the involvement of the deeper two-thirds of the reticular dermis and significant involvement of the adnexal structures with naevus cells. Using this de-

finition, Rhodes *et al* [87] have recently carried out a study on 243 melanomas and have found in this series that as many as 19% showed evidence suggesting origin from a pre-existing small congenital naevus. This figure is higher than many people would have suspected and, if confirmed, is powerful evidence to suggest that surgical excision of these smaller congenital lesions as a preventative measure is certainly justified.

The other group of naevi associated with an increased risk of malignant change are the recently recognized atypical or dysplastic naevi [61]. These were described almost simultaneously by Lynch and Clark. The terms originally used were the familial atypical mole malignant melanoma syndrome (FAMMM) by Lynch [58, 59] and the BK mole syndrome by Clark [17, 86]. These terms were both used to describe familial conditions, but subsequently it has been recognized that a sporadic form of the condition does occur. Affected patients have large numbers of naevi, some of which are relatively large (more than 2 cm in diameter), and have an irregular border, sometimes with an associated inflammatory flare. On histological examination these lesions may show signs of 'dysplasia' [28]—defined as irregular proliferation of atypical melanocytes in and around the basal layer, a lymphocytic infiltrate and a fibrillary change in the collagen of the papillary dermis. Patients with this type of naevus tend to develop multiple primary melanomas of the superficial spreading type, and there is some evidence that these patients have a generalized systemic melanocytic disorder with increased numbers of large melanocytes.

A lesion which should not be confused with malignant melanoma is the spindle cell naevus described by Reid [85]. This lesion appears to occur most commonly on the thighs of females and clinically is a dense black lesion. Biopsy reveals a well-demarcated lesion with aggregates of spindle-shaped cells around the dermal–epidermal junction. There is no upward movement of atypical melanocytes through the epidermis, and no downward invasion. Pigment is frequently present in fairly large quantities. It is not known whether or not these lesions, if left untreated, would develop into true malignant melanoma, but there is no doubt that in the past examples of this condition have been incorrectly labelled malignant melanoma.

The benign naevus which even more frequently causes diagnostic confusion is the Spitz naevus (juvenile melanoma, benign epithelioid or spindle cell naevus). In young patients these lesions are usually recognized because of their red dome-shaped appearance, but they are much less typical in their clinical features in older patients. The features of value in identifying a Spitz naevus [95] from a Spitzoid malignant melanoma are the regularity and symmetry of the lesion, the clear demarcation of the lesion from surrounding normal epidermis, the large plump melanocytic cells in an oedematous papillary dermis, dilated capillaries around and within the lesion, and the lymphocytic infiltrate admixed with the lower melanocytic cells. These features in combination make the diagnosis of a Spitz naevus highly likely, but any one can be found in isolation in a malignant melanoma. This distinction between true Spitz naevus and malignant melanoma mimicking Spitz naevus is one of the most difficult problems facing the dermatopathologist.

Immunological considerations [18, 75, 101] For many years it has been considered on clinical grounds that host responsiveness may play some part in controlling the rate of spread of malignant melanoma. This view is mainly based on observations of spontaneous regression of both primary and secondary tumour deposits [32], and has led to intensive immunological investigation to determine the nature of this immune response. At the present time there appears to be no gross non-specific humoral or cell-mediated immunological abnormality in malignant melanoma patients other than those with terminal disease, but studies looking at humoral and cell-mediated phenomena directed specifically against melanoma-derived material have yielded interesting and at times conflicting results.

Apparently melanoma-specific antibodies were first reported by Lewis in Uganda [55] and have since been observed by many other workers [67, 79, 80, 82]. These antibodies are directed against antigens on specific sites of the tumour cell—the cell membrane, the cytoplasm and the nucleolus. There is some controversy over the relationship between the presence of such an antibody and the clinical stage of disease. Some workers report loss of demonstrable antibody in advanced disease [55], while others record high melanoma antibody titres in the presence of a large tumour volume and disseminated disease. These conflicting results may in part be attributable to technical variations, but they emphasize the fact that the use of immunofluorescence as a diagnostic or prognostic test in malignant melanoma is at present a research technique [1]. The only benign pigmented lesion in which similar cytoplasmic antibodies are demonstrable is the halo naevus, and this observation has given rise to speculation that the halo naevus may be a very early malignant melanoma undergoing self-destruction [19].

Cell-mediated immunological responses to malignant-melanoma-associated products have also been recorded [35]. *In vivo* work using melanoma extracts as skin test material has been reported by Fass *et al* [33] and showed positive 48 h results using autologous extracts in three of eight patients. The three reactive patients were all those with early disease, and the five non-reactive patients had disseminated disease but demonstrated positive skin tests to recall antigens. Other workers find no such clear relationship between skin test reactivity and stage of disease or total tumour burden.

In vitro tests have utilized antigen-mediated lymphocyte transformation, leucocyte migration inhibition and lymphocyte-mediated cytotoxicity as tests of lymphocyte sensitization to melanoma products [39, 81].

Guides to prognosis [7, 21–24, 26, 27, 89] (Table 64.4). A large number of studies published on melanoma in the last 5 yr are concerned with the identification of those histological features which are of the greatest value in assessing prognosis for the individual patient. The most important by far of these is the Breslow thickness measurement [9–12] (p. 2448) as virtually all published studies show an inverse linear correlation between 5 yr survival and tumour thickness obtained by this measurement. The assessment of the Clark level of invasion is also of value in this respect (p. 2448). All patients entering any trial of therapy should have both these measurements performed before entering the studies. Once correction is made for Breslow thickness a few histological features may be useful additional guides to prognosis. Day's multifactorial analysis suggests that ulceration, mitotic rate and the presence of microscopic satellites are all independent variables once adjustment is made for Breslow thickness [22–27].

The histogenetic type of lesion does not at present appear to affect prognosis, and other features such as cell type and peritumoral inflammatory flare are not of prognostic significance. Early reports that the presence of evidence of tumour regression in thin tumours which otherwise have a 'good prognosis' [40] is an adverse sign have not been confirmed.

Balch's group also report that microscopic evidence of ulceration is a poor prognostic factor independent of Breslow thickness [8]. This feature has not been found to be an independent variable in other series. A recent report by Friedman *et al* [34] suggests that histological evidence of a pre-existing naevus is an independent prognostic variable associated with a better 5 yr survival than lesions of equal thickness with no such feature.

TABLE 64.4. Clinical and pathological features claimed to be of prognostic significance in primary cutaneous malignant melanoma

Features	Comment
Clinical	
Sex	In many series females do better than males
Age	In general, 5 yr survival declines with advancing age
Body site	Recent unconfirmed claims for certain poor prognosis sites, e.g. BANS area, midline lesions
Pathological	
Breslow thickness	In all series by far the most important prognostic feature
Clark levels of invasion	Claimed in some series to add information to Breslow thickness in certain situations
Ulceration	A poor prognostic feature in many series
Angio-invasion	A poor prognostic feature in many series
Evidence of regression	Early claims of poor prognosis not well substantiated; lack of agreement over definition of regression
Mitotic rate	High mitotic rate appears to be an independent variable in some series
Pre-existing naevus	Recent claims that this is a good prognostic sign
Cell type	No significance for cutaneous melanoma; contrasts with the observations in ocular melanoma

A more recent study has been an attempt to identify clinical features of prognostic significance. It has long been recognized that females had a better prognosis than males [90], but this advantage appears to be lost in older females over the age of 50, suggesting that changing hormonal influences around the menopause may affect the tumour–patient balance. The site of the lesion is also reported as an independent variable in some series, with Day *et al* [25] suggesting that lesions in the BANS area (back, upper arm, neck and shoulder) have a poorer prognosis than lesions of equal thickness on other sites. In general, truncal lesions, particularly those adjacent to the midline, have a poorer prognosis than limb lesions.

Treatment [5, 43, 60, 74, 100]. Early recognition of cutaneous malignant melanoma is essential, as, if recognised and excised before the tumour has invaded deeply, melanoma is a curable disease. All patients with lesions clinically suspected to be melanoma should have the lesion excised for histological confirmation. In the majority of early melanomas the size of the lesion permits an excision biopsy. There is little hard data to support the idea that incisional biopsy has a deleterious effect on the patient's subsequent course, but many clinicians are reluctant to perform such a biopsy in case

tumour cells are dislodged into lymphatics. In fact, the situation rarely arises as larger lesions are usually clearly melanomas and definitive therapy can be planned. In cases of real clinical doubt over the diagnosis, histological confirmation with 'rapid paraffin' section material is preferable to frozen section as the finer points of melanoma histology may not be immediately apparent on frozen section. Accurate measurement of the Breslow thickness is not possible on frozen sections, and for this reason also paraffin-processed material is preferred.

Once the histological diagnosis is confirmed and the Breslow thickness measurement known, decisions can be made concerning the extent of surgical excision considered necessary. Lesions under 1 mm in thickness on any body site may only require a margin of 1 cm of normal skin around the lesion and may therefore not require grafting. Thicker lesions, particularly those on the trunk [25], almost certainly require wider excision with a margin of 3 cm or more of normal skin and skin grafting. It appears that, while adequate depth of excision is essential, the removal or retention of the deep fascia does not alter prognosis [88]. At the present time there are a number of trials in progress tailoring width of excision of primary tumours to Breslow thickness. Results of these studies should help to clarify whether or not all tumours thicker

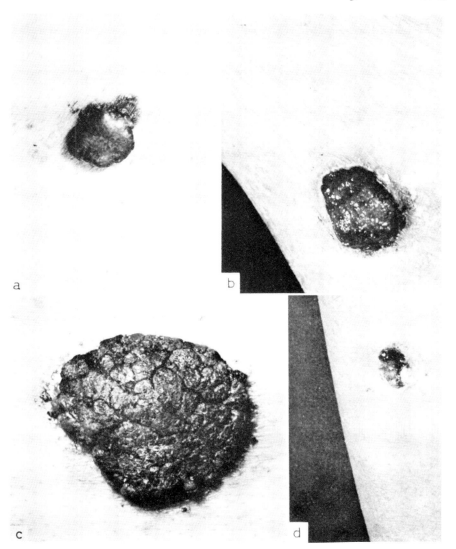

FIG. 64.48. Diagnosis of malignant melanoma: (a) malignant melanoma; (b) pigmented cystic basal cell carcinoma; (c) pigmented seborrhoeic keratosis; (d) inflamed and ulcerated seborrhoeic keratosis. (St. John's Hospital.)

than 1 mm require grafting. It has long been the practice in lentigo maligna melanoma to excise only a fairly narrow margin of normal skin because of the anatomical considerations involved when dealing with facial skin.

In the case of patients with thicker poor prognosis primary tumours, there is a lack of agreement over the need for further surgical therapy [29, 30]. The case for prophylactic or elective dissection of lymph nodes for patients with melanoma of thickness 2·0 mm or greater on a limb has been made by Balch [6] and others who report improved 5 yr survival in patients with tumours 2–3·5 mm thick after elective node dissection. Patients with thicker tumours appear not to benefit from this procedure, and the suggested explanation for this is that these patients already have microscopic disseminated disease. In contrast with this observation, a W.H.O. trial [98] found no survival difference between patients with poor prognosis tumours who had elective node dissection and those who only underwent dissection once the nodes were clinically involved. Lymph node dissection carries a degree of morbidity and this should also be considered. At the present time few patients in the U.K. undergo elective node dissection, but a high proportion of patients in North America with intermediate or thick tumours do have elective dissections. Further well-documented trials are needed to clarify which approach is associated with greatest 5 yr survival.

An alternative method of managing patients with thick poor prognosis tumours on a limb is the use of arterial perfusion with a cytotoxic drug, usually melphalan. This type of therapy has been practised for many years by Krementz and more recently by other groups [20, 48, 96]. The reported 5 yr survival figures are encouraging, but no controlled trial has been carried out comparing perfusion either with elective node dissection or with simple observation after surgical excision of the primary tumour.

Patients with clinical evidence of involvement of the draining lymph nodes should have full node dissection carried out. The number of nodes removed and the percentage of those involved by tumour should be counted as this is a guide to prognosis. Patients with only one node involved have a prognosis very little different from those with no nodal involvement but those with three or more, and with tumour invasion beyond the node capsule, have a poorer prognosis. Trials of adjuvant chemotherapy or immunotherapy in this group of patients with stage II disease do not at present show any significant benefit. A large W.H.O. study of over 1,000 patients revealed no improved 5 yr survival for patients treated with DTIC, BCG or a combination of the two for a period of 2 yr after full node dissection.

The management of patients with advanced stage III disease is difficult and unrewarding [94]. Melanoma responds poorly to chemotherapy, and results with the two most widely used single agents, DTIC and videsine, indicate a response rate of 20–26% in most series with remissions of 6 months or less [14, 57]. Combination chemotherapy appears to be slightly more effective, with better response rates of 40–50% reported for VBM (vindesine, bleomycin and methotrexate), BOLD (bleomycin, vincristine, CCNU and DTIC) [91] or BELD (bleomycin, vindesine, CCNU and DTIC). Toxicity with these regimes is significant and a decision must be made as to whether or not it is justified in view of the relatively short remissions reported for most patients.

Malignant melanoma is traditionally regarded as a radioresistant tumour. Radiotherapy has little part to play in the management of primary tumours although it has been recorded in the past that the lentigo maligna melanoma variant is 'relatively' radiosensitive, and radiotherapy has been used to

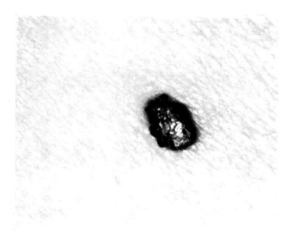

FIG. 64.49. Capillary aneurysm. (see p. 2452) (St. George's Hospital.

treat elderly and infirm patients with these lesions [42]. Radiotherapy can, however, be of considerable value in the palliation of metastatic disease. Low doses of irradiation can dramatically relieve pain from secondary deposits in bone, and intracerebral metastases may benefit from X-irradiation used in combination with systemic steroids. Recent radiobiological studies have indicated that there is a large 'shoulder' effect when melanoma cells are irradiated [102]. This feature may partly explain the poor results of X-ray therapy in the past, and the current use of large fraction doses of X-irradiation may overcome this problem.

Despite numerous publications there is little evidence that any form of immune stimulation is of value in the management of malignant melanoma. Non-specific therapy in the past has included the use of BCG, *Corynebacterium parvum* and levamisole. No controlled trial has demonstrated benefit from these agents. Similarly, specific immunotherapy using melanoma-related products has shown no lasting benefit.

REFERENCES

1 ABEL E. A. & BYSTRYN J. C. (1976) *J Invest Dermatol* **66**, 117.
2 ACKERMAN A. B. (Ed) (1981) *Pathology of Malignant Melanoma*. New York, Masson.
3 ALLEN A. B. & SPITZ S. (1953) *Cancer* **6**, 1.
4 ANDERSON D. E., *et al* (1967) *JAMA* **200**, 741.
5 BAAB G. H. & McBRIDE C. M. (1975) *Arch Surg* **110**, 896.
6 BALCH C. M., *et al* (1979) *Cancer* **43**, 883.
7 BALCH C. M., *et al* (1979) *Surgery* **86**, 343.
8 BALCH C. M., *et al* (1980) *Cancer* **45**, 3012.

9 BALCH C. M., *et al* (1982) *Ann Surg* **188**, 732.

10 BRESLOW A. (1970) *Ann Surg* **172**, 902.

11 BRESLOW A. (1975) *Ann Surg* **182**, 502.

12 BRESLOW A. & MACHT S. H. (1977) *Plast Reconstr Surg* **144**, 327.

13 BRODSKY I., *et al* (1965) *Cancer* **18**, 1048.

14 CARMICHAEL J., *et al* (1982) *Eur J Cancer Clin Oncol* **12**, 1293.

15 CLARK W. H., *et al* (1969) *Cancer Res* **29**, 705.

16 CLARK W. H., *et al* (1975) *Semin Oncol* **2**, 83.

17 CLARK W. H., *et al* (1978) *Arch Dermatol* **114**, 732.

18 COCHRAN A. J., *et al* (1976) *Int J Cancer* **18**, 298.

19 COPEMAN P. W. M., *et al* (1973) *Br J Dermatol* **88**, 127.

20 CREECH O. (1958) *Ann Surg* **148**, 616.

21 DAY C. L., *et al* (1981) *Am J Surg* **142**, 247.

22 DAY C. L., *et al* (1981) *Surgery* **89**, 599.

23 DAY C. L., *et al* (1981) *Cancer* **47**, 955.

24 DAY C. L., *et al* (1981) *Ann Surg* **194**, 108.

25 DAY C. L., *et al* (1982) *Ann Surg* **195**, 30.

26 DAY C. L., *et al* (1982) *Ann Surg* **195**, 35.

27 DAY C. L., *et al* (1982) *Ann Surg* **195**, 44.

28 ELDER D., *et al* (1981) *Cancer* **46**, 1787.

29 ELDH J., *et al* (1979) *Scand J Plast Reconstr Surg* **13**, 341.

30 ELIAS E. G., *et al* (1981) *Surg Gynecol Obstet* **153**, 67.

31 EPSTEIN E. (1965) *AMA Arch Dermatol* **91**, 335.

32 EVERSON T. C. & COLE W. H. (1966) *Spontaneous Regression in Cancer.* Philadelphia Saunders.

33 FASS L., *et al* (1970) *Lancet* **ii**, 583.

34 FRIEDMAN R. J., *et al* (1983) *Arch Dermatol* **119**, 455

35 FRITZ, *et al* (1976) *Arch Dermatol* **255**, 203.

36 GELLIN G. A., *et al* (1969) *Arch Dermatol* **99**, 43.

37 GEORGE P. A., *et al* (1960) *Cancer* **13**, 854.

38 GREELEY P. A., *et al* (1965) *Plast Reconstr Surg* **36**, 26.

39 GREEN A. (1982) *Aust J Dermatol* **23**, 105.

40 GROMET M. A., *et al* (1978) *Cancer* **42**, 2282.

41 HAPPLE R., *et al* (1975) *Hautarzt* **26**, 120.

42 HARMER C. L. (1976) *Clin Exp Dermatol* **1**, 29.

43 HEPPNER G. H., *et al* (1973) *Int J Cancer* **11**, 245.

44 KLEPP O. & MAGNUS K. (1979) *Int J Cancer* **23**, 482.

45 KOPF A. W., *et al* (1975) *Arch Dermatol* **111**, 1291.

46 KOPF A. W., *et al* (1976) *Cutis* **17**, 873.

47 KORTING G. W., *et al* (1969) *Z Haut GeschlKrankh* **44**, 87.

48 KREMENTZ E. T. & CAMPBELL M. (1982) In *Malignant Melanoma.* Ed. Costanzi J. J. Boston, Nijhoff.

49 KUHNL-PETZOLDT C. (1974) *Arch Dermatol Forsch* **250**, 309.

50 LANE BROWN M. M. & MELIA D. F. (1973) *Pigment Cell* **1**, 229.

51 LEE J. A. H. (1982) *Epidemiol Rev* **4**, 110.

52 LEE J. A. H. & MERRIL J. M. (1970) *Med J Aust* **2**, 846.

53 LEE J. A. H. & STORER B. E. (1980) *Lancet* **ii**, 1337.

54 LEE J. A. H. & STRICKLAND D. (1980) *Br J Cancer* **41**, 757.

55 LEWIS M. G. (1971) *Br Med J* **ii**, 547.

56 LORENTZEN M., *et al* (1977) *Scand J Plast Reconstr Surg* **11**, 163.

57 LUCE J. K. (1975) *Semin Oncol* **2**, 175.

58 LYNCH H. T., *et al* (1981) *Br J Cancer* **44**, 553.

59 LYNCH H. T., *et al* (1983) *Cancer Genet Cytogenet* **8**, 325.

60 MACKIE R. M. (1982) *Clin Exp Dermatol* **7**, 231.

61 MACKIE R. M. (1982) *Br J Dermatol* **107**, 621.

62 MACKIE R. M. & AITCHISON T. C. (1982) *Br J Cancer* **46**, 955.

63 MACKIE R. M. & HUNTER J. A. A. (1982) *Br J Cancer* **46**, 75.

64 MACKIE R. M. & YOUNG D. (1984) *Int J Dermatol* **23**, 433.

65 MAGNUS K. (1977) *Int J Cancer* **20**, 477.

66 MARK G. J., *et al* (1973) *Hum Pathol* **4**, 395.

67 MCBRIDE C. M., *et al* (1972) *Surg Forum* **23**, 92.

68 MCGOVERN V. J. (1970) *Pathology* **2**, 85.

69 MCGOVERN V. J. (1983) *The Pathology of Melanoma* (Biopsy Pathology Series). London, Saunders.

70 MCGOVERN V. J. & LANE BROWN M. M. (1969) *The Nature of Melanoma.* Springfield, Thomas.

71 MCGOVERN V. J., *et al* (1973) *Cancer* **32**, 1446.

72 MIHM M. C. (1975) *Semin Oncol* **2**, 104.

73 MIHM M. C., *et al* (1973) *N Engl J Med* **289**, 989.

74 MILTON G. W., *et al* (1982) *Br J Surg* **69**, 108.

75 MISGELD V. (1973) *Hautarzt* **24**, 511.

76 MISHIMA Y. (1964) *J Histochem Cytochem* **12**, 784.

77 MISHIMA Y. (1967) *Cancer* **20**, 632.

78 MISHIMA Y. & MATSUNAKA M. (1975) *J Invest Dermatol* **65**, 434.

79 MORTON D. L., *et al* (1968) *Surgery* **64**, 233.

80 MUNA N. M., *et al* (1969) *Cancer* **23**, 88.

81 NAGEL G. A., *et al* (1971) *Eur J Cancer* **71**, 41.

82 NAIRN R. C. (1972) In *Melanoma and Skin Cancer.* Ed. McCarthy W. H. Sydney, Government Printer.

83 PACK G. T. (1958) *Surgery* **46**, 447.

84 PATHAK D. R., *et al* (1982) *Cancer* **50**, 1440.

85 REID R. J., *et al* (1975) *Semin Oncol* **2**, 119.

86 REIMER R., *et al* (1978) *JAMA* **239**, 744.

87 RHODES A. R., *et al* (1982) *J Am Acad Dermatol* **6**, 230.

88 ROMSDAHL M. M. & COX I. S. (1970) *Arch Surg* **100**, 491.

89 SCHMOEKEL C. & BRAUN-FALCO O. (1978) *Arch Dermatol* **114**, 871.

90 SCHREIBER M. M., *et al* (1981) *Arch Dermatol* **117**, 6.

91 SEIGLER H. F., *et al* (1980) *Cancer* **46**, 2346.

92 SEIJI M. & TAKAHASHI M. (1982) *Hum Pathol* **13**, 607.

93 SHAW H. M., *et al* (1980) *Cancer* **46**, 2731.

94 SKOV-JENSEN T., *et al* (1966) *Cancer* **19**, 620.

95 SPITZ S. (1948) *Am J Pathol* **24**, 591.

96 SUGARBAKER E. V. & MCBRIDE C. M. (1976) *Cancer* **37**, 188.

97 SWERDLOW A. J. (1979) *Br Med J* **ii**, 1324.

98 VERONESI U., *et al* (1982) *Cancer* **49**, 2420.

99 WANEBO H. J., *et al* (1975) *Cancer* **35**, 666.

100 WEAVER P. C., *et al* (1975) *Clin Oncol* **1**, 45.

101 WEESBACH H. W., *et al* (1972) *Arch Dermatol Forsch* **245**, 346.

102 WHELDON T. (1979) *Br J Radiol* **52**, 417.

MESODERMAL TUMOURS

The different derivatives of the mesoderm interact to a greater degree and are more plastic in structure than those of the ectoderm. The mesenchymal cell gives rise to a range of daughter cells which can, within limits, interchange their function and their microscope appearance. The character of the mesoderm, therefore, makes an orderly histogenic classification of tumours arising from it difficult. The position is further complicated by the traditional inclusion in this group of some conditions which are not true neoplasms. Granuloma telangiectaticum and histiocytoma are in many, if not all, instances exaggerated repair reactions. Xanthoma is the result of metabolic disturbance, and most of the benign angiomatous conditions are either malformations or the result of degeneration of the subendothelial supporting tissue. Such conditions are discussed at length elsewhere. They will be touched on here only as far as is necessary to clarify the diagnosis of true neoplasms.

Certain fibrous tissue tumours of the skin and soft tissues are particularly likely to occur in children and a large series of such tumours has been reviewed [5].

TUMOURS OF FIBROUS TISSUE

The following tumours are considered here or elsewhere in the book.

Dermatofibroma (histiocytoma) (p. 1706)
Disseminated dermatofibroma (p. 1825)
Cheloids and hypertrophic scars (p. 1831)
Elastofibroma (p. 1829)
Juvenile fibromatosis (p. 1823)
Fibrous hamartoma of infancy (p. 1825)
Nodular fasciitis
Desmoid tumour
Dermatofibrosarcoma protuberans
Fibrosarcoma
Epithelioid cell sarcoma
Atypical fibroxanthoma
Malignant fibrous histiocytoma

Myxoma and myxosarcoma are not considered as separate tumours. Mucin is produced by fibroblasts and the tumours which show large amounts of mucin in their stroma are essentially fibromas or fibrosarcomas. They are comparatively rare, and even the benign tumours tend to recur after excision.

Dermatofibroma is, in most instances, a histiocytoma (p. 1706) with maturation of the cells towards fibroblasts. Occasionally, the cells may be relatively immature and show evidence of rapid division. Fibroblasts, by their nature, spread between the collagen bundles, and all these features may make histological differentiation from a fibrosarcoma difficult [30]. The architecture of a dermatofibroma is more orderly, with a regular network of fine capillaries each surrounded by radiating slightly whorled fibroblasts. The fibroblasts appear to be acting in a more individual way and lack the concerted invasion by strands and columns which is usual in fibrosarcomas. Some of the cells may contain iron pigment or fat [10]. The epidermis is separated from the tumour by a narrow band of papillary dermis.

The small number of reports of malignant histiocytomas has recently been reviewed [16]. Whether this rare tumour represents malignant change in a histiocytoma or a primary malignant tumour microscopically resembling a histiocytoma is not obvious, but in many of the patients widespread metastases made the malignant nature unquestionable [32].

Nodular fasciitis (proliferative fasciitis [28]; subcutaneous pseudosarcomatous fibromatosis [14]).
Definition. An enlarging tumour in the subcutaneous or deeper tissues which is due to a benign reactive proliferation of fibroblasts which has a superficial resemblance to a sarcoma.

Incidence and aetiology [12, 28]. A number of quite large series have been published in the last 10 yr [12, 22, 28], suggesting that the condition is not uncommon. It is most frequent in middle age, but has been reported in patients from 5 months to 75 yr. There is no predilection for either sex. It is not associated with other diseases. There is no evidence that trauma initiates the lesions.

Pathology [12, 18]. The tumour is composed of fibroblasts, multinucleate cells, capillaries and a constant but scanty round-cell infiltrate in a myxoid or collagenous stroma. The fibroblasts vary in size and shape from tapered or stellate to large rounded cells. The cytoplasm may be pink and granular, the nuclei vesicular and mitoses may be numerous. The majority of cells are spindle cells haphazardly arranged in a myxoid stroma and accompanied by proliferating vessels. At the periphery compact bundles of fibroblasts and capillaries probe the fascial planes and may infiltrate fat or muscle bundles. Perineural extension can occur. It is not surprising that this histological picture was considered suggestive of a fibrosarcoma before its benign nature was recognized.

Clinical features. The majority of tumours appear as tender rapidly growing masses beneath the skin. The average size is 1–3 cm in diameter. The commonest situation is the forearm, but the lesion can occur anywhere including the orbit and the mouth [27]. In nearly half the patients the tumour has been noticed for only 2 weeks or less when they come for advice. Prolonged follow-up has shown that the condition is benign.

Treatment. Resolution has followed incomplete surgical removal. It is desirable, however, to carry out complete, but not radical, excision [12].

Desmoid tumour. This soft tissue tumour occurs principally in parous women, and in the subumbilical paramedian region. It is most common in the third to fifth decade. It has been reported in association with familial multiple polyposis (Gardner's syndrome) [26] and in two families without Gardner's syndrome [2].

The tumour usually arises from the muscular aponeurosis of the lower abdominal wall and infiltrates the adjacent muscles. It may occur in musculoaponeuroses elsewhere [7]. It is not encapsulated and may spread widely and become very large. It does not metastasize, but local recurrence follows inadequate removal. Microscopically, there is fibroblast proliferation and infiltration, often with areas of mucoid degeneration. The clinical picture is of a firm irregular tumour, deep to the subcutaneous tissue, attached to the muscles of the abdominal wall or elsewhere. A wide surgical excision is required to cure the condition.

Dermatofibrosarcoma protuberans
Definition. A locally malignant tumour arising in the dermis and composed of more or less mature fibroblasts.

Incidence and aetiology. It is an uncommon tumour of equal frequency in males and females. Some cases have been preceded by trauma.

Pathology [3, 10, 16, 30]. The tumour is usually a solitary multinodular mass and is essentially a well-differentiated fibrosarcoma. The structures within the dermis are replaced by masses of uniform fibroblasts. These extend right up to the dermo–epidermal junction and down into the subcutaneous fat or deeper. Laterally they infiltrate widely between collagen bundles of the deeper dermis and

blend into the normal dermis. In many instances there is little mitotic activity. The central cells are rather plump, and those at the periphery are rather compressed and attenuated. They usually form quite definite bands which interweave or radiate like spokes of a wheel [30]. The interstitial tissue contains collagen fibres, except in the most cellular parts of the tumour. It is exceptional for histiocytes containing iron pigment or lipid to be found. Blood vessels are hard to see unless special stains are employed, when they are seen in numbers. The large older lesions may show central mucoid degeneration. Metastases resembling Hodgkin's disease and reticulum-cell sarcoma have been seen in two cases [8]. Electron microscopy suggests a neural origin for the tumour [11], though other studies have supported its histiocytic nature [20].

Clinical features. The tumour is more often situated on the front of the trunk, particularly in the flexural regions, than the extremities or the head. It may begin in early adult life with one or more small firm painless flesh-coloured or red dermal nodules.

These grow slowly, coalesce and extend, becoming redder or bluish as they enlarge. The surface is raised by irregular protuberant swellings, and a hard indurated plaque of irregular outline forms the base. In the later stages a proportion of lesions become painful and there may be rapid growth, ulceration and discharge. Metastasis is extremely rare [30]; spread to regional lymph glands and more distant sites has been reported [10, 23].

Diagnosis. In the early stages it may be impossible to distinguish this tumour from a histiocytoma or a cheloid. The slow progression, deep red or bluish-red and characteristic irregular contour and extended plaque-like base separate the older tumour from most others.

Treatment. The tumour should be excised completely, with a generous margin of healthy tissue. Local recurrence invariably follows inadequate removal, and surgeons often underestimate the clearance necessary to cure the tumour.

Fibrosarcoma [4, 10, 29]
Definition. A malignant tumour of connective tissue composed of cells which resemble fibroblasts.

Aetiology. This is an uncommon tumour of the skin in humans, though frequently seen in rodents painted with carcinogens or exposed to UV radiation. Males are affected more often than females, and it may arise at any age from birth onwards. It may occur, after a long interval, following intensive irradiation [21, 24] in scars of lupus vulgaris, tertiary syphilis and burns, and in xeroderma pigmentosum.

Many pathologists consider that most of the tumours previously described as fibrosarcomas of the skin must now be regarded as benign proliferations ['fasciitis'], as sarcomas arising from other tissues such as fat or synovium or as malignant histiocytomas and related tumours. This view can be accepted without excluding the possibility of a more malignant tumour than dermatofibrosarcoma protuberans, as some pathologists are doing. Histological appearances can be misleading, and biological evidence of malignancy from the clinical facts is desirable to confirm the diagnosis of fibrosarcoma of the skin. It must be admitted, however, that the fibrosarcomas and 'pseudosarcomas' are not yet clearly defined.

Pathology. The tumour is composed of atypical fibroblasts, usually large, often pleomorphic and having frequent mitotic figures. They are disposed in a disorderly fashion, but tend to stream and eddy in bands. There is more or less evidence of collagen and reticulin formation, and compression of adjacent tissue may give a suggestion of encapsulation. The blood supply is copious. The less well-differentiated tumours are best described as anaplastic sarcomas, and may be difficult to distinguish from anaplastic carcinomas and malignant melanomas. Some produce large amounts of mucin ('myxosarcoma'). The tumour readily metastasizes through the lymphatic and blood streams.

Clinical features. The tumour is usually a relatively slowly growing smooth-surfaced, reddish or purple and firm nodule. The more anaplastic examples grow faster and feel softer. Ulceration usually occurs sooner or later, and the more superficially placed lesions may become pedunculated. Haemorrhage or necrosis within the mass may cause it to feel fluctuant. The more invasive lesions can produce extensive local destruction and metastasize by the blood stream. The tumour can occur anywhere on the body surface, but is less common on the trunk than elsewhere.

Diagnosis. The early slow growing fibrosarcoma is similar to a histiocytoma, but exhibits progressive growth and becomes more vascular as it enlarges. There is no sharp line of division between this tumour and dermatofibrosarcoma protuberans. The more aggressive tumours must be differentiated histologically from amelanotic-malignant melanoma,

squamous or basal cell carcinoma of the invasive type, secondary deposits in the skin and atypical fibroxanthoma.

Treatment. Surgical excision with a wide margin laterally and beneath the tumour is the treatment of choice. Radiotherapy alone is probably ineffective [10].

Epithelioid cell sarcoma [6, 17, 25]

Definition. A malignant tumour of connective tissue of the skin, subcutaneous tissues or fascial sheaths whose cells have an epithelioid appearance.

Incidence. It is an uncommon tumour, affecting males more often than females and tending to begin in early adult life.

Pathology. The tumour is composed of firm nodules 5–50 mm in diameter surrounded by fibrous tissue and fat, and it is often closely associated with fascia, periosteum, tendon or nerve sheaths. The cut surface is greyish-white and flecked or mottled with yellow or brown. Microscopically there are masses of large, round, polygonal or spindle cells with acidophilic cytoplasm. The larger nodules have necrotic centres. Mitotic figures are common and binucleate cells occur, but there is little cellular pleomorphism. Intercellular hyalinized collagen increases the acidophilia, while calcification, with osteoid or bone formation, may take place in the necrotic areas. The tumour spreads along dense fibrous structures and may ulcerate in areas with little subcutaneous fat. Local recurrence after excision is common, and metastasis, principally to lung and pleura, may occur. The histogenesis is not clear.

Clinical features. The presenting sign can be a dermal nodule, which grows outwards and may ulcerate early, a nodule or lobular subcutaneous tumour which is painless and grows slowly, or a tumour attached to deeper structures which is rather poorly defined and causes pain, paraesthesiae or muscular wasting when growing along a large trunk nerve. The extremities are the usual situation for the tumour, particularly the flexor aspect of the finger and the palm. It may grow at a deceptively slow rate.

Diagnosis. Superficial lesions can easily be mistaken for an ulcerating squamous cell carcinoma and the deeper ones are usually regarded as inflammatory in nature. Histological diagnoses have varied, with granulomatous inflammation and synovial sarcoma being the commonest benign and malignant diagnoses, respectively.

Prognosis and treatment. Complete removal by surgical excision is essential if local recurrence and eventual metastasis are to be avoided, and the earlier this is done the less likely is the process to spread along fascial planes. Before the tumour was defined, the pathologist often underestimated its potential hazard and at least 18% of the original cases have died of metastases.

Atypical fibroxanthoma [5, 9, 13, 15] (syn. pseudo-sarcoma, paradoxical fibrosarcoma [1], pseudo sarcomatous dermatofibroma). In the majority of cases described under these titles an enlarging tumour has arisen in the exposed skin of elderly people, most of whom have either undergone radiotherapy or have a fair complexion which has been exposed to excessive sunlight. The lesions occur most frequently on the ears and cheeks, and have a red fleshy granulomatous appearance; they are often ulcerated but rarely exceed 30 mm in diameter, and are usually of less than 6 months' duration. In a smaller proportion of cases the patient is younger and the lesions may occur on covered parts undamaged by radiant energy [9]. Many of the tumours have been misdiagnosed clinically as granuloma telangiectaticum and, treated by curettage and cauterization, have been cured. Local recurrence has occasionally been seen, and spread to lymph nodes is reported [9, 19].

The remarkable and paradoxical feature of the tumour is its histological resemblance to a malignant connective tissue neoplasm. It arises in the dermis and may extend into the fat. It is composed of large fibroblastic and histiocytic cells which may be atypical multinucleate giant cells, lymphocytes and ectatic vascular spaces. The cells are arranged in a haphazard fashion and mitotic figures may be frequent. The histiocytic cells may contain lipid or haemosiderin.

The benign behaviour of the tumour enables it to be treated by limited local removal. Radiotherapy is undesirable.

REFERENCES

1 BOURNE R. G. (1963) *Med J Aust* i, 504.
2 BRANZOVSKY T. (1974) *Arch Geschwulstforsch* **43**, 277.
3 BURKHARDT B. R., *et al* (1966) *Am J Surg* **111**, 638.
4 DAHL I. (1976) *Acta Pathol Microbiol Scand (A)* **84**, 183.
5 DEHNER L. P. & ASKIN F. B. (1967) *Cancer* **38**, 888.
6 ENZINGER F. M. (1970) *Cancer* **26**, 1029.
7 ENZIGER F. M. & WEISS S. W. (1983) *Soft Tissue Tumours.* St Louis, Mosby.
8 FISHER E. R. & HELLSTROM H. R. (1966) *Cancer* **19**, 1165.
9 FRETZEN D. F. & HELWIG E. B. (1973) *Cancer* **31**, 1541.
10 GENTELE H. (1951) *Acta Derm Venereol (Stockh)* **31** (Suppl. 27).
11 HASHIMOTO K., *et al* (1974) *Arch Dermatol* **110**, 874.
12 HUTTER R. V. P., *et al* (1962) *Cancer* **15**, 992.
13 KEMPSON R. L. & McGAVRAN M. H. (1964) *Cancer* **17**, 1463.
14 KONWATER B. E., *et al* (1955) *Am J Clin Pathol* **25**, 241.
15 KROE D. J. & PITCOCK J. A. (1969) *Am J Clin Pathol* **51**, 487.
16 MACKENZIE D. H. (1970) *The Differential Diagnosis of Fibroblastic Disorders.* Oxford, Blackwell, p. 44.
17 MACKENZIE D. H. (1971) *Br J Cancer* **25**, 458.
18 MEHREGAN A. H. (1966) *Arch Dermatol* **93**, 204.
19 MENDELOW B. V. & RIPPEY J. J. (1975) *S Afr Med J* **49**, 402.
20 OZZELLO L. & HAMELS J. (1976) *Am J Clin Pathol* **65**, 136.
21 PETTIT V. D., *et al* (1954) *Cancer* **7**, 149.
22 PRICE E. B. JR., *et al* (1961) *Am J Clin Pathol* **35**, 122.
23 PRZYBORA L. A. & WOJNEROWICZ C. (1959) *Oncologia (Basel)* **12**, 236.
24 RACHMANINOFF N., *et al* (1961) *Am J Clin Pathol* **36**, 427.
25 SANTIAGO H., *et al* (1972) *Hum Pathol* **3**, 133.
26 SMITH W. G. (1959) *Proc Staff Meet Mayo Clin* **34**, 31.
27 SOLOMON M. P., *et al* (1974) *Oral Surg* **38**, 264.
28 SOULE E. H. (1962) *Arch Pathol* **73**, 437.
29 STOUT A. P. (1948) *Cancer* **1**, 30.
30 TAYLOR H. B. & HELWIG E. B. (1962) *Cancer* **15**, 717.
31 VARGAS-CORTES F., *et al* (1973) *Mayo Clin Proc* **48**, 211.
32 WASSERMAN T. H. & STUARD I. D. (1975) *Cancer* **33**, 141.

Malignant fibrous histiocytoma [2, 7]. This entity was first recognized in 1964 [5] and named malignant fibrous xanthoma. In 1972 the term malignant fibrous histiocytoma [3] was first used. It is now recognized as the commonest tissue sarcoma of late adult life.

Definition. A malignant soft tissue tumour of uncertain histogenesis.

Pathology. The tumour consists of an aggregate of cells in the dermis. Five distinct subtypes are recognized. These are the pleomorphic, myxoid [6], giant cell, inflammatory [4] and angiomatoid [1] variants, although two different areas of the tumour may show two distinct types of differentiation. There may be patches of spindle cells arranged in a storiform (rush-mat-like) pattern. Abnormal mitoses are frequent.

The precise histogenesis is not established. Ultrastructural studies suggest a mixture of cells of histiocytic and fibroblast derivation.

Clinical features. These tumours are rarely diagnosed prior to excision and pathological study. The majority are found in the extremities in older patients, although the angiomatoid variant is seen in younger patients [1] aged 15–25. Clinically the lesion is a nodule usually with considerable extension in the underlying dermis. There is a recent report of a malignant fibrous histiocytoma developing in a burn scar [8].

Treatment. Wide excision is recommended as local recurrence has been observed in 44% and metastases, most commonly to the lungs, in 42%. The inflammatory variant is said to be the most aggressive and most likely to be fatal.

REFERENCES

1 ENZINGER F. M. (1979) *Cancer* **44**, 2147.
2 FLETCHER C. D. M. & MCKEE P. H. (1984) *Clin Exp Dermatol* **9**, 451.
3 KEMPSON R. L. & KYRIAKOS M. (1972) *Cancer* **29**, 976.
4 KYRIAKOS M. & KEMPSON R. L. (1976) *Cancer* **37**, 1584.
5 O'BRIEN J. E. & STOUT A. P. (1964) *Cancer* **17**, 1445.
6 WEISS S. W. & ENZINGER F. M. (1977) *Cancer* **39**, 1672.
7 WEISS S. W. & ENZINGER F. M. (1978) *Cancer* **41**, 2250.
8 YAMAMURA T., *et al* (1984) *Br J Dermatol* **110**, 725.

Liposarcoma [3, 8, 9]

Definition. A malignant tumour composed of mesenchymal cells tending to differentiate into fat cells.

Incidence. It is a rare tumour in the skin. Most cases have occurred in the middle-aged or elderly. It is rather more common in males than females [8], in contrast with the greater frequency of benign lipomas in females [1].

Pathology. The tumour consists of a mixture of undifferentiated sarcoma cells and uniglobular and multiglobular fat cells. Frozen sections stained for fat are necessary to confirm the diagnosis. The more anaplastic tumours may be composed of bizarre cells containing little fat. Type C virus particles have been found in tissue cultures of human liposarcoma [7].

Clinical features. The tumour is a diffuse nodular infiltration of the subcutaneous fat up to 20 cm in size [10], and is usually situated on the lower limb or buttock. It may arise in a pre-existing lipoma [11]. Multiple primary growths occur and similar tumours arise in the retroperitoneal and mesenteric fat [8, 10]. It may metastasize by the blood stream.

Treatment. Wide surgical excision is necessary. The tumour is relatively radiosensitive, but radiotherapy alone gives disappointing results [8].

Alveolar soft-part sarcoma (malignant non-chromaffin paraganglioma)

Definition. A malignant tumour of muscles or fascial planes which occurs mainly in young adults and which has characteristic histological features.

Pathology [2]. The tumour is composed of cells arranged in a pseudo-alveolar pattern, with numerous vascular channels and delicate septa in close relationship. There are no reticulin fibres between the cells, and groups of them may bud into the vascular channels. The cells are large, oval or polyhedral, with a distinct boundary and finely granular cytoplasm. The histological pattern overlaps ganglioneuroma, phaeochromocytoma and other tumours of structures of neural crest origin, suggesting that the tumour arises from undifferentiated neural cells [4]. It must be differentiated from metastatic adenocarcinoma or malignant granular cell myoblastoma.

Clinical features. The majority of patients are between 15 and 25 yr old. The tumour is usually situated deep to the skin on the arm or leg. It is well circumscribed and is usually symptomless. The size varies from 4 to 23 cm in diameter. There is a considerable risk of local recurrence after conservative excision, and metastases to lungs, brain and elsewhere can follow.

Treatment. Wide excision is required.

Embryomal rhabdomyosarcoma.

In the last 10 yr several large series of tumours with this designation have been described [5, 6]. The great majority of patients are children, of either sex, and most tumours occur on the head and neck, though the site may be in the soft parts of the limbs and retroperitoneum. The tumours on the head arise principally in the orbit, nasopharynx or nose. The first symptom may be a painless swelling, blockage of the nose or nasal bleeding, or proptosis and swelling of the eyelids. Metastasis is common, first to the regional lymph nodes and later to lungs, bone, etc. Extensive local spread is common.

The majority of tumours in recent series have not shown evidence of cross-striation, which is proof of the histogenesis. The distinctive features, on which the diagnosis has been made, are a small-cell sarcoma with acidophilic granular cytoplasm, a tendency to alveolar arrangement, within a fine reticulin network, and a fibrous or myxoid stroma.

The prognosis is poor. The majority of tumours recur after excision, and neither radiotherapy nor chemotherapy has proved effective although the tumour is radiosensitive [6].

REFERENCES

1 ADAIR F. E., *et al* (1932) *Am J Cancer* **16**, 1104.
2 CHRISTOPHERSON W. M., *et al* (1952) *Cancer* **5**, 100.
3 ENTERLINE H. T., *et al* (1960) *Cancer* **13**, 932.
4 KARNAUCHOW P. N. & MAGNER D. (1963) *J Pathol Bacteriol* **86**, 169.
5 LAWRENCE W. JR., *et al* (1964) *Cancer* **17**, 361.
6 MASSON J. K. & SOULE E. H. (1965) *Am J Surg* **100**, 585.
7 MORTON D. L., *et al* (1969) *Surgery* **66**, 152.
8 PACK G. T. & PIERSON J. C. (1954) *Surgery* **36**, 687.
9 RESZEL P. A., *et al* (1966) *J Bone Joint Surg Am* **48**, 229.
10 SIEGMUND H. (1934) *Virchows Arch Pathol Anat Physiol* **293**, 458.
11 STERNBERG S. S. (1952) *Cancer* **5**, 975.

TUMOURS OF VESSELS

The systematic classification of tumours of vessels is unsatisfactory for several reasons. It is difficult to draw exact lines separating vascular malformations and reactive hyperplasias from neoplasms. With undoubted neoplasms, the traditional system of finding a benign and malignant tumour for each cell type, which works quite well with epithelial tumours for instance, is difficult to apply because vasoformative cells are labile, pluripotent and hard to categorize. Microscopic morphology is insufficiently precise to cope with their variability, and electron microscopic and histochemical features are helping to clarify the situation. It has, for instance, been shown that the cells of the glomus tumour have the fine structure of transected smooth-muscle cells [22, 25]. The attempt to fill every cell of a 'periodic table' of tumours creates false problems with vascular tumours, and the method of fitting a number of tumours, or even different phases of a single tumour [6, 11, 27], into a spectrum of change gives a much more intelligible picture of the malignant group. These more recent studies have thrown some doubt on the validity of the histogenetic attributions and, possibly, even of the individuality of some named tumours. In this section the various tumours will be described under their currently accepted titles.

Certain vascular lesions are undoubted malformations or are due to abnormalities of the endothelial cells or supporting structures. The 'port-wine' type of naevus, lymphangioma circumscriptum, angiokeratoma corporis diffusum and angioma serpiginosum, are examples. Others, such as spider naevi and granuloma gravidarum of the oral cavity, appear to be under hormonal influence. The various types of capillary aneurysm and venous lake are the result of weakening of the perithelial supporting structures. None of these conditions needs be considered here as they are not, in any sense, neoplastic. There are, however, problems concerning granuloma telangiectaticum and capillary-cavernous ('strawberry') naevus which must be discussed.

The two common types of vascular naevus are so different that it is unfortunate that they are usually considered together. The 'strawberry naevus' is initially a haemangioma, a benign neoplasm of vasoformative tissue, which usually begins so soon after birth that the circulatory changes consequent upon leaving the uterus seem likely to act, in some way, as a stimulus. In the early stages of its evolution there are masses of immature vasoformative cells occupying the dermis with more or less evidence of maturation of capillary channels through them, the maturation tending to occur first in the papillary dermis. Examination of specimens removed at different stages shows increasing maturation to capillary or cavernous channels with the passage of time, and a reciprocal decrease in the proportion of immature cells. Formed channels become filled with thrombus from time to time and, although partial recanalization occurs, the end result is intravascular fibrosis and obliteration of the haemangioma. The unusual features of this benign tumour are not the ability of the cells to mature, but their incapacity to sustain the pool of immature cells and, more particularly, the tendency for the mature structures to be eliminated by the extrinsic clotting mechanism.

Granuloma telangiectaticum resembles the strawberry naevus in being composed of masses of vasoformative tissue in its earlier stages, but differs in the oedematous mucin-rich nature of the stroma and the presence of inflammatory cells, suggesting a reactive rather than neoplastic origin. This concept would be more persuasive if the stimulus to the vascular reaction were to be found.

In this section the following tumours are described.

Granuloma telengiectaticum
Glomus tumour
Multiple progressive angioma
Haemangiopericytoma
Kaposi's sarcoma

Lymphangiosarcoma of Stewart and Treves
Malignant angio-endothelioma
Diffuse malignant proliferation of vascular endothelium

Granuloma telangiectaticum (Syn. pyogenic granuloma, botriomycome) [14].
Definition. A vascular nodule which develops rapidly, often at the site of a recent injury, and is composed of proliferating capillaries in a loose stroma.

Incidence and aetiology. It is a common lesion affecting both sexes and occurring at any age. It is seen quite often in children and young adults, but is unusual in the elderly [11]. In a minority of cases a minor injury, usually of a penetrating kind, has occurred a few weeks before the nodule appears. In other cases the patient can remember no injury, but his occupation and the situation of the lesion make minor trauma a likely happening. There is no evidence that micro-organisms initiate the vascular proliferation.

The balance of evidence favours a reactive rather than neoplastic basis, although some workers incline to the latter view [9]. Comparison of the condition with Kaposi's sarcoma suggested that both are responses to a similar stimulus modified by genetic or hormonal factors [11]. It differs in its behaviour from the vascular naevi of infancy, the vascular malformations of adult life, and benign and malignant angiomas. Its histological appearance, despite statements to the contrary, is characteristic in the majority of cases and unlike other vascular tumours.

Three conditions with a similar histology have been separately described: urethral caruncle, granuloma gravidarum of the oral cavity and juvenile angiofibroma, which is a nasopharyngeal tumour of young men.

Pathology. There is considerable proliferation of small blood vessels which erupt through a breach in the epidermis to produce a globular pedunculated tumour. The epidermis forms a collarette at the base of the lesion and covers part, or all, of the tumour in a thin layer. The proliferating vessels are set in a gelatinous stroma, lacking in collagen in the earlier stages and relatively rich in mucin. The endothelial cells are plump, as in new granulation tissue, lining the vessels in a single layer, and surrounded by a mixed cell population of fibroblasts, mast cells, plasma cells and, where the surface is eroded, polymorphonuclear leucocytes. The older lesions tend to organize and partly fibrose, and at this stage distinction from an angioma may be difficult. In rare

instances, sometimes following injudicious treatment, satellite lesions which have a similar pathology to the primary lesion may develop around a granuloma telangiectaticum and respond to simple destructive measures, thus indicating that they are not malignant metastases [26].

Clinical features. The tumour is vascular, of bright red to brownish-red or blue-black colour. It is partially compressible, but cannot be completely blanched and does not show pulsation. The surface of the earlier and bright red lesion is usually thin intact epidermis. The older and darker ones are frequently eroded and crusted, and may bleed very easily. Occasionally, the surface is raspberry like or even verrucous. The size commonly varies between 5 and 10 mm, but at times it may reach 50 mm. The outline is rounded. The base is often pedunculated and surrounded by a collar of acanthotic epidermis; the lesion may be sessile. The common sites are the hands (especially on the fingers), the feet, lips, head and upper trunk, and the mucosal surfaces of the mouth and perianal area. The initial evolution is rapid and after a few weeks the growth ceases. Spontaneous disappearance rarely occurs. There is no pain, and the patients mainly complain of the appearance or of recurrent bleeding.

Diagnosis. In most cases the history and clinical appearance leave little doubt about the diagnosis, and microscopic confirmation is easily obtained. In 38% of one series of cases the clinical diagnosis of granuloma telangiectaticum proved to be wrong [18]. The errors included kerato-acanthoma and other epithelial neoplasms, inflamed seborrhoeic keratoses, melanocytic naevi, juvenile and malignant melanoma, virus warts, molluscum contagiosum, angioma, glomus tumour and a variety of inflammatory conditions [13, 18]. To this list must be added eccrine poroma, Kaposi's sarcoma and metastatic carcinoma as conditions easily mistaken for granuloma telangectaticum.

Treatment. The pedunculated lesions are easy to treat by curettage and cauterization or diathermy coagulation of the base. A considerable proportion of granulomas recur after such treatment because the proliferating vessels in the base extend in a conical manner into the deeper dermis. In some areas, for instance in the nail fold or on the palmar aspect of a finger, it may be reasonable to carry out curettage and hope for the best. Wherever possible it is desirable to excise a narrow, but deep, ellipse of skin beneath the lesion and close the wound with sutures. Radiotherapy may be effective in a dose of

500 rad repeated in a week if necessary, but is rarely used in most countries.

Glomus tumour [25] (Syn. glomangioma)
Definition. A tumour of the neuromyo-arterial glomus composed of vascular channels surrounded by proliferating glomus cells and by nerve fibres.

Incidence and aetiology. Glomus tumours are comparatively uncommon. Some are present at birth; they rarely appear during infancy, but from the age of 7 onwards the incidence increases gradually [16]. Multiple tumours are, relatively, 10 times more frequent in children than in adults [10, 20]. The occurrence of familial cases with an autosomal dominant type of inheritance [5, 19, 24] and the association of multiple tumours with malformation of the same limb [16] suggest that a genetic factor may be involved. A history of trauma preceding the tumour may be given [23].

Pathology. The tumour may vary in size from a few millimetres to several centimetres in diameter. It is round, encapsulated and situated in the dermis. The proportion of glomus cells to vascular spaces varies. The smaller painful lesions tend to be mainly cellular. The larger, multiple and often painless ones are angiomatous, with only a band of cells around the dilated vascular channels. The glomus cell is cuboidal with a well-marked cell membrane and a round central nucleus. The cells align themselves in rows around the single layer of endothelial cells of the vascular spaces and in a somewhat less orderly fashion further out. Numerous non-myelinated nerve fibres course through the cellular masses. Electron microscopy [15, 22, 25] suggests that glomus cells are transversely cut smooth-muscle cells and there are many mast cells around the tumour, but that nerve fibres are not associated with the glomus cells. It is possible that glomus tumours are related to the arterial side, and that haemangiopericytoma comes from the capillary or venous side of the peripheral vessels [22].

Clinical features. The solitary tumour is a pink or purple nodule varying in size from 1 to 20 mm; it is conspicuously painful [8]. Pain may be provoked by direct pressure, by change in skin temperature or may be spontaneous. The common sites are the extremities, and those tumours beneath the nail are particularly painful and are brought for treatment whilst still very small. The affected nail has a bluish-red flush. They have also been reported on the head, neck and penis. The multiple tumours are larger and usually dark blue in colour, and are situated deep in the dermis. They are less restricted to the extremities, may be widely scattered and are not usually painful [20]. In some cases grouped multiple tumours may be painful, and pain, intermittent discoloration and sweating of a limb may precede the development of a palpable tumour. Malignant change does not occur [10], but there are reports of multiple glomus tumours associated with other malignancies.

Diagnosis. The solitary tumour is to be distinguished from other painful tumours such as leiomyoma, eccrine spiradenoma and neuromatoid hyperplasia. The multiple glomangioma may be indistinguishable clinically from a cavernous haemangioma, and is possibly identical with 'blue rubber bleb' naevus [19].

Treatment. Surgical excision cures, but local recurrence may occur if the whole tumour is not removed.

Multiple progressive angioma [1, 3, 4]. This condition, first described by Darier, has received relatively little attention. The tumours arise in the subcutaneous tissue on the face or extremities of children or adolescents. They are bluish compressible nodules, sometimes disposed along the course of a vein, and are of different sizes and different ages. The histological picture is that of a cavernous angioma. They may disappear after months or years. Local destructive measures may speed the resolution [1]. The condition is probably a malformation rather than a neoplasm.

Haemangiopericytoma
Definition. A tumour with malignant potentialities composed of vascular channels and proliferating pericyte-like spindle cells.

Incidence. It is a very uncommon tumour. This may be because some pathologists regard it as a highly vascular fibrosarcoma. It has been reported at all ages, and a series of 31 tumours in children has been described [7]. In some of these cases it had been present at birth. The sexes are equally affected. The usual situation is in the subcutaneous or intramuscular tissues, and on the lower trunk, head and neck or thigh [5].

Pathology [12]. There are branching capillaries, with normal endothelium but often containing few red blood cells, surrounded by masses of round or spindle cells which are embedded in a network of reticulin. The cells may exhibit pleomorphism and mitotic activity. A proportion, varyingly reported as 11·7% [21] or 56·5% [17], metastasize to the lung and elsewhere.

Clinical features. The tumour is a firm, often circumscribed and nodular, mass varying in size up to 8 cm in diameter with normal skin over it [2]. In most cases it is flesh-coloured and is not painful. The growth rate may be slow or quite fast. It is unlikely to be diagnosed clinically.

Treatment. As many of the tumours have eventually proved to be malignant, complete surgical removal is desirable. Radiotherapy is ineffective [17].

REFERENCES

1 AUKEN G. (1951) *Acta Derm Venereol (Stockh)* **31**, 304.
2 BIANCHI O., *et al* (1968) *Ann Dermatol Syphiligr* **95**, 269.
3 BRAUN-FALCO O. (1953) *Dermatol Wochenschr* **127**, 321.
4 CHEVRANT-BRETON J., *et al* (1984) *Dermatologica* **168**, 290.
5 ENZINGER F. M. & SMITH B. H. (1976) *Hum Pathol* **7**, 61.
6 GORLIN R. J., *et al* (1966) *Arch Dermatol* **82**, 776.
7 JONES E. W. (1964) *Br J Dermatol* **76**, 21.
8 KAUFFMAN S. L. & STOUT A. P. (1960) *Cancer* **13**, 695.
9 KNOTH W. & EHLERS G. (1962) *Arch Klin Exp Dermatol* **214**, 394.
10 KOHAUT E. & STOUT A. P. (1961) *Cancer* **14**, 555.
11 LEE F. D. (1968) *J Clin Pathol* **21**, 119.
12 LIDHOLM S. O. (1956) *Acta Pathol Microbiol Scand* **38**, 186.
13 MARTENS V. E. & MACPHERSON D. J. (1956) *AMA Arch Pathol* **61**, 120.
14 McGEOCH A. H. (1961) *Aust J Dermatol* **6**, 33.
15 MURAD T., *et al* (1968) *Cancer* **22**, 1239.
16 OBERDALHOFF H. & SCHÜTZ W. (1951) *Chirurg* **22**, 145.
17 O'BRIEN P. & BRASFIELD R. D. (1965) *Cancer* **18**, 249.
18 ROWE L. (1958) *AMA Arch Dermatol* **78**, 341.
19 DE SABLET M. & MASCARO J. M. (1967) *Ann Dermatol Syphiligr* **94**, 35.
20 SLUITER J. T. F. & POSTMA C. (1959) *Acta Derm Venereol (Stockh)* **39**, 98.
21 STOUT A. P. (1949) *Cancer* **2**, 1027.
22 TARNOWSKI W. M. & HASHIMOTO K. (1969) *J Invest Dermatol* **52**, 474.
23 TORCHI M. (1960) *Atti Soc Med Bolzano* **4**, 545.
24 TOURAINE A., *et al* (1936) *Bull Soc Fr Dermatol Syphiligr* **43**, 736.
25 VENKATACHALUM M. A. & GREALLY J. G. (1969) *Cancer* **23**, 1176.
26 WARNER J. & WILSON JONES E. (1968) *Br J Dermatol* **80**, 218.
27 WEIDNER F. & BRAUN-FALCO O. (1970) *Hautarzt* **21**, 60.

Classical Kaposi's sarcoma (syn. idiopathic haemorrhagic sarcoma)

Definition. A tumour composed of proliferating capillary vessels and perivascular connective-tissue cells which is multifocal and may metastasize.

Incidence and aetiology [9, 34]. This was originally considered a rare disease, largely restricted to Central and Eastern European Jews. It is now known to occur in Italy, Sweden and, with much greater frequency than anywhere else, in certain parts of Africa [37, 39]. The African cases have a geographical distribution, the disorder being most prevalent in eastern Zaire, becoming rare where forest gives way to savanna to the north and occurring with rather less frequency in the countries to the east, west and south. In Uganda all the African tribal groups are affected but no cases have been seen in Indian or European inhabitants [55]. It affects Negro children as well as adults. In Europeans it is a disease of later adult life. It is more than 10 times as common in males as females. There are two families recorded with a high incidence of the disease.

The cause of the tumour, its true nature and its proper classification have been discussed many times without any definite conclusions being reached [4, 12, 53]. It has been attributed to an infectious agent (possibly tick borne), and considered to be a genetically determined disorder analogous to von Recklinghausen's disease, a hamartoma, a benign neoplasm of vascular endothelium or perithelial cells, or a malignant tumour (fibrosarcoma or angiosarcoma). It is probably best regarded as a malignant tumour of a primitive mesenchymal cell whose incidence is partly influenced by genetic factors and by some environmental circumstance (possibly a virus), and perhaps by lymphatic stasis and sex hormones.

Pathology [37, 53, 54]. The process begins in the mid-dermis and extends upwards to raise the epidermis, which may be thinned, or acanthotic and verrucose. Interweaving bands of spindle cells embedded in a network of reticulin, eventually replacing the collagen, and a maze of vascular spaces are invariable features of the tumour. The vascular component is formed partly by delicate capillaries and partly by cleft-like spaces between the spindle cells. Extravasated erythrocytes may be seen. Around the cellular masses there are haemosiderin-laden macrophages and an inflammatory reaction, which is lymphocytic and most vigorous in earlier lesions. The process often extends along veins. The blood vessels around the tumour may show proliferative endarteritis. Foci of necrosis occur in some of the masses. Similar changes are found in lymph glands and viscera in cases that metastasize. The spindle cells do not have the histochemical characteristics of blood vessel endothelium or of neurilemma [35], and electron microscope studies suggest that they are derived from perithelial fibroblasts [21].

Clinical features [4, 32, 44, 54]. The lesions have a dark blue or purplish colour. Initially, they may be almost macular, and when they become tumid pressure may produce partial blanching to reveal a brown tinge. The process usually begins on the extremities, most commonly on the feet and occasionally on the hands, ears or nose. Individual tumours enlarge to a diameter of 10–30 mm and stop growing. The process is multifocal and adjacent areas may fuse to form a plaque or tumour. Oedema of the limb may follow, or at times precede [4, 39], the appearance of the tumour. There are few subjective symptoms; pain may be felt in nodules on pressure areas. The lesions may involute to leave pigmented scars, or become eroded, ulcerated or fungating. New lesions may appear along the course of superficial veins, and in time most patients have both limbs involved more or less symmetrically. The rate of spread is remarkably variable. It tends to be slow in Europeans and more rapid in Africans, where oedema is often the first sign. Lymph nodes, mucosal surfaces and internal organs, particularly the small intestine [54], may all be involved as the disease progresses. Kaposi's sarcoma may at times start in other organs and run its course without skin manifestation. Three cases with fever, weight loss, lymphadenopathy, hepatosplenomagaly, anaemia and hypergammaglobulinaemia have been reported [45] in the U.S.A. Visceral involvement is the common pattern in African children, with lymph nodes as the main tissue involved. An association with lymphomas [4] and other malignancy [36] has been reported.

Diagnosis. The early lesion is most likely to be confused with a telangiectatic granuloma [10, 43]. It must also be distinguished from histiocytoma or from other types of sarcoma. Its evolution from a macular lesion and its characteristic colour, slow development and multifocal distribution make the diagnosis likely in most instances. Cases where the tumour is preceded by oedema may cause difficulty, as lymphangiosarcoma may arise in chronic lymphoedema. In prolonged venous hypertension of the lower legs, nodules with a close resemblance to Kaposi's sarcoma may develop [31]; they differ, however, in lack of progression, and

spindle cell proliferation is not seen in the histological sections.

Treatment. Where a small area is involved, excision or radiotherapy can be used. Superficial radiotherapy is rapid and effective, and is the treatment of choice for the majority of patients with nodular disease of the extremities. Extensive disease can be treated by cytotoxic drugs such as chlorambucil [11], cyclophosphamide, vinblastine [47] or actinomycin [26].

Kaposi's sarcoma and the acquired immunodeficiency syndrome (AIDS) [14, 15, 20]. In the past 4 yr there has been a sudden and dramatic increase in the number of cases of Kaposi's sarcoma occurring in young patients with the acquired immunodeficiency syndrome (AIDS). The first patients described with this condition were all young homosexual males and were mainly from the areas of New York and San Francisco [18]. Since this time geographical pockets of the disease have been found in the Caribbean [25, 58] and also in Africa [1, 8, 28]. The form of Kaposi's sarcoma affecting these patients appears to be particularly virulent, with five of the first nine patients reported dying of their disease within 2 yr of diagnosis. Since this time the number of cases reported has risen dramatically [6]. In the U.S.A. the numbers appear to double over a 6 month period. The death rate continues to be high at around 70%, and although a high proportion (around two-thirds) of the patients are homosexual, the majority of the remainder are drug abusers. A small number of homosexuals (haemophiliacs and others who have received multiple blood transfusions) have also developed the syndrome. Around 50% of AIDS patients develop Kaposi's sarcoma and the remaining 50% have evidence of severe immunodeficiency. Both groups are at risk for other opportunistic infections such as *Pneumocystis carinii* pneumonia.

There is very good evidence to suggest that there is an aetiological association between AIDS and a virus isolated almost simultaneously by French and American workers. The French group, headed by Montagnier, term the virus lymphadenopathy-associated virus (LAV) [59], and the American group, headed by Gallo, use the term human T-cell lymphoma/leukaemia virus III (HTLV-III) [16]. There is a very low prevalence of HTLV-I or HTLV-II in patients with AIDS-related problems [42, 52].

Clinical features. Patients presenting with Kaposi's sarcoma associated with severe immunodepression have subtle lesions which may well be missed by the unwary [14]. They may have only one or two lesions scattered over the body and these may resemble slight areas of trauma or a simple bruise. The lesions are therefore quite dissimilar from the classic florid lesions developing on the lower limbs of the older patients from central Europe.

Pathology. At the present time the pathological features of this condition are poorly described. The important early feature appears to be a slit-like development of angioproliferation with little or no lymphocytic infiltrate such as is associated with the original type of Kaposi's sarcoma.

Therapy. At the time of writing there appears to be no effective therapy for this condition. Cytotoxic chemotherapy, interferon and interleukin-2 have all been tried with very limited success. The prognosis for these patients is very poor, with 70% mortality within 2 yr of diagnosis.

Lymphangiosarcoma of Stewart and Treves [13, 21, 23, 29, 49]

Definition. A malignant tumour of vascular endothelium arising in an area of chronic lymphoedema, usually in an arm following radical mastectomy.

Incidence and aetiology. The tumour occurred in 0·45% of patients who survived mastectomy for more than 5 yr [45]. The mean age at appearance of the lymphangiosarcoma is 62, and the mean interval between mastectomy and the appearance of the tumour is 10·5 yr [22]. Two cases have been reported in men following mastectomy [38]. Not all patients have received radiotherapy in association with the mastectomy, and not all have had axillary nodes removed. Lymphoedema is not invariably present, or may be late in appearing and antedate the tumour by only a short time. The incidence and cause of postmastectomy lymphoedema have been reviewed [56]. In the majority of cases the clinical course and autopsy findings have shown that the treatment of the breast carcinoma was successful and the patients have had less frequent involvement of the axillary nodes than usual [38]. A small number of cases have arisen in lymphoedema of the lower limb, or in the upper limb without breast cancer and mastectomy [46]; most of these patients were women.

Multiple primary malignancies have occurred in 8% of cases [13] and a systemically acting carcinogen has been suggested [22, 49]. There is no factual evidence to support this.

Pathology [51]. In the early stages, or at the edge of a lesion, there are proliferating, and sometimes dilated, vascular spaces lined by hyperplastic endothelium. They are surrounded by a focal infiltration of lymphocytes, and there may be extravasation of red blood cells into the dermis. These changes may be continuous with frankly malignant tissue. Bizarre vascular channels are lined by one or more layers of typical endothelial cells. The channels are well outlined by reticulin and contain exfoliated endothelial cells and lymphocytes, but few erythrocytes. Pleomorphic or anaplastic cells may form in sheets around the channels. Haemosiderin-laden macrophages can often be found at the periphery.

Clinical features [48]. The first sign may be an area of bruising in the lymphoedema, thought to be traumatic by the patient. Dusky blue or red nodules develop and grow rapidly, and fresh discrete nodules appear nearby. In some cases blisters are a prominent feature [13]. The arm is the usual site first affected, suggesting that irradiation promotes the neoplasm indirectly through lymphoedema, if at all. As the tumours proliferate, the oedema may increase and the older lesions ulcerate. Dissemination occurs early, with the first visceral deposits usually being in the lung and pleural cavity.

Diagnosis. Although similar in many ways to Kaposi's sarcoma, the sex ratio is reversed in favour of females, lymphoedema has been present for a number of years and most cases occur after mastectomy. Microscopically, the proliferative change is in, rather than around, the endothelial cells. Malignant melanoma, pyogenic granuloma and metastatic carcinoma may have to be excluded at the early stages. The tumour does not arise in the lymphoedema of filariasis [46].

Treatment. Single cases have been reported to have survived for long periods after external radiotherapy and intra-arterial ⁹⁰Y in ceramic microspheres. In the early stages radical amputation of the limb may offer hope of cure. In later cases the prognosis is hopeless.

Malignant angio-endothelioma (syn. angiosarcoma, angioplastic reticulosarcoma [60, 64])

Definition. A malignant tumour [27] of vasoformative cells, arising from either lymphatic [7] or blood vessels. Some reported tumours classified in this group are probably cases of highly vascular anaplastic carcinomas and sarcomas [62].

Incidence. This is a rare tumour in any form. One variety affects mainly the elderly of either sex, occurring on the scalp or face [17, 37]. Another type is seen in children, affecting soft tissues or the paranasal region. The majority of these cases are lethal, but there exist other examples of more questionable malignancy.

Pathology [60, 63]. In the well-differentiated tumour, vascular channels infiltrate the normal structures in a disorganized fashion as if trying to line every available tissue space by a layer of endothelial cells. The cells may be plumper than normal, double-layered in places, and form solid intravascular buds. The pattern of growth is more suggestive of lymphatic than blood vessels, but both probably take part. Less well-differentiated tumours show atypical endothelial cells which may be heaped into several layers or become syncytial. Advancing malignancy may be associated with loss of vascular pattern and proliferation of cell masses embedded in a reticulin network, justifying the title angioplastic reticulosarcoma. It is possible that cases of haemangiopericytoma come within the spectrum of these tumours [60].

Clinical features [17, 60, 63]. In the skin, malignant angio-endothelioma is invariably a livid or dusky red colour, even when there are blebs exuding fluid with the characteristic protein profile of lymph [30, 60]. The least malignant are hyperaemic macules which slowly spread and can only be recognized histologically. A more malignant variety, seen on the scalp [3] or face of elderly patients, has a more oedematous, erysipeloid or frankly tumid appearance. The margin is usually irregular and less raised; nodules and tumours may be multiple.

The malignant angiosarcoma of children is said to occur more frequently in those of Jewish or Italian stock, with equal sex incidence [64]. It is predominantly a tumour of soft tissues with a capacity to invade muscle, fat and veins. The extremities are affected chiefly, but examples also occur in the paranasal region. Several cases have arisen in vascular naevi some years after treatment [17]. There is a high risk of dissemination, and death is almost inevitable. A papillary endovascular angio-endothelioma with a bizarre microscopic picture but a good prognosis after adequate excision has been described [9].

Treatment. In the less malignant types wide excision and grafting has controlled some cases. The response to radiotherapy is disappointing.

Diffuse malignant proliferation of vascular endothelium [5] (syn. angio-endotheliomatosis proliferans systemisata [33, 50]). A small number of cases of this disorder are on record. The histological features of all are similar. The capillaries of the dermis and subcutis are dilated, increased in number and stuffed with cells that in some instances obstruct the lumen. The proliferating cells appear to come from the endothelium and may be arranged in a reticular fashion, forming nests within the lumina and dilating the vessels to a coil-like shape. Many of the cells show mitoses, some of which are abnormal. In one patient who died the same intravascular proliferation was observed in the heart, uveal tract, brain, thyroid and bone, and extravascular atypical mononuclear cells were found in these organs and elsewhere. The cell is regarded as a malignant endothelial cell [5].

The skin manifestations are brownish-red to purplish plaques or nodules up to 5 cm or more in diameter on the trunk and limbs. They may be tender and are mainly subcutaneous, being firm to the touch and tethered to the tissue beneath. Annular lesions [50] and poikiloderma-like changes [5] have been seen. General malaise and weakness may occur, and neurological signs may result from involvement of cerebral vessels. The cases have almost all been rapidly fatal.

The exact nature of this disease, and its range of clinical and pathological variations, must remain uncertain until a larger number of cases are reported.

Angiolymphoid hyperplasia with eosinophils (syn. Kimura's disease)
Definition. An apparently benign locally proliferating lesion composed of vascular channels with a surrounding infiltrate of lymphocytes and eosinophils. A recent paper [25] has suggested that Kimura's disease is distinct from angiolymphoid hyperplasia with eosinophils, but in general the conditions are considered synonymous.

Incidence and aetiology. These lesions have now been reported from many parts of the world but appear very much more common in Japan than in other countries. The cause is unknown, but antigenic stimulation following insect bites has been postulated.

Clinical features [2, 19, 40, 57, 65]. Affected individuals are commonly young adults who present with a cluster of small translucent nodules around the ear or the hairline. These rarely exceed 2–3 cm in diameter, but occasionally deeper extensions and larger subcutaneous nodules are associated. Spontaneous regression is seen in the majority of cases after a variable period of time. Peripheral blood eosinophilia may be present.

Pathology [24, 61]. A poorly organized lesion is seen. Clusters of proliferating capillaries are lined with plump swollen endothelial cells, and a cellular infiltrate composed mainly of lymphocytes and of large numbers of eosinophils is seen around these vessels.

Treatment. The natural history of the lesion is such that if a confident diagnosis is made on a small lesion, it is reasonable to observe the lesion for 3–6 months and await spontaneous regression. Both surgery and radiotherapy have been employed and both appear to be satisfactory.

REFERENCES

1 Arnoux E., *et al* (1983) *Lancet* ii, 110.
2 Baker G. R. (1981) *J Dermatol Surg Oncol* 7, 229.
3 Bardwil J. M., *et al* (1968) *Am J Surg* 116, 548.
4 *Bluefarb S. M. (1957) *Kaposi's Sarcoma. Multiple Idiopathic Haemorrhagic Sarcoma.* Springfield, Thomas.
5 Braverman I. M. & Lerner A. B. (1961) *Arch Dermatol* 84, 22.
6 Centre for Disease Control (1983) AIDS Update 1983. MMWR 32, 309.
7 Chen K. T. K. & Gilbert E. F. (1979) *Arch Pathol* 103, 80.
8 Clumack N., *et al* (1983) *Lancet* i, 642.
9 Dabska (1969) *Cancer* 24, 503.
10 Degos R., *et al* (1964) *Ann Dermatol Syphiligr* 91, 113.
11 Degos R., *et al* (1967) *Dermatologica* 135, 345.
12 *Dupont A. (1951) *L'Angio-reticulomatose Cutanée.* Thesis, University of Louvain.
13 *Eby C. S., *et al.* (1967) *Arch Surg* 94, 223.
14 *Friedmann-Kien A. E., *et al.* (1982) *Ann Int Med* 96, 693.
15 Friedmann-Kien A. E., *et al* (1983) *Int Conf on Cutaneous Oncology, The Hague, September* 15, 1983.
16 Gallo R., *et al* (1984) *Science* 224, 500.
17 Girard C., *et al* (1970) *Cancer* 26, 868.
18 Gottlieb G. J., *et al* (1981) *Am J Dermatopathol* 3, 111.
19 Grimwood R., *et al* (1979) *Arch Dermatol* 115, 205.
20 Groopman J. E. (1984) *Nature* 308, 769.
21 Hashimoto K. & Lever W. F. (1964) *J Invest Dermatol* 43, 539.
22 *Herrman J. B. (1965) *Surg Gynecol Obstet* 121, 1107.
23 Hori Y. (1981) *J Dermatol Surg Oncol* 7, 130.
24 Inada S., *et al* (1977) *J Dermatol (Tokyo)* 4, 207.
25 Kung I. T. M., *et al* (1984) *Pathology* 16, 39.
26 Kyalwazi S. K., *et al* (1971) *E Afr Med J* 48, 16.
27 Lambert D., *et al* (1977) *Ann Dermatol Vénéréol* 104, 549.
28 Liataud B., *et al* (1983) *Ann Dermatol Vénéréol* 110, 213.
29 Mackenzie D. H. (1971) *J Clin Pathol* 24, 524.
30 Maddox J. C. & Evans H. H. (1981) *Cancer* 48, 1907.
31 Mali J. W. H., *et al* (1966) *Ned Tijdschr Geneeskd* 110, 749.
32 Martinotti L. (1938) *Arch Ital Dermatol Sifilogr Venereol* 14, 367.
33 Midana A. & Ormea F. (1965) *Ann Dermatol Syphiligr* 92, 229.
34 Murray J. F. & Lothe F. (1962) *Union Int contra Cancrum*, 18, 413.
35 Niemi M. & Mustakallio K. K. (1965) *Acta Pathol Microbiol Scand* 63, 567.
36 O'Brien P. H. & Brasfield R. D. (1966) *Cancer* 19, 1497.
37 Oettle A. G. (1962) *Union Int contra Cancrum* 18, 330.
38 Oettle A. G. & Van Blerk P. J. P. (1963) *Br J Surg* 50, 736.
39 Olowasanmi J. O., *et al* (1969) *Br J Cancer* 23, 714.
40 Reed R. J. & Terazekis N. (1972) *Cancer* 29, 489.
41 *Reynolds W. A., *et al* (1965) *Medicine (Baltimore)* 44, 419.
42 Robert-Guroff M., *et al* (1984) *Lancet* ii, 128.
43 Ronchese D. & Kern A. B. (1957) *AMA Arch Dermatol* 75, 418.
44 Rothman S. (1962) *Union Int Contra Cancrum* 18, 364.
45 Rywlin A. M., *et al* (1966) *AMA Arch Dermatol* 93, 554.
46 *Scott R. B., *et al* (1960) *Am J Med* 28, 1008.
47 Scott W. P. & Voight J. A. (1966) *Cancer* 19, 557.
48 Shirger A. (1962) *Med Clin North Am* 46, 1045.
49 Stewart F. W. & Treves N. (1948) *Cancer* 1, 64.
50 Tappeiner J. & Pfleger L. (1963) *Hautarzt* 14, 67.
51 Taylor J. F., *et al* (1971) *Int J Cancer* 8, 112.
52 Tedder R. S., *et al* (1984) *Lancet* ii, 125.
53 *Tedeschi C. G. (1958) *AMA Arch Pathol* 66, 656.
54 Templeton A. C. (1976) In *Cancer of the Skin.* Ed. Andrade R., *et al.* Philadelphia, Saunders, p. 1183.
55 Templeton A. C. & Viegas O. A. C. (1970) *Trop Geogr Med* 22, 431.
56 Treves N. (1957) *Cancer* 10, 444.
57 Vazquez-botet M. B. & Sanchez J. L. (1978) *J Dermatol Surg Oncol* 4, 931.
58 Viera J., *et al* (1983) *N Engl J Med* 308, 125.
59 Vilmer E., *et al* (1984) *Lancet* i, 753.
60 Weidner F. & Braun-Falco O. (1970) *Hautarzt* 21, 60.
61 Wells G. C. & Whimster I. W. (1969) *Br J Dermatol* 81, 1.
62 Willis R. A. (1960) *Pathology of Tumours.* London, Butterworths.
63 Wilson Jones E. (1964) *Br J Dermatol* 76, 21.
64 Wilson Jones E. (1976) *Clin Exp Dermatol* 1, 287.
65 Wilson Jones E. & Bleehen S. S. (1969) *Br J Dermatol* 81, 804.

TUMOURS OF NERVES AND NERVE SHEATHS

There are no true neuromas of the skin. The tumours that are usually given this title are composed of proliferating axons and sheaths, but do not contain nerve cells. The correct term for such lesions is neuromatoid hyperplasia, but in conformity with past usage they will be described under the title 'neuroma'.

Tumours of nerve sheath are composed of either neurilemmal or connective-tissue cells, and may occasionally become malignant.

Cutaneous meningioma and Merkel cell tumours are also included in this section.

Neuroma cutis
Neurofibromatosis (p. 119)
Neurofibroma
Neurilemmoma
Neurofibrosarcoma
Cutaneous meningioma
Merkel cell tumour

Neuroma

Definition. A tumour composed of nerve cells and elements of their sheaths.

Amputation-stump 'neuroma' is a response to injury, and not a tissue tumour. An accessory digit (p. 222) may, at times, be composed principally of neuroid arborization, but being a defect of development cannot be classed as a neuroma. We are left with a small number of cases of 'neuroma' reported some decades ago, which are of somewhat dubious authenticity as true tumours, with 'multiple ganglioneuroma of the skin', a single case in which the tumours underwent spontaneous involution [7], and with the unique case of Knauss [3] with multiple subcutaneous ganglioneuromas. The unequivocal demonstration of nerve cells within a tumour justifies the title of ganglioneuroma. The demonstration of only axons and neurofibromatous tissue suggests a neuromatoid hyperplasia [4]. It seems reasonable, therefore, to consider that neuroma does not exist as a neoplasm of the skin.

The spontaneous 'neuroma cutis' of the older writers is a condition which occurs more commonly in men than women, usually in adult life, and takes the form of areas of small painful nodules situated on the trunk or proximal parts of the limbs. The individual lesions are discrete and disseminated rounded nodules varying from 1 to 10 mm in diameter which are pink to purple or brown in colour. The skin over them may be dry and scaly. They are firm and fibrous and fixed in the dermis, distributed at random, and do not follow the course of a nerve trunk. The nodules are tender, usually from an early stage of evolution, and may be subject to periodic episodes of excruciating pain provoked by contact, change of temperature or emotion. The pain may radiate and its quality, together with the colour and texture of the skin, is reminiscent of causalgia. A similar, but apparently painless, condition on the face and conjunctiva has been reported [11].

The histological picture is similar to that of other neuromatoid hyperplasias. Numbers of myelinated and non-myelinated nerve fibres lie embedded in a mass of connective tissue in the dermis. It differs from amputation-stump 'neuroma', which is situated in the deeper tissues.

Neuroma cutis must be a very uncommon condition. The writer has heard of one case, but not seen it. The differential diagnosis from leiomyoma would be difficult clinically. The advice of a neurosurgeon might be necessary to help control the pain by nerve root or sympathetic block.

A condition which should arouse suspicion of associated malignancy is that of true neuroma of mucous membranes, commonly of oral mucosa or conjunctiva, which may be found preceding or in association with medullary carcinoma of thyroid or phaeochromocytoma (see below). The suggested explanation for this association is of a general disorder of neural crest development [5, 8].

A case of asymptomatic carcinoma of the thyroid has been found at prophylactic thyroidectomy following discovery of such oral mucosal neuromas [1].

Multiple mucosal neuromata, endocrine disturbance and medullary thyroid carcinoma (Sipple's syndrome) [4]. In this disorder multiple neuromata of the oral mucosa may be associated with phaeochromocytoma, parafollicular thyroid cysts secreting calcitonin, medullary thyroid carcinoma and opaque nerve fibres on the cornea. The condition is inherited as an autosomal dominant, and the patients may have a 'Marfanoid' habitus and thick lips which make them all look alike [1]. The mucosal lesions may be present in childhood and should be regarded as a warning of the more serious later complications.

Neurilemmoma (Schwannoma)
Definition. A tumour of nerve sheaths composed of cells resembling Schwann cells.

Incidence. The tumour is relatively uncommon. It arises most frequently from the acoustic nerve. In the peripheral nervous system it is usually found in association with one of the main nerves of the limbs, usually on the flexor aspect near the elbow, wrist or knee, the hands or the head and neck [10].

It may be seen on the tongue. Other sites include the wall of the gastrointestinal tract and the posterior mediastinum. It may occur at any age, but is most common in the fourth and fifth decades. Females are affected more often than males [2]. Neurilemmoma may be found in von Recklinghausen's disease, and is often multiple.

Pathology [9, 10]. The tumour is rounded, circumscribed and usually encapsulated. It is situated in the course of a nerve, usually in the subcutaneous fat. The cells are spindle shaped and are enclosed by a stringy meshwork of argyrophilic intercellular fibrils. They are arranged in bands which stream and interweave. The nuclei are elongated and plump, and characteristically arrange themselves side by side in ranks. This arrangement is not always well shown, and some tumours closely resemble leiomyomas. In other tumours there is mucous secretion, producing a vacuolated stroma; fibrils are scanty and the cells are more polymorphic. Electron microscopy shows evidence of association with Schwann cells [12]. There is no proliferation of nerve fibrils. Malignant change may occur rarely, usually in cases associated with von Recklinghausen's disease.

Clinical features [6]. The tumours are rounded or ovoid circumscribed nodules varying in size up to 5 cm, and firm (or, sometimes soft and cystic) in consistency. The colour is pink-grey or yellowish. Small lesions may be intradermal, but larger ones are subcutaneous in situation. The tumours may sometimes be painful. When multiple, a careful search should be made for evidence of von Recklinghausen's disease. They are usually slow growing.

Diagnosis. Of the various nodular dermal and hypodermal tumours it is most likely to be mistaken for a glomus tumour when painful, and for a lipoma, 'sebaceous' cyst, synovial ganglion, juxta-articular node or neurofibroma when not. The diagnosis can be suspected when it is in the course of a nerve; otherwise, histological examination is necessary.

Treatment. Surgical excision will cure the lesion, though recurrence may occur if this is incomplete. When the tumour is arising from the sheath of a large nerve care must be taken not to damage this. The malignant tumour is particularly likely to recur locally, but metastasis is rare.

Neurofibromatosis. This condition is dealt with in another section (p. 119). Solitary neurofibromas occur which resemble the lesions seen in von Recklinghausen's disease in their range of clinical and microscopic features and which may be a manifestation of occult neurofibromatosis. Neurofibromas may occasionally undergo malignant change, usually when the lesion is associated with one of the larger or more proximal nerves and only in manifest von Recklinghausen's disease.

Neurofibrosarcoma

Definition. A malignant tumour arising from the nerve sheath, usually in patients with neurofibromatosis.

Aetiology. Although the tumour usually arises in patients with multiple neurofibromatosis, this is not invariably the case. Whether the tumour begins in a benign neurofibroma is questionable [2].

Incidence. It is an uncommon tumour. It occurs in young adults, or even children, when it complicates multiple neurofibromatosis.

Pathology. The basic pattern is that of a fibrosarcoma, sometimes with myxosarcomatous areas, and sometimes pleomorphic and anaplastic. There is usually little trace of the characteristic fine wavy fibrils of the neurofibroma. The tumour disseminates.

Clinical features. The diagnosis should be suspected when a previously static tumour in a patient with neurofibromatosis begins to enlarge or becomes painful. The pain may become radicular as the lesion progresses. The commoner sites are the flexor aspects of the limbs. The tumours are not always associated with nerve trunks.

Treatment. Wide local excision or amputation is necessary because of the aggressive behaviour of the tumour, and even then the prognosis is not good. The tumour is not radiosensitive.

REFERENCES

1 BARTLETT R. C., *et al* (1971) *J Oral Surg* 31, 206.
2 DAS GUPTA T. K., *et al* (1969) *Cancer* 24, 355.
3 KNAUSS K. (1898) *Virchows Arch Pathol Anat Physiol* 153, 29.
4 LUDY J. B. (1930) *Arch Dermatol Syphilol* 21, 419.
5 MARQUES C., *et al* (1975) *Med Clin (Barc)* 64, 526.
6 MERCANTINI E. S. & MOPPER C. (1959) *AMA Arch Dermatol* 79, 542.
7 MONTGOMERY H. & O'LEARY P. A. (1934) *Arch Dermatol Syphilol* 29, 26.
8 MURRAY-WALKER D. (1973) *Br J Dermatol* 88, 599.

9 *RUSSELL D.S. & RUBENSTEIN L.J. (1971) *Pathology of Tumours of the Nervous System.* 3rd ed. London, Arnold.
10 STOUT A.P. (1935) *Am J Cancer* 24, 751.
11 THIES W. (1964) *Arch Klin Exp Dermatol* 218, 561.
12 WAGGENER J.D. (1966) *Cancer* 19, 699.

Granular-cell myoblastoma (syn. Abrikossoff's tumour)

Definition. A tumour composed of cells with a characteristic granular cytoplasm; the histogenesis is debatable.

Incidence. This is a rare tumour, occurring in the tongue as well as in the skin, and also in a variety of deeper situations. Males and females are equally affected, and it is common in the third to fifth decade of life. It can occur in childhood [2, 5].

Pathology. The tumour is formed by large polyhedral cells arranged in sheets, which infiltrate the dermal connective tissue and subcutaneous fat. The cytoplasm is pale and contains brightly acidophilic granules. The nuclei are relatively small and round, and tend to be vesicular. The epithelium over the area may show pseudo-epitheliomatous hyperplasia. The original suggestion that the cells are myoblasts probably arose from examination of tumours of the tongue in which infiltration between the striated muscle bundles gave the impression of origin from the muscle. The general belief now is that the cells are of neural or nerve sheath origin [2, 4, 6, 8] or are lipid-containing histiocytes [3]. Histochemical and enzyme studies favour the former derivation [1]. It has been suggested that the condition is a reactive rather than a neoplastic process [10].

Clinical features. The tumour is usually solitary, situated in the skin or beneath the epithelium of the tongue. It is firm rounded but with rather indefinite margins, sessile or pedunculated and between 5 and 20 mm in diameter, although larger tumours may be seen. The colour may vary from flesh colour to pink or greyish-brown. It is most common in the tongue, where the epithelium over it may be thickened. On the skin surface the epithelium covering the tumour is usually normal, although it may thicken or at times ulcerate. There is no particular site of election on the skin. Multiple tumours may occur and several have been reported in children, one of whom also had axillary freckling [2]. The tumour grows slowly.

A malignant type of granular-cell myoblastoma which metastasizes has been reported [7, 11].

Among the internal sites reported are muscle, lip, jaws, parotid gland, pharynx, larynx, trachea, bronchus, lung, chest wall, breast, lacrymal sac, orbit, heart, oesophagus, common bile duct, urinary bladder, spermatic cord, male urethra, perineum, anal region, vulva and ovary [5, 9].

Diagnosis. Histological examination is usually necessary to separate this from other tumours of the deeper dermis.

Treatment. Unless the tumour is widely excised, local recurrence is likely.

REFERENCES

1 ALKEK D.S., *et al* (1968) *Arch Dermatol* 98, 543.
2 APTED J.H. (1968) *Br J Dermatol* 80, 257.
3 AZZOPARDI J.G. (1956) *J Pathol Bacteriol* 71, 85.
4 *BANGLE R. (1952) *Cancer* 5, 950.
5 CAVE V.G., *et al* (1955) *AMA Arch Dermatol* 71, 579.
6 FUST J.A. & CUSTER R.P. (1949) *Am J Clin Pathol* 19, 522.
7 GAMBOA L.G. (1955) *AMA Arch Pathol* 60, 663.
8 GARANCIS J.C., *et al* (1970) *Cancer* 25, 542.
9 PUGH J.I., *et al* (1967) *Br J Surg* 54, 590.
10 SHEAR M. (1960) *J Pathol Bacteriol* 80, 225.
11 SVEDJA J. & HORN V. (1958) *J Pathol Bacteriol* 76, 343.

Cutaneous meningioma [1–3]

A number of cases have been reported of a tumour with the histological characteristics of a meningioma arising in the skin. The tumour occurs over the scalp or in the paraspinous region of the trunk of children and young adults. The lesions resemble 'soft naevi' or are covered with small mamillary excrescences. On the scalp the area may be bald or contain hair. The skin is adherent to the mass, which is dermal or subcutaneous, and there may be a central depression with epidermal atrophy or ulceration. The size ranges from 2 to 10 cm. The histological appearance is similar to intracranial meningioma, and psamoma bodies are present. Dermal nerves traverse the tumour and may form a conspicuous element. One case [3] died of uraemia complicating hypertension. Autopsy showed no intracranial tumours, but revealed a phaeochromocytoma. Meningiomas may occur ectopically in deeper tissues (type II) or, rarely, erode through the skull and appear within the scalp (type III) [2].

REFERENCES

1 BAIN G.O. & SHNITKA T.K. (1965) *AMA Arch Dermatol* 74, 590.
2 LOPEZ D.A., *et al* (1974) *Cancer* 34, 728.
3 SHNITKA T.K. & BAIN G.O. (1959) *AMA Arch Dermatol* 80, 410.

Merkel cell tumours (trabecular cell carcinoma of skin)

Definition. A tumour thought to arise from the cutaneous Merkel cell.

Incidence. The first definitive report of the Merkel cell tumour dates from 1977, although there are reports in 1972 of 'trabecular cell carcinoma of skin' which is almost certainly synonymous. To date, around 53 cases have been recorded [7] and the female:male incidence at present is 4:1. The Merkel cell [3] itself is currently thought to be a secondary sensory cell, perhaps acting as a mechanoreceptor which transforms mechanical to neural stimuli [2, 4, 8].

Pathology. The cells comprising the tumour may be either a solid mass or a more diffuse collection of cells. On light microscopy they may resemble small lymphocytes or a poorly differentiated metastatic deposit. The cells are argyrophilic [1], with sparse cytoplasm, dispersed chromatin and inconspicuous nucleoli [5, 6].

Electron microscopy is required for positive identification of the multiple round secretory granules which pack the cytoplasm of these cells.

Clinical features. The lesions appear to have few distinctive features and are described as raised reddish-blue nodules which may develop on any body site. Six of the first 15 cases described [1] occurred on the lower limb, but lip, scalp and eyelid are also recorded as sites of origin. Surgical excision has been commonly used therapy, but the prognosis is poor with 11 of 15 in the largest series quoted developing secondary spread and six of these dead of metastases within 2 yr.

REFERENCES

1 *FRIGERIO B., *et al* (1983) *Histopathology* 7, 229.
2 GARCIA P. R., *et al* (1980) *Am J Anat* 157, 166.
3 MERKEL F. (1875) *Arch Mikrosk Anat Entwicklungsmech* 11, 636.
4 PEARSE A. G. E. (1980) *Am J Dermatopathol* 2, 121.
5 TANG C. K. & TOKER C. (1979) *Mt Sinai J Med* (NY) 46, 516.
6 TOKER C. (1972) *Arch Dermatol* 105, 107.
7 WARNER T. F. C. S., *et al* (1983) *Cancer* 52, 238.
8 DE WOLF-PEETERS C., *et al* (1980) *Cancer* 46, 1810.

LEIOMYOMA

Definition A benign tumour of smooth muscle derived from the arrector pili muscle, from the media of blood vessels, or from smooth muscle of the scrotum, labia majora or nipples.

Incidence The tumour occurs in three main types, all of them uncommon. Leiomyoma cutis originates in the pilomotor muscle and is the most frequent. It can occur at any age from birth onwards, but appears usually in early adult life. It has been reported in identical twins [7], in siblings and in several generations of a family [3]. The cases with a familial background have all had multiple tumours. The sexes are affected equally.

Dartoic myoma arises in the smooth muscle of the genitalia and areola of the nipple. It can occur at any age. This type is less common than the cutaneous variety, occurring probably in the ratio of 1:6 [3].

Angiomyoma arises from the muscular coat of veins, and is seen mainly in middle age or later as a solitary nodule on a limb. It is rather more prevalent than glomus tumour in published series [4] and markedly so in Ugandan Africans [8]. Females are more commonly affected than males.

Pathology [2]. The smooth-muscle cells proliferate, to produce interweaving bundles of spindle-shaped cells which are strongly eosinophilic. The nuclei are long and thin, and the general appearance of the mass in ordinary sections may suggest a hypertrophic fibrous reaction. The smooth-muscle cells can be distinguished from collagen by their different reaction with trichrome stains, and by the presence of myofibrils, which stain with phosphotungstic acid haematoxylin, and by their blunt-ended nuclei.

The tumour of pilomotor origin (leiomyoma cutis, multiple cutaneous leiomyomas) is usually composed of numerous dermal nodules with vague margins where the cells penetrate the surrounding collagen bundles and an upper border which approaches the papillary body. Dartoic myomas are nodular tumours with a similar appearance. The angiomyomas are related to veins in the subcutaneous tissue, and are rounded and encapsulated [4].

Clinical features [1, 4, 5]. Cutaneous leiomyoma generally presents as a collection of pink, red or dusky brown firm dermal nodules of varying size but usually less than 15 mm across. The nodules are often subject to episodes of pain and may be tender. The pain can be provoked by touching or chilling the skin, or by emotional disturbance. It is often worse in winter. Some lesions contract and become paler when painful [3, 6]. The condition has usually begun with the appearance of one small nodule which has gradually increased in size, and further similar lesions have appeared nearby or at some other area. Adjacent tumours may coalesce to form a plaque. The areas most commonly affected are the extremities, with the proximal and extensor aspects somewhat favoured. The trunk is involved more often than the head and neck. Multiple lesions may be regional and unilateral, or more than one region can be affected. Solitary lesions may occur, apart from the dartoic type.

Dartoic myoma is a solitary dermal nodule occurring most commonly in the scrotum, but also appearing on the penis, labia majora and nipple area. Pain is less frequent than with leiomyoma cutis. Contraction in response to stimulation by touch or cold can occur.

Angiomyoma is usually a solitary flesh-coloured rounded subcutaneous tumour up to 40 mm in diameter. It is more frequent on the lower limb than the upper and may appear on the trunk or face. About half the reported cases have been painful [4].

Diagnosis. The multiple type should cause little difficulty and even without pain it is fairly distinctive. Hidrocystoma may have a similar appearance. The solitary painful lesion may be mistaken for a glomus tumour, and a history of contraction is helpful. In practice the diagnosis can be elusive [3].

Treatment. Surgical excision cures the solitary tumour. The severity of the pain may make the patient demand treatment, and extensive lesions require plastic surgery. Excision of an area containing multiple tumours is often followed by their appearance in the neighbourhood of the treated area.

REFERENCES

1 *ABULAFIA J & GRINSPAN D. (1956) *Arch Argent Dermatol* **6**, 1.
2 DUHIG J. T. & AYER J. P. (1959) *AMA Arch Pathol* **68**, 424.
3 FISHER W. C. & HELWIG E. B. (1963) *Arch Dermatol* **88**, 510.
4 MACDONALD D. M. & SANDERSON K. V. (1974) *Br J Dermatol* **91**, 161.
5 MALOTELA-RUIZ E. (1963) *Ann Dermatol Syphiligr* **90**, 289.
6 MONTGOMERY H. & WINKELMANN R. K. (1959) *AMA Arch Dermatol* **79**, 32.
7 RUDNER E. J., *et al* (1964) *Arch Dermatol* **90**, 81.
8 TEMPLETON A. C. (1972) *E Afr Med J* **48**, 521.

LEIOMYOSARCOMA

Definition. A malignant tumour of smooth muscle.

Incidence. It is a rare tumour and probably of equal incidence in men and women. It can occur at any age from infancy [4] onwards, but is most frequent over the age of 60.

Pathology [1, 2, 7]. The lesion is distinguished from other dermal malignant tumours composed of spindle-shaped cells by the presence of myofibrils within the cells. In other respects it may resemble an anaplastic malignant melanoma or fibrosarcoma. Some lesions show relatively little microscopic evidence of malignancy, and there may be palisading of nuclei similar to neurilemmoma.

Clinical features. The tumour may be situated in the dermis, when it is reddish in colour and may bleed on trauma. It is usually larger than a leiomyoma, and is not tender or painful. The majority of tumours have, however, arisen in the subcutaneous or deeper tissues as nodular tumours or diffuse swellings [6]. It may invade underlying muscle fascia or spread along subcutaneous veins [5]. It is most common on the thigh, followed by the head and neck, arm and trunk [7], and may arise from the penis [3]. It is unlikely to be diagnosed clinically. Metastases to the regional lymph nodes, and by the blood stream, may occur. Multiple tumours may be secondary to a retroperitoneal leiomyosarcoma.

Treatment. Wide surgical excision is necessary, as local recurrence follows inadequate excision.

REFERENCES

1 AKERS W. A., & PRAZAK G. (1960) *Arch Dermatol* **81**, 953.
2 DAHL I & ANGERVALL L. (1974) *Pathol Eur* **9**, 307.
3 GREENWOOD N., *et al* (1972) *Cancer* **29**, 481.
4 HEIECK J. T. & ORGAN C. H. (1970) *Arch Dermatol* **102**, 213.
5 JERNSTROM P. & GOWDY R. A. (1975) *Am J Clin Pathol* **63**, 25.
6 PHELAN J. T., *et al* (1962) *N Engl J Med* **266**, 1027.
7 STOUT A. P. & HILL W. J. (1958) *Cancer* **11**, 844.

OSTEOMA CUTIS

Definition. A true bony new growth arising within the skin from bone-forming tissue and showing no tendency to invade.

Incidence and aetiology. Osteoma cutis is a rare tumour. Most osseous nodules in the skin are not true neoplasms but result from metaplastic ossification, which usually occurs in a focus of calcification, and the initiating lesion is frequently an inflammatory granuloma or scar. Osteomas have been reported in scleroderma, in old acne cysts, and at the sites of puncture of the skin and of haematomas. They may be found in melanocytic naevus, pilomatricoma (p. 2401), histiocytoma, chondroid syringoma and may be secondary to basal cell carcinoma [5, 11]. Another cause is Albright's hereditary osteodystrophy in which cutaneous ossification has recently been recognized with increasing frequency [2, 6, 8]. Multiple miliary osteomas of the skin occur after acne [1, 3], sometimes with neurotic excoriations or after dermabrasion [10]. There remain a minority of reported cases which appear to be primary osteomas, the majority of which are multiple and on the face or scalp [7, 10, 12].

There is no point in trying to estimate the age and sex incidence for so heterogeneous a group as the secondary osteomas of the skin. It seems likely that primary osteomas will become even more rare if hereditary osteodystrophy and other causes are sought.

Pathology [11]. Whether metaplastic or primary, the microscopic picture is of a small circumscribed nodule of osseous tissue with trabeculae enclosing fat and, occasionally, marrow cells.

Clinical features. Metaplastic osteomas are frequently small and clinically undetectable in the primary lesion. They are usually situated deep in the dermis or subcutaneous tissue. They may be seen when radiographs of the area are taken, but are most commonly first noticed by the histology technician as a hard body that damages the knife edge. The distinguishing feature, if the tumour is found clinically, is the stony-hard texture on palpation, similar to pilomatricoma. A case of osteoma cutis associated with diaphyseal aclasis has been reported [4].

Treatment. If required, a simple excision cures the lesion.

REFERENCES

1 BASLER R. S. W., *et al* (1974) *Arch Dermatol* **110**, 113.
2 BROOK C. G. D. & VALMAN H. B. (1971) *Br J Dermatol* **85**, 471.
3 DELANEY T. J. & GOLD S. C. (1974) *Br J Dermatol* **91**, 68.
4 DONALDSON E. M. & SUMMERLY R. (1962) *Arch Dermatol* **85**, 141.
5 DUPERRAT B. (1961) *Ann Dermatol Syphiligr* **88**, 11.
6 EYRE W. G. & REED W. B. (1971) *Arch Dermatol* **104**, 636.
7 HELM F., *et al* (1967) *Arch Dermatol* **96**, 681.
8 PETERSEN W. C. & MANDEL S. L. (1963) *Arch Dermatol* **87**, 626.
9 REICHENBERGER M. & LOHNERT J. (1971) *Hautarzt* **22**, 73.
10 ROSSMAN R. E. & FREEMAN R. G. (1964) *Arch Dermatol* **89**, 68.
11 ROTH S. L., *et al* (1963) *Arch Pathol* **76**, 44.
12 ZABEL R. (1970) *Dermatol Monatsschr* **156**, 798.

Cutaneous calculus [1, 3]. This small tumour, which is not very uncommon, has a characteristic yellowish white colour and is situated in the subepidermal tissue. It is seen most commonly on the face in children; it varies in size up to 10 mm or so, but may occasionally be larger and plaque like, and it has a hard consistency. The epidermis over it may be verrucose. Episodes of inflammation and shedding of a portion of the lesion may occur. Microscope examination shows calcareous bodies in the superficial part of the dermis. A histiocytic or foreign body reaction often surrounds some of the calcified bodies. The exact histogenesis is uncertain. Calcification of naevus cells has been suggested [2]. The lesion can be removed easily by curettage.

REFERENCES

1 HUNTER G. A. & DONALD G. F. (1963) *Aust J Dermatol* **7**, 23.
2 STEIGLEDER G. K. & ELSCHNER N. (1957) *Hautarzt* **8**, 127.
3 WOODS B. & KELLAWAY T. D. (1963) *Br J Dermatol* **75**, 1.

CHAPTER 65

General Aspects of Treatment

D. S. WILKINSON & R. H. CHAMPION

Much of the material that was included in this chapter in previous editions, under the title of 'Principles of Treatment' is now dealt with in other chapters in this book. We shall therefore consider only those aspects of treatment that are not covered elsewhere.

PRINCIPLES OF TREATMENT

The general principles of dermatological therapy differ in no way from those of any other branch of medicine. The dictum *primum non nocere* has an especial significance in relation to the vulnerability of damaged skin to sensitization reactions to applied medicaments. To seek 'short cuts' by the use of 'blunderbuss' agents is to imperil the patient by risking a secondary eruption. There is a particular temptation to be overzealous in treatment when visible disease resists initial therapy; visual evidence of failure is hard to accept with equanimity. The dermatologist, particularly, must follow the maxim of using a few safe and well-tried remedies and regard his ability to persuade, console and counsel his chief weapon. Patients with persistent and pruritic skin disease easily become anxious and depressed and the relief of these symptoms must often play an important part in therapy.

Inflammation of the skin is similar to that occurring elsewhere and follows the same rules of pathology. But the nature of the skin imposes particular difficulties on the dermatologist which are not present to the same extent in other branches of medicine. These involve its close relationship with the environment, the accessibility of its lesions, the special quality of itching and the psychological importance of the skin itself. In addition, we should note the vulnerability of the skin to irritants in the presence of eczema elsewhere [1] and the prolonged period of time required for restitution of functional normality after an irritant insult [4].

The environment. The adaptation of the skin to varying environmental conditions is so well balanced that any failure as a result of disease may be overlooked in treatment. Loss of heat and fluid are considerable in erythroderma; rapid changes of temperature or exposure to an atmosphere of low humidity increase the pruritus of eczema in the aged with dry skins, and are also of occupational importance. Advice and simple protection against these environmental extremes form an essential part of therapy and are often more effective than active therapeutic agents. Friction and chafing from clothes must be minimized. These considerations are poorly understood by patients, who retain a belief that skin disease is a manifestation of dirt or bacteria, to be expunged with vigour and exorcized by soap and water. The provision of an equable external milieu is one of the most cogent reasons for treatment in hospital.

Accessibility of lesions. Self-treatment and interference by the patient may invalidate the best efforts of the physician. This must always be assumed to occur even when denied. Sedatives and antipruritic agents may fail to stop nocturnal scratching and may sometimes increase it. Occlusive paste bandages and firm tubular gauze dressings may be used with success to overcome this.

The presence of a skin lesion which is constantly in the 'mind's eye' even if scarcely visible, may create a situation in which the patient seeks to hasten cure; less commonly, as in factitious dermatitis, it will serve a useful purpose and be perpetuated despite the strongest denials. The ability of young children with atopic dermatitis to exacerbate their lesions in order to gain attention or impose an emotional dominance is well known; some patients with chronic leg ulcers find that these also serve a similar purpose and will unconsciously resist their cure.

The quality of itching. Those who have suffered both pain and itching frequently assert that the latter is harder to bear and more distressing. Though this may be doubted, it seems likely that itching has a particularly distressing quality that is not easily borne with equanimity. Drugs are available to lessen pain but severe pruritus is less amenable to such therapy and the automatic response of scratching or rubbing often increases the severity of the underlying disease. This perpetuation of the 'itch–scratch' cycle is responsible for the chronicity of many eczematous and pruriginous conditions and plays an important role in the management of atopic dermatitis. The subject is dealt with more fully in Chapter 60.

The psychological importance of the skin. It requires little reflection or knowledge of folklore and mythology to appreciate this. From the earliest written records to the present day the skin has held a particular place in man's emotional life. Testimony to this lies in everyday expressions. The long association of two dreaded diseases—leprosy and syphilis—with the skin has not been quite forgotten and may contribute to the strong repugnance felt by patients to disease of this organ. The sexual importance of the skin requires no emphasis but further influences the outlook and attitude of the patient. The dermatologist may thus be faced with a situation that complicates rational treatment and which may alter an otherwise favourable prognosis. He should be aware of the strength of such feelings even when they are not expressed. The management of alopecia demands an understanding of the symbolism of the 'crown' and the persistence, even in 'civilized' communities, of the belief of the magical property of hair. The story of Job illustrated the association of a repugnant skin disease with a depressive illness and strong feelings of guilt. The implications for therapy have been dealt with by several authors [3, 5, 6] and in Chapter 61.

The timing of treatment. A dermatosis can never be regarded as a static event. The interrelationships discussed above, the effect of the patient's actions and attitudes, the frequent development of anxiety or depression and the daily variations in the internal and external milieu require constant reappraisal and adjustment of treatment. Topical corticosteroids should be reduced in strength as the disease recedes. The timing of a return to work often involves a difficult decision; even the return of a patient from hospital to his environment may be misjudged. In either case a relapse may cause the patient to lose confidence. In all dermatological therapy Napoleon's dictum may be remembered with advantage: '*la puissance ne consiste pas à frapper fort ou à frapper souvent, mais à frapper juste*'.

Qualities of the eczematous skin. Features of the behaviour of eczematous or irritated skin that have a bearing on treatment have not received as much attention as they should in relation to therapy. Björnberg [1] showed that the skin affected by eczema in one area became unduly susceptible to the effects of irritants in other apparently normal areas. This may explain some cases of unexpected irritant dermatitis, say of the hands, in a worker who has an eczema of the leg or elsewhere. The concept has not yet been extended to other diseases causing epidermal skin damage, such as seborrhoeic dermatitis, but it might be advantageous to do so.

The second example has even more important implications for therapy. Malten [4] has shown that a single irritant insult to the skin damages the water-holding capacity of the stratum corneum for several weeks—long after apparent 'anatomical' and visual recovery is evident. The importance of this observation on the relapse of eczematous conditions and irritant dermatitis needs no underlining. But the obvious inference—that topical treatment and avoidance of irritants to previously affected areas must be continued long after apparent 'cure'—is not generally recognized.

FOUR-DIMENSIONAL APPROACH

Many minor or localized skin disorders can be dealt with expeditiously by appropriate topical measures or drugs. In most cases cure will follow after a varying time and, although recurrences may take place, these can be considered as separate events. In more extensive conditions, however, or in those in which the natural history does not conform to an assured pattern, therapeutic measures must be based on broader considerations. Widespread physiological or biochemical changes may involve other systems and demand attention to general medical principles; the course of the disease varies in time as well as intensity, and therapy must be adjusted to waves of progression and regression; the effect of the disease on the individual may lead to a distortion of the body image and give a different quality to the same intensity of disease from one patient to another. Such dermatological disorders, therefore, can be said to have four dimensions, each of which must be considered in planning therapy: intensity, extent, time and perceptive quality.

Intensity. A patient whose psoriasis or atopic dermatitis becomes severe or generalized poses problems quite different from those usually involved in these diseases. His working life will be interrupted, reactive depression may occur and even a previously well-adjusted relationship with his environment may break down. The housewife with severe hand eczema or the industrial worker with a protracted dermatitis is in a similar position. The first need of therapy is to regain the former position of functional parity and to re-establish a *modus vivendi*.

Extent. Involvement of other organs, either the cause or the result of a skin disorder, may have graver consequences to the patient than the disorder itself. Cardiac death from hypercholesterolaemia is a more important risk that the skin lesions. The recognition of cardiac changes in systemic sclerosis or sarcoidosis, neuropathy in Behçet's syndrome, nephropathy in various forms of vasculitis or hypocalcaemia in pustular psoriasis will govern the therapeutic approach. The effects of erythroderma on cardiac function and nutritional needs must be allowed for in treatment.

Time. Failure to appreciate the natural history of disease has been responsible for much unnecessary therapy and for a wrong assessment of therapeutic needs. In lichen planus and alopecia areata specific therapy is lacking and the average duration is unaffected by empirical measures. Infantile eczema tends to improve with the passage of time; nummular eczema 'burns itself out' in months or years. In these diseases the patient is ill served by measures that can only alter the immediate situation without an additional planned campaign to sustain him over this prolonged period. A diminishing concentration of topical corticosteroids, measures designed to distract his attention from the disease and manoeuvres designed to help his morale are necessary parts of the whole treatment. In diseases with a short-lived though hectic course, such as erythema multiforme exudativum, oral steroids, if given at all, should be 'tailed off' once the expected peak of the disease is past. In the chronic diseases such as psoriasis, systemic sclerosis, lichen sclerosus of the vulva, ichthyosiform erythroderma or dermatitis herpetiformis, therapy should be on the lines of a siege operation or, sometimes, as a deliberately planned retreat in which the disease is contained and held in check. It is a wise precaution to hold a therapeutic reserve whenever possible, for periods of exceptional activity of the disease process.

Perception. Health is a state of mind in which we are not conscious of our bodies. Unfortunately, diseases of the skin are usually visible to the patient and to others, even when there is no pain, itching or discomfort. This endows them with a particular quality of being 'perceived objects', lying almost outside the body proper and easily detached from the natural absorption of the body image into 'self'. Psychological distortions referable to the skin are part of man's history and myth and the 'faith-healer' is often more adept at recognizing this and correcting it than the physician, who sometimes forgets that there is a distinction between the actual state and what is perceived [1]. This distortion of perception is a quality of altered awareness in which the patient's and the doctor's assessment of the disease differ and which may be manifested within the bounds of psychological normality as a lowered itch threshold or a bizarre estimation of the significance or consequences of the disease. The concept of a 'private perceptual space' [2] may serve to explain the very great differences in the extent of itching experienced by different subjects with identical diseases, of similar severity. The psychological aspects of skin disease are dealt with in Chapter 61.

To summarize, therefore, any chronic or extensive skin disease must be treated not only in its own right but with an understanding of its effect on other bodily systems, its variability in time and the special effect or perceptive quality it holds for the particular patient.

REFERENCES

1 BJÖRNBERG A. (1968) *Skin Reactions to Primary Irritants in Patients with Hand Eczema.* Goteborg, Oscar Isaacson.
2 BRAIN Lord (1959) *The Nature of Experience.* London, Oxford University Press.
3 COTTERILL J.A. (1981) *Br J Dermatol* **105**, 311.
4 MALTEN K.E. (1981) *Contact Dermatitis* **7**, 238.
5 NOVAK M. (1979) *Cutis* **23**, 528.
6 WHITLOCK F.A. (1976) *Psychological Aspects of Skin Disease: Major Problems in Dermatology* ed. Rook A.J. London, Saunders, Vol. 8.

DRESSINGS [5, 17, 27]

The type of dressing to be used for covering the skin during topical treatment should be related to the physiological state and requirements. Wet dressings lower the temperature of the treated area, occluded dressings increase it [11]. The purpose of a dressing is to keep the agent used in close apposition to the skin and, normally, to allow the free evaporation of sweat. It should prevent or minimize friction, chafing and damage from rubbing and scratching and be comfortable for the patient. It should enable him, whenever possible, to carry on his normal life while retaining in place the applications used, without undue soiling or staining of clothing.

Cool, light dressings should be used for covering

wet dressings or creams in acute eczematous conditions; cotton gloves should be worn at night to keep ointments and pastes in place. In particular circumstances paste bandages covered with tubular gauze may be applied for several days at a time in chronic eczema or atopic dermatitis, and polyethylene occlusive dressings may be used to increase penetration of corticosteroids.

When creams or oily lotions are used, dressings should preferably be of rag or linen torn into strips and laid over the affected areas. When wet dressings are applied, several layers of rag soaked in the solution are kept constantly damped by removing the outer layers and soaking them in a fresh solution. Such dressings can be kept in place with a loose outer covering if the patient is at rest in bed. Otherwise tubular gauze is useful. Pastes may be applied on strips of rag or linen and laid over the affected area but are best applied directly to the skin and covered with a stockingette firm tubular gauze or elasticated tubular net.

In certain areas of the body, e.g. the groins, specialized forms of dressing are needed [26].

Gauze and lint should be avoided. If the lesion is exudative these stick to the skin and are painful to remove; if creams or pastes are being applied, contact with the skin is reduced by leakage through the gauze mesh. In any raw or exuding lesions plain paraffin gauze or non-adherent gauze is preferable and can be removed without discomfort. This in its turn may be covered with ordinary gauze, rag, linen or other dressings as appropriate.

Tubular gauze. By ingenious techniques of folding and cutting, this closely woven, fine tubular gauze provides a covering in the shape of sandals, stockings, helmets, vests, etc. An experienced nurse can very rapidly cover the whole surface of the body, and the dressings will stay in place for 12–24 h. A 'suit' of Tubegauz may be worn as underclothing beneath ordinary clothes (Fig. 65.1). Oozing of pastes through the gauze is prevented by the insertion of greaseproof or tissue paper which the dressing holds in place, or by dusting with an inert powder. Surgical stockingette, which is thicker, is also widely used for the same purpose.

Paper 'jumpsuits' have also been used successfully [7] but, although an attractive idea, we did not find them wholly satisfactory.

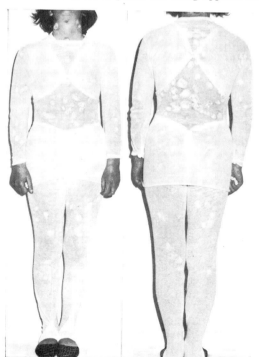

Fig. 65.1. Tubular gauze dressings. Complete 'suit' used for a patient with psoriasis (Stoke Mandeville Hospital).

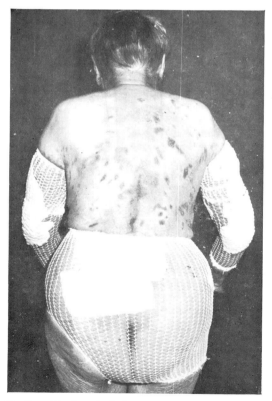

Fig. 65.2. Elasticated tubular net retaining dressings in a patient with pemphigoid (Stoke Mandeville Hospital).

Elasticated tubular net (Figs 65.2 and 65.3). This type of bandage is increasingly used in a wide variety of situations. It has the advantage of simplicity, adaptability and easy removal. It is relatively long-lasting and can be washed without significant loss of elasticity. Ingenious adaptations consist in covering wide areas of solar keratoses being treated with 5-fluorouracil, particularly on the back, and of holding in position irrigation needles in the treatment of leg ulcers.

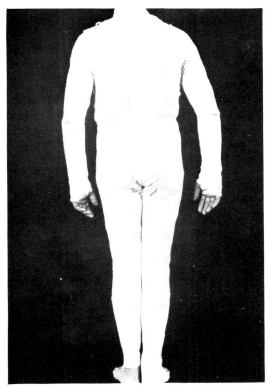

Fig. 65.3. Elastic tubular net over a paper suit (Wycombe General Hospital).

Occlusive dressings. Initial enthusiasm for polyethylene occlusion over topical corticosteroids has been tempered by a recognition of its limitations and adverse effects. However, used judiciously, it remains a very valuable technique. A piece or tube of polyethylene, particularly of the self-clinging film type, is secured over the treated area and left in place for 8 h or longer. In psoriasis, for which it was originally chiefly used, the immediate results are good but relapse occurs rapidly after its use is discontinued. We believe that its main value in this disease is as a preliminary short-term treatment before passing on to traditional therapy.

Certain side effects should be noted. The rustling is aesthetically disturbing to some patients or their spouses and a disagreeable odour accompanies prolonged occlusion. Folliculitis may occur, especially on hairy limbs and in the inguinogenital region. This may induce further lesions of psoriasis. The risk can be reduced by restricting the occlusion to 8–12 h a day, by thorough cleansing before application, by the concomitant use of antibacterial bath additives or emulsions, or by steroid-antibacterial preparations. In hospital wards there is the added risk of contamination of the polyethylene by *Pseudomonas aeruginosa* [20].

Absorption of corticosteroids may occur to a significant degree under widespread occlusion. In extensive psoriasis the danger of approaching a significant systemic dose is evident. Local atrophy, usually reversible after some months, may occur, usually affecting the normal skin adjacent to the treated area. We have noticed, with others, the reduced tolerance to dithranol or tar in patients treated even for short periods by this method.

Occlusive therapy remains of value in the treatment of chronic eczematous or psoriatic conditions of the hands, feet and scalp, where polyethylene gloves, bags or contrived helmets are used overnight. Modified occlusion is provided by unsealed polyethylene or the use of greasy ointments or pastes (Chapter 67).

Leg dressings (Fig. 65.4) Crêpe or elastic net bandaging may be used over applications. Women, and sometimes men, can be persuaded to wear an old pair of nylon stockings instead. Old pyjama trousers or long underpants are of value underneath ordinary trousers to prevent staining of the clothes. Tubular elastic bandages or elastic webbing bandages, 'blue-line' (cotton–rubber) or 'red-line' (nylon–rubber), give more support. An acrylic self-adhesive bandage needs careful application but is well tolerated by rubber-sensitive patients.

The indications for pressure bandaging include hypertrophic lichen planus and chronic eczema in patients with leg oedema or varicosities. Their use in leg ulcer treatment is dealt with in Chapter 32. We use a non-elastic 'ventilated' diachylon bandage, alone or over paste bandages. Although sensitization reactions occur, they are far less frequent than with most rubber-based elastic adhesive bandages. Such diachylon bandages, with interspersed polyethylene, applied directly over corticosteroid ointments, are particularly useful for chronic hyperkeratotic eczema of the heels.

In the application of compressive leg bandaging the experience of the dresser matters more than the

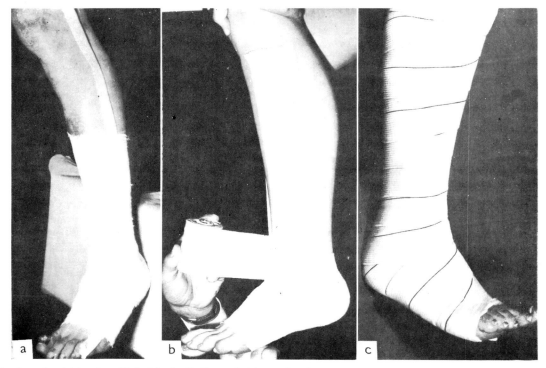

Fig. 65.4. Special dressings (Stoke Mandeville Hospital). (a) Paste bandage with unopened tubular gauze strip inserted to facilitate removal. (b) Method of application of diachlyon leg bandage (using lateral slats). (c) Elastic webbing bandage with protective pad inserted at the vulnerable site.

form of bandaging used. Pressure must be carefully and evenly applied from the base of the toes to below the knees. Selective pressure, with or without foam pads or slats of paste bandage, may be concentrated at the blow-out site in the form of a pad. In general, the mistake is to exert too little, rather than too much, pressure. The technique can be learnt only by experience.

Leg ulcer dressings. These are discussed in more detail in Chapter 32 and will be mentioned only briefly here. Because of the chronicity of most leg ulcers, a wide variety of dressings has been used; each has its own advocate. Non-adhesive gauzes are pleasant for the patient but abundant exudate may spread beneath them. Silicone foam sponges [29] may be useful for deep ulcers, and collagen sponges [6, 22] are said to encourage the development of granulation tissue. We have found gold leaf [14] quite useful in the later stages of ulcer healing.

Porcine skin or lyophilized porcine dermis are useful and the latter was found to reduce the healing time significantly compared with standard 'Bisgaard' treatment, but we found them of little value in arterial type ulcers. Human amnion has also been used [4, 8, 24].

Proteolytic enzymes [19] are theoretically able to hydrolyse collagen fibres. They are applied after cleaning the ulcer and removing any loose debris. Various forms are available. We have not found them to be of great value in our patients (who are usually admitted because their ulcers are, in any case, recalcitrant).

Small dextranomer beads provide an ingenious way of drawing up exudates and their contents, thus removing bacteria and degradation products to the surface [9, 12]. Our experience has been limited. They do often appear to produce a clean, dry ulcer bed but the drying effect may occasionally cause some pain. It requires further evaluation.

Felt, Sorbo and plastic foam. These can be used to supplement pressure or to protect areas vulnerable to trauma or friction. Foam pads to localize pressure over intercommunicating veins are more effective if extended some way up the saphenous vein and beneath the malleolus ('sickle pad').

Adhesive tape compression [10]. Thin strips of adhesive tape (or diachylon bandage) are applied very closely together with moderate pressure across a leg ulcer, to half encircle the leg, and are left for 3–5 days. A dressing or gauze pack may be applied on top. The leg is then bandaged conventionally.

Compression stockings. Graduated compression stockings based on sound pathophysiological principles [13, 25] are now available to match the ankle pressure required in any individual case. They were found to be more effective than standard 'two-way stretch stockings [25].

Medicated dressings. While plain paraffin gauze (tulle gras) or non-adherent gauze dressings fulfil most needs, there is a place for the short-term use of medicated dressings in open infected lesions. Several varieties are now available but should be used with discretion over leg ulcers, where the risk of sensitization is high [28].

Medicated paste bandages. Of the several types available, the zinc paste, coal tar paste and iodo-hydroxyquinoline bandages are most frequently used. They should be cut frequently and moulded to the skin while being applied, avoiding constriction at the bends of the knees and elbows. They are useful in atopic dermatitis, discoid and other forms of chronic eczema, lichen simplex, hypertrophic lichen planus, prurigo, artefacts and gravitational eczema and ulceration. They are covered by any conventional form of dressing appropriate to the site. Corticosteroids can be applied beneath these, if required.

Miscellaneous dressings. Adhesive foam or felt pads or rings are used around warts and calluses or to prevent pressure on small painful malleolar ulcers, but they should not be used on eczematous areas. Polyethylene foam mesh dressings aid sweat evaporation and do not stick to the skin. Wide excision of hidradenitis suppurativa without grafting was possible with the use of Silastic elastomer foam dressings [18, 30]. Foam elastomer dressings provided cosmetic and functional advantages in the surgical treatment of facial carcinoma [23].

Plastic adhesive films. Collodion retains its place in wart treatment but plastic-type aerosol sprays have superseded it for other purposes. They are non-occlusive and peel off in 2–3 days. They are convenient and non-sensitizing but may cause temporary smarting and are not suitable for very young children.

Attempts to incorporate active ingredients to simplify the treatment of psoriasis and chronic eczema have not so far been satisfactory.

These films have a limited though useful range of function in dermatology and dermatological surgery. They are also useful for preserving skin markings at sites of patch or intradermal tests.

Corticosteroid-impregnated tapes. An acrylic-backed adhesive tape impregnated with flurandrenolone, 4 mcg/cm², offers a cosmetically attractive and simple form of occlusive dressing (Cordran, Haelan tape) for lichen simplex, hypertrophic lichen planus, etc. We have also found it useful in treating hyperkeratotic palmar eczema, local patches of lupus erythematosus and some cases of localized palmoplantar pustulosis.

Colostomy dressings. These come to the notice of dermatologists only if sensitization or irritant dermatitis has developed (see p. 620). A mass formed of pectin, gelatin, sodium carboxymethylcellulose and polyisobutylene [5, 15, 16] has considerable advantages. Without the polyethylene backing it has been adapted for use in leg ulcers [1–3].

Allergic contact dermatitis. Patients with ulcers or eczema of the leg appear to be particularly prone to develop sensitization reactions to colophony, parabens and antibiotics. This may limit the choice of dressings used. They may also become sensitized to rubber chemicals in elasticated supports; this imposes a considerable restriction in the choice of supporting devices used to control oedema. In some cases the liberal use of a non-perfumed talcum powder may be sufficient to prevent irritation, at least for a few hours, but in others such form of support may be quite impractical.

REFERENCES

1 ALLEN S. (1973) *Curr Med Res Opin* **1**, 603.
2 ASHURST P.J. (1945) *Practitioner* **215**, 353.
3 BAXTER R. (1980) *Aust Fam Physician* **9**, 599.
4 BENNETT J.P. *et al.* (1980) *Lancet* **i**, 1153.
5 BICKERTON J. & SMALL J. (1982) *Bandaging.* London, Heinemann.
6 COLLINS J. *et al* (1976) *Surg Forum* **27**, 551.
7 DOWNHAM T.F. (1979) *Cutis* **23**, 869.
8 EGAN T.J. *et al* (1983) *Angiology* **34**, 197.
9 FRANK D.H., *et al* (1979) *Ann Plast Surg* **3**, 395.
10 GILGE O. (1949) *Acta Derm Venereol* (Suppl) (Stockh) **22**, 29.
11 HAWKINS K. (1978) *Nursing* **8**, 64.
12 JACOBSON S., *et al* (1976) *Scand J Plast Reconstr Surg* **10**, 65.

13 Jones N.A.G., *et al* (1980) *Br J Surg* **67**, 569.

14 Kanof N.M. (1976) *Cutis* **18**, 395.

15 Knighton D.R., *et al* (1976) *Surg Gynecol Obstet* **143**, 449.

16 Kyte E.M. & Hughes E.S.R. (1970) *Med J Aust* **ii**, 186.

17 *Lawrence J.C. (1982) *Injury* **13**, 500.

18 Morgan W.P., *et al* (1980) *Br J Surg* **67**, 277.

19 Nierman M.M. (1978) *Drugs* **15**, 226.

20 Noble W.C. & Savin J.A. (1966) *Lancet* **i**, 347.

21 Rundle J.S.H., *et al* (1976) *Br Med J* **iii**, 216.

22 Shekter A.S., *et al* (1975) *Acta Chir Plast (Prague)* **17**, 159.

23 Shukla H.S. (1982) *Br J Surg* **69**, 435.

24 Somerville P.G. (1982) *Phlebologie* **35**, 223.

25 Stemmer R., *et al* (1980) *Hautarzt* **31**, 355.

26 Wilkinson D.S. (1969) *Practitioner* **202**, 27.

27 Wilkinson D.S. (1977) *Nursing and Management of Skin Diseases*, 4th ed. London, Faber & Faber.

28 Wilkinson J.D., *et al* (1980) *Acta Derm Venereol (Stockh)* **60**, 245.

29 Wood R.A.B. & Hughes L.E. (1975) *Br Med J* **iv**, 131.

30 Wood R.A.B., *et al* (1977) *Br J Surg* **64**, 554.

THE AIMS AND LIMITATIONS OF DRUG THERAPY IN DERMATOLOGY

Drug therapy may be specific, empirical, or placebo in its effect. Dermatology has suffered more than most specialties from an abundance of empirics and placebos. It has not been shown that dermatological patients respond more to placebos than others, but the presence of an obvious and visible disease and the anxiety that this engenders endows all forms of treatment with an aura of suggestibility that often confuses the judgement of the patient and physician alike. The past records of dermatological therapy give abundant evidence of the 'wish to believe'. The results of 'double-blind' trials have destroyed the edifice of this belief. Care and concern for the patient demand a middle course; drugs should not be despised if they help the patient, but they should never be regarded as pharmacologically active without unequivocal evidence of their effectiveness when tested against an inert substance. There must be no confusion in the dermatologist's mind. He has at his command a few specific remedies, a number of empirical ones and many placebos (p. 2488). The first are accepted because their action is known. The second are effective in 'double-blind' trials, although their mode of action remains unknown. The third are often effective in a manner that bears no relation to the pharmacology of the drug or the pathogenesis of the disease; often, the physician endows them with his personality.

Advances in pharmacology are now so rapid that any list of effective drugs that are widely used in the general management of patients with skin lesions will soon be outdated. Moreover, individual and national differences in prescribing habits are so variable that a detailed discussion of particular drugs would be inappropriate. The subject is discussed in Chapter 66. Here, we shall consider only briefly some drugs of a general nature that may be used in dermatology.

Psychopharmacological agents [9, 10, 14]. In recent years there has been a marked trend, in the U.K. at least, away from reliance on these drugs or willingness to take them on the part of the patient. This stems from four sources: the virtual proscription of barbiturates as potentially addictive drugs, the influence of the media and 'health' groups, the emotive interpretation of the term itself and the widespread publicity given to the side effects of drugs in general (e.g. thalidomide, benoxaprofen). Even the conservative dermatologist, who may feel, on occasions, that the short-term administration of sedatives or hypnotics would be of help in reducing itching or restoring normal sleep patterns, may encounter unexpected resistance by the patient. Unfortunately, reasonable alternatives—discussion, the encouragement of the development of relaxation or autosuggestive techniques (p. 2494)—are time consuming and seldom carried out by busy general practitioners. Thus, anxiety may intensify until the acute 'emergency' situation, so well known to dermatologists, develops. In such cases rest, adequate sleep and some form of sedation become imperative and may be obtained only by removal of the patient from his environment to hospital.

The two situations in which the rational use of psychopharmacological agents may be necessary are anxiety and depression. There are now a vast number of agents available for the treatment of these conditions. National differences in prescribing are as widespread as are the individual preferences of prescribers. One drug often replaces another for reasons of fashion or commercial pressure, rather than for reasons of improved efficacy. The dermatologist is best advised to choose two or three, preferably having short- and medium-term and more prolonged effects, and to use them appropriately.

Anxiety. Environmental levels of anxiety and tension have increased in modern industrialized life. Anxiety, not always recognized or acknowledged by the patient, may be an essential driving force in some individuals ('trait' anxiety [19]); only when this increases, as a result of extra stresses or the presence of disease, may it become marked ('state' anxiety). Then the symptoms themselves, e.g. the intensity of pruritus, may become part of 'a general stress response characterized by emotional over-arousal' [14].

The benzodiazepines [1, 9, 14] are the safest, most effective anxiolytics at present in use. A large number are available; the only real difference lies in their different plasma half-lives [14]. They are equally effective for treating both anxiety and in-somnia although the causes of the latter should be examined before recourse to drug therapy [5]. They are widely used, especially by older females in the lower socio-economic groups [13]. Diazepam and chlordiazepoxide are the best known. Nitrazepam, used as a hypnotic, has a half-life of about 30 h and may thus accumulate on repeated use. A single dose of diazepam is frequently given to allay appre-hension in young children before minor operative procedures [11, 12]. When appropriate, a suitable analgesic should be given before the diazepam [4]. The intravenous use of benzodiazepines carries a risk of thrombosis or ischaemia [6]. They should be diluted with blood and given slowly [3]. The ben-zodiazepines have no antidepressive effect and may, in fact, enhance depression. The side effects are those of any drug affecting the central nervous sys-tem, including over-sedation [8]. Alcohol is poten-tiated [15]. Long-term use may lead to tolerance or, occasionally, to dependence [16]. Withdrawal symptoms have occurred [18].

Depressive states. These are common in dermatolog-ical practice but, like myxoedema, may develop in-sidiously and pass unrecognized by those seeing the patient frequently. If accompanied by anxiety, the depressive element may be marked. The distinction between the two is not always easily made but may become apparent if a patient fails to respond to anx-iolytics. The *tricyclic compounds* such as amitripty-line and imipramine are drugs of choice in such situations and, because they also have some seda-tive properties, are more useful than pure anxioly-tics in cases with mixed features, but they are not appropriate for patients with pure primary anxiety [14].

Other drugs in use [10]. Butyrophenone derivations such as *haloperidol* are also used for anxiety, depres-sion and alcohol withdrawal symptoms. Chloral hy-drate (0·3–2 g) should not be despised as a hypnotic, particularly in children. The unpleasant taste of paraldehyde has limited its oral use but it is an effective and quick-acting hypnotic, especially for hypomanic states, given by intramuscular injection (5–10 ml). Beta-adrenoceptor antagonists ('beta

blockers') have not found much place in dermatol-ogy, although symptoms mediated by the β-division of the sympathetic nervous system have been helped by propranolol [20]. A number of side effects have been reported [2].

Clonidine, which appears to reduce the vasolabil-ity of the cranial vessels in migraine, may have a more extended use: we have found it useful in con-trolling the flush of rosacea; its effect on peripheral and vasolability is less certain. *Pimozide* is of promis-ing value in parasitophobia and related states (p. 2260); *thalidomide* (with reservations) for severe prurigo and for leprosy. *Naoxone* and related opioid antagonists have recently emerged as drugs with interesting properties [7, 17] e.g. an ability to block some forms of flushing (p. 2241). They are still being investigated; so far, their dermatological value is limited.

REFERENCES

1 Committee on the Review of Medicines (1980) *Br Med J* **280**, 910.
2 Clerens A., et al (1981) *Dermatologica* **163**, 5.
3 Driscoll E.J., et al (1979) *J Oral Surg* **37**, 809.
4 *Drug Ther Bull* (1976) **14**, 20.
5 *Drug Ther Bull* (1978) **16**, 21.
6 *Drug Ther Bull* (1981) **19**, 9.
7 *Drug Ther Bull* (1981) **19**, 81.
8 Edwards J.G. (1981) *Drugs* **22**, 495.
9 Garattini S., et al (1973) *The Benzodiazepines.* New York, Raven Press.
10 *Goodman L.S. & Gilman A. (1980) *The Pharmacolog-ical Basis of Therapy.* 6th ed. New York, Macmillan.
11 Gordon N.Y. & Turner D.J. (1968) *Br J Anaesth* **41**, 136.
12 Haq L.V. & Dundee J.W. (1968) *Br J Anaesth* **40**, 972.
13 Lader M. (1978) *Neuroscience* **3**, 159.
14 *Lader M. & Petursson H. (1983) *Drugs* **25**, 514.
15 Linnoila M., et al (1979) *Drugs* **18**, 299.
16 Marks J. (1978) *The Benzodiazepines. Use, Overuse, Misuse, Abuse.* Lancaster, MTP Press.
17 McNicolas L.F. & Martin W.R. (1984) *Drugs* **27**, 81.
18 Petursson H. & Lader M.H. (1981) *Br Med J* **283**, 643.
19 Spielberger C.D. (1972) In *Anxiety, Current Trends in Therapy and Research Vol 1.* Ed Spielberger C.D. New York, Academic Press
20 Tyrer P. (1980) *Drugs* **20**, 300.

Antihistamines. These are discussed in Chapter 66. As with anxiolytics, it is preferable that the derma-tologist has an intimate knowledge of a very few of the many available. He requires a short-, medium-and long-acting variety. Individual variations in the main side effect, drowsiness, may call for alterna-tives. New drugs appear to be free of this but may need to be given in higher than the standard recommended doses, especially for chronic urticaria.

Hydroxyzine is mentioned her, rather than with the neuroleptics, because it is chiefly used for relief of pruritus, for which it is generally regarded as being more valuable than other antihistamines and neuroleptics [1].

REFERENCE

1 Arnold A.J., *et al* (1979) *J Am Acad Dermatol* 1, 509.

THE PLACEBO

The placebo ('I shall please') has long been a cause of dissension among doctors and of benefit to patients. Those who extolled its virtues were accused of deceit and those who did not were led into errors of judgement on the effects of the drug they were prescribing. Trials of new therapeutic agents are still often poorly controlled and neglect of the placebo effect [2] has led to unwarranted optimism. Too little attention has been given to the response of itching to inert drugs despite the excellent early classical studies on the subject [1].

Any relationship between a physician and a patient creates a situation in which the placebo response may occur; the degree depends upon the personality and optimism of the physician or of the patient, the setting or nature of the communication [6, 8], fatigue and concentration. Every prescription written has a placebo effect in the signature. The physical and emotional act of giving and receiving creates a psychological bond. Primitive modes of religious or magical therapy leaned heavily on hieratical manipulation of the placebo situation.

The occurrence of adverse effects—including rashes—in the course of placebo therapy is well attested in clinical trials of many agents. Even true addiction and dependence have occurred [9]. Every drug is also a placebo and every placebo exerts some drug-like effects. In one trial, 14% of 69 patients were found to react consistently with placebo responses [5]; an additional 55% were inconsistent reactors. Variations in the placebo response to tablets of different colours—green is best for anxiety—have been demonstrated [7]. Minor aberrations of normal physiological function may occur for many placebo effects. When an inert preparation was given to three groups with widely differing advice about the nature of the drug, those who believed it to resemble amphetamines were found to have a significantly raised pulse rate [3].

It is now accepted that the efficacy of a new drug or local preparation must be shown to be statistically and consistently superior to a matched 'dummy'. Regrettably, this is not always clear in published reports.

Whenever the mode of action of a drug is not established, the effects of a placebo may predominate early in a clinical trial if that of the active agent is slow to show itself. Conversely, if the action of the drug is retarded by enzyme production or other mechanisms, the longer-term comparison may be weighted against it. In the comparison [10] of a 'dummy' tablet and sedatives, drowsiness and nausea occurred equally with all, but certain specific side effects, such as vivid dreams, occurred only with one active agent.

The placebo response in dermatology. The less effective any existing treatment is, the more likely are any favourable effects to be of placebo type. Lichen planus, alopecia areata and chronic urticaria have been 'cured' in the past with many different preparations, which have not been shown to be pharmacologically effective in these diseases. But the patient has been sustained through their natural course by receiving a potion or a lotion which at least sustains the faith and the hope and, at most, is free from potential toxicity. The placebo effect is also apparent in the control of insomnia and pruritus and extends to physical methods of treatment, notably acupuncture (p. 2491) and even UV light [9, 11].

Ethics [8]. Most but not all physicians would agree that the administration of a placebo as a therapeutic measure is justifiable if no known effective treatment exists. In any case it is less likely to harm the patient than a poorly tested or a powerful 'new' drug of uncertain value. In some cases the deliberate use of a placebo initially may be valuable in ensuring rapport with a patient who claims to be prone to all the side effects known for all drugs taken; and to assess the placebo response reactions. It also gains time for the anxious patient to accept a prolonged or incurable condition while a situation of rapport is being built up. This presupposes, of course, that no widely accepted active agent is available that is likely to be more beneficial.

In all cases—particularly in drug trials—the overriding consideration must always be the benefit to the patient. The doctor is always in a particularly authoritative position and must not abuse this authority. The patient's fully informed consent (with a witness) must always be obtained if a 'controlled' trial is embarked on. It is doubtful whether the use of 'dummy' preparations is ever justified in children, even with the parents' consent.

Preparations [4]. Placebos must be harmless. Many drugs that are *not* harmless are really only being given as placebos. Lactose tablets are commonly given but even this substance is not totally harmless. Aspirin should be avoided. Carefully worded instructions may reinforce a placebo effect [1] as may an unusual size or shape of tablet.

No official placebo is included in the British National Formulary but many manufacturers will supply inert preparations matched to their own products.

REFERENCES

1 BEECHER H.K. (1959) *Measurement of Subjective Responses*. New York, Oxford University Press, p. 389.
2 BENSON H. & EPSTEIN M.D. (1975. *JAMA* **232**, 1225.
3 BRODEUR D.W. (1965) *Psychopharmacologica* **7**, 444.
4 *Drug Ther Bull* (1965) **3**, 58.
5 LASAGNA L. (1952) *Proc R Soc Med* **55**, 773.
6 LASAGNA L., *et al* (1954) *Am J Med* **16**, 770.
7 SHAPIRA K., *et al* (1970) *Br Med J* ii, 446.
8 SHEPHERD M. (1968) *Clinical Psychopharmacology*. London, English University Press.
9 SIMPSON N.B. & DAVIDSON A.M. (1979) *Proc Eur Dial Transplant Assoc* **16**, 743.
10 VINAR O. (1969) *Br J Psychol* **115**, 1189.
11 WINKELMANN R.K. (1982) Symposium on Clinical Pharmacology of Symptom Control. *Med Clin North Am* **66**, 1119.

THE PATIENT AND THE DRUG [7, 8]

In company with all practitioners of medicine, but perhaps more than most, dermatologists must achieve rapid rapport with their patients and be seen either to be able to assuage the symptoms and reduce the signs of visible disease or to bring the patient—and his relatives or parents—to accept chronicity or irreversible changes. Dermatology has been called an 'applied intuitive art' [8]. If so, an easy understanding must be achieved between the artist and his sitter. Allowance must be made for symptoms of anxiety—aggression, lack of faith, mistrust. Little by little, if necessary, the dermatologist must overcome these and gain the ascendance in the situation. The various manoeuvres employed by patients in the consultation 'gamesmanship' have been well described by Cotterill [2].

Increasingly, patients ask for an explanation of their disease and of any therapy offered. They may be well-informed or misinformed, but they are informed. Recourse to the *Book of Proverbs* or *Job* is not received with the understanding it used to command. It is never easy to explain autoimmune diseases or the mechanism of psoriasis in easily comprehensible terms. The intelligence of the patient must be gauged; a suitable metaphor or simile is often apt. In any case, the patient's questions must be answered. In seeking clues to the causation of conditions such as contact dermatitis or chronic urticaria, one should always listen attentively to the patient's explanation. He may well be wrong; but occasionally he is right, however unexpected the answer. However, his account of the onset and course of the disease may have become distorted by time of for medico-legal reasons and can never be believed in cases of dermatitis artefacta. His memory (or suppression) of drug or topical medicaments given is usually defective, especially if they were self-administered. Intensive probing was needed to obtain acknowledgment of the self-use of strong topical corticosteroids in some patients with perioral dermatitis (p. 1613). This was especially seen in medical and paramedical personnel.

Drug compliance [4]. It is too easily assumed that the patient will take or has taken the medicines prescribed. A thrice-daily routine is difficult, especially for those who travel to work. This has led drug manufacturers to attempt to find once-daily substitutes, e.g. for antibiotics. The reasons for non-compliance cannot easily be evaluated [4] but levels of anxiety, degree of motivation and the patient's attitude to the doctor and the disease, and that of others in his social environment, are important factors.

In poorer countries the cost of treatment and, in developed countries, more complex socio-economic issues may determine the degree to which treatment is continued as long as is necessary [5].

Side effects of drugs. Because of the public's greater awareness of the side effects of drugs, bolstered by exuberant presentation by the media, any doctor is put in a difficult position. The patient needs basic information [3, 6]. If the doctor does not explain possible major side effects, he is guilty of neglect; if he over-stresses these, he will invite non-compliance. If he includes too many of the minor possible side effects he will invite a placebo-type reaction (p. 2488). He must assess the patient's common sense and exert his own. Care must be taken with those with compromised hepatic or renal function and the elderly, who easily become confused with dosage. Various aids to overcome this have been devised [1].

REFERENCES

1 ATKINSON L., *et al* (1978) *Gerontology* **24**, 225.
2 COTTERILL J.A. (1981) *Br J Dermatol* **105**, 311.

3 *Drug Ther Bull* (1981) **19**, 73.
4 EVANS L. & SPELMAN M. (1983) *Drugs* **25**, 63.
5 GOODMAN L.J. & SWARTWOUT J.E. (1981) *J Am Acad Dermatol* **5**, 711.
6 HERMANN F., *et al* (1978) *Br Med J* **ii**, 1132.
7 JOSSAY M. (1981) *101 Conseils du Dermatologie: Peau, Cheveux, Jambes, Silhouette.* Paris, Hachette.
8 REES B. (1979) *Cutis* **23**, 625.

TOPICAL THERAPY

Simple remedies [1, 7]. Advances in the science of formulation of topical agents have resulted in a number of very sophisticated applications that are available to cover almost every need in topical prescribing, but these may be expensive or not in worldwide supply. It may therefore be useful to remember the benefits that may still be obtained from the judicious use of simple, cheap agents that are readily available. They are not as elegant and may not be quite as effective in all cases; but they have a considerable overall value, especially in remote areas.

The almost forgotten pumice stone [2], used alone when the skin is wet or after applying a simple salicylic acid–propylene glycol gel [3], is very valuable for hyperkeratotic conditions and, of course, for removing the protective coating of verrucae. One of our patients with considerable hyperkeratosis of the heels preferred a 'hoof rasp' to all keratolytics. A simple aid for applying creams to inaccessible areas has been designed [4].

Various combinations of powder, glycerine, water and alcohol will produce shake lotions or 'cooling pastes' (Chapter 67). Zinc paste with 1% phenol is an effective and safe antipruritic and protective agent for pruritus ani. Potassium permanganate crystals can be diluted to form antiseptic soaks or wet dressings (see Formulary). The triphenye methane dyes and Castellani's paint, used correctly, may not be aesthetic but they are effective, particularly for mixed or fungal infections. Simple non-steroidal creams, pastes and lotions are still useful for inflammatory dermatoses [6].

Leg ulcers are often as satisfactorily treated with Eusol or Eusol and paraffin as by the many, more expensive, applications and dressings now available. 'Samaritan mixture' (Formulary) combines acetic acid with oil; we have used it as a home dressing for leg ulcers, particularly if infected by *Pseudomonas pyocyaneus*. 'Black wash' (0·5% aqueous silver nitrate) is also used for leg ulcers and for burns (although its hypotonicity makes it unsuitable for large burned areas).

Zinc cream, zinc and castor oil or a zinc paste are very effective in 'napkin dermatitis' provided the occlusive effect of plastic covering is removed [5].

Sodium chloride 0·9% with a preservative has been held to be a non-painful local anaesthetic [8] (though of short duration).

REFERENCES

1 ARNDT K.A. (1978) *Manual of Dermatologic Therapeutics.* 2nd ed. Boston, Little Brown.
2 BADEN H.P. (1980) *J Am Acad Dermatol* **2**, 29.
3 BADEN H.P., *et al* (1973) *Cutis* **12**, 787.
4 GOOLAMALI S.K. (1979) *Br J Dermatol* **10**, 723.
5 MALEVILLE J., *et al* (1982) *Rev Pediatr* **18**, 601.
6 PERRER W.J. (1980) *Cutis* **26**, 172.
7 POLANO M.K. (1984) *Topical Skin Therapeutics.* Edinburgh, Churchill Livingstone.
8 WIENER S.G. (1979) *Cutis* **23**, 342.

Topical medication in neonates and young children [7]. The neonate is particularly susceptible to the effects of drugs, whether these are given orally or absorbed percutaneously. There are important physiological differences [3] between the infant and the adult, e.g. a greater proportion of brain, liver and body fluid per unit weight, decreased plasma protein binding, immature metabolic pathways in the liver and inadequate conjugative and synthetic pathways affecting the disposal and conversion of drugs. Infants have a relatively large surface area which maximizes the effect of topical agents and the barrier function of the skin is impaired in premature babies. The absorption of hexachlorophane, for instance, caused the deaths of several infants [2].

Accepted rules for drugs based on body surface area are laid down for older infants but even these are fallacious for pre-term infants and neonates [7]. The greatest caution should be observed in applying active topical agents to these very young subjects, especially if they are repeated or capable of being rapidly absorbed.

Effects of some specific agents. The following examples serve to illustrate these limitations. *Boric acid* should not be used on the skin of infants because of its general toxicity after percutaneous absorption. Similarly, the absorption of *salicyclic acid* was responsible for 13 deaths, 10 of which were in children under the age of 3 yr [6]. The effects of the use of too frequent or too strong hexachlorophane are now well known and precautions for its use in infants have been stressed [5]. Potent *topical corticosteroids* must also be used with great discretion in young children [1], especially in the napkin and other occluded and flexural areas [4]. Suppression of the pituitary-adrenal axis is slower to return to normal than in adults.

REFERENCES

1 BURTON J.L. (1983) *Res Clin Forums* **5**, 61.
2 GOUTIERES F. & AICARDI J. (1977) *Br Med J* ii, 663.
3 MORSELLI P.L. (1976) *Clin Pharmacokinet* **1**, 81.
4 MUNRO D.D. (1976) *Br J Dermatol* **94** (Suppl. **12**) 67.
5 TRYALA E.E., *et al* (1977) *J Pediatr* **91**, 481.
6 WEISS J.F. & LEVER W.F. (1964) *Arch Dermatol* **90**, 614.
7 WEST D.P., *et al* (1981) *J Invest Dermatol* **76**, 147.

HOME HOSPITALIZATION ('MINIHOSPITALIZATION' [1]): 'HOSPITALISATION Á DOMICILE'

The increasing cost of hospital in-patient therapy and its social and domestic consequences have prompted the concept of reproducing, as far as possible, hospital conditions in the home. This implies rigid control of visitors and activities and regular supervision by a doctor and nurse. It has found favour in France and has been commended in the U.S.A. [1]. However, in the U.K. at least, the practical and logistic difficulties are considerable, e.g. supervision, elimination of house dust mite, responsibility for complications, etc. A controlled study would be of interest.

REFERENCE

1 ROTH H.L. (1981) *J Am Acad Dermatol* **5**, 239.

PHYSIOTHERAPY

Physiotherapy embraces a great number of different therapeutic procedures of which only a few have a direct application to dermatology. The alleviation of symptoms of disease by physical manoeuvres or manipulation of the environment has a long and honoured history but has become obscured and to some extent diverted from its original purpose by the attraction of drug therapy with its well-attested pharmaceutical effect.

The role of the physiotherapist has assumed greatly increased potential in recent years. Her duties have extended far from the massage and simple forms of heat and light therapy of the past; she has become an extremely experienced member of a team devoted to a wide range of physiotherapeutic manoeuvres and to rehabilitation in the widest context.

In dermatology, the physiotherapist is probably not sufficiently invited to participate in the overall management of the patient with chronic or disabling diseases. Rehabilitation is discussed below but techniques of relaxation are of undoubted bene-fit to many tense patients with irritable or vasolabile skin disease. Muscular relaxation is a key that opens the door to emotional relaxation but it requires some experience and training to use the key effectively. Relaxation techniques [13] are a valuable adjunct to drug therapy and may even supplant this. Massage and re-education in limb movement are of great practical value in patients with deforming linear scleroderma, for which we have so little to offer. The influence of communal participation of physiotherapeutic activities, in which warmth, touch and encouragement combine to create an ambience conducive to relaxation and to a feeling of positive activity should not be underestimated.

There has been renewed interest in the value of massage [3] in the treatment of lymphoedema (p. 1236) and in rosacea.

Some physiotherapists have specialized in the physiological aspects of venous leg ulceration and can with advantage participate in treatment from an early stage and continue active movement and encouragement through the period of rehabilitation.

Other modes of physical medicine such as short-wave diathermy play a small part in dermatological management. *Ultrasound* has found a secure place in the treatment of soft-tissue disease and injury [1, 2] and may occasionally be of adjuvant value in conditions such as scleroderma [10], panniculitis and other dermatological conditions affecting deeper tissues.

Acupuncture. The empirical basis on which this rested for so long has been changed by the discovery of the endorphins. Although anecdotal reports of success in the treatment of some skin disease—notably atopic dermatitis—are numerous, there have been few properly controlled studies. No acceleration of healing was found in one group of 21 patients but itching was relieved and sleep patterns improved [5]. Further studies are required.

Biofeedback techniques. These involve the induction of a learned response aimed at controlling or modifying vascular responses [4] or inappropriate bodily responses to various centrally mediated stimuli. They may reduce emotional intensification of emotional erythema and have been used to control flushing, for patients with dysidrosis whose disease flared with stress [8, 9] and in patients with atopic dermatitis [7]. However, there is considerable individual variability in responses [12] and their main value may lie in anxiety reduction [6] and in the active involvement of the patient in helping himself. It has been suggested that the techniques may be the 'ultimate placebo' [11] and their place in dermatology may remain limited by the time and patience required. Nevertheless, further developments in these methods may prove rewarding in specific dermatological situations, given a highly motivated and suitable subject.

REFERENCES

1 DYSON M. & SUCKLING J. (1978) *Physioth* **64**, 105.
2 DYSON M., *et al* (1976) *Ultrasonics* **14**, 232.
3 FOLDI M. & CASLEY-SMITH J.R. (1983) *Lymphangiology* Schattauer, p. 677.
4 FRIAR L.R. & BEATTY J. (1976) *J Consult Clin Psychol* **44**, 46.
5 GOLDSCHMITT D. & HEIBREDER G. (1981) *Med Welt* **32**, 158.
6 GREEN E.E., *et al* (1973) *Ann NY Acad Sci* **233**, 157.
7 HAYNES S.N., *et al* (1979) *Biofeedback Self Regul* **4**, 193.
8 KELLUM R.E. (1976) *Consultant* **16**, 111.
9 KOLDYS K.W. & MEYER R.P. (1979) *Cutis* **24**, 219.
10 RUDOLPH R.I. & LEYDEN J.J. (1976) *Arch Dermatol* **112**, 995.
11 STROEBEL C.F. & GLUECK B.C. (1973) In *Biofeedback: Behavioural Medicine.* Ed. Birk L. New York, Grune & Stratton.
12 VOLOW M.R., *et al* (1979) *Biofeedback Self Regul* **4**, 133.
13 WEINSTEIN D.J. (1976) *Behav Res Ther* **14**, 481.

Heliotherapy and actinotherapy [2, 4, 13, 15].
Exposure to natural sunlight has an established place in dermatological therapy. The use of artificial UV radiation was pioneered by Finsen at the turn of the century but its study has received a great stimulus in the past decade with the advent of PUVA therapy, with the increasing popular demand for a 'healthy' tan and with the increasing realization of the potential harm from any form of UV radiation. Artificial sources of UV radiation are unable to simulate natural sunlight precisely, but this should in theory give the opportunity of choosing wavelengths that are wanted for any particular purpose—if they are known.

The type of UV lamp will not be discussed in detail. PUVA is discussed on p. 1505. The carbon arc lamp is now little used. The main source of UV radiation is the mercury vapour lamp, the radiation emitted depending on the pressure within the lamp, the phosphors coating the tube and other variables, which help to provide a more continuous spectrum like that of sunlight. The Kromayer lamp was designed mainly for contact therapy. It emits considerable amounts of shorter UV radiation and is not now used very much for therapeutic purposes. Alpine sunlamps and Theraktin lamps are examples of mercury vapour lamps which have been available for many years. Recently a comparison of Philips T1-12 and Sylvaner UV6 and UV21 tubes showed them to be equivalent in effect [14]. The xenon lamp [1] emits a more continuous spectrum which makes it valuable for experimental and testing purposes but expense limits its therapeutic use.

UV lamps provide a much more powerful source of UV light than natural sunlight, although a properly designed therapeutic course of UV radiation may give an amount of radiation comparable with that from a fortnight's sunny holiday.

Dermatological uses. Where natural sunlight is lacking [3] actinotherapy may be simulated with the Alpine sunlamp or with banks of fluorescent UVB lamps. The role of UVB in the treatment of psoriasis is traditional and has been disputed but now seems to be gaining favour again (Chapter 37). Acne vulgaris may be helped by spaced exposure to E_2–E_3 doses of UVB but the effect is less dramatic than that of natural sun (p. 1928). Chilblains and erythrocyanosis respond to doses of four or more minimal erythema doses of UVB repeated three or more times (p. 626). In some clinics very short-wave (bactericidal) doses of UV radiation, given conveniently by the contact Kromayer lamp, are used for leg ulcers. The dose must be many times that of the minimal erythema dose [2].

Phototherapy is used also to treat neonatal icterus and may be helpful in controlling the pruritus of primary biliary cirrhosis [8] and uraemia [7]. Traditionally, it has been used empirically to speed resolution (or perhaps disguise the lesions) of pityriasis rosea. We also find it of definite value in pityriasis lichenoides chronica. Carefully graded exposure to natural sunlight, UVB, UVA or PUVA can also be used to cause increased pigmentation and tanning for the treatment or prophylaxis of light-sensitive dermatoses, especially polymorphic light eruption.

The influence of UV radiation on the immune system is important [4, 6].

Sun beds [5, 9]. These have achieved a considerable popularity in recent years. Some sun beds and sun tan parlours provide UVB. In England many now emit mainly or entirely UVA. As UVA is biologically very much less active than UVB, small traces of UVB in a light source can be very significant. UVA is much less effective in producing a durable tan but may achieve some [10, 11, 12]. There is little evidence that this does much towards positive health. UVA cannot be exonerated completely from causing long-term side effects and it also seems able to potentiate the harmful effects of UVB. Caution must be taken by patients with any form of light sensitivity as well as by those on photosensitizing drugs or in contact with topical photosensitizers.

REFERENCES

1 BERGER D.S. (1969) *J Invest Dermatol* **53**, 192.
2 *DIFFEY B.L. (1982) *Ultraviolet Radiation in Medicine*, Medical Physics Handbooks 11. Bristol, Adam Hilger.
3 DIFFEY B.L., *et al* (1982) *Br J Dermatol* **106**, 33.
4 Editorial (1983) *Lancet* **i**, 566.
5 EPSTEIN J.H. (1981) *South Med J* **74**, 837.
6 FOX I.J., *et al* (1980) *Clin Immunol Immunopath* **17**, 141.
7 GILCHREST B.A., *et al* (1977) *N Engl J Med* **297**, 136.
8 HANID M.A. & LEVI A.J. (1980) *Lancet* **ii**, 530.
9 HAWK J.L.M. (1982) *Br Med J* **286**, 329.
10 KAIDBEY K.H. & KLIGMAN A.M. (1976) *Arch Dermatol* **109**, 674.
11 KAIDBEY K.H. & KLIGMAN A.M. (1978) *Arch Dermatol* **114**, 46.
12 LANGNER A. & KLIGMAN A.M. (1972) *Arch Dermatol* **106**, 338.
13 *MAGNUS I.A. (1976) *Dermatological Photobiology*. Oxford, Blackwell Scientific.
14 SCHOTHORST A.A., *et al* (1984) *Br J Dermatol* **110**, 81.
15 WADSWORTH H. & CHANMUGAM A.P.P. (1980) *Electrophysical Agents in Physiotherapy*. Australia, Science Press.

Hypothermia and hyperthermia. Cooling of the scalp to 25° with ice turban packs or chemical coolants has been used to prevent or reduce hair loss during the critical period after administration of chemotherapeutic drugs [2].

Because of the demonstration of the potential of hyperthermia as an antitumour agent [1, 5], there have been occasional reports of its value in treating deep mycoses [6], leishmaniasis and mycobacterial infections [8]. The similarity between the kinetics of tumour cells and of psoriasis cells have prompted its use in the form of ultrasound in this disease [3, 4]. More recently, chemically generated heat in exothermic bags was used in 22 psoriatics in a comparison with Goeckerman's regime [7], with apparent success and without side effects. This convenient form of therapy requires further study.

REFERENCES

1 CALALIERE R., *et al* (1967) *Cancer* **20**, 1351.
2 GUY R., *et al* (1982) *Lancet* **i**, 937.
3 ORENBERG E.K., *et al* (1979) *J Invest Dermatol* **72**, 199.
4 ORENBERG E.K., *et al* (1980) *Arch Dermatol* **116**, 893.
5 SUIT H.D. & SHWAYDER M. (1974) *Cancer* **34**, 122.
6 TAGAMI H., *et al* (1979) *Arch Dermatol* **115**, 740.
7 URABE H., *et al* (1981) *Arch Dermatol* **117**, 770.
8 YAMAMOTO T., *et al* (1977) *Jpn J Clin Dermatol* **27**, 951.

CLIMATOTHERAPY [4, 5]

The influence of a calm and restful environment is of undoubted value in the treatment of disease in which emotional factors may be playing a part—even a secondary one. When this environment includes constant sunshine, particularly at the seaside [3], conditions such as acne and psoriasis will usually benefit. Where high altitude sanitoria or convalescent homes are readily available, as in many parts of continental Europe, a reduction in airborne allergens can be expected to help some atopic patients [2]. Psoriatics have undoubtedly benefited greatly by visits to the Dead Sea [1] and other specialized centres in Europe (p. 1493). It is difficult for those of us who do not have the advantages of these retreats to assess realistically the more specific claims made for them in relation to alterations in enzymes, vitamin levels [7] and cutaneous reactivity [6], but the psychological benefits are undoubted and may be long lasting.

REFERENCES

1 AVRACH W.W. & NIORDSEN A.M. (1974) *Ugeskr Laeger* **136**, 2687.
2 CABARIEU G., *et al* (1974) *Rev Fr Allergol* **14**, 63.
3 MOLIN L. (1972) *Acta Derm Venereol (Stockh)* **52**, 152.
4 POPCHRISTOV P. & BALEVSKA N. (1966) *Hochgebirgsklimatherapie und Thalasotherapie Hautkranker in Bulgarien*. Sofia, Med. Fiskultura.
5 PÜRSCHEL W. (1973) *Dermatologica* **146** (Suppl. 1) 1.
6 PÜRSCHEL W., *et al* (1980) *Z Hautkr* **55**, 193.
7 ZLATKOV N.B., *et al* (1976) *Dermatol Monatsschr* **162**, 746.

ABREACTIVE THERAPY

This technique, used widely after the last war [1] to explore and exteriorize tensions in patients suffering from a number of diseases thought to be causally related, appeared to be of value at the time. However, it has been little used in recent years [3]. Interested readers are referred to the earlier texts [1, 2].

REFERENCES

1 SHORVON H.J., *et al* (1950) *Br Med J* **ii**, 1300.
2 SLATER E. & ROTH M. (1969) *Clinical Psychiatry*. London, Balliere.
3 WHITLOCK F.A. (1976) *Psychophysiological Aspects of Skin Disease*. Vol. 8. *Major Problems in Dermatology*. Ed. Rook A.J. London, Saunders.

HYPNOTHERAPY [6, 15]

In contrast, this has become a more acceptable and more widely used mode of therapy in recent years, particularly since the discovery of endorphins [12]. Hypnosis is defined as 'an unusual or altered state of consciousness in which distortions of perception ... occur as uncritical responses of the subject to notions from an objective source ... or a subjective source ... or both [7]. As such, it has an honourable and long history in European culture, as shown in the rites of Dionysus and the catharsis associated with them. Hypnotic experiences resemble those seen in subjects who may normally have a heightened capacity for dissociation, e.g. from pain, or for the production of pseudoparalyses of hysterical type. Similar, though milder, distortions of perception occur spontaneously, like those occuring just before sleep or as the result of repetitive monotonous or rhythmical sensory stimuli [3]. No absolute physiological definition is possible—and this has been one reason for the reluctance to accept hypnotherapy as a valid therapeutic act—but EEG changes occur on entry into and during the maintenance of hypnosis [4]. Another reason for reservations about the value of hypnotherapy lies in the unproven [14] and rather vague claims of the role of the 'neurovegetative' system in the aetiology of a number of chronic skin diseases of unknown pathology [12]. A balanced view is that, while organic lesions cannot be expected to alter, the tolerance to pain or discomfort can be raised and anxiety about the diease alleviated [6, 9]. When the technique of autohypnosis has been mastered—and this is not difficult—the patient develops an increasing tolerance to somatic problems and 'the quality of existence is thereby improved' [6]. Its main value, therefore, may lie in teaching this to patients with diseases which have a large quotient of anxiety—asthma, hyperventilation, enuresis, trigeminal neuralgia, migraine, etc. [1]. Autohypnosis is to be distinguished from suggestion given in the conscious state to influence the effect of conventional treatment or to modify symptoms, and from relaxation techniques [13].

Claims of the value of hypnotherapy in dermatological disorders are based on its supposed ability to modify the perception of itching and to influence peripheral vascular reactivity. Earlier reports of its success in the treatment of warts [5, 10, 11] and in the suppression of tuberculin reactions have not led to any further significant advances in this field, perhaps because the technique is seldom used by dermatologists and has not been subjected to repeated critical assessment.

Undoubtedly, hypnotherapy and autohypnosis, under proper conditions, can help reduce dependence on drugs [15], can aid the restoration of sleep patterns and can improve abnormal behavioural patterns in blushing, nail-biting and—perhaps—trichotillomania [3, 8]. Single case reports are not fully convincing, however. Psychosexual problems are probably helped [2] in so far as the anxiety surrounding them is concerned.

A valid objection to hypnotherapy is that it allays symptoms without removing their cause, but this is equally true of much other therapy. However, until properly controlled and long-term follow-up studies are available, judgement must be reserved.

REFERENCES

1 ANDERSON J., *et al* (1975) *Int J Clin Exp Hypn* **23**, 48.
2 FABBRI R. (1976) *Am J Clin Hypn* **19**, 5.
3 GAISKI T.J. (1981) *Am J Clin Hypn* **23**, 198.
4 HILGARD E. & HILGARD J. (1975) *Hypnosis in the Relief of Pain*. Los Altos, California, Kaufmann.
5 JOHNSON R.F. & BARBER T.X. (1978) *Am J Clin Hypn* **20**, 165.
6 *MAYER-LOUGHMAN G.P. (1980) *Br J Hosp Med* **23**, 447.
7 MELLETT P. (1980) *Br J Hosp Med* **23**, 441.
8 ROWEN R. (1981) *Am J Clin Hypn* **23**, 195.
9 SCHAFER D.W. (1975) *Int J Clin Exp Hypn* **23**, 1.
10 SHEEHAN D.V. (1978) *Am J Clin Hypn* **20**, 160.
11 SINCLAIR-GIEBEN A.H.C. & CHALMERS D. (1969) *Lancet* **ii**, 480.
12 TOBIA L. (1982) *Minerva Med* **73**, 531.
13 WEINSTEIN D.J. (1976) *Behav Res Ther* **14**, 481.
14 WHITLOCK F.A. (1976) *Psychophysiological Aspects of Skin Disease*. Vol. 8. *Major Problems in Dermatology*. Ed. Rook A.J. London, Saunders, p. 237.
15 *WILKINSON J.B. (1981) *J R Soc Med* **74**, 525.

OCCUPATIONAL THERAPY AND REHABILITATION [1, 3, 6, 16]

Occupational therapy. A person conditioned to an active life does not take kindly to bed-rest. Patients with skin diseases should be encouraged to become mobile as soon as their state allows it. Those with leg ulcers should not be kept in bed for long periods but should be subjected to active and passive leg exercises to reduce the risk of thrombosis, foot drop and atrophy of the leg muscles. They should be encouraged to walk for increasing periods with re-education of their leg movements, rather than to sit. The elderly patient with exfoliative dermatitis or pemphigus should be stimulated to pass his time without boredom, which passes imperceptibly in the aged into depression and despondency. In the alien milieu of a hospital ward he very quickly deteriorates mentally and physically. Subsequent discharge or rehabilitation may then be extremely difficult. An effort of imagination and will is needed by the dermatologist and his staff to recognize the particular needs and limitations of old age. Occupational therapy should not only engage manual skill but also satisfy the emotional and intellectual needs of the patient.

The young breadwinner of the family in hospital becomes anxious about his ability to return to work. The medical social worker, as part of the dermatological team, should make contact with him and, if necessary, with his family. Whatever his disease, he may not have had any full explanation of it and its probable future course. His stay in hospital will be doubly worthwhile if he is helped to adjust to it, rather than brooding on it. Group therapy for those with chronic skin diseases if of distinct value [1] but difficult to organize under the usual conditions of practice. However, with the current increasing emphasis on community medicine, there is scope for a greater awareness and provision of facilities of this type. The mutual aid and advice given by the Eczema Society and the National Psoriasis Association and similar bodies [11–13] in other countries can be invaluable. Jopling [11–13] has pointed out the social disadvantages and anxieties felt (though perhaps not openly expressed) by those with persistent psoriasis. Such social considerations should be as much in the mind of the dermatologist as is the essential treatment of the condition. Psychosocial factors are also prevalent amongst patients with severe or persistent facial lesions, although often concealed by them [3]. We shall now consider some specific groups of patients in whom problems of readjustment or rehabilitation may be important.

The young manual worker [9, 17]. He is often anxious about his future working capacity. This should be assessed after all relevant investigations have been carried out. With his consent, contact with his firm's medical officer, as well as his general practitioner, should be routine and the results of patch tests etc. should be conveyed with an interpretation that is relevant to his occupation. The medical social worker will be able to help in advising him and his family; ideally, a case conference should be held on each such patient. It is easy for a doctor to regard chronic hand dermatitis as a minor condition for which repetition of a corticosteroid cream is the only remedy, but to a worker its existence may mean the difference between a livelihood or disablement. His anxieties may not be readily revealed and may require patience to uncover. Re-education in working procedures, an ex-

planation of irritant (or allergic) dermatitis and attention to the causes of persistence and relapse [17] should be part of the normal procedure of 'treatment'. Readjustment of work may be possible, by contact with the personnel officer of his factory; advice to 'leave the job' may not only be demoralizing but, in some instances [7], ineffective. After suffering a severe attack of dermatitis a patient is likely to be suspicious of any agent he handles on return to work, but he should be encouraged to persist at work during the first critical weeks in which non-specific factors may temporarily exacerbate the condition. He should be seen at intervals for at least 3 months after return to work. The employers should be willing to grant him time to attend hospital for this purpose.

The disabled patient. There are two categories.

With occupational dermatitis [1, 9, 15]. When a worker's skin has irrevocably broken down, a course of retraining may enable him to learn a new craft. The value of such courses, however, is limited by the age, intelligence and adaptability of the patient and the extent of the residual disability. The difficulties are considerable and the ultimate prognosis in many cases remains poor [2, 9], especially among dichromate-sensitive patients [4, 7]. An attempt should be made to assess each patient's disability as accurately as possible [5]. The subject is discussed further in Chapter 16.

With other diseases. The elderly patient admitted with leg ulcers, particularly those of arterial type or those in rheumatoid patients, poses extremely difficult problems for rehabilitation at home. This is easier in countries that still have a culture of strong family ties. In others, the medical social worker and the geriatricians should always be involved. Similar conditions apply to patients disabled with multiple sclerosis, systemic sclerosis, etc. There, however, special State provisions and the support of national societies afford considerable help.

The housewife. Her anxieties centre round her family responsibilties and home commitments. The more obsessional she is, the more anxious she will be. Relatives must play their part in her recovery by reassurance and a show of competence in managing in her absence. Depression may occur as a reaction to immobilization and isolation. Anxiety, itching and sleeplessness contribute to this and adequate sedation is always helpful in the early days of in-patient treatment. As the dermatitis improves, increasing rehabilitation should be started. The causes of persistence or relapse in her everyday life should be explained [9]. 'Give-out' explantory sheets can be valuable reminders.

The young atopic patient. The problems here are often those of personality and environmental stresses rather than of working conditions. Apparent resolution in the protected environment of a hospital ward does not always survive exposure to the harsher emotional winds of outside life. However, a temporary withdrawal from an adverse environment is always helpful.

Children with infantile eczema. The main need is for dialogue with the parents [8] and sustained contact to help relieve the inevitable tensions and emotional stresses that the condition imposes on them. Special problems arise in the rare cases in which hospital admission is required [14]. This is best dealt with in children's units. A joint control, with the nursing staff equipped with the special requirements of sick children and the expertise in basic dermatological therapy, is invaluable. The mother should usually be encouraged to participate in the ward activity and will gain confidence in helping in the management of the problem.

The older dermatologically ill child. Children with disabling or disfiguring diseases demand special attention towards adjustment to the various epochs of their life—relationships with other children, the first school, and the passage through puberty. Play and companionship in the early years mark the transition from maternal social relationships. Disfigurement or disease is always a source of childish cruelty, and integration into the social group requires much skilled help from nursing staff and 'mother figures'. It can be greatly helped by a dermatologist aware of the problem. The transition to school and the pressure of examinations call for guidance and careful management. The difficulties of a spastic child or a deaf mute are evident enough to arouse sympathy. The emotionally volatile, scratching atopic or the obviously disfigured child receives less sympathy and attention, though his needs are as great and his potentialities often greater.

The psoriatic patient. The stigma attached to the patient with evident plaques of psoriasis is evident especially in public places and his confidence is undermined by his appearance. The National Psoriasis Association have done a great deal to break down this 'taboo' [11, 13]. The ability to learn to live with the disease [11, 12] is paramount but a great deal of support is often needed to achieve this. The dermatologist has his part to play but this must be supplemented by nurses, physiotherapists and the community at large. The concept of the 'day centre' combines effective therapy with personal and communal participation but is unfortunately available in only a few countries. It would be in the interest of all those suffering from this disease if such facilities were expanded.

REFERENCES

1 ADAMS R.M. (1983) *Occupational Skin Disease*. New York, Grune & Stratton, p. 174.
2 BANDMANN H.J. & AGATHOS M. (1982) In *Occupational and Industrial Dermatology*. Eds. Maibach H.I. & Gellin G.A. Chicago, Year Book Medical Publishers, p. 157.
3 BERSCHEID B., *et al* (1983) *Clin Plast Surg* 9, 289.
4 BREIT B. & TURK B.M. (1976) *Br J Dermatol* 94, 349.
5 CHURCH R. (1985) In *Essentials of Industrial Dermatology*. Eds. Griffiths W.A.D. & Wilkinson D.S. Oxford, Blackwell Scientific 85.
6 COLES R.B. (1959) *Almoner* ii, 466.
7 CZARNECKI N. (1979) *Hautarzt* 30, 80.
8 EMMERSON R.W. (1979) In *Modern Topics in Paediatric Dermatology*. Ed. Verbov J. London, Heinemann, p. 55.
9 FREGERT S. (1975) *Contact Dermatitis* 1, 96.
10 GRIFFITHS A. (1985) In *Essentials of Industrial Dermatology*. Eds. Griffiths W.A.D. & Wilkinson D.S. Oxford, Blackwell Scientific 1.
11 JOPLING R. (1976) *Clin Exp Dermatol* 1, 233.
12 JOPLING R.G. (1977) In *Medical Encounters*. Eds. Davis A. & Horobin G. London, Helm.
13 JOPLING R. & COLES R.B (1984) In *Psoriasis*. Eds. Roenick H.H. & Maibach H.I. New York, Dekker.
14 MACCARTHY D., *et al* (1962) *Lancet* i, 603.
15 SAMITZ M.H. (1982) In *Occupational and Industrial Dermatology*. Eds. Maibach H.I. & Gellin G.A. Chicago, Year Book Medical Publishers, p. 165.
16 WILKINSON D.S. (1977) *The Nursing and Management of Skin Disease*. 4th ed. London, Faber.
17 WILKINSON D.S. (1985) In Essentials of Industrial Dermatology. Eds Griffiths W.A.D. & Wilkinson D.S. Oxford, Blackwell Scientific 111.

DIETARY REGIMES

The value of dietary regimes in the treatment of most skin diseases has not been proven. Some exceptions to this rule are discussed below but even these are not universally accepted. There has been a renewed interest in this subject in recent years in Western Europe and the U.S.A., stimulated in part by the media and in part by a general trend towards reduced dependence on drugs and a return to a belief in 'simplistic' medicine. Sensible advice on diet, aimed chiefly at the obese or those overweight for their age and height plays an obvious part in the treatment of conditions such as intertrigo and gravitational eczema or leg ulceration.

The effects of malnutrition, unfortunately still prevalent in many parts of the world, need no underlining or emphasis in this text. But relative malnutrition may occur in any patient with anorexia nervosa, carcinomatosis and, especially, carcinoma of the throat or oesophagus. Bowel-shortening operations, total parenteral nutrition and pre-colectomy dietary regimes have led to selective deficiencies, e.g. of fatty acids or zinc [16, 17, 21], but this has now been recognized and corrected.

Even in advanced industrial communities, quite marked malnutrition is seen in elderly people living alone, in whom financial stringency, apathy, boredom or immobility lead to a diet deficient in folic or ascorbic acid or even in protein itself. Chronic alcoholics may suffer from avitaminosis or from general malnutrition. A growing group of 'food faddists' (and a smaller group of those believing themselves to suffer from 'total allergy') may also become deprived of essential vitamin or protein requirement.

Although the dermatologists in Europe and the U.S.A. do not generally need to concern themselves with vitamin therapy, elderly alcoholics or misguided patients are still admitted to dermatological wards with scurvy or gross vitamin B complex deficiency, both of which may be unrecognized.

Whenever there is doubt, it is simpler and cheaper to give ascorbic acid than to attempt to measure serum levels; a gradual return to a full and balanced diet may, in the apathetic, require sip-feeds with protein-containing supplements and possibly added vitamins. Intramuscular high potency vitamin supplements and vitamin B_{12} are of value, especially in alcoholics. Nasal drip feeding is sometimes indicated.

Food metabolites and toxins [4]. Technical advances in recent years have greatly extended our knowledge of foods and their metabolites. It has been suggested [15] that some food peptides can act as exogenous 'hormones'. Such 'exorphens', e.g. those derived from milk or wheat protein, have an opiate-like activity, which will be lacking in patients on a gluten-free diet. The importance of trace elements such as zinc is now fully established but there is increasing interest in plant-derived toxins and 'microtoxins' [11] such as protease inhibitors, haemagglutinins, goitrogens, cyanogens (? cause of tropical ataxic neuropathy), glossypol, etc. Fortunately, cooking destroys many of these but they are not without importance in poorer countries, where

the diet may be heavily biased towards one plant product.

Special dietary regimes. These are obligatory in some genetic conditions and in some diseases of metabolic origin, useful in the control of a few important dermatological conditions, and of disputed value in some others.

Genetic conditions. Phenylketonuria and Refsum's disease are well-known examples, the control of tyrosinaemia II a more recent one [13]. They are discussed in Chapter 62.

Metabolic diseases. Diabetes is, of course, the best-known example. Hypercholesterolaemic xanthomatosis benefits from a strict limitation of dietary cholesterol. Patients with carotinaemia must avoid carotenoids.

Atopic eczema [1, 2]. There has been a revival of interest in dietary factors in this disease in recent years, particularly on the part of allergists. The RAST test and the scratch-chamber technique [9] have given this interest further stimulus, although the difficulty of relating the results of these tests to the history has not been completely resolved [3]. The subject is extremely complicated and still under intense investigation. It is discussed in detail in Chapter 13.

Chronic urticaria (see Chapter 29). The extent of food allergens in the causation of chronic urticaria is still disputed. In the management of a condition that is so tedious and prolonged, it is always worthwhile considering carefully planned exclusion diets.

Sensitivity to *food dyes* and *preservatives* is responsible for a modest proportion of cases of chronic urticaria [5, 14, 18, 20]. If the history, supplemented by a diary, fails to incriminate the cause, a diet free from these agents [3, 14] may be used as a diagnostic manoeuvre. Intolerance to other drugs or foodstuffs may coexist [18], a complicating factor in assessment.

Yeasts, another possible cause [12], are present in bread, sausage, wine, beer, Marmite and yeast tablets [3]. Other responsible chemical substances or constituents include salicylates [14], sulphur dioxide, quinine, menthol and possibly food flavourings.

Dermatitis herpetiformis [7, 8, 10]. Despite initial doubt, withdrawal of dietary gluten appears to be of definite benefit in patients with this disease. Of 42 patients treated with a gluten-free diet, 71%

were able to discontinue drugs after a mean period of 29 months, although a reduction in dose became possible after a mean period of 8 months. Only five of 30 patients on a normal diet (14%) were able to do so [8]. But the improvement in the skin condition and the intestinal intra-epithelioid lymphocyte count were closely related to the strictness with which the diet was carried out.

A dietician's advice is invaluable as is the advice and encouragement given by belonging to the Coeliac Society. Very rarely it may be necessary to add a milk-free diet [6, 7].

Drug regimes. Patients taking monoamine oxidase inhibitors must avoid foods containing amines. Corticosteroids are catabolic and extra milk and protein (and possibly anabolic steroids) may be needed in elderly patients on long-term treatment.

Claims made for special diets in a number of common diseases such as psoriasis and acne have not been convincing, though there was some reduction of pain and frequency of aphthous ulcers in patients on a gluten-free diet [19]. This requires further investigation. Although a fasting diet gave some temporary benefits to patients with atopic eczema, rosacea and palmoplantar pustulosis [12], change to a vegetarian diet caused regression. The authors of this study believed that the improvement during fasting might be related to neutrophil leukocyte turnover as reflected by the serum concentration of lactoferrin.

REFERENCES

1 ATHERTON D.J., *et al* (1978) *Lancet* i, 401.
2 ATHERTON D.J., *et al* (1982) In *Food Allergy. Clinics in Immunology and Allergy*, Eds. Brostoff J. & Challacombe S.J. 2nd ed. London, Saunders, p. 77.
3 AUGUST P.J. (1980) In *Proc. First Food Allergy Workshop, 1980*. Oxford, Medical Education Services, Medicine, p. 76.
4 CROUNSE R.G. (1982) *J Am Acad Dermatol* 7, 400.
5 DOEGLAS H.M.G. (1975) *Br J Dermatol* 93, 135.
6 ENQUIST A. & POCK-STEEN O.C.L. (1971) *Lancet* ii, 438.
7 FRY L. (1982) *Clin Exp Dermatol* 7, 633.
8 FRY L., *et al* (1982) *Br J Dermatol* 107, 631.
9 HANNUKSELA M. (1980) *Acta Derm Venereol* (Suppl) (Stockh) 92, 44.
10 KATZ S.I. (1980) *Ann Intern Med* 93, 857.
11 LIENER I.E. (1980) *Toxic Constituents of Plant Foodstuffs*. 2nd ed. New York, Academic Press.
12 LITHELL H., *et al* (1983) *Acta Derm Venereol* (Stockh) 63, 397.
13 MACHINO H., *et al* (1983) *J Am Acad Dermatol* 9, 533.
14 MICHAELSSON G. & JUHLIN L. (1983) *Br J Dermatol* 88, 525.
15 MORLEY J.E. (1982) *JAMA* 247, 2379.
16 PROTTEY C., *et al* (1975) *J Invest Dermatol* 64, 228.
17 RIALLA M.C., *et al* (1975) *Ann Intern Med* 83, 786.
18 RUDZKI E., *et al* (1980) *Dermatologica* 161, 57.
19 WALKER D.M., *et al* (1980) *Br J Dermatol* 103, 111.
20 WARIN R.P. & SMITH R.J. (1976) *Br J Dermatol* 94, 401.
21 WEISMANN K., *et al* (1976) *Clin Exp Dermatol* 1, 237.

Parenteral nutrition. Since this is a regulated form of feeding, it should be mentioned in the context of diets. Although chiefly used as a form of therapy, it may serve as a form of nutrition in some countries. Advances in nutritional expertise in the last decade have demonstrated the importance of incorporating vitamins and trace elements in the basic solutions of dextrose, soya bean oil emulsion, synthetic L-amino acids, etc. The metabolism of these constituents varies in normal, starved and semi-stressed subjects [2]. Lipids have been introduced as a source of calories and newer substrates. such as branched chain amino acids, their keto analogues and synthetic glycerides and maltose, are being developed.

Different techniques have been applied to particular circumstances [3], but the indications are almost entirely confined to surgical or medical situations in which the gastrointestinal canal is unable to function properly and the dermatological indications are likely to be few and oblique. Monitoring is essential and complications—of which there are many—are best avoided by a team approach [1].

REFERENCES

1 NEHME A.E. (1980) *JAMA* 243, 1906.
2 PHILLIPS G.D. & ODGERS C.L. (1982) *Drugs* 23, 276.
3 SELTZER M.H., *et al* (1981) *J Parenter Ent Nutr* 5, 70.

THE EMERGENCY TREATMENT OF ANAPHYLAXIS [1]

Anaphylaxis is unpredictable and is liable to occur at any time as the result of the introduction of an antigen into the blood stream of a sensitized person. Its severity is determined by the sensitivity of the recipient and the amount and rate of absorption of the antigen. Whenever there is a possibility of anaphylaxis occurring during tests or desensitization, particularly of atopic subjects, with 'prick' or injected antigens, adequate measures must be at hand for immediate treatment. Anaphylaxis develops with alarming speed, the patient becoming unconscious within a minute or two of the onset. Death can occur almost instantaneously.

Anaphylactoid reactions have occurred with epidermal occlusive and open testing of contact-urticaria-eliciting agents [4, 5] and after exercise in patients with cholinergic urticaria [3].

It has also occurred by exercise induction of cholinergic urticaria [3], a diagnostic test sometimes used in hospital.

Two precautions can be taken. Skin testing in atopic subjects or in those suspected of being acutely sensitive to an antigen should be carried out with great discretion, the weakest available strength being used and the procedure confined to prick testing. Care in desensitization should follow the accepted sequence of intracutaneous, subcutaneous and then intramuscular injections, increasing the dose steadily and never exceeding initially, when changing to a new route of injection, the highest dose attained by the preceding one.

An emergency tray containing the following items must always be at hand: *adrenaline* 1/1000 as individual dose phials (with a glass scourer if needed); *injectable antihistamine* such as diphenhydramine hydrochloride; *hydrocortisone hemisuccinate* for intravenous or intramuscular injections; *aminophylline* for intravenous injection; an *anaesthetic airway*; a *sterile scalpel and forceps* for cutting down on veins or, in an emergency, for tracheotomy; a *tourniquet*. Oxygen and suction apparatus should always be within call.

At the onset of anaphylactic shock an airway is inserted, a tourniquet applied above the point of entry and 0·5 ml adrenaline 1/1000 injected into and around the site. The remainder of the dose of 1 ml should be given subcutaneously or, if the attack is severe, 0·1 ml intravenously, given during 1 min. The subcutaneous dose may be repeated in 5–15 min. Rubbing the injection site hastens absorption [2]. An antihistamine is given intramuscularly or intravenously and hydrocortisone hemisuccinate prepared for intravenous injection if the patient shows no sign of responding within 2–3 min. The veins will be collapsed and it may be necessary to cut down on them. If the attack is not too severe the injection may be given intramuscularly. But if it is needed at all it is usually needed rapidly.

REFERENCES

1 AUSTEN K.F. (1965) *JAMA* **192**, 108.
2 ** Drug Ther Bull* (1965) 3, 93.
3 KAPLAN A.P., *et al* (1981) *J Allergy Clin Immunol* **68**, 319.
4 VON KROGH G. & MAIBACH H.I. (1982) *Semin Dermatol* 1, 59.
5 VON PEVNY I., *et al* (1981) *Dermatosen* **29**, 123.

CHAPTER 66

Systemic Therapy

R.J. PYE, S.O.B. ROBERTS & R.H. CHAMPION

INTRODUCTION

Although many patients consider that topical therapy is a feeble way to treat the skin, this remains the most logical way to treat many skin diseases and with a minimal risk of systemic toxicity. However, there are a number of drugs where an adequate effect can be achieved only by the systemic route. Some of these drugs, e.g. antibiotics, are used in specific ways by dermatologists. A brief survey of some of the more important drugs or those used in special ways in dermatology will be given here, with no attempt to describe the pharmacology in detail. Other drugs are described elsewhere in these volumes.

The important subject of drug interaction is referred to on p. 1241. The particular problems of prescribing for special groups, such as children, pregnant women, lactating women and the elderly are dealt with in some detail in the *British National Formulary* [3] (and other national formularies), as are the difficulties in prescribing for patients with liver failure, renal failure and diseases affecting other organs. Where there is any doubt the advice of a clinical pharmacologist, a pharmacist or the drug manufacturer should be sought or information obtained from such reference works as *Martindale* [5] and Goodman and Gilman [4] or specialized monographs [2]. The *ABPI Data Sheet Compendium* [1] is also valuable. The dosage for children is often calculated roughly on the basis of age, but should more accurately be based on body weight or, even better, body surface [3].

REFERENCES

1 Association of British Pharmaceutical Industry (1984–5) *ABPI Data Sheet Compendium*. London, Datapharm.
2 BICKERS D.R., *et al* (1984) *Clinical Pharmacology of Skin Disease*. New York, Churchill Livingstone.
3 *British National Formulary No 11* (1986) London, British Medical Association, and the Pharmaceutical Society of Great Britain.
4 GILMAN A.G., *et al* (1985) *Goodman & Gilman's The Pharmacological Basis of Therapeutics*. 7th ed. New York, MacMillan.
5 REYNOLDS J.E.F. (1982) *Martindale. The Extra Pharmacopoeia*. 28th ed. London, Pharmaceutical Press.

CORTICOSTEROIDS

Adrenocorticortrophic hormone (ACTH): corticotrophin. In general, the effects are those of adrenocortical hormones including mineralocorticoids, but since the stimulation is on the gland itself the response is inevitably more varied and complex than that of a single glucocorticoid.

Corticotrophin and its synthetic analogue tetracosactrin have little therapeutic advantage and are mainly used as diagnostic agents in endocrinology. The theoretical advantages of corticotrophin and its analogues include the fact that the adrenal cortex is not suppressed (although the pituitary is) and that growth in children may proceed normally. However, these are outweighed by the limited and unpredictable response of the adrenals.

Adverse effects. The injection may occasionally be painful and generalized allergic reactions may occur with ACTH or rarely with tetracosactrin [1]. Otherwise, their side effects are those of corticosteroids (see below) except that they also exert a mineralocorticoid effect with sodium retention, oedema and hypertension. Increased pigmentation may occur and increased amounts of weak androgens are secreted. It is possible that the reported absence of dermal atrophy in patients treated with ACTH for prolonged periods [5] may be because androgens exert a protective action and prevent the inhibitory effects of glucocorticoids on fibroblasts [7].

Dose and method of use. Depot preparations of corticosteroids (20–100 i.u.) or tetracosactrin (0·5–2 mg) are given intramuscularly or subcutaneously every 2–4 days and the dose and frequency of injection are reduced as soon as the patient responds.

No specific dose can be recommended as being equivalent to a given dose of corticosteroids and it is usual to titrate the dose against the clinical response, although the plasma cortisol may be monitored instead.

Adrenocortical steroids (corticosteroids). In contrast with ACTH, these are well absorbed from the gastrointestinal tract. Intravenous injection produces immediate and dramatic effects.

These steroid hormones are used in dermatology in four ways: parenterally, orally, topically and intralesionally. The last two modes are dealt with on p. 2559 and 2598. Unless a very rapid effect is needed, or gross malnutrition or inability to swallow is present, the corticosteroids are normally given orally.

The plasma cortisol is at its highest in the morning and at its lowest around midnight. The hypothalamic–pituitary–adrenal (HPA) axis is controlled by the night value and, if this is high, then the increase in plasma ACTH which would normally follow is suppressed. A single morning dose therefore causes less adrenal suppression than the same dose divided throughout the day [9]. Indeed, alternate day therapy greatly reduces undesirable side effects and numerous workers have obtained disease control at least as good as that with daily treatment in a wide variety of conditions, including steroid-responsive dermatoses [4, 11]. Almost normal ACTH responsiveness was found when 80 mg prednisone was given on alternate days [6] and children's growth continued normally on alternate day doses of prednisone up to 14 mg [12]. However, there are no conclusive studies in skin diseases to show that side effects are reduced by alternate day therapy without some loss of therapeutic activity.

For routine oral use, prednisolone (or prednisone which is converted to prednisolone in the liver) is preferred. Enteric-coated tablets are available but absorption from them may be less reliable. Dexamethasone and betamethasone have a longer action and cause adrenal suppression more readily. Triamcinolone seems to be more effective in psoriasis than other non-fluorinated steroids; however, it is rare for such therapy to be indicated, if at all. It also causes more muscle wasting than other steroids [3].

Dose of corticosteroids. This varies greatly with the condition being treated. In pemphigus the initial dose is usually high (80–180 mg a day). There are also enthusiasts who use pulse therapy of 1,000–2,000 mg prednisolone or equivalent intravenously for the treatment of severe dermatoses. In self-limiting conditions the usual oral dose is of the order of 20–40 mg daily, declining over 10–21 days in slowly reducing doses. In 'tailing-off' prednisolone, the dose should be reduced gradually.

When an immediate effect is required, as in anaphylactic reactions, 50–200 mg of hydrocortisone is injected intravenously or intramuscularly and repeated, if necessary, but adrenaline subcutaneously or intramuscularly is usually to be preferred for a quick action.

Adverse effects [10]. These are numerous and are so well known that they need only be summarized here.

Carbohydrate metabolism. Hyperglycaemia and glycosuria may occur especially in 'latent diabetics'.

Lipid metabolism. Deposition of fat in the form of the 'buffalo hump' and 'moon face' may occur. The mechanism is obscure.

Electrolytes. There is sodium retention and potassium loss. The plasma proteins may concentrate. An increased blood viscosity may induce thrombosis. The renal tubules reabsorb more water, leading to oedema. The normal diuretic response to the administration of water is reduced.

These effects of corticosteroids require continuous observation and biochemical assessment. In prolonged courses, or with high doses, potassium salts may need to be given.

Other effects. The skin may develop red or purple striae; hirsutism occurs or is increased by large doses; there is delayed healing of wounds, due to reduced fibroblastic activity. Inhibition of connective tissue cell reaction prevents the normal 'walling-off' of infective foci and predisposes to spread of infection. Osteoporosis, hypertension and cardiac failure may occur. Increased vascular fragility is not dangerous but venous thrombosis may cause pulmonary infarction and death. An increase in the incidence of gastric ulceration occurs; 'silent' bleeding presents a particular hazard. The central nervous system may show EEG abnormalities; convulsions may occur in children and psychotic episodes in adults. Myopathy particularly occurs with triamcinolone. Posterior subcapsular cataracts, aseptic necrosis of bone and arteritis are all further hazards.

The short-term administration of adrenocorticosteroids may be life-saving or afford a considerable amelioration of the misery of an acutely ill patient, and the risks are usually small; long-term administration should be undertaken only after weighing up the balance of the advantages and the possible dangers.

Indications for systemic corticosteroids. The main dermatological uses of oral and parenteral corticosteroids are as follows:

(i) as a short cover for acute and severe reactions running a defined course, e.g. severe erythema multiforme of Stevens Johnson type, acute urticaria of known cause, autosensitization eczema, lichen planus, severe drug eruptions and, rarely, acute contact sensitivities, particularly those due to *Rhus toxicodendron*;

(ii) for certain acute allergic or anaphylactic reactions carrying danger to life, e.g. anaphylactic shock (after adrenaline), multiple bee or wasp stings, poisonous bites;

(iii) in severe or generalized immunological disorders, e.g. systemic lupus erythematosus, active dermatomyositis and pyoderma gangrenosum;

(iv) in certain generalized vascular disorders of supposed immunological pathogenesis, e.g. polyarteritis nodosa, temporal arteritis, Wegener's granulomatosis, thrombocytopenic purpura and some cases of allergic vasculitis when vital organs are involved;

(v) for certain chronic disorders otherwise fatal or disabling, e.g. pemphigus, pemphigoid, benign mucous membrane pemphigoid and exfoliative dermatitis;

(vi) with rather variable efficacy in some miscellaneous conditions such as epidermolysis bullosa in childhood or persistent aphthosis accompanied by great pain;

(vii) in sarcoidosis, when the posterior uveal tract is involved or when progressive pulmonary or renal disease is present.

Relative indications. These depend on the degree or site of involvement and the particular circumstances of each patient. They should be given, hesitantly, as a supplement to other treatment and, usually, as a temporary measure. In self-limiting conditions, such as severe lichen planus or erythema multiforme, they may be of limited value and are easily discontinued; in chronic conditions, such as the lymphomas, they may be continued as long as they suppress the disease. But in the remainder their effect is inconstant or doubtful and the problem of successful withdrawal may become a serious test of therapeutic skill. Such conditions include severe eczema, Reiter's disease and Sjögren's syndrome. Very occasional cases of severe acne and hidradenitis suppurativa may benefit.

Corticosteroids are very seldom indicated in pityriasis rosea, erythema nodosum, chronic urticaria, lichen simplex, prurigo and alopecia areata. The use of corticosteroids in psoriasis is generally condemned except occasionally in acute generalized pustular psoriasis, acute psoriatic erythroderma with metabolic consequences, fulminating psoriatic arthritis or, rarely, intractable disabling palmoplantar pustular psoriasis (see p. 1523). Subsequent withdrawal may be difficult and may precipitate severe relapses. Methotrexate may be needed temporarily to facilitate such withdrawal [2].

Surgical procedures in steroid-treated patients [8]. Any patient who has had corticosteroid treatment of more than a few days' duration during the 12 months preceding any major surgical procedure may be incapable of reacting to the stress of operation by the normal increase in adrenocortical activity.

It has been found that the stress of a major operation causes the production of up to 300 mg of cortisol over 24 h. It is therefore necessary to give an equivalent dose of hydrocortisone to a patient whose adrenals cannot respond normally.

Hydrocortisone sodium succinate 100 mg is given intramuscularly with the premedication and repeated every 8 h. This dose is halved every 24 h until it is equivalent to the pre-operative steroid dosage. Any serious postoperative complications may, of course, require extra dosage.

It is essential that all patients be given 'steroid cards' to carry with them; these give exact details of the drug given and its dose.

REFERENCES

1 ALMEYDA J. (1971) *Br J Dermatol* **84**, 298.

2 BAKER H. (1976) *Br J Dermatol* **94** (Suppl. **12**), 83.

3 BOLAND E.W. (1962) *Ann Rheum Dis* **21**, 176.

4 *Drug Ther Bull* (1976) **14**, 49.

5 GRAHAME R. (1969) *Ann Phys Med* **10**, 130.

6 HARTER J.G., *et al* (1963) *N Engl J Med* **269**, 591.

7 HARVEY W. & GRAHAME R. (1973) *Ann Rheum Dis* **32**, 272.

8 KEHLET H. & BINDER C. (1973) *Br J Anaesth* **45**, 1043.

9 MYLES A.B., *et al* (1971) *Ann Rheum Dis* **30**, 149.

10 RAAB W. (1963) *Excerpta Medica (Dermatol)* XIII, 17, 63.

11 BABHAN N.B. & KOPF A.W. (1971) *Arch Dermatol* **103**, 615.

12 REINER L.G., *et al* (1976) *J Allergy Clin Immunol* **55**, 224.

SEX HORMONES

Androgens. Testosterone is the most potent and important androgen and is used only for replacement therapy. Many derivatives of testosterone have been prepared which seek to minimize the masculinizing effect in women whilst retaining the anabolic action—the so-called anabolic steroids. It is a matter of debate whether the dissociation is entirely possible.

Anabolic steroids
Danazol, 100–600 mg daily [7]. The mode of action of danazol is not just to inhibit gonadotrophin production. It is used for the treatment of endometriosis and cystic disease of the breast, with a number of other non-dermatological indications. It is of value to dermatologists for its very gratifying influence on hereditary angio-oedema HAE (p. 1107). It stimulates the liver to produce more of the deficient C1 esterase inhibitor.

Stanazolol, 2·5–10 mg daily. This achieves a similar effect in HAE and is less expensive. An increase in fibrinolysis activity may lead to reduced pain in liposclerosis of the legs [2, 3]. There are some problems with androgen effects in women, and on the liver. The drug should not be given during pregnancy.

Anti-androgens. The place of these drugs in dermatological practice has yet to be established.

Cyproterone acetate is a potent anti-androgen, which also possesses progestogenic activity. It may prove to be of value in female balding [6] and in hirsuties [1, 4, 5] although the long-term side effects are unknown. For its use in acne see p. 1924.

REFERENCES

1 ANDERSON J.A.R. & BROWNING M.C.K. (1977) *Br J Dermatol* **97** (Suppl. **15**), 20.
2 BROWSE N.L., *et al* (1977) *Br Med J* ii, 434.
3 BURNAND K., *et al* (1980) *Br Med J* **280**, 7.
4 DEWHURST C.J., *et al* (1977) *Br J Obstet Gynaecol* **84**, 119.
5 HAMMERSTEIN J. & CUPCEANN B. (1969) *Germ Med Mon* **14**, 599.
6 HAMMERSTEIN J., *et al* (1975) *J Steroid Biochem* **6**, 827.
7 MADANES A.E. & FARBER M. (1982) *Ann Intern Med* **96**, 625 (and 672).

Oestrogens. Prevention of postmenopausal vaginitis and atrophy have been observed following both systemic [5] and topical [2] therapy. The contraceptive pill may be used in Fox–Fordyce disease [3]. The potential hazards of oestrogen therapy restrict their use in the regular treatment of acne. Clearly, oestrogens should not be given where there is a previous history of thrombo-embolism, obstructive jaundice, carcinoma of the breast [1, 4], herpes gestationis or porphyria cutanea tarda.

Ethinyloestradiol 10–12 µg daily may be given for menopausal symptoms. Dienoestrol cream 0·01%, stilboestrol pessaries or conjugated oestrogens may be used topically but are readily absorbed and so may cause systemic effects.

REFERENCES

1 ARON-BRUNETIÈRE & ROBIN J. (1967) *Bull Soc Fr Dermatol Syphiligr* **75**, 47.
2 GOLDZIEHER M.A. (1946) *J Gerontol* **1**, 196.
3 KRONTHAL H.L., *et al* (1965) *Arch Dermatol* **91**, 243.
4 KUMMEL J. (1966) *Med Welt (Stuttg)* **3**, 294.
5 RAURAMO L. & PUNNONEN R. (1973) *Front Hormone Res* **2**, 48.

ANTIHISTAMINES

Antihistamines should not be the automatic prescription for all itchy rashes or even worse, as used by some non-dermatologists, the automatic prescription for all skin rashes, even though antihistamines are among the more harmless of placebos. In the early 1950s antihistamines were used to treat almost every disorder characterized by any inflammation anywhere—spending in the U.S.A. in 1951 amounted to $100,000,000. They are valuable remedies for skin disorders which are mediated by histamine and they also have other properties. They also have some central antipruritic effect. The recent introduction of relatively non-sedative antihistamines has made it essential to understand what one is attempting to achieve, a central or a peripheral effect.

Physiological antagonists. Adrenaline and related drugs can be used to counteract the action of histamine e.g., in anaphylaxis or acute angio-oedema. Adrenaline by injection (subcutaneous, intramuscular, only very rarely intravenous) is the treatment of choice for life-threatening emergencies of this type. The usual dose is 0·35 ml of a 1 in 1000 solution, if necessary followed by a further 0·35 ml given slowly over 10 min. Ephedrine and terbutaline, which are likewise β-adrenergic agonists but can be administered by mouth, are of some value in the management of urticaria.

Antihistamines: competitive inhibitors [5, 8]. These drugs have a $CH_2CH_2CH{<}$ grouping resembling the histamine molecule and thus allowing them to block histamine receptors. There are two (at least) types of histamine receptors. H_1 antagonists mediate the well-known effects of vasodilatation, increased permeability of small blood vessels, smooth muscle contraction and itching. H_2 receptors are best known for mediating the effects on gastric acid production. However, they also play a role in skin blood vessels, as well as having an effect on the immune system somewhat resembling that of levamisole.

H_1 antihistamines. Their main therapeutic effect is a peripheral one antagonizing the action of histamine and is therefore particularly valuable in urticaria and angio-oedema, even though other mediators are also involved in these disorders. There is little reason to think that antihistamines are of value by their peripheral action in the management of most other inflammatory skin diseases where the role of histamine is much in doubt. The role of histamine as a peripheral mediator of itching is discussed in Chapter 60. Antihistamines are frequently prescribed as antipruritic drugs but it seems that most of such action is either central or a placebo one. It is therefore important that, when a central antipruritic effect is looked for, the newer less sedative antihistamines should be avoided [6].

Other actions of antihistamines include anticholinergic effects which may at times be therapeutically useful or more often may cause side effects.

The drugs are absorbed from the gut, their action commencing within 15–30 min; intramuscular or intravenous injections may not work much more rapidly. Although often stated to be excreted within a few hours, recent investigations have shown that even short-acting antihistamines may take over 24 hr to be eliminated from the blood, and tissue levels may be maintained even longer [7].

Side effects vary greatly from patient to patient and include especially drowsiness, potentiated by alcohol. Some patients are stimulated by the drugs and may be unable to sleep. Convulsions may occur with overdosage. The anticholinergic action may cause dry mouth, blurring of vision, difficulty in micturition and impotence.

The number of antihistamine preparations containing tartrazine or other azo-dyes potentially harmful in urticaria is diminishing [1].

The main site of metabolism is the liver and so caution should be exercised in patients with impaired hepatic function.

Antihistamines should not be taken for the first time before driving or other hazardous occupations and the patient should be warned of this possible hazard.

In Britain there are over 30 antihistamines currently available, many of them with only minor differences in action. Usually if a disease is somewhat resistant to one antihistamine it may respond no better to others, but most dermatologists find it useful to be able to change the drugs around and to be familiar with the mode of action of several. The *British National Formulary* states that there is no evidence that any antihistamine is better than any other. Certainly it is necessary to be fully familiar with one or more short-acting and long-acting drugs, and with sedative and non-sedative drugs. Some antihistamines are said to have special beneficial properties by virtue of other pharmacological effects (anticholinergic, antiserotonin); others are claimed to have special benefits by lacking these other actions.

The dosage and frequency of administration of antihistamines are those recommended by the manufacturers and are usually based on the inhibition of experimental histamine weals. Many dermatologists at times feel constrained cautiously to exceed these doses. In general it is prudent to begin with a modest dose, increasing the dose stepwise until either the condition comes under control or significant side effects preclude a larger dose. At that stage an alternative preparation may legitimately be tried, again starting with low or moderate dosage.

All drugs are best avoided in pregnancy if possible, especially in the first trimester, but it is sometimes highly desirable to be able to administer antihistamines. It can be said that there is no convincing evidence to incriminate such older antihistamines as chlorpheniramine [4], although this is not the same as saying that they have been proved innocuous. Data may never be accumulated for recently introduced drugs because so many thousands of cases may have to be treated in pregnancy before an increase in birth defects, etc., can be excluded.

Where side effects or lack or clinical efficacy occur it is useful to be able to change to a drug with an unrelated chemical structure. Antihistamines have long been subdivided into six or more groups as follows:

Alkylamine
Chlorpheniramine 4 mg three times daily (long acting also available)
Brompheniramine 4 mg three times daily (long acting also available)
These are short-acting, somewhat sedative, cheap, good all-purpose antihistamines.
Phenothiazine
Promethazine 25 mg twice daily

Trimeprazine 10 mg at night or up to five times
    daily
These are long-acting, more sedative, also more
    anti-emetic drugs.
Ethylene diamine
Mepyramine 100 mg three times daily
Ethanolamine
Diphenhydramine 50 mg three times daily
Piperazine
Cyclizine, Chlorcyclizine
Others
Hydroxyzine 25 mg three times daily
Mebhydrolin 50 mg three times daily
Cyproheptadine 4 mg three times daily; also has
    antiserotonin properties
Terfenadine 60 mg twice daily
Astemizole 10 mg once daily

The newer antihistamines, terfenadine and his-
manal, have less action on the central nervous system and this makes them valuable for urticaria, hay
fever and selected cases of atopic dermatitis, but less
useful as central antipruritics [3]. They are more
costly.

H₂ antagonists. These drugs have an enormous sale
for the control of gastric acid secretion. Their role
in dermatology is still uncertain [2, 5]. They may
be of some value in histamine-mediated disorders
which fail to respond to H₁ antagonists. Combined
with an H₁ antagonist they have a modest action
on dermographism and a more doubtful one in
other types of urticaria. Their use as an antipruritic
in disorders without wealing, e.g. renal disease, polycythaemia, lymphoma, is based on anecdotes
rather than firm data from studies of large numbers
of patients. They have been used as immune stimulants in chronic fungus infections but seem to
lack any adverse immune stimulant effect on
patients with renal transplants or autoimmune disease. Their anti-androgen effect does not seem to be
powerful enough to represent a major break-
through in this field. The most widely used drug is
cimetidine, the usual dose of which is 600–
1,600 mg daily. Ranitidine has similar actions but
seems to lack the hormonal effects.

REFERENCES

1 ALDRIDGE R.D., *et al* (1984) *Br J Dermatol* **110**, 351.
2 DILLER G. & ORFANOS C.E. (1982) *Hautarzt* **33**, 353.
3 *Drug Ther Bull* (1984) **22**, 21.
4 GREENBERGER P. & PATTERSON R. (1978) *Ann Intern Med*
    89, 234.
5 KERDEL F. & SOTER N. (1983) In *Recent Advances in Der-
    matology*. Eds. A.J. Rook & H.I. Maibach. Edinburgh,
    Churchill Livingstone, Vol. 6.
6 KRAUSE L. & SHUSTER S. (1983) *Br Med J* **287**, 1199.
7 SIMONS F.E.R., *et al* (1984) *J Allergy Clin Immunol* **73**,
    69.
8 WARIN R.P. & CHAMPION R.H. (1974) *Urticaria*. London,
    Saunders.

OTHER ANTI-ALLERGIC DRUGS

Cromoglycate (Intal, Nalcrom, Rynacrom). This is a
remarkable drug, almost devoid of toxicity, which
inhibits the release of histamine and other inflammatory mediators from mast cells. It is especially
effective on mast cells in the lung but also on those
in the nose and gut. It seems to have little action
on cutaneous mast cells. For dermatologists this
drug is mainly of interest in controlling the respiratory or gut symptoms which may be associated
with atopic dermatitis. Its use in atopic dermatitis
itself is still not clarified. It appears to be genuinely
helpful in mastocystosis.

Doxantrazole, Ketotifen, Oxatamide. These are all
antihistamine-like drugs but they also have other
properties somewhat comparable with those of
cromoglycate. They have some popularity as treatments for difficult urticaria.

NON-STEROIDAL
ANTI-INFLAMMATORY DRUGS

A large number of these drugs have been introduced in the past two decades, mostly on the basis
of their ability to inhibit the cyclo-oxygenase (or
possibly the lipoxygenase) involved in the production of prostaglandins. Their use is mainly for rheumatic complaints but dermatologists may find them
useful in such inflammatory disorders as erythema
nodosum. They are also of some value in inhibiting
the physiological responses to insect stings. They
seem to have little action on such disorders as
eczema but one of these drugs, benoxaprofen
showed promise in psoriasis, perhaps through
anti-lipoxygenase activity, before it was withdrawn
because of side effects (p. 1511). Early interest in
these drugs for topical use has not yet been re-
warded. Many of them share with aspirin a harmful
effect on urticaria—probably based on pharmacology rather than immunology.

REFERENCE

1 KOCH-WESER J. (1980) *N Engl J Med* **302**, 1179; 1237.

RETINOIDS [4, 30, 31,]

This class of compounds covers both the synthetic and the natural forms of vitamin A (the term vitamin A includes the preformed vitamin A alcohol retinol, its aldehyde retinal and its acid *trans*-retinoic acid, as well as the provitamin β-carotene). Chemical manipulation of retinol has led to numerous new compounds which are less toxic than the parent molecule. The mode of action of the retinoids has not been completely elucidated but they have profound effects on differentiation, cell growth and immune response. The potential for their use in tumour prevention, cancer chemotherapy and dermatology is now undisputed.

Effect on differentiation. It has been known for many years that vitamin A deficiency results in epithelial squamous metaplasia and that vitamin supplements reverse this effect. Retinoids have now been shown to reduce differentiation in a number of cell types, e.g. mouse teratocarcinoma [9, 29, 32] and human myeloid leukaemia cells [6], and to cause regression of bronchial metaplasia in heavy smokers [13]. Epidermis undergoes profound changes and shows hypergranulosis and hyperplasia with decreased numbers of tonofilaments and desmosomes and widening of intracellular spaces [10, 11]. The effect on desmosomes appears to contribute to the keratolytic effect of retinoids in hyperkeratotic disorders.

Effect on cancer. In models of carcinogenesis the induction of the enzyme ornithine decarboxylase occurs during transformation [2]. The enzyme induction is inhibited by retinoids and this inhibition has been used to test the anticarcinogenic effect of new retinoids. Topical retinoic acid has been shown to prevent both the induction of ornithine decarboxylase and the formation of skin tumours in mice [17]. This effect may be of value in the treatment of sun-induced neoplasms in man.

Tumour growth. The growth of a number of human tumour cell lines, e.g. melanoma, seems to be inhibited by retinoids but the response may be variable [16]. A similar regression of tumours has been shown in an *in vitro* mouse model [18]. High concentrations of retinoids cause cytotoxicity through membrane labilization, although at lower doses membrane stabilization may occur.

Receptors. There are specific retinol and retinoic acid receptors. The activity of retinoids is mediated through these in a similar manner to steroid hormones [21]. The receptors have a more significant effect on differentiation [14] than on the inhibition of tumour growth.

Cell-surface effects. Retinoids affect transformed cell surfaces and lead to loss of anchorage-independent growth, cell adhesiveness and density-dependent growth [5]. It is not clear whether these effects are exerted directly by the retinoid involvement in glycosyl transfer reactions or through changes in gene expression.

Immunostimulation. In animal models retinoids may act as an adjuvant and stimulate antibody formation to antigens that were previously not immunogenic [7, 30]. In addition retinoids may stimulate cell-mediated cytotoxicity [16].

Neutrophil migration. The migration of neutrophils is reduced by retinoids both in experimental models of inflammation [8] and in patients with acne [20]. The mode of action is unknown.

Isotretinoin (13-*cis*-retinoic acid). Isotretinoin has been shown to be very effective in the treatment of severe, recalcitrant cystic acne unresponsive to antibacterial agents [15, 25] and to be superior to etretinate. Dose ranges have varied considerably from 2·0 to 0·1 mg/kg per day, but the most widely used regime at present is 0·5–1·0 mg/kg per day as a 16-week course. This produces prolonged remission in the majority of patients (see Chapter 52). Isotretinoin 0·2% topically also appears to suppress acne [27]; however, these observations need confirmation. In addition to acne isotretinoin has been used in the treatment of Gram-negative folliculitis, rosacea and hidradenitis suppurativa [31].

In acne the major therapeutic effect seems to be a profound reduction in sebaceous gland activity [15]. There are reductions in bacterial flora, but it is likely that these changes are secondary to the reduction in sebum secretion. The anti-inflammatory and desquamating effects of retinoids may also play a beneficial role.

A wide range of disorders of keratinization have been found to be responsive to isotretinoin [24]. In Europe this group of disorders is now usually treated with etretinate.

Etretinate [4]. Etretinate in doses of 20–75 mg/day has been shown to be effective in the treatment of erythrodermic and generalized pustular psoriasis [30]. Chronic plaque psoriasis is less responsive and higher doses are usually required [12]. A retinoid sparing effect has been achieved by the use of UVB,

PUVA, topical treatment and even cytotoxic agents [31]. Palmoplantar pustular dermatosis, especially when associated with marked hyperkeratosis, and psoriatic arthropathy are also improved by treatment with etretinate.

A wide variety of disorders of keratinization are somewhat responsive to etretinate: epidermolytic hyperkeratosis, keratoderma, X-linked ichthyosis, ichthyosis vulgaris, erythrokeratoderma variabilis, pityriasis rubra pilaris and lichen planus. Darier's disease, lamellar ichthyosis and non-bullous ichthyosiform erythroderma are equally responsive to both etretinate and isotretinoin [31]. Long-term treatment is required as worthwhile remissions following cessation of treatment have not been reported. Toxicity therefore may prove to be a problem in these patients.

A range of skin tumours may sometimes clear with either isotretinoin or etretinate. These include solar keratoses, keratoacanthoma, epidermodysplasia verruciformis and basal cell epithelioma. However these preparations may be of particular value in the prevention of tumours in those patients with high risk disorders such as xeroderma pigmentosum, porokeratosis of Mibelli, familial self-healing squamous epithelioma of the skin and in those transplantation patients with extensive sunlight-damaged skin.

Malignant melanoma and mycosis fungoides appear to be sensitive to retinoids but the role of retinoids in cancer chemotherapy has not been fully established.

Toxicity [4]. A number of side effects are common to both drugs. These appear to be dose related and are largely cutaneous. They include cheilitis, conjunctivitis, dryness of mucous membranes and epistaxis, desquamation of hands and feet, pruritus, myalgia, arthralgia, lethargy and alopecia [31, 34]. Facial dryness appears to be greater with isotretinoin and alopecia is greater with etretinate. In order to minimize alopecia it has been suggested that women should not receive more than 50 mg of etretinate a day [22].

Patients may develop abnormal liver enzyme levels during therapy with etretinate. Not all values have returned to normal on cessation of the drug [31, 33].

Increase in VLDL cholesterol and reduction in HDL cholesterol have been reported with etretinate therapy [19]. Many patients receiving isotretinoin have been reported with elevated serum VLDL triglyceride in the absence of a preceding hyperlipoproteinaemia. These levels have returned to normal on cessation of treatment, but all patients should be screened for hyperlipoproteinaemia prior to treatment with either isotretinoin or etretinate [31, 33].

An ossification disorder resembling idiopathic skeletal hyperostosis has been reported in four patients receiving long-term isotretinoin [26].

Teratogenicity. Both preparations are known to be teratogenic in animals. Maternal ingestion of isotretinoin early in pregnancy can lead to fetal abnormalities [28] and the infants seem to have a characteristic appearance [1, 3].

It is important that women are not pregnant prior to starting treatment. Effective contraception is mandatory during and after a course of treatment. Isotretinoin has a short half-life and therefore contraceptive measures need to be taken for only 1 month after cessation of treatment, but etretinate has a long half-life, of approximately 100 days. Significant plasma levels are present at 140 days [23] and therefore post-treatment contraception is necessary for at least 1 yr after this drug.

REFERENCES

1 BENKE P. (1984) JAMA **251**, 3267.
2 BOUTWELL R.K., et al (1982) J Am Acad Dermatol **6**, 796.
3 CRUZ E., et al (1984) Pediatrics **74**, 428.
4 CUNLIFFE W.J. & MILLER A.J. (1984) Retinoid Therapy. Lancaster, MTP Press.
5 DION D.L., et al. (1978) Exp Cell Res **117**, 15.
6 DOVER D. & KOEFFLER H.P. (1982) J Clin Invest **69**, 277.
7 DRESSER D.W. (1968) Nature **217**, 527.
8 DUBERTRET L., et al (1982) Br J Dermatol **107**, 681.
9 EDWARDS M.K.S. & McBURNEY M.W. (1983) Dev Biol **98**, 187.
10 ELIAS P.M. & WILLIAMS M.I. (1981) Arch Dermatol **117**, 160.
11 FRITSCH P. (1981) Int J Dermatol **20**, 314.
12 GOERZ G. & ORFANOS C.E. (1978) Dermatologica **157**, (Suppl. 1) 38.
13 GOUVEIA J., et al (1982) Lancet ii, 710.
14 JETTEN A.M. & JETTEN M.E.R. (1979) Nature **278**, 180.
15 JONES D.H., et al (1982) Br J Dermatol **108**, 333.
16 LOTAN R. (1980) Biochim Biophys Acta **605**, 33.
17 LOWE N.J. & BREEDING J. (1982) J Invest Dermatol **78**, 121.
18 MAYER H., et al (1978) Experimentia **34**, 1105.
19 MICHAELSSON G., et al (1981) Br J Dermatol **105**, 201.
20 NORRIS D.A., et al (1983) Clin Res **31**, 593A.
21 ONG D.E. & CHYTIL F. (1975) Nature **255**, 74.
22 ORFANOS C.E., et al (1981) Hautarzt **32**, 275.
23 PARAVICINI U. et al (1981) Ann NY Acad Sci **359**, 54.
24 PECK G.L. & YODER F.W. (1976) Lancet ii, 1172.
25 PECK G.L., et al (1979) N Engl J Med **300**, 329.
26 PITTSLEY R.A. & YODER F.W. (1983) N Engl J Med **308**, 1012.

27 PLEWIG G., *et al* (1983) *J Invest Dermatol* **80**, 357.
28 ROSA F.W. (1983) *Lancet* **ii**, 513.
29 SPEERS W.G. (1982) *Cancer Res* **42**, 1843.
30 SPORN M.B. *et al* (1984) *The Retinoids.* New York, Academic Press, Vols. 1 and 2.
31 STRAUSS J.S., *et al* (1982) *J Am Acad Dermatol* **6**, 573.
32 STRICKLAND S. & MAHDAVI V. (1978) *Cell* **15**, 393.
33 THUNE P. & MORK N.J. (1980) *Dermatologica* **160**, 405.
34 WARD A., *et al* (1984) *Drugs* **28**, 6.

IMMUNOSUPPRESSIVE AND CYTOTOXIC DRUGS

These drugs, which have been primarily developed for use in oncology, must be approached with great caution when they become part of a dermatologist's armamentarium; it is essential that the treatment is not more disabling than the disease. A complete understanding of the clinical pharmacology of these drugs and their possible side effects is required for the proper management of patients [3–5]. Brief details are given below of those drugs that may be of value in dermatological practice.

Alkylating agents. Although the effect of these drugs is not cell cycle dependent, it is dependent on proliferation and is expressed only when cells enter the S phase. Alkylation of DNA by these drugs leads to impaired replication.

Cyclophosphamide: Dose, 1–3 mg/kg body weight daily in two or three divided doses. Cyclophosphamide is inactive *in vitro* but is metabolized to an active antimitotic agent which also has profound immunosuppressive activity. It has been successfully used together with corticosteroids in the treatment of pemphigus [8, 11, 15] and pemphigoid [11], Wegener's granulomatosis [9, 19], systemic lupus erythematosus [7], polymyositis [7], mycosis fungoides [1] and histiocytosis X [18].

Chlorambucil: Dose, 0·1–0·2 mg/kg per day in one or two doses. Chlorambucil is slow acting and rather less toxic than cyclophosphamide. It has been successfully used in the treatment of mycosis fungoides [14], Behçet's disease [13], lupus erythematosus [17], Wegener's granulomatosis [2], steroid-resistant sarcoidosis [10] and in combination with prednisone for Sézary syndrome [21].

Mustine injection. This is the original nitrogen mustard and has little to commend it except speed of action. It may be used topically in mycosis fungoides (p. 1745); one method of desensitization for topical therapy involves intravenous injection of gradually increasing doses [20].

Dacarbazine injection: (DTIC) Doses, 2–4·5 mg/kg intravenously daily for 10 days. This is an imidazole derivative whose mode of action is unknown. It is used particularly for the treatment of metastatic malignant melanoma [6, 12, 16] (p. 2458).

REFERENCES

1 AUERBACH R. (1970) *Arch Dermatol* **101**, 611.
2 BERGHIND G., *et al* (1972) *Acta Med Scand* **191**, 5.
3 CALABRESI P. & PARKS R.E. (1980) In *The Pharmacological Basis of Therapeutics* Ed Gilman A.G., *et al.* 7th ed. New York, Macmillan, ch. 55.
4 CARTER S.K., *et al* (1977) *Chemotherapy of Cancer.* New York, Wiley Medical.
5 DANTZIG P.I. (1974) *Arch Dermatol* **110**, 393.
6 *Drug Ther Bull* (1976) **14**, 39.
7 FRIES J.F., *et al* (1973) *Arthritis Rheum* **16**, 154.
8 GLICKMAN F.S. (1973) *Arch Dermatol* **107**, 467.
9 HAYNES B.F. & FAUCI A.S. (1978) *N Engl J Med* **299**, 764.
10 ISRAEL H.L. (1971) *Thorax* **20**, 57.
11 KRAIN L.S., *et al* (1972) *Arch Dermatol* **106**, 657.
12 LUCE J.K. (1975) *Semin Oncol* **2**, 179.
13 MAMO J.C., *et al* (1970) *Arch Ophthalmol* **84**, 446.
14 MANTE C., *et al* (1968) *Acta Derm Venereol* (Stockh) **48**, 60.
15 MCELVEY E.N., *et al* (1971) *Arch Dermatol* **103**, 198.
16 NATHANSON L., *et al* (1971) *Clin Pharmacol Ther* **12**, 955.
17 SNAITH M.I., *et al* (1973) *Ann Rheum Dis* **32**, 279.
18 STARLING K.A., *et al* (1972) *Am J Dis Child* **123**, 105.
19 STEINMAN T.I., *et al* (1980) *Am J Med* **68**, 458.
20 VAN SCOTT E.J. & KALMANSON J.D. (1973) *Cancer* **32**, 18.
21 WINKELMANN R.K., *et al* (1973) *Am J Med* **55**, 192.

Antimetabolites

Methotrexate [13, 22a]. This folic acid antagonist binds to dihydrofolate reductase and prevents the production of tetrahydrofolic acid, the active coenzyme form of folic acid. It is cell cycle specific, acting in the S phase, and is also a powerful immunosuppressive, but with little anti-inflammatory activity.

Low doses are well absorbed from the gastrointestinal tract. The majority of the drug is excreted unchanged in the urine within 24 h. Care should therefore be taken in the elderly and in other circumstances where there is renal impairment.

For its use in psoriasis [2] see p. 1500. It has also been employed in a wide variety of other diseases, including Reiter's disease [33], pityriasis rubra pilaris [15], ichthyosiform erythroderma [9] and keratoacanthoma [25]. It is effective in pemphigus vulgaris [17] and foliaceus [23], pemphigoid and corticosteroid-resistant dermatomyositis [29]. Leucovorin (folinic acid) is a potent antidote in methotrexate overdose [3].

Azarabine (triacetyl azauridine). This is an inhibitor of pyrimidine synthesis which has been used in mycosis fungoides [19] and for psoriasis [20, 35]. It is of proven efficiency, and the serious neurotoxicity was found to be avoidable by using lower dosages (125 mg/kg per day instead of 200 mg/kg). However, it remains uncertain whether it precipitates serious thrombo-embolic events [34].

Azathioprine: Dose, 1·5–3.0 mg/kg per day. It is converted in the body to mercaptopurine, an inhibitor of purine synthesis and an immunosuppressive; in addition it has powerful anti-inflammatory properties. It appears to be inferior to methotrexate in the treatment of psoriasis [2, 8, 10] but may be useful for psoriatic arthritis (see p. 1518). Azathioprine is of value in producing steroid sparing in pemphigus vulgaris [5, 24], pemphigoid, systemic lupus erythematosus [27, 32], dermatomyositis [16], Wegener's granulomatosis [22], perhaps pityriasis rubra pilaris [12] and rarely in intractable eczema in adults.

Mycophenolic acid [31]: Dose, 30–96 mg/kg per day. This drug is an inhibitor of purine synthesis. After oral administration it is converted to an inactive glucuronide in the liver and activated by a glucuronidase present in the skin. It has a beneficial effect in psoriasis [14, 18] but careful individualization of dose is required; acute side effects include gastrointestinal and genito-urinary problems and chronic toxicity remains to be evaluated [34].

Bleomycin [4]. This is a group of polypeptide antibiotics given parenterally which have no immunosuppressive action and with toxicity confined to the skin [6] and lungs. It is effective against squamous cell carcinoma of the skin and in inducing remission in mycosis fungoides [30]. It has been used intralesionally for the treatment of intractable virus warts [28].

Hydroxyurea [21]: Dose, 500 mg two or three times daily. Hydroxyurea blocks pyrimidine synthesis; it causes much more short-term marrow suppression than methotrexate, necessitating frequent blood counts [7]. However, it is less effective than methotrexate and has little effect on psoriatic arthropathy. Combination with methotrexate confers no advantage [26].

Razoxane (ICRF 159). This antimitotic agent has been found to be particularly effective for the treatment of some tumours where blood vessels are primarily affected. It has been shown to be very effective in the treatment of psoriasis and the associated arthropathy [1]. However, there have been a number of reports that acute myeloid leukaemia develops in patients who have received chronic low dose razoxane for the treatment of malignant conditions or psoriasis. Sixteen cases had been reported by 1986 [36]. The mean dose, duration of treatment and time from the beginning of treatment to the diagnosis of leukaemia are 195 g, 38·4 months and 42·2 months, respectively.

In many cases, particularly of psoriasis, patients have been exposed to other treatments which may have contributed to the development of leukaemia. Although razoxane is highly effective and reasonably well tolerated in the treatment of severe disabling psoriasis, the reports of an association between the chronic administration of this drug and the later development of acute leukaemias dramatically alters the perceived risk to benefit ratio. The treatment of psoriasis or any other non-malignant condition with razoxane is therefore contra-indicated.

REFERENCES

1 ATHERTON D.J., *et al* (1980) *Br J Dermatol* **102**, 307.
2 BAKER H. (1975) *Dermatologica*, **150**, 136.
3 BERTINO J.R., *et al* (1971) *Ann NY Acad Sci* **186**, 486.
4 BLUM R.H., *et al* (1973) *Cancer* **31**, 903.
5 BURTON J.L., *et al* (1970) *Br Med J* iii, 84.
6 COHEN I.S., *et al* (1973) *Arch Dermatol* **107**, 553.
7 DAHL M.C.G. & COMAISH J.S. (1972) *Br Med J* iv, 585.
8 DU VIVIER A., *et al* (1974) *Br Med J* i, 49.
9 ESTERLEY N.B. (1971) *Pediatrics* **48**, 995.
10 GREAVES M.W., & DAWBER R., (1970) *Br Med J* ii, 237.
11 GREAVES M.W., *et al* (1971) *Br Med J* i, 144.
12 HUNTER G.A. (1972) *Br J Dermatol* **87**, 42.
13 JOLIVET J., *et al* (1983) *N Engl J Med* **309**, 1094.
14 JONES E.L., *et al* (1975) *J Invest Dermatol* **65**, 537.
15 KNOWLES W.R., *et al* (1970) *Arch Dermatol* **102**, 603.
16 LEVER W.F. (1972) *Arch Dermatol* **105**, 771.
17 LEVER W.F. (1972) *Arch Dermatol* **106**, 491.
18 MARINARI R., *et al* (1977) *Arch Dermatol* **113**, 930.
19 McDONALD C.J., *et al* (1971) *Arch Dermatol* **103**, 158.
20 MILSTEIN H.G., *et al* (1973) *Arch Dermatol* **108**, 43.
21 MOSCHELLA S.L. & GREENWALD M.A. (1973) *Arch Dermatol* **107**, 363.
22 PICKERING J.G. (1972) *Proc R Soc Med* **65**, 592.
22a RAU R. (Ed.) (1986) *Low dose methotrexate in Rheumatic Diseases*, Karger, Basel.
23 RIVITTI E.A., *et al* (1973) *Int J Dermatol* **12**, 119.
24 ROENIGK H.H. JR., *et al* (1973) *Arch Dermatol* **107**, 353.
25 RUTKIN L. (1968) *Dermatologica* **137**, 373.
26 SAUER G.C. (1973) *Arch Dermatol* **107**, 369.
27 SCHUR P.H., *et al* (1968) *N Engl J Med* **278**, 277.
28 SHUMACK P.H. & HADDOCK M.J. (1979) *Aust J Dermatol* **20**, 41.

29 SOKOLOFF M.C., *et al* (1971) *Lancet* i, 14.
30 SPIGEL S.C. & COTTMAN C.A. (1973) *Cancer* 32, 767.
31 SWEENEY M.J., *et al* (1972) *Cancer Res* 32, 1803.
32 SZTENJNBOK M., *et al* (1971) *Arthritis Rheum* 14, 639.
33 TOPP J.R., *et al* (1971) *Can Med Assoc J* 105, 1168.
34 VAN SCOTT E.J. (1976) *JAMA* 235, 197.
35 VOGLER W.R. & OLANSKY S. (1970) *Ann Intern Med* 73, 951.
36 WALTON P.L. (1986) Personal communication.

Adverse effects. Most of these agents have certain unwanted effects in common, as would be expected from their antimitotic action upon rapidly dividing cells. Thus, all of them except bleomycin cause bone marrow depression. This is usually manifest as leucopenia or thrombocytopenia; mild hypoplastic anaemia is common with azarabine and megaloblastic anaemia occurs with hydroxyurea and rarely with methotrexate.

Mucosal irritation occurs with the production of nausea, vomiting and ulceration; gastrointestinal side effects are uncommon with hydroxyurea and azathioprine. Methotrexate has a higher incidence of these and is also hepatotoxic [7, 8], though less so when given in intermittent weekly dosage [1]. A diffuse anagen alopecia is very common with cyclophosphamide but is much less frequent with other agents.

The reproductive system is also affected. All these agents cause azoospermia and anovulation; they are all potential teratogens, hydroxyurea being one of the most potent teratogenic agents known. It is therefore mandatory to institute effective contraceptive measures. Sterile haemorrhagic cystitis occurs in up to 10% of patients on cyclophosphamide and may even be fatal [4]. The immunosuppressive action gives rise to an increased liability to infection. Banal virus infections such as measles, varicella, vaccinia and herpes simplex may become generalized and cause death. Bacterial, fungal and yeast infections may also disseminate with fatal results. There is an increased incidence of non-Hodgkin's lymphoma and cutaneous squamous cell carcinoma in patients with renal transplants receiving immunosuppression (corticosteroids, azathioprine, cyclophosphamide or chlorambucil) [5]. Other immunosuppressives are less strongly associated with the promotion of malignancy, though several cases of squamous cell carcinoma of the nasopharynx have been reported with metotrexate [3].

Bleomycin appears to cause no immunosuppression but it does produce significant and unique adverse reactions in the skin and lungs. When the total dose exceeds 150 mg, many patients develop a variety of cutaneous manifestations including infiltrated plaques, nodules and bands on the hands

with gangrene of the fingertips and hyperpigmentation on the trunk [2]. Up to 10% develop progressive pulmonary fibrosis [6] which may be reversible with high dose steroid therapy if detected early. This combination of changes suggests the possibility of a drug-induced systemic sclerosis [2].

REFERENCES

1 ALMEYDA J., *et al* (1972) *Br J Dermatol* 87, 623.
2 COHEN I.S., *et al* (1973) *Arch Dermatol* 107, 553.
3 DANTZIG P.I. (1974) *Arch Dermatol* 110, 393.
4 HALL T.C. (1967) *Cancer Chemother Rep* 51, 335.
5 KINLEN L.J., *et al* (1979) *Br Med J* ii, 1461.
6 MOSHER M., *et al* (1972) *Cancer* 30, 56.
7 WARIN A.P., *et al* (1975) *Br J Dermatol* 93, 321.
8 ZACHARIAE H., *et al* (1975) *Acta Derm Venereol (Stockh)* 55, 291.

LEVAMISOLE [1, 2]

Levamisole was introduced because of its activity against a whole range of nematodes. It was later found to be an immunostimulant, enhancing depressed cell-mediated immunity. It has been used for the treatment of many disorders in general medicine and dermatology in which some often ill-characterized modulation of the immune system is desired. Many of the studies have been of considerable interest but so far the drug has not established a place for itself in the regular armamentarium to justify the very real toxic side effects.

REFERENCES

1 DE CREE J. & SYMOENS J. (1979) In *Drugs and Immune Responsiveness*. Eds. Turk J.L. & Parker D. London, MacMillan, ch. 6.
2 RENOUX G. (1980) *Drugs* 19, 89.

HEAVY METALS

Arsenic. This is now almost never used for psoriasis because of its toxic effects. Antimony salts have been dealt with in Chapter 26.

Zinc sulphate capsules: Dose, 220 mg three times a day. An effervescent preparation is available (Solvazinc), which appears to cause fewer gastrointestinal symptoms. The various uses of zinc to replace deficiencies, promote healing of leg ulcers, etc. are discussed on p. 2335.

Gold (sodium aurothiomalate): Dose, 10 mg [1] intramuscularly as a test dose, followed by 50 mg at weekly intervals. Although this regime was devised for the treatment of rheumatoid arthritis it has been successfully used in the treatment of pemphigus [2]. If there has been no improvement by the time the total dose reaches 1 g treatment should be stopped. If improvement dose occur, the frequency of the injections is reduced to every 2–3 weeks. Renal, hepatic and marrow damage must be looked for and rashes are common (see p. 1258).

REFERENCES

1 GOTTLIEB N.L. (1977) *Bull Rheum Dis* **27**, 912.
2 PENNEYS N.S., *et al* (1976) *Arch Dermatol* **112**, 185.

CHELATING AGENTS

Chelating agents are available which form complexes with a number of heavy metals. They are only occasionally of use in dermatology.

D-*Penicillamine* [4]. This is a degradation product of penicillin and chelates copper, mercury, zinc and lead. It is used for Wilson's disease, lead poisoning, cystinuria and rheumatoid arthritis [5]. Its dermatological interest lies in its ability to cause a variety of serious diseases, including systemic lupus erythematosus-like syndrome and pemphigus-like bullous eruptions [1, 2, 6], and its possible benefit in scleroderma [3].

Desferrioxamine. This is used in the treatment of various iron storage diseases. In general, acute iron overload seems to respond much more satisfactorily. However, it is logical to use it in porphyria cutanea tarda as long as iron overload is present, though its value has yet to be proved (see p. 2282).

REFERENCES

1 HEWITT J., *et al* (1971) *Med Int* **122**, 1003.
2 HEWITT J., *et al* (1975) *Br J Dermatol* **93** (Suppl. 11), 12.
3 JAYSON M.I.V., *et al* (1977) *Proc R Soc Med* **70** (Suppl. 3), 82.
4 LEADING ARTICLE (1975) *Lancet* **i**, 1123.
5 MULTI-CENTRE TRIAL GROUP (1973) *Lancet* **i**, 275.
6 TAN S.G. & ROWELL N.R. (1976) *Br J Dermatol* **95**, 99.

ANTIBIOTICS AND ANTIBACTERIAL AGENTS

Antibiotics are substances synthesized by microorganisms which are toxic to others at high dilution [1]. This action is directed chiefly against bacteria. Many antibiotics are now synthetic or semisynthetic. They are usually divided into bacteriostatic

and bactericidal groups, though the distinction is not complete; erythromycin, for example, may be either bactericidal or bacteriostatic depending on the nature of the infecting organism and the drug concentration achieved [2].

In clinical use, antibiotics are divided into those with a narrow spectrum of activity and those broad spectrum drugs which act against Gram-positive and Gram-negative organisms. In the laboratory, antibiotics can be divided into four main groups [2]:

(1) those which interfere with bacterial cell synthesis, e.g. the penicillins and cephalosporins;
(2) agents affecting bacterial cell membrane permeability, e.g. the polymyxins (and nystatin and amphotericin);
(3) antibiotics which inhibit bacterial protein biosynthesis, e.g. the tetracyclines, aminoglycosides, macrolides, lincosamides and chloramphenicol;
(4) those which affect bacterial nucleic acid metabolism, e.g. the rifamycins.

Drug resistance. Bacterial resistance can occur in three ways. When all sensitive bacteria have been eradicated, any remaining inherently resistant bacteria are free to multiply; this is the commonest form of resistance. Less frequently, bacteria may acquire resistance to a drug to which they were initially sensitive. The third form, which currently gives rise to concern, is transferable drug resistance. Here a resistance (R) factor is transferred from one bacterium, which may be non-pathogenic, to another previously susceptible bacterium. This usually takes place in the bowel and involves mainly Gram-negative organisms; a single R factor may transfer multiple drug resistance.

REFERENCES

1 GARROD L.P., *et al* (1981) *Antibiotic and Chemotherapy*, 5th Ed. Edinburgh, Churchill Livingstone.
2 Symposium on Mode of Action of Antibiotics on Microbial Walls and Membranes (1974) *Ann NY Acad Sci* **235**, 1.

Sulphonamides. These antibacterial drugs heralded a new era when they were introduced into clinical practice in Germany in 1935. They were then active against a wide range of bacteria but today the problems of acquired resistance have reduced their role, when used alone, to a very minor one. The combination of a sulphonamide (usually sulphamethoxazole) with trimethoprim, however, is a potent and valued antimicrobial weapon important in dermatology.

Sulphonamides are derivatives of *para*-aminobenzenesulphonamide; several thousand of them were synthesized but only a few are of clinical significance [4]. They act by inhibiting the bacterial enzyme dihydrofolic acid synthetase which converts *para*-aminobenzoic acid (PABA) to dihydrofolic acid. Mammalian cells and resistant bacteria do not synthesize folic acid and are unaffected.

Sulphonamides are bacteriostatic and are inhibited by pus. Most are well absorbed orally. They are distributed through all body tissues, metabolized in the liver and excreted mainly by the kidneys. Crystalluria is a serious risk and a high fluid intake should be maintained, though the risk is minimal with sulphadimidine.

Adverse effects. Millions of patients have been safely treated with these drugs but all sulphonamides should be regarded as potentially dangerous drugs [4]. Besides crystalluria, they may rarely cause blood dyscrasias (Negroes being especially susceptible to acute haemolytic anaemia), fever, serum sickness and a great variety of skin manifestations (see p. 1264) including erythema nodosum and erythema multiforme. Fatal cases of the Stevens–Johnson syndrome have followed the use of long-acting sulphonamides [1]. Because of the relatively high incidence of this reaction, the long-acting sulphonamides are no longer available in America [6] and are little used in Britain.

Uses. There are now very few situations where they are drugs of first choice. They are of value in lymphogranuloma venereum, chancroid and nocardiosis and in toxoplasmosis (combined with pyrimethamine). Sulphapyridine is now used only as an alternative to dapsone in dermatitis herpetiformis and allied conditions. The use of sulphasalazine in acute generalized morphoea has been reported [5].

Sulphadimidine: Dose, 3 g initially followed by up to 6 g daily in divided doses. For urinary tract infections, two-thirds of these doses are given.

Sulphapyridine: Dose, 0·5–1·5 g daily as an alternative to dapsone in dermatitis herpetiformis.

Silver sulphadiazine has a role as a topical non-absorbable antimicrobial with a broad spectrum.

Trimethoprim [3]. Trimethoprim is a synthetic antimicrobial agent in its own right. It is a potent inhibitor of bacterial dihydrofolic acid reductase which converts dihydrofolic acid to tetrahydrofolic acid but has many thousand times less effect on the comparable mammalian enzyme. Trimethoprim is very well absorbed orally, distributed widely through most body tissues and excreted almost completely by the kidney. Although now available as a separate drug it has been used mainly in combination with sulphamethoxazole in the proportions 1 to 5 as cotrimoxazole. This is entirely logical as these drugs inhibit successive stages in bacterial folate metabolism and it is not surprising that their combined effect is synergistic. Both drugs used singly are bacteriostatic but cotrimoxazole appears to be bactericidal.

Cotrimoxazole Tablets B.P. These contain sulphamethoxazole 400 mg and trimethoprim 80 mg. The dose is two tablets twice daily. Double strength cotrimoxazole (960 mg) is also available. It is effective against a wide range of Gram-positive and Gram-negative bacteria as well as nocardia and is in general well tolerated. It is best avoided in pregnancy, however, and in infants under 6 weeks and therefore in lactating mothers feeding young babies. Typical sulphonamide skin reactions may occur in up to 8% of patients. It is not believed to cause folate deficiency in man but evidence suggests it should be used with caution in those who might be folate deficient and whose marrow may be depressed by disease or other drugs [3].

It is much prescribed for urinary tract and respiratory infections but is of value in brucellosis, chancroid, atypical mycobacterial infections [2] and mycetoma. It is often effective used long term and in low dose in tetracycline-failed acne.

REFERENCES

1 BAKER H. (1968) *Br J Dermatol* **80**, 844.
2 BARROW G.I. & HEWITT M. (1971) *Br Med J* i, 505.
3 KUCAS A. & BENNETT N. McK. (1979) *The Use of Antibiotics.* 3rd ed. London, Heinemann.
4 MANDELL G.L. & SANDE M.A. (1985). In Goodman & Gilman's *The Pharmacological Basis of Therapeutics* 7th ed. Eds. Gilman A.G., *et al.* New York, MacMillan. Ch. 49.
5 STAVA Z. & KOBIKOVA M. (1977) *Br J Dermatol* **96**, 541.

Penicillins. The basic structure of a penicillin consists of a rhiazolidine ring, a β-lactam ring and a variable side chain. 6-Aminopenicillamic acid is the starting point for the semisynthetic penicillins of which there are now many. It is convenient to divide the penicillins into four main groups according to their antibacterial properties and consequent clinical usage.

1. Penicillinase-sensitive penicillins ('penicillin'), e.g.
   (a) Benzyl penicillin (penicillin G)
   (b) Phenoxymethyl penicillin (penicillin V)

2. Penicillinase-resistant penicillins, e.g.
   Flucloxacillin
3. Broad spectrum penicillins (vulnerable to penicillinase) (β-lactamases). By combining clavulanic acid, a potent β-lactamase inhibitor, with amoxycillin (Augmentin) the spectrum of activity has been broadened to cover penicillin-resistant staphylococci, e.g.
   (a) Ampicillin
   (b) Amoxycillin
4. Antipseudomonal penicillins, e.g.
   (a) Carbenicillin
   (b) Azlocillin

Toxicity. The penicillins as a whole are remarkably non-toxic to man [4]. The main problems with their use are hypersensitivity reactions which are not uncommon; an incidence between 1 and 10% is usually accepted [2] and there is little doubt that the oral route is safer [5]. Anaphylaxis from any one penicillin means that all penicillins must be permanently withheld.

Penicillinase-sensitive penicillins (penicillin). Penicillin is the drug of choice against *Streptococcus pyogenes* group A, *Treponema pallidum* and *Bacillus anthracis* as it is in yaws and diphtheria. Notwithstanding the emergence of resistant strains of organism, it remains an important first line drug against gonorrhoea. In most serious infections penicillin is given by injection as benzyl penicillin but treatment may be continued with oral penicillin V and this drug has a small but important role in prophylaxis against streptococcal cellulitis in lymphoedema.

Benzyl penicillin injection B.P. (penicillin G): Dose, 300 mg (0·5 mega-units) four times daily up to 1·8 g (3 mega-units) daily. If higher blood levels are required, probenecid may be given to block renal tubular excretion of penicillin. Long-acting injectable preparations are available.

Phenoxymethyl penicillin (penicillin V): Dose, 250–500 mg every 6 h.

Penicillinase-resistant penicillins. For practical purposes this means flucloxacillin, which is resistant to staphylococcal β-lactamase and is the drug of choice against penicillin-resistant straphylococci. It is somewhat less effective against other Gram-positive infections. Adequate levels are achieved by the oral route but parenteral administration is preferred in serious infections.

Flucloxacillin: Dose, 250–500 mg every 6 h and at least 30 min before food.

Broad spectrum penicillins. Ampicillin is the much used example with a spectrum of activity against Gram-negative bacteria. It is acid stable and therefore absorbed orally but is not resistant to penicillinase. It is little used in dermatology but is important as a cause of drug rashes. These occur in about 5–10% of all patients treated but in a majority of those with infectious mononucleosis, cytomegalovirus infections or lymphatic leukaemia [2] (see p. 1261). The typical morbilliform rash is thought to be toxic in nature and unrelated to true penicillin hypersensitivity. Amoxycillin is almost identical, is twice as well absorbed as ampicillin but is currently much more expensive. It should probably only replace ampicillin in the patient known to be susceptible to antibiotic-induced diarrhoea [3]. Where an even broader spectrum is needed, perhaps in the treatment of heavily infected leg ulcers with surrounding cellulitis, amoxycillin with clavulanic acid (Augmentin) is worth consideration [1, 6]. Its role in dermatology is likely to be a limited one.

Ampicillin: Dose, 250 mg to 1 g every 6 h and at least 30 min before a meal.

Amoxycillin capsules: Dose, 250–500 mg every 8 h.

Amoxycillin 250 mg and clavulanic acid (Augmentin) tablets: Dose, 1–2 tablets every 8 h.

Antipseudomonal penicillins. Carbenicillin, its successor ticarcillin, and azlocillin must all by given by injection or infusion and have little place in dermatology. A safe effective orally absorbed antipseudomal drug is still awaited.

REFERENCES

1 ANONYMOUS (1982) *Drug Ther Bull* **20**, 21.
2 BEELEY L. (1984) *Br Med J* **288**, 511.
3 DYAS A, & WISE R. (1983) *Br Med J* **286**, 583.
4 GARROD L.P., *et al* (1981) In *Antibiotic and Chemotherapy.* 5th ed. Edinburgh, Churchill Livingstone.
5 INTERNATIONAL SYMPOSIUM (1974) *J Infect Dis* **129** (Suppl. 121).
6 ROLINSON G.N. & WATSON A. (1980) Augmentin: Proceedings of First Symposium. Amsterdam, Excerpta Medica.

Cephalosporins [1]. These are derivatives of 7-aminocephalosporamic acid and are similar in structure and properties to the penicillins. They are bactericidal, acting on bacterial cell walls, and have wide spectra of activity encompassing Gram-negative organisms and staphylococci—penicillin-resistant staphylococci are generally susceptible but the degree of effectiveness varies from cephalosporin to cephalosporin. Most are administered parenterally but some orally effective ones are available, e.g.

cefaclor. They are all excreted by the kidney but unlike penicillin may cause tubular damage. Their main role is perhaps as alternative therapy in penicillin hypersensitivity but this is not without risk as some 8–10% of all penicillin-allergic patients react to cephalosporins. Apart from this they have little dermatological interest.

REFERENCE

1 ANONYMOUS (1982) *Drug Ther Bull* **20**, 85.

Antileprotics. The sulphones remain drugs of choice for all forms of leprosy. They are derivatives of 4,4-diaminodiphenyl sulphone (dapsone); they are related to the sulphonamides, and probably act in the same way. *Mycobacterium leprae* is usually extremely sensitive [13] but may become resistant. Sulphones are bacteriostatic, not bactericidal.

Dapsone. This drug is orally absorbed and is available as 50 and 100 mg tablets. The usual adult dose in leprosy is 50–100 mg/day although much smaller doses used to be given. It is excreted mainly in the urine [1]. Some degree of haemolysis is an extremely common adverse reaction [2, 4]. In pregnancy and lactation there is clearly a risk of haemolysis and methaemoglobinaemia in the baby but the presence of dapsone in breast milk may have prophylactic value against leprosy [5]. Leprosy apart, dapsone is a well-established means of suppressing the cutaneous lesions of dermatitis herpetiformis [6, 9] and several other diseases. Most dermatologists are more familiar with the use of the drug in this way and further details are described on p. 2525.

Clofazimine [7, 10, 12]. This synthetic drug is given orally. The usual dose is 100 mg three times a week or 100 mg daily in combination with rifampicin if sulphone resistance has occurred [14]. It has an anti-inflammatory effect which may prevent erythema nodosum from developing [3]. For lepra reactions 300 mg/day is recommended. Clofazimine has a very long half-life: 70 days or more. It accumulates in the tissues and is slowly excreted in urine, sweat, sebum and milk.

The main side effect is red–brown to black discoloration of skin and conjunctivae but urine and sputum become red too and breast milk may be discolored. Milk gastrointestinal reactions may occur and ichthyosiform rashes [11]. In general clofazimine is a well-tolerated drug which may be prescribed in pregnancy and during lactation. In renal and hepatic impairment biochemical tests of function

are recommended from time to time but the drug may be used. Clofazimine may be valuable in treating pyoderma gangrenosum [8] and perhaps also in discoid lupus erythematosus.

Rifampicin. This drug will be discussed later (under tuberculosis therapy). It seems to be bactericidal for *M. leprae* in very low dosage and acts much more rapidly than dapsone, rendering the patient noncontagious in a few days or weeks [3]. It does not shorten the total duration of treatment, which should be continued with dapsone.

Thiambutosine. This is a diphenylthiourea, useful as a second-line drug when dapsone cannot be used. Resistance may develop, especially after 1 yr of treatment.

Long-acting sulphonamides. These appear to have no particular advantages and are expensive.

REFERENCES

1 ALEXANDER J.O'D., *et al* (1970) *Br J Dermatol* **83**, 620.
2 ANONYMOUS (1981) *Lancet* ii, 184.
3 BROWNE S.G. (1975) *Practitioner* **215**, 493.
4 CREAM J.J. & SCOTT G.L. (1970) *Br J Dermatol* **82**, 333.
5 FORREST J.M. (1976) *Med J Aust* ii, 138.
6 FRY L., *et al* (1980) *Br J Dermatol* **102**, 371.
7 KARAT A.B.A., *et al* (1971) *Br Med J* iv, 514.
8 KARK E.C., *et al* (1981) *J Am Acad Dermatol* **4**, 152.
9 KATZ S.I., *et al* (1980) *Ann Intern Med* **93**, 857.
10 LEVY L. (1974) *Am J Trop Med Hyg* **23**, 1097.
11 MICHAËLSSON G., *et al* (1976) *Arch Dermatol* **112**, 344.
12 RODRIGUEZ J.N. (1974) *Int J Lepr* **42**, 276.
13 SHEPARD C.C. *et al* (1969) *Am J Trop Med Hyg* **18**, 258.
14 YAWALKAR S.J. & VISCHER W. (1979) *Lepr Rev* **50**, 135.

Tetracyclines [26]. These are orally effective broad spectrum antibiotics with relatively low toxicity. The original three tetracyclines were chlortetracycline, oxytetracycline and tetracycline. Later derivatives include demethylchlortetracycline, methacycline, doxycycline and minocycline (the last three being synthetic). They act by inhibition of protein synthesis [27]: with the exception of minocycline they all have similar spectra of activity differing, however, in their absorption, distribution and excretion.

Many streptococci are resistant to tetracyclines [11]. Interestingly, fewer staphylococci are now tetracycline resistant [26] and even these strains are sensitive to minocycline [7]. Strains of *Escherichia coli* may show transferable drug resistance.

The tetracyclines are bacteriostatic against many Gram-positive and Gram-negative bacteria and are also active against rickettsiae, Mycoplasma [2, 5], Chlamydia [28] which cause lymphogranuloma venereum, psittacosis and trachoma, as well as amoebae [16].

It is important to note that absorption is impaired by the simultaneous taking of milk, aluminium, calcium or magnesium salts or iron preparations due to chelation [19]. However, food does not interfere with the absorption of doxycycline or minocycline. All tetracyclines are concentrated in the liver and excreted into the bile, whence they enter an enterohepatic circulation. Urinary excretion is significant and renal failure may be exacerbated [22] by all except doxycycline [17, 20].

Side effects [1, 3, 12]. A variety of rashes has been described (p. 1262) including the phototoxicity especially shown by demethylchlortetracycline [6, 18, 24]. Glossitis, cheilitis and persistent pruritus ani may occur. Gastrointestinal disturbances are dose dependent [10] and are much more common with daily doses of 2 g or more, which are rarely used in dermatology. Nausea and vomiting are direct irritant effects; diarrhoea may be the result of superinfection, resistant staphylococci being especially dangerous. Tetracyclines are deposited in growing teeth (see p. 2121) and bones [25] and their use should be avoided in pregnancy, during lactation [14] and in childhood. Rarely, there may be diffuse fatty degeneration of the liver. An uncommon dermatological problem is the development of Gram-negative folliculitis after tetracycline therapy of acne [9, 13].

Dermatological uses. Apart from the infections mentioned above, tetracyclines are rarely drugs of first choice. The exception, of course, is the treatment of acne vulgaris [4, 8] (p. 1921) and rosacea [21] (p. 1610). It is estimated that 10% of the tetracycline produced for human use in the U.S.A. is prescribed by dermatologists for treating acne [1].

Tetracycline, Chlortetracycline, Oxytetracycline. Daily dosages range from 500 mg (for acne) up to 3 g.

Doxycycline, Minocycline: Daily dosages, 100–200 mg. Doxycycline is the ordinary tetracycline of choice in patients with renal impairment. Minocycline is usually effective against staphylococci resistant to other tetracyclines and often in tetracycline-failed acne.

Preparations are also available as syrups, injections for intramuscular, intravenous or intralesional use, ointments and creams.

REFERENCES

1 Ad hoc Committee Report (1975) *Arch Dermatol* **III**, 1630.
2 Chanock R.M., *et al* (1962) *Proc Nat Acad Sci USA* **48**, 41.
3 Clendenning W.E. (1965) *Arch Dermatol* **91**, 628.
4 Crounse R.G. (1965) *JAMA* **193**, 906.
5 Eaton M.D. (1950) *Proc Soc Exp Biol Med* **72**, 24.
6 Falk M.S. (1960) *JAMA* **172**, 1156.
7 Finland M. (1974) *Clin Pharmacol Ther* **15**, 3.
8 Fry L. & Ramsay C.A. (1966) *Br J Dermatol* **78**, 653.
9 Fulton J.E., *et al* (1968) *Arch Dermatol* **98**, 349.
10 Garrod L.P., *et al* (1981) *Antibiotic and Chemotherapy.* 5th ed. Edinburgh, Churchill Livingstone, p. 169.
11 Gopalkrishna K.V. & Lerner P.I.(1973) *Am Rev Respir Dis* **108**, 1007.
12 Kunin C.M. (1968) *Pediatr Clin North Am* **15**, 43.
13 Leyden J.L., *et al* (1973) *Br J Dermatol* **88**, 533.
14 Macaulay J.C. & Leistyna J.A. (1964) *Pediatrics* **34**, 423.
15 Marples R.R., *et al* (1971) *J Invest Dermatol* **56**, 127.
16 Martin G.A., *et al* (1953) *JAMA* **151**, 1055.
17 Merier G., *et al* (1969) *Helv Med Acta* **35**, 124.
18 Morris L.E. (1960) *JAMA* **172**, 1155.
19 Neuvonen P.J., *et al* (1974) *Br Med J* **iv**, 532.
20 Ribush N. & Morgan T. (1972) *Med J Aust* **i**, 53.
21 Rook A.J. (1966) *Practitioner* **197**, 442.
22 Shils M.E. (1963) *Ann Intern Med* **58**, 389.
23 Smith E.L. & Mortimer P.R. (1967) *Br J Dermatol* **79**, 78.
24 de Verber L.L. (1962) *Can Med Assoc J* **86**, 168.
25 Wallman I.S. & Hilton H.B. (1962) *Lancet* **i**, 827.
26 Weinstein L. (1975) In *The Pharmacological Basis of Therapeutics.* Eds. Goodman L.S. & Gilman A. New York, Macmillan, p. 1183.
27 Weisblum B. & Davies J. (1968) *Bact Rev* **32**, 493.
28 Wright L.T., *et al* (1948) *JAMA* **138**, 408.

Macrolides

Erythromycin: Dose, 1–2 g daily in divided doses. This is the only significant member of the macrolide group of antibiotics. It is active mainly against Gram-positive organisms such as staphylococci and streptococci. Staphylococci may rapidly develop resistance, especially in hospital, where up to 50% of strains may be resistant; streptococci are occasionally resistant. There may be cross-resistance with lincomycin.

Side effects are not common, the only serious problem being an allergic cholestatic hepatitis which occurs only with erythromycin estolate. Erythromycin is an extremely useful drug for the out-patient treatment of staphylococcal or streptococcal pyodermas, especially in the penicillin-allergic patient. It may also be used for atypical mycobacterial infections. Particular dermatological uses are for erythrasma and acne; it may safely be given in renal failure as less than 5% is excreted in the urine.

Aminoglycosides. This group includes streptomycin (see below), kanamycin, neomycin, gentamicin and tobramycin. They are but little used in dermatological practice, their chief use being against Gram-negative infections. They inhibit protein synthesis; bacteria may rapidly become resistant and cross-resistance occurs within the group. Normally there is almost no absorption by mouth. They are ototoxic and, to a lesser degree, nephrotoxic.

Dermatological uses. These are few. Streptomycin is still used for tuberculosis, is dramatically effective in tularaemia and is used as an alternative to tetracyclines in granuloma venereum. The topical use of neomycin is discussed in Chapter 69.

Gentamicin [4]. This is the most important of the aminoglycosides [3]. Although it has a broad spectrum of activity, its use should be restricted to the treatment of serious Gram-negative infections, especially those due to *Pseudomonas aeruginosa* [1, 2]. It has a synergistic effect with carbenicillin against *Pseudomonas* and other Gram-negative organisms. It should not be used in pregnancy and should preferably be controlled by measurements of its plasma concentration, which should be kept below 10–12 µg/ml.

REFERENCES

1 BULGER R.J., *et al* (1963) *Ann Intern Med* **59**, 593.
2 JAO R.L. & JACKSON G.G. (1964) *JAMA* **189**, 817.
3 MANDELL G.L. & SANDE M.A. (1985). In Goodman & Gilman's *The Pharmacological Basis of Therapeutics* 7th ed. Eds. Gilman A.G., *et al.* New York, MacMillan. Ch. 51.
4 SECOND INTERNATIONAL SYMPOSIUM ON GENTAMICIN (1971) *J Infect Dis* **124** (Suppl. S.I.).

Lincosamides. Lincomycin and its derivative clindamycin (which ought to be used in preference to lincomycin [3]) act against Gram-positive cocci including some penicillin-resistant staphylococci. They are highly active against bacteroides infections and penetrate well into bone.

Side effects. Diarrhoea may occur in up to 20% of cases; pseudomembranous colitis may supervene and may last for weeks after the drug has been withdrawn [4, 5]. There have been a number of deaths from this complication; one severe case has been reported in a patient treated for acne [6].

Clindamycin. This is an effective alternative drug for

the treatment of acne [2]; however, in view of its known toxicity, it is now rarely used systemically for this condition [1].

REFERENCES

1 AD HOC COMMITTEE REPORT (1975) *Arch Dermatol* **111**, 1630.
2 CHRISTIAN G.L. & KREUGER G.G. (1975) *Arch Dermatol* **111**, 997.
3 GARROD L.P., *et al* (1973) *Antibiotic and Chemotherapy.* Edinburgh, Churchill Livingstone.
4 TEDESCO F.J., *et al* (1974) *Ann Intern Med* **81**, 429.
5 VITERI A.L., *et al* (1974) *Gastroenterology* **66**, 1137.
6 WOLFE M.S. (1974) *JAMA*, **229**, 266.

Chloramphenicol. This would be a useful drug for a number of infections were it not for the bone marrow aplasia which occurs in 1 in 40,000 courses of treatment [1]. This has been known for 25 yr, and yet a survey of 576 cases of blood dyscrasia due to chloramphenicol concluded that in most cases there had been no indication to justify its use [2]. Nevertheless, it probably remains the treatment of choice for typhoid fever and *Haemophilus influenzae* meningitis.

REFERENCES

1 POLAK B.C.P., *et al* (1972) *Acta Med Scand* **192**, 409.
2 MANDELL G.L. & SANDE M.A. (1985). In Goodman & Gilman's *The Pharmacological Basis of Therapeutics* 7th ed. Eds. Gilman A.G., *et al.* New York, MacMillan. Ch. 52.

Rifampicins. See below: antituberculous therapy (p. 2519).

Polymyxins. Polymyxin B and polymyxin E (Colistin) are relatively toxic drugs which are not absorbed from the gastrointestinal tract. Their use for Gram-negative infections has been largely superseded by gentamicin and carbenicillin. Polymyxin B is used topically.

Fusidic acid. This interesting antibiotic is produced by a strain of *Fusidium coccineum* and has the basic structure of a steroid, though it shows little in the way of metabolic effects. It is a very safe drug, primarily used for staphylococcal infections, though it is also active against other Gram-positive bacteria and the Gram-negative cocci. Nearly all strains of staphylococci are outstandingly sensitive to fucidin but there may be a few resistant mutants which can multiply rapidly. However, concomitant administration of penicillin can be used to kill any resistant mutants as they emerge [1]. It is available for oral use, as an injection and for topical application. Its indiscriminate prescription for minor infections should be discouraged for fear of encouraging resistant strains.

REFERENCE

1 O'GRADY F & GREENWOOD D. (1973) *J Med Microbial* **6**, 441.

Antibiotic combinations [1]. Antibiotic combinations are frequently used, often irrationally. Some combinations are contra-indicated because they lead to antibacterial antagonism. Examples are between penicillin and tetracycline [3], between penicillin and chloramphenicol [5] or between ampicillin and carbenicillin [4]. However, two bactericidal antibiotics are often synergistic, whereas a combination of a bactericidal and a bacteriostatic antibiotic often shows antagonism, but there are important exceptions to this rule [2].

In dermatological practice combinations of systemic antibiotics are rarely needed except in serious staphyloderma due to resistant organisms. Combined therapy should always be based on sensitivity testing.

REFERENCES

1 BRUMFIT W. & PERCIVAL A. (1971) *Lancet* **i**, 387.
2 JAURETZ E. (1967) *Pharm Physns* **1**, 1.
3 OLSSON R.A., *et al* (1961) *Ann Intern Med* **55**, 545.
4 SELIGMAN S.J. (1968) *Clin Res* **16**, 335.
5 WALLACE J.F., *et al* (1967) *J Lab Clin Med* **70**, 408.

Metronidazole [1]. Metronidazole is a synthetic agent active against protozoa and anaerobic bacteria. It is particularly useful in trichomoniasis, amoebiasis and giardiasis and has proved extremely valuable against bacteroides species. For the dermatologist it has a limited role in the treatment of tetracycline-failed rosacea [2]. Metronidazole is well absorbed by the oral or rectal route and may also be given intravenously. It is available as 200 and 400 mg tablets, the usual adult dose by mouth being 200 mg twice daily for rosacea, 200 mg every 8 h for trichomonas infections, 400 mg every 8 h for anaerobic bacterial infections and 800 mg every 8 h for amoebiasis. The suppositories contain 500 mg and in anaerobic infections are prescribed in the adult dose of 1 g every 8 h at first, dropping to 1 g every 12 h. The fate and mode of excretion of metronidazole are not fully understood [3]; it is generally regarded as safe in hepatic and renal disease. There is no evidence that it is a human teratogen, and it may be given to lactating mothers although it causes darkening of milk and may give it a bitter taste. In normal doses and for short periods it is generally a remarkably safe drug but minor gastrointestinal side effects such as nausea, an unpleasant taste in the mouth and black hairy tongue are not uncommon. Vomiting, abdominal pain and diarrhoea may follow. Darkening of urine, headache and drowsiness also occur and leucopenia may be noted. Much less common adverse reactions are peripheral neuropathy, particularly associated with prolonged treatment, and central nervous system effects (dizziness, ataxia and fits) from high dosage. Fears that metronidazole might be a carcinogen are not to date supported by factual evidence. The only important interaction is with alcohol, giving a disulphiram-like reaction in some patients.

REFERENCES

1 PHILLIPS I. & COLLIER J. (Eds.) (1979) *Metronidazole. Royal Society of Medicine International Congress & Symposium Series No. 18*. London.
2 SAIHAN E.M. & BURTON J.L. (1980) *Br J Dermatol* **102**, 443.
3 SOMOGYI A.A., *et al* (1984) *J Antimicrob Chemother* **13**, 183.

Antituberculous drugs (see also Chapter 22). The important first line drugs for the treatment of *Mycobacterium tuberculosis* infections are isoniazid, rifampicin, ethambutol and streptomycin [4, 9]. In the initial period of treatment, usually 60 days or until sensitivities are available, three of these drugs are used concurrently. For the continuation phase of therapy two drugs to which the organism is sensitive are sufficient for cure without the occurrence of resistant strains. (For details see Chapter 22.)

Second line drugs such as pyrazinamide, ethionamide, cycloserine, *para*-aminosalicylic acid or thiacetazone may be required where drug resistance or adverse reactions preclude the use of more than one of the four first line agents.

Isoniazid. This is a synthetic orally absorbed bactericidal agent usually given in a dose of 300 mg/day to adults (5–10 mg/kg every 24 h). It is excreted mainly by the kidney after acetylation and further metabolism. It is permissible in pregnancy [12] but during lactation should be supplemented with pyridoxin because of the theoretical risk of toxic side effects (see below). In severe renal failure the adult dosage should be reduced to 200 mg/day. Adverse reactions may be divided into toxic and allergic. Toxic reactions are more common in slow acetylators and include most commonly peripheral neuropathy but also convulsions, mental disturbances and a pellagra-like rash [8]. They are usually reversible on cessation of therapy. Pyridoxin 10 mg/day given prophylactically will reduce the incidence of these problems where high doses are used. The main allergic reactions are rashes, agranulocytosis and hepatitis, this last being apparently more common in patients with pre-existing liver disease [6].

Rifampicin. This is a synthetically modified antibiotic of the rifamycin group, bactericidal and very effective against *M. tuberculosis*, many atypical myobacteria and Gram-positive cocci. It is also useful in leprosy. To counter the emergence of resistant strains it is always used in combination with other antimicrobials. Unfortunately (because it would be of great value in the Third World), it remains a very expensive drug.

Rifampicin is well absorbed orally and is available as 150 mg capsules and a 100 mg/5 ml mixture. In adults it is usual to prescribe 450–600 mg daily as a single dose before breakfast (10 mg/g per day) (see p. 820 for duration of therapy and further details). Excretion is predominantly in the bile and so hepatic impairment is an indication for avoidance or at least lower dosage. In pregnancy rifampicin is best avoided but where it has been used the incidence of abnormalities noted at birth has not been excessively high—4·3% compared with 1·8% in tuberculous controls [16]. If used in late pregnancy it may cause haemorrhagic problems in neonates. Rifampicin is generally regarded as a relatively non-toxic antituberculous drug but many different adverse reactions have been described: mild gastrointestinal disturbances, rashes—particularly flushing [5, 7]. Transient impairment of liver function as revealed by elevation of transaminase levels is common but need not usually interrupt therapy. Orange–red discoloration of urine, saliva and sweat may be noticed. Thrombocytopenia, however, is an uncommon side effect which must not be ignored. Three other serious adverse reactions are a 'flu-like illness, a syndrome of dyspnoea, wheezing and hypotension and the occurrence of renal failure, all of which are characteristically associated with intermittent or irregular medication [3]. Drug interactions occur with warfarin (diminished anticoagulant effect), oral contraceptives (possibly) and corticosteroids (diminished steroid effect [13]).

Streptomycin. This is an aminoglycoside antibiotic used mainly in the treatment of tuberculosis. It must be administered parenterally and is commonly given in a dose of 500–1000 mg/day by intramuscular injection, the lower doses being preferred in patients over 40 [11]. Excretion is by the kidney so

that dosage should be reduced in renal impairment. Dose reduction is also important in the premature infant. Of the important side effects the most common is vertigo which is especially troublesome in the elderly. Deafness may also develop and both these eighth nerve effects are dose related [1]. These two adverse reactions provide a strong contra-indication to the use of streptomycin in pregnancy and lactation as the infant may be affected, and of course in patients with pre-existing vestibular or auditory impairment. Allergic reactions include skin eruptions from the trivial to exfoliative dermatitis, eosinophilia and drug fever. Contact sensitization to streptomycin is a well-recognized hazard among nurses, justifying precautions to avoid skin contamination, e.g. by wearing gloves. Because streptomycin is a neuromuscular blocking agent it may increase the effects of suxamethonium and other similar drugs and should be used only with extreme caution in myasthenia gravis.

Ethambutol. This is a synthetic agent effective only against *M. tuberculosis* and some atypical mycobacteria. It is orally absorbed and is available on its own as 100 and 400 mg tablets and in combination with isoniazid in a variety of strengths. The usual initial dose is 15 mg/kg per day in adults and 25 mg/kg per day in children, reducing later in that age group to 15 mg/kg per day. It may also be used as intermittent treatment in a dose of 45–50 mg/kg twice weekly. Excretion is mainly via the kidney necessitating reduction of dosage in renal impairment. Optic (retrobulbar) neuritis with diminished visual acuity and red–green colour blindness slowly reversible on cessation of therapy was a relatively common side effect of higher dose schedules but should be rare with currently recommended levels [2, 10]. It seems to be more effective to train patients to check their own vision regularly when on this drug than to rely on periodic ophthalmic examinations. Ethambutol may also, though rarely, cause peripheral neuropathy and renal damage, and may precipitate attacks of gout. It appears not to be a teratogen in humans [14] and is not contra-indicated during lactation.

Para-aminosalicylic acid. This drug is much less active than the above drugs but has a role in preventing the emergence of resistant strains of *M. tuberculosis*. It is given in the large dose 10–20 g/day and unfortunately is associated with a high incidence of minor but unpleasant side effects [15]—gastrointestinal symptoms occur in nearly all patients. Allergic reactions with rashes and fever are common and there seems to be either cross-hypersensitivity with streptomycin or potentiation of streptomycin allergy. Though once a valued drug in triple therapy its use is now largely restricted to poorer countries where its low cost is a major consideration.

Reserve drugs [9]. A number of other antituberculous drugs are available and may be required if resistance or hypersensitivity reactions preclude the use of standard treatment. They include pyrazinamide, capreomycin, ethionamide and cycloserine.

REFERENCES

1 BALLANTYNE J. (1970) *J Laryngol Otol* **84**, 967.
2 CLARKE G.B.M., *et al* (1972) *Br J Dis Chest* **66**, 272.
3 FLYNN C.T., *et al* (1974) *Br Med J* ii, 482.
4 GARROD L.P., *et al* (1981). In *Antibiotic and Chemotherapy*. 5th ed. Edinburgh, Churchill Livingstone, ch. 23.
5 GIRLING D.J. (1977) *J Antimicrob Chemother* **3**, 115.
6 GIRLING D.J. (1978) *Tubercle* **59**, 13.
7 GIRLING D.J. & HITZE K.L. (1979) *Bull WHO* **57**, 45.
8 HORNE W. (1972) *Practitioner* **208**, 263.
9 KUCERS A. & BENNETT N. McK. (1979). In *The Use of Antibiotics*. 3rd ed. London, Heinemann, Part III.
10 LEES A.W., *et al* (1971) *Tubercle* **52**, 182.
11 LINE D.H., *et al* (1970) *Tubercle* **51**, 76.
12 LUDFORD J., *et al* (1973) *Am Rev Respir Dis* **108**, 1170.
13 McALLISIER W.A.C., *et al* (1983) *Br J Dermatol* **286**, 923.
14 PYLE M.M. (1970) *Med Clin North Am* **54**, 1317.
15 ROSSOUW J.E. & SAUNDERS S.J. (1975). *J Med* **44**, 1.
16 STEEN J.S.M. & STAINION-ELLIS D.M. (1977) *Lancet* **2**, 604.

ANTIFUNGAL DRUGS [3, 15, 18]

The drugs available for systemic use against fungal diseases are few in number. Griseofulvin is for practical purposes an anti-ringworm agent only and is considered elsewhere (p. 929). Of the polyene antibiotics amphotericin is the only one suitable for systemic use, though nystatin tablets are effective within the bowel. Both drugs have a very broad spectrum but one which excludes the dermatophytes. Among the imidazoles, with their wide range of activity, ketoconazole, which may be given orally, and miconazole, which must be administered parenterally, are important systemic agents. The pyrimidine analogue, flucytosine, is effective against yeasts and in chromomycosis, while potassium iodide is an elderly but effective remedy in sporotrichosis and subcutaneous phycomycosis.

Polyenes [12]

Nystatin [12]. Nystatin was the first polyene antibiotic discovered (in 1951) and is still valuable today as a topical anti-candida agent. It is not absorbed from the gut in significant amounts and it proved to be too toxic for systemic use when given parenterally. By mouth it is, in effect, a topical agent for the gastrointestinal tract and used in this manner is almost entirely without adverse effects. Intestinal irritation may accompany large doses but allergic reactions are almost unknown. One case of fixed drug eruption has been reported [13].

Amphotericin B [3, 12]. This is a polyene antibiotic derived from *Streptomyces nodosum*. It has a very wide range of activity against *Candida* sp. and almost all deep fungal pathogens. Resistance is rare. Absorption from the gut is negligible and so as with nystatin tablets and lozenges are for practical purposes topical therapy for the gut. For systemic use amphotericin B must be given by slow intravenous infusion in 5% dextrose. The solution thus diluted is unstable; it should be used promptly and other drugs should not be added—except heparin or hydrocortisone. The definitive adult dose range is normally in the range of 0·4–1 mg/kg per day but toxicity is minimized if a very small dose (1 mg) is infused on the first day, somewhat more (10 mg) on the second, building up to full dosage by day 5. Clearly in the gravely ill patient this preferred approach is not feasible.

The fate of amphotericin in the body is not fully understood [1]. Only small amounts appear in urine; much is probably bound to sterol-containing membranes. As amphotericin B is often the drug of first choice in life-threatening situations, renal failure demands dose reduction and extreme caution; it is not an absolute contra-indication. Adverse reactions are common, initially: fever, rigors, hypotension, nausea, vomiting, tinnitus and bronchospasm. Phlebitis at the site of infusion is also frequent. Hypokalaemia and hypochromic anaemia may occur and, rarely, liver function abnormalities. Nephrotoxicity is of great importance; renal clearance may be decreased and tubular damage may develop. These are particularly a problem of extended treatment but are potentially reversible. If renal impairment is severe, therepy must therefore be interrupted and should be restarted at a lower dosage.

Flucytosine [4, 17]. This is a synthetic cytosine analogue which is converted to 5 fluorouracil in the body. It is effective against yeasts, including *Candida* sp., *Cryptococcosis neoformans* and many of the fungi involved in chromomycosis. It is orally absorbed but may be given intravenously too. The tablets contain

500 mg, the usual adult dose being 150 mg/kg per day. Lower doses are necessary in renal failure. It is important to monitor serum levels, aiming to achieve 40–60 mg/l and to avoid toxic levels—above 120 mg/l. Because resistance, both primary and secondary, is well recognized, sensitivity testing initially and at intervals is strongly recommended. In cryptococcosis, flucytosine is usually given with amphotericin to prevent resistant strains developing.

The main side effects are nausea, vomiting, diarrhoea and rashes, but thrombocytopenia and neutropenia may also occur.

Imidazoles

Miconazole. This is a much used topical imidazole poorly absorbed by the oral route. It may be administered intravenously by slow intravenous infusion three times in 24 h, the usual adult dose being 1·8–3 g per day. Side effects are not particularly common. They include pruritus, rashes, fever, faintness and venous thrombosis at the infusion site. Anorexia, nausea, vomiting and diarrhoea occur and anaphylaxis is a rare but genuine problem. Hyperlipidaemia and haematological abnormalities should also be recognized [20] and eruptive xanthomas have occurred [2]. The place of systemic miconazole remains uncertain but some patients with systemic candidiasis, coccidioidomycosis [10] and paracoccidioidomycosis not responding to first choice drugs may benefit from its use.

Ketoconazole [7, 15]. This broad spectrum, orally absorbed imidazole has few side effects apart from its hepatotoxicity (see below) and has been claimed as a major advance in antifungal chemotherapy. Its precise value in the classical systemic mycoses and in opportunist infections is not yet clear but in paracoccidioidomycosis [7] and in chronic mucocutaneous candidiasis [8, 22] it has an undoubted role. In rare griseofulvin-resistant ringworm, particularly extensive tinea corporis, it appears to be extremely effective [6, 11]. Pityriasis versicolor responds well though it is not yet clear if late relapses—a problem in tropical climates—are less common than with topical therapy or whether this drug should be used routinely for this minor infection [21]. The place of ketoconazole in vulvovaginal candidiasis and minor cutaneous candida infections has not yet been fully elucidated but its effectiveness against all but a few rare resistant isolates of *C. albicans* [16] is not in doubt. *Candida* (Torulopis) *glabrata* and possibly *Trichophyton concentricum* seems to show primary resistance. A report that nearly 90% of patients with onychomycosis were cured by ketoconazole [5] is at variance with our experience with a small number of griseofulvin-failed cases of tinea of the nails.

Ketoconazole is available in 200 mg tablets and in superficial mycoses is usually given in the adult dose of 200–400 mg/day with food, but 800 mg/day may be required in severe infections. Antacids, cimetidine, ranitidine and anticholinergic drugs may all reduce absorption. Ketoconazole should be avoided in pregnancy.

Common minor side effects are headache and nausea. Itching and rashes are rare, although a case of exfoliative dermatitis has been reported [14]. Gynaecomastia may occasionally develop, and the levels of liver enzymes, both transaminases and alkaline phosphatase, may rise. Often these changes in liver function tests are transient but persistent elevation to three times normal is an indication for cessation of treatment as drug-induced hepatitis is now recognized as a rare adverse reaction to this drug and one which in a few cases has been fatal [9]. The frequency is currently thought to be approximately 1:10,000 patients but even this low level of hepatotoxicity does justify warning the patient to be alert for hepatic symptoms, careful monitoring of hepatic function during prolonged therapy and avoidance of the drug when there is a history of serious hepatic disease [19]. Ketoconazole is not contra-indicated in renal disease.

Potassium iodide [18]. In the form of a saturated aqueous solution (100 g in 100 ml water) this is the preferred treatment for lymphocutaneous sporotrichosis and subcutaneous phycomycosis (basidiobolomycosis). It is administered orally starting with 0·6 ml three times a day and gradually increasing until a level of four or five times the dose is attained in an adult. The mode of action is obscure and potassium iodide does not inhibit *Sporothrix schenkii in vitro*. Progress must be expected to be slow and treatment should be continued until 4 weeks after apparent cure. Iodides are best avoided in pregnancy because of the risk of goitre and hypothyroidism in the infant. Adverse reactions include iododerma, salivary and lactimal gland swelling and hypersecretion, and gastrointestinal disturbances, as well as anxiety, depression and hypothyroidism.

REFERENCES

1 ATKINSON A.J. & BENNETT J.E. (1978) *Antimicrob Agents Chemother* **13**, 271.
2 BARR R.J., *et al* (1978) *Arch Dermatol* **114**, 1544.
3 BENNETT J.E. (1974) *N Engl J Med* **290**, 30.
4 BENNETT J.E. (1977) *Ann Intern Med* **86**, 319.

5 BOTTER A.A. & NUIJTEN S.T.M. (1981) *Mykosen* **24**, 156.

6 COX F.W., *et al* (1982) *J Am Acad Dermatol* **6**, 455.

7 GRAYBILL J.R. (Ed.) (1983) Symposium on New Developments in Therapy for the Mycoses. *Am J Med* **74** (Suppl. **18**).

8 GRAYBILL J.E., *et al* (1980) *Arch Dermatol* **116**, 1137.

9 HEINBERK J.K. & SVEJGAARD E. (1981) *Br Med J* **183**, 825.

10 HOEPRICH P.D., *et al* (1980) *JAMA* **243**, 1923.

11 JONES H.E., *et al* (1981) *Arch Dermatol* **117**, 129.

12 MEDOFF G. & KOBAYASHI G.A. (1980). In *Antifungal Chemotherapy*. Ed. Speller D.C.E. Chichester, Wiley, ch. 1.

13 PAREEK S.S. (1980) *Br J Dermatol* **103**, 679.

14 RAND R., *et al* (1983) *Arch Dermatol* **119**, 97.

15 ROBERTS D.T. (1982) *Br J Dermatol* **106**, 597.

16 RYLEY J.F., *et al* (1984) *Sabouraudia* **22**, 53.

17 SCHOLER H.J. (1976) *Chemotherapy* **22**, 103.

18 SPELLER D.C.E. (Ed.) (1980) *Antifungal Chemotherapy*. Chichester, Wiley.

19 STEM R.S. (1982) *J Am Acad Dermatol* **6**, 544.

20 SUNG J.P. & GRENOAHL J.G. (1977) *N Engl J Med* **297**, 786.

21 URCUYO F.G. & ZAIAS N. (1982) *J Am Acad Dermatol* **6**, 24.

22 VALDIMARSSON H. & HAY R.J. (1981) *J R Soc Med* **74**, 152.

ANTIVIRAL AGENTS

In spite of great efforts to find effective antiviral agents the armamentarium of drugs useful against viruses remains pitifully small [9]. The interferons disappointingly have not yet proved to be of practical value in human viral infections and the available preparations are associated with unpleasant side effects when given intravenously. Since the third edition of this book one major new agent of proven merit, acyclovir, has appeared. Others are promised. It is clear, however, that several of the drugs previously regarded as useful systemic antiviral agents are best abandoned in this role because they lack convincing activity in properly controlled trials, because they are too toxic or both.

Cytarbine. A large number of controlled studies have failed to substantiate the earlier claims that this drug had useful antiviral effects in man and its value seems to be restricted to the treatment of leukaemia.

Amantidine. This was recommended for A_2 influenza prophylaxis. Its use is now confined to the treatment of Parkinsonism and its importance to the dermatologist lies in recognizing that it can cause livedo reticularis (and ankle oedema) [15].

Vidarabine (adenosine arabinoside, ARA-A). This purine nucleoside acts by inhibiting viral DNA synthesis. It has effects mainly against the herpes group of viruses and appears to be effective in early cases of herpes simplex encephalitis and in varicella/zoster infections of immunocompromised subjects. At a dose of 10 mg/kg per day intravenously it causes mainly mild gastrointestinal side effects and in 5% of subjects rashes. Central nervous system and haematological side effects have also been reported [13]. A 3% ointment has an established place in the topical treatment of herpes simplex keratoconjunctivitis.

Idoxuridine. This synthetic nucleoside is effective against DNA viruses, particularly the herpes group. Its use is now restricted to topical application because of severe bone marrow and hepatic toxicity when given intravenously.

Methisazone. This thiosemicarbazone has been used as a prophylactic treatment of contacts of smallpox and variola minor. Early trials were encouraging but further studies have revealed no convincing reduction of mortality. It has been advocated for the treatment of various complications of vaccination but is probably only worth considering in the case of vaccinia gangrenosa [11]. Oral absorption is irregular and vomiting common and often severe enough to prevent completion of therapy. In a world hopefully free from smallpox there should be little need for this drug.

Acyclovir [1, 5, 7, 10, 12, 14]. This is a very active agent against herpes viruses. In serious infections it has been used intravenously but it is also available as 200 mg tablets, as an ophthalmic ointment and as a cream [6]. Unfortunately it has no effect on the latent phase of either herpes simplex or zoster and is apparently ineffective in clinical practice against other viruses. The dose intravenously for series systemic herpes simplex infections is 5 mg/kg every 8 h by slow infusion (over 1 h). In herpes zoster 10 mg/kg every 8 h is advised. Orally 200 mg every 4 h (five times a day) is effective and remarkably safe treatment for severe vulvovaginal herpes simplex [2], for example.

The main route of excretion is renal [4]. Side effects include elevation of blood urea and creatinine which may rarely progress to acute renal failure. In patients with established renal impairment lower doses are indicated. Although animal and human evidence shows no teratogenic activity, as acyclovir is a relatively new drug it is best avoided in pregnancy. There is currently no information about drug levels in human milk when given during lactation. Although some strains of herpes simplex virus have shown evidence of resistance, this appears to be uncommon and of minor degree [3, 8].

REFERENCES

1 BRIGDEN D. & SUTTON R.N.P. (Eds.) (1983) Symposium on Acyclovir *J Infect* **6** (Suppl. 1).
2 BRYSON Y.J. (1984) *J Antimicrob Chemother* **12** (Suppl. B), 61.
3 DEKKER C., *et al* (1983) *J Antimicrob Chemother* **12** (Suppl. B), 137.
4 DE MIRANDA P. & BLUM M.R. (1983) *J Antimicrob Chemother* **12** (Suppl. B), 29.
5 ELION G.B. (1983) *J Antimicrob Chemother* **12** (Suppl. B), 9.
6 FIDDIAN A.P., *et al* (1983) *J Infect* **6** (Suppl. 1), 41.
7 FIELD H.J. & PHILLIPS I. (Eds.) (1983) Symposium on Acyclovir. *J Antimicrob Chemother* **12** (Suppl. B).
8 FIELD H.J., *et al* (1982) *Am J Med* **73** (Suppl. 1), 369.
9 HIRSCH M.S. & SWARTZ M.N. (1980) *N Engl J Med* **302**, 903 and 949.
10 KING D.H. & GALASSO G. (Eds.) (1982) Symposium on Acyclovir. *Am J Med* **73** (Suppl. 1).
11 KUCERS A. & BENNETT N. McK. (1979) *The Use of Antibiotics.* 3rd ed. London. Heinemann, p. 965.
12 OXFORD J.S. (1979) *J Antimicrob Chemother* **5**, 333.
13 ROSS A.H., *et al* (1976) *J Infect Dis* **133** (Suppl. A), 192.
14 SPRUANCE S.L., *et al* (1977) *N Engl J Med* **297**, 69.
15 VOLLUM D.I., *et al* (1971) *Br Med J* ii, 627.

DRUGS TO IMPROVE THE PERIPHERAL CIRCULATION

Vasodilators. Vasodilators are amongst the more disappointing drugs which should in theory be of value in dermatology. They are of great value for cardiac failure. Extensive clinical trials with several different groups of drugs have seldom justified their widespread use. The diseases treated, such as intermittent claudication, are notorious for spontaneous improvement. Several drugs are able to cause some flushing of the face and some increase in total blood flow through the limbs, without necessarily increasing the nutritional flow through the capillary bed where it is needed.

Oxpentifylline [6]. This lowers blood viscosity by improving red cell deformability. It is of some value in the treatment of intermittent claudication and perhaps also of arterial ulcers.

Hydroxyethyl rutosides (Paroven) [7]. These are bioflavonoids and have effects on capillary permeability and on other tissue activities. They have been advocated for many vascular disorders, including gravitational disorders, and although they do have some demonstrable activity they are not widely used.

Fibrinolytic therapy. The integrity of blood vessel function depends on an appropriate balance between fibrin deposition and fibrin removal, both within the lumen and in the tissues. Drugs which enhance fibrinolysis are sometimes used where the balance is excessively towards fibrin deposition. They are of special value in some variants of the gravitational syndrome, particularly with the clinical pictures of lipodermatosclerosis or atrophie blanche (Chapter 32). They are also used sometimes to treat vasculitis and Raynaud's phenomenon. Phenformin with ethyloestrenol has now been replaced by stanozolol, a modified androgen with anabolic properties. The usual dose is 5 mg twice daily. Side effects include mild androgenicity, occasional cholestatic liver damage and fluid retention. The drug is usually given for some months and liver function tests every month or two are appropriate. Stanozolol, like danazol, is also used to treat hereditary angio-oedema (see p. 1107).

Drugs which alter platelet function [2, 3]. A wide variety of drugs have been claimed to have such actions. Small doses of aspirin together with dipyrimadole are most often used.

Low molecular weight dextrans (Rheomacrodex). Dextrans are glucose polymers with average molecular weights of 40,000–110,000. Low molecular weight dextran (Dextran 40) is rapidly excreted but should not be used in severe cardiac or renal failure. The recommended dose is 1,000 ml daily at first and later 500 ml daily [5].

It is claimed that they reduce intravascular cell aggregation and lower blood viscosity, thus increasing capillary flow and tissue perfusion [1].

They have been claimed to be of value in systemic sclerosis and Raynaud's phenomenon of late onset [4], but this has been disputed [1]. Livedo reticularis with ulceration has been successfully treated [5].

REFERENCES

1 ALANI M.D. (1970) *Acta Derm Venereol (Stockh)* **50**, 137.
2 *Br Med Bull* (1978) **34**, 183.
3 DRUCKER C.R. & DUNCAN W.C. (1982) *J Am Acad Dermatol* **7**, 359.
4 HOLTI G. (1965) *Br J Dermatol* **77**, 560.
5 ISSTOFF S.W. & WHITING D.A. (1971) *Br J Dermatol* **85** (Suppl. 7), 26.

6 PORTER J.M., *et al* (1982) *Am Heart J* **104**, 66.
7 PULVERTAFT T.B., *et al* (1981) *Royal Society of Medicine International Congress and Symposium Series No 42.*

4 *Drug Ther Bull* (1984) **22**, 33.
5 POLLITT N. (1975) *Br J Detmatol* **93**, 721.
6 ROBERTS H.J. (1981) *JAMA* **246**, 129.
7 THOMAS R, *et al* (1982) *Arch Dermatol* **118**, 891.

VITAMINS

The pharmacology of vitamins and their deficiencies are discussed in Chapter 62. They are used very widely in medicine and even more often are irrationally self-prescribed [4]. Often their use is a reflection of the excitement the vitamins engendered when they were discovered in the first half of this century and is based on neither clinical evidence nor clinical trials. More often than not they are given as non-specific 'tonics', dare one say it, as placebos, usually harmless, but vitamins A, D and E in excess can cause serious toxicity. Dermatologists need to be familiar with vitamins:

1. to correct specific deficiencies such as scurvy;
2. as a supplement in general malnutrition states (the use of vitamins in this way is discussed in Chapter 62);
3. for other pharmacological effects, often not clearly related to the vitamin action and in doses very much larger.

Vitamin A. The theoretical basis for the use of vitamin A in severe ichthyosis, Darier's disease and other abnormalities of keratinization was that deficiency of vitamin A causes hyperkeratosis. However, there in no evidence of vitamin deficiency in these patients. Used in enormous and potentially toxic doses of 200–400,000 units daily some therapeutic effect could be achieved [7]. However, the use of vitamin A in this way has now been replaced by the use of retinoic acid and more particularly of the retinoids (p. 2507).

Beta carotene. A dose of 150 mg daily is of some value in certain photodermatoses, notably congenital porphyria and erythropoietic protoporphyria [5].

Vitamin E. This has been used in a large number of common and rare diseases. Although there are enthusiasts for its use [1, 2, 3, 5], there are no clearcut indications in dermatology based on appropriate trials and it is not without toxicity [6].

REFERENCES

1 AYRES S. & MIHAN R. (1975) *Cutis* **16**, 1017.
2 AYRES S. & MIHAN R. (1982) *J Am Acad Dermatol* **7**, 521.
3 BIERI J.G., *et al* (1983) *N Engl J Med* **308**, 1063.

MISCELLANEOUS DRUGS USED IN SPECIAL WAYS IN DERMATOLOGY

Antimalarials. A variety of drugs have been used in the treatment of malaria, a description of which is unnecessary here. However, for over 30 yr it has been well-known that several of these drugs may have other useful properties in the management of skin diseases [1, 2]. There was a vogue for the use of chloroquine in particular for the treatment of many diseases but the initial hopeful results were not followed by subsequent properly conducted trials on larger numbers of patients, and their use for such conditions as lichen planus, lichen sclerosus and rosacea has now rightly been abandoned. However, there are several diseases where there is an undoubted beneficial effect—discoid and systemic lupus erythematosus (p. 1301 and 1332), polymorphic light eruption (p. 642) and solar urticaria. They are of some value in rheumatology, where there is a resurgence of their use, as well as their more obvious application in diseases caused by some protozoa. Their use in sarcoidosis (p. 1781) and pophyria cutanea tarda (p. 2282) is discussed elsewhere.

The mode of action of antimalarials is complex and still largely empirical. They can interfere with many biological processes. They bind to DNA, stabilize membranes, inhibit hydrolytic enzymes, interfere with prostaglandin synthesis and block chemotaxis [1, 2].

The major problem with chloroquine is the retinopathy and potential blindness [3, 4]. There are considerable problems in defining the criteria for the diagnosis of retinopathy and the estimate that 3–5% of patients who receive the drug may develop this complication is almost certainly too high. A number of questions remain unanswered. It is generally agreed that the risk to the retina of giving chloroquine sulphate 250 mg daily for 3 months is virtually negligible although the drug is cumulative to some extent from one year to another.

Hydroxycloroquine has been used less and therefore has caused fewer cases of retinopathy. There is no evidence that it is intrinsically safer. Mepacrine (50–100 mg daily) lacks the ocular toxicity but stains the skin and causes more drug eruptions so that it is not an ideal replacement. It is still uncertain whether regular ophthalmological examinations will predict the onset of retinopathy from chloroquine at a stage before it has become irreversible. At present it seems safest to recommend that the drug should not be used for more than 3 months but, if the clinical indications are strong enough to continue the drug, ophthalmological follow-up should be undertaken every 4–6 months.

REFERENCES

1 ISAACSON D., *et al* (1982) *Int J Dermatol* 21, 379.
2 KORANDA F.C. (1981) *J Am Acad Dermatol* 4, 650.
3 OLANSKY A.J. (1982) *J Am Acad Dermatol* 6, 19.
4 PORTNOY J.Z. & CALLEN J.P. (1983) *Int J Dermatol* 22, 273.

Dapsone [1–4]. Dapsone (DDS) first came into medicine as an antibacterial agent but was found to be less effective and more toxic than sulphonamides. Likewise its activity against tuberculosis was disappointing. Nevertheless, it has been the mainstay in the treatment of leprosy for many years (see Chapter 23). It also has some action against malaria and other parasites.

However, it has also proved a very valuable drug in the management of a wide range of mainly uncommon dermatoses. Its mode of action is not fully understood. Although many of the diseases found empirically to respond to this drug have in common the involvement of either polymorphs or immune complexes, the metabolic action of dapsone cannot yet be explained simply in these terms. The diseases for which dapsone is particularly effective are dermatitis herpetiformis and erythema elevatum diutinum. Other diseases also favourably but not invariably influenced include other bullous diseases (pemphigoid, mucous membrane pemphigoid, linear IgA disease, chronic bullous disease of childhood, bullous eruption of systemic lupus erythematosus, subcorneal pustular dermatosis), pyoderma gangrenosum, rheumatoid arthritis and collagen diseases, relapsing polychondritis, acne conglobata, leukocytoclastic vasculitis and granuloma faciale.

Toxicity is a considerable problem with dapsone but overall the drug has probably fewer long-term side effects than do corticosteroids or sulphapyridine. The main toxic side effect is haemolysis which is not usually dependent on glucose 6-phosphate dehydrogenase deficiency, although that enzyme defect may compound the problem. Some haemolysis is almost invariably found on therapeutic doses. Methaemoglobinaemia is also common and is responsible for the bluish lips, etc., so common in patients on this drug. A level of 3% methaemoglobinaemia is often unnoticed, of 12% may be acceptable, but 20% usually not. Regular blood checks of haemoglobin and reticulocytes but also

including white cells and platelets should therefore be undertaken in all patients for the first few months after starting dapsone. Dapsone has several other but less common side effects, including bone marrow damage, peripheral neuropathy, drug, rashes, renal damage, hypoalbuminaemia, cholestasis, psychoses and reversible male infertility. A dose of 100 mg daily is often used as a starting dose. Many patients with dermatitis herpetiformis can be controlled on very much less. Some diseases can only be controlled by larger doses, but the incidence of side effects then rises very sharply and most dermatologists prefer not to exceed a dose of 100–150 mg daily.

Other drugs which share some of the useful assets of dapsone include sulphapyridine and, to a lesser extent, sulphamethoxypyridazine. Others are less commonly used [3]. Sulphapyridine is in general less effective than dapsone and, in doses which are effective, tends to cause more side effects, especially marrow suppression although not haemolysis. The usual dose is 0·5 g twice or three times daily.

Clofazamine. This antileprotic drug (see p. 2515) has also been used especially in pyoderma gangrenosum and in lupus erythematosus.

REFERENCES

1 BERNSTEIN J.E. & LORINCZ A.L. (1981) *Int J Dermatol* 20, 81.
2 KATZ S.I. (1982) *Arch Dermatol* 118, 809.
3 LANG P.G. (1979) *J Am Acad Dermatol* 1, 479.
4 SAMSOEN M., *et al* (1981) *Ann Dermatol Syphil* 108, 911.

Thalidomide [4]. Thalidomide is an interesting drug whose name is linked with the causation of severe birth defects so that its use, if any, is very restricted and it must never be allowed to be given to pregnant women. It also has other toxic side effects, notably causing peripheral neuropathy [1, 3, 4], so that the manufacturers advise against its use. It can be helpful in severe leprosy reactions (p. 836). It can also be helpful in some, but by no means all, patients with nodular prurigo [1], and more particularly with the type of light-sensitive prurigo seen especially in South America [5]. Lupus erythematosus [5, 6], light-sensitive dermatoses and even aphthosis [2], Behçet's disease and Weber–Christian disease have apparently been helped, although other treatments are to be preferred. It is a drug whose use must always be kept under the strictest control and it must be used only by patients who are able to understand the problems. Drugs chemically similar to thalidomide but without the fetal toxicity seems also to lack the therapeutic efficacy.

REFERENCES

1 ARONSON I.K., *et al* (1984) *Arch Dermatol* **120**, 1466.
2 BOWERS P.W. & POWELL R.J. (1983) *Br Med J* **287**, 800.
3 CLEMMENSEN O.J., *et al* (1984) *Arch Dermatol* **120**, 338.
4 Editorial (1985) *Lancet* **ii**, 80.
5 HASPER (1983) *Arch Dermatol* **119**, 812.
6 KNOP J., *et al* (1983) *Br J Dermatol* **108**, 461.
7 WULFF C.H., *et al* (1975) *Br J Dermatol* **112**, 475.

Colchicine [3, 4]. Colchicine has been used in the treatment of gout for many centuries and is still a valuable remedy. It is also of use in familial Mediterranean fever. It has an antimitotic action (for which it is sometimes used topically) but its good effects in skin diseases probably depend more on its suppression of various aspects of polymorph activity, notably chemotaxis. This confers on it an anti-inflammatory effect. It may also inhibit histamine release from mast cells. Its use is somewhat restricted by its side effects, especially those on the gastrointestinal tract, but the bone marrow and kidney may also be affected. It should be avoided in pregnancy. It is not therefore a first line drug but can prove of value in Behçet's disease, pustular psoriasis [1] and perhaps even in psoriasis vulgaris, relapsing polychondritis [2], leucocytoclastic vasculitis and Sweet's syndrome—all diseases in which polymorphs are presumed to play a role. A common dose is 0·5–1 mg by mouth daily, although larger doses are used by rheumatologists.

REFERENCES

1 ARAM H. (1983) *Int J Dermatol* **22**, 566.
2 ASKARI A.D. (1984) *J Am Acad Dermatol* **10**, 507.
3 MALKINSON F.D. (1982) *Arch Dermatol* **118**, 453.
4 TAKIGAWA M., *et al* (1982) *Arch Dermatol* **118**, 458.

TRANSEPIDERMAL ADMINISTRATION OF DRUGS
(See also p. 234)

Absorption of drugs into the skin in order to have an effect on the skin is an integral part of the action of most pharmacologically active local applications. Occasional systemic toxicity has been known for many years (Chapter 11). More recently percutaneous absorption has been used by general physicians to achieve a slow and steady release of certain drugs into the body [1]. Although this is not primarily of concern to dermatologists they may well wish to be informed of how other people are using the skin. The drugs currently being evaluated include nitroglycerine for angina, clonidine for hypertension and hyoscine for motion sickness. The development is a good stimulus to the study of percutaneous absorption.

REFERENCE

1 SHAW J.E. & URQUHART J. (1981) *Br Med J* **283**, 875.

VACCINATIONS AND IMMUNIZATIONS

The term vaccination is often loosely applied to any process of active or even also of passive immunization, although *sensu strictu* it should be kept for vaccination against smallpox. Protection against infections can be provided by both active and passive immunization. Active immunization can be by attenuated live organisms, by killed organisms or by modified toxin. Passive immunization may be by relatively unpurified human immunoglobulin, by specific human immunoglobulins or by antisera produced in animals. Full details of the indications, recommendations and side effects are found in standard publications [1, 3–5]. Recommendations do vary from country to country.

Active immunization. Smallpox vaccination is now a thing of the past. It was strongly (but not absolutely) contra-indicated in patients with atopic dermatitis and to some extent in patients with any active skin disease, but notably Darier's disease, and also in patients who were immunosuppressed.

Tuberculosis. BCG vaccination (see p. 801).

Routine immunization procedures. In the U.K. there are against diphtheria, tetanus, pertussis, poliomyelitis, measles and, in older girls, rubella. Active immunization against yellow fever and cholera may also be necessary for international travel, and immunization against typhoid and poliomyelitis are often recommended. Other active immunization procedures available are those against influenza, hepatitis B, mumps, pneumococcus, haemophilus influenzae, meningococci, anthrax, rabies, plague and an ever-growing list. Great advances can be expected in the near future, perhaps allowing active immunization with synthetic peptides which carry the antigenic message of the proteins of the infecting organisms, and/or using genetically engineered organisms [5].

Passive immunization of short duration. This can be provided by immunoglobulins of human origin or of animal origin which are now much more pure than they used to be, but there is still a theoretical risk of allergic reactions to them. Such vaccines are available against measles, hepatitis A and B, varicella zoster, mumps and rabies and against the toxins of diphtheria and gas gangrene. Again in the not too distant future we can expect monoclonal antibodies prepared against the antigenic proteins or even peptides.

In general apart apart from the hazards of smallpox vaccination there are few major dermatological contra-indications to these immunization processes, though there are various general medical contra-indications, e.g. live vaccines in pregnancy or immunosuppressed patients and the current pertussis vaccine in infants who have had convulsions.

A decreasing number of virus vaccines are now prepared on chicken or duck egg (e.g. influenza vaccine) and could contain traces of egg antigen which are a potential problem with injected vaccines. Information on this is available in the manufacturers' literature. Most virus vaccines are now prepared on tissue culture where this risk is minimal. The risk is a small one in atopic patients and indeed in other patients who are very sensitive to eggs. Traces of antibiotics, e.g. penicillin and neomycin, are also found in some vaccines. Where there is any doubt, information should be sought either from the individual manufacturer's literature or from the manufacturers themselves. Also when there is any doubt with injected vaccines it can never do any harm to give test doses of, for example, one-hundredth and then one-tenth the full dose at hourly intervals before the main dose.

Non-specific reactions to immunization procedures with both living and killed vaccines include fever, convulsions (a much discussed and emotive subject) and local swelling. Because of these there is much to be said for avoiding routine inoculations at times when infantile eczema is in exacerbation. More obvious immunological reactions include urticaria (both ordinary and serum sickness type), various toxic erythemas and erythema multiforme. These may or may not be reproduced with repeat doses.

Specific desensitization. Specific desensitization for allergic reactions [2] impinges on the dermatologist most often in the management of atopic patients with hay fever or perhaps asthma, occasionally atopic dermatitis and following anaphylactic reactions to insect stings. The indications for drug reactions and delayed hypersensitivity contact dermatitis are few, the efficacy and safety often dubious.

REFERENCES

1 *British National Formulary No 11* (1986) London, British Medical Association & Pharmaceutical Society of Great Britain.
2 CHAMPION R.H. & LACHMANN P.J. (1985) In *Recent Advances in Dermatology*. Ed. Champion R.H. Edinburgh, Churchill Livingstone, Vol. 7.
3 DHSS (1982) *Immunisation against Infectious Diseases*.
4 LACHMANN P.J. & PETERS R. (1982) *Clinical Aspects of Immunology*. 4th ed. Oxford, Blackwell.
5 YOUNG C.R. (1984) *J R Soc Med* 77, 261.

CHAPTER 67

Topical Therapy*

W.A.D. GRIFFITHS, F.A. IVE & J.D. WILKINSON*

GENERAL CONSIDERATIONS [1, 4, 15]

The empirical nature of much of the topical therapy used in the past, and the fact that physicians often had to rely on a purely subjective assessment of its value, gave rise to a confused and complicated dermatological pharmacopoeia. Although the formulations listed in the official monographs had been tried and tested over many years, a properly controlled evaluation led to major deletions in more recent editions of these pharmacopoeias [4, 5, 14, 16, 18]. In earlier times, there were only a few 'active' ingredients, and most traditional dermatological treatments relied on physical rather than chemical properties for their effect. Such active ingredients as did exist were mixed together, according to the physician's prescription, in a suitable carrier substance, vehicle or base. The influence exerted by the vehicle was often underestimated, especially its effect on drug penetration and performance [2, 7, 11, 15]. Even specific remedies were used in a somewhat random and haphazard way and might, at times, be incorporated into totally inappropriate vehicles. The importance of the vehicle is now well recognized [13, 17], not only for its physical properties but also as a delivery system for the many new active topical drugs that have been developed over the last 50 yr. These new drugs are far more active than their predecessors and include both specific therapeutic agents and drugs with more general effects. The vehicles are frequently tailor-made and chosen as carefully as the drug for which they are intended. Many of these new drugs are unstable unless used in the prescribed concentration and vehicle and attempts at modifying or altering these complex drug–vehicle systems will often adversely affect penetration, absorption and performance.

When dilutions are required, reference may be made to the *External Diluent Directory* [6]. There are many topical preparations, however, where dilution

*We should like to express our gratitude to Dr. M. Whitefield for his help with this Chapter.

is neither practical nor possible after manufacture and packaging. Where a patient finds the lowest strength still too potent, the physician will then have to advise the use of smaller quantities applied at less frequent intervals.

Although extemporaneous formulations are now less frequently recommended and several traditional treatments have been discarded because of toxicity, sensitivity or lack of demonstrable effect, new remedies have not entirely replaced older ones [1, 8, 15] which are often still very effective and whose side effects are at least familiar and well recognized. The complexity of modern formulations, coupled with stricter safety and efficacy requirements, increased legislative controls and a reluctance among some pharmacists to prepare extemporaneous formulations, however, will make it increasingly difficult for the physician to obtain traditional or 'personalized' prescriptions. One notable disadvantage of proprietary preparations is the limited description of the constituents that is generally given.

The nature of the skin barrier has been fully discussed in Chapter 11. In general, drugs penetrate at rates determined largely by their lipid–water coefficients [2, 7, 11], water-soluble ions and polar molecules (except for the very smallest) being excluded. In diseased skin, where the stratum corneum is improperly formed, drug absorption may be far more efficient but, as clinical improvement occurs and a normal stratum corneum emerges, absorption may slow down and incomplete healing may occur unless steps are taken to increase the efficacy of drug penetration.

Treatment by topical application means that there is intimate contact between the drug and the target tissue and side effects are minimized. It is often difficult, however, for the clinician to regulate the amount of drug applied and patient compliance may at times be a problem.

Complex physical laws govern the absorption of substances through the skin [2, 3, 7] (Chapter 11) but a major stimulus to research into the penetration of active agents was the recognition that the absorption of corticosteroids produces vasoconstriction and that this can be used as a 'marker' of penetration [11, 12]. Permeability of the skin can also be increased by the use of 'accelerants', e.g. the addition of tetrafurfuryl alcohol or propylene glycol to a weak corticosteroid produces a vasoconstrictive effect equivalent to that of a stronger corticosteroid. Among many such agents dimethyl sulphoxide (DMSO) is outstanding in this ability [9, 10]. In practice, the degree of penetration depends on the nature of the vehicle used, the behaviour of the active agent in this vehicle and the method of application employed, e.g. occlusion and hydration enhance penetration.

The basic principles of prescribing and formulating topical applications are unfortunately often neglected in the medical curriculum. However, a doctor today not only must ensure that treatment is in the right form and contains the most appropriate active ingredient but also must be able to instruct the patient how to use the treatment and advise as to any likely side effects [15].

REFERENCES

1 *Arndt K.A. (1978) Manual of Dermatologic Therapeutics. 2nd ed. Boston, Little, Brown.

2 *Barry B.W. (1983) Dermatological Formulations: Percutaneous Absorption in Drugs and The Pharmaceutical Sciences. Ed. Swarbrick J. New York, Marcel Dekker, Vol. 18.

3 Blank I.H. & Scheuplein R.J. (1969) In Handbook of Cosmetic Science. Ed. Hibbott H.W. Oxford, Pergamon, p. 47.

4 *British National Formulary No. 6 (1983) London, British Medical Association and The Pharmaceutical Society of Great Britain.

5 British Pharmacopoeia Commission (1980) 13th ed. London, HMSO.

6 External Diluent Directory (1982) London, The National Pharmaceutical Association.

7 Flynn G.L. (1979) Modern Pharmaceutics in Drugs and The Pharmaceutical Sciences. Eds Barker G.S. & Rhodes C.T. New York, Marcel Dekker, Vol. 7, p. 263.

8 Hellier F.F. (1969) Practitioner 202, 23.

9 Jacob S.W. & Herschler R. (Eds.) (1975) Biological Actions of Dimethyl Sulphoxide. In Ann NY Acad Sci 23, 243.

10 Martin D. & Hauthal H.G. (1976) Dimethyl Sulphoxide. New York, Van Nostrand Reinhold.

11 Mauvais-Jarvis P., et al (Eds.) (1980) Percutaneous Absorption of Steroids. New York, Academic Press.

12 McKenzie A.W. & Stoughton R.B. (1962) Arch Dermatol 86, 608.

13 Munro D.D. & Wilson L. (1969) Br J Dermatol 81, (Suppl. 4).

14 Pharmaceutical Society of Great Britain (1979) Pharmaceutical Codex. 11th ed. London, Pharmaceutical Press.

15 *Polano M.K. (1984) Topical Skin Therapeutics. Edinburgh, Churchill Livingstone.

16 Reynolds J.E.F. & Presad A.B. (Eds.) (1982) Martindale: The Extra Pharmacopoeia. 28th ed. London, Pharmaceutical Press.

17 Sarkany I. & Hadgraft J.W. (1969) In Handbook of Cosmetic Science. Ed. Hibbott H.W. Oxford, Pergamon, p. 98.

18 United States Pharmacopoeia National Formulary (1980) USP XX; NF XV. Rockville, Md, United States Pharmacopoeial Convention.

THE VEHICLE
(SYN. BASE)

In dermatology, a drug is very rarely, if ever, applied to the skin in the form of a pure chemical substance but is normally incorporated into a vehicle. The term 'vehicle' is now preferred to the older term 'base' for the sum of the excipients in which an active agent is offered to the skin. An 'ideal' vehicle should be easy to apply and remove, non-toxic, non-irritant, non-allergenic, chemically stable, homogeneous, bacteriostatic, cosmetically acceptable [8, 20] and pharmacologically inert [4, 14]. In addition, one has to consider the properties of the vehicle in relation to the active agent. For effective drug delivery a vehicle should ensure chemical stability of the active drug, its efficient release from the formulation, its easy partition into the outer layer of the skin and the efficient permeation of the drug through the epidermis.

Many attempts have been made to produce a comprehensive classification of external formulations but the most simple system consists of an initial division into liquid, semisolid and powder (Table 67.1) [3]. The liquid preparations may be divided into monophasic solutions, emulsions and suspensions. Solutions can be usefully separated into aqueous, alcoholic, alcoholic–aqueous and oily. The emulsions are classified into oil in water (O/W) and water in oil (W/O). The semisolid preparations divide into water-free and water-containing systems, highly concentrated non-aqueous systems being called ointments and water-containing semisolid preparations being classified as either hydrogels, creams or emulsions. Semisolid suspensions are called pastes. Ointments can be classified as non-polar (generally tenside-free systems), polar (containing tensides with a hydrophilic–lipophilic balance (HLB) of less than 10) and strongly polar systems (with tensides with an HLB value of over 10). In the aqueous system, monophasic and multiphasic systems are differentiated with aqueous gels being placed with the monophasics. The multiphasic systems are termed creams. They are

TABLE 67.1. Classification system for external preparations

A. Liquid
    1. Monophasic = solutions
        (a) Pure aqueous
            (i) Low viscosity   Lotions
            (ii) High viscosity, psuedoplastic   Gels
        (b) Alcoholic, alcoholic–aqueous   Paints
        (c) Oily   Oils
    2. Emulsions
        (a) Oil in water (O/W)
        (b) Water in oil (W/O)
    3. Suspensions
B. Semisolid
    1. Water-free ointments
        (a) Non-polar
        (b) Polar (tensides up to HLB 10)
        (c) Strongly polar (HLB of greater than 10)
    2. Containing water
        (a) Monophasic (hydrogels)
        (b) Multiphasic (emulsions, creams)
            (i) Washable (O/W)   Aqueous creams
            (ii) Non-washable (W/O)   Oily creams
            (iii) Intermediate type   Ambiphilic
    3. Highly concentrated suspensions   Pastes
C. Powders

similar to emulsions and so, here again, classification into O/W or W/O is possible, depending upon whether they can be washed off with water or not. Ambiphilic creams are intermediate, combining some features of both. All commonly used external preparations fit into one of the categories listed in Table 67.1 and are shown, figuratively, in Fig. 67.1.

BASIC MATERIALS [2, 4, 5, 18, 19]

These are discussed fully in specialized texts, such as that of Polano [14] and will only be mentioned briefly here.

Powders. Inorganic powders are an important component of many dermatological treatments and include zinc oxide, titanium dioxide, talc, bentonite and calamine. Organic powders include various starches and zinc stearate. *Zinc oxide* is widely used as a component of many dusting powders, shake lotions and pastes. It has covering and protective properties, gives consistency to creams and pastes and is said to have cooling and slightly astringent properties. *Titanium dioxide* is chemically very inert and for this reason it can be used instead of zinc oxide in pastes containing salicylic acid. It is also superior to zinc oxide in its UV-reflecting properties. *Talc* is inert magnesium polysilicate, with a very

low specific gravity. It contributes 'slip' and has a cooling effect. *Calamine* may be either zinc carbonate or zinc oxide, coloured with a little ferric oxide, and has bland, soothing and antipruritic properties. *Starch* is more absorbent than inorganic powders but tends to deteriorate and is prone to microbiological decomposition. Some powders, e.g. *bentonite* (collodial hydrated aluminium silicate), *aluminium magnesium silicate*, *tragacanth*, *methyl cellulose* and *carbomer* are used in gels or as stabilizers in shake lotions.

Grease. These can be divided into true fats and oils, waxes, mineral greases and macrogols. *True fats and oils* are the triglycerides of saturated and non-saturated fatty acids with a small amount of free fatty acid. There are many varieties, e.g. arachis oil, olive oil, lanolin, cetyl and stearyl alcohol, etc. *Wool fat B.P., Anhydrous lanolin U.S.P., Purified wool fat* [7, 9], is a mixture of higher fatty acids esterified with monohydric alcohols including cholesterol esters and related alcohols. It may be mixed with other fats or greases to improve its flow properties and enable it to emulsify water. Although still widely used, patients may become sensitized to the wool alcohol fraction and therefore the use of a purified, less sensitizing, lanolin extract has been proposed [6]. *Hydrous wool fat B.P., Lanolin U.S.P.,* is wool fat with 25–30% water. It is used both as an emollient

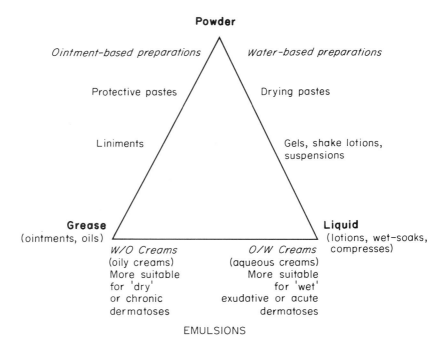

FIG. 67.1. A practical guide as to the choice and performance of dermatological vehicles (adapted from Polano [14]).

and as a protective. *Eucerin (Wool Alcohols* B.P.) is the wool alcohol fraction of wool fat and contains cholesterol and isocholesterol. It is mixed with liquid, soft and hard paraffin to form *Ointment of Wool Alcohols* B.P. which, on the addition of water, produces *Hydrous Ointment* B.P., a vehicle for many W/O creams. *Theobroma oil* B.P., *Cocoa Butter* U.S.P., consists chiefly of the triglycerides of palmitic, stearic and oleic acids. It is a solid fat which melts at between 30 and 35°C. Other true fats include *Cetyl Esters Wax* N.F., *Stearyl Alcohol* N.F. and *Cetostearyl alcohol* B.P. They are mainly used as stabilizing agents in creams.

Waxes include *Beeswax* B.P., used to stiffen ointments for salve pencils, and *Emulsifying wax* B.P., *Lanette Wax* S.X., which is a mixture of one part sodium lauryl sulphate and nine parts cetostearyl alcohol. It is an important emulsifying agent in anionic O/W creams.

Mineral greases may be fluid, soft or solid [17].

Fluid greases include *Liquid Paraffin* B.P., *Mineral Oil* U.S.P. or low molecular weight *macrogols* such as polyethylene glycol 300. They can be used to soften ointments and pastes or to clean debris and crust from the skin.

Soft greases include *Yellow* and *White Soft Paraffin* B.P., *Petrolatum* U.S.P., *Vaseline, Plastibase*—a suspension of mineral oil in polyethylene—and mixed

liquid and *solid macrogols* (having molecular weights of 300 and 4000 respectively). *Cetomacrogol 1000* B.P. is a condensation of cetostearyl alcohol with ethylene oxide. It is useful as a non-ionic emulsifying agent.

Liquids in common use include *Purified water* B.P., U.S.P., *Glycerol* B.P., *Glycerine* U.S.P. (a thick hygroscopic liquid used in some lotions and gels), *Ethanol* B.P., U.S.P. (which is 95–96% ethyl alcohol) and other solvents such as *Ether* B.P., U.S.P., and *Chloroform* B.P., U.S.P. Industrial *Methylated Spirits* B.P. or *Rubbing Alcohol* U.S.P. or *Isopropyl Alcohol* B.P. can be substituted. *Calcium Hydroxide Solution* B.P., U.S.P., or *limewater* is a 0.15% aqueous solution of calcium hydroxide. It is considered to have anti-inflammatory and soothing properties and is used in cooling pastes and other soothing preparations. *Sorbitol Solution* B.P., U.S.P., is a 70% solution of *Sorbitol* B.P., a polyalcohol, in water. It is often used as a humectant in O/W creams. *Propylene Glycol* B.P., U.S.P., is a useful solvent and good penetrant, especially for corticosteroid creams and ointments [13, 15, 16]. It may also act as a keratolytic and preservative water-containing creams. At high concentration, it is hygroscopic and may be irritant [1, 12]. It may also, albeit rarely, sensitize [10, 11].

REFERENCES

1 ANGELINI G. & MENINGHINI C.L. (1981) *Contact Dermatitis* 7, 197.
2 ARNDT K.A. (1978) *Manual of Dermatologic Therapeutics.* 2nd ed. Boston, Little, Brown.
3 BRANDAU R. & LIPPOLD B.H. (1982) *Dermal and Transdermal Absorption.* Stuttgart, Wissenschaftliche Verlagsgesellschaft, p. 16.
4 *British National Formulary No. 6* (1983) London, British Medical Association and The Pharmaceutical Society of Great Britain.
5 British Pharmacopoeic Commission (1980) *British Pharmacopoeia.* 13th ed. London, HMSO.
6 CLARKE E.W., *et al* (1977) *Contact Dermatitis* 3, 69.
7 CONRAD L.I., *et al* (1966) *J Soc Cosmet Chem* 17, 149.
8 CUSSLER E.L. (1978) In *Cosmetic Science.* Ed. Brewer M.M. London, New York, Academic Press, Vol. 1, p.117.
9 GUILLOT J.P., *et al* (1980) *Int J Cosmet Sci* 2, 1.
10 HANNUKSELA M., *et al* (1978) *Contact Dermatitis* 1, 112.
11 HANNUKSELA M., *et al* (1979) *Contact Dermatitis* 2, 105.
12 HJORTH N. (1980) *Br J Dermatol* 103 (Suppl. 18), 19.
13 OSTRENGA J. *et al* (1971) *J Invest Dermatol* 56, 392.
14 *POLANO M.K. (1984) *Topical Skin Therapeutics.* Edinburgh, Churchill Livingstone.
15 PONEC N. (1976) *Dermatological* (Suppl) 152, 37.
16 REINSTEIN J., *et al* (1972) *Acta Derm Venereol (Stockh)* 52, (Suppl. 67), 13.
17 SEVILLE R.H. (1975) *Br J Dermatol* 93, 205.
18 *United States Pharmacopoeia National Formulary* (1980) USP XX; NF XV. Rockville, MD, United States Pharmacopoeial Convention.
19 WADE A. (Ed.) (1977) *Martindale: The Extra Pharmacopoeia.* 27th ed. London, Pharmaceutical Press.
20 WEINSTEIN S. (1978) *J Soc Cosmet Chem* 29, 99.

PRINCIPLES OF FORMULATION AND CHOICE OF VEHICLE FOR DERMATOLOGICAL USE [1–9]

Only the most general principles of pharmaceutical formulation will be dealt with here. For more detailed information readers are referred to the work of Polano [9] or other standard reference books [1, 2, 3, 4, 8, 10, 12].

All topical preparations can be considered as being either *monophasic* (e.g. lotions, powder or grease), *biphasic* (e.g. creams and protective or drying pastes) or *triphasic* (e.g. cream pastes or cooling pastes) (Fig. 67.1).

Monophasic vehicles. Powders, now mainly used as toiletries or for prophylaxis, absorb moisture, reduce friction, have good covering properties and can be used to increase surface area. They are best applied to normal skins and therefore have limited dermatological use. *Greases* are emollient, protective and hydrating. They are the principal component of ointments and salve pencils; their occlusiveness tends to enhance penetration of active ingredients. Some ointments have added emulsifiers to improve drug incorporation and to help them emulsify sweat and sebum. Simple Ointment B.P., for example, contains wool fat and cetostearyl alcohol. White Ointment U.S.P. contains 5% beeswax and is therefore useful for those who are lanolin sensitive. Oils can be used as emollients or as a means of removing grease or fatty pastes from the skin or, with added surfactant, as bath emollients. *Liquids* evaporate and tend therefore to be cooling, soothing and drying. Alcoholic or hydro-alcoholic solutions are, in addition, astringent and antiseptic. These basic elements can be combined to form biphasic or triphasic preparations.

Biphasic vehicles. The combination of powder with water gives either a drying paste or a shake lotion, according to the proportion of each component. Grease or oil and powder will form either a liniment or a protective (fatty) paste. Water and grease, however, will mix to form stable or semistable emulsions only in the presence of a surfactant or emulsifier. These then form O/W or W/O creams according to the type of emulsifier used and the relative proportions of the two components. In general the characteristics of a biphasic vehicle are those of its continuous phase modified by its disperse phase.

Triphasic vehicles. These are represented by cream pastes or cooling pastes and are often simply referred to as creams in the U.K., e.g. Zinc Cream B.P. They combine some of the advantages of all their ingredients and can be used in even the most acute dermatoses.

Choice of vehicle. It is a basic dermatological precept that the more acute the dermatosis the more bland should be the treatment. The application of a cooling paste or paste bandage and the use of frequent wet compresses, with or without topical steroids, remains an indispensible part of the management of acute or exudative dermatoses. The principle of 'wet on wet' and the use of occlusive ointments for dry or chronic dermatoses is also axiomatic. As the condition improves a 'wet' dermatosis may subsequently be treated with either a drying paste or an O/W cream and a 'dry' dermatosis may have a hydrous ointment or W/O cream applied. The additional powder in liniments or protective pastes allows the skin to 'breathe' and makes them less occlusive than plain ointments.

Coldcreams and *cooling pastes* rely for their effect

on their inherent instability, the water tending to separate out and evaporate. Cream pastes and ordinary W/O (oily) creams are more stable and hence less cooling.

Aqueous or water-based preparations (Fig. 67.1), e.g. lotions, O/W creams, gels and drying pastes, tend to be cooling, soothing and drying due to their evaporative water loss.

Lotions, wet soaks, wet compresses and O/W creams can be used to clean or redissolve dried exudate and crust and may, at times, be antiseptic and mildly astringent (e.g. dilute Potassium Permanganate Solution B.N.F.). Aqueous-based preparations need to be used frequently if they are to retain their physical effects. They are particularly helpful in the initial management of acute dermatoses and intertrigos.

Shake lotions, such as Calamine Lotion B.P., are able to cover large areas of the body with a thin coating of powder and, because of the increased evaporative surface, are even more soothing and cooling than ordinary lotions. The well-established anti-inflammatory and soothing effects of calamine are therefore simply a reflection of its physical characteristics. However, it would not be the rational treatment for those with xerotic pruritus.

Gels are semisolid preparations gelled with high molecular weight polymers, e.g. carboxypolymethylene (Carbomer B.P.) or methylcellulose, and can be regarded as semiplastic aqueous lotions. They are non-greasy, water miscible, easy to apply and wash off and are especially suitable for treating hairy parts of the body.

Ointments have oil or grease as their continuous phase (Fig. 67.1). They are semisolid anhydrous substances and are occlusive, emollient and protective. They restrict trans-epidermal water loss and are therefore hydrating and moisturizing. Ointments can be divided into two main groups—*fatty*, e.g. White Soft Paraffin B.P. (Petrolatum, Vaseline), and *water soluble*, e.g. Macrogol (polyethylene glycol) Ointment B.P. The latter have the advantage of being less greasy with good solvent properties and are easily washed off. Both types of ointment are emollient and lubricant but the fatty bases are obviously more occlusive and as a result have greater protective and hydrating properties.

Creams are semisolid emulsion systems containing both oil and water. *Oil in water* (aqueous or vanishing) creams are water miscible, cooling and soothing and are well absorbed into the skin. They are not occlusive but, because of their dispersed lipid phase, they also have a mild moisturizing and emollient effect, e.g. Aqueous Cream B.P. *Water in oil* (oily) creams are immiscible with water and, there-

fore, more difficult to wash off. They are emollient, lubricant, moisturizing and mildly occlusive (but less so than ointments), e.g. Oily Cream B.P. Both systems require the addition of either a natural or a synthetic detergent or emulsifier. O/W creams always contain a preservative to prevent secondary bacterial and fungal colonization. Many W/O creams contain lanolin.

Pastes are semisolid stiff preparations containing a high proportion of finely powdered material. The characteristic features of a paste are substantivity, 'inertness' and 'blandness'. There are drying pastes, cream pastes and protective pastes. They can also be used as a delivery system for drugs and because of their substantivity the drug effect can be limited to a well-defined area. *Protective* (fatty) pastes are greasy and therefore messy and water insoluble. They are difficult to apply and remove but their very stiffness permits accurate localization. They are occlusive, protective and hydrating. *Drying* (nongreasy) pastes are water miscible and more easily removed. They are drying and soothing and are often used in conjunction with dressings as paste bandages or as vehicles for active medicaments. Pastes can be 'softened' by the addition of 10% arachis oil or 'hardened' by the addition of hard paraffin [11]. *Cream* pastes combine some of the features of powders, liquids and fats, and can be used on acute conditions, e.g. Zinc Cream B.P.

Dusting powders usually contain a mixture of two or more substances in fine powder form, free from grittiness. They are normally only applied to normal intact skin as a preventative or protective measure. They are used to reduce friction (talc) or excessive moisture (starch) and tend therefore to be used in areas prone to moisture and friction, e.g. intertriginous areas, feet, etc. They have a slightly drying and lubricating effect but are nowadays regarded as a somewhat inefficient means of delivery of active drugs.

Paints are liquid preparations, either aqueous, hydro-alcoholic or alcoholic (tinctures), which are usually applied with a brush to the skin or mucous membranes. They evaporate and are therefore cooling as well as astringent and antiseptic. Alcoholic paints often sting.

Collodions, e.g. Flexible Collodion B.P. are liquid preparations consisting of pyroxylin (cellulose nitrate) in a mixture or organic solvents, usually ether or ether–alcohol. They evaporate to leave a flexible film which can hold medicaments in contact with the skin. They may also be used as protectives to seal minor cuts and abrasions. They are easy to apply and water repellent but also highly inflammable, irritant to the eyes and mucous membranes and only really suitable for small areas.

REFERENCES

1 ARNDT K.A. (1978) *Manual of Dermatologic Therapeutics*. 2nd ed. Boston, Little, Brown.

2 BARRY B.W. (1983) *Dermatological Forumulations: Percutaneous Absorption in Drugs and The Pharmaceutical Sciences*. Ed. Swarbrick J. New York, Marcel Dekker, Vol. 18.

3 *British National Formulary No. 6* (1983) London, British Medical Association and The Pharmaceutical Society of Great Britain.

4 British Pharmacopoeia Commision (1980) *British Pharmacopoeia*. 13th ed. London, HMSO.

5 FUHRER C. (1982) In *Dermal and Transdermal Absorption*. Eds Praudau R. & Lippold B.H. Stuttgart, Wissenschaftliche Verlagsgesellschaft.

6 KATZ M. (1973) In *Drug Design*. Ed Ariens E.J. Academic Press, New York, p. 117.

7 NURNBERG E. (1978) *Hautarzt* **29**, 61.

8 Pharmaceutical Society of Great Britain (1979) *Pharmaceutical Codex* 11th ed. London, Pharmaceutical Press.

9 POLANO M.K. (1984) *Topical Skin Therapeutics*. Edinburgh, Churchill Livingstone.

10 REYNOLDS J.E.F. & PRESAD A.B. (Eds.) (1982) *Martindale: The Extra Pharmacopoeia*. 28th ed. London, Pharmaceutical Press.

11 SEVILLE R.H. (1975) *Br J Dermatol* **93**, 205.

12 *United States Pharmacopoeia National Formulary* (1980) USP XX; NF VX. Rockville, MD, United States Pharmacopoeial Convention.

EMULSIONS [2, 4, 5, 8–10, 14–16]

An emulsion is a two-phase system consisting of two immiscible components, one (the dispersed or inner phase) being suspended in the other (the continuous or outer phase) as small droplets 0.2–50 μm in size. One phase is aqueous, the other oily. Stable emulsions remain in this form; unstable emulsions, with a large droplet size, tend to separate as cream does from milk. Emulsions can be diluted with the outer (continuous) phase only. When the diameter of the droplets of the dispersed phase is very small, microemulsions ('transparent systems') are formed with different properties [4, 16].

Emulsification of immiscible phases is produced by the addition of an emulsifying agent which is a large molecule with both strongly polar (i.e. water soluble) and non-polar (i.e. oil soluble) groups allowing it to bridge the gap between polar and non-polar substances.

W/O systems result from the dispersion of an aqueous in an oily phase, as in Oily Cream B.P. O/W systems are formed when oil is the disperse phase and water the continuous phase, as in Aqueous Cream B.P. The former constitute, in general, oily creams or 'coldcreams', the latter aqueous or 'vanishing creams'. It is sometimes possible to produce both types of emulsion in the same system [4]. These are called ambiphilic creams. A simple method of determining the nature of an emulsion is to interpose on a filter paper a drop of the emulsion between one of oil and one of water. In 15 min the continuous phase will mix with, or be dispersed by, one or other of the neighbouring drops. Alternatively, it may be tested by adding a larger quantity of water. If the emulsion separates, it is of W/O type; if not, it is of O/W type, the continuous phase being (within limits) able to expand and still retain its contained disperse phase.

General theory of emulsions [1, 4, 9, 12, 16]. This is a highly specialized and complicated branch of pharmaceutics. The brief outline given here relates to those emulsions likely to be encountered in dermatological rather than cosmetic practice, but it is in the latter field that the art of emulsification has become specially developed.

All molecular substances possess electrical charges. When the molecules are symmetrical these are balanced and the molecule is electrically neutral (non-polar), e.g. benzene. Non-polar substances are insoluble in water but soluble in other non-polar solvents. They are referred to as being hydrophobic since they cannot be mixed with water. Polar substances, in contrast, have asymmetrical formulae with unbalanced electrical charges and are soluble in water (hydrophilic) but insoluble in organic solvents and oils, e.g. acetic acid and alcohols. Some substances, however, have dual characteristics, being hydrophobic at one end and hydrophilic at the other. As they dissolve partly in water and partly in oil they act as emulsifying agents by binding the two phases together. Depending on the attractive force of the two portions of the molecule one or other phase will predominate. If the hydrophilic attraction is dominant an O/W emulsion results; if hydrophobic forces are dominant then a W/O emulsion is formed. These forces also determine their relative solubility in oil or water. On balance sodium stearate (soap) is hydrophilic and thus mixes with water and forms an O/W emulsion whereas calcium strearate, which contains two long-chain fatty acids, is hydrophobic, mixing with fats and oils to form W/O emulsions. In general, the ease of emulsification and thus the stability of the emulsion depends on the interfacial tension existing between the two phases involved in the emulsion, those with a low interfacial tension emulsifying easily and those with a high interfacial tension requiring considerable mechanical energy to enlarge the surface area between the dissimilar molecules;

small droplets, having considerably less surface tension, are therefore less likely to conglomerate or precipitate out of suspension. The ionic situation at the interface and the electrical properties of repulsion and attraction are of fundamental importance in the theory of emulsification [4]. Concentration, temperature and the addition of electrolytes have a critical effect on this balance and the stability of the emulsion. These considerations are of special practical importance when emulsions are used as bases for ionic and electrically active preparations in topical dermatological therapy.

The properties of emulsions. The term 'emulsion' is sometimes used loosely. The aqueous phase may vary from water to a solid gel and the oily phase from a liquid to a solid. The emulsifier may be regarded as a third, interfacial phase. Added ingredients may considerably modify the properties. Emulsions are easily disturbed by an excess of the dispersed phase. Thus, Oily Cream B.P. may separate in the presence of excess water. Even perfume and preservatives may act as surface-active agents and destabilize the emulsion. The degree of homogenization and particle dispersion are obviously important. In dermatological practice stability and incompatibility with additives are paramount. 'Creaming', flocculation and coalescence may occur. Phase inversion may occur from the addition of bivalent- or trivalent-phase electrolytes. Less attention has been paid to the rheological properties of dermatological as opposed to cosmetic preparations but an even flow of the emulsion on the skin is obviously desirable in both cases [1].

Choice of emulsion. Emulsions follow the characteristics of the external phase, O/W emulsions being readily diluted with water, W/O emulsions with oil. O/W emulsions are generally more acceptable on the skin than W/O emulsions. Aqueous Cream B.P. is the standard example of such an O/W emulsion. Emulsification greatly increases the surface area of the dispersed phase and thus may alter its chemical or pharmaceutical properties. Apart from the question of incompatibilities, W/O emulsions are used to provide a greasy residue with some 'cooling' effect; O/W emulsions aid penetration of lipophilic substances [12] and apart from their cosmetic acceptability and cooling and soothing properties also leave a thin film of lipid on the surface as an emollient.

Emulsifying agents [2, 3, 8, 11, 13, 15]. The activity of an emulsifying agent depends upon its ability to alter the interfacial angle of physically dis-

similar substances (the contact or wetting angle). This in turn depends upon the strength of the relative cohesive forces involved. In dermatology three-part systems also occur, i.e. water–oil–solid (skin or hair), but these are modified by the natural surface emulsion of amino and fatty acids derived from sweat and sebum. An extreme example of emulsifying action is seen in cleansers, shampoos and detergents.

Hydrophilic–lipophilic balance value [6, 7]. The relative affinity of an emulsifier for water (hydrophilic) and for oil (lipophilic) has a value in denoting its emulsification tendency. Emulsifiers having an HLB value of 3–6 tend to give W/O systems and those with higher values O/W systems (Table 67.2). The HLB value only indicates this one character of the emulsifier and has no other relevance.

TABLE 67.2. Some common emulsifiers [4, 16]

Producing W/O systems (HLB 3-6)
Polyvalent metallic soaps
(Oil-soluble quaternary ammonium cationics)
Propylene glycol fatty acid esters and monostearate
Sorbitan monopalmitate and monooleate
Glyceryl monostearate
Producing O/W systems (HLB 7–17)
Alkyl sulphates and sulphonates
Synthetic phosphoric acid esters
Cationic emulsifiers
Sorbitan monolaurate
Most polyoxyethylene compounds
Triethanolamine oleate

Amphipathic agents [11]. These are substances with molecules or ions part of which have an affinity and part a repulsion for the medium in which they are dissolved. They form the great bulk of emulsifying agents and consist of five groups, based on the character of the polar attachment to the hydrophobic portion of the molecule.

These are:

(i)   Anionic
(ii) Cationic
(iii) Non-ionic (these do not dissociate in water)
(iv) Ampholytic, the activity depending on the pH of the solution
(v)   Miscellaneous.

Anionic emulsifiers. These include the soaps and the sulphated compounds. The hydrophilic portion of the molecule provides the anion.

Soaps. O/W emulsions are formed from the monovalent alkaline salts of long-chain fatty acids and have the general formula RCOOM (alkali soaps), e.g. sodium stearate. Metallic soaps have the general formula $(RCOO)_N M$ where M is a polyvalent metal and N is valency. The most common metals are calcium or magnesium and these form W/O emulsions. Calamine Liniment B.P.C. is such a 'soap', calcium oleate being formed by the action of lime water on the oleic acid. Organic soaps are formed by the substitution of hydrogen ions in fatty acids by organic basic groups, e.g. triethanolamine stearate. They produce stable O/W emulsions, little affected by acids or calcium ions. If the amines are volatile the emulsion dries out and cannot be re-emulsified by water. They thus produce water-resistant coatings.

Sulphates and sulphonated emulsifiers. A sulphate compound results from esterification of a fatty alcohol with sulphuric acid followed by neutralization with an alkali, e.g. sodium lauryl sulphate, triethanolamine lauryl sulphate. A slightly different process produces sulphonated derivatives, e.g. sodium secondary dodecyl sulphonate (Teepol). Both types of preparation are widely used as emulsifiers for O/W systems and have the advantage of being tolerant to calcium, thus avoiding the creation of a scum with hard water. For emulsification, a stabilizer has to be added and this is normally a fatty alcohol, e.g. cetostearyl alcohol as in Emulsifying Wax B.P., a self-emulsifying anionic wax for emulsions containing 10% sodium lauryl sulphate and 90% cetostearyl alcohol. Sulphonated compounds are less used for emulsions but, being effective wetting agents, find an important place in detergents.

Cationic emulsifiers. Here the cation provides the surface activity (reverse soaps) and the compounds used are quaternary ammonium salts. They are less efficient than anionic emulsifiers and are chiefly used where antiseptic properties of the formulation are required as they inhibit the growth of many microorganisms.

Non-ionic emulsifiers. These are esters or ethers with balanced hydrophilic and hydrophobic groups, and as they do not dissociate they show considerable stability to acids and alkalis. They are derived from alcohols, e.g. cetyl alcohol, glycerol, mannitol, sorbitol, and include cetomacrogol, Spans and Tweens. Their physical behaviour and chemistry varies with individual members of the groups. Cetomacrogol 1000 B.P. is an ether of cetyl alcohol and polyethylene oxide containing 20–24 units. It is a component of Cetamacrogol Emulsifying Wax B.P. which contains 10% cetomacrogol 1000 and 90% cetos-

tearyl alcohol; polyoxethylene sorbitol monooleate (polysorbate 80 or Span 80) is an ester of sorbitol containing polyethylene oxide (about 20 groups) and oleic acid. Both these preparations are widely used for O/W emulsions.

Ampholytic emulsifiers. Their behaviour depends on the pH of the emulsion. They are anionic above pH 9, cationic below pH 5 and non-ionic at pH 7. They tolerate electrolytes and are compatible with phenols and quaternary ammonium agents.

Other emulsifiers. These include the older animal and vegetable emulsifiers such as gum acacia, tragacanth, starches, dextrins and lecithin. The wool fats and alcohols are of especial importance as W/O emulsifiers.

REFERENCES

1 BARRY B.W. (1983) *Dermatological Formulations: Percutaneous Absorption in Drugs and The Pharmaceutical Sciences.* Ed. Swarbrick J. New York, Marcel Dekker, Vol.18.
2 BECHER P. (1957) *Emulsions: Theory and Practice.* New York, Reinhold.
3 *BICKERMAN J.J. (1958) *Surface Chemistry.* New York, Academic Press.
4 *CLARK R. (1963) In *Handbook of Cosmetic Science.* Ed. Hibbot H.W. Oxgord, Pergamon.
5 *FLYNN G.D. (1979) In *Modern Pharmaceutics: Drugs and The Pharmaceutical Sciences.* Eds. Banker G.S. & Rhodes C.T. New York, Marcel Dekker, Vol.7, pp.1, 26.
6 GRIFFIN W.C. (1949) *J Soc Cosmet Chem* 1, 311.
7 GRIFFIN W.C. (1954) *J Soc Cosmet Chem* 5, 249.
8 HOLLIS G.L. (1980) *Directory of Surface Active Chemicals: Surfactants U.K.* 2nd ed. Darlington, U.K., Tergo-Data.
9 *JELLINET J.S. (1970) *Formulation and Function of Cosmetics.* New York, Wiley, pp. 32, 133.
10 KATZ M. (1973) *Drug Design* (*Medicinal Chemistry.* Ed. Ariens E.J. Vol.4) New York, Academic Press, p.93.
11 MOILLIET J.L., *et al.* (1969) *Surface Activity.* 2nd ed. London, Spon.
12 POLANO M.K. (1984) *Topical Skin Therapeutics.* Edinburgh, Churchill Livingstone.
13 SCOTT B.A. (1963) In *Handbook of Cosmetic Science.* Ed. Hibbott H.W. Oxford, Pergamon, p.145.
14 SUMNER G.G. (1954) *Clayton's The Theory of Emulsions and their Technical Treatment.* London, Churchill.
15 WHITE R.F. (1964) *Pharmaceutical Emulsions and Emulsifying Agents.* 4th ed. London, Chemist & Druggist.
16 *WILKINSON J.B. (Ed.) (1979) *Harry's Cosmeticology.* 6th ed. London, Hill.

PRESERVATIVES [2, 12, 16, 27, 41]

Mineral oils, greases and W/O creams with oil as the continuous phase do not usually require preservatives. Lotions, O/W creams and gels, however, since they have water as their continuous phase, are easily contaminated with both moulds and bacteria, and animal and vegetable oils, unless protected from biological decomposition, may deteriorate or become rancid [36]. The ideal preservative should be non-toxic, non-irritant, non-sensitizing, odourless, colourless and effective even at very low concentrations and under conditions of normal usage [31]. In addition, it must be compatible with both the vehicle and the active ingredients [13]. Although topical preparations do not need to be sterile they should be free from pathogens and contain only acceptable numbers of non-pathogenic microbes [20].

The *parahydroxybenzoic acid esters* are effective and widely used preservatives [15]. They can be used singly [35] or in combination. Considering their widespread use their sensitizing potential appears to be low [24]. Since, individually, they are only sparingly water soluble and since their effects are additive, mixtures are usually preferred. This also increases their spectrum of activity and lowers the risk of sensitization. As little as 0.4% parabens may be enough to preserve an O/W cream [14]. Their activity is reduced in the presence of oils and non-ionic emulsifiers.

Chlorocresol is a widely used preservative especially in the U.K. It is more effective in acid than in alkaline solution. It has a low sensitizing potential but may cross-react with chloroxylenol [5, 26]. It was for many years the preservative in Aqueous Cream B.P. but has now been replaced by phenoxyethanol. It is the preservative in a widely prescribed range of topical corticosteroids.

Sorbic acid (2,4 hexadienoic acid) is also a good preservative which maintains its activity in the presence of non-ionic detergents. It has a low sensitization index [25] and is now being used increasingly. It can only be used, however, in preparations with a pH of less than 6.5. Sensitivity, although rare, has been reported [4, 21, 37].

Propylene glycol at higher concentrations can inhibit the growth of moulds and fungi and can therefore be used as a preservative. *Organic mercurials* are used as preservatives in many ophthalmic preparations and in some vaccines and skin test solutions [16] but may rarely also be incorporated in some topical preparations [42]. *Ethylenediaminetetraacetate* is a widely used preservative in ear, nose and eye drops. *Gallates* and other antioxidants such as *butylhydroxyanisole* (BHA) and *butylhydroxytoluene* (BHT) are used to prevent rancidity in oily and fatty preparations.

Other preservatives, including those mainly used in cosmetic products, are discussed on pp. 494 and 540.

Sensitization. [19, 32]. Although the incidence of sensitization to preservatives is low when compared with their widespread usage, the cases of sensitivity that do occur appear to be the result more of medicament than cosmetic usage [12, 43]. Sensitivity to an ingredient of the vehicle may be 'occult' and is easily overlooked [18].

Other components of the base may also at times sensitize. These include ethylenediamine [17], lanolin [3], propylene glycol [22], emulsifiers [23] and fragrance [28, 33].

LANOLIN [3, 10, 38]

Lanolin resembles the sebaceous secretion of the human skin and will absorb about 30% of water. It is therefore a useful W/O emulsifier and is widely used in many therapeutic and cosmetic preparations [10]. Its composition varies qualitatively and quantitatively with humidity, temperature and method of collection. It is composed of alcohol and acid esters and a very variable proportion of free fatty alcohols and acids. Small quantities of anionic detergent may also be present [6]; the amount in 20 samples of wool grease varied from 0.55 to 2.4% [1]. These may increase the detectable incidence of hypersensitivity significantly [8].

The proportion of free fatty alcohols found in over 30 different samples of lanolin varied from 6.1 to 12.6% [8]. Lanolin derivatives result from acetylation, ethoxylation, solvent fractionation, saponification and acidolysis. They are highly effective wetting agents for finely ground solids in liquid vehicles, powerful emulsifiers, solubilizers of colloidal dispersal systems and spreading agents.

Nomenclature [40]. The nomenclature of the various types of lanolin is confusing and is discussed on p.2531. Wool fat and wool alcohols both contain small quantities of BHA or BHT as antioxidants.

Amerchols are a proprietary range of surface-active emulsifying agents based on wool fat and containing free sterol and higher alcohols.

Lanesta is the name given to a range of isopropyl esters of wool fat alcohols.

Solulan comprises a range of polyoxyethylene derivatives of wool fat or wool alcohols, some wholly or partly acetylated.

Lanolin sensitivity [12, 19, 30, 32]. Most cases of lanolin sensitivity are a result of medical rather than cosmetic usage [12, 43]. Patients with chronic stasis eczema or leg ulcers appear to be particularly susceptible [3, 41, 43]. Although still therefore a relatively infrequent sensitizer in the general population [7], it may occur unexpectedly in dermatological practice and is frequently overlooked [11], especially in atopics and those with hand eczema, who may use large quantities of lanolin-based emollients over long periods of time. Sensitivity to lanolin is usually relevant [19] and most cases will be detected by patch testing with 30% wool alcohols [29]. The incidence of lanolin sensitivity in any series will depend on the proportion of leg ulcers and other susceptible groups in the test material [43]; this currently appears to be about 3% of patients tested in Europe [19] and North America [32]. Although the actual sensitizing agents in lanolin have long been in doubt, the consensus of opinion has been that the alcohol constituents are responsible [3, 10]. Recent studies [8] showed that removal of both the detergent and the free fatty alcohols from lanolin reduced the incidence of sensitivity capable of detection by standard patch test procedures almost to zero. Acetylated lanolin also shows a reduced sensitization capacity [8, 10], but the situation is less clear with hydrogenated lanolin [34, 39]. Further studies are under way to determine the extent to which reduction in the detergent and free fatty alcohol component of lanolin would be a satisfactory and commercially viable proposition.

Lanolin-containing preparations [9, 15]. Nearly 200 proprietary preparations containing lanolin were listed in Great Britain in 1966 [9]. It is a very common ingredient of cosmetic formulations [10]. Unfortunately, since there is still as yet no product labelling in Europe, and since even topical medicaments only list 'active' ingredients, it is still often very difficult to advise a patient with lanolin sensitivity. It is well to remember that even many 'safe' official topical preparations may contain wool fat or other lanolin ingredients, e.g. Oily calamine lotion B.P.C., Hydrous Wool Fat Ointment B.P.C., Hydrocortisone Ointment B.P., Salicylic Acid Ointment B.P., etc.

Lanolin-free bases. Among bases free of lanolin may be mentioned Emulsifying Wax and Ointment B.P., lanette wax, Macrogol Ointment B.P. and the paraffins. Lanolin has also been removed from many proprietary corticosteroid ointments in recent years.

REFERENCES

1 ANDERSON C.A., *et al.* (1966) *J Pharm Pharmacol* **18**, 809.
2 BLOOMFIELD S.F. (1978) *J Appl Bacteriol* **45**, 1.
3 BREIT R. & BANDMANN H.J. (1973) *Br J Dermatol* **88**, 414.
4 BROWN R. (1979) *Contact Dermatitis* **5**, 268.
5 BURRY J.N. *et al.* (1975) *Contact Dermatitis* **1**, 41.
6 CLARKE E.W. (1971) *J Soc Cosmet Chem* **22**, 421.
7 CLARKE E.W. (1975) *J Soc Cosmet Chem* **26**, 323.
8 CLARKE E.W., *et al.* (1977) *Contact Dermatitis* **3**, 421.
9 CONRAD L.I. (1966) *J Soc Cosmet Chem* **17**, 149.
10 *CRONIN E. (1966) *Br J Dermatol* **78**, 167.
11 CRONIN E. (1972) *Trans St Johns Hosp Dermatol Soc* **58**, 153.
12 *CRONIN E. (1980) *Contact Dermatitis*. Edinburgh, Churchill Livingstone.
13 CROWSHAW B. (1977) *J Soc Cosmet Chem* **28**, 3.
14 DOORNE H.V. & DUBOIS F.L. (1980) *Pharm Weekbl* **2**, 19.
15 EVANS S. (1970) *Br J Dermatol* **82**, 625.
16 FISHER A.A. (1973) *Contact Dermatitis*. 2nd ed. Philadelphia, Lea & Febinger.
17 FISHER A.A. (1974) *Cutis* **13**, 27.
18 FISHER A.A., *et al.* (1971) *Arch Dermatol* **104**, 286.
19 FREGERT S., *et al.* (1969) *Trans St Johns Hosp Dermatol Soc* **55**, 17.
20 GAY M. (1980) *Pharm Weekbl* **115**, 769.
21 HANNUKSELA M. (1979) *Int J Cosmet Sci* **1**, 257.
22 HANNUKSELA M., *et al.* (1975) *Contact Dermatitis* **1**, 112.
23 HANNUKSELA M., *et al.* (1976) *Contact Dermatitis* **2**, 201.
24 HJORTH N. (1980) *Br J Dermatol* **103** (Suppl. **18**), 19.
25 HJORTH N. & TROLLE-LARSEN C. (1962) *Am Pressman* **77**, 146.
26 HJORTH N. & TROLLE-LARSEN C. (1963) *Trans St Johns Hosp Dermatol Soc* **49**, 127.
27 KATZ M. (1973) *Drug Design (Medicinal Chemistry*. Ed. Ariens E.J. Vol.4) New York, Academic Press, p. 93.
28 LARSEN W.G. (1977) *Arch Dermatol* **113**, 623.
29 MORTENSEN T. (1979) *Contact Dermatitis* **5**, 137.
30 NEWCOMB E.A. (1966) *J Soc Cosmet Chem* **17**, 149.
31 NOBLE W.C. & SAVIN J.A. (1966) *Lancet* **i**, 347.
32 North American Contact Dermatitis Group (1973) *Arch Dermatol* **108**, 537.
33 NOVAK M. (1974) *Cesk Dermatol* **49**, 375.
34 OLEFFE J.A., *et al.* (1978) *Contact Dermatitis* **4**, 233.
35 O'NEILL J.J., *et al.* (1979) *J Soc Cosmet Chem* **30**, 25.
36 POLANO M.K. (1984) *Topical Skin Therapeutics*. Edinburgh, Churchill Livingstone.
37 SAIHAN E.M. & HARMAN R.R.M. (1978) *Br J Dermatol* **99**, 583.
38 SCHLOSSMAN M.C. & McCARTHY J.P. (1979) *Contact Dermatitis* **5**, 65.
39 SUGAI T. & HIGASKI J. (1975) *Contact Dermatitis* **1**, 146.
40 WADE A. (Ed.) (1977) *Martindale: The Extra Pharmacopoeia*. 27th ed. London, Pharmaceutical Press.
41 *WILKINSON D.S. (1972) In *Mechanisms in Drug Allergy*. Eds. Dasch C.H. & Jones H.E.H. Edinburgh, Churchill Livingstone, p.75.
42 WILKINSON D.S. (1978) *Contact Dermatitis* **5**, 58.
43 WILKINSON J.D., *et al.* (1980) *Acta Derm Venereol (Stockh)* **60**, 245.

THE INCORPORATION OF ACTIVE INGREDIENTS [6, 7]

The effect of any topical application is the sum of the non-specific effects of the vehicle and the specific effects of the active ingredients. The response to any topically applied drug is dependent on three factors [1, 4].

1. *Availability for absorption*. The drug must be readily released from the vehicle. Concentration and partition coefficients are important.
2. *Penetration*: penetration and permeation of the drug through the skin.
3. *Interaction and degradation*: the effect of the active drug on its target receptors and the rate at which it is degraded or removed from the skin.

An active drug and its vehicle must be compatible. An unsuitable combination may either inactivate the active drug or prevent its efficient release from the vehicle. If an active drug is to be added to a vehicle then the final formulation should be adjusted so as not to upset the liquid:solid balance of the preparation. If a liquid active agent is added then the liquid component of the vehicle should be proportionately reduced; if a solid agent is added then the solid phase should be adjusted accordingly. In this way the consistency of the final product will remain unaltered [6].

Some active agents are rapidly degraded if mixed in an inappropriate base. Thus a proportion of the salicylic acid in Lassar's paste may be rapidly converted to inactive zinc salicylate. This has little specific effect on its own but is able to 'protect' dithranol from being oxidized by the zinc oxide [6].

Suitable vehicles for dilution of ionic agents. A dilution of a topical formulation containing ingredients which are anionic or cationic must be made in a non-ionic vehicle to avoid upsetting the activity or stability of the preparation. Among such substances are triphenylmethane dyes, polyvalent metals, many antibiotics and corticosteroids.

Suitable emulsifying agents and bases which can be used for this purpose are detailed in the pharmacopoeias [2, 7]. W/O emulsions may be prepared with sorbitan monostearate and O/W emulsions with sorbitan esters and polyoxyethylene derivatives. Cetomacrogols are commonly used in the U.K. (see Formulary).

Some commonly used agents and preservatives [3, 5] are incompatible with non-ionic bases, e.g. phenols, resorcinol and salicylic acid.

When dilution or mixing of ionic agents is desirable, the advice of a pharmacist should be sought.

REFERENCES

1 BARRY B.W. (1983) *Dermatological Formulations: Percutaneous Absorption in Drugs and The Pharmaceutical Sciences.* Ed. Swarbrick J. New York, Marcell Dekker.
2 *British National Formulary No. 6* (1983) London, British Medical Association and The Pharmaceutical Society of Great Britain.
3 BROWNE M.R.W. (1966) *J Soc Cosmet Chem* **17**, 185.
4 KATZ M. (1973) *Drug Design* (*Medical Chemistry*. Ed. Ariens E.J. Vol. 4) New York, Academic Press.
5 PATEL N.K. & FOSS N.E. (1964) *J Pharm Sci* **53**, 94.
6 POLANO. M.K. (1984) *Topical Skin Therapeutics.* Edinburgh, Churchill Livingstone.
7 WADE A. (Ed.) (1977) *Martindale: The Extra Pharmacopoeia'.* 27th ed.

MODIFYING FACTORS [2, 5, 9, 12, 17, 27, 29, 33, 42]

The absorption of drugs can be influenced in various ways, e.g. by chemical modification of the drug to obtain a more favourable lipid–water partition coefficient, by modification of the size of the molecule, by micronization (to increase the rate of dissolution), by suitable choice of the point of application and the form in which the drug is applied and by the use of absorption promoters. Propylene glycol [26, 28], urea [8], salicylic acid [25, 28] and DMSO and related drugs [6, 25, 37, 38] have all been shown to be promoters of drug penetration. The mechanism by which these drugs work remains unclear, although they may act as marginal irritants [4] and hence facilitate penetration through the stratum corneum.

Dimethylsulphoxide [3, 14, 15, 18, 19, 21]. DMSO is a highly polar, stable substance with exceptional solvent properties. It releases histamine *in vivo* and induces weals when applied topically. It reacts with water, liberating heat.

DMSO acts as a penetrant, enhancing the penetration of drug substances through the skin [1, 21, 39], and it can induce the formation of a steroid reservoir [37]. The stratum corneum retains significant amounts of DMSO and, since most drugs are more soluble in DMSO than water, the high concentration of drug attained within the stratum corneum tends to further promote percutaneous absorption [18]. This quality has been shown to be of especial value in increasing the effectiveness of idoxuridine in herpes simplex [22] and zoster [16]. It may similarly enhance the action of antiperspirants, antipruritics and local anaesthetics. In the past toxicological considerations have precluded its more widespread use.

Dimethyl formamide and dimethyl acetamide act similarly but are less effective [1, 6, 30]. These and many other penetration enhancers are fully discussed by Barry [2].

Physiological factors affecting the delivery of active drug [2, 13, 24, 32]. Epidermal hydration and occlusion significantly increase drug penetration [10, 32, 40] and other factors such as age [20, 30], skin condition [31, 36], temperature [35], skin type [11, 41] and site of application are also important [7, 23, 34] and have a significant effect on absorption rates. These and other factors are discussed in more detail in Chapter 11.

REFERENCES

1 BAKER H. (1968) *J Invest Dermatol* **50**, 283.
2 *BARRY B.W. (1983) *Dermatological Formulations: Percutaneous Absorption in Drugs and The Pharmaceutical Sciences*. Ed. Swarbrick J. New York, Marcel Dekker, Vol. 18.
3 *BEGER I. & HAUTHAL H.G. (1976) In *Dimethyl Sulphoxide*. Eds. Martin D. & Hauthal H.G. New York, Van Nostrand Reinhold.
4 CHAUDRASEKARAU S.K. & SHAW J.E. (1978) *Curr Probl Dermatol* **7**, 142.
5 DUGARD P. (1977) *Adv Mod Toxicol* **4**, 525.
6 FELDMAN R.J. & MAIBACH H.I. (1966) *Arch Dermatol* **94**, 649.
7 FELDMAN R.J. & MAIBACH H.I. (1967) *J Invest Dermatol* **48**, 181.
8 FELDMAN R.J. & MAIBACH H.I. (1974) *Arch Dermatol* **109**, 58.
9 *FLYNN G.L. (1979) In *Modern Pharmaceutics*. Eds. Banker G.S. & Rhodes C.T. New York, Marcel Dekker.
10 FRITSCH W.C. & STOUGHTON R.B. (1963) *J Invest Dermatol* **41**, 307.
11 FROSCH P.J. & KLIGMAN A.M. (1977) *Br J Dermatol* **96**, 461.
12 HIGUCHI T. (1977) In *Design of Biopharmaceutical Properties through Pro Drugs and Analogy*. Ed. Rocher B. Washington, DC American Pharmaceutical Association, p. 40.
13 IDSON B. (1978) *Curr Probl Dermatol* **7**, 132.
14 *JACOB S.W. & HERSCHLER R. (Eds.) (1975) *Biological Actions of Dimethyl Sulphoxide*. In *Ann NW Acad Sci* **23**, 243.
15 JACOB S.W., et al. (1964) *Curr Ther Res* **6**, 134.
16 JUEL-JENSEN B.E., et al (1970) *Br Med J* **iv**, 776.
17 *KATZ M. (1973) *Drug Design (Medicinal Chemistry*. Ed. Ariens E.J. Vol. 4) Academic Press, New York, p.93.
18 *KATZ M. & POULSEN B.J. (1971) In *Handbook of Experimental Pharmacology*. Eds Brodie B.B. & Gillette J. New York, Springer, Vol. 28, p. 103.

19 KLIGMAN A.M. (1965) *JAMA* **193**, 923.
20 KLIGMAN A.M. (1978) *Curr Probl Dermatol* **7**, 1.
21 *LANDAHU G. & SCHLOSS HAUER H.J. (Eds.) (1965) *Dimethyl Sulphoxide—DMSO Symposium Berlin, 1965*. Berlin, Saladruck.
22 MACCALLUM F.O. & JUEL-JENSEN B.E. (1966) *Br Med J* **ii**, 85.
23 MAIBACH H.I., et al (1971) *Arch Environ Health* **23**, 208.
24 MCKENZIE A.W. & STOUGHTON R.B. (1962) *Arch Dermatol* **86**, 608.
25 MUNRO D.D. & STOUGHTON R.B. (1965) *Arch Dermatol* **92**, 585.
26 OSTRENGA J., et al (1971) *J Invest Dermatol* **56**, 392.
27 *POLANO M.K. (1984) *Topical Skin Therapeutics*. Edinburgh, Churchill Livingstone.
28 POLANO M.K. & PONEC M. (1976) *Arch Dermatol* **112**, 675.
29 *POLANO M.K. & PONEC M. (1980) In *Percutaneous Absorption of Steroids*. Eds Mauvais-Jarvis P. *et al*. New York, Academic Press, p. 67.
30 RASMUSSEN J.E. (1979) In *The Year Book of Dermatology 1979*. Ed. Dobson R.L. Chicago, Year Book Medical Publishers, p.15.
31 SCHAEFER H. (1979) In *Percutaneous Absorption of Steroids. Int. Symposium, Paris 1979*.
32 SCHEUPLEIN R.J. (1978) In *Physiology and Pathophysiology of the Skin*. Ed. Jarret. New York, Academic Press, Vol. 5, p. 1669.
33 *SCHEUPLEIN R.J. (1980) In *Percutaneous Absorption of Steroids*. Eds. Mauvais-Jarvis P., *et al*. New York, Academic Press, p. 1.
34 SCHEUPLEIN R.J. & BLACK I.H. (1971) *Physiol Rev* **51**, 702.
35 SHAW J.E., et al (1980) In *Current Concepts in Cutaneous Toxicity*. Eds. Drill V.A. & Lasar P. New York, Academic Press.
36 SOLOMON A.E. & LOWE N.J. (1979) *Br J Dermatol* **100**, 717.
37 STOUGHTON R.B. (1965) *Arch Dermatol* **91**, 657.
38 STOUGHTON R.B. (1966) *Arch Dermatol* **94**, 646.
39 STOUGHTON R.B. & FRITSCH W.C. (1964) *Arch Dermatol* **90**, 512.
40 SULZBERGER M.B. & WITTEN V.H. (1961) *Arch Dermatol* **84**, 1027.
41 WEIGAND D.A., et al (1980) In *Current Concepts in Cutaneous Toxicity*. Eds. Drill V.A. & Lasar P. New York, Academic Press.
42 WESTER R.C. & MAIBACH H.I. (1977) In *Cutaneous Toxicity*. Eds. Drill V.A. & Lasar P. New York, Academic Press, p. 63.

DOSAGE [2, 6, 8]

In dermatology an active ingredient is usually prescribed as a per cent of the total prescription while the quantities used are governed by the total surface area to be covered and the likely duration of treatment. The total dose, however, still has to be considered, especially with regard to possible toxicity,

TABLE 67.3. A guide to suitable quantities of a topically applied drug for 1 week's treatment

	To use sparingly	To use liberally	Lotions
Whole body	100 g	250–500 g	500 ml
Localized disease	15–30 g	50–100 g	25–100 ml

e.g. phenol, podophyllin and the local and systemic effects of topically applied steroids.

Important variables include concentration, the total amount applied, the frequency of application and the total area treated. Other factors such as drug penetration, site, hydration and occlusion have already been discussed. It should be noted, however, that dose–response curves are frequently non-linear and penetration and clinical effect depend less on the total amount of drug applied and more on the actual amount of active drug in contact with the skin [13, 14]. Penetration of steroid creams and ointments is not enhanced by simply increasing the amount applied above an optimum thickness [9, 10] and change in concentration is not always reflected by a parallel change in efficacy. For instance 2.5% hydrocortisone preparations are no more effective than those containing 1% and extemporaneously diluted steroids cannot be presumed to produce a pro rata decrease in effect. Some dilutions may show very little reduction in efficacy because of their dose–response curve and depot effect [4] whereas others may have far less effect than anticipated especially if they are incorporated into an inappropriate base [7].

Frequency of application. Very little is known about optimal frequency of application. Bland applications obviously have to be applied frequently enough to maintain their physical effect but most active preparations are usually applied just once or twice daily. With topical steroids, because of their depot effect, it may be possible to reduce this to alternate days or less.

Steroid creams and ointments should be applied sparingly. Dilute or less potent steroids can be used when larger areas of the body need to be covered. Non-steroid creams, liniments and pastes, however, are used thickly to allow for their different physical modes of action.

Quantitative aspects of topical prescribing [3, 5, 12]. This is often overlooked. The amount prescribed should last the patient until his next visit or should be adequate for the intended duration of treatment. Polano [8] recommends 10 g cream or ointment per application per day as the minimum

amount feasible for whole body application. Schlagel [11] and Katz [6] both found 12 g per day the minimum amount necessary and 'liberal' applications of emollients may entail using more than 100 g per day. A 'thick' layer of cream or ointment is usually 0.05–0.1 mm in thickness and a 'thin' layer 0.005–0.01 mm [1, 8]. The *British National Formulary* [2] makes some suggestions as to appropriate quantities of topical applications to be prescribed for both regional or whole body use. The quantities that we find to be adequate in general for 1 week's treatment are given in Table 67.3.

REFERENCES

1 ARNDT K.A. (1978) *Manual of Dermatologic Therapeutics.* 2nd ed. Boston, Little, Brown, p. 11.
2 *British National Formulary No. 6* (1983) London, British Medical Association and The Pharmaceutical Society of Great Britain.
3 FREDRICKSON T., *et al* (1980) *Br J Dermatol* **102**, 575.
4 GIBSON J.R., *et al* (1982) *Br J Dermatol* **106**, 445.
5 HRADIL E., *et al* (1979) *Acta Derm Venereol (Stockh)* **58**, 375.
6 KATZ M. (1973) *Drug Design (Medicinal Chemistry.* Ed. Ariens E.J. Vol. 14) New York, Academic Press.
7 MEHTA A.C., *et al* (1982) *Br J Pharmacol Prac* **3**, (10), 10.
8 POLANO M.K. (1984) *Topical Skin Therapeutics.* Edinburgh, Churchill Livingstone.
9 PONEC M. (1977) In *Chemical and Biochemical Aspects of Topical Psoriasis Treatment.* Thesis, Leiden, p. 49.
10 SCHALLA W., *et al* (1980) *Aktuel Dermatol* **6**, 3.
11 SCHLAGEL C.A. & SANBORN E.C. (1964) *J Invest Dermatol* **42**, 253.
12 VAN DER HARST C.A., *et al* (1982) *Acta Derm Venereol (Stockh)* **62**, 270.
13 WESTER R.C. & MAIBACH H.I. (1976) *J Invest Dermatol* **67**, 518.
14 WESTER R.C., *et al* (1977) *Arch Dermatol* **113**, 620.

TOPICAL AGENTS USED IN DERMATOLOGICAL THERAPY [19, 27]

The substances discussed below are not intended to provide a complete dermatological formulary but merely a brief guide to those traditional agents and their derivatives that are in common topical use.

Drugs with specific or particular activities or indications are discussed in separate sections later.

Details of preparations are found in the Formulary (p. 2609).

Aluminium. As a thin foil it has been used as a protective dressing. It is used in Baltimore paste as an inert protective application and as aluminium acetotartrate (subacetate) for wet dressings or as non-sensitizing eardrops in moist and exudative otitis externa. 20% solutions of the chloride and chlorhydrate in alcohol are now commercially available as axillary antiperspirants [24]. Bentonite, widely used as a gelling agent in shake lotions and emulsions, is colloidal hydrated aluminium silicate. Aluminium oxide in a graded particulate form is used as an abrasive cleanser in some cases of acne.

Benzoic acid. This is an antiseptic, preservative and antifungal agent. Benzoic acid compound ointment B.N.F. (Whitfield's ointment) contains 6% benzoic acid and 3% salicylic acid in emulsifying ointment. It is also used as a tincture. Benzoic acid is a permitted food preservative.

Benzyl benzoate, as a 25% emulsion, is the standard treatment for scabies.

Ethyl *p*-aminobenzoate (benzocaine) is best avoided on account of its sensitization risk. The parahydroxybenzoates are widely used as preservatives in topical applications (p. 2538).

Bismuth. The subgallate is used in suppositories. Bismuth salts have been used as inert powders but darken on exposure to light.

Boron. Though boric acid has been used extensively in the past, there is no evidence that it has any advantage over other, safer preparations or is of any value in dermatological practice.

Calcium. This is used as a calcium hydroxide (lime water) in the preparation of several local preparations, e.g. zinc cream and oily calamine lotion. With oleic acid it forms a soap.

Camphor. It is sometimes added to lotions for its antipruritic and cooling effect. It is widely used in proprietary chilblain preparations.

Ichthammol. Originally a shale oil treated with sulphuric acid and ammonia, ichthammol (ammonium ichthysulphonate) is a viscous black substance containing no less than 10% organically combined sulphur. It is soluble in water and glycerin but becomes viscous and hard on standing. Its physical properties lead to difficulties in formulation [3]. It is still used as an anti-inflammatory and vasoconstrictive agent for eczema, seborrhoeic dermatitis and rosacea, although without indisputable evidence of its effectiveness. It also used with glycerin in external otitis and in treating boils and cellulitis.

Iodine (see p. 2553). An antiseptic.

Lead. It is an astringent and antipruritic, as Lead lotion B.P.C. Since it is not in the *British National Formulary* it is little used. Lead oleate is an ingredient in diachylon plasters.

Magnesium. The oxide is used in dusting powders and, as the hydrous polysilicate (talc), in shake lotions and pastes. It adds 'slip' to the former and adhesive qualities to the latter. Magnesium sulphate in 25% solution or as a paste is used in inflammatory lesions for its osmotic effect.

Menthol [29]. It has been added to calamine and other lotions and creams to relieve pruritus. The sensation of cold it induces is thought to suppress itching by competitive stimulation of the nerve receptors.

Mercury. Though mercury has been much used in the treatment of psoriasis and eczema, we are not convinced of its value. Toxic effects from absorption are frequent. It is a parasiticide, however, and has some antibacterial action. The biniodide and perchloride are occasionally used as wet dressings, and organic mercurial compounds such as phenylmercuric acetate as preservatives. Sensitization to all these preparations is not uncommon. We have obtained a positive patch test to 1×10^{-7} in such a case.

Hydragraphen, a phenylmercuric dinaphthylmethane disulphonate (Penotrane) is now only available as pessaries. These must not be used in the presence of copper intra-uterine devices.

Phenol. This is a potent but toxic bactericide. In a strength of 0.5–1% it is often added to calamine or other lotions for its antipruritic effect. It exerts an analgesic effect on the pain receptors. It is used as phenol hydrate for its caustic action (p. 2591). It is absorbed through the skin especially in infancy [23] and excreted in the urine. It has caused severe toxic effects and death when used to excess.

Pyrogallic acid (1,2,3-trihydroxybenzene). It is a reducing agent which has been used in treating psoriasis of the scalp. It darkens on oxidation. It is little used in the U.K.

Resorcinol (*m*-dihydroxybenzene). This is isomeric with catechol and hydroquinone. In alkaline solutions it has a strong affinity for oxygen and is a reducing agent. Though it is still used by some in treating acne and is a constituent of magenta paint, it not infrequently causes irritant and allergic reactions. Methaemoglobinaemia, toxicity in children and myxoedema have been reported from percutaneous absorption, especially from ulcerated surfaces. As its advantages are less apparent than its dangers there is little justification for its continued use.

Selenium disulphide. This is used for the treatment of seborrhoea of the scalp and the control of pityriasis versicolor. Though absorption was found to occur through prolonged contact with normal skin [27] no significant absorption occurred after shampooing diseased scalps [25].

It is also used, as an intermittent overnight shampoo, for the suppression of pityriasis versicolor [9] and in treating confluent and reticulate papillomatosis [10]. The risk of toxicity is low [8].

Silver. The nitrate is used in solid form as a caustic and haemostatic. Solutions of 0·5–2·0% inhibit the growth of *Pseudomonas aeruginosa* [22]. It has returned to favour in recent years because of its antibacterial action [14], simplicity and apparent freedom from sensitization. It is used particularly for burns [3] and is a safe and convenient dressing for leg ulcers. Argyria may follow its prolonged administration to eyes and mucosae.

Silver sulphadiazine [21]. First introduced [6] over 18 yr ago, this compound has established itself as a safe and convenient dressing for burns [7]. Even when applied over wide areas systemic absorption is minimal and the risk of renal damage is thought to be slight [4]. It appears to have a low potential for sensitization and is useful in the management of stasis ulceration where it gives good prophylaxis against *Staphylococcus aureus* and some Gram-negative organisms. It is applied as a 1% cream. It has also been used in a tulle gras formulation [11]. When sulphonamide-resistant Gram-negative bacilli were present a silver nitrate–chlorhexidine cream was found of value [14].

Sulphur. Is still widely used for acne, seborrhoeic conditions and rosacea despite some disbelief in its activity [20] and even allegations of comedogenicity [17] though these have lacked subsequent confirmation [26]. Sodium thiosulphate 20% in a 1%

cetrimide solution is a useful treatment for extensive pityriasis versicolor infections.

Tars. See below.

Titanium. Used as a dioxide it is chemically inert and a useful substitute for zinc oxide when salicylic acid is also required [5]. It has been recommended as the active ingredient of some light-protective creams [16].

Urea B.P. (carbamide) [1, 13]. It accelerates the digestion of fibrin at about 15% and is proteolytic at 40% strength, solubilizing and denaturing protein. This property, together with its antibacterial activity, has encouraged its use in infected and crusted or necrotic sloughs [15], but its most popular current use is as 10% O/W cream for ichthyosis [28] and dry skin conditions requiring emollients. Combinations with hydrocortisone are useful for the dry itching skins of atopics or those with asteatotic eczema. It has also been used as a 40% aqueous solution for the treatment of black hairy tongues [18] and for acne conglobata [30]. Pretreatment with urea enhanced the subsequent effect of 5-fluorouracil in treating keratoses [31]. This was due to an epidermal thinning which may equally enhance the absorption of many other topically applied substances.

Zinc oxide. This is present in a large number of dermatological and cosmetic formulations. Zinc peroxide 50% in water, freshly prepared, constitutes Meleney's paste.

The calamine now in use consists of zinc carbonate coloured with ferrous oxide, although many naturally pink zinc ores have been used in the past 350 yr.

Zinc pyrithione (zinc omadine) is a fungicide and bactericide. It is incorporated in shampoos [2] as an antidandruff agent. Some, but by no means all, of its success may be due to the prevention of aggregation of horn cells into visible flakes [12]. Zinc undecylenate is also used.

Oral zinc sulphate is discussed elsewhere (p. 2335.

REFERENCES

1 Ashton H., *et al* (1971) *Br J Dermatol* **85**, 194.
2 Brauer E.W., *et al* (1966) *J Invest Dermatol* **47**, 174.
3 Cason J.S., *et al* (1966) *Br Med J* ii, 1288.
4 Delaveau P. & Friedrich-Nove P. (1977) *Therapie* **32**, 563.
5 De Vries H.R. (1961) *Br J Dermatol* **73**, 371.
6 Fox C.L. (1978) *Arch Surg* **96**, 184.

7 Fox C.L. (1978) *Recent Advances in Dermato Pharmacology*. Eds Frost, *et al*. New York, Spectrum.
8 Henschler D. & Kirschner W. (1969) *Arch Toxikol* **24**, 341.
9 Hersle K. (1971) *Acta Derm Venereol (Stockh)* **51**, 476.
10 Kirby J.D. & Borrie P.F. (1975) *Proc R Soc Med* **68**, 532.
11 Lawrence J.C. (1977) *Burns* **3**, 186.
12 Leyden J.J., *et al* (1975) *J Soc Cosmet Chem* **26**, 573.
13 Lorenzetti O.J. & Thomas E. (1972) *Cutis* **12**, 782.
14 Lowbury E.J.L., *et al* (1976) *Br Med J* i, 493.
15 Kligman A.M. (1957) *Acta Derm Venereol (Stockh)* **37**, 155.
16 Main R.A. (1966) *Practitioner* **196**, 654.
17 Mills O.H., jr & Kligman A.M. (1972) *Br J Dermatol* **86**, 620.
18 Pegum J. (1971) *Br J Dermatol* **84**, 602.
19 *Polano M.K. (1952) *Skin Therapeutics*. Amsterdam, Elsevier.
20 Pullman H., *et al* (1977) *Arch Dermatol Res* **257**, 327.
21 Richards R.M.E. & Mahlangu G.N. (1981) *J Clin Hosp Pharm* **6**, 233.
22 Ricketts C.R., *et al* (1970) *Br Med J* ii, 444.
23 Rogers S.C.F., *et al* (1978) *Br J Dermatol* **98**, 559.
24 Scholes K.T. (1978) *Br Med J* ii, 84.
25 Slinger W.N. & Hubbard D.M. (1951) *Arch Dermatol* **64**, 41.
26 Strauss J.S., *et al* (1978) *Arch Dermatol* **114**, 1340.
27 Suskind R.R. (1964) In *The Evaluation of Therapeutic Agents and Cosmetics*. Eds. Sternberg T.H. & Newcomer V.D. New York, McGraw-Hill, p.171.
28 Swanbeck G. (1968) *Acta Derm Venereol (Stockh)* **48**, 123.
29 Symposium on Menthol (1967) *Proc. Int. Symp. Paris, 1966*. Stuttgart, Theime.
30 Williamson D.M. (1977) *Clin Exp Dermatol* **2**, 351.
31 Wohlrab W. (1977) *Dermatologica* **155**, 97.

Dyes. The acridine dyes proflavine and acriflavine are to be condemned because of their high sensitizing potential. The triphenylmethane (rosaniline) dyes still continue to be widely used, despite the development of colourless and therefore more acceptable alternative agents. They have excellent anti-candidal properties and are effective against Gram-negative organisms. They are cheap and rarely sensitize [2]. Methylrosaniline chloride (crystal, gentian violet) and *p*-diethylamine triphenylmethanol (brilliant green) are normally used as 0·5–1% aqueous or alcoholic solutions or in pastes, gels or cetomacrogol creams. Vaginal pessaries are also available. The colour may be disguised by covering with a suitable powder or paste. They have their uses also as indelible skin markers prior to surgery [1] or for marking patch-test sites for later reference.

Necrotic lesions induced by triphenylmethane dyes on stripped skin or scarification were investigated by Mobacken *et al* [3, 4, 7], who found a reduced synthesis of protein and collagen and of DNA, with delay in fibroplasia and collagen formation. This may account for some reports of ulcer formation in infants' mouths being treated for thrush [5, 6]. Despite this they have recently been commended for use in neonates on umbilical stumps [9].

The triphenylmethane dyes were found to interact with cellular DNA [8] and thus to be mutagenic and, by inference, possibly carcinogenic. The degree to which this finding can be extrapolated to clinical experience still awaits further study.

REFERENCES

1 Asscher A.W., *et al* (1968) *Lancet* ii, 638.
2 Bielicky T. & Novak M. (1969) *Arch Dermatol* **100**, 540.
3 Bjornberg A. & Bobacken H. (1972) *Acta Derm Venereol (Stockh)* **52**, 476.
4 Bobacken H. *et al* (1974) *Acta Derm Venereol (Stockh)* **54**, 343.
5 Horsfield P., *et al* (1976) *Br Med J* iii, 520.
6 John R.W. (1968) *Br Med J* i, 157.
7 Norby K. & Mobacken H. (1972) *Acta Derm Venereol (Stockh)* **52**, 476.
8 Rosenkranz H.S. & Carr H.S. (1971) *Br Med J* iii, 702.
9 Wald E.R., *et al* (1977) *Am J Dis Child* **131**, 178.

Benzoyl Peroxide. Benzoyl peroxide is a powerful oxidizing agent, used also as a catalyst for resins and a bleaching agent for flour. Topical applications have been shown to be absorbed in considerable amounts [10]. However, the drug has been reported as non-toxic to humans [6] although unconfirmed reference has been made to its tumour-promoting activity in mice [13]. Its effectiveness as a peeling agent and comedolytic is the main basis for its successful use in the treatment of acne [9, 14]. It has been shown to be germicidal [7] and the reduction in facial microbial flora is equal to that attained by systemic tetracycline [5]. Autoradiographic studies have shown that it also has a direct sebostatic effect on the sebaceous gland [4]. It is available in lotion or gel form, alone, with sulphur and with hydrocortisone. Though a potential irritant, it is well tolerated by most patients if applied with care in the early stages of treatment. Improved formulation may lessen the irritancy [8]. Sensitization may occur [12] and bleaching of the hair [2] and, to a lesser extent, the skin [3] may follow its use.

A 20% lotion has been found to promote rapid re-ephithelialization of wounds [1]. It has also been found helpful in the desloughing of leg ulcers and pressure sores [11]. We have found it surprisingly well tolerated by most if not all patients.

REFERENCES

1 Alvarez O.M., *et al* (1983) *Arch Dermatol* **119**, 22.
2 Bleiberg J., *et al* (1973) *Arch Dermatol* **108**, 583.
3 Buskell L.L. (1974) *Arch Dermatol* **110**, 461.
4 Fanta D. & Jurecka W. (1978) *Acta Derm Venereol (Stockh)* **58**, 361.
5 Fulton J.E., *et al* (1977) *J Cutan Pathol* **1**, 191.
6 Holzman J., *et al* (1979) *Arzneimittelforsch* **29**, 1180.
7 Leyden J.J., *et al* (1979) *J Invest Dermatol* **72**, 165.
8 Lovenzetti O.J., *et al* (1977) *J Soc Cosmet Chem* **28**, 533.
9 Lyons R.E. (1978) *Int J Dermatol* **17**, 246.
10 Nacht S., *et al* (1981) *J Am Acad Dermatol* **4**, 31.
11 Pace W.E. (1976) *Can Med Assoc J* **115**, 1101.
12 Poole R.L. (1970) *Arch Dermatol* **102**, 635.
13 Slaga T.H., *et al* (1981) *Science* **213**, 1023.
14 Vasarinsh P. (1968) *Arch Dermatol* **98**, 183.

TARS

A tar is a product of the destructive distillation of organic substances. Four groups of substances are concerned as sources of therapeutic tars: wood, coal, bitumen and crude petroleum.

Wood tars. Oils of cade, beech, birch and pine are widely used, particularly in Scandinavian countries. Wood tars lack certain basic chemical structures characteristic of coal tars, such as pyridine, quinoline and quinaldine rings [11]. They may sensitize (p. 562) but do not photosensitize.

These tars are normally applied in 1–10% strength in ointments or pastes, or as a paint in 95% alcohol.

Bituminous tars. These were originally obtained from the distillation of shale deposits containing fossilized fish, hence 'ichthyol', ammonium ichthosulphonate. The sulphur content of ichthyol (about 10%) is present as compounds of thiopen, which is itself inert. Bituminous tars are less effective than coal tars and may have a different mode of action. They are not photosensitizers [7].

Petroleum tars. These are of no therapeutic importance.

Coal tar [10, 24]. Coal tar is a black viscous fluid with a characteristic smell. Attempts to remove the colour, odour, photosensitizing property and carcinogenicity have not been entirely successful [20] and variations in this natural product have made the assessment of active ingredients particularly difficult [22]. Of some 10,000 different constituents believed to make up coal tar, only 400 have been identified [4]. These constitute 55% of the whole.

All coal tars are products of different distillates of heated coal. The content of the tar depends on the type used and the temperature of the distillation. 'Low temperature' tar was found to contain a greater number of components but to be less effective in producing orthokeratosis in mouse tail skin than 'high temperature' tar [21, 22]. It was also more irritating. However, a comparison of high and low temperature tars showed no eventual difference in effect in the treatment of psoriasis itself, though crude (high temperature) coal tar gave quicker results [2]. This suggests that the reversal of parakeratosis is only one factor in the control of psoriasis. The authors of this study point out that dithranol was not very effective in the mouse tail test [24].

The hydrocarbons, which constitute about half the composition of tar, include benzol, naphthalene and anthracene. The high boiling point tar acids (phenolics) include isomers of substituted polyhydroxyphenols [23] and it seems likely that it is such phenols that may be responsible for the therapeutic effect of tar [6, 23]. However, the exact mechanism by which tar exerts its effect remains unknown. These high temperature fractions may have a direct effect on the granular layer by release of *lysosomes* followed by mitotic stimulation. Low temperature extracts appeared to cause epidermal thickening without restitution of the granular layer [22, 23] and may be the reason for the indifferent action of some synthetic and proprietary tar preparations [24, 25].

Until a more suitable preparation is available many dermatologists will continue to believe that crude tar remains therapeutically superior [1, 25].

The combination of tar with UV light (the Goerckerman regime) has long been known to be helpful in psoriasis. In recent years attempts have been made to identify the critical wavelengths of light involved [3, 18]. Generally UV-B light has been found to be more effective than UV-A [14]. Refined tars are less phototoxic than the crude product and phototoxicity is directly related to therapeutic efficacy [7]. UV-A is effective in combination with tar in psoriasis but the dose of energy involved must be of the order of 100 times greater than the dose of UV-B needed to produce the same therapeutic benefit [12].

Laboratory studies have shown that this regimen reduces epidermal DNA synthesis [17, 19]. This may be related to the undoubted formation of cross-links between opposite strands of the DNA double helix [13].

A cytostatic effect of crude coal tar has also been postulated [9] following the findings that prolonged application to normal skin produces epidermal thinning associated with retention hyperkeratosis. More studies are still required particularly to identify the more active fractions of tar distillates.

Carcinogenicity. The well-established carcinogenicity of pitch and heavy tar fractions has aroused renewed interest in the current climate of therapeutic conservatism and consumer protection [26], fuelled perhaps by reports such as that which shows urine from psoriatics using crude coal tar to be mutagenic to certain bacterial strains [20]. Reports of malignant tumours in man in relation to tar therapy are surprisingly extremely rare. Rook reported five cases [16] and Greither 13 [5]. Most had genital or groin involvement, but these are now unlikely sites for tar application when corticosteroids are so readily available. A recent series with a 25 yr follow-up has shown reassuringly no increased incidence of skin tumours [15].

Uses [8, 10]. The chief use of coal tar preparations lies in their keratoplastic and antipruritic activity in atopic dermatitis and chronic eczema and in psoriasis, where it is the basis of the Goeckerman regime (p. 1493). Wood tars are widely used for much the same purpose in some continental countries but are not enhanced by UV light. Oil of cade is particularly used in scalp preparations (see Formulary).

REFERENCES

1 CHAMPION R.H. (1966) *Br Med J* ii, 993.
2 CHAPMAN R.S. & FINN O.R. (1976) *Br J Dermatol* **94**, 71.
3 FISCHER T. (1971) *Acta Derm Venereol (Stockh)* **57**, 345.
4 FRANK H.G. (1963) *Ind Eng Chem* **55**, 38.
5 GREITHER A., *et al* (1967) *Z Haut Geschlkrankh* **42**, 631.
6 HELLIER F.F. & WHITEFIELD M. (1967) *Br J Dermatol* **79**, 491.
7 KAIDBEY K.H. & KLIGMAN A.M. (1977) *Arch Dermatol* **112**, 592.
8 KINMONT P.D.C. (1957) *Practitioner* **179**, 598.
9 LARKER R.M., *et al* (1981) *Br J Dermatol* **105**, 77.
10 *MULLER S.A. & KIERLAND R.R. (1964) *Proc Staff Meet Mayo Clin* **39**, 275.
11 OBERMEYER M.E. & BECKER S.A. (1935) *Arch Dermatol Syphil* **31**, 796.
12 PARRISH J.A. *et al* (1978) *J Invest Dermatol* **70**, 111.
13 PATHAK M.A. & BISWAS R.K. (1977) *J Invest Dermatol* **68**, 236.
14 PETROZZI J.W., *et al* (1978) *Br J Dermatol* **98**, 437.
15 PITTELKOW M.R., *et al* (1981) *Arch Dermatol* **117**, 465.
16 ROCK A.J. (1956) *Br J Cancer* **10**, 17.
17 STOUGHTON R.B., *et al* (1978) *Arch Dermatol* **114**, 43.
18 TANNENBAUM L., *et al* (1975) *Arch Dermatol* **111**, 476.
19 WALKER J.F., *et al* (1978) *Br J Dermatol* **99**, 89.
20 WHEELER L.A., *et al* (1981) *J Invest Dermatol* **77**, 181.
21 WINKELMANN R.K., *et al* (1964) *Proc Staff Meet Mayo Clin* **39**.
22 WRENCH R. & BRITTEN A.Z. (1975) *Br J Dermatol* **92**, 569.
23 WRENCH R. & BRITTEN A.Z. (1975) *Br J Dermatol* **92**, 575.
24 WRENCH R. & BRITTEN A.Z. (1975) *Br J Dermatol* **93**, 75.
25 YOUNG E. (1970) *Br J Dermatol* **82**, 510.
26 ZACKHEIM H.S. (1978) *Arch Dermatol* **14**, 126.

DITHRANOL [16]
(ANTHRALIN; CIGNOLIN)

Dioxyanthranol

$C_{14}H_{10}O_3$

These differ only in the position of the hydroxy group and are comparable in effect.

Dithranol is similar in its irritating and staining properties to chrysarobin but is stronger in effect. It is used in ointments, pastes, creams, or as a paint in acetone and benzene.

The mechanism of the action of dithranol is still uncertain. It inhibits glycolytic enzymes *in vitro* [12]. It has been suggested that enzyme inactivation may result from lipoid peroxidation leading to cross-linkage of enzyme proteins [3]. Mitotic inhibition [4] appears to be preceded by a paradoxical acanthogenic effect [1, 2]. Mitochondrial DNA production is reduced in the animal model [7, 17] and this antimitotic effect has been shown to be equipotent with methotrexate [6]. *In vitro* studies with human skin showed decreased oxygen consumption and inhibition of the pentose phosphate shunt [10]. The level of cyclic guanosine monophosphate is known to be increased in psoriasis. Dithranol has been shown to restore cyclic nucleosides in skin to normal levels [14].

There is no evidence that the use of dithranol or anthralin in paste vehicles causes systemic toxicity. Nor is dithranol a carcinogen in man although it induced respiratory-deficient mutants in yeast [20]. Whatever its mode of activity it is well recognized that dithranol must be kept in its reduced state until delivered to the skin where oxidation is allowed to occur and therapeutic effect attained. Dithranol, especially when incorporated in zinc oxide, is slowly oxidized by alkaline impurities to an inactive pink anthrone [18].

The effect of salicylic acid in preventing this has been known for a long time but has only recently been studied [8, 9, 11]. Salicylic acid neutralizes hydroxyl ions in an alkaline medium and perhaps reacts with free zinc ions to form an inactive zinc-dithranol complex. It was also found [10] that zinc ions and salicylic acid, as well as dithranol itself, inhibit glucose-6-phosphate dehydrogenase, thus justifying the time-honoured combination of these three agents.

An improved formulation of dithranol in zinc and salicylic acid paste (see Formulary) is claimed to have a longer shelf-life and may be easier for patients to apply [15].

The use of a water-soluble antioxidant, ascorbic acid, has allowed the production of a series of stable dithranol cream preparations [18]. These are not as therapeutically potent as equivalent strengths of pastes or ointments but show much greater patient acceptability for home usage [19].

Recent advocacy of short-duration applications of strong dithranol pastes on an out-patient basis should reduce patient's resistance to the home use of these preparations [13].

REFERENCES

1 BRAUN-FALCO O., et al (1971) Arch Dermatol Res 241, 217.
2 COX A.J. & WATSON W. (1972) Arch Dermatol 106, 503.
3 DIEZEL W., et al (1975) Dermatologica 150, 154.
4 FISHER L.B. & MAIBACH H.I. (1975) J Invest Dermatol 64, 338.
5 HODGSON C. & HELL E. (1970) Br J Dermatol 83, 397.
6 KLEM E.B. (1977) J Invest Dermatol 70, 27.
7 LOWE N.J. & BREEDING J. (1981) Arch Dermatol 117, 698.
8 LUCKACS S. & BRAUN-FALCO O. (1973) Hautarzt 24, 304.
9 PANEC-WAELSH M. & HULSEBOTSCH H.J. (1974) Arch Dermatol Res 249, 141.
10 RAAB W.P. (1976) Br J Dermatol 95, 193.
11 RAAB W. & GMEINER B. (1974) Arch Dermatol Res 251, 87.
12 RASSNER G. (1972) Arch Dermatol Res 243, 47.
13 RUNNE V. & KUNZE J. (1982) Br J Dermatol 106, 135.
14 SAIHAN E.M., et al (1980) Br J Dermatol 102, 565.
15 SEVILLE R.H. (1966) Br J Dermatol 78, 269.
16 SHROOT B., et al (1981) Br J Dermatol 105 (Suppl. 20), 3.
17 WALKER J.F., et al (1978) Br J Dermatol 99, 89.
18 WHITEFIELD M. (1981) Br J Dermatol 105 (Suppl. 20), 28.
19 WILSON P.D. & IVE F.A. (1980) Br J Dermatol 103, 105.
20 ZETTERBERG G. & SWANBECK G. (1971) Acta Derm Venereol (Stockh) 51, 45.

VITAMIN A ACID [38]
SYN. TRETINOIN; RETIN-A;
β-trans-RETINOIC ACID

Vitamin A has been used topically for over 20 yr but originally in the form of the alcohol or ester. The results were not impressive and it was not until Stuttgen [36] reported good effects from a 0·1% concentration of vitamin A acid that interest was re-awakened. Even then, it was some years before the full potentials of this preparation were fully realized. It was inevitable that this swing of opinion should have led to overenthusiasm and the publication of a number of poorly controlled clinical trials that have not always stood the test of time.

Mode of action [25, 32, 38]. Different forms of isomers of vitamin A acid have similar effects on the epidermis but vary in activity [34]. Its main action lies in restoring normal keratinization in conditions in which this is disturbed. It enhances DNA synthesis in the germinative epithelium and increases the mitotic rate. It also has a regulating effect on epidermal cell differentiation, leading to a thickening of the granular layer and a normalization of parakeratosis.

A number of molecular mechanisms have been advanced to explain its activity. The most widely held theory is that like steroid hormones the molecules bind initially to cytosol receptors which then translocate to the nucleus, thereafter altering protein synthesis via messenger RNA [29]. Other theories of action relate to possible effects on glycoprotein production [7] and on inhibition of polyamine synthesis [3]. Electron microscopy studies showed a decrease in desmosome and tonofilament formation, an increase in keratinosomes and a selective stimulation of gap junction proliferation [8, 30]. The predominance of one or other of these effects depends on the concentration used. Much of the difficulty of assessing the preparation in practice stems from this and from the erythema and irritance to which the higher concentrations may give rise.

Uses. Vitamin A acid has been used for a number of skin disorders characterized by follicular plugging, parakeratosis and hyperkeratosis.

Acne. The first studied and pre-eminent use of topical vitamin A acid is in the treatment of acne.

Numerous reports attest to its value [4, 5, 23, 26, 41]. It is normally applied at a concentration of 0·025–0·5% in a lotion or gel (though stronger preparations have been tolerated in dark-skinned races). After an initial exacerbation [31] it causes the softening and expulsion of comedones in 3–4 weeks and will prevent these reforming if its use is continued. Neither erythema nor peeling are necessary for this to be achieved [15]. It is also effective in steroid-induced acne and other acneiform eruptions [27, 33].

Psoriasis. Despite theoretical indications of potential value, local applications of vitamin A acid have not been particularly impressive in their effect on psoriasis [14].

Other conditions. A number of other conditions have been treated with varying success, usually in concentrations of 0·1–0·3%. We can confirm its value in the treatment of senile comedones [22]. Comedonic and other warty naevi also show some response [6, 13].

Darier's disease was an obvious candidate for vitamin A therapy in topical form. Some cases have responded well [10, 12, 16], especially if mild or localized. Keratosis pilaris often responds well and we have found it better than other conventional measures though some care is required in application. Of the ichthyoses, the lamellar variety appears to be helped most [1, 31], though ichthyosis vulgaris was also responsive in a four-centre trial [28], as was erythrokeratoderma variabilis [40] although a personal case did not show improvement.

Vitamin A acid has also been used with success in lichen planus but we have not found it of practical value except in oral lesions [13] where it is surprisingly well tolerated. Similar observations have been made on its usefulness in geographic tongue, a disorder which has always been resistant to therapeutic approach [17].

Fox-Fordyce disease (apocrine miliaria) has been effectively treated with a 0·1% solution [39]. Hydrocortisone cream (1%) has been recommended to control the associated axillary discomfort [11]. Hypertrophic scars and keloids respond in most cases to a daily application of a 0·05% solution [18].

A related effect on fibroblasts may account for the improvement in wound healing induced by topical retinoids [20].

Chloasma has been bleached successfully with a combination of vitamin A acid 0·1%, hydroquinone 5% and dexamethasone 0·1% in a fatty acid propylene glycol base applied daily to affected areas [21]. The mechanism of action remains unknown but all the ingredients appear to be necessary to make it effective.

Cancer chemoprophylaxis and chemotherapy. Retinoids have been shown to exert control over the differentiation of abnormal epithelial cells in animals [35]. In humans, senile (solar) keratoses of the face were found to respond well [2, 36] although in general currently available retinoids are less effective anticancer agents than other available procedures [9]. Application to carcinoma *in situ* of the cervix has produced significant reduction in size of the lesions in 33% of patients [37] and regression has been seen in cutaneous metastases of malignant melanoma [2, 24].

Sensitization. Despite very widespread use, the risk of sensitization seems to be very small, though it may be masked by irritant reactions. Two cases, in volunteer test subjects, have been reported [19] but had unusual features.

REFERENCES

1 BADEN H.P. & GOLDSMITH L.A. (1972) *Prog Dermatol* **6**, 7.
2 BOLLAG W. & OTT F. (1971) *Cancer Chemother Rep* **55**, 5960.
3 BOUTWELL R.K. & VERMA A.K. (1979) *Pure Appl Chem* **51**, 857.
4 BROOKES D.B., *et al* (1978) *Br J Clin Pract* **32**, 349.
5 DE BERSAQUES J. (1972) *Arch Belg Dermatol Syphiligr* **28**, 315.
6 DECHERED J.W., *et al* (1972) *Br J Dermatol* **86**, 578.
7 DE LUCA L.M., *et al* (1979) *Fed Proc* **38**, 2535.
8 ELIAS P.M. & FRIEND D.S. (1976) *J Cell Biol* **68**, 173.
9 ELIAS P.M., *et al* (1981) *Cancer* **48**, 932.
10 FULTON J.E., *et al* (1968) *Arch Dermatol* **98**, 396.
11 GIACCOBETTI R., *et al* (1979) *Arch Dermatol* **115**, 1365.
12 GEOTTE D.K. (1973) *Arch Dermatol* **107**, 113.
13 GUNTHER S. (1973) *Arch Dermatol* **107**, 277.
14 GUNTHER S. (1973) *Br J Dermatol* **89**, 515.
15 GUNTHER S. (1974) *Dermatol Wochenschr* **160**, 215.
16 GUNTHER S. (1975) *Acta Derm Venereol (Stockh)* **55** (Suppl. 74), 146.
17 HELFMAN R.J. (1979) *Cutis* **24**, 179.
18 JANSSEN DE LIMPENS A.M.P. (1980) *Br J Dermatol* **103**, 319.
19 JORDAN W.P., JR. *et al* (1975) *Contact Dermatitis* **1**, 306.
20 KLEIN P. (1975) *Acta Derm Venereol* **55** (Suppl. 74), 171.
21 KLIGMAN A.M. & WILLIS I. (1975) *Arch Dermatol* **111**, 40.
22 KLIGMAN A.M., *et al* (1971) *Arch Dermatol* **104**, 420.
23 KLIGMAN A.O.C., *et al* (1969) *Arch Dermatol* **99**, 469.
24 LEVINE N. & MEYSKENS F.L. (1980) *Lancet* **ii**, 224.
25 LOGAN W.S. (1972) *Arch Dermatol* **105**, 748.

26 LYONS R.E. (1978) *Int J Dermatol* 17, 246.
27 MILLS O.H., *et al* (1973) *Arch Dermatol* 108, 381.
28 MULLER S.A., *et al* (1977) *Arch Dermatol* 113, 1052.
29 ONG D.E., *et al* (1975) *Science* 190, 60.
30 PAPA C.M. (1976) *Cutis* 17, 575.
31 PECK G.L. (1977) *JAMA* 238, 472.
32 PLEWIG G., *et al* (1971) *Arch Klin Exp Dermatol* 239, 390.
33 PLEWIG G.L. & KLIGMAN A.M. (1975) *Acta Derm Venereol (Stockh)* 55 (Suppl. 74), 119.
34 SPEARMAN R.I.C. & JARRETT A. (1974) *Br J Dermatol* 90, 553.
35 SPORN M.B. & NEWTON D.C. (1979) *Fed Proc* 38, 2528.
36 STUTTGEN G. (1962) *Dermatologica* 124, 65.
37 SURWIT E.A., *et al* (1982) *Am J Obstet Gynecol* 143, 821.
38 Symposium (1975) *Acta Derm Venereol (Stockh)* 55 (Suppl. 74), 145.
39 TKACH J.R. (1979) *Arch Dermatol* 115, 1285.
40 VAN DER WATEREN A.R. & COROCANE R.H. (1977) *Br J Dermatol* 97, 83.
41 ZACHARIAE H. (1980) *Acta Derm Venereol* (Suppl) 89, 65.

MISCELLANEOUS AGENTS

Antihistamines. There is scarcely any dermatological indication for their topical use [3]. Contact sensitization is frequent and they do no more than suppress temporarily the sensation of itching. Phenol, menthol, crotamiton or lignocaine are safer. Antihistamines will doubtless continue to be prescribed and used widely by the public, however.

Bufexmac (*p*-butoxyphenylacethydroxamic acid). Earlier reports of the effectiveness of this non-steroid anti-inflammatory agent [1, 10] have not been borne out [4] though it does appear to exert some mild anti-inflammatory effect. Some cases of sensitization have been reported [16, 21].

Crotamiton (Eurax). If this acaricide is used as a 10% cream or lotion in treating scabies, the skin must be thoroughly dried before applying it. A second application is made 24 h later. Crotamiton is also an antipruritic and a bacteriostatic. Sensitization may occur [17] though this is uncommon in our experience.

Glutaraldehyde. This is most widely used as a 2% buffered solution for the sterilization of endoscopic instruments. A 10% solution can be used as a twice daily application for viral warts of the feet and hands. It should not be used on facial or ano-genital warts. It is anhidrotic [8] and is thus also used for plantar hyperhidrosis [11] and, in weaker strength (as it stains the skin brown), for palmar sweating.

It has been advocated for bullous eruptions of the hands and feet [6] in a 10% solution buffered with 5% sodium bicarbonate. It is an irritant and a sensitizer, however.

Monosulfiram (tetraethylthiuram monosulphide). This is a parasiticide and fungicide. A 25% emulsion is diluted with three parts of water immediately before use in treating scabies. A soap containing 5% is also available (Tetmosol). Antabuse-like reactions have been noted with alcohol because of its similarity to disulfiram [7] and a case of toxic epidermal necrolysis occurred in a patient sensitive to tetramethylthiuram disulphide [5].

Salt. Salabrasion is a term that has been applied [15] to the abrasion of tattooed skin by the vigorous use of salt with manual abrasion or in conjunction with dermabrasion.

Sulphacetamide. This continues to be a useful preparation for blepharitis and conjunctival infections. It can also be used as a 15% alcoholic solution for chronic paronychia and onycholysis.

Sunflower seed oil [18]. This oil, rich in linoleic acid, has been used topically to correct the skin manifestations of essential fatty acid deficiency. 250 mg of the oil were rubbed gently into the flexor surface of the forearms with improvement of the scaling and a reduction of trans-epidermal water loss.

Thymol. This is used as a solvent stabilizer in foodstuffs. In medicine it finds its most common usage in mouthwashes and occasionally in aural formulations. It is regarded as having some antifungal effect but is a poor bactericide [19]. It has been used to afford symptomatic relief from the pain of genital herpes [14].

Caffeine. In a concentration of 30% in a cream base caffeine has been used in the treatment of atopic eczema [12]. It is claimed that it has a marked antipruritic effect and when used in combination with 0·5% hydrocortisone is apparently equal in efficiency to 0·1% betamethasone [13]. It has been suggested that its presence improves the bioavailability of the steroid [20].

Aminonicotinamide. This is a potent antagonist of nicotinamide and has been reported as being helpful in patients with psoriasis [22]. So far these reports remain unconfirmed but claims of success with this drug in pityriasis rubra pilaris [2] have now been refuted [9].

REFERENCES

1 ACTEN G., *et al* (1973) *Dermatologica* **146**, 1.
2 BINNICK S.A. (1978) *Arch Dermatol* **114**, 1348.
3 BURROWS D., *et al* (1968) *Br J Dermatol* **79**, 497.
4 CHRISTIANSEN J.V., *et al* (1977) *Dermatologica* **154**, 177.
5 COPEMAN P.W.M. (1968) *Br J Med* i, 623.
6 DES GROSEILLERS J.P. & BRISSON P. (1974) *Arch Dermatol* **109**, 70.
7 GOLD S. (1966) *Lancet* ii, 1417.
8 GORDON B.J. & MAIBACH H.I. (1969) *J Invest Dermatol* **53**, 436.
9 GRIFFITHS A. & RALFS I. (1981) *Arch Dermatol* **117**, 127.
10 GRIGORIOUS D. (1972) *Med Hyg* **1004**, 491.
11 JUHLIN L. & HANSSON H. (1968) *Arch Dermatol* **97**, 327.
12 KAPLAN R.J., *et al* (1977) *Arch Dermatol* **113**, 107.
13 KAPLAN R.J., *et al* (1978) *Arch Dermatol* **114**, 60.
14 KNIGHT V. & NOALL M.W.N. (1976) *N Engl J Med* **294**, 337.
15 KOEBER W.A. & PRICE N.M. (1978) *Arch Dermatol* **114**, 884.
16 LACHAPELLE J.M. (1975) *Contact Dermatitis* **1**, 201.
17 MORGAN J.K. (1968) *Br J Clin Pract* **22**, 261.
18 PROTTEY C., *et al* (1975) *J Invest Dermatol* **64**, 288.
19 Report by Public Health Laboratory Services Committee on the Testing and Evaluation of Disinfectants (1965) *Br J Med* i, 408.
20 SIEGEL F.P., *et al* (1978) *Arch Dermatol* **114**, 1717.
21 SMEENK G. (1973) *Dermatologica* **147**, 334.
22 ZACKHEIM H.S. (1978) *Arch Dermatol* **114**, 1632.

KERATOLYTICS

The limited effectiveness of standard keratolytics has prompted some recent research into this group of topical agents. New substances have been investigated and new formulations propounded.

α-Hydroxy acids. Among a large number of substances studied for their antikeratinogenic effect, α-hydroxy acids were found to be the most effective [14]. Most forms of ichthyosis benefitted from the thrice daily application of citric, glycolic, lactic, malic, pyruvic or glucuronic acids, 5% in hydrophilic ointment or other convenient bases. Other hyperkeratotic conditions have also responded. Lactic acid, 3–5%, is an ingredient of some proprietary and cosmetic emollients and we and others [4] have found it of value in a wide range of conditions in which 'dry skin' is a feature.

Salicylic acid (*o*-hydroxybenzoic acid). This time-honoured keratolytic and keratoplastic is used

CO$_2$H
OH

C$_7$H$_6$O$_3$

alone, in ointment, oil and alcoholic vehicles or in combination with tar and other topical agents. It has been advocated in a 60% propylene glycol gel [1]. Together with benzoic acid, it constitutes Whitfield's ointment or lotion, a logical and effective fungicide. In zinc paste, it prevents the oxidation of dithranol to danthron.

The application of salicylic acid to extensive areas, particularly in children, may involve a risk of toxic symptoms from absorption [10]. Toxicity has now been recorded following external treatment in adults [6] and we have encountered symptoms of salicylism in its extensive use in a patient with psoriasis.

At the concentration normally used, salicylic acid may exert a direct solubilizing effect on the stratum corneum with dissolution of the intercellular cement [5, 9]. A 3% solution reduced epithelial hyperplasia [17] by 15% and was equivalent in this respect to 0·1% hydrocortisone. In a penetrating vehicle epithelial proliferation was inhibited. Salicylic acid appears to be antihyperplastic only on pathological epidermal proliferation [19]. However, its main effect appears to be a reduction of intercellular stickiness, perhaps by an action on the cement substance [8]. This results in enhanced shedding of corneocytes and has no recordable effect on mitotic activity [12].

The addition of 10% salicylic acid has been shown to increase the rate of passage of steroids across a membrane [11]. Clinically this effect has been confirmed when strong steroids are used [16] but not with hydrocortisone [15]. A direct anti-inflammatory effect has also been claimed [18] but has yet to be confirmed.

Propylene glycol. It was found [3] that a 40–60% aqueous solution of propylene glycol was effective, under occlusion, in softening the skin of patients with ichthyosis. An ethanol–cellulose gel was also effective [2] and more acceptable cosmetically. Applied twice daily as a 50% solution it is reported to clear pityriasis versicolor in 2 weeks [7].

REFERENCES

1 BADEN H.P. (1974) *Arch Dermatol* **110**, 737.
2 BADEN H.P. & ALPHER J.C. (1973) *J Invest Dermatol* **61**, 330.

3 BADEN H.P. & GOLDSMITH L.A. (1972) *JAMA* **220**, 579.
4 DAHL M.V. (1983) *Arch Dermatol* **119**, 27.
5 DAVIES M.G. & MARKS R. (1976) *Br J Dermatol* **95**, 187.
6 DAVIES M.G., et al (1979) *Br Med J* i, 661.
7 FAERGEMAN J. & FREDRIKSSON T. (1980) *Acta Derm Venereol (Stockh)* **60**, 92.
8 HUBER C. & CHRISTOPHERS E. (1977) *Arch Dermatol Res* **257**, 293.
9 MARKS R., et al (1975) *J Invest Dermatol* **64**, 283.
10 PASCHER F. (1978) *Int J Dermatol* **17**, 768.
11 POLANO M.K. & PONEC M. (1976) *Arch Dermatol* **112**, 675.
12 ROBERTS D.L., et al (1980) *Br J Dermatol* **103**, 191.
13 SCHUPPLI R., et al (1972) *Dermatologica* **144**, 248.
14 VAN SCOTT E.J. & YU R.J. (1974) *Arch Dermatol* **110**, 586.
15 WEBSTER R.C., et al (1978) *Arch Dermatol* **114**, 1162.
16 WEINERT V. & BLAZEK V. (1981) *Arch Dermatol Res* **271**, 19.
17 WEIRICH E.G., et al (1975) *Dermatologica* **151**, 321.
18 WEIRICH E.G., et al (1976) *Dermatologica* **152**, 87.
19 WEIRICH E.G., et al (1978) *Dermatologica* **156**, 89.

GERMICIDES AND ANTIBACTERIAL AGENTS [4, 15, 38, 41]

Disinfectants and antiseptics are generally used to destroy or inhibit the growth of pathogenic organisms in the non-sporing or vegetative state. An antiseptic (or germicide) kills or prevents the growth of microorganisms, usually in relation to living tissue. A disinfectant destroys pathogens in the environment. Germicides are more closely defined as bactericides, fungicides, etc. Bacteriostatic agents inhibit the growth of bacteria; bactericidal agents kill them. Most bactericidal substances are bacteriostatic in low concentrations but some bacteriostatics are never bactericidal.

There is considerable literature on the properties required for good germicides and their evaluation [40, 41]. Their efficiency *in vivo* may not correspond with that obtained *in vitro* because of tissue toxicity and inhibition by serum, tissue proteins and pus. Chlorine, metals and certain dyes are highly effective in low concentrations but their action is depressed in the presence of proteins. The use of otherwise efficient agents may also be limited by toxicity, sensitization [9], staining or odour. Disinfectants should be rapidly effective, non-corrosive, able to penetrate well, compatible with soaps and not inhibited by serum or faeces. Antiseptics may be allowed a less rapid action, except in pre-operative preparation of the skin; a sustained action is important. Bactericidal agents with a broad spectrum of activity are preferred.

Antiseptic agents of value on the normal skin may be inhibited or even detrimental when applied to broken skin or under particular conditions of moisture or occlusion [9, 47].

Principles of selection and use. It is better to use two or three antiseptic agents well than to change them frequently. They should be used for the purpose for which they were designed, in the recommended strength and vehicle and for no longer than is necessary to achieve their purpose. The emergence of microorganisms against which they have no activity may be as deleterious as the original bacteria they were used to suppress. Sensitization reactions may follow prolonged use; their frequency varies with different groups. The inclusion of antiseptics in cosmetics is now common practice [33] and, despite careful testing, sensitization may occur unexpectedly and take unusual forms (p. 491) [48].

Classification [10, 15]. The following groups contain substances of dermatological importance:

Phenols, halogenated phenols, alkyl-substituted phenols and resorcinols
Alcohols
Aldehydes
Acids
Halogens and halogenated compounds
Oxidizing agents
Heavy metals and their salts
Surface-active agents
Dyes
Hydroxyquinolines
Miscellaneous agents

Phenols and chlorinated phenols. These have a bactericidal action in appropriate concentrations but they rapidly lose their effect either on dilution or in the presence of organic matter. Though phenol itself is the prototype of this group several of its compounds are more effective and less toxic.

Phenol (carbolic acid). Liquefied phenol consists of an 80% wt/wt solution of phenol in water. It is widely used as a skin caustic. It is soluble in oils and fats and may rapidly be removed from the skin with glycerin, vegetable oils or 50% alcohol. The addition of salt increases its action by reducing its solubility in water; alcohol has the opposite effect. It is readily absorbed through the skin [24, 35] and has been found in the urine of infants treated with Castellani's paint (carbo–fuchsin solution) [42]. If the arterial supply is diminished it may cause gangrene [14]. It is clinically bacteriostatic in a strength of 1% and fungicidal at 1·3%. In a strength of 1–2% it has a reputation as an antipruritic.

Cresol. This is a mixture of *o-*, *m-* and *p*-cresol, alkyl derivatives of phenol with similar but more powerful bactericidal activity than phenol. Saponated cresol solutions such as Lysol are much used as disinfectants (50% in saponified linseed oil).

Thymol. Thymol, also an anthelmintic, is traditionally used as an oral antiseptic.

Other phenolics include benzoic acid, used as a fungicide and food preservative, its derivatives the parahydroxybenzoates, and the tars.

Chloroxylenol. This is marketed in the U.K. as Dettol and is probably the commonest British household antiseptic. A 5% solution dissolved in soap and perfumed with terpineol forms Chloroxylenol Solution B.P. This can be applied undiluted to the skin. Sensitivity reactions to terpineol are common. *Pseudomonas pyocyanea* has been isolated from the corks of bottles containing chloroxylenol [3]. Enhancement of its activity against pseudomonas can be achieved by the addition of 0·1% edetic acid [43].

Hexachlorophane (H-1; G-11) [30, 37]. This chlorinated bisphenol was until recently used extensively in medicinal and toiletry products. It owed its popularity to its effective, though slow, action against Gram-positive organisms and its tenacity and persistence in the stratum corneum [7, 28], particularly when applied in bath oils or non-soap detergent preparations. It has fallen into disfavour, however, to some extent undeservedly, because of its toxicity from absorption when used in exceptional conditions. In 1968 vacuolar degeneration of the white matter of the brain was found in two children with burns and two with ichthyosis who died in hospital after routine bathing with hexachlorophane [22]. Similar changes were found after the daily washing of newborn rhesus monkeys [25] and in seven out of 69 infants who died in the perinatal period, having had a 3% emulsion used in and around the umbilicus for up to 19 applications [39]. Other studies suggested that appreciable blood levels could occur in infants from even modest exposure, but no neurotoxicity was found among nearly 30,000 infants in a hospital in South Australia in which 3% hexachlorophane was used routinely, and blood levels never approached one-fifth the minimal neurotoxic level for rats or newborn monkeys [37]. The benefits of hexachlorophane in the control of staphylococcal sepsis in the newborn were considered to outweigh its potential toxic effects [13, 37]. Though it should not be used in premature infants or in those with burns or badly excoriated skin, there is no evidence that the mod-

erate and sensible use of this agent is harmful to adults. Prolonged use, especially in obsessional washers, should be discouraged and there seems little justification for its regular use as a face and body cleanser in patients with acne [3].

Inadvertent contact with undissolved concentrate has caused severe scrotal irritation [5, 49]. Primary sensitization is rare [12].

Alcohols. The bacericidal activity of the aliphatic alcohols increases with the molecular weight. Seventy per cent ethyl alcohol is effective, the isopropyl slightly more so.

Aldehydes. Conversely, the simpler are the more active.

Formaldehyde solution (formalin). Formalin contains about 40% formaldehyde gas. It has a high degree of chemical reactivity with proteins and has the property of converting toxins to toxoids, enabling the antigenic reactions to be retained. Though employed chiefly as a disinfectant, it has also been used in fungus infection, hyperhidrosis and in the treatment of verrucae. Sensitization is not uncommon.

Hexamethylenetetramine. This liberates formaldehyde and is sometimes used in dusting powders for the feet.

Acids. Benzoic acid is the only one commonly used, though acetic acid retains a reputation for a bactericidal effect on *Ps. aeruginosa*.

Halogens and halogenated compounds. Iodine and chlorine are powerful germicidal agents.

Iodine. Its mode of action is unknown. Effective concentrations also kill spores. Its action is rapid, most bacteria being killed within 1 min of exposure to a 1:20,000 concentration [15]. A 1% aqueous solution of iodine has been shown to be viricidal when used as a hand wash [18].

Weak Iodine Solution B.P. contains 2·5%, with 2·5% potassium iodide in an alcoholic solution.

If sodium iodide, 0·3–2 g, is taken by mouth it is excreted in the urine and can be detected by the addition of chlorine water, turning starch paper blue or giving a red colour with chloroform. This can be utilized in the diagnosis of iodide drug eruptions and to test patients' reliability in the taking of drugs.

Iodoform (CHI_3). It releases iodine and has a mild

antibacterial action. It is incorporated in bismuth–iodoform paste, now little used.

Iodophors. These are complexes of iodine and a solubilizer or carrier that liberates iodine in solution.

Povidone–iodine (Betadine). This is an iodophor, being a complex of iodine which slowly liberates inorganic iodine onto the skin or mucous membranes. The activity of the iodine is preserved without the irritative effects of the free tincture. It was found to be effective in reducing postoperative sepsis [6, 34] and has replaced hexachlorophane in the U.K. in many areas of use. It is well tolerated and easily removed with water. Despite some favourable reports, it is probably of less value in preventing sepsis in burns [16, 29]. Severe metabolic acidosis has been reported in two patients with extensive burned areas [36]. We have found it an acceptable treatment for leg ulcers and it has been recommended as a skin cleanser in acne [19, 32]. It can also be used as a shampoo in cases of seborrhoeic dermatitis. It is preferable to hexachlorophane for use on areas of inflamed and broken skin, e.g. in the perianal and perigenital regions, and can be used as a spray under plasters [8] and tar bandages.

Povidone–iodine has a low rate of sensitization, although four out of seven patients sensitive to potassium iodide reacted to a 2–5% aqueous solution.

It is available in several forms.

Cadexomer iodine (iodophor). Cadexomers differ from iodophors in that no chemical bond exists between the carrier and the active agent. A three-dimensional lattice of cross-linked glucose chains entraps the iodine molecule and releases it only in the presence of moisture. This compound has been found useful in absorbing moist exudates from the surfaces of chronic venous ulcers and in reducing bacterial contamination [44].

Chlorine. Chlorine is easily bound by organic matter and its use is clinically limited to hypochlorite solutions. Eusol, a solution of calcium hypochlorite, is still used extensively, alone or with paraffin.

Chloramines. These are chloramide derivatives of toluene. They are also used for water sterilization.

Chlorhexidine. This became the natural successor to hexachlorophane. It has been particularly studied by Lowbury and his colleagues [26, 27] who found it more effective in reducing skin flora, especially in

a detergent or alcoholic vehicle. In powder form it has been shown to be as effective as hexachlorophane in preventing colonization of the skin of neonates with coagulase positive staphylococci [1]. As a skin preparation solution it proved the equal of povidone–iodine in the prevention of postoperative infections [6]. Sensitization appears to be infrequent. It is inactivated by soap and by the tannin of corks.

Hydroxyquinolines. See p. 2556.

Oxidizing agents. Only three need be considered.

Hydrogen peroxide. Hydrogen peroxide 5–7% in water (Hydrogen Peroxide Solution B.P.) gives up to 20 times its volume of oxygen (20 vol). At this strength it bleaches hair and kills most organisms. The effervescence caused helps remove slough and tissue debris. It is now available as a 1·5% cream for use in the treatment of leg ulcers. In the very rare condition of acatalasia the addition of hydrogen peroxide to the patient's blood causes a darkening instead of the normal exuberant effervescence. Hydrogen peroxide is used in the treatment of anaerobic infection, especially Vincent's infection.

Zinc peroxide. It releases oxygen slowly. A 20–50% suspension, freshly prepared with water, has been used for anaerobic infections [31].

Potassium permanganate. It is used as mildly antiseptic application in the form of wet dressings or irrigations with a 1:6,000–1:8,000 freshly prepared solution.

Heavy metals. They have poor bactericidal properties and are relatively toxic. Though strong protein precipitants, their activity may be due to sulphydryl enzyme inhibition.

Mercury. Mercury has largely fallen into disuse. Sensitization reactions were common and toxic reactions such as nephrotic syndrome, acrodynia [35] and aplastic anaemia [45] have been recorded.

Silver. See above.

Surface-active agents (cationic surfactants). These are quaternary ammonium or pyridinium compounds with bactericidal activity against many Gram-positive and some Gram-negative organisms. They are inhibited by anionic agents and are thus incompatible with soaps. They are absorbed by cotton and other porous materials [20] and by surgical rubber gloves. Experimentally, they have been shown to exert toxic effects on the microcirculation [9] and should be used with caution on abraded skin.

Benzalkonium chloride (Roccal, Zephiran) is freely soluble. It is used as a sterlizing and preoperative solution or tincture, as lozenges and as a proprietary cream.

Cetrimide solution is used as a cleansing agent but may cause sensitization.

Domiphen bromide can be used as a lotion and is incorporated in lozenges (Bradosol).

Dequalinium chloride was a widely and successfully used cream and lotion [11] but necrotic reactions in naturally occluded body areas were found to occur [28] (p. 2192). The lozenges, however, are safe.

Other members of the group, such as cetylpyridinium chloride, have not been widely used in the U.K. Outbreaks of pseudomonas infection in hospital have been attributed to insufficient concentration of these antiseptics or the inhibitory effect of substances to which they adhere [23, 46].

Miscellaneous. The following may be mentioned.

Nitrofurazone (Furacin). It is a bactericidal and bacteriostatic agent effective against Gram-positive and Gram-negative organisms. Sensitization occurs and although used widely by surgeons for burns and ulcers its dermatological value is limited; it has been claimed as effective against the Louisiana fire ant bite [50].

Polynoxylin [2, 17], polyoxymethylene (Anaflex, Ponoxylan). It is a condensation product of formaldehyde and urea and is used (10%) in paste, cream, powder or gel form or as oral lozenges and eardrops. Sensitization has not yet been reported.

Cyclic salicylanilides. The halogen and trifluoromethyl-substituted [21] salicylanilides have received much attention in recent years. Though little is yet known about the clinical effects of the trifluoromethyl compounds, the halogenated salicylanilides, notably tetrachlorosalicylanide (T_4CS), were found to produce photodermatitis when incorporated in a soap (p. 513) [48]. Trichlorocarbanilide, a related non-fluorescing compound, is without this risk [12].

REFERENCES

1 ALDER V.G., *et al* (1980) *Arch Dis Child* **55**, 277.
2 ALEXANDER J. O'D. (1962) *Br J Dermatol* **74**, 364.
3 Annotations (1964) *Br Med J* **ii**, 1513.
4 AYLIFFE G.A.J. (1980) *J Hosp Inf* **1**, 111.
5 BAKER H., *et al* (1969) *Arch Dermatol* **99**, 693.
6 BERRY A.R., *et al* (1982) *J Hosp Inf* **3**, 55.
7 BLACK J.G., *et al* (1974) *Toxicology* **2**, 127.
8 BORODA C. & MONZAS G.J. (1974) *Surgery* **75**, 638.
9 BRANEMARK P.I. (1966) *Acta Clin Scand* (Suppl) **357**, 166.
10 *CADE R.A. & GEUMP W.S. (1957) In *Antiseptics, Disinfectants, Fungicides and Chemical and Physical Sterilisation.* Ed. Reddish G.F. Philadelphia, Lea & Febiger, ch. 14.
11 COLES R.B., *et al* (1958) *Br Med J* **ii**, 1014.
12 CROW K.D., *et al* (1969) *Br J Dermatol* **81**, 180.
13 DE SOUZA S.W., *et al* (1975) *Lancet* **i**, 860.
14 DIECHMANN W.B. (1949) *J Ind Hyg Toxicol* **31**, 146.
15 *ESPLIN D.W. (1965) In *The Pharmacological Basis of Therapeutics.* Eds. Goodman L.S. & Gilman A. New York, MacMillan, p. 1021.
16 GALLAND R.B., *et al* (1977) *Lancet* **ii**, 1043.
17 HALER D. (1963) *Nature* **198**, 400.
18 HENDLEY J.O., *et al* (1978) *Antimicrob Agents Chemother* **14**, 690.
19 HUDSON A.L. (1973) *Clin Trials J* **1**, 23.
20 KUNDSIN R.B. & WALKER C.W. (1957) *Arch Surg* **75**, 1036.
21 LANGE W.E. & ANDERSON J.C. (1966) *J Soc Cosmet Chem* **17**, 355.
22 LARSON D.L. (1968) *Hospitals* **42**, 63.
23 LEE J.C. & FAILKOW P.J. (1961) *JAMA* **177**, 708.
24 LEWIN J.F. & CLEARY W.T. (1982) *Forensic Sci Int* **19**, 177.
25 LOCKHART J.D. (1972) *Pediatrics* **50**, 229.
26 LOWBURY E.J.L. & LILLY H.A. (1973) *Br Med J* **i**, 510.
27 LOWBURY E.J.L., *et al* (1974) *Br Med J* **iv**, 369.
28 MANOWITZ M. & JOHNSTON V.D. (1967) *J Soc Cosmet Chem* **18**, 527.
29 McCLUSKIE B. (1976) *Aust NZJ Surg* **44**, 254.
30 McKENZIE A.W. & WILKINSON D.S. (1977) In *Recent Advances in Dermatology.* Ed. Rook A. Edinburgh, Churchill Livingstone, p. 285.
31 MELENEY F.L. (1952) *JAMA* **149**, 1450.
32 MILLIKAN L.E. (1976) *Cutis* **17**, 394.
33 MOLNER N.H. (1969) *J Soc Cosmet Chem* **20**, 103.
34 MORGAN W.J. (1978) *Lancet* **i**, 769.
35 PASCHER F. (1978) *Int J Dermatol* **17**, 768.
36 PIETSCH J. & MEAKINS J.L. (1976) *Lancet* **i**, 280.
37 PLUEKHAHN V.D. & DOLLINS R.D. (1976) *Med J Aust* **1**, 860.
38 POLANO M.K. (1952) *Skin Therapeutics.* Amsterdam, Elsevier.
39 POWELL H.A., *et al* (1973) *J Paediatr* **82**, 976.
40 PRICE P.B. (1957) In *Antiseptics, Disinfectants, Fungicides and Chemical and Physical Sterilization.* Ed. Reddish G.F. Philadelphia, Lea & Febiger, ch. 17.
41 *REDDISH G.F. (Ed.) (1957) *Antiseptics, Disinfectants, Fungicides and Chemical and Physical Sterilisation.* Philadelphia, Lea & Febiger.
42 ROGERS S.C.F., *et al* (1978) *Br J Dermatol* **98**, 559.
43 RUSSELL A.D. & FURR J.R. (1977) *J Appl Bacteriol* **43**, 253.

44 Skog E., *et al* (1983) *Br J Dermatol Update* **109**, 77.
45 Slee P.H.T.J. (1979) *Acta Med Scand* **205**, 463.
46 Stratford B.C. (1963) *Med J Aust* **ii**, 309.
47 Tilsely D.S. & Wilkinson D.S. (1965) *Trans St Johns Hosp Dermatol Soc* **51**, 49.
48 Wilkinson D.S. (1962) *Br J Dermatol* **74**, 295.
49 Wilkinson D.S. (1978) *Contact Dermatitis* **4**, 172.
50 Young R.W. & Pullig R.M. (1981) *J La State Med Soc* **133**, 10.

Hydroxyquinolines. This important group has a wide range of antibacterial activity. Many members are used also as intestinal antiseptics. They are very poorly absorbed. On the skin the more powerful compounds have the disadvantage of staining; sensitization reactions are probably becoming more common. By and large, however, they are safe and an acceptable alternative to antibiotics, especially when used in combinations with topical steroids [1]. The nomenclature is confusing:

Potassium hydroxyquinoline sulphate	Chinosol
Chlorohydroxyquinoline (65% dichlorohydroxyquinoline)	Halquinol
Dichlorohydroxyquinaldine	Chlorquinaldol
Diiodohydroxyquinoline	Floraquin
	Diodoquin
Hydroxyiodoquinoline	Chiniofon
Iodochlorohydroxyquinoline	Clioquinol
	Chinoform
	Vioform

These compounds have good antibacterial activity and a definite, though less-marked, activity against skin dermatophytes. The association of cases of subacute myelo-optic neuropathy in Japan after the ingestion of clioquinol [2, 3] prompted some anxiety about the use of this substance in infants in conditions in which absorption might occur, e.g. in the napkin area. No indication of any such adverse effect has come to light, however, although raised levels of protein-bound iodine have been found in these infants and may give rise to confusion in the determination of thyroid indices [4].

REFERENCES

1 Maibach H.I. (1978) *Arch Dermatol* **114**, 1773.
2 Toyokura Y. & Takasu T. (1975) *Jpn J Med Sci Biol* **28** (Suppl.), 87.
3 Nakae K., *et al* (1973) *Lancet* **i**, 171.
4 Upjohn A.C., *et al* (1971) *Postgrad Med J* **47**, 515.

TOPICAL ANTIBIOTICS

The scope, choice and indications for antibiotics in skin disease are fully discussed in Chapter 66. Whenever possible the sensitivity of the infecting organism should be determined before treatment. Where this is not possible the choice will depend on the nature of the infection and the prevailing patterns of drug resistance. Staphylococcal resistance to tetracyclines is well known, but it is estimated that 30% of group A haemolytic streptococci in the general population of the U.K. are also resistant [14]. Since glomerulonephritis may complicate streptococcal skin infection in children [12] a non-antibiotic antibacterial agent is preferred by some [15] for treatment of impetigo.

The value of many topical antibiotics is limited by their marked tendency to sensitize the skin, e.g. chloramphenicol and neomycin [8]. Cross-reactions occur within the aminoglycoside group [13].

Penicillin and streptomycin. Though solutions and powders containing these are successfully used by surgeons, they are potent sensitizers of the skin. Incautious handling by nurses was once a frequent cause of a disabling dermatitis until a 'no-touch' technique was enforced.

Tetracyclines [17]. These are not widely used alone as topical agents but are present in several proprietary corticosteroids. 250 mg chlortetracycline in 5 ml water held in the mouth for 2 min four times a day is sometimes of value in recurrent oral aphthosis [7].

Neomycin and framycetin (soframycin). Thirty-three preparations containing one or other of these are marketed in Great Britain and are widely used, though sensitization reactions are common, especially around leg ulcers, under occlusion or in ointment bases [8].

Sodium fusidate (p. 2517). Derived from *Fusidium coccineum*, it is active against staphylococcal infections and effective in erythrasma [11]. It has an exceptional ability to penetrate the stratum corneum [18].

Resistant strains of organisms have now been found in dermatology wards. It is advisable not to use this valuable antibiotic topically on in-patients [1].

Gentamicin sulphate. Its particular dermatological value lies in its broad spectrum of activity, including *Ps. aeruginosa* [2]. However, epidemics of bacterial gentamicin resistance in dermatological units [20] have led to the exclusion of the topical preparations from many hospital pharmacopoeias. Sensitization reactions are becoming fairly common in patients with leg ulcers and ototoxicity has followed topical use on denuded skin surfaces [6].

Tyrothricin. This is a mixture of gramicidin and tyrocidine. It is unsuitable for systemic use but has been used, usually in combination with other antibiotics, in the treatment of mouth and skin infections. It should not be instilled into the nose to combat staphylococcal carriage since it can cause anosmia.

Bacitracin. This is also too toxic for systemic use. Its antibacterial action is principally against Gram-positive organisms, so it is usually used topically in combination with other antibiotics such as neomycin or polymixin B. Allergic reactions of an anaphylactoid nature have been recorded [16].

Polymixin B. This has no activity against Gram-positive organisms but is effective against most Gram-negative organisms. Ototoxicity has followed its use in otitis externa associated with drum perforation [4].

Mupirocin (pseudomonic acid) [3]. This is a new and interesting topical antibiotic derived from *Ps. fluorescens*. It is chemically unrelated to other antibiotics and its mode of action in arresting bacterial protein synthesis is novel [9]. Cross-resistance with other antibiotics is therefore not seen. It is active against a wide range of Gram-positive organisms and some Gram-negative organisms [19]. Its usefulness in the elimination of staphylococcal nasal carriage has been demonstrated [5]. It would appear to be as clinically active against staphylococci as sodium fusidate but without the problems of emergent resistant bacterial strains [10].

REFERENCES

1 AYCLIFFE G.A.J., et al (1977) J Clin Pathol **30**, 40.
2 BARBER M. & WATERWORTH P.M. (1966) Br Med J i, 203.
3 CHAIN E.B. & MELLOWS G. (1977) J Chem Soc Perkin Trans 1, 294.
4 Committee on Safety of Medicines (1981) Curr Probl Ser No. 5.
5 DACRE J.E., et al (1983) Lancet ii, 1036.
6 DAYAL V.S., et al (1974) Arch Otolaryngol **100**, 338.
7 GRAYKOWSKI E.A., et al (1967) JAMA **196**, 637.
8 HJORTH N. & THOMSEN K. (1968) Br J Dermatol **80**, 163.
9 HUGHES J. & MELLOWS G. (1980) Biochem J **191**, 209.
10 LEWIS-JONES C.A., et al (1984) R Soc Med Int Congr Symp Ser **80**, 103.
11 MACMILLAN A.L. & SARKANY I. (1970) Br J Dermatol **82**, 507.
12 MARKOWITZ M., et al (1965) Pediatrics **35**, 293.
13 PIRILA U., et al (1967) Acta Derm Venereol (Stockh) **47**, 419.
14 ROBERTSON M.H. (1968) Br Med J iii, 349.
15 SCOTT O.L.S. & JOHNSON M.L. (1969) Practitioner **202**, 37.
16 VALE M.A., et al (1978) Arch Dermatol **114**, 800.
17 VERBOV J.L. (1969) Trans St Johns Hosp Dermatol Soc **55**, 78.
18 VICKERS C.F.H. (1969) Br J Dermatol **81**, 902.
19 WHITE A.R., et al (1984) R Soc Med Int Congr Symp Ser **80**, 42.
20 WYATT T.D., et al (1977) J. Antimicrob Chemother **3**, 213.

Topical antibiotics in acne [16]. The good effect of oral antibiotics on acne must be weighed against the risks and possible adverse effects of long-term administration [2]. Even though the tetracyclines in particular appear to be very safe drugs [1], it was logical to investigate the topical use of these agents. In the U.K. only neomycin and chloramphenicol have been employed as topical antiacne agents and then only when combined with steroid preparations. Both drugs are fairly potent sensitizers and have not gained wide acceptance by dermatologists although the chloramphenicol-containing preparation has been shown to be as effective as vitamin A acid [6].

In general terms topical antibiotics work about as well as benzoyl peroxide or tretinoin in acne and in view of the increase in bacterial resistance now being found a degree of caution should be exercised in their use [7]. Generally attention has centred on three topical antibiotics all of which are commercially available in the U.S.A.

Tetracycline hydrochloride. Various topical preparations have been used in the past [11, 12]. Most observers noted a reduction in free fatty acids. In a recent small trial [10] this was enhanced by DMSO. In a multigroup study [8] 300 patients were treated with 0·22% tetracycline hydrochloride solution and over half the patients improved moderately. Slightly better results were achieved at a 0·5% level [5].

Erythromycin. Only the lipid soluble forms, e.g. the base, propionate or stearate, are effective. At a strength of 2% in a propylene glycol–ethanol base, applied four or five times a day, it has a rather slow beneficial effect [9]. It also works in rosacea [13].

Clindamycin. There seems little doubt that 1% solutions of this drug are more effective than tetracycline or erythromycin [15]. Research data remain contradictory both on the mechanism of action of the drug and on its overall safety. Some researchers claim suppression of *P. acnes* [15]; others deny it [17] but find reduction of free fatty acids in the sebum. Some find no evidence of systemic absorption [3] while others can detect it [18]. A few cases of drug-related diarrhoea [4, 18] and one case of pseudomembranous colitis [14] have been reported. Further studies are still required to evalute this drug adequately. The major objection to all topical antiacne antibiotics remains the emergence of bacterial resistance patterns [7]. This fear combined with the clinical problems of slowness of response and difficulties in penetration appear to be the main reasons for their failure to achieve wide acceptance.

REFERENCES

1 *Ad hoc* Committee on the Use of Antibiotics in Dermatology (1975) *Arch Dermatol* 111, 1630.
2 AKERS W.A. & MAIBACH H.I. (1976) *Cutis* 17, 531.
3 ALGRA R.J., *et al* (1977) *Arch Dermatol* 113, 1390.
4 BECKER L.E., *et al* (1981) *Arch Dermatol* 117, 482.
5 BLANEY D.J. & COOK C.H. (1976) *Arch Dermatol* 112, 971.
6 BROOKES O.B., *et al* (1978) *Br J Clin Pract* 32, 349.
7 EADY E.A., *et al* (1982) *Br J Dermatol* 107, 235.
8 FRANK S.B., *et al* (1982) *Br J Dermatol* 107, 235.
9 FULTON J.E. JR. & PABLO G. (1974) *Arch Dermatol* 110, 83.
10 GLOOR M., *et al* (1974) *Hautarzt* 25, 391.
11 KRANTNER V. & SASKO E. (1970) *Cesk Dermatol* 45, 45.
12 KRAUS S.J. (1968) *J Invest Dermatol* 51, 431.
13 MILLS O.H. & KLIGMAN A.M. (1976) *Arch Dermatol* 112, 553.
14 MILLSTONE E.B., *et al* (1981) *Arch Dermatol* 117, 154.
15 RESH W. & STOUGHTON R.B. (1976) *Arch Dermatol* 112, 182.
16 STOUGHTON R.B. (1979) *Arch Dermatol* 115, 486.
17 THOMSEN R.J., *et al* (1980) *Arch Dermatol* 116, 1031.
18 VORON D.A. (1978) *Arch Dermatol* 114, 798.

ANTIFUNGAL AGENTS

These are discussed in detail in Chapters 25 and 66. One relatively new group, however, deserves mention here because of its broader range of activity.

Imidazoles [5, 11, 16, 19]. Among this large group, long used in toiletries and cosmetics because of their non-irritant properties, three in particular have emerged in recent years as potent and well-tolerated antifungal agents. These are miconazole 1[2,4- dichloro- β -dichlorobenzyloxy(phenethyl)imidazole nitrate], clotrimazole (bis-phenyl(2-chlorophenyl-1-imadozyl methane) and econazole 1-[2(4-dichlorophenyl)(4-chlorbenzyloxy) - ethyl]imidazole nitrate. They have a wide range of activity against both yeasts and dermatophytes. They are used exclusively as topical applications principally on the skin and in the female genital tract. They are equally effective, and are as effective as, but less irritating than, Whitfield's ointment [7, 8] in superficial fungal infections of the skin. Several other reports [10, 13, 17, 22] have testified to their value and acceptability. As usual, tinea pedis is apt to be more resistant than other forms [13]. Nevertheless, a mycological cure rate of 60% was obtained in 4 weeks using miconazole cream and powder in 45 young sportsmen regularly using showers and gymnasia. There is evidence to suggest that after 4 days of application a depot builds up in the skin which exerts a prophylactic effect against experimentally induced fungal disease [21]. The imidazoles are also effective against pityriasis versicolor [7, 8] erythrasma [7] and candida [20].

The use of an imidazole spray to control pityriasis capitis reduced pruritus in 47 out of 63 patients [1]. A suggestion that miconazole applied to nails will clear onychomycosis [4] has not been confirmed.

A fourth compound known as tioconazole will soon be on the market. This has been shown to have similar antifungal effects on animal models [18]. Initial clinical study [9] suggests that it may be more effective than existing preparations.

Sensitization appears to be very rare and only sparse reports have appeared [12, 15].

Thiabendazole (2-(thiazol-4-yl)benzimidazole). This has long been known as a fungicide, particularly in S. America. At a concentration of 10% in a vanishing cream base it was found effective in tinea corporis and tinea capitis [3], or it can be used at 1% in ethyl alcohol [21]. It has also cleared tinea nigra palmaris [6]. In the experimental situation it lacks the depot prophylactic antifungal effect of other imidazoles [21].

Its major use is as an anthelmintic and at a concentration of 15–20% in a hydrophilic ointment under occlusion, or as a 2% solution in 90% DMSO it is very effective for larva migrans infestation [2, 14]. Depending on availability, the oral suspension applied directly to skin under polyethylene occlusion is equally effective.

REFERENCES

1 ARON-BRUNETIERE R., *et al* (1977) *Acta Derm Venereol (Stockh)* **57**, 77.
2 BATTISTINI F. (1969) *Tex Rep Biol Med* **27** (Suppl. 2), 645.
3 BATTISTINI F., *et al* (1974) *Arch Dermatol* **109**, 695.
4 BOTTER A.A. (1970) *Mykosen* **14**, 187.
5 BRUGMANS J., *et al* (1972) *Eur J Clin Pharmacol* **5**, 93.
6 CARR J.F. & LEWIS C.W. (1975) *Arch Dermatol* **111**, 904.
7 CLAYTON Y.M. & KNIGHT A.G. (1976) *Clin Exp Dermatol* **1**, 225.
8 CLAYTON R., *et al* (1977) *Arch Dermatol* **113**, 850.
9 CLAYTON Y.M., *et al* (1982) *Clin Exp Dermatol* **7**, 543.
10 COMAISH J.S. (1975) *Postgrad Med J* **50** (Suppl. 50), 73.
11 VAN CUTSEM J.M. & TRIENPOINT D. (1972) *Chemotherapy* **17**, 392.
12 DEGREEF H. & VERHOEVE L. (1975) *Contact Dermatitis* **1**, 269.
13 DEGREEF H., *et al* (1975) *Dermatologica* **150**, 103.
14 KATZ R. & WOOD R.W. (1968) *Arch Dermatol* **94**, 643.
15 VAN KETEL W.G. (1974) *Contact Dermatitis Newsletter* No. 16, 517.
16 KUNICKI A. (1974) *Arzneimittelforsch* **24**, 534.
17 MACKIE R.M. (1980) *Practitioner* **224**, 1311.
18 ODDS F.C. (1980) *J Antimicrob Chemother* **6**, 749.
19 SAWYER P.R., *et al* (1975) *Drugs* **9**, 406.
20 SPIEKERMANN P.H. & YOUNG M.D. (1976) *Arch Dermatol* **112**, 350.
21 WALLACE J.M., *et al* (1977) *Arch Dermatol* **113**, 1539.
22 ZAIAS N. & BATTISTINI F. (1977) *Arch Dermatol* **113**, 307.

TOPICAL STEROIDS

The revolution brought about in dermatological therapy by the introduction of topical steroids, which started with Compound F or hydrocortisone in 1952 [18] is well known. Cortisone itself had been shown to be effective in some dermatoses when given systemically. It was found to be inactive when applied topically. During the 1950s further derivatives were produced with enhanced topical activity. The basic structure of the steroid moiety is given in Fig. 67.2. Modification of both the ring structure and the side chains produced dramatic

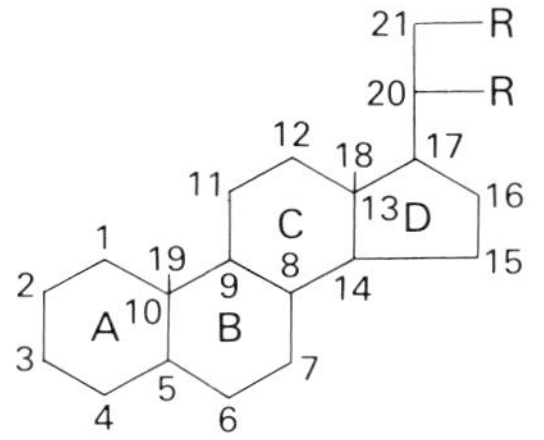

FIG. 67.2. The configuration of the basic corticosteroid structure.

changes in the effectiveness of the steroid. Thus fluorination of the 9 position, the introduction of an unsaturated bond between the first two carbon atoms and the nature of the side chains particularly in the 21 position enhanced activity [5].

During the 1960s the full therapeutic possibilities of topical steroids were explored and those dermatoses most responsive to them were identified. In the next decade the adverse effects of treatment were encountered with increasing frequency. The greater the efficacy of the topical steroid in treating the inflammatory dermatoses the greater appeared to be the side effects. The first need demonstrated was a suitable method for ranking topical steroids in order of potency [14]. This may be assessed by therapeutic trial but the method is slow and expensive and is not suitable for predicting the effect of newer products. The introduction of the vasoconstrictor assay [13] and its subsequent modifications [1] has proved of great value. The assay depends upon the property of glucocorticosteroids to produce transient vasoconstriction. The degree of pallor produced following application of a steroid in varying dilution for a standard length of time increases with the concentration of the steroid.

Despite the fact that this assay depends upon only one of the numerous biological effects of corticosteroids it has been repeatedly demonstrated to correlate well with clinical effectiveness. This and other aspects of steroid assessment have been discussed in detail [1]. Another method of assessing steroid potency employs the Duhrung chamber [6].

The second need has been for a product which retained its therapeutic effectiveness while diminishing the adverse effects [3]. Despite numerous claims to the contrary, such a product has not appeared.

Percutaneous absorption. The application of a corticosteroid to the surface of the skin is followed by absorption through the skin (percutaneous absorption) during which time it must exert all its beneficial effects. In theory the absorbed steroid distributed in the circulation may affect the skin 'on a second pass' by perfusion from the cutaneous capillaries outwards to the skin. This is rarely of clinical importance but must be considered in side-to-side comparisons in therapeutic trials. The percutaneous absorption of topical steroids is a multistage process. Barry [1] has indicated 17 different stages between the application of the steroid and its effect on the skin cell. A considerable body of data has accumulated on the various stages of absorption. The essential features are that the corticosteroid is normally crystalline and must be suspended in a suitable vehicle (see below).

The steroid diffuses into the stratum corneum or its constituents. Interaction with any other skin treatment which may have been applied is of obvious importance. It appears that the whole stratum corneum contributes to the barrier through which the steroid must penetrate, representing the probable rate-limiting step. Vickers [19] introduced the concept of a reservoir for corticosteroids within the stratum corneum which permits the absorption of steroid up to a certain level but not more. The rate of penetration into the stratum corneum is greater the more hydrophilic the steroid, i.e. water solubility favours rapid penetration. Within the viable epidermis the converse holds true. Penetration into the living keratinocytes is fastest with lipophilic steroids. Hydrocortisone has low solubility in lipids and fluocinolone acetonide relatively high lipid solubility. In experimental assays it generally holds true that the higher lipid-soluble steroids are clinically the more potent. The dichotomy between the rapid rate of penetration into the stratum corneum with low lipid solubility and the slow rate of intracellular penetration with low lipid solubility explains why there can be such wide differences in clinical effectiveness between individual steroids. Receptor binding by the cytoplasm is also greater with increasing lipid solubility. Studies to determine the strength of binding indicate that clinical potency is also related to high receptor binding. Furthermore binding appears to be specific for glucocorticoids without cross-binding of other steroids such as β-oestradiol or nandrolone. Receptor binding affinity is rather sensitive to structural alterations in the steroid. Thus the introduction of a double bond in the A ring, esterification in the 17α position and fluorination at position 9α increase binding affinity while esterification in the 21 position reduces binding affinity (see Fig. 67.2). The steroid–receptor complexes are translocated to the nucleus where they modulate messenger RNA production.

Exposure to UV light enhances percutaneous steroid absorption [11]. The mechanism of anti-inflammatory activity of glucocorticoids is still incompletely understood. Two proteins with antiphospholipase activity have similar effects on the inhibition of arachidonic acid release from various cells. Macrocortin with a molecular weight of 16,000 and lipomodulin (molecular weight 40,000) appear to be distinct and to be closely involved in the mediation of the effects of glucocorticoids in macrophages and neutrophils respectively [10]. The reader is also referred to the work of Ponec [16].

Vehicle. The choice of vehicle is of the greatest importance in the formulation of topical steroids [15]. The foregoing discussion should make it apparent that solubilities and partition coefficients profoundly alter bioavailability. It also follows that disturbance of the physicochemical composition of the vehicle will alter bioavailability [20]. This is of particular importance to the *extempore* dilution of a proprietary manufactured product. The practice of diluting or of adding other medicaments should be discouraged [8]. If dilution is considered necessary the manufacturer's own recommended diluent should be used. A further problem arises regarding alteration of the formulation of a manufacturer's product. Taking the example of betamethasone-17 valerate the addition of tar, salicylic acid or extemporaneous dilution, hastens isomerization to the 21 valerate which is considerably less potent as a corticosteroid [17]. The importance of this finding to other steroids has recently been re-examined and discussed [7]. The stability of the steroid in relation to the additives used is a subject of much research. Some, e.g. propylene glycol, may according to the manufacturer enhance penetration without impairing steroid stability.

Alteration of the vehicle of the potent steroid clobetasol propionate significantly reduced percutaneous absorption and the potential for producing systemic toxicity without reducing the vasoconstrictor assay parameters [9].

Clinical dermatologists and perhaps more frequently patients are impressed that a topical steroid is more active at the beginning of treatment than later. To achieve the same effect the patient may need to apply the steroid after ever shortening intervals. The question of whether this process of tachyphylaxis occurs with topical steroids has been discussed [4]. Evidence has been presented that intermittent application may avoid tachyphylaxis [2, 12].

REFERENCES

1 BARRY B.W. (1983) *Dermatological Formulations.* Basel, Dekker.
2 CLEMENT M., *et al* (1985) *Clin Exp Dermatol* **10**, 22.
3 DIPETRILLO T. (1984) *Arch Dermatol* **120**, 878.
4 DU VIVIER A. (1976) *Arch Dermatol* **112**, 1245.
5 ELKS J. (1976) *Br J Dermatol* **94** (Suppl. **12**), 3.
6 FROSCH P.J., *et al* (1981) *Br J Dermatol* **104**, 57.
7 GIBSON J.R., *et al* (1983) *Clin Exp Dermatol* **8**, 489.
8 GIBSON J.R., *et al* (1984) *Br J Dermatol* **111** (Suppl. 27), 204.
9 HARDING S.M., *et al* (1985) *Clin Exp Dermatol* **10**, 13.
10 HIRATA F. (1983) In *Advances in Prostaglandins, Thromboxane, and Leukotriene Research.* Eds. Samuelsson B., *et al.* Vol. II New York, Raven.

11 LAMAUD E. & SCHALLA W. (1984) *Br J Dermatol* **111**, (Suppl. **27**), 152.

12 MARGHESCU S. (1983) *Hautarzt* **34**, 114.

13 McKENZIE A.W. & STOUGHTON R.B. (1962) *Arch Dermatol* **86**, 608.

14 *Monthly Index of Medical Specialities* (1986) London, Medical Publications.

15 POLANO M.K. & PONEC M. (1976) *Arch Dermatol* **112**, 675.

16 PONEC M. (1984) *Int J Dermatol* **23**, 11.

17 RYATT K.S., *et al* (1982) *Br J Dermatol* **107**, 71.

18 SULZBERGER M.B. & WITTEN W.H. (1952) *J Invest Dermatol* **19**, 101.

19 VICKERS C.F.H. (1963) *Arch Dermatol* **88**, 20.

20 WOODFORD R. & BARRY B.W. (1982) *J Invest Dermatol* **79**, 388.

Unwanted effects of topical steroids [11, 21].

The unwanted effects of topical steroids are directly related to their potencies. So far it has not proved possible to dissociate side effects from potency. Avoidance of side effects can therefore only be avoided either by relying on weaker steroids or by acquiring a clear appreciation of how, when and where to use the more potent preparations.

The side effects can be considered at several levels.

Epidermal effects

1. Epidermal thinning is associated with a decrease in epidermal kinetic activity [18], a decrease in mean keratinocyte thickness, and a general flat-tening of the epidermo-dermal convolutions (Fig. 67.3).

2. Melanocyte inhibition, a vitiligo-like condition, has been described. This complication is more likely to occur with steroids under occlusion or with intracutaneous steroid injections [1, 19].

Dermal effects [15, 29]. Collagen synthesis is reduced, and there is a reduction in ground substance. This results in the formulation of *striae* from poor support of dermal vasculature leading to easy rupture on trauma or shearing (Fig. 67.4). The resulting intradermal haemorrhage spreads relatively unimpeded to produce a *blot haemorrhage*. This resolves with the formation of a stellate scar (Fig. 67.5). The appearance is that of prematurely aged skin (Fig. 67.3).

Vascular effects

Fixed vasodilation. Corticosteroids at first produce vasoconstriction of the superficial small vessels followed by a phase of rebound vasodilation which in later stages is fixed (Fig. 67.6) [27].

Rebound phenomenon. As vasoconstriction wears off the small vessels overdilate allowing oedema, enhanced inflammation and sometimes pustulation (Fig. 67.7).

Systemic absorption. Inhibition of the pituitary–adrenal axis by excessive application of moderately potent topical steroids or by relatively modest use of

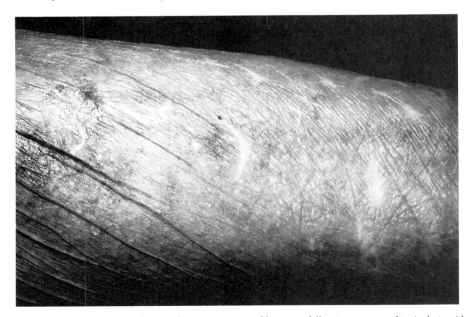

FIG. 67.3. Severe thinning of the skin and scars of tears in a 50-yr-old woman following overuse of topical steroids.

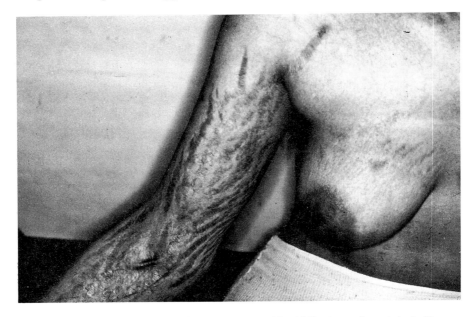

FIG. 67.4. Thinning of the skin and the formation of striae in a 19-yr-old girl following prolonged plastic film occlusion of topical steroids for psoriasis.

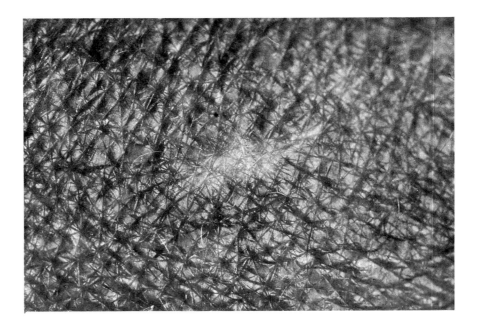

FIG. 67.5. Stellate scar following a spontaneous blot haemorrhage.

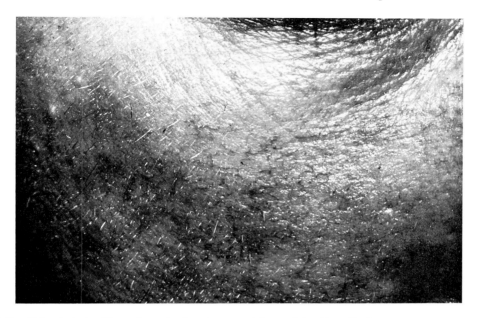

FIG. 67.6. Fixed telangiectasia of the malar region from inappropriate use of steroids on the face.

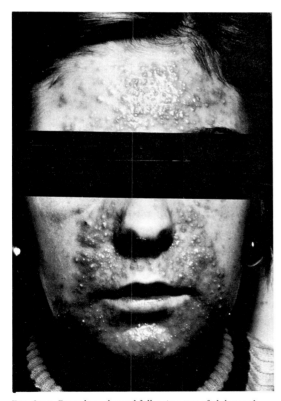

FIG. 67.7. Pustular rebound following use of clobetasol propionate (courtesy of Dr. I. Sneddon).

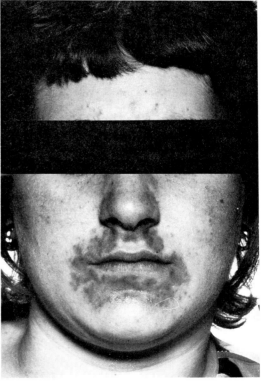

FIG. 67.8. Perioral dermatitis from prolonged use of topical steroids.

stronger steroids is well documented [6, 7, 22, 26]. Cushingoid features may be seen in infants inappropriately treated [4]. Severe medical problems are fortunately rare despite alarmingly abnormal biochemical parameters. Stunting of growth in a child treated with long-term fluorinated steroids has been observed but the weaker steroids are considered safe in children [22].

Posterior subpolar cataracts in the eye and the precipitation of glaucoma [10, 23, 30] are other hazards.

A number of iatrogenic clinical syndromes have been defined as largely due to the use of topical steroids.

1. *Perioral dermatitis q.v.* (Fig. 67.8).
2. *Tinea incognito* [14]. Topical steroids reduce the inflammation and itching of tinea without clearing

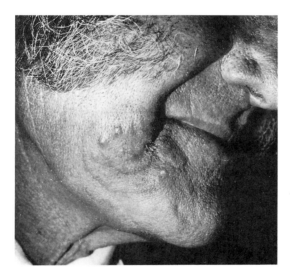

FIG. 67.9. Tinea incognito–steroid-treated fungal infection in a gardener.

the fungus (Fig. 67.9). The clinical signs of fungal infections are confusingly obscured.

3. *Infantile gluteal granuloma* [3] (See pp. 244 & 956). This curious condition is only found in infants who wear napkins—an alteration of host response to candida under the influence of steroids has been suggested.

4. *Pustular psoriasis* In the U.K. topical steroids are used much less than elsewhere for treating chronic plaque psoriasis, because the rebound phenomenon following withdrawal or reduction of the topical steroid may in a few patients be followed by the onset of an acute pustular stage [5].

Clinical experience in Europe, where tar and/or dithranol have been used by many dermatologists in preference to topical steroids, suggests that the plaques of psoriasis in a patient treated with topical steroids appear very unstable and less well defined at the margins, becoming more likely to spread as sheets. The author has also found patients less easy to treat subsequently with dithranol than non-steroid treated cases.

Comedones were induced by the application of fluorinated steroids to the perianal skin [24]. The symptoms of anogenital pruritus may change to marked soreness under the influence of topical steroids. All cutaneous infections may be exacerbated by the injudicious application of topical steroids [17]. The combination of a steroid with an antibiotic is discussed below.

Precautions. Care should be exercised in prescribing topical steroids and especially in repeating prescriptions. Plain hydrocortisone 1% in white soft paraffin is safe to use in most circumstances. The more potent steroids are more hazardous. Facial skin is especially susceptible to steroid damage [28]. The more potent steroids should be reserved for treating severe facial dermatoses such as chronic discoid lupus erythematosus or facial psoriasis.

The corticosteroids are assessed for potency on the basis of the vasoconstrictor assay [28] (see p. 2559) and in clinical trials and atrophogenicity assays [11]. A combination of these and other methods is used to produce a grouping of steroids of roughly equivalent potency. Such groupings are clinically very helpful but can be regarded as only a rough guide [13]. Individual response, the circumstances of use and occasional case reports of adverse reactions in the literature make the assessment of the relative strengths of topical steroids uncertain.

The classification recommended in the *British National Formulary* contains only four categories of potency which in the American classification expands to seven groups. The more comprehensive classification provided in the *Monthly Index of Medical Specialities* (MIMS) is widely adopted in the U.K. Further discussion is given by Polano [25]. The classification suggested (Table 67.4) is based on the MIMS list and generally reflects the authors' clinical experience. More objective assay studies indicate that some degree of reclassification may ultimately be necessary. Occlusion enhances percutaneous absorption. Children and babies have delicate easily damaged skin and having a high surface area to body volume may easily show pituitary adrenal suppression from systemic absorption.

TABLE 67.4. A suggested classification of topical corticosteroids according to their potencies

Mild

Fluocinolone acetonide 0.00025%
Hydrocortisone base or acetate 0.1–2.5%
Methylprednisolone 0.25%

Medium

Clobetasone butyrate 0.05%
Desoxymethasone 0.055%
Fluocinolone acetonide 0.000625%
Fluocinolone acetonide 0.01%
Fluocortolone hexanoate 0.1%
Fluocortolone pivalate 0.1%
Flucortolone 0.25%
Flucortolone hexanoate 0.25%
Flurandrenolone 0.0125%
Flurandrenolone 0.05%
Hydrocortisone 1% + urea

Strong

Beclomethasone dipropionate 0.025%
Betamethasone dipropionate 0.05%
Betamethasone valerate 0.025%
Betamethasone valerate 0.1%
Desonide 0.05%
Desoxymethasone 0.25%
Difluocortolone valerate 0.1%
Flucortolone acetonide 0.025%
Fluocinolone acetonide 0.025%
Fluocinonide 0.05%
Fluprednylidene 0.1%
Hydrocortisone butyrate 0.1%
Triamcinolone acetonide 0.1%

Very strong

Beclomethasone dipropionate 0.5%
Clobetasol dipropionate 0.05%
Difluocortolone valerate 0.3%
Fluocinolone acetonide 0.2%
Halcinonide 0.1%

Infection and topical steroids. Topical corticosteroids may impair the host's immunological response against the infection while obscuring other clinical signs of inflammation.

Combinations of steroid–antimicrobial agents [16]. Such combinations have not been readily accepted by dermatologists because the broad spectrum of therapeutic activity encourages sloppy diagnosis or perhaps no diagnosis at all. Antimicrobial agents are notorious topical sensitizers. The admixture of any chemical to a steroid may prejudice the stability and potency of the steroid, the vehicle or both. The flexural areas of the body, for which combination treatments are often advocated, are just those in which the conditions for the occurrence of adverse effects are increased. The case is much stronger in treating eczemas with evidence of secondary infection [16, 17], although many dermatologists would prefer to give an antibiotic systemically.

Additives, preservatives, fragrances, stabilizers and antioxidants are a necessary fact of life for any topical preparation. Adverse reactions to any of them should be considered in a patient with poor response to a usually responsive dermatosis. True allergy to the steroid itself occurs very rarely [9].

Occlusion and topical corticosteroids [12]. The incorporation of a corticosteroid such as flurandrenolone into the adhesive of a plastic tape with high occlusiveness enhances the potency of the topical steroid by encouraging hydration of the stratum corneum. A similar effect is obtained using a sheet of plastic film. Whole body occlusion formerly widely used was attended by so many adverse reactions that it should not be used.

Intralesional steroids. A few recalcitrant dermatoses (e.g. nodular prurigo, lichen simplex) may respond to repeated injection of steroid into the lesion. Triamcinolone is often used—dermal atrophy and leukoderma may occur. Blindness was reported following intralesional injection of the eyebrow skin [2].

The individual conditions for which topical steroids are used are numerous and are therefore considered elsewhere in this work.

REFERENCES

1 ARNOLD J (1975) *Dermatologica* **151**, 274.
2 BARAN R.L. (1974) *Arch Dermatol* **110**, 465.
3 BOMIFAZI E. (1981) *Clin Exp Dermatol* **6**, 23.
4 BORZYSKOWSKI M., *et al* (1976) *Clin Exp Dermatol* **1**, 337.
5 BOXLEY J.D., *et al* (1975) *Br Med J* ii, 255.
6 CARRUTHERS J.A., *et al* (1975) *Br Med J* iv, 203.
7 CORNELL R.C. & STOUGHTON R.B. (1981) *Br J Dermatol* **105**, 91.
8 COTTERILL J.A. & SWALLOW R. (1982) *Br J Dermatol* **107**, 71.
9 CRONIN E. (1980) In *Contact Dermatitis* 1st ed., Edinburgh, Churchill Livingstone, p. 246.
10 CUBEY R.B. (1976) *Br J Dermatol* **95**, 207.
11 DYKES P.J. & MARKS R. (1979) *Br J Dermatol* **101**, 599.
12 FISHER L.B., *et al* (1978) *Arch Dermatol* **114**, 384.
13 GIBSON J.R., *et al* (1983) *Clin Exp Dermatol* **8**, 489.
14 IVE F.A. & MARKS R. (1968) *Br Med J* iii, 149.
15 LETTMANN P., *et al* (1983) *J Invest Dermatol* **81**, 169.
16 LEYDEN J.J. & KLIGMAN A.M. (1977) *Br J Dermatol* **96**, 179.

17 MARPLES R.R., *et al* (1973) *Arch Dermatol* **108**, 237.
18 MARSHALL R.C. & DU VIVIER R.A. (1978) *Br J Dermatol*
       98, 355.
19 MCCORMACK P.G., *et al* (1984) *Arch Dermatol* **120**,
       708.
20 MCKENZIE A.W. & STOUGHTON R.B. (1962) *Arch Der-
       matol* **86**, 608.
21 MILLER J.A. & LEVENE G.M. (1982) *Br J Hosp Med* **28**,
       331.
22 MUNRO D. (1976) *Br J Dermatol* **94** (Suppl. 12), 67.
23 NIELSEN N.W. & SORENSEN P.N. (1978) *Arch Dermatol*
       114, 953.
24 OLIET E.J. & ESTES S.A. (1982) *J Am Acad Dermatol* **7**,
       407.
25 POLANO M.K. & AUGUST P.J. (1984) In *Topical Skin
       Therapeutics*. Ed. Polano M.K. Edinburgh, Churchill
       Livingstone, p. 101.
26 SCOGGINS R.B. & KLIMAN B. (1965) *J Invest Dermatol*
       45, 347.
27 SMITH J.G., *et al* (1976) *Arch Dermatol* **112**, 1115.
28 STANKLER L. & EWEN S.W.B. (1972) *J Invest Dermatol*
       59, 394.
29 TAN C.Y., *et al* (1981) *J Invest Dermatol* **76**, 126.
30 ZUGERMAN C., *et al* (1976) *Arch Dermatol* **112**, 1326.

TOPICAL CYTOTOXIC THERAPY

Topical application of cytotoxic drugs. A number of
cytotoxic agents have been used topically for the
eradication of superficial malignant conditions of
the skin. These are discussed in Chapters 64 and
66. We are concerned here with the use of these
agents in proliferative but benign conditions.

Aminonicotinamide. A 1% cream of this potent antagonist of nicotinamide has been used with success
in treating psoriasis [46] and in pityriasis rubra pilaris [2] but failed in a further two cases [16].

Azelaic acid. Following studies on the melanotoxic
effect of the dicarboxylic acid isolated from *Pityrosporum* yeasts trials of a 15% topical preparation reported clearing of lentigo maligna in 90 days with
a follow-up of over 2 yr [29]. Its value could not be
confirmed by other studies [9, 32]. More potent derivatives may be produced. The effect of azelaic acid
on acne is under study.

Bleomycin. A number of reports have appeared on
the successful treatment of recalcitrant viral warts
with intralesional injections of 0·1% bleomycin
[6, 20, 31]. Two large double-blind placebo-con-
trolled trials gave similar results [5, 37]. 75–95% of
warts on the hands and 60% of plantar warts
cleared following one to three injections. Local pain
is significant but tolerated by patients who had previously received many unsuccessful treatments.

Bleomycin has antitumour, antibacterial and antiviral activity. It binds to DNA, causing strand scis-
sion and elimination of pyrimidine and purine
bases. The mechanism of action in warts is not yet
known. The small volumes used do not cause systemic toxicity. Treatment of a periungual wart resulted in a permanent nail dystrophy [26]. The
compound must be handled with care.

Cantharidine. This highly toxic vesicant is derived
from the dried blister beetle *Cantharis vesicatoria*. It
is used to raise experimental blisters and as a 0·7%
solution to treat viral warts. 103 of 158 common
warts on the hands and fingers cleared without adverse effects [35] but the drug has not proved very
popular.

Methotrexate. This has been used topically in resistant psoriasis [13] but has not become an established treatment.

Colchicine and its derivatives. These alkaloids are derived from the seeds or corms of the Autumn Crocus
Colchicum autumnale. The alkaloid is readily soluble
in water; 1% in an ointment base has been used for
recalcitrant psoriasis [23]. Results in the treatment
of viral warts are variable [40]. In one study only
30% of warts cleared with 2, 4 and 8% alcoholic
solutions [43]. Two of nine patients with alopecia
totalis responded to a 0·1% solution but it was more
successful in patients with less severe alopecia
areata [47].

Dinitrochlorobenzene and Minoxidil. The potent topical sensitizer dinitrochlorobenzene (DNCB) 0·1% in
acetone has been used to treat alopecia areata [17]
and viral warts [4, 36] by inducing an inflammatory response containing a high proportion of
immunocompetent lymphocytes. Doubts over the
mutagenicity potential of DNCB led to the use of
other agents such as squaric acid dibutylester [18],
Primula [34] and diphencyprone [19, 45]. The reaction in alopecia areata was compared with that
induced by a simple irritant croton oil, which did
not induce regrowth of hair [39]. Phenolics, ca-
tharides, camphor and other irritants have been
used for many years, mostly without controlled
trials. These and the use of the vasodilator Minoxidil
1% have been reviewed [27, 44]. The development
of hypertrichosis during treatment for hypertension
suggested investigation of its use in alopecias.
Results have been variable with approximately half
the patients with alopecia areata obtaining acceptable regrowth [10] and 32% of male patients with
androgenetic alopecia showing a good to excellent
response [7].

5-Fluorouracil [14, 22]. In the form of a 5% cream it has been established as an effective treatment for multiple solar keratoses [1, 3]. Lesions on the scalp and face respond more readily than lesions on the limbs. The cream is applied twice daily for 2 weeks. A brisk inflammatory response should occur within the keratoses, otherwise clearing is incomplete. Severe ulcerative reactions result in a few patients. Combination with a fluorinated steroid limited the intensity of the inflammatory response without reducing the efficacy of the 5-fluorouracil [3]. Some patients require longer periods of treatment and others are cleared only by occlusion of the agent with polyethylene film. The complications of treatment have been reviewed [24]. Viral warts have been treated with success rates approaching those of other methods [21]. The combination of 5-fluorouracil with 10% salicylic acid was found superior to the keratolytic alone [15]. Limited plaque lesions of psoriasis may be treated with 5-fluorouracil under occlusion [25, 42]. The lesions ulcerated but remained clear from 6 to 13 months. Psoriasis of the nails responded to a 1% solution [12]. Less favourable results are seen in porokeratosis, Kyrle's disease, Darier's disease and pityriasis rubra pilaris.

Nitrogen mustard (Mechlorethamine, HN_2). Mechlorethamine has been used widely in the treatment of mycosis fungoides (q.v.). A small double-blind study in psoriasis was encouraging [8]. The solution must be freshly made up before treatment. Frequent sensitization may be a problem but desensitization can be achieved [28]. Local hyperpigmentation is a complication [33]. Nitrogen mustard has also been used in the treatment of acrodermatitis continua [30].

Podophyllin [41]. This is an extract of the dried rhizome and the roots of *Podophyllum peltatum* (N. America) or of *Podophyllum emodi* (India) commonly known as the Mandrake or May-apple. The chief constituents of the resin are lignans which are C18 compounds. The most important ones are podophyllotoxin and B-peltatin. Podophyllin resin 10–40% depending on the source is available in various vehicles such as compound benzoin tincture, alcohol or flexible collodion and is effective in clearing anogenital warts. It should not be used on the buccal mucosa or tongue or in pregnancy [11]. Adverse reactions include polyneuropathy, coma, urticaria, leukopaenia and thrombocytopaenia. Severe ulcerative local reactions are not uncommon and it is considered unwise to allow the patient to treat himself. Podophyllin in liquid paraffin spreads too readily and should not be used. A test dose of 5–

10% washed off after 1 h is an advisable precaution. The cytotoxic effect may cause confusion in the histological picture of treated warts, with some cells appearing like a squamous carcinoma [38].

REFERENCES

1 BELISARIO J.C. (1964) *Acta Derm Venereol (Stockh)* **44** (Suppl. **56**).
2 BINNICK S.A. (1978) *Arch Dermatol* **114**, 1348.
3 BREZA T., *et al* (1977) *Arch Dermatol* **112**, 1256.
4 BUCKNER D. & PRICE N.M. (1978) *Br J Dermatol* **98**, 451.
5 BUNNEY H.H., *et al* (1984) *Br J Dermatol* **110**, 197.
6 CORDERO A.A., *et al* (1980) *Cutis* **26**, 319.
7 DE VILLEZ R.L. (1985) *Arch Dermatol* **121**, 197.
8 EPSTEIN E. & UGEL A.R. (1970) *Arch Dermatol* **102**, 504.
9 ERTLE T., *et al* (1981) *Arch Dermatol Res* **271**, 197.
10 FENTON D.A. & WILKINSON J.D. (1983) *Br Med J* **287**, 1015.
11 FISHER A.A. (1981) *Cutis* **28**, 233.
12 FREDRIKSSON T. (1974) *Arch Dermatol* **110**, 735.
13 FRY L. & MCMINN R.M.H. (1967) *Arch Dermatol* **96**, 483.
14 GOETTE D.K. (1981) *J Am Acad Dermatol* **4**, 633.
15 GONCALVES J.C.A. (1975) *Br J Dermatol* **92**, 89.
16 GRIFFITHS A. & RALFS I. (1981) *Arch Dermatol* **117**, 127.
17 HAPPLE R., *et al* (1978) *Arch Dermatol* **114**, 1629.
18 HAPPLE R., *et al* (1980) *Dermatologica* **161**, 289.
19 HAPPLE R., *et al* (1983) *Acta Derm Venereol* **63**, 49.
20 HUDSON A.I. (1976) *Arch Dermatol* **112**, 1179.
21 HURSTHOUSE M.W. (1975) *Br J Dermatol* **92**, 93.
22 JANSEN G.T. (1983) *Arch Dermatol* **119**, 785.
23 KAIDBEY K.H., *et al* (1975) *Arch Dermatol* **111**, 33.
24 KURTIS B. & ROSEN T. (1979) *J Dermatol Surg Oncol* **5**, 394.
25 LJUNGGREN B. & MOLLER H. (1972) *Arch Dermatol* **106**, 263.
26 MILLER R.A.W. (1984) *Arch Dermatol* **120**, 963.
27 MITCHELL A.J. & KROLL E.A. (1984) *J Am Acad Dermatol* **11**, 763.
28 MONK B.E., *et al* (1984) *Clin Exp Dermatol* **9**, 243.
29 NAZZARO-PORRO M., *et al* (1979) *J Invest Dermatol* **72**, 296.
30 NOTOWICZ A.K., *et al* (1978) *Arch Dermatol* **114**, 129.
31 OLSEN R.L. (1977) *JAMA* **237**, 940.
32 PATHAK M.A., *et al* (1979) *J Invest Dermatol* **72**, 266.
33 PRICE N.M. (1977) *Arch Dermatol* **113**, 1387.
34 RHODES E.L., *et al* (1981) *Br J Dermatol* **104**, 339.
35 ROSENBERG E.W., *et al* (1977) *Arch Dermatol* **113**, 134.
36 SANDERS B.B. & SMITH K.W. (1981) *Cutis* **27**, 389.
37 SHUMER S.M. & O'KEEFE E.J. (1983) *J Am Acad Dermatol* **9**, 91.
38 SULLIVAN M. & KING L.S. (1947) *Arch Dermatol* **56**, 30.
39 SWANSON N.A., *et al* (1981) *Arch Dermatol* **117**, 384.
40 TOURAINE R. & REVUZ J. (1978) *Dermatologica* **157**, 397.

41 TREASE G.E. & EVANS W.C. (1983) In *Pharmacognosy*, 12th ed. London, Bailliere Tindall.

42 TSUJI T. & SUGAI T. (1972) *Arch Dermatol* **105**, 208.

43 VON KROGH G. & RUDEN A.C. (1980) *Acta Derm Venereol* **60**, 87.

44 WEISS V.C. & WEST D.P. (1985) *Arch Dermatol* **121**, 191.

45 WILKERSON M.G., *et al* (1984) *J Am Acad Dermatol* **11**, 802.

46 ZACKHEIM H.S. (1975) *Arch Dermatol* **111**, 880.

47 ZISIADIS S.K., *et al* (1980) *Dermatologica*, **161**, 365.

ANTIPERSPIRANTS

Aluminium salts have long been used for topical control of hyperhidrosis. Weaker preparations are rarely helpful for the more severely affected patient. A series of papers [5, 7, 9, 10] demonstrated the effectiveness of 20% aluminium chloride hexahydrate in alcohol applied under occlusion at night, provided the skin is thoroughly dried before application and if necessary the patient is mildly sedated. The mechanisms of action is probably by inducing blockage of the sweat ducts [6]. Irritation can be a problem but usually responds promptly to a weak to medium strength topical steroid.

Aldehydes have a similar mode of action. Aqueous glutaraldehyde solution (10%) can be applied on a swab to the soles of the feet [3, 8]. The keratin stains orange-brown. Formaldehyde Solution B.P. (1–3%) used as a twice daily soak helps mild cases. It is a frequent sensitizer and unsuitable for prolonged use.

Zinc, starch and talc dusting powder dries moist skin by adsorption and absorption. The formulation also provides some measures of lubrication of the surfaces. Too much starch in the formulation risks the formation of cement-like particles with an effect opposite to that intended. Most over-the-counter antiperspirant preparations contain aluminium chlorhydroxide. Some also contain potential sensitizing antiseptic agents, triclosan, zinc phenosulphonate or quarternary ammonium preparations. Fragrances are usually included. These preparations should not be applied to the recently shaved skin.

Anticholinergic agents are best applied topically to minimize systemic side effects. Poldine methylsulphate [4] and glycopyrronium bromide [1] can be very effective for up to 1 month. The latter has fewer central effects than atropine but some difficulty in swallowing and difficulty in accommodation of the eyes is usual for 24–48 h following treatment. It is given by immersing the hand or foot in a solution while a weak current is passed (iontophoresis). Iontophoresis of tap water alone is also effective by an unknown mechanism [2, 11] which does not appear to be due to ductal occlusion.

Surgical treatments are considered on pp 1889 and 2581.

REFERENCES

1 ABELL E. & MORGAN K. (1974) *Br J Dermatol* **91**, 87.

2 GRICE K., *et al* (1972) *Br J Dermatol* **86**, 72.

3 JUHLIN L., *et al* (1968) *Arch Dermatol* **97**, 327.

4 HILL B.H.R. (1976) *Aust J Dermatol* **17**, 92.

5 HOLZLE E. & KLIGMAN A. (1978) *Br J Dermatol* **99**, 117.

6 HOLZLE E. & KLIGMAN A. (1979) *Br J Dermatol* **30**, 279.

7 PAPA C.M. & KLIGMAN A.M. (1967) *J Invest Dermatol* **49**, 139.

8 SATO K., *et al* (1969) *Arch Dermatol* **100**, 564.

9 SHELLEY W.B. & HURLEY H.J. (1958) *Br J Dermatol* **70**, 75.

10 SHELLEY W.B. & HURLEY H.J., JR. (1975) *Acta Derm Venereol (Stockh)* **55**, 241.

11 SHRIVASTAVA S.N. & SINGH G. (1977) *Br J Dermatol* **96**, 189.

COOLING SPRAYS

Ethyl chloride spray reduces surface temperature by evaporation. Temporary local anaesthesia is induced, which may be useful in children to avoid the use of needles, and in post herpetic neuralgia. Pressurized fluoroalkanes have wider application in providing an anaesthetized firm skin during dermabrasion [1]. Worries about the ecological dangers to the Earth's ozone layer have prompted moves to limit the use of these compounds.

REFERENCE

1 STEGMAN S.J. & TROMOVITCH T.A. (1984) In *Cosmetic Dermatologic Surgery* Chicago, Year Book Medical Publishers, p. 61.

DEPIGMENTING AGENTS [5]

The search for more effective depigmenting agents in the wake of cultural as well as medical demand [2] has been limited by the sensitization potential of many of the new agents studied, e.g. 4-isopropylcatechol [2] and *p-tert*-butylphenol [10]. Hydroquinone, 2–5% has long been used with varying and inconsistent effect. Irritation is not infrequent [1, 3, 7] and exogenous ochronosis and pigmented colloid milium have been reported [6]. Monobenzyl ether of hydroquinone damages the melanocytes irreversibly [13], is a potent sensitizer and can cause an unpleasant confetti-like melanoleukoderma in some patients [4]. A burning sensation after use is common [12].

Mercury, once widely used, persists as a 'folk-lore' remedy in 'skin-bleach' creams in some countries. The daily uptake from absorption has been calculated as 20 times that taken in food [11]. A case of membranous neuropathy has been reported [8].

Based on observations made in the treatment of other diseases, an apparently synergistic mixture of hydroquinone, vitamin A acid and a topical steroid gives excellent results in melasma [9] but is less effective in post-inflammatory pigmentation (see Formulary).

REFERENCES

1 ARNDT K.A. & FITZPATRICK T.B. (1965) *JAMA* **194**, 117.
2 BLEEHEN S.S., et al (1968) *J Invest Dermatol* **50**, 103.
3 BLEEHEN S.S., et al (1977) *J Soc Cosmet Chem* **28**, 407.
4 BECKER J.W., JR & SPENCER R.C. (1962) *JAMA* **180**, 279.
5 ENGASSER P.G., et al (1981) *J Am Acad Dermatol* **5**, 143.
6 FINDLAY G.H., et al (1975) *Br J Dermatol* **93**, 613.
7 FISHER A. (1983) *Cutis* **31**, 240.
8 KIBUKAMUSOKE J.W., et al (1974) *Br Med J* **ii**, 646.
9 KLIGMAN A.M. & WILLIS I. (1975) *Arch Dermatol* **111**, 40.
10 MALTEN K.E., et al (1971) *Trans St Johns Hosp Dermatol Soc* **57**, 115.
11 MARZULLI F.N. & BROWN D.W.C. (1972) *J Soc Cosmet Chem* **23**, 875.
12 MOSHER D.B., et al (1977) *Br J Dermatol* **97**, 669.
13 RILEY P.A. (1970) *J Pathol* **101**, 163.

EPILATORIES AND DEPILATORIES

Epilation refers to complete removal of the hair from the follicle, depilation to removal of the hair at the skin level [3]. Epilation can be brought about only by plucking or wax epilatories. These are based on resin and beeswax. X-rays in a dose sufficient to cause permanent epilation should always be condemned. Electrolysis and short-wave diathermy destruction of individual hairs can, in skilled hands [1], be very effective but may otherwise cause pitting. Focal post-inflammatory pigmentation is troublesome in Black and Latin skins. As vellus hair follicle density on the face is approximately 400 per square centimetre and about 100 hairs are usually treated at one sitting, treatment may have to be prolonged. Some patients find local pain unbearable. Local anaesthesia may be necessary.

An effective depilatory must, in theory, damage the skin to the same extent as the·hair. The formulation of depilatories is a cosmetic matter and one undertaken with care. They are widely used and, in persons with healthy skins, cause little trou-

ble. These consist of strontium or barium sulphide 20% (for instance, in a talc, methyl cellulose, glycerine and water base) or thioglycollic acid [2]. The latter are becoming more widely used but are slower in action and less effective on coarse axillary hairs.

Bleaching with 10–20 vol hydrogen peroxide and enough ammonia to turn litmus blue is a simple and safe alternative to these measures.

REFERENCES

1 GALLANT A. (1983) *Principles and Techniques for the Electrologist*. Cheltenham, Stanley Thorne.
2 JELLINEK J.S. (1970) *Formulation and Function of Cosmetics*. New York, Wiley, p. 504.
3 SPOOR H.J. (1978) *Cutis* **21**, 283.

INSECT REPELLENTS AND PARASITICIDES [2, 3, 7, 11, 14]

These are also discussed in Chapter 27.

Repellents. Despite considerable research in recent years, the ideal repellent has not yet been discovered. It must combine seemingly opposed qualities—persistence on the skin, sustained volatility and lack of toxicity [3]. A high ambient temperature, washing and sweating, clothing friction and exercise all limit effectiveness [3, 5] but the most important factor remains the variability of individual 'attractiveness' to mosquitos.

A mixture of *Oil of spike lavender* and *Oil of citronella* is pleasant to use but may cause sensitization [1].

Dimethylphthalate 30–70% is still widely used. It should not be used round the eyes or lips or come into contact with plastic spectacle frames. It is being supplanted by *diethyltoluamide* (Deet) [4] which provides protection, in theory at least, for up to 4 h. *Dibutylphthalate* is also used.

Lotions of *3-Ethyl-hexanediol-1,3* (Indalone) should contain less than 10% water. It is also an UV barrier.

Among other repellents tested one can mention *triethylene glycol monohexyl ether*, *hexamethyleneimine butane sulphonamide* and various mixtures of these and others, none of which offers any particular advantage.

For repelling ticks, butopyronoxyl is effective [11].

Ectoparasiticides

These fall into two groups: *parasiticides*, used in the treatment of the affected patient, and *insecticides*, used primarily for environmental control. The distinction, however, is an arbitrary one.

Parasiticides. The most commonly used parasiticide against *Sarcoptes scabiei* in the U.K. remains benzyl benzoate. It may sting in infants and small children. γ-Benzene hexachloride (γ-BHC) (Lindane) in a 1% cream is less irritating but fears that sufficient may be absorbed in infants to cause central nervous system toxicity have been recorded and discussed [10, 12, 13]. Resistance of head lice to γ-BHC has also been noted [9]. Carbaryl has been recommended as a non-toxic effective treatment for head lice [8]. Dicophane in powder form has been withdrawn in the U.K. γ-BHC is effective but remains under suspicion for toxicological reasons. *Monosulfiram (Tetmosol)*, 25% in a lotion diluted with two to three parts of water before use, is useful and is also effective against fleas, lice and ticks. A soap is also available. Alcohol should not be taken at the same time because of its Antabuse-like action. *Crotamiton* is of some value, chiefly as a 'follow-up' preparation. *Malathion*, 0·5% in an alcoholic base, is increasingly popular for killing head lice. It is one of the least toxic of the organophosphorus agents [8].

Insecticides. Advice on safe and effective insecticides is restricted by toxicological and environmental considerations, as these are commonly used more widely in the form of powders or aerosols and may affect other than their intended victims.

Nicotine, pyrethrum and derris are used in pest control and general insect suppression. Pyrethrum is virtually devoid of toxicity but must be present in adequate strengths, e.g. 0·25% of pyrethrin, to be effective. They are available combined with piperonyl butoxide (2–4%) as a safe over-the-counter preparation in the U.S.A. [6].

Many of the repellents already mentioned, and γ-benzene hexachloride, are used as insecticides.

A number of new *organophosphorus* compounds have attracted increasing interest. They can be used to spray the environment as well as the animal vectors and include dichloros with fluitrothion ('Nuvan Top') and iodofenphos ('Nuvanol N'). Preliminary veterinary studies have been encouraging but the limits of safety in animal life and the extent of their value in human flea and mite infestation are still to be decided.

REFERENCES

1 CRONIN E. (1980) In *Contact Dermatitis*. 1st ed. Edinburgh, Churchill Livingstone, p. 159.

2 DETHIN V.C. (1947) *Chemical Insect Attractants and Repellents*. London, Lewis.
3 FELDMAN R.J. & MAIBACH H.I. (1970) *J Invest Dermatol* 54, 399.
4 GOUK H.K. (1966) *Arch Dermatol* 93, 112.
5 KHAN A.A., et al (1973) *J Econ Entomol* 66, 433.
6 LYNFIELD Y.K. & O'DONOGHUE M.N. (1982) *J Am Acad Dermatol* 6, 949.
7 MAIBACH H.I., et al (1974) *Arch Dermatol* 109, 32.
8 MAUNDER J.W. (1981) *Clin Exp Dermatol* 6, 605.
9 POLANO M.K. (1983) *J Am Acad Dermatol* 8, 120 ff.
10 RASMUSSEN J.E. (1981) *J Am Acad Dermatol* 5, 507.
11 REYNOLDS J.E.F. & PRESAD A.B. (Eds.) (1982) *Martindale: The Extra Pharmacopoeia*. 28th ed. London, Pharmaceutical Press, p. 828.
12 SHACTER B. (1981) *J Am Acad Dermatol* 5, 517.
13 SOLOMON L.M., et al (1977) *Arch Dermatol* 113, 353.
14 WORLD HEALTH ORGANIZATION (1970) *Insecticide resistance and vector control. W.H.O. Tech Rep Ser 443*.

SUNSCREENS

The last few years have seen an enormous growth of interest in and sales of sunscreens. This is related in part to wider knowledge on the ageing and carcinogenic effects of sun exposure. The use of PUVA has highlighted the importance of assessing the individual susceptibility of the skin to UV light. This varies with the skin type. Protection from UV radiation can be by complete avoidance or relative avoidance, by wearing protective clothing where the weave is more important than the thickness of the material or its colour [14] or by topical applications. These are of two types.

Physical barriers ('Sun blocks'). These consist of titanium dioxide, zinc oxide or similar finely ground powders in an oily base. They have the effect of reflecting and scattering the light. Their effectiveness is dependent on the amount applied, which makes them cosmetically unattractive. They are useful, however, for skiers, mountaineers and sailors exposed to intense UV. *Extempore* formulations are no longer necessary as a wide range of commercial preparations are available.

Chemical UV absorbers. These are generally less effective than physical barriers but are cosmetically more acceptable. The efficiency of each agent is related to the spectrum of wavelengths absorbed and to the resistance of the vehicle to washing off during swimming or sweating [2, 7, 8]. They are assessed *in vivo* by determining a sun protection factor (SPF) using a standardized source of UV light [1, 4, 10]:

$$SPF = \frac{\text{Dose UV radiation to produce minimal erythema with sunscreen}}{\text{Dose UV radiation to produce minimal erythema without sunscreen}}$$

The use of animal models complements this testing procedure. The reduction of the rise of ornithine decarboxylase levels in hairless mice irradiated with and without a sunscreen [5] and the prevention of carcinogenesis [15] show good correlation with sun protection factors but indicate that protection is incomplete. Assessment of resistance to water has been attempted by several methods [7, 12].

A wide range of chemical sunscreens are available commercially. These include para-aminobenzoic acid and derivatives, salicylates, anthranilates, cinnamates, benzophenones, camphor derivatives and others. Roelandts *et al* [11] have reviewed the chemistry and Hawk *et al* [6] have tested the efficacy in volunteers, on the basis of sun protection factors and transmission spectra of 55 commercially available products. Protection is more difficult to achieve in the UV-A range than in the UV-B range [3]. Contact dermatitis can occasionally occur with chemical sunscreens [13].

REFERENCES

1 BICKERS D.R. (1982) *J Am Acad Dermatol* 7, 402.
2 CATALANO P.M. & FULGHUM D.D. (1977) *Clin Exp Dermatol* 2, 127.
3 DIFFEY B.L. & FARR P.M. (1985) *Br J Dermatol* 112, 83.
4 FARR P.M. & DIFFEY B.L. (1985) *Br J Dermatol* 112, 113.
5 GANGE R.W. & MENDELSON R. (1982) *Br J Dermatol* 107, 215.
6 HAWK J.L.M., *et al* (1982) *Clin Exp Dermatol* 7, 21.
7 KAIDBEY K.H. & KLIGMAN A.M. (1981) *J Am Acad Dermatol* 4, 566.
8 KRAFT E.R., *et al* (1982) *J Soc Cosmet Chem* 23, 383.
9 MACLEOD T.M. & FRAIN-BELL W. (1975) *Br J Dermatol* 92, 417.
10 RAPAPORT M.J. (1983) *Int J Dermatol* 22, 293.
11 ROELANDTS R., *et al* (1983) *Int J Dermatol* 22, 247.
12 SAYRE R.M. (1979) *Arch Dermatol* 115, 46.
13 THOMPSON G., *et al* (1977) *Arch Dermatol* 113, 1252.
14 WELSH C. & DIFFEY B. (1981) *Clin Exp Dermatol* 6, 577.
15 WULF H.C., *et al* (1982) *J Am Acad Dermatol* 7, 194.

DISGUISING AND COVERING PREPARATIONS

Disfiguring lesions of the exposed skin may cause psychological 'crippling' and social ostracism [3].

When such lesions are not amenable to therapy the dermatologist must advise on the best method of covering or disguising them. Port-wine naevi and scars are rendered less conspicuous in this way, but darkly pigmented and hairy naevi are less easily dealt with. Depigmented areas may be disguised by dihydroxyacetone, pickled walnut juice, potassium permanganate or a mixture of these.

To achieve a satisfactory camouflage, two or more creams have usually to be blended on the skin and then covered with face powder [2]. Expert advice on the cosmetic aspects is desirable, since a compensatory make-up elsewhere on the face distracts from the lesion. A good covering power must be allied to good spreading. In most Western European countries certain pharmaceutical and cosmetic firms who have taken a special interest in these problems are willing to advise on individual cases. In the U.K. the Red Cross provides a service in hospitals to give help and advice in suitable cases.

The composition of one such cream is based on a brown and white masking cream combined with a red and honey-coloured toning product to blend with normal make-up. The results of the application of this cream, the full formula for which is given by Arndt and Fitzpatrick [1], were considered very good in the conditions in which it might usefully be employed.

REFERENCES

1 ARNDT K.A. & FITZPATRICK T.B. (1965) *JAMA* 194, 965.
2 CALNAN C.D. (1963) *Br Med J* i, 437.
3 *Drug Ther Bull* (1965) 3, 45.

CLEANSING AGENTS [6, 10]

Cleansing primarily implies the removal of dirt or grease from the skin but has acquired the implication of the removal of surface bacteria and, in an odour-conscious civilization, the elimination of glandular secretions and the effects of bacterial activity. Both the cosmetic and the pharmaceutical industries now regularly incorporate germicides in cleansing agents and antiperspirants [5, 8].

Soaps. These may cause irritant reactions under experimental conditions but they need seldom be avoided in patients with dermatoses [2], although in hard water areas their use in excess may be irritating in acute eczematous conditions. This does not appear to be due to their alkalinity [1]. Sensitization may occur to the perfume and—but very rarely in modern practice—to a germicide, colouring or other additive.

'Simple soap' contains no perfume or colour. Soft soap (Sapo Mollis B.P.C.) is a jelly-like soap from which the glycerol has not been 'salted' out. It makes up 65% of Soap Spirit B.P.C., which may be used as a shampoo.

'Medicated' soaps may cause sensitization. 4% povidone iodine, a widely used antiseptic cleanser, sensitizes less than the older tincture of iodine.

Emollient cleansers. Aqueous cream and emulsifying ointment can be used as a substitute for soap in patients with active scaly or inflammatory dermatoses. Several commercial preparations based on soya bean oil are cosmetically more acceptable but are more expensive. Liquid paraffin (Mineral oil U.S.P.) forms the basis of many emollient cleansers.

Medicated shampoos. Shampoos containing antiseptic preparations such as selenium sulphide, coal tar, hexachlorophane, piroctone and pyrithrione have for long been used empirically for dandruff and related scaly disorders of the scalp. Re-examination of the role of *Pityrosporum* yeasts in the aetiology of dandruff may provide some rationale for their use [4, 9].

Detergents. These excellent degreasers are widely used in various guises in dermatology, e.g. as the basis of medicated shampoos. *Cetrimide Solution* B.N.F. contains 1% of a cationic detergent. As it is a quarternary ammonium disinfectant, it is also used as a cleanser for impetigo and other crusted infective lesions due to Gram-positive organisms. It should not be used after 7 days of opening. *'Teepol'* is an aryl alkyl sulphonate with a non-ionic phenolethylene oxide condensate. *Emulsifying Ointment* B.N.F. contains almost 3% sodium laural sulphate. It is less drying than most cleansers and can be used as an after-cleansing emollient. It is very well tolerated and is frequently prescribed as a substitute for soap in the treatment of infantile and asteatotic eczema.

Detergent 'cakes', erroneously termed 'soaps', are excellent cleansers. A tablet of this type, consisting essentially of sulphated anionic long-chain fatty alcohols, was well tolerated by all but those with very dry skins [7] but did not provide enough advantages to displace soap in general use. Sulphonated castor oil preparations have good cleansing properties but do not foam and are therefore less attractive to the user.

Industrial cleansers [4]. The removal of machine oil, resin and other industrial contaminants cannot be considered in detail here. Workers still frequently resort to hydrocarbon solvents to achieve this. Waterless cleansers are now widely available but not yet sufficiently used. There is no perfect cleanser in this field, for obvious reasons. Soap powder-wood flour mixtures [3] are still useful and well tolerated. The removal of resins and paints poses particular difficulties.

Incidental cleansers. Where heavy soiling is not a problem, the use of hand creams or emollients alone may be sufficient to remove superficial dirt and grease and are frequently thus used. Cosmetic cleansing creams are widely used by women for facial cleansing. Medicated preparations such as pHiso-MED are frequently prescribed for the control or prophylaxis of infective conditions such as folliculitis, furunculosis and infective perianal dermatitis; many soaps now contain a 'built-in' germicide. There is no conclusive evidence that 'superfatted' soaps are less drying to the skin or leave more lipid behind [2].

REFERENCES

1 BETTLEY F.R. & DONOGHUE E. (1969) *Br J Dermatol* **72**, 67.
2 BLANK I.H. (1969) *Practitioner* **202**, 147.
3 CRUIKSHANK C.N.D. (1965) *Trans St John's Hosp Dermatol Soc* **51**, 241.
4 FUTTERER E. (1981) *J Soc Cosmet Chem* **32**, 327.
5 HARTMANN A.A. (1980) *Arch Dermatol Res* **267**, 161.
6 HODGSON G.A. (1965) *Trans St Johns Hosp Dermatol Soc* **51**, 202.
7 JACKMAN P.J.H. (1982) *Semin Dermatol* **1**, 143.
8 MOLNAR N.M. (1969) *J Soc Cosmet Chem* **20**, 103.
9 SHUSTER S. (1984) *Br J Dermatol* **111**, 235.
10 Symposium on Skin Cleansing (1965) *Trans St Johns Hosp Dermatol Soc* **51**, 133.

Medicated baths. Hexachlorophane concentrate (10%) is available in Great Britain but is not recommended for children under 2 yr. If not mixed thoroughly before immersion, an irritant dermatitis of the scrotum may occur [6]. Chlorhexidine is an alternative. Coal tar solution is used for psoriatics but a proprietary tar emollient has the advantage of not staining the bath. Preparations of colloidal oatmeal, with or without liquid paraffin, are also acceptable for pruritic and eczematous conditions. Germicides added to shower baths had a marked effect on skin flora [2].

Bath oils [4]. The recognition of the importance of hydration of the skin has led to an increased interest in the application of mineral oils [1, 5] during or after bathing to reduce the rate of water loss through the epidermis. Such bath oils are found to be beneficial by most patients with dry skins, particularly the elderly with asteatotic eczema and children with a dry skin associated with atopic dermatitis. In a trial in a hard-water area, there was a marked preference for the use of such mineral oils; whether this is true of soft-water areas is not yet known.

Bath oils are of spreading or dispersable type. Their dispersion and effectiveness depend on the viscosity and other physical properties of the mineral oil used, those with a lower naphthenic content having a greater affinity for the skin. An excess of surfactants above 4% reduces this [1]. 10% alkyl arylpolyether alcohol in mineral oil was the best of several tested [3]. Bubble baths which are based on detergents should be avoided by patients with dry or pruritic skins.

REFERENCES

1 KNOX J.M., *et al* (1958) *Arch Dermatol* **78**, 642.
2 BLANK H. (1969). *Practitioner* **202**, 147.
3 OGURA R. (1969) *J Soc Cosmet Chem* **20**, 109.
4 STOLAR R.E. (1966) *J Soc Cosmet Chem* **17**, 607.
5 TAYLOR E.A. (1966) *J Invest Dermatol* **37**, 69.
6 WILKINSON D.S. (1978) *Contact Dermatitis* **4**, 172.

CHAPTER 68
Physical and Surgical Procedures

R.P.R. DAWBER & J.D. WILKINSON

The extent to which the dermatologist bestrides both medicine and surgery is well shown in his approach to the treatment of benign and malignant tumours of the skin. Some will devote a great deal of time and thought to surgical techniques and to them dermatological surgery becomes almost a speciality in its own right. The number of books and articles devoted to this subject alone testifies to its importance [2, 4, 8–11]. Others, with different interests or outlooks, will restrict themselves to those minor procedures at which they have become adept and prefer to refer more complicated problems to other specialists. These attitudes are, of course, greatly influenced by national habits and customs. In many countries the dermatologist is his own plastic surgeon. Traditionally, in Great Britain the tendency has been to refer cases requiring more extensive surgery to the general or plastic surgeons. The comprehensive network of centres of plastic surgery developed during and since the last world war, and the ease of referral within the National Health Service, have often made it more convenient to send technically demanding cases to those permanently engaged in carrying out advanced plastic and reconstructive surgery. For this reason and because of limitations of space, we shall not discuss skin surgery in any great detail. The interested reader will already be aware of the literature, including those journals devoted wholly to this subject, such as the *Journal of Dermatologic Surgery and Oncology*. The Epsteins' textbook [4] is, of course, of particular value are other recent monographs, *Basics of Dermatologic Surgery* [12] and *Simple Skin Surgery* [2], which could reasonably be regarded as defining the range of dermatological surgery as at present practised in the United Kingdom. Other books deal more specifically with cosmetic dermatological surgery [9, 11] or other more general aspects of plastic surgery [3, 5, 7, 10]. Baer and Kopf [1], in their thorough introductory monograph on this subject, have laid down a number of sensible dicta to be observed before the dermatologist undertakes local surgical procedures. It is obviously im-

portant that he should have acquired the necessary skill and competence to carry them out satisfactorily and that his staff are fully experienced in the techniques and aware of the dangers of each procedure. A simple technique done well will frequently give a better result than a more advanced technique performed badly. There is much to be said, therefore, for the dermatologist carrying through as many of the minor surgical techniques as he can, providing that he knows his limitations. Specializing as he does in one body organ, he is more likely to be aware of the various diagnostic and therapeutic possibilities. He is also able to concentrate his surgical skills to include only those techniques relevant to dermatological practice. Finally, as a physician, he is probably better able than most surgeons to assess the importance of medical factors such as diabetes, bleeding tendencies, etc. in relation to any surgical procedure carried out.

Referrals for surgical treatment now account for at least 20% of a dermatologist's workload, even in the United Kingdom [5]. This is a trend that is likely to continue and the acquisition of basic dermatological surgical skills is certain to become an increasingly important component of dermatological training.

REFERENCES

1 *Baer R.L. & Kopf A.W. (1964) *Year Book of Dermatology, 1963–64*. Chicago, Year Book Medical Publishers.
2 Burge S. & Rayment R. (1986) *Simple Skin Surgery*. Oxford, Blackwell Scientific Publication.
3 Converse J.M., *et al* (1977) *Reconstructive Plastic Surgery*. Philadelphia, W.B. Saunders.
4 *Epstein E. & Epstein E. J. (1982) *Skin Surgery*. 5th ed. Springfield, Thomas.
5 Grabbe, W.C. & Smith J.W. (1979) *Plastic Surgery*. 3rd ed. Boston, Little, Brown.
6 Hunter J.A.A. & Benton E.C. (1984) *Brit J Derm* **110**, 195.
7 McGregor I.A. (1975) *Fundamental Techniques of Plastic Surgery and Their Surgical Applications*. New York, Churchill Livingstone.

8 PETRES J. & HUNDEIKER M. (1978) *Dermatosurgery.* New York, Springer.
9 *REES T.D. (1980) *Aesthetic Plastic Surgery.* Philadelphia, W.B. Saunders.
10 SISSON G.A. & TARDY M.J. (1977) *Plastic and Reconstructive Surgery of the Face and Neck.* New York, Grune & Stratton.
11 STEGMAN S.J. & TROMOVITCH T.A. (1984) *Cosmetic Dermatologic Surgery.* Chicago, Year Book Medical Publishers.
12 *STEGMAN S.J., et al (1982) *Basis of Dermatologic Surgery.* Chicago Year Book Medical Publishers.

LOCAL ANAESTHESIA [1, 4, 5, 7, 9]

The prime considerations are effectiveness, rapid action and relative freedom from toxicity and sensitization. These qualities are found in lignocaine hydrochloride, which is the local anaesthetic of choice of dermatologists in Great Britain. Procaine (an amine ester) is recommended [7] chiefly by anaesthetists because of its lower toxicity, but the amounts used by dermatologists in standard procedures are usually small and its cross-reactivity to other drugs of the para-aminobenzoic acid ester type is a strong disincentive to its use. Of three other preparations of the same general amino group as lignocaine [9] mepivicaine and bupivicaine are similar but have a more sustained action whereas prilocaine has a rather quicker effect [3]. Most local anaesthetics also contain parabens preservative.

Adrenaline (Epinephrine) 1/80,000 to 1/200,000 is added to prolong anaesthesia and to reduce immediate bleeding. It also, by reducing absorption, reduces the risk of systemic toxicity. It should never be used, however, for operations on fingers and toes or in other areas where the blood supply is likely to be impaired. If a larger amount of local anaesthetic is to be used, the concentration of both local anaesthetic and adrenaline should be reduced and adrenaline should be avoided entirely in patients with hypertension, cardiac disease and in those on psychotropic drugs, especially phenothiazines or monoamine oxidase inhibitors.

Toxic reactions [9, 13]. Toxic reactions to local anaesthetics are rare with small quantities. They are likely to occur if the injection is inadvertently given intravenously. Amide (amine ether) type anaesthetics should be used with care in those with hepatic disease and amine esters, such as procaine, with caution in those with renal impairment or in those with a history of allergy to benzocaine, sulphonamides, PPD or other *para*-type chemicals. Amide ether type anaesthetics such as lignocaine are nowadays generally preferred because of the very low incidence of allergic reactions to this type of anaesthetic. For patients genuinely sensitive to this group of anaesthetics, local anaesthesia may be obtained using injection of antihistamine (see below) or normal saline [14].

Overdosage usually presents itself as a sensation of numbness or tingling. Systemic reactions include vasodilation, cardiac or respiratory depression or central nervous system symptoms such as dizziness, drowsiness, tinnitus, slurred speech, muscle twitching and tonic seizures; these side effects are to some extent reversible with diazepam (Valium).

The use of adrenaline may be associated with mild tachycardia and an excited state and its use should also be avoided during pregnancy, in combination with inhalation anaesthesia and in patients suffering from glaucoma.

Allergic or anaphylactic reactions are sometimes unexpected and always disconcerting; they require immediate countermeasures (p. 2498). Patients should always be asked if they have had any untoward reactions to local anaesthetics, e.g. in dental procedures. These may have been nothing more than fainting but in cases of doubt a test dose can be given or an alternative method of anaesthesia chosen. In any event, the necessary equipment for dealing with anaphylaxis should always be at hand. Vasovagal attacks associated with the use of anaesthesia are, of course, common and should not be confused with the more serious toxic or allegic reactions.

Local complications include bruising and a temporary sensation of stinging or burning, which is quite common. More persistent sensory anaesthesia or temporary motor nerve palsies may occur. Very rarely, there may be tissue necrosis.

Methods of local anaesthesia. Local anaesthesia may be achieved *topically* [8]—although this usually requires both time and occlusion—or by *local infiltration.* Other methods of anaesthesia include *field* blocks or *regional anaesthesia* [1, 2, 10] with temporary interruption of sensory nerve conductivity in a given area; employing either field block with infiltration of local anaesthetic around the lesion to be excised or a nerve block with infiltration close to the nerve supplying the operative field. The choice of which type of local anaesthetic to use depends not only on the method of anaesthesia and the site and expected duration of operation but also on the patient's general condition and the physician's own preference and experience.

The maximum recommended dosage for lignocaine with adrenaline (epinephrine) is 7 mg/kg or approximately 50 ml of a 1% lignocaine solution or

4.5 ml/kg or 30 ml of a plain 1% lignocaine solution. In practice most dermatologists use substantially less. Children should receive smaller or more dilute preparations. Before injecting any local anaesthetic it is a wise precaution always to aspirate first. This should be mandatory when attempting nerve blocks, especially on the head and neck. Commonly used nerve blocks in dermatology include supraorbital, supratrochlear, infraorbital and mental blocks. Simple combination blocks also exist for the nose and ear [11]. When attempting 'ring blocks' such as digital nerve blocks or when anaesthetizing circumferentially around a structure such as the ear, adrenaline should never be used.

Other anaesthetic agents

(i) Ethyl chloride, dichlorotetrafluorethane (Freon) and solid carbon dioxide snow give short-lived periods of anaesthesia with refrigeration. They are suitable for the incision of small cysts, abscesses or superficial skin lesions and for the curettage of multiple small warts or milia.

(ii) The anaesthetic effect of *antihistamines* can be used when hypersensitivity to other agents is present. Diphenhydramine hydrochloride as a 1% solution is suitable.

(iii) The injection of *normal saline* into the skin sufficient to cause a weal may be used to produce an anaesthetic effect [14].

(iv) Intravenous *diazepam* (2.5–10 mg) is useful, particularly for children to allay anxiety, but it is not in itself anaesthetic at this dose. Small procedures, however, such as the removal of mollusca contagiosa can often be carried out with less distress following its administration.

(v) *Hypnosis* and acupuncture may be useful, given an experienced practitioner and a suitable subject. Apparently painless minor surgery can be carried out on difficult sites, particularly in those sensitive to local anaesthetics.

(vi) *General anaesthesia* will not be discussed here. An anaesthetist's advice will normally be sought. Patients requiring this, especially children, are best admitted to hospital either as a day case or overnight. Written consent should always be obtained.

Some reassurance about the relative painlessness of the planned procedure should always be given, particularly to those anxious or fearful of injections. Young children should not have their trust abused, however, by being told that 'it will not hurt'. They are notably braver when their mothers are not present. Time, patience and gentleness are the guiding principles for successful anaesthesia. Preliminary sedation is often helpful. In older children who have not been taught a reasonable amount of self-control and stoicism, firmness may have to be allied to kindness and tricks of distraction.

REFERENCES

1 ADRIANI J. (1970) *Pharmacology of Anaesthetic Drugs.* Springfield, Thomas.
2 ADRIANI J. (1970) *Regional Anaesthesia—Techniques in Clinical Applicaton.* Springfield, Thomas.
3 BROWN G. & WARD N.L. (1969) *Br Dent J* **126**, 557.
4 COVINO B.F. & VASALLO H.G. (1976) *Local Anaesthetics: Mechanism of Action and Clinical Use.* New York, Grune & Stratton.
5 DE JONG R.H. (1977) *Local Anaesthetics.* 2nd ed. Springfield, Thomas.
6 EPSTEIN E. & EPSTEIN E. JR. (1982) *Skin Surgery.* 5th ed. Springfield, Thomas.
7 FABER G.A. (1982) In *Skin Surgery.* Eds. Epstein E. & Epstein E., Jr. 5th ed. Springfield, Thomas, p. 54.
8 JUHLIN L., *et al* (1980) *Acta Derm Venereol* **60**, 544.
9 MARTINDALE W.A. (Ed.) (1977) *The Extra Pharmacopoeia.* 27th ed. London, Pharmaceutical Press, p. 857.
10 MOORE D.C. (1973) *Regional Block: Handbook for Use in Clinical Practice in Medicine and Surgery.* 4th ed. Springfield, Thomas.
11 PANJE W.R. (1979) *J Dermatol Surg Oncol* **5**, 311.
12 PANJE W.R. (1982) In *Skin Surgery.* Eds. Epstein E. & Epstein E. Jr. 5th ed. Springfield, Thomas, p. 65.
13 VERRILL P.J. (1975) *Practitioner* **214**, 380.
14 WIENER S.G. (1979) *Cutis* **23**, 342.

EXCISION [2, 5, 16]

The aim of an excision should be to remove completely the lesion in question and to leave as inconspicuous a scar as possible. The nature of the lesion and the probable effects of alternative treatment help to determine the amount of scarring that is acceptable. An ugly scar may be justified if the patient has a malignant melanoma but not if he has a benign naevus. Most lesions fall well within these extremes, and the choice of excision or other forms of treatment is a matter of judgement, experience and, to some extent, convenience.

Preparation. The practical aspects of equipment and sterilization will not be discussed here. Proper sterilization of instruments is obviously essential [12].

Patients should be aware of the limitation of surgery and the fact that complications may and do occur and that these cannot always be predicted or avoided. The patient's informed consent [10] should be obtained in writing. Parental consent should be obtained in the case of minors. Prior to surgery, the patient should have had the procedure fully explained to them and the probable benefits and potential risks of the operation should be discussed. Most patients attending for surgery are anxious and they will require reassurance. For particularly anxious patients, a pre-operative sedative may be useful.

Re-examination and palpation of the lesion will reveal its extent, probable depth and proximity to large blood vesels, nerves or other important structures. Langer's lines of skin tension [11] were previously used as a guide to incision but the best cosmetic results are usually obtained by following the wrinkle lines [2, 7] which run perpendicular to the major underlying muscles. The two often coincide, as on the neck. When they do not, as on the limbs, the choice depends on other factors. Small excisions on the lower leg, for instance, can be more securely apposed and kept free of tension if they are longitudinal. Testing for skin laxity with the fingers usually clarifies the best direction in which to make an excision. The size and type of excision made will also depend upon many factors including the site and nature of the lesion to be excised and the nature of the planned skin closure.

The skin surface should be cleaned prior to operation with either a detergent—antibacterial combination, preferably one containing chlorhexidine [6] or an iodophor (povidone–iodine) scrub, or with a surface antiseptic skin preparation such as 0.5% chlorhexidine in 70% isopropyl alcohol or an iodine paint [1, 8, 9, 17]. The purpose of the skin preparation is to remove transient pathogens and to reduce the resident flora so that the risk of surgical infection is slight [13]. The surgeon will also normally use a pre-operative surgical scrub containing chlorhexidine, an iodophor or hexachlorophane. In view of the risk of hepatitis and AIDS, all surgeons should nowadays wear gloves [15].

The borders of any lesion likely to be obscured by local anaesthetics can be marked with light scoring of the skin or with an aniline dye or a mixture of aniline dyes as in Bonney's Blue.

General technique [5, 16]. A syringe containing local anaesthetic fitted with a secure, fine, flexible needle is necessary for infiltration of anaesthetic into the skin. Normally this would be 1–2% lignocaine hydrochloride with or without adrenaline (see p. 2576). The addition of adrenaline reduces bleeding but may obscure polar outlines. In some countries, e.g. Denmark, it is *required by law* for operations on the face and neck. It is to be avoided on the fingers and toes and at any site where the blood supply is impaired, especially in the elderly. A topical 'caine' anaesthetic may be applied pre-operatively (see p. 2576) in children, and on sensitive regions such as the genitalia. 1–4% cocaine can be used topically as a local anaesthetic on mucosal surfaces.

Sensitization to lignocaine is exceedingly rare. Occasional cases of toxicity and death are reported [4] but are not to be expected with the quantities normally used in routine dermatological practice. In patients allergic to lignocaine alternative methods of anaesthesia may be used (see p. 2577) but chemically closely related preparations such as procaine or prilocaine may be tolerated [3]. A preparatory sedative may be required for anxious children. Diazepam (0.2 mg/kg) intravenously has been found helpful.

A small round-ended blade (Gilette no. 15) is best used for the excision, which should be performed with two elliptical incisions perpendicular through the skin. The length of the wound should be at least three times its breadth so that the angles at the tips of the excision should never exceed 30°. The lesion is held firmly but gently with toothed iris forceps or a skin hook and separated from its base. Ideally, for histological purposes, it should contain at least some subcutaneous fat.

The specimen is placed immediately in a formol–saline specimen bottle or, for immunofluorescence or frozen section studies, on aluminium foil and suspended in liquid nitrogen. To prevent curling of small biopsy or excision samples, these may be placed on small squares of filter paper and floated into the formalin solution.

Venous bleeding is staunched initially by pressure. Any persistent bleeding points can be sealed using bipolar electrocoagulation or ball-point cautery. Chemical styptics such as ferric subsulphate (Monsel's) solution, 20–50% trichloroacetic acid, 30–50% aluminium chloride in spirit or silver nitrate are commonly used for open wounds. Oxidized cellulose is also sometimes helpful. Arterial bleeding may require clamping and suturing with plain 4.0 or 5.0 catgut.

If the skin is lax, nothing further is required, but undercutting of the skin is normally carried out as the first of several procedures to reduce wound tension. In regions such as the thigh and leg, excess fat may have to be removed to facilitate wound closure. In these areas, and whenever a wound is likely to be infected or avascular, an antibiotic powder spray may be used once bleeding has stopped.

Subcutaneous absorbable sutures made of Vicryl (polyglactin), Dexon (polyglycolic acid) or chromic catgut are used for large excisions or at sites of probable tension. The final procedure is to appose the wound edges exactly and neatly with interrupted nylon or silk sutures.

Good cosmetic results depend on careful suturing.

The operator should be conversant with the various necessary suturing techniques [5, 14]. A double first loop (surgeon's knot) and a second 'square knot' will prevent slipping.

REFERENCES

1 ALTEMEIER W.A. (1977) In *Surgical Antiseptics in Disinfection, Sterilization and Preservation.* Ed. Block S.S. Philadelphia, Lea & Febiger, p. 641.

2 *BAER R.L. & KOPF A.W. (1964) *Year Book of Dermatology, 1963–64.* Chicago, Year Book Medical Publishers, p. 7.

3 VON BAHR V. & ERICKSSON E. (1962) *Swenska Läkartidn* **59**, 2221.

4 DEACOCK A.R. DE S. & SIMPSON W.T. (1964) *Anaesthesia* **19**, 217.

5 *EPSTEIN E. & EPSTEIN E. JR (Eds.) (1982) *Skin Surgery.* 5th ed. Springfield, Thomas.

6 KAUL A.F. & JEWITT J.F. (1981) *Surg Gynecol Obstet* **152**, 677.

7 *KRAISSL C.J. (1951) *Plastic Reconstr Surg* **8**, 1.

8 LOWBURY E.J.L. & LILLY H.A. (1973) *Br Med J* i, 510.

9 PETERSEN A.F., *et al* (1978) *Surg Gynecol Obstet* **146**, 63.

10 REDDEN E.M. & BAKER D.C. (1984) *J Dermatol Surg Oncol* **10**, 111.

11 RIDGE M.D. & WRIGHT V. (1966) *J Invest Dermatol* **46**, 341.

12 SEBBEN J.B. (1984) *J Am Acad Dermatol* **11**, 301.

13 SELWYN S. & ELLIS H. (1972) *Brit Med J* i, 136.

14 SMITH J.G. & CHALKER D.K. (1982) *South Med J* **75**, 129.

16 STEGMAN J.J., *et al* (1982) *Basis of Dermatologic Surgery.* Chicago, Year Book Medical Publishers.

17 TAOAGALI J.L. (1978) *NZ Med J* **88**, 97.

Biopsy techniques. Tissue for diagnosis may be obtained in one of several ways [1, 2]. For small lesions, or for those in which excision would be expected to be curative, *excision biopsy* is obviously preferred. When performing *incisional* or *excisional* biopsy of a lesion it is important to include some normal adjacent skin. This helps greatly with histological interpretation. *Punch biopsy* [2], by its very nature, is less representative than either of the above two methods of tissue sampling but is a useful office technique in appropriate circumstances or when multiple samples are required. If the tissue to be sampled is first stretched at 90° to the proposed line of excision, the resultant defect will be semi-elliptical and easier to close [3]. Punches normally vary from 0.2 to 0.5 mm in diameter.

The *shave biopsy* involves making a tangential cut parallel to the skin surface. The technique is perhaps best reserved for protuberant lesions such as squamous cell papillomas or for non-pigmented cellular naevi where formal excision would leave an unacceptable scar. It is obviously an unsatisfactory technique when knowledge of the depth of the histological process is required. Being superficial, however, these biopsies heal quickly with good cosmetic result, usually only requiring superficial skin styptics to stop bleeding. In general, for histological purposes complete specimens are preferred, but when this is not possible the sample should include both normal adjacent skin and a representative cross-section of the lesion to be examined. If there are lesions in various stages of development then either more than one biopsy must be taken or the earlier lesion should be preferred.

REFERENCES

1 BEERMAN H. & WOOD M.G. (1982) In *Skin Surgery.* Eds. Epstein E. & Epstein E., Jr. 5th ed. Springfield, Thomas, p. 370.

2 STEGMAN J.J., *et al* (1982) *Basis of Dermatologic Surgery.* Chicago, Year Book Medical Publishers.

3 WHITE H.S. & PERRY H.O. (1960) *Arch Dermatol* **81**, 520.

Sutures [2, 3, 9, 10]. Skin sutures are of two main types, *absorbable* and *non-absorbable*. Both types of suture should ideally have very low tissue reactivity, high tensile strength and good knot security and should provide easy handling.

Absorbable sutures are represented by plain and chromic catgut, Vicryl (polyglactin-910) and Dexon (polyglycolic acid). *Plain catgut* loses its strength in 4–5 days and is nowadays mainly used for haemostasis. *Chromic catgut*, to all intents and purposes, has been replaced by the newer *synthetic absorbable sutures* (Vicryl, Dexon) which cause very little by way of tissue reaction and which are dissolved completely in 90–120 days. Absorbable sutures are used exclusively as 'deep' suture materials, e.g. subcutaneous or subcuticular.

Non-absorbable sutures include silk, nylon and polypropylene (Prolene). Again, the newer synthetic sutures have better tensile strength and cause less tissue reactivity but silk sutures are easier to tie and have better knot security. Braided nylon and Dacron (also braided) have better knot-tying properties but there is possibly, as with silk, an increased risk of infection due to the braided nature of the suture material. A coated braided polyester suture is also available and possibly has the best overall characteristics but it is expensive. For wounds which are likely to remain under constant pressure, such as those on the back or shoulders, one can use non-absorbable suture material such as nylon to close the deep subcutaneous layer. Most dermatologists, however, continue to prefer absorbable sutures.

In general, skin suture needles are of the reverse-cutting type. Suture size usually varies from 3/0 to 6/0 depending on site and function.

Suture technique [3, 8, 9]. Several suture techniques are necessary if one is to become proficient in dermatological surgery. A *simple interrupted suture* is usually the preferred method of final skin closure, although some surgeons prefer to use a *running subcuticular stitch* with a broad piece of porous or semiporous tape applied to the skin surface to give extra support and stability to the wound. The tape can be left in place after the subcuticular suture has been removed and will continue to keep the skin edges approximated until it peels off. Interrupted non-absorbable nylon sutures, however, are normally preferred. Skin sutures should not need to be applied under any tension and are normally 4/0 to 6/0 and placed close to the skin edge for fine approximation. If the wound tends to invert, then the deeper component of the suture can be placed more laterally to help evert the edges. For most superficial biopsies or excisions, interrupted skin sutures are all that are required.

If there is tension across the wound, or a significant tendency to inversion, then it may be advisable to place one or two *vertical mattress* sutures first. A modification of this suture, the *half-buried mattress* is also useful as a corner stitch when anchoring the apices of flaps. The *horizontal mattress* (with bolsters) [6] can also be used to approximate long wounds or wounds under tension. There is a risk of tissue necrosis or scarring, however, if the suture is pulled too tight or left in too long.

There are various forms of *buried suture* that are used to close off 'dead space' in a deep wound. Normally one would use interrupted *deep subcutaneous* or buried dermal sutures [1] but a variant of the horizontal mattress known as a 'purse-string' suture can also be used with similar effect. *Running sutures*, both cutaneous and subcutaneous, can be used to save time but are less secure than interrupted sutures. The *running subcuticular* suture—in reality a running superficial horizontal mattress—is difficult to do well but is an elegant suture for shallow wounds or when there are already deep subcutaneous sutures in place.

Tape closures may be used in conjunction with interrupted sutures or on their own if there is good approximation and adequate subcutaneous or subcuticular support. They are not suitable for wounds under tension. Another use of tape closures is as an additional skin support both whilst skin sutures are in place and for the 2–3 weeks following their removal. We ourselves like to immobilize the treated area by using a 'protective box' of semiporous tape to prevent excessive movement of tissues around the wound [12]. Cyanoacrylates have also been used in the past [4, 5, 11].

Stainless steel staples are a fast and effective way to suture longer skin incisions. They are strong and incite very litle tissue reaction but are perhaps not fine or flexible enough to cope with the contours and irregularities of surgical excisions on the face [7, 10].

REFERENCES

1   ALBOM M. (1977) *J Dermatol Surg Oncol* 3, 504.
2   ASTON S.J. (1976) *J Dermatol Surg Oncol* 2, 57.
3   DINGMAN R.O., *et al* (1982) In *Skin Surgery*. Epstein E. & Epstein E. Jr. 5th ed. Springfield, Thomas, p. 74.
4   MATUSOMOTO T., *et al* (1967) *Arch Surg* 94, 861.
5   MATUSOMOTO T., *et al* (1969) *Arch Surg* 98, 266.
6   SIMMONDS W.L. (1977) *J Dermatol Surg Oncol* 3, 281.
7   STEGMAIER O.C. (1982) *J Am Acad Dermatol* 6, 305.
8   STEGMAN J.J., *et al* (1982) *Basis of Dermatologic Surgery*. Chicago, Year Book Medical Publishers.
9   STEGMAN S.J. (1978) *J Dermatol Surg Oncol* 4, 63.
10   SWANSON N.A. & TROMOVITCH T.A. (1982) *Int J Dermatol* 21, 273.
11   WILKINSON D.S. (1972) *Arch Dermatol* 106, 834.
12   WILKINSON D.S. (1985) *Personal Communication*.

Particular forms of excision. Variations in detail and technique apply to particular lesions and areas of the body. A few examples only are given.

Pilar or epidermoid cysts [4, 14]. Small cysts are often deeper than they appear and may be difficult to locate after infiltration with local anaesthetic. Larger, tense epidermoid cysts of the scalp often extend deeply and their removal is frequently accompanied by arterial bleeding, which must be located and dealt with. Most cysts are best removed by traditional elliptical incision and blunt dissection with scissors or a haemostat, while pulling gently on the ellipse and the attached cyst. If the cyst ruptures, the remaining contents should be expressed and the whole of the cyst wall removed.

Lesions on the shoulder and upper back. Dermatologists are frequently consulted about lesions in these areas. Though excision is simple, the greatest care should be taken to appose the wound with the least tension and to apply firm anti-tension dressings. Subcutaneous or subcuticular sutures may be required and movement and tension across the scar should be restricted as far as possible. When the lesion is large, or when there is any reason to suspect an unsightly scar, the patient should be warned of this and excision performed only if absolutely necessary.

Benign moles are best left alone. The patient or parent should be told that the results of intervention may well be worse than the original blemish.

Basal cell and squamous cell carcinomas [4]. Small basal cell carcinomas are often easily excised; the best choice of treatment, however, depends on age, site, extent and type of lesion. A clear margin should always be obtained and prior skin marking may be advisable. Histological control is mandatory.

In patients with chronic actinic damage, some keratoses justify biopsy excision, especially if they are beginning to 'heap up' or if there is a suspicion of malignant change. Again, all specimens should be sent for histological examination. Squamous cell carcinomas that require excision and grafting would generally, in Great Britain, be referred to a surgeon unless they were small and on a site where a reasonably wide primary excision could easily be performed. In some cases a preliminary biopsy may be necessary to confirm the diagnosis. If this or local excision reveals an anaplastic or undifferentiated carcinoma, further wide excision would have to be considered and regional glands kept under close observation.

Cure rates for basal cell carcinoma, treated by surgical excision vary from 90 to 98% [3, 6, 12, 13]. Some sites such as the lips, ear, scalp and periocular and nasolabial areas have a higher rate of recurrence [1, 6].

Chondrodermatitis nodularis helicis. A thick elliptical incision is made around the lesion, the skin is eased back gently and the nodule and underlying cartilage are removed by a shave excision. The surrounding skin is then gently undermined and reapposed with fine skin sutures and tape closures.

Mucous membranes. Excision of lesions in the mouth and on the tongue, lips and genitalia is difficult only in that access may be restricted and bleeding profuse. If a semicircular suture needle is inserted first, the excision (or biopsy) may be conveniently carried out onto this as a base and the edges of the excised wound brought quickly together. Electrodiathermy on cut or cut-coagulation mode is also of use when performing surgery in the mouth. Good pressure on surrounding tissues by an assistant, the use of adrenaline in the local anaesthetic and tongue or tissue clamps are all helpful.

Excision of axillary vault [4, 7, 8]. This very satisfactory form of treatment for severe axillary sweating is simple to carry out under local anaesthesia. A transverse elliptical excision is made in the dome of the axilla to remove 4.5 cm × 1.5 cm of tissue. It should be deep enough to remove the main bulk of the glands, which lie up to 0.6 cm below the surface. Apposition without tension can usually be achieved without much undercutting. A light pressure dressing is applied for 24–48 h and the wound is then left undressed and cleansed daily with a bactericidal antiseptic.

A more extensive surgical removal [15, 16] gives better long-term results but is normally best performed by the plastic surgeons. A radical excision of all the sweat glands with Z-plasty repair was successful in all but 7 of 123 cases [2].

Keratoacanthoma. If it cannot be excised *in toto*, a biopsy for confirmation of the diagnosis must include the centre, edge and a portion of normal adjacent skin.

Excision of pigmented lesions (Chapter 64). Pigmented lesions demand diagnostic acumen, skill and decisiveness in action. Blue naevi, pigmented basal cell carcinomas or seborrhoeic warts, and histiocytomas are usually easily recognizable, though diagnostic difficulties occasionally occur. If any doubt at all exists in the mind of the dermatologists the lesion should be excised locally, if it is small enough, with a request for an urgent histopathological opinion. Frozen section examination is usually not definitive enough in the doubtful—and thus most important—cases. When the lesion is too large to excise without grafting, the dermatologist may have to decide whether to biopsy or not. Such evidence as exists suggests that this does not adversely influence the prognosis. The subject is discussed fully by Epstein [5]. It is better to err on the safe side and to treat the lesion as malignant until subsequently proved otherwise. The best protection for the patient's cosmetic appearance is the clinical judgement of the dermatologist, but the best protection for his life is an occasional error on the side of safety.

The great majority of black lesions of the skin are benign [5]. In the rare case where a lesion is obviously a malignant melanoma, it is the duty of the dermatologist to act rapidly. If he does not himself practise surgery, it behoves him personally to see that the patient is in the hands of a surgeon without delay. It is our experience that many of these patients know the significance of the lesions without admitting it and have often delayed consultation for fear of the truth. They may then attempt to evade further decisive action.

Hypertrophic scars. These will often resolve with time. Intralesional steroid injections are helpful. They may be treated—and could often be prevented—by Z-plasty techniques [11] or by sustained pressure.

REFERENCES

1 BART R.S., *et al* (1978) *Arch Dermatol* **114**, 739.
2 BRETTEVILLE-JENSEN G., *et al* (1975) *Acta Derm Venereol (Stockh)* **55**, 73.
3 CHERNOSKY M.E. (1978) *South Med J* **71**, 802.
4 *EPSTEIN E. & EPSTEIN E. JR (Eds.) (1982) *Skin Surgery.* 5th ed. Springfield, Thomas.
5 EPSTEIN E., *et al* (1969) *JAMA* **298**, 1369.
6 HELM J. (1980) *Cancer Dermatology.* Springfield, Thomas.
7 HURLEY H.J. (1982) In *Skin Surgery.* Eds. Epstein E. & Epstein E., Jr. 5th ed. Springfield, Thomas.
8 HURLEY H.J. & SHELLEY W.B. (1963) *JAMA* **186**, 209.
9 HURLEY H.J. & SHELLEY W.B. (1966) *Br J Dermatol* **78**, 127.
10 KETCHAM A.S. (1982) In *Skin Surgery.* Eds. Epstein E. & Epstein E., Jr. 5th ed. Springfield, Thomas.
11 LONGACRE J.J. (1972) *Scar Tissue. Its Use and Abuse.* Springfield, Thomas.
12 MARCHAC D., *et al* (1982) *J Dermatol Surg Oncol* **8**, 379.
13 PORTE A., *et al* (1979) *Ann Chir Plast* **24**, 253.
14 ROXBURGH R.A. (1969) *Br J Hosp Med* **2**, 866.
15 SKOOG T. & THYRESSON N. (1962) *Acta Chir Scand* **124**, 531.
16 SKOOG T. & THYRESSON N. (1966) *Br J Dermatol* **78**, 551.

Special diagnostic techniques [1]

(a) The *shave* technique or *scrapings* from the affected skin or mucosal surface may be useful in obtaining material for cytological diagnosis in suspected cases of pemphigus or herpes (Tzanck smear) or for confirming the presence of fungal hyphae.

(b) *Punch biopsy* has already been discussed (p. 2579).

(c) *Aspiration technique* (needle biopsy) consists of withdrawing from a lymphatic gland or deep lesion a small sample for cultural or cytological examination. A trocar and cannula, 1.5–2 mm in diameter, or a wide-bored needle and a 50-ml syringe are used; a small amount of sterile normal saline is injected and an equal quantity of material withdrawn. Larger tissue fragments are fixed and treated by standard histopathological measures; small ones are used for smears.

By this method spirochaetes may be found in the inguinal gland when they have not been recovered from the chancre.

The technique of obtaining material for the diagnosis of leprosy is discussed n Chapter 23.

REFERENCE

1 BEERMAN H. &. WOOD M.G. (1982) In *Skin Surgery.* Eds. Epstein E. & Epstein E. Jr. 5th ed. Springfield, Thomas.

Nail biopsy [1–3, 5, 6]. A thin longitudinal incision is made through the nail plate and into the nail bed. This is extended proximally to include nail matrix and distally to include a small piece of skin from the finger tip. The specimen should not exceed 2 mm in width otherwise the patient may be left with a permanently split nail. Sutures are normally placed proximally and distally and the nail plate itself can be held in position using butterfly plasters and suitable dressings. Strict antisepsis must be observed.

For lesions involving only the distal portion of the nail, punch biopsy [4] or biopsy of the nail bed following nail avulsion may be used instead.

REFERENCES

1 BARAN R. & SAYAG J. (1976) *J Dermatol Surg Oncol* **2**, 322.
2 BENNETT R.G. (1976) *J Dermatol Surg* **2**, 325.
3 FOSNAUGH R.P. (1982) In *Skin Surgery.* Eds. Epstein E. & Epstein E. Jr. 5th ed. Springfield, Thomas.
4 SCHER R. (1978) *J Dermatol Surg Oncol* **4**, 528.
5 STONE O.J., *et al* (1977) *Curtis* **21**, 257.
6 ZAIAS N. (1967) *J Invest Dermatol* **49**, 406.

Muscle biopsy [4, 5]. The dermatologist will normally only require muscle biopsies in suspected cases of dermatomyositis. The value of this investigation is limited by the patchy nature of the pathological changes. The traditional open biopsy, which is still indicated when large samples or special investigations are required, may be replaced by needle biopsy [2, 6] in some instances. This causes less scarring and has given adequate material with minimal complications [1, 5, 6].

An intermediate technique using Weil–Blakely conchotome forceps through a skin incision 8 mm long is also popular in some countries [3].

REFERENCES

1 BERGSTROM J. (1975) *Scand J Clin Lab Invest* **35**, 609.
2 CURLESS R.G. & NELSON M.B. (1975) *Dev Med Child Neurol* **17**, 542.
3 DIETRICHSON P. (1975) *Tidsskr Nor Laegeforen* **32**, 1856.
4 DUBOWITZ V. & BROOKE M.H. (1973) *Muscle Biopsy: A Modern Approach.* Philadelphia, Saunders.
5 EDWARDS R.H.T. & MAUNDER C.A. (1977) *Hosp Update* **3**, 569.
6 EDWARDS R.H.T. *et al* (1973) *Lancet* **ii**, 1070.

Nail plate avulsion [1]. It is sometimes necessary to remove diseased or damaged nails. This can easily be done with a dental spatula in conjunction with digital nerve block.

In-grown toe nails. A simple method to treat in-grown toe nails is to remove the lateral portion of the nail plate under digital nerve ring block and then to phenolize the angle of the nail to prevent this recurring [5]. It is important that the phenol is in contact with the dry nail matrix for approximately 3 min. The 80–90% phenol should be fresh and can be neutralized subsequently by rinsing with a 70% alcohol solution. The leading edge of the nail plate should have a small pledglet of wool placed under it and the patient should be instructed on how to cut the nail correctly and to prevent pressure on the toe. Excess granulation tissue can be removed either by curettage and cautery or by the use of a silver nitrate pencil.

Recurrent in-grown toe nails can be treated either by wedge resection [4, 8] or by removing the lateral portion of the nail plate and destroying the lateral nail matrix using a teflon-coated electrocautery tip.

Myxoid (mucoid) cysts. Myxoid (mucoid) cysts of the nail may be managed by a variety of simple techniques including the injection of steroid into the cysts [6, 7], simple needling or de-roofing with or without electrodesiccation, the injection of sclerosant [3], with cryotherapy [2, 4], or by a variety of other surgical techniques [2, 4]. Recently [9] excision of the proximal and lateral nail fold has been suggested as being a successful way to deal with these.

REFERENCES

1 ALBOM M.J. (1977) *J Dermatol Surg Oncol* **3**, 35.
2 ARMIJO M. (1981) *J Dermatol Surg Oncol* **7**, 317.
3 AUDEBERT C. (1985) *Personal Cummunication.*
4 BARAN R. (1984) *Dermatologic Clinics* **2**(2), 271.
5 CAMERON P.F. (1981) *Brit Med J* **283**, 821.
6 EPSTEIN E. (1965) *JAMA* **194**, 98.
7 EPSTEIN E. (1979) *Arch Derm* **115**, 1315.
8 FOSNAUGH R.P. (1982) In *Skin Surgery.* Eds. Epstein E. & Epstein E. Jr. 5th ed. Springfield, Thomas.
9 SALASCHE J.J.S.J. (1984) *J Dermatol Surg Oncol* **10**, 36.
10 SONNEX T.S., *et al* (1982) *Br J Dermatol* **107**, (Suppl. 22), 21.

Wound closure [1, 12, 13]. A fundamental requirement of those involved in dermatological surgery is the ability to repair the surgical wound that they induce. Their surgery should, in addition, leave the least conspicuous scar possible. Although 'open wounds' left to heal by 'primary intent' do so surprisingly well, especially when small and superficial, the dermatological surgeon should have a range of closure techniques at his disposal so as to be able to cope with all but the most unexpected situations.

The *side-to-side* closure is the most frequently used and often the most cosmetically satisfying technique for the majority of surgical repairs. The basic method of closing a simple wedge biopsy or ellipse is, of course, well known to all doctors. *Undermining* of the free skin edges will assist in bringing the skin edges together without undue tension. This is normally best done at the level of the superficial fat but deeper planes may be required on the scalp and elsewhere. It is obviously important for all dermatologists who practise surgery to have sufficient knowledge of anatomy [6] and to be aware of the various danger areas such as those relating to the facial nerve, the superficial peroneal nerve (in the popliteal space), and the spinal accessory nerve (in the posterior triangle of the neck) [13].

Closure may require additional buried (absorbable) sutures if the wound is deep or if there is excessive movement or tension across the wound.

Where histological confirmation of clearance is required, it is often advisable to 'colour code' or otherwise mark the surgical specimen on removal. This helps to plan re-excision if this later proves necessary.

Suture removal depends on site and the amount of tension across the wound. With additional supporting surface tapes and buried sutures where appropriate, 4–5 days is usually enough for skin sutures on the face, 5–7 days for scalp and neck and 10–14 days elsewhere.

More advanced closure techniques [1, 2, 3, 8, 13]. The basic concept of a *side-to-side* closure can be extended to include *advancement and rotation* flaps and even *free skin grafts*. Details of such techniques are beyond the scope of this chapter but are useful skills for those involved in a substantial amount of cutaneous surgery. For details of the various flaps and grafts relevant to dermatology, the reader is referred elsewhere [1–3, 7, 10, 11, 13, 15].

Several techniques however, are of general use, even for those restricting their surgery to simple elliptical excisions.

The M-plasty [13, 14]. Sometimes it is not possible to complete an ellipse without crossing an important anatomical or cosmetic line. In this situation an M-plasty will help to reduce the overall length of excision required by bringing the apex of the excision back within the original area to be excised.

Obviously, for malignant lesions, there should still be an adequate margin of clearance at the inverted apex.

'Dog-ear' repairs [5, 13]. 'Dog-ears' occur when the length to width ratio of an excision is insufficient to prevent the skin at the poles from buckling when the opposing skin edges are brought together. It occurs more commonly when there is insufficient laxity or movement in the surrounding tissues. Excisions where the angle at the apex exceeds 30° are also liable to produce 'dog-ears'. Pseudo 'dog-ears' occur if too much fat is left at the poles of an excision.

There are three ways in which this problem can be surmounted [13]. First, the excision can be extended and the redundant overlapping skin excised. Second, one side of the pucker can be cut back flush with the skin and the excess skin from the other side identified by drawing it across the wound. This can then be cut off. Finally, the 'dog-ear' can be converted into a 'T' and the excess skin removed as in a T-plasty. This is a useful technique when the length of the wound cannot be extended. Other techniques have also been reported [9].

Wound edges of unequal lengths. The problem can frequently be overcome simply by using a *halving technique* whereby a suture is placed across the centre of the wound and subsequent sutures continue to divide the resultant defects into ever smaller compartments. Because of local skin elasticity, the shorter side tends to stretch to match the longer. For more disproportionate edges a wedge may have to be removed from the longer side so as to make the sides of the resultant ellipse more equal, or, finally, the wound can be sutured in the normal way and a 'dog-ear' repair done at the end to remove the excess skin from one side.

REFERENCES

1 CHERNOSKY M.E. (1982) In *Skin Surgery*. Eds. Epstein E. & Epstein E., Jr. 5th ed. Springfield, Thomas, p. 189.
2 CONVERSE J.M. (1982) In *Skin Surgery*. Eds. Epstein E. & Epstein E., Jr. 5th ed. Springfield, Thomas, p. 245.
3 CRABBE W.C. & MEYERS M.B. (Eds.) (1975) *Skin Flaps*. Boston, Little, Brown.
4 EPSTEIN E. & EPSTEIN E. JR. (1982) *Skin Surgery*. 5th ed. *Springfield, Thomas*.
5 GORMLEY D.E. (1977) *J Dermatol Surg Oncol* **3**, 194.
6 HOLLINGSHEAD W.H. (1968) *Anatomy for Surgeons: Head and Neck*. 2nd ed. Hagerstown, Harper & Row, Vol. 1, pp. 1–187.
7 KNOWLES W.R. (1976) *J Dermatol Surg* **2**, 141.
8 McGREGOR I. (1972) *Fundamental Aspects of Plastic Surgery*. 5th ed. Baltimore, Williams & Williams, p. 166.
9 SALASCHE S.J. & ROBERTS L.C. (1984) *J Dermatol Surg Oncol* **10**, 478.
10 SIMONDS W.L. (1970) *Cutis* **6**, 221.
11 SIMONDS W.L. (1978) *J Dermatol Surg Oncol* **4**, 383.
12 STEGMAN S.J. (1978) *J Dermatol Surg Oncol* **4**, 390.
13 STEGMAN S.J. et al (1982) *Basics of Dermatologic Surgery*. Chicago. Year Book Med Publ.
14 WEBSTER R.C. & DAVIDSON T.M. (1976) *J Dermatol Surg Oncol* **2**, 393.
15 WEBSTER R.C. & SMITH R.C. (1978) *J Dermatol Surg Oncol* **4**, 397.

Surgical dressings [6]. Dressings, if dry, should be non-adherent for otherwise they are liable to become incorporated in the eschar and this may lead to damage to new epithelium when the dressing is changed. Totally occlusive dressings, whilst retaining moisture, tend to encourage infection. They are therefore probably less suitable for closed (sutured) wounds but may be useful for open superficial wounds. Paraffin gauze is still a safe and useful dressing of this type, being hydrating and non-adherent. It may be used in conjunction with an antibacterial ointment in the initial management of superficial or open wounds. Later, when the operative site is clean, an occlusive or semipermeable film may be used to good effect.

Most modern dressings are either semipermeable or vapour-permeable or occlusive in type. The vapour-permeable dressings can be used not only on closed surgical wounds but also on split skin graft donor sites and other wounds. They have been shown to speed healing and to reduce pain [3, 15, 34]. They also appear to give superior cosmetic results [7].

Some wounds require pressure dressings, e.g. following grafts, flaps, hair transplants, etc. In reality these are used more to give support than as true pressure dressings since it is obviously important that, whilst they should exert sufficient pressure to prevent the formation of serum or blood clots under the wound, they should not impede re-vascularization of the tissues. Some surgeons employ a 'tie-down' dressing with rolls or layers of cotton wool and others use special bandaging techniques. Self-adhesive or conforming bandages are a useful type of dressing in this kind of situation.

The use of anti-tension strips or vapour-permeable adhesive dressings to prevent scar distortion has already been discussed (see above). Additional 'grip' can sometimes be obtained by pretreating the area with a volatile plastic dressing. Wounds or excisions on the lower leg will, in addition, require support bandages since wound healing at this site is always very slow and without support there is a risk that the operative site may break down to form an ulcer.

Wound healing with respect to surgical scars [2, 8, 10, 12, 14, 25, 29]. The process of normal wound healing is reviewed elsewhere (p 591) and will not be discussed here [16, 26, 27]. Surgical wounds may heal either by regeneration (with reconstruction of the original architecture as happens after superficial cryotherapy) or with variable degrees of scarring during the process of repair. All wounds are followed by some degree of inflammation with tissue swelling, fibrin formation and subsequent inflammatory cell, macrophage and epidermal activity. Superficial crusts usually develop in the first 12–24 h in open wounds and this is followed by a burst of epidermal basal cell mitotic activity, usually starting 12–14 h following injury with migration of epidermal cells into the wound 6–72 h later [17].

The studies of Gillman and his colleagues on wound healing have served to emphasize the sequence of events involved and to stress the importance of dermal stability, freedom from tension and control of bleeding. Blood clots do not 'provide a scaffolding' for granulation tissue; they may retard healing. Epithelialization of suture wounds [12, 23] further distorts the integrity of dermal and adnexal structures. Suture tracks also provide a portal of entry for infection [4, 11]. Sutureless apposition of small wounds is therefore ideal [33] particularly on the face [31] where the tissues are lax. When sutures are used, they should be removed as soon as possible.

The mechanical strength of the wound in the first few days is largely due to the new epidermis and stratum corneum. The *rate* of increase in tensile strength of the wound rises to a maximum in 10–15 days but full restoration of absolute strength takes several months. Even 2–3 weeks following incision the skin has only regained 20% of its original strength [9, 18]. Epithelial migration is enhanced by a humid microenvironment [30].

In areas subject to tension, adequate anti-tension devices should be employed and continued as long as practicable, particularly in the 'cape' area of the upper trunk.

Zinc [21], oxygen [10, 24] and other factors [16, 26] may influence the rate of healing but their role remains conjectural and is in any case far less important than expertise and care in the performance of the operation and its aftercare.

Full thickness wounds undergo a lot of remodelling and some contracture. Even simple linear scars

tend to contract and this may cause significant distortion in scars that are long.

Delay or failure in wound healing. Some causes of this are shown in Table 68.1. Poor blood supply, haemorrhage, infection and excess movement or tension all inhibit wound healing. Most surgical incisions will have regained only 3–4% of their tensile strength at 2 weeks, and unless subcutaneous or subcuticular sutures have been used it is over the next 2–6 weeks that a wound is at greatest risk of 'splaying' or dehiscing. Hypertrophic scars also tend to form from the fourth to sixth week onwards if there is insufficient support or chronic inflammation within the wound.

Although healing by 'secondary intent'—as in Mohs' fresh tissue technique—gives better cosmetic results than one would expect, results are usually better with sutured wounds [28]. Wounds that break down or which cannot be completely closed will normally have to heal by 'secondary intention' and will leave a splayed and possibly hypertrophic scar. Obviously the texture of the skin at this site will be abnormal and will lack skin appendages.

Transected appendages or implanted epidermis may lead to milia formation or dermal inclusion cysts. The response of a pigmented skin to any form of surgery is unpredictable and where there are multiple lesions a test area should always be treated first. Hypertrophic scars need to be differentiated from true cheloids. Despite all efforts to prevent tension, some splaying of the scar or cheloid formation may occur following excision on the upper trunk and shoulders.

Painful scars (common on the hands and feet) are due to abnormal proliferation or involvement of nerve endings at the scar site. There may be hyperaesthesia or even some loss of sensation following any operation due to destruction of superficial nerves. Care should always be taken to avoid the more major or functionally important nerves wherever possible.

Subsequent procedures. Sutures are conventionally removed after 4–5 days on the face, 5–7 days on the scalp, 7–14 days on the trunk and limbs. The longer they remain, the greater danger of sepsis or of unsightly epithelialization of suture tracts. Alternate sutures may be removed early and further anti-tension dressings applied.

After the sutures have been removed the area can be resprayed with a plastic adhesive film or a semipermeable adhesive dressing applied.

Where anti-tension devices have been required, these must be replaced after the sutures have been

TABLE 68.1. Complications in wound healing

Complications	Predisposing factors	Prevention
Infection [1]	Infected lesions	Careful pre-operative and operative techniques
	Poor sterility	Sutureless closure
	Steroids	Antibiotic sprays
	Adjacent infectious source	Prophylactic antibiotics for infected or potentially infected wounds [13, 19, 32]
	Occlusive dressings	
	Poor blood supply	
	Fat, haematoma and foreign material	
	Sutures	
	Poor technique	Layered closure
	Excessive devitalized tissue from careless handling or electrocoagulation	Gentle tissue handling
		Minimize devitalization of tissues
Delay in closure	Poor blood supply	Care in decision to operate
	Excess movement	Warmth
	Infection	Careful postoperative dressings
	Tension	
	Steroids	
	Debilitated patient	
	Poor nutritional status	
'Gaping scar'	Inadequate apposition	Careful apposition
	Dermal instability	Subcutaneous or subcuticular sutures
	Excess movement	
	Infection	Adequate postoperative support, e.g. anti-tension dressings
	Tension	
Painful scars	Feet and fingers especially	Avoid pressure sites if possible
		Dressings to reduce subsequent pressure and/or movement
		Careful apposition
Hypertrophic scars	Site	Avoid 'cape' area if possible
	Tension	Good surgical technique including undermining of edges where necessary
	Reaction to embedded material	
	Trauma	
	Individual susceptibility	
Cheloids	Previous history	Avoid surgery where possible
	Black skin	
	Upper half of body	Anti-tension measures for 3 weeks
	Tension	
		Watch and prepare to treat
'Railroad tracks'	Skin sutures under too much tension	Good suture technique
		Use of 'non-reactive' suture material
Stitch marks, stitch 'abscess'	Sutures left in too long	Early suture removal
Wound edge inversion	Poor technique	Good surgical technique
		Occlusive or semi-occlusive dressings
Bleeding and/or haematoma formation	Bleeding tendency	Pre-operative screening
	Aspirin	Good haemostasis
	NSAI drugs	Use of adrenaline in local anaesthetic
	Alcohol	

removed. The 2 weeks that follow are critical and in regions such as the thigh and shoulders it is advisable to persuade the patient to continue with such dressings for at least this length of time, preferably longer.

Fortunately, sepsis is uncommon. It has been shown [22] that the incidence of infection can be reduced to 2% under ordinary dermatological outpatient conditions.

REFERENCES

1 ALTMEIER W. (1972) *Bull M Surg* **57**, 7.
2 *BAER R.L. & KOPF A.W. (1964) *Year Book of Dermatology, 1963–64.* Chicago, Year Book Medical Publishers, p. 32.
3 BARNETT A., *et al* (1983) *Am J Surg* **145**, 379.
4 CONNOLLY W.B., *et al* (1969) Am J Surg **117**, 379.
5 DUNPHEE J. & VAN WINKLE W. (1968) *Nutritional Aspects of Wound Healing in Repairs and Regeneration* New York, McGraw-Hill.
6 EAGLESTEIN W.H. (1983) *J Am Acad Dermatol* **12**, 434.
7 EATON A.C. (1980) *Br J Surg* **67**, 857.
8 EPSTEIN E.H. JR (1982) In *Skin Surgery*. Eds. Epstein E. & Epstein E., Jr. 5th ed. Springfield, Thomas, p. 108.
9 FORRESTER J.C., *et al* (1968) *Bull Soc Ins Chir* **1**, 1.
10 GIBSON E.W. & VAN DER MEULEN J.D. (1975) *International Symposium on Wound Healing, Rotterdam, 1975*, Montreux Foundation International.
11 GIBSON E.W. & POATE W.J. (1968) *Br J Plast Surg.* **17**, 265.
12 *GILLMAN T. (1968) In *An Introduction to the Biology of the Skin*. Eds. Champion R.H., *et al.* Oxford, Blackwell.
13 GOLDMAN P.L. & PERESDORF R.G. (1979) *Drug Ther* **9**, 80.
14 HAYES H. (1977) *J Dermatol Surg Oncol* **3**, 188.
15 HINMAN C.C. (1962) *Nature* **200**, 377.
16 HUNT T. & ZEDERFELDT B. (1968) In *Nutritional Aspects of wound Healing in Repairs and Regeneration*. Eds. Dunphee J. & Van Winkle W. New York, McGraw-Hill.
17 KRAWCZYK W.S. (1972) In *Epidermal Wound Healing*. Eds. Maibach H.I. & Rovee D.J. Chicago, Year Book Medical Publishers, p. 123.
18 MADDEN J.W. & PEACOCK E.E. JR (1971) *Ann Surg* **174**, 511.
19 MILES A.A. (1957) *Br J Exp Pathol* **39**, 79.
20 NIINITOSKI J (1969) *Acta Physiol Scand*, (Suppl. **334**).
21 OBERLEAS D., *et al* (1971) *Am J Surg* **121**, 566.
22 OLIVER J.O. (1966) *Trans St Johns Hosp Derm Soc* London **48**, 174.
23 *ORDMAN L.J. & GILLMAN T. *Arch Surg* **93**, 883.
24 PAI M.P. & HUNT T.K. (1972) *Surg Gynaecol Obstet* **135**, 756.
25 *PEACOCK E.E. JR & VAN WINKLE W. (1970) *Surgery and Biology of Wound Repair*. Somerville, NJ, Ethicon.
26 POLLACK S. (1979) *J Dermatol Surg Oncol* **5**, 389.
27 POLLACK S. (1979) *J Dermatol Surg Oncol* **5**, 477.
28 ROBBINS P., *et al* (1979) *J Dermatol Surg Oncol* **5**, 329.
29 *ROTHNIE N.G. (1965) *Triangle* **7**, 157.
30 ROVEE D.T., *et al* (1972) *Epidermal Wound Healing*. Eds. Maibach H.I. & Rovdee D.J. Chicago, Year Book Medical Publishers, p. 150.
31 SHEPHERD M.P. (1976) *Br J Surg* **53**, 445.
32 STONE H.H. (1979) *Am Surg* **189**, 691.
33 WATTS G.T. (1970) *Br Med J* i, 502.
34 WINTER G.D. (1962) *Nature* **193**, 293.

Flaps [3, 5, 14]. A flap is a section of full thickness skin in which one portion, the flap pedicle, remains attached to the skin whilst the distal portion of the flap is undermined and moved by rotation or advancement to cover an adjacent defect. The blood supply of any flap is therefore, at least initially, supplied via its pedicle. Those with broad pedicles thus tend to do better. An adequate blood supply is essential. The length to width ratio of a flap should rarely exceed 3:1. Good haemostasis is also important to allow neurovascularization to occur and to facilitate lymphatic drainage. Not all movement has to be by the flap itself. The surrounding tissues, when undermined, can also be moved to help accommodate a flap and to reduce tension when it comes to suturing.

Flaps commonly used in cutaneous surgery include simple rotation, rhomboid and advancement flaps with various modifications to create O to Z closures [7], nasolabial fold flaps, A to T flaps, etc. The technique of Z-plasty, Burrow's wedge flaps and wedge resections of the lip are also useful additional techniques for the dermatological surgeon [2, 4, 6, 8, 14].

Grafts [4, 6, 8, 11–13]. These are divided according to their type and thickness. Composite grafts do not concern us here. The three main categories of grafts used in dermatology are *full thickness*, *split-skin* and *pinch grafts.*

Full thickness grafts are used to cover wounds which cannot easily be closed primarily or by using a flap. Sometimes a wound can be partially closed with interrupted sutures and a free graft used to cover the residual defect. Morbidity tends to be less with grafts than flaps but the donor area also requires repair. Post-auricular, supraclavicular and eyelid skin is often used to repair defects on the face.

Split-skin grafts are more commonly used to cover large surgical defects or where there is a compromised blood supply. It is a relatively simple technique but colour and texture match is not usually as good as with full thickness grafts.

Pinch grafts [4, 14] are small, 5–10 mm, split-skin grafts harvested under local anaesthetic by picking up small amounts of skin with a needle and shaving the tented skin off with a scalpel or razor blade. The grafts are then placed on moistened gauze and transferred to the recipient skin surface. The technique is particularly useful for leg ulcers [1] where cosmetic appearance is not so important and where other grafts often fail due to pockets of pus or exudate forming under the grafted skin. This is less of a problem with pinch grafts. Also, being so small, their metabolic demands are minimal. Modifications of this technique have been to *mesh* split-thickness skin grafts [9] or to cut them up into pieces the size of a postage stamp prior to application.

Punch grafts are often used in hair transplant work [10, 15, 16] (see p. 2596).

REFERENCES

1 CEILLEY R.I., *et al* (1977) *J Dermatol Surg Oncol* **3**, 303.
2 CHERNOSKY M.E. (1982) In *Skin Surgery*. Eds. Epstein E. & Epstein E., Jr. 5th ed. Springfield, Thomas, p. 189.
3 CONVERSE J.M. (1982) In *Skin Surgery*. Eds. Epstein E. & Epstein E., Jr. 5th ed. Springfield, Thomas, p. 245.
4 CONVERSE J.M., *et al* (1977) *Reconstructive Plastic Surgery*. Philadelphia, W.B. Saunders, Vol. 1, p. 595.
5 CRABBE W.C. & MYERS M.B. (1975) *Skin Flaps*. Boston, Little, Brown.
6 CRABBE W.C. & SMITH W. (1973) *Plastic Surgery: A Concise Guide to Clinical Practice*. Boston, Little, Brown, p. 1085.
7 HAMMOND R.F. (1979) *J Dermatol Surg Oncol* **5**, 205.
8 MCGREGOR I.A. (1975) *Fundamental Techniques of Plastic Surgery and their Surgical Applications*. New York, Churchill Livingstone, p. 30.
9 NAPPI J.F., *et al* (1984) *J Dermatol Surg Oncol* **10**, 380.
10 NORWOOD O.T. & SHIELL R.C. (1984) *Hair Transplant Surgery*. 2nd ed. New York, Springfield, Thomas.
11 PETREZ J & HUNNEIKER M. (1978) *Dermatosurgery*. New York, Springer p. 152.
12 REES T.D. (1980) *Aesthetic Plastic Surgery*. Philadelphia, W.B. Saunders.
13 SISSON G.A. & TARDY M. JR. 1977) *Plastic and Reconstructive Surgery of the Face and Neck*. New York, Grune & Stratton, p. 236.
14 STEGMAN J.J., *et al* (1982) *Basis of Dermatologic Surgery*. Chicago, Year Book Medical Publishers.
15 UNGER W.P. (1979) *Hair Transplantation* New York, Marcel Dekker.
16 WILLIAMS J.P.G., *et al* (1972) *Arch Dermatol* **106**, 595.

CURETTAGE [2, 14]

Curettage is the destruction or enucleation of skin lesions by means of a sharp spoon. Many varieties of curette are available. Whatever size or type is used, the edge must be kept sharp. A small ophthalmic curette is used to enucleate milia or small cysts and to probe for deep tumour projections [6], but for most purposes a strong single- or double-ended oval curette from 4 to 12 mm in length is used. The handle should be solid, bevelled and near enough to the spoon to give firm leverage.

Uses. The following may be mentioned as examples:
Verrucae and warts, especially when periungual, can be treated using curettage and cautery. On the palms and soles preliminary incision of the skin around the wart or verruca prevents tearing and makes curettage easier. Local anaesthetic (plain) is required. A 'double technique' using a clean curette to remove debris and residual wart virus reduces the risk of recurrence. Weight-bearing areas and skin overlying joints, nerves or nail matrix should be treated with caution.

Keratoses, mollusca contagiosa and other superficial lesions such as milia and sebaceous hyperplasia can be easily removed—often without the use of local anaesthetic—and this can be combined with simple skin styptics such as 30–50% trichloroacetic acid or Monsel's solution to coagulate the skin surface.

Basal cell papillomas ('seborrhoeic warts') are usually easily removed by the curette alone, often without anaesthetic, with subsequent application of a skin styptic or some oxidized cellulose [8] to prevent bleeding. Rather more fibrotic basal cell papillomas such as often occur round the neck may require electrodiathermy in addition. The lesions of dermatitis papulosa nigrans can be treated in the same way.

Small sebaceous cysts and inclusions and foreign body cysts can be enucleated and chronic pyodermatous sinuses can be scraped out, with or without subsequent phenolization. In calcinosis cutis and for gouty tophi the curette has a place in the removal of individual lesions. In curetting pyogenic granulomas, it is important to scrape and cauterize the edges thoroughly and always to have the specimen checked histologically. The curette may be used to remove dead tissue and slough from indolent ulcers and the hard adherent hyperkeratotic skin that impedes healing.

Malignant tumours. Squamous cell carcinomas are usually best excised or dealt with by traditional means, but small well-defined squamous cell carcinomas can be curretted in combination with electrodesiccation or thorough cauterization in the elderly or bed-ridden patient [4]. Curettage also forms part of chemosurgical techniques [1].

Curettage followed by cauterization or electrodesiccation has become a common method of treatment for basal cell carcinomas in the U.K. following the demonstration [13, 15] of low recurrence rate and good cosmetic results. Its speed and convenience commend it. It has long been used as a routine treatment in other parts of the world [1]. It is not, however, the method of choice for infiltrative or large lesions or those situated around the ears, eyes or nose [3, 7, 12].

Method. The curette should be grasped firmly with the thumb close to the head of the curette and with the skin around the lesion held firm. Seborrhoeic warts and solar keratoses will scrape flush with the skin and heal with little or no scarring.

The aim of curettage is to destroy the offending lesion as completely as possible. Where histology is required, the first 'bite' should encompass as much of the lesion as possible including the base, or alternatively a shave biopsy can be performed first. For verrucae or skin cancers, the curette should be used with a firm 'in-up-and-out' movement. As much of the lesion as possible should be curetted by 'feel' and the edges should then be scraped and scalloped, preferably with a clean curette (or the other end of a double-ended one) to remove any tissue which might contain virus or residual malignant cells. In treating basal cell carcinomas the affected tissue is soft and 'mushy'. Once the friable tissue has been removed, thorough scraping in all planes should continue before cauterization or electrodesiccation. The procedure should then be repeated using a smaller curette to probe for tumour extensions. At least 3 mm of 'normal skin' should be destroyed at the edges of the lesion.

Results. For superficial lesions and skin cancers less than 1 cm in diameter, the cosmetic results are very good. Treatment of deeper or more extensive lesions with curettage and cautery may lead to less acceptable scarring or scar contracture.

With proper selection and good technique a 95% cure rate can be achieved using curettage and cautery or electrodesiccation as the primary treatment of basal cell carcinoma [5, 10, 16]. The technique is not suitable, however, for morphoeic or recurrent basal cell carcinoma [3, 11], for high risk sites [3, 9] or for lesions which have previously had an incisonal biopsy.

REFERENCES

1 *BELISARIO J. (1959) *Cancer of the Skin*. London, Butterworths, p. 151.
2 BURNS R.E. (1961) *Arch Dermatol* **84**, 662.
3 HELM F.E. (1984) *Dermatol Wochenschr* **150**, 451.
4 KNOX J.M., et al (1960) *Arch Dermatol* **82**, 197.
5 KOPF A.W., et al (1977) *Arch Dermatol* **113**, 439.
6 KRULL E.A. (1978) *J Dermatol Surg Oncol* **4**, 656.
7 LEVINE H.J. & PAILIN P.L. (1980) *Laryngoscope* **90**, 955.
8 MOHS F.E. (1978) *J Dermatol Surg Oncol* **4**, 106.
9 PANJE W.R. & CEILLEY R.I. (1979) *Laryngoscope* **89**, 1914.
10 POPKIN G.L. & BART R.S. (1975) *J Dermatol Surg Oncol* **1**, 33.
11 REYMANN F. (1980) *Dermatologica* **161**, 217.
12 SALASCHE S.J. (1983) *J Dermatol Surg Oncol* **8**, 496.
13 SIMPSON J.R. (1966) *Br J Dermatol* **78**, 147.
14 STURM H.M. & LEIDER M. (1979) *J Dermatol Surg Oncol* **4**, 656.
15 *SWEET R.D. (1963) *Br J Dermatol* **75**, 137.
16 WILLIAMSON G.S. & JACKSON R. (1962) *Can Med Assoc J* **86**, 855.

CHEMOSURGERY

The term 'chemosurgery' has come to include not only 'superficial' chemotherapy [1, 2], e.g. the application of cauterizing chemicals to evoke peeling and destruction of superficial lesions, but also the use of chemical cautery combined with surgery for deeper and more destructive processes. Skin peeling procedures, which are not practised widely by British dermatologists, are discussed on p. 2590. We are concerned here with the second definition.

Monochloroacetic acid, dichloroacetic acid and trichloroacetic acid may be used in conjunction with curettage and intead of, or in addition to, thermal cauterization in the treatment of keratoses, warts and various other superficial skin lesions.

Zinc chloride is an escharotic and fixative which enables cells to be examined by the frozen section technique after removal of successive layers of tissue. By using a marking technique, complete removal of all projections of malignant tissue can be obtained. The technique is particularly applicable to invasive and infiltrative basal cell carcinomas and other such tumours.

Microscopically controlled surgery (chemosurgery; Mohs' technique) [9–11]. The principle of microscopically controlled serial excision surgery is that maximum confidence as regards tumour clearance is combined with minimal loss of normal viable tissue. Removal of a skin cancer, layer by layer, with histological control allows unsuspected ramifications of cancer to be detected and ablated. Originally defects were allowed to heal by primary intent but now, for those cancers where the risk of recurrence is judged to be slight, immediate repairs are often preferred since the cosmetic and functional results are thereby improved [13, 14]. There are two basic techniques.

The fixed tissue technique, using zinc chloride paste, is now mainly reserved for deeply invasive or multiply recurrent tumours [8, 12]. Tissue handling and marking is easier with the fixed tissue technique.

The fresh tissue technique is the method of choice for cancers of the eyelid and is nowadays the chief method used for less complicated skin cancers.

The results of Mohs' technique are impressive with a 98–99% 5-yr cure rate for basal cell carcinomas and a 94.4% 5-year cure rate for squamous cell carcinomas [9, 10]. It is nowadays regarded as the treatment of choice for multiple recurrent skin cancers, with a 5-yr cure rate of 96.8% [9, 10] compared with a cure rate of 50% with conventional methods [5].

Dichloroacetic acid is used both as a skin styptic and to aid the initial penetration of the zinc chloride paste.

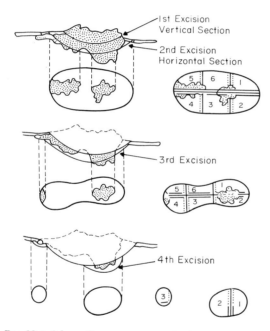

Fig. 68.1. Schematic representation of a skin cancer (shaded areas). Vertical and horizontal projections are shown at three stages of excision. The areas of cancer are located by microscopic examination of the undersurface of each of the excised layers. (Illustrated by courtesy of Helm F., *et al*, 1964.)

Essentially the technique involves excising and examining sequentially premarked oriented slices of tissue to determine the site and depth of malignant invasion [6, 9–11] (Fig. 68.1).

It is of obvious advantage in the complete extirpation of basal cell carcinomas in areas such as the alae nasi or eyelids [9–11] and has been extended

to squamous cell carcinomas of the ear, penis and elsewhere. In the vulval area it is said to eliminate the need for radical vulvectomy. Mohs also claims good results in malignant melanomas [7, 8]. When carried out by a team experienced in the technique and the interpretation of the histology, it is undoubtedly of great value.

The fixed technique is not without pain to the patient and both methods are time-consuming for the physician and pathologist. The good results obtained by traditional methods of treatment in the great majority of cases is likely to restrict the technique to cases of particular difficulty.

Chemosurgery has also been advocated [3, 6] as a rational way of treating gangrene in order to preserve as much viable tissue as possible, providing an alternative to conventional surgery.

REFERENCES

1 Ayres S. (1960) *Arch Dermatol* **82**, 578.
2 Ayres S. III (1977) In *Skin Surgery*. Eds. Epstein E. & Epstein E. Jr. 5th ed. Springfield, Thomas.
3 Bailin P.L. (1978) *Cutis* **21**, 476.
4 Helm F., *et al* (1964) *Dermatol Wochenschr* **150**, 451.
5 Menn H. (1971) *Arch Dermatol* **103**, 628.
6 Mohs F.E. (1956) *Chemosurgery in Cancer, Gangrene and Infections*. Springfield, Thomas.
7 Mohs F.E. (1977) In *Skin Surgery*. Eds. Epstein E. & Epstein E. Jr. 4th ed. Springfield, Thomas, p. 526.
8 Mohs F.E. (1977) *Arch Dermatol* **113**, 285.
9 Mohs F.E. (1978). *Chemosurgery Microscopically Controlled Surgery for Skin Cancer*. Springfield, Thomas.
10 Mohs F.E. (1978) *J Dermatol Surg Oncol* **4**, 1.
11 Mohs F.E. (1982) In *Skin Surgery*. Eds. Epstein E, & Epstein E. Jr. 5th ed. Springfield, Thomas.
12 Mohs F.E. & Sahl W.J. (1979) *J Dermatol Surg Oncol* **5**, 303.
13 Robins P., *et al* (1979) *J Dermatol Surg Oncol* **5**, 329.
14 Smith J.D. (1977) *J Dermatol Surg Oncol* **3**, 184.

CAUSTICS, CHEMICAL PEELING [5, 12]

In experienced hands caustics provide a simple and readily available means of destroying many superficial skin conditions. Used with electrocautery or diathermy, they constitute one form of chemosurgery for basal cell and squamous cell carcinomas. The operator should be well acquainted with the action and degree of penetration of individual caustics and the toxic effects that may result from absorption, especially if they are to be used more extensively, and particularly when applied to the face [14].

In treating individual lesions caustics are usually applied by means of a cotton-bud applicator or a wool-tipped orange stick, pointed if necessary.

Silver nitrate. This is used in the form of a pencil or as a strong solution to suppress exuberant granulation. It is haemostatic and may be used to arrest bleeding after curettage. Repeated use tends to lead to unsightly staining of the skin.

Phenol (liquified phenol). This is a valuable superficial caustic which should, however, be used cautiously. It should *not* be diluted as this increases its absorption and potency [14] and thus also its nephrotoxicity, hepatoxicity and cardiotoxicity. Ochronosis may occur from prolonged absorption. It is not a haemostatic and bleeding limits its effectiveness. When used as a treatment for in-grown toe nails it is important that the phenol is applied to a 'dry' nail bed and that sufficient time is allowed for it to take effect.

Potential toxicity remains a major concern especially with more extensive use and it should not, of course, be used during pregnancy. It is particularly useful, however, applied to cyst linings after lancing and expressing the contents of acne cysts and also for individual lesions of hidradenitis suppurativa. The cosmetic results are excellent even with large acne cysts on the face. Phenol is also used in a soap–croton oil–water mix for chemical face peels (see below). A glycol–spirit solution can be used for neutralization if required.

Trichloroacetic acid. This is an effective haemostatic caustic which has many uses. The 30–50% concentration can be used as a styptic and is frequently employed in conjunction with superficial curettage in the treatment of solar keratoses, seborrhoeic warts, etc. The supersaturated solution can also be used on its own to treat many benign and dysplastic skin lesions. 50% trichloroacetic acid is similar to phenol in its destructive effect on the epidermis.

We have also found trichloroacetic acid to be a useful treatment for xanthelasmas (Fig. 68.2) and solar lentigos. It must be applied with great care, however, especially around the eyes. Its action is rapid and a white 'frosting' occurs within a few seconds. The effect can be partially neutralized by applying alcohol, water or sodium-bicarbonate-soaked gauze, but in reality it is unlikely to make much difference once the acid has penetrated the skin.

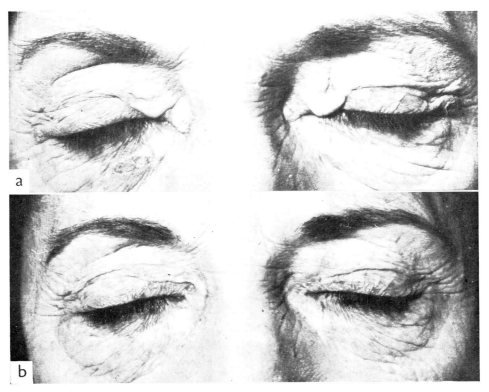

FIG. 68.2. Trichloroacetic acid. Effect of four applications on xanthelasmata: (a) before treatment; (b) after treatment. (Stoke Mandeville Hospital.)

Excess grease should first be removed using detergent, ether or acetone. Trichloroacetic acid should then be applied with an 'almost dry' cotton applicator. The concentration to be used will vary according to site, the condition to be treated and whether the trichloroacetic acid is being used as a styptic or a superficial skin caustic.

Weaker solutions of trichloroacetic acid are sometimes used for treating wider areas of skin (see below). Because of deliquescence, trichloroacetic acid should be kept in a closed, coloured and corrosion-resistant bottle.

Dichloroacetic acid . This is also a powerful caustic and skin styptic.

Monochloroacetic acid. This should not be considered as a superficial caustic. It penetrates rapidly and may remove the whole epidermis by blister formation. We use it in this way for mosaic warts and it can also be used for resistant periungual warts.

Zinc chloride. This is a very powerful caustic (see p. 2589).

Chemical peeling [1, 3, 5, 12, 13]. This is essentially a cosmetic procedure, used to improve the appearance of ageing, wrinkled or sun-damaged skin. It is less effective in dealing with acne scars but is a valid dermatological manoeuvre for these and other superficial lesions on the face. In Great Britain it is usually carried out by plastic surgeons and it will therefore not be considered in any great detail here. Those interested are referred to the main references cited.

Chemical face peeling is used in conjunction with, or as an alternative to, dermabrasion [1, 2, 7]. Patients with a dry skin and a fair complexion are the best subjects [13]. One technique makes use of a phenol–soap–croton mixture [3–5, 13] the other a 30–50% solution of trichloroacetic acid [3, 10]. The effect is enhanced by tape occlusion. The neck should not be included as the skin in this area is more liable to scarring and hyperpigmentation [10, 11]. Weaker preparations, e.g. 20% trichloroacetic acid, are generally used on eyelids and care must be taken not to cause hypertrophic scars which may occur around the mouth or mandible.

Prolonged erythema and increased sensitivity to sunlight and pigmentary changes (both hyperpigmentation and hypopigmentation) may follow the procedure. Phenol is also associated with a risk of systemic toxaemia and particularly cardiac arrythmias [14] if used in too large a quantity or applied too quickly (especially on the face).

In spite of all these problems, most cosmetic surgeons still regard the phenol peel as a very worthwhile procedure giving a genuine long-lasting improvement in those with sun-damaged skin.

REFERENCES

1 AYRES S. III (1982) In *Skin Surgery*. Eds. Epstein E. & Epstein E. Jr. 5th ed. Springfield, Thomas, p. 711.
2 BAKER T.J. & GORDON H.L. (1971) *Surg Clin North Am* 51, 387.
3 BAKER T.J. & GORDON H.L. (1973) In *Cosmetic Facial Surgery.* Eds. Rees T.D. & Wood-Smith D. Philadelphia, Saunders, p. 345.
4 BAKER T.J. & GORDON H.L. (1974) *Plast Reconstr Surg* 53, 522.
5 *BAKER T.J. & GORDON H.L. (1982) In *Skin Surgery*. Eds. Epstein E. & Epstein E. Jr. 5th ed. Springfield, Thomas, p. 768.
6 BROWN V.K.H., *et al* (1975) *Arch Environ Health* 30, 1.
7 BURKS J. & FARBER G. (1979) *Dermabrasion and chemical peel.* In *The Treatment of Certain Cosmetic Defects and Diseases of the Skin.* Springfield, Thomas.
8 CHUPMAN E.S. & ELLERBERG J.D. (1979) *Plast Reconstr Surg* 63, 44.
9 CONNING D.M. & HAYES M.J. (1970) *Br J Ind Med* 27, 155.
10 RESNIK S.S. & LEWIS L.A. (1976) *Cutis* 17, 127.
11 SPIRA M., *et al* (1970) *Plast Reconstr Surg* 45, 247.
12 STEGMAN S.J. & TROMOVITVH T.A. (1984) *Cosmetic Dermatologic Surgery.* Chicago, Year Book Medical Publishers.
13 STOUGH D.B.(1976) *Cutis* 18, 239.
14 TRUPPMANN E.S. & ELLENBERG J.D. (1979) *Plast Reconstr Surg* 63, 44.

ELECTROSURGERY
[5, 7, 9, 11, 15, 18, 20, 21]

Destruction of tissue utilizing electrical currents is achieved in several ways. In *electrolysis* [2] a direct current is employed to cause the liberation of chemicals around the follicle. Most epilation is, in fact, now performed using *thermolysis* (fine needle diathermy or electrocoagulation) [23, 25]. The *cautery* [9] uses heat resulting from conversion of the current by the resistance of platinum tips, using a step-down transformer and a variable rheostat. Monopolar electrosurgical machines such as the hyfrecator can be used for *electrodesiccation* and *fulguration*. Bipolar machines can also be used for *cutting* and *electrocoagulation* [9]. In the former, a spark action is used (fulguration) and in the latter a needle is inserted directly into the lesion for electrocoagulation. In both instances the tips remain cold and they can both be used without local anaesthesia if the lesions to be treated are small, e.g. skin tags, etc.

Oscillations from old-fashioned spark-gap machines were 'damped' and therefore particularly good for electrocoagulation. Vacuum tube (triode) machines produce 'undamped' oscillations with excellent cutting characteristics. Most modern machines combine features of both [6]. Bipolar instruments require the patient to be attached to a larger dispersive electrode. It is important that this is in good contact with the patient, otherwise low frequency burns may occur.

Machines available for hospital use or for use in theatre usually have isolated circuitry and are enclosed in a gas-proof case. The anaesthetist must avoid all inflammable gases when the sparking current is being used. Smaller wall-hanging machines, especially designed for dermatological use, are not so enclosed and should not be used in theatres or in conjunction with inflammable gases or liquids. *Caution.* Before using any high-frequency equipment, the dermatologist must make sure that the patient does not have an implanted cardiac pacemaker [17, 22]. Ventricular fibrillation may develop even if the patient is only in close proximity to a diathermy machine. This was pointed out many years ago [26] and has recently been the subject of an official reminder in Great Britain.

Histological and tissue effects. The effect of desiccation is to shrivel the cells in contact with the current, condensing and elongating their nuclei. Histological death of the cell and thrombosis of the smaller blood vessels occur. There is little haemorrhage.

Healing takes place with crust formation, mild exudation and sloughing of the crust in 7–21 days. Even with extensive electrodesiccation, scars tend to be minimal and to improve with time. The healing of electrocautery crusts is slower.

Uses. The uses of the various methods of electrosurgery are fully described in the main texts cited and have been well summarized [8, 14]. Most dermatologists will develop their own particular technique and establish, by experience, the indications for each method of electrosurgery. In Great Britain, the cautery is probably still more widely used than diathermy. Only an outline of the main uses will be given here.

Electrolysis (fine needle and low current electrodiathermy). Electrolysis is used for the destrucion of hair follicles and for small vascular lesions, e.g. telangiectases and small spider naevi.

The cautery [9, 12]. This can be used alone for desiccation or in conjunction with curettage in the management of warts, verrucae, pyogenic granulomas and other superficial benign tumours of the skin. It is also widely used (see p. 2588) in the treatment of superficial skin cancers, mainly basal cell carcinoma. The vigorous use of the cautery after curettage has become established as a recognized and reliable method of treating basal cell carcinoma in appropriate areas (p. 2588). Though healing is slow, the resulting scar is often minimal and far less conspicuous than would result from radiotherapy or grafting.

The 'ball-point cautery' is a very effective haemostatic and can be used in conjunction with scissors to 'snip and cauterize' skin tags and condyloma acuminata [24]. A 'spade' tip is normally used after curettage or other ablative measures. A 'cold-point' cautery tip is particularly useful for angiomas of the lip (or elsewhere) and for large spider telangiectases.

Slow healing is the main disadvantage of this form of electrosurgery [12].

In the United States electrodesiccation has tended to be used instead of electrocautery.

Electrodesiccation and coagulation [6, 14, 20, 21]. The main uses are as follows.

(i) The destruction of benign superficial lesions such as keratoses, seborrhoeic warts, virus warts [19], mollusca contagiosa, areas of sebaceous hyperplasia, small keratoacanthomas and other superficial dermal and epidermal lesions.

(ii) The ablation of angiomas, telangiectases (using low current), senile angiomas of the lips, mucous cysts and other vascular lesions such as rhinophyma and condyloma. The loop electrode can be used to remove polyps or provide tissue specimens. It is especially useful for lesions in the mouth or on the genitalia.

(iii) The coagulation of sebaceous and epidermoid cysts. The needle is inserted into the centre of the cyst and the contents are coagulated until the skin is hot to the touch. The coagulation causes the cyst contents and sac to be extruded after some days through the coagulated punctum which enlarges, leaving a depressed scar. This technique may be of value for very small cysts which are not amenable to surgery but has been generally very unreliable in the authors' hands. Electrodiathermy has also been used to marsupialize hidradenitis suppurativa tracts and to 'debulk' cheloids prior to injection with steroid [6].

(iv) The destruction of skin tags. A very large number may be removed at one sitting without anaesthetic. The needle may be used for electro-coagulation or the 'ball-point' tip for fulguration.

(v) The destruction of malignant tumours [3, 4, 13, 20] usually in conjunction with curettage [1, 27]. As with all methods of treatment of these lesions that depend on personal expertise in a particular field, the results depend on the experience of the operator. This probably explains the different views expressed [20] on the cure rate obtained. The destructive power of electrocoagulation is equal to that of any other method of tissue destruction; the results obtained reflect, therefore, both patient selection and the operator's experience rather than the apparatus itself. In general, the cure rate is comparable with those obtained with surgery or radiotherapy so long as certain anatomical sites and types of lesion are avoided [10, 16].

Morphoeic basal cell carcinoma should not be treated with electrodiathermy. Also, because the limits of invasion of squamous cell carcinoma are often ill-defined, we do not, ourselves, regard electrocoagulation or electrodesiccation as an entirely safe method except for small or very early lesions.

One important disadvantage of electrosurgery is that it is often not possible to obtain a complete histological specimen. It is important, however, even with apparently benign lesions to take a representative specimen for histological examination whenever possible.

REFERENCES

1 ALBRIGHT & SPENCER D. (1982) *J Am Acad Dermatol* **17**, 2.
2 BARBER K.A. & JACKSON R. (1982) In *Skin Surgery*. Eds. Epstein E. & Epstein E. Jr. 5th ed. Springfield, Thomas, p. 427.
3 BELISARIO J.C. (1959) *Cancer of the Skin*. London, Butterworths, p. 155.
4 BELISARIO J.C. (1964) *Acta Derm Venereol (Stockh)* **44** (Suppl. 56).
5 BLEKENSHIP M.L. (1979) *Int J Dermatol* **18**, 443.
6 *BODIAN E.L. (1978) *J Dermatol Surg Oncol* **4**, 235.
7 *BURDICK K.H. (1966) *Electrosurgical Procedures In Dermatology*. Springfield, Thomas.
8 BURDICK K.H. (1975) In *Current Dermatologic Management*. Ed. Maddin S. 2nd ed. St Louis, Mosby, p. 18.
9 BURDICK K.H. (1982) In *Skin Surgery*. Eds. Epstein E. & Epstein E. Jr. 5th ed. Springfield, Thomas, p. 419.
10 CRISSY J. (1971) *J Dermatol Surg Oncol* **3**, 287.
11 ELLIOTT J.A. (1966) *Arch Dermatol* **94**, 340.
12 EPSTEIN E. (1982) In *Skin Surgery*. Eds. Epstein E. & Epstein E. Jr. 5th ed. Springfield, Thomas, p. 405.
13 FREEMAN R.G. & KNOX J.M. (1967) *Treatment of Skin Cancer. Recent Results in Cancer Research*. New York, Springer.
14 FRITSCH W.C. (1975) In *Current Dermatologic Management*, Ed. Maddin S. 2nd ed. St Louis, Mosby, p. 20.
15 GRUMAY H.M. (1978) *Alternating Current: Electrosurgery in Physical Modalities in Dermatologic Therapy, Radiotherapy, Electrosurgery, Phototherapy, Cryotherapy*. New York, Springer, p. 203.
16 HELM J. *Cancer Dermatology*. Springfield, Thomas.
17 KRULL E.A., *et al* (1975) *J Dermatol Surg Oncol* **1**, 41.
18 JACKSON R. (1970) *Can J Surg* **13**, 354.
19 MAHRLE G. & ALEXANDER W. (1983) *J Dermatol Surg Oncol* **9**, 445.
20 POPKIN G.L. (1982) In *Skin Surgery*. Eds. Epstein E. & Epstein E. Jr. 5th ed. Springfield, Thomas, p. 385.
21 SCHOCH E.P., JR (1982) In *Skin Surgery*. Eds. Epstein E. & Epstein E. Jr. 5th ed. Springfield, Thomas, p. 414.
22 SEBBEN J.E. (1983) *J Am Acad Dermatol*, **9**, 457.
23 SPOOR H.J. (1978) *Cutis* **21**, 283.
24 THOMPSON J.P.S. & GRACE R.H. (1978) *J R Soc Med* **71**, 180.
25 WAGNER R.F., *et al* (1985) *J Am Acad Dermatol* **12**, 441.
26 WAJSCZUK K., *et al* (1969) *N Engl J Med* **290**, 34.
27 WHELAN C.S. & DECKERS P.J. (1981) *Cancer* **47**, 2280.

MINOR SURGICAL TECHNIQUES

The sterile needle. A sterile needle, preferably of the long, thin, 'cutting' type, flamed or otherwise sterilized before use, can be used red-hot (or as nearly so as possible), for the destruction of stellate naevi and the perforation of nail plates in cases of subungual haematomas, and cold, for the removal of splinters and as an aid in the identification of acari.

The pointed orange stick. Slightly broader and less sharp than a needle, it is used to enucleate small molluscum bodies. The other end of the orange stick may be lightly tipped with wool and used to touch the lesions with phenol or iodine. Mollusca contagiosa can also be eradicated by 'pricking' with phenol. A very sharply pointed orange stick dipped in trichloroacetic acid may also be used to treat stellate naevi although fine needle electrocoagulation is usually better.

The comedone expressor. The comedone expressor is a single- or double-ended small spoon with a central hole used to express comedones in acne or small milia. A firm, consistent levering motion is required, preferably after the area has been softened with keratolytics, washing or a hot bath.

Intelligent patients learn to use this instrument themselves to advantage but an obsessional attachment to it should be avoided.

Scarification. Scarification of the skin has been used for the removal of superficial blemishes and naevi, foreign-body particles and tattoos. Unfortunately the latter lie too deeply for this to be done without subsequent scarring unless they are small, when excision is usually preferable. Many of its previous uses have been supplanted by dermabrasion (see below). Light scarification or scraping of a finger web, after the application of 10% potassium hydroxide, is a useful way of revealing acari or eggs in scabetic patients.

Acne cysts, if inflamed, respond well to the injection of some half-strength intralesional steroid. Larger more indolent cysts can be treated by lancing and phenolization following extrusion of the cyst contents.

SURGICAL PARING

The procedure of paring away the surface of the epithelium is commonly used in the treatment of rhinophyma. Excess tissue can be removed until the normal shape of the nose is restored. Tulle gras or dry dressings are applied and re-epithelialization takes place without scarring from the abundant pilosebaceous follicles extending deeply into the dermis. This simple procedure is a most satisfactory one for this disfiguring condition.

Less dramatically, but more commonly, the paring away of hyperkeratosis is carried out for corns, verrucae and especially plantar verrucae in the course of treatment, particularly in combination with salicylic acid plaster, monochloroacetic acid, podophyllin and other cytotoxic agents. It is advisable to use a round-bladed scalpel to avoid cutting the skin. Paring of corns in the diabetic patient must be carried out with caution and strict asepsis. Infection following such paring when carried out by the patient or an inexperienced operator may lead to cellulitis of the foot or leg.

The bulk of a keratoacanthoma may be removed by paring or curettage followed by the application of a cytotoxic agent, cryotherapy, electrodiathermy or radiotherapy.

A similar destruction of excess tissue, particularly in rhinophyma, may be obtained by electrosurgery [1, 2].

REFERENCES

1 NIEDELMAN M.L. (1959) *Arch Dermatol* **70**, 91.
2 SCOTT M.J. (1956) *Northwest Med Seattle* **55**, 46.

DERMABRASION (SURGICAL SKIN PLANING) [1, 3]

The abrasive technique for the removal of superficial vascular and pigmentary lesions, rhinophyma [3], pitted or depressed scars, tattoos and foreign bodies was first practised by Kromayer [4]. Its chief value lies in treating lesions on the face where regeneration of the epidermis proceeds rapidly, generally without scarring, because of the abundance of pilosebaceous structures from which repair occurs as long as destruction does not extend to the subcutis. It has been used with success in the treatment of superficial skin epitheliomas [1, 5], although it is not the treatment of choice [3].

Considerable advances in the technique have taken place in the last 20 yr, due especially to the high-speed rotary drill and the use of more efficient refrigeration [3]. Care must be taken to follow details of the technique rigidly to avoid damage to the patient or operator. Briefly, the technique (allowing for many individual modifications) is as follows [3].

(i) The patient is sedated.
(ii) The area is prechilled with cold packs.
(iii) The skin is cleansed with spirit or some suitable substitute after washing with soap and water.
(iv) The ears and nostrils are plugged with ointment-impregnated gauze and the hair and ears are carefully protected by clipped towels.
(v) The eyes are carefully protected, e.g. by ointment and lead shields, by gauze in thickness held by an assistant, or by the plastic cups used by sunbathers to protect the eyes.
(iv) The area to be treated is frozen by a continuous stream of Freon (dichlorotetrafluoroethane) and the skin abraded with the drill to the required depth and area. The degree of freezing and of drilling necessary is obviously a matter only to be learnt by experience. The abrading wheels ('brushes') may be of stainless steel wires or diamond fraizes.

Bleeding occurs for 15–30 min after treatment. Paraffin gauze, dry dressings, non-adherent gauze or nylon dressings are applied and removed in 1–24 hr, the crusts separating in 7–10 days. Healing is usually completed within 3 weeks, particularly if the wound is left open and dry.

Infection following dermabrasion is rare. Mild irritation or discomfort from sunlight or cosmetics may occur for a few weeks. Milia, persistent erythema, hyperpigmentation, hypertrophic scars and dermatitis are occasional complications. The treatment can be repeated on the same area at any time after 4 weeks and the technqiue may be combined with chemosurgery [2].

Dermabrasion has received much attention in the U.S.A. and elsewhere but has only found limited application in the U.K. It can be considered as a very useful part of cosmetic dermatological practice. Its value in the minimizing of pitted acne scars of the face is undoubted (though the small 'ice-pick' scars respond less satisfactorily than coarse irregular scars). It has a place in the treatment of some superficial port-wine angiomas. Facial tattoos are obviously a rare but legitimate indication, but superficial tumours, keratoses and warty lesions can usually be dealt with better by other methods. It has been combined with topical steroids in hypertrophic lichen planus and lichen simplex.

REFERENCES

1 Ayres S. III (1975) In *Curent Dermatology Therapy.* Ed: Maddin S. 2nd ed. St Louis, Mosby, p. 11.
2 Ayres S. III (1975) In *Skin Surgery* Eds. Epstein E. & Epstein E. Jr. 4th ed. Springfield, Thomas, p. 573.
3 Epstein E. & Epstein E. Jr. (1979) *Techniques in Skin Surgery.* Philadelphia, Lea & Febiger, p. 171.
4 Kromayer E. (1930) *The Cosmetic Treatment of Skin Complaints.* London, Oxford University Press.
5 Ridley C.M. (1958) *Br J Dermatol* 70, 293.

HAIR TRANSPLANTATION [1,2]

The punch autograft remains the major procedure in this field but many other surgical techniques have been developed which may sometimes be used alone or as adjuncts to punch grafting. These include strip and fusiform grafting, scalp reduction of balding areas, supra-, pre- and post-auricular transposition scalp flaps and the controversial 'Juri' flap [1]. The major condition for which these techniques are used remains androgenic alopecia in its various forms.

Careful pre-operative assessment of the mental and physical status of the patient is crucial. It is imperative to exclude those subjects with known functional psychoses, those who are dysmorphophobic or cannot comprehend the nature of the treatment and its effects, and those with physical illness that might compromise healing or satisfactory hair regrowth, e.g. bleeding disorders, steroid therapy and previous hypertrophic or cheloid scars. Every patient accepted for transplantation or other surgical corrective treatment *must* have received clear instructions on the details of the operation and its potential side effects.

Punch autografts [2]. The details of the technique will not be considered here. In treating androgenic alopecia, the order of grafting will depend on the hair pattern, but in general punches are inserted from the frontal margin, working towards the crown. Improvements in technique now allow from 60 to 150 punch transfers to be carried out per session with relatively few graft failures. Some

patients are happy with frontal density correction and less dense grafting on other more posterior vertex areas. In any one donor session it is usual to leave a minimum of 4 mm between punched donor sites. With successive treatment sessions, previously treated sites may require 'blender' and 'filler' grafts.

In general most patients detect early hair growth in the eighth to twelfth week after treatment, good hair usually being established at about the sixth month after graft insertion.

Complications are rare and include arterial bleeding, A–V and venous aneurysms, foreign-body reactions, infection, poor graft survival and hypertrophic scarring.

Some surgeons use punch grafting for focal scarring alopecia, but dense hair growth is always difficult to achieve in scar tissue.

Other procedures. It is now commonplace for skilled scalp surgeons to use punch grafting with other grafting, reduction and flap procedures. For details of these methods the reader is referred to more detailed texts [2].

In the U.K. many dermatologists remain nihilistic with regard to surgical correction of alopecia but with careful patient selection and adequate surgical skill good results can be obtained.

REFERENCES

1 *Norwood O.T. & Shiell R.C. (1984) *Hair Transplant Surgery.* 2nd ed. Springfield, Thomas.
2 Unger W.P. (1979) *Hair Transplantation.* New York, Marcel Dekker.

CRYOTHERAPY [17, 21]

The earliest freezing agent used in the treatment of skin diseases was the salt–ice mixture ($-20\,°C$) advocated by Arnott in 1851; by 1913, the clinical effectiveness of liquid air and solid carbon dioxide (CO_2 snow) was well known [17]. Increasing knowledge in the field of cryobiology, together with the development of sophisticated cryoprobes and liquid gas jets, has led to a great increase in the use of cryotherapy during the last 20 years [19].

Liquid nitrogen and carbon dioxide snow are now most commonly used, their boiling points being $-196\,°C$ for liquid nitrogen and $-79\,°C$ for carbon dioxide.

Nitrous oxide gas is also used as a refrigerant in closed probe systems (applying the Joule–Thomson effect), giving a working temperature of $-70\,°C$.

Histopathology. Histological changes are evident within 30 min of freezing [20]. Cells show pyknotic nuclei, oedema and coarsely granular and often vacuolated cytoplasm. At the edge of the frozen area the cells have eosinophilic cytoplasm with small basophilic nuclei. By 1 h, dermal vascular damage and oedema appear. Later changes are those seen in any acutely ischaemic area. The cellular infiltrate is mainly of polymorphonuclear leukocytes, with some lymphocytes and plasma cells most obvious at the edge of the frozen area. Resolution begins within 3 days and healing usually occurs without scarring or contraction [17].

Clinical methods [19]. Carbon dioxide snow is made by releasing gas from a cylinder into a chamois leather bag, the solid 'snow' then being transferred to a plastic funnel tube in which it is compressed; alternatively, small cylinders of gas may be discharged through a narrow opening into a collecting tube. Such apparatus is useful for superficial lesions; deeper destruction can only be produced by applying greater pressure with special applicators.

Liquid nitrogen is universally available owing to its widespread use in industry, hospital and research establishments. It is very cheap. The liquid is unstable at room temperature; however, one litre stored in an unsealed (Dewar) flask will last a full day and treat 50–60 patients. Cotton wool swabs or copper discs are dipped into the liquid and applied to the skin for 5–30 s. Liquid nitrogen cryoprobes and jets are now commercially available for use when greater tissue destruction is required.

Nitrous oxide cryoprobes are also available. The gas is easily obtained because of its use in anaesthetics, but it is more expensive and less convenient than liquid nitrogen.

Clinical uses. A wide spectrum of skin lesions have been treated with freezing. Table 68.2 shows a list of many of the conditions in which cure has been obtained. The simplicity and speed of cryotherapy treatment make it particularly attractive for dermatological practice. It must be stressed that, for most lesions in Table 68.2, other modes of treatment are equally effective but are often less convenient and give inferior cosmetic results.

Lesions that are superficial, benign or flat can be treated by the liquid nitrogen swab or carbon dioxide snow method. To obtain cure of pre-neoplastic and neoplastic conditions the lower temperature and more destructive properties of a cryoprobe or

TABLE 68.2. Skin conditions responsive to cryotherapy

Naevi [18]	Pigmented
	Epidermal
Lentigo [11]	Benign and malignant
Vascular lesions [11]	Telangectasia
	Spider naevus
	Pyogenic granuloma
	Pseudo-pyogenic granuloma
	Kaposi's sarcoma
	Haemangioma
	Lymphangioma
Keratotic and pre-neoplastic	Viral warts [4, 9]
	Molluscum contagiosum
	Seborrhoeic keratosis
	Solar keratosis
	Cutaneous horn
	Keratoacanthoma
	Bowen's disease [7]
Carcinoma [13]	Basal cell epithelioma
	Squamous cell epithelioma
Cysts	Epidermal
	Synovial
	Acne [12]
Oral Lesions [5]	Mucous cyst
	Leukoplakia
	Vascular lesions
Axillary hyperhidrosis [2]	
Scarring	Acne (CO_2 snow; acetone 'slush')
	Cheloid

Biopsy can be taken without local anaesthetic.

jet equipment are desirable. Cryosurgical treatment of basal cell epitheliomas gives cure rates which compare favourably with other modes of therapy [10, 15, 21]. No doubt exceptions, experience and choice of site are important—the eyelids, scalp and alae nasi are unfavourable sites. The temperature reached [8] and the number of freeze–thaw cycles are also critical. Repeat freeze–thaw cycles give more reliable cell death, whichever method is adopted [20].

Side effects. Pain is minimal compared with surgery and is usually transient, due to the anaesthetizing effect of freezing. Pronounced oedema is not uncommon in the lax tissue around the eyes, lips, tongue and labia. Haemorrhagic blisters may occur. It is important to note that blister formation is not necessary for the cure of lesions such as viral warts [3]. Sun-damaged and senile atrophic skin, and areas previously treated with topical steroids or X-irradiation, are more likely to blister or become necrotic from freezing. Skin necrosis is a desirable part of the treatment of neoplastic and many pre-neoplastic lesions; several weeks may elapse before healing is complete. Hypopigmentation is common after low temperature liquid nitrogen cryotherapy (probe or jet), particularly in dark-skinned patients [18]. Temporary postinflammatory hyperpigmentation is to be expected following less severe freezing. Paraesthesiae and, rarely, anaesthesia occur and may be troublesome because of the local effect of freezing on nerve endings. Care must be taken to avoid damage to major nerves since distal anaesthesia and motor paralysis may occur. Similarly, deep freezing over the lacrimal or tear ducts may lead to permanent ductal obstruction. Adventitious glands are sensitive to freezing and temporary hair loss and hypohidrosis are common; both can occasionally be permanent. In the treatment of axillary hyperhidrosis, the depilation was regarded by the patients as a 'bonus' [2].

REFERENCES

1 ABLIN R.J., *et al* (1981) *Tumor Diagnostik* **2**, 246.
2 ASHBY E.C. & WILLIAMS J.L. (1976) *Br Med J* ii, 1173.
3 BARR A. & COLES R.B. (1969) *Trans St Johns Hosp Dermatol Soc* **52**, 69.
4 BUNNEY M.H. (1975) *Br J Hosp Med* **13**, 567.
5 CHAPIN M.E. (1977) *J Dermatol Surg Oncol* **3**, 428.
6 DAWBER R.P.R. & WILKINSON J.D. (1979) *Br J Dermatol* 47.
7 DAWBER R.P.R., *et al* (1983) *Br J Dermatol* **8**, 153.
8 GAGE A.A., *et al* (1982) *Cryobiology* **19**, 273.
9 GHOSH A.K. (1977) *Br J Vener Dis* **53**, 49.
10 GRAHAM G.F. (1982) *J Dermatol Surg Oncol* **9**, 238.
11 GRAHAM G.F. & STEWART R. (1977) *J Dermatol Surg Oncol* **3**, 437.
12 LEYDEN J., *et al* (1874) *Br J Dermatol* **90**, 335.
13 LUBRITZ R.R. (1977) *J Dermatol Surg Oncol* **3**, 414.
14 LUBRITZ R.R. & SMOLEWSKI S.A. (1982) *J Am Acad Dermatol* **7**, 631.
15 McINTOSH G.S., *et al* (1983) *Postgrad Med J* **59**, 698.
16 SHEPHERD J.P. & DAWBER R.P.R. (1982) *Plast Reconstr Surg* **70**, 677.
17 SHEPHERD J.P. & DAWBER R.P.R. (1982) *Clin Exp Dermatol* **7**, 321.
18 TORRE D. (1976) *Cutis* **17**, 452.
19 TORRE D. (1977) In *Cryosurgical Advances in Dermatology and Tumours of the Head and Neck*. Ed. Zacarian S.A. Springfield, Thomas, p. 51.
20 UEDA K., *et al* (1982) *J Dermatol (Tokyo)* **9**, 93.
21 *ZACARIAN S.A. (1985) *Cryosurgery for Skin Cancer and Cutaneous Disorders*. St Louis, Mosby.

INTRALESIONAL THERAPY [4]

In dermatological usage this term is now virtually confined to the practice of injecting corticosteroid directly into the skin lesions, but it can also correctly be applied to certain other techniques:

(i) *Mepacrine* A 5–10% solution, diluted with an equal part of lignocaine, in the treatment of leishmaniasis, repeated weekly or fortnightly.

(ii) *Local cytotoxic agents.* These have been used intralesionally, e.g. in the destruction of basal cell carcinomas (see p. 1591).

(iii) *Phenol.* The phenolization of acne cysts. In experienced hands, this (p. 1591) gives good results.

(iv) *Antibiotics.* These may be injected directly into infected cysts, abscesses and localized areas of pyoderma.

Corticosteroids. Several preparations for intralesional use are available. An aqueous suspension of triamcinolone acetonide, 10 mg/ml, is commonly used, sometimes diluted to half its strength with saline or lignocaine. A suspension of triamcinolone hexacetonide is also available at a strength of 5 mg/ml and we find this convenient and sufficiently strong for all conditions except cheloids, when a 40 mg/ml concentration of triamcinolone acetonide or 20 mg/ml concentration of triamcinolone hexacetonide may be required.

Depending on the size of the lesion, an injection of 0·1–2·0 ml is normally given with a 25–30 gauge needle. Our personal preference is to use a disposable 1 ml insulin syringe with fused-on needle.

It is important that the injection is placed in the

deep dermis neither subcutaneously nor too superficial, otherwise atrophy is likely to ensue.

Systemic side effects are rare unless relatively large amounts are injected frequently. Apart from the usual risks of any intralesional injection, depigmentation, atrophy and telangiectasia may occur. Atrophy is less common with weaker suspensions and, when it occurs, is usually reversible. It can occasionally persist, however, causing a cosmetic defect as undesirable as the original condition. For this reason it may be advisable to use a weaker strength of triamcinolone for facial lesions that are not very thick or infiltrated. It is important to check that the needle has not entered a vessel before injecting, especially when in the vicinity of the supra-orbital nerve.

Intralesional therapy is appropriate in many conditions, especially when they are localized or few in number. Most obvious indications include lichen simplex, lupus erythematosus, lymphocytoma cutis, lichen planus (especially hypertrophic lesions) and granuloma annulare. Tufts of hair will grow in patches of alopecia areata that are not in a refractory phase; the treatment boosts the patient's morale but does not affect the course of the disease. Localized patches of psoriasis respond well but may recur. Necrobiosis lipoidica may improve but we have also seen ulceration follow in some diabetic patients. Small lesions of sarcoidosis will also respond to injection of steroid.

Intralesional corticosteroid therapy is a most useful and satisfying form of treatment for inflammatory acne cysts and nodules. The success rate in myxoid cysts is much less but it is a reasonable first choice of therapy in a difficult situation. Steroid injections can also be used as a first line of treatment of chondrodermatitis nodularis.

Cheloids may require even stronger suspensions—up to 40 mg/ml triamcinolone acetonide—repeated at intervals of a few weeks. Considerable resistance may be met with the first injections but this diminishes as the cheloid softens and flattens. The treatment may be combined with cryotherapy [5].

High pressure jet therapy [2, 9]. The injection of agents under high pressure enables penetration of the skin to take place without significant damage and, generally, without pain (except in the scalp and on the fingertips). An evenly distributed concentration of the agent required can be directed at the site required. Its main uses are for initiating local anaesthesia in children and for prophylactic inoculations. It has the following particular dermatological uses:

(i) The deposition of IDU into herpetic lesions [7].
(ii) The deposition of corticosteroids into nodular or cystic acne. We have found this to be effective and quick.
(iii) The treatment of localized areas of lichen simplex or pustulosis.
(iv) The treatment of cheloids [9].
(v) To speed the regrowth of hair in alopecia areata.
(vi) The treatment of granuloma annulare. Complete resolution was achieved in 68% of cases in one series [10].
(vii) The treatment of psoriasis of the nails [1–3]. In a large series of patients [2, 3] in whom nail fold injections of up to 0·2–0·3 ml were given at intervals of 2–3 weeks, a high success rate was obtained when the matrix was involved; onycholysis was less responsive. Unfortunately, the lesions recurred in one-third to one-half of those treated. Nevertheless, patients appreciate the treatment, which remains the best available for nail involvement by this disease.

The Port-o-Jet apparatus [9, 11] enables intralesional treatment to be given in multiple areas or to many patients quickly and efficiently. A smaller apparatus, the Dermojet, can also be used but must be cleaned meticulously after use to avoid blocking. If equipment is not well maintained, there is a risk if implanting particles of nickel or rubber [8]. Implantation dermoids may also occur.

REFERENCES

1 ABELL E. (1972) *Br J Dermatol* **86**, 79.
2 BLEEKER J.J. (1974) *Br J Dermatol* **91**, 97.
3 BLEEKER J.J. (1975) *Br J Dermaol* **92**, 479.
4 CALLEN J.P. (1981) *J Am Acad Dermatol* **4**, 149
5 CEILLY R.I. & BABIN R.W. (1979) *J Dermatol Surg Oncol* **5**, 54.
6 DU FOURMENTEL C., *et al* (1973). *Bull Soc Fr Dermatol Syphiligr* **80**, 238.
7 JUEL-JENSEN B.E. & MACCALLUM F.O. (1965) *Br Med J* **i**, 901.
8 LA CHAPELLE J.M., *et al* (1982) *Contact Dermatitis* **8**, 122.
9 MOYNAHAN E.J. & BOWYER A. (1965) *Br Med J* **ii**, 1541.
10 SPARROW G. & ABELL E. (1975) *Br J Dermatol* **93**, 85.
11 VERBOV J.L. & ABELL E. (1970) *Trans St Johns Hosp Dermatol Soc* **56**, 49.

Silicone [6, 7]. The dermatological use of medical grade silicone is now mainly restricted to its use as a 'cushion' in patients with persistent or painful corns or calluses [2–4]. In most other dermatological situations, it has been replaced by injectable collagen (see below). It is still used by plastic surgeons, however, in patients requiring more extensive tissue contouring and augmentation as, for example, in patients suffering from facial hemiatrophy [1, 5].

REFERENCES

1 ASHLEY F.L., *et al* (1965) *J Plast Reconstr Surg* **35**, 640.
2 BALKIN S.W. (1972) *Clin Orthop* **87**, 235.
3 BALKIN S.W. (1975) *Arch Dermatol* **11**, 1143.
4 BALKIN S.W. (1977) *J Dermatol Oncol* **3**, 612.
5 EDGERTON M.T. & WELLS J.H. (1976) *J Plast Reconstr Surg* **58**, 157.
6 LE VAN P. (1978) *J Dermatol Surg Oncol* **4**, 378.
7 SELMANOWITZ V.J. & ORENTREICH N. (1977) *J Dermatol Surg Oncol* **3**, 597.

Injectable collagen [1–3]. Over many years, attempts have been made to develop an inert type of injectable material to correct contour defects of the skin. During the last 6 yr, purified injectable bovine collagen has been available and has been widely used in clinical practice. Good success rates have been reported with this substance in the treatment of scars (e.g. acne vulgaris) and age and sun-induced rhytides and folds. Correct injection technique is crucial to obtain satisfactory results. The rate of adverse effects such as local inflammation, arthralgia, urticaria, myalgia and anti-collagen antibodies is low. Repeat implantations at intervals of 6–24 months are often needed to maintain correction of contour defects. This mode of treatment is expensive.

REFERENCES

1 CASTROW F.F. & KRULL E.A. (1983) *J Am Acad Dermatol* **9**, 889.
2 TROMOVITCH T.A., *et al* (1984) *J Am Acad Dermatol* **10**, 273.
3 WATSON W., *et al* (1983) *Cutis* **31**, 543.

MISCELLANEOUS PHYSICAL AND SURGICAL PROCEDURES

A number of diverse physical and surgical procedures are described that do not fit easily into the main categories discussed in this chapter.

Polyester fibre-web sponges. This convenient means of inducing mechanical exfoliation (epidermabrasion) in acne and other disorders involving pilosebaceous occlusion has considerable consumer appeal [1] and may be a useful aid to cleansing [2, 4]. There is at least a theoretical danger of inducing

acne mechanica with over enthusiastic use and a cumulative irritant effect may occur if it is used simultaneously with other topical anti-acne medication or topical keratolytics. We have found it helpful in keratosis pilaris. It has also been recommended for helping to remove scales in psoriasis [3].

REFERENCES

1 DUTT N.P. & ORENTREICH N. (1976) *Cutis* **17**, 604.
2 JAMES M.B. (1974) *Cutis* **14**, 432.
3 SHELLORD W.V.D. (1978) *Cutis* **21**, 415.
4 SIBLEY M.J., *et al* (1974) *Cutis* **14**, 269.

Hyperbaric oxygen [2–4]. Originally introduced as an aid to open-heart surgery, its potentialities have increased with experience [3].

The uptake of oxygen in all tissues is vastly enhanced by subjecting the body to increased atmospheric pressure. The function of oxyhaemoglobin can be supplemented by the oxygen physically dissolved in solution at a pressure of 3 atm, when the amount rises from 0·3 vol% to over 6 vol%. Intermittent hyperbaric oxygen therapy can be used to gain time and prevent peripheral tissue death when the circulation is temporarily impeded, as after fractures, with ergotamine poisoning or with severe spasm. It has been used successfully in *Clostridium welchii* infections by arresting α-toxin production [4] and in the treatment of burns [1].

Its chief use in dermatology is for the treatment of ischaemic ulceration of the legs [5], in conditions in which collateral vessels can be expected, but not in atherosclerosis [4], except for relief of pain. The specialized equipment and technique required and the risks of this form of therapy restrict its use, at least in the U.K. [2].

REFERENCES

1 GROSSMAN A.R. & YANDA R.L. (1973) In *Proc 5th Int Hyperbaric Congress*. Ed. Trapp W.G., *et al*. Burnaby, Simon Frazer University.
2 Leading Article (1978) *Br Med J* **i**, 1012.
3 *LEDINGHAM I.McA. (1965) *Proc 2nd Int Congress on Hyperbaric Oxygenation, Glasgow*, (1964). Edinburgh, Livingstone.
4 SMITH G. (1964) *Proc R Soc Med* **57**, 818.
5 SMITH G., *et al* (1962) *Lancet* **i**, 816.

Heparin. This is used in two ways in dermatology. It may be given intravenously by continuous infusion, as for disseminated intravascular coagulation states [5] or severe vasculitis progressing to gangrene [3], or it may be given subcutaneously in a dose of 5,000 units twice a day, normally injected into the skin of the abdominal wall. This has been found effective in preventing deep vein thrombosis [2, 4, 7] and can be given with advantage to recumbent patients at risk from infected leg ulcers, cellulitis, etc. This method is simple and normally requires no laboratory control—unless surgery is contemplated. It may be of value in relieving the pain of vasculitis or arteriolar types of leg and foot ulcers.

Other uses of heparin are discussed by Ryan [6].

The dose given in one series was from 45 to 135 USP units/kg body weight per day. Failure may be due to inadequate dosage [1].

REFERENCES

1 COLMAN R.W., *et al* (1974) In *Controversies in Internal Medicine.* Ed. Inglefinger F.J. Philadelphia, Saunders.
2 GALLUS A.S., *et al* (1973) *N Engl J Med* **288**, 545.
3 KISKER C.T., *et al* (1968) *J Pediatr* **73**, 748.
4 NICHOLAIDES A.N., *et al* (1972) *Lancet* **ii**, 890.
5 ROBBOYS S.J., *et al* (1973) *Br J Dermatol* **88**, 221.
6 *RYAN T.J. (1976) Microvascular Injury. Major Problems of Dermatology.* Ed. Rook A. Philadelphia, Saunders, Vol. 7, p. 383.
7 VAN VROONHOVEN T.J.M.V., *et al* (1974) *Lancet* **i**, 375.

Low molecular weight dextrans. These have been discussed on p. 1523.

Venesection (phlebotomy). The withdrawal of 500 ml blood once or twice a month leads to a considerable clinical and biochemical improvement in patients with porphyria cutanea tarda [1–4]. The decrease in photosensitivity correlates with rapid lowering of urinary uroporphyrin levels but clinical improvement is not apparent for some months. A somewhat more rapid improvement has been claimed for more frequently repeated venesections [2]. In either case these are continued until the haemoglobin level approaches 11–12 g/100 ml.

The mechanism remains uncertain and may not be due simply to reduced iron stores.

REFERENCES

1 EPSTEIN J.H. & REDEKER R.G. (1968) *N Engl J Med* **279**, 13101.
2 HARPER L.C. & BICKERS D.R. (1975) In *Year Book of Dermatology.* Eds. Malkinson F.D. & Pearson R.W. Chicago, Year Book Medical Publishers p. 34.
3 *RAMSAY C.A., *et al* (1974) Q J Med* **43**, 1.
4 WALSH J.R., *et al* (1970) *Arch Dermatol* **101**, 167.

Plasmapheresis. The technique of plasma exchange has been developed from renal transplant surgery. It is increasingly used in dermatology but is at present limited to those centres that are equipped to carry it out. Its particular value lies in the removal of circulating immune complexes and paraproteins. The disadvantage of the removal of normal immunoglobulins [1] was overcome by the use of an IBM continuous flow blood cell separator [4]. Apart from its value—often life-saving—in patients with macroglobulinaemia and cryoglobulinaemia, it has been used successfully in patients with lupus erythematosus who had disturbances of complement [6]. The exchange of 5–8 litres of plasma weekly was followed by a fall in DNA binding and loss of joint pains and proteinuria. It has also been used to remove intercellular antibodies in pemphigus [5] and in porphyria cutanea tarda [2].

Leukopheresis has been advocated in patients with malignant melanoma after sensitization to B.C.G. [3].

REFERENCES

1 GODAL H.C. & BORCHGREVINK C.F. (1965) *Scand J Clin Lab Invest* **17** (Suppl. **84**), 133.
2 HARPER L.C. & BICKERS D.R. (1975) In *Year Book of Dermatology.* Eds. Malkinson F.D. & Pearson R.W. Chicago, Year Book Medical Publishers, p. 35.
3 LEVY N.L., *et al* (1974) *Cancer* **34**, 1548.
4 POWLES R., *et al* (1971) *Br Med J* **iii**, 664.
5 RUOCCO V., *et al* (1978) *Br J Dermaol* **98**, 237.
6 VERRIER-JONES, J., *et al* (1976) *Lancet* **i**, 709.

CYTOTOXIC THERAPY [2, 5, 14, 23]

A number of different cytotoxic agents have been used topically in the treatment of malignant and pre-malignant lesions of the skin. Their use in the therapy of non-malignant conditions, e.g. condylomas, is discussed on p. 2566.

5-Fluorouracil [7, 11]. This has a long-established record [4] that has stood the test of time. Not only does it effectively destroy keratoses but it also appears able to deal with less obvious areas of actinic damage giiving a 'hold effect' [20] around treated lesions. It is used in a 1–5% cream or lotion applied once or twice a day. A propylene glycol vehicle has been recommended [11]. This can easily be compounded from an ampoule of the 5% solution. Its effect can also possibly be enhanced by the addition of sodium hydroxide, 2–5% [11]. An erythematous reaction appears in 4 or 5 days and increases in extent, with some crusting or oozing for a further 10 days. Treatment may be continued longer if necessary, or repeated at a later date. Provided that the patient persists with the treatment despite the reaction it causes, the results are excellent, though less impressive on the hands and forearms than on the face and scalp. We agree with others [2] that the addition of keratolytics or topical vitamin A acid may be of value in this situation. 5-Fluorouracil may also be combined with cryotherapy [1, 10].

Allergic contact and photosensitivity reactions have occurred from 5-fluorouracil [18]. Onycholysis followed its application around nails [19].

It is also of value in superficial malignancies of the skin such as Bowen's disease [6, 12, 22] and erythroplasia of the penis [13] but it should only be used for the most superficial type of skin malignancy [2, 17]. Even when applied with occlusion [6], recurrences are frequent [17], but reasonable results have been obtained, particularly with strengths of 5% or more [21]. There is a risk even when treating superficial basal cell carcinomas that deep tumour 'rests' will remain and lead to late and initially occult recurrence [5, 15].

Colchicine. Derivatives of the parent substance are less toxic; N-desacetylmethyl colchicine (Colcemid, omacine) has been used in strengths of 0·25–1% or more [2]. It inhibits mitosis in the metaphase. It is applied, once or twice a day, for 4 weeks, covered by an adhesive dressing, and has been used for basal cell carcinomas, Bowen's disease, leukoplakia and solar keratoses. Keratoacanthomas also apparently respond [2, 8]. We have used it as an accessory treatment after curettage and cauterization of basal cell carcinomas in situations where recurrences might be expected. Its use leads to more scarring than would otherwise occur but it may be a useful adjunct to therapy. Thiocolsiran is similar.

Methotrexate. This drug interferes with the synthesis of deoxyribonucleic acid and it may therefore be combined with colcemid to produce a synergistic effect. It is nowadays little used topically, however, in tumour therapy.

Nitrogen mustard (mechlorethamine). It has been used topically in patients suffering from mycosis fungoides (see p. 1745) [9, 24], histiocytosis X [16] and multicentric reticulohistiocytosis [3].

REFERENCES

1 ABADIR D.R. (1982) *J Dermatol Surg Oncol* **9**, 403.
2 *BELISARIO J.C. (1982) In *Skin Surgery*. Eds. Epstein E. & Epstein E., Jr. 5th ed. Springfield, Thomas, p. 667.
3 BRANDT F., *et al* (1982) *J Am Acad Dermatol* **6**, 260.
4 DILLAHA C.J., *et al* (1963) *Arch Dermatol* **88**, 247.
5 EPSTEIN E. & EPSTEIN E. JR. (Eds.) (1982) *Skin Surgery*. 5th ed. Springfield, Thomas.
6 FULTON J.E., *et al* (1968) *Arch Dermatol* **97**, 178.
7 GOETTE D.K. (1981) *J Am Acad Dermatol* **6**, 33.
8 GOETTE D.K., *et al* (1982) *Arch Dermatol* **118**, 309.
9 HAMMINGA B., *et al* (1982) *Arch Dermatol* **118**, 150.
10 HEISING R.A. (1979) *Cutis* **24**, 871.
11 JANSEN G.T. (1982) In *Skin Surgery*. Epstein E. & Epstein E., Jr. 5th ed. Springfield, Thomas, p. 661.
12 JANSEN G.T., *et al* (1967) *South Med J* **60**, 185.
13 LEWIS R.J. & BENDL B.J. (1971) *Can Med Assoc J* **104**, 148.
14 MARRON-GASCA J. (1979) *Actas Dermosilogr* **70**, 383.
15 MOHS F.E., *et al* (1978) *Arch Dermatol* **114**, 1021.
16 NETHERCOTT J.R., *et al* (1983) *Arch Dermatol* **119**, 157.
17 REYMANN F. (1972) *Dermatologica* **144**, 205.
18 SAMS W.M. (1968) *Arch Dermatol* **97**, 14.
19 SHELLEY W.B. (1972) *Acta Derm Venereol (Stockh)* **52**, 320.
20 SIMMONDS W.L. (1973) *Cutis* **12**, 615.
21 STULL H.L., JR., *et al* (1967) *J Invest Dermatol* **49**, 219.
22 STURM H.M. (1979) *J Am Acad Dermatol* **1**, 513.
23 DU VIVIER A. (1982) *Clin Exp Dermatol* **7**, 89.
24 DU VIVIER A. & VOLLUM D.I. (1980) *Br J Dermatol* **102**, 319.

LASERS
N.P.J. WALKER

Lasers of various types are now being used for the treatment of many cutaneous lesions [2]. The therapeutic application of a laser depends on its wavelength and power output, which in turn depend on the active medium—gas, solid or liquid. The choice of laser depends on the desired effect and the absorption characteristics of the target tissue.

General principles. *Laser* is an acronym for *l*ight *a*mplification by the *s*timulated *e*mission of *r*adiation. Stimulated emission occurs when a photon causes an excited atom to return to a lower energy state and release a second photon in phase and of the same wavelength as the stimulating photon. The resultant output is characterized by certain properties that make laser radiation potentially useful:

Monochromaticity ⎫
Coherence   ⎬ spatial
Collimation   ⎭ temporal

The very high degree of coherence and the lack of divergence of the beam enable extremely high and precise power densities to be achieved. Tissue effects depend on wavelength, power density (W/cm²), length of exposure and tissue absorption. Most lasers in current use have a continuous output although, if required, shuttering allows for accurate pulsing. Low power lasers are reported as being biostimulative and have been advocated for the treatment of leg ulcers and other chronic wounds. There is a paucity of controlled work and evidence for their usefulness is slight [1, 12].

Safety. Lasers are powerful energy sources which can scar and maim if used incorrectly. They should be used only in properly controlled sites by trained personnel who are taking all the necessary precautions to protect themselves and their patients from accidental exposure.

Types of laser.
Ruby (wavelength 694 nm, pulsed). This was the first laser, developed in 1960. It has been used for the treatment of pigmented and vascular lesions with some success but for mainly practical reasons it has not been widely used clinically. These practical difficulties are not insurmountable and with repeated treatments blue–black tattoos can be removed without significant scarring [11].

Argon (wavelength 488–514 nm, continuous). The blue–green visible light produced by the argon laser is absorbed by haemoglobin. This absorption is the basis for its use in the treatment of vascular lesions, especially capillary haemangiomas. The therapeutic effect, lightening in colour, depends on the radiation causing a coagulative necrosis of the blood vessels with relative sparing of the upper dermis and the epidermal appendages. For a haemangioma to be amenable to treatment the radiation must cause sufficient damage to the vessels without scarring the epidermis. To assess whether a lesion is suitable, test patches are treated. The effect is assessed after several weeks and, if satisfactory lightening without scarring has been achieved, treatment can proceed. Suitability for treatment can usually be assessed on clinical grounds. Lesions which normally respond well are deep in colour and blanch poorly on pressure. These are relatively mature lesions and are commonest in adults. The morphological features correlate with the histology. It would seem that to have a sufficient difference of absorption between the vessels and the surrounding tissues the fraction of dermis occupied by the ectatic vessels should be more than 5%, the mean vessel area should be more than 2500 μm^2 and the percentage of vessels containing erythrocytes more than 15% [9]. Pink lesions which blanch readily, commonest in young patients, respond poorly, though chilling the surface and measures to slow down the circulation may improve the response rate. Overall about 60% of adult patients can expect a definite improvement.

The argon laser is used for the treatment of other vascular lesions where selectivity of absorption may help and for the removal of tattoos and other lesions where selectivity may be less important and the relatively low power output a disadvantage [5].

Neodymium yttrium aluminium garnet (wavelength 1064 nm, continuous). This invisible radiation in the near IR is not selectively absorbed and has much greater tissue penetration than the argon laser. This permits more effective coagulation and it is used for the endoscopic treatment of haemorrhage. It offers an alternative to the carbon dioxide laser for surgical work [6].

Carbon dioxide (wavelength 10600 nm continuous). This invisible radiation, in the IR, is rapidly absorbed by water and therefore by body tissue. There is no selectivity of effect. When a beam of CO_2 laser radiation strikes body tissue the cells are vaporized almost instantaneously. Although vaporization is limited to those cells immediately in the path of the beam there is a narrow band of thermal damage to the side of the beam 30–50 μm wide. Blood vessels of less than 0·5 mm are sealed, producing a dry, almost bloodless, field. Nerve endings are also sealed; postoperative pain and morbidity are slight. Skin takes slightly longer to heal than after scalpel incision but there is little tendency to scar or stricture formation. The CO_2 laser is an extremely precise destructive device. With continuous output, via a focusing handpiece, the operator, using a high power density, can vary the depth of an incision by the speed with which he moves the beam over the surface, performing excisions as easily as with a scalpel. Lower power densities can be achieved by holding the handpiece away from the surface, defocusing the beam. This allows a variety of skin lesions to be treated. Small amounts of tissue can be vaporized with single or multiple pulses, larger amounts by repeated traverses of the beam with continuous output. The CO_2 laser has been used to treat many conditions with good effect (Table 68.3) [3, 7, 13]. For some, such as recalcitrant warts and tattoos, it might be considered to be the treatment of choice. For certain capillary haemangiomas it is better than the argon laser. In the pink lesion the CO_2 laser can be used to produce a very precise superficial burn with coagulation of the superficial capillary plexus. Marked lightening of the lesion may result but great care must be taken to avoid scarring.

TABLE 68.3. Some therapeutic applications of CO_2 laser radiation

Capillary Haemangiomas	Other vascular lesions	Cheloids
Epidermal Naevi	Warts, Condylomatas	Tattoos
Seborrhoeic Keratoses	Tumours	

Tunable dye lasers. These and other lasers, such as the xenon fluoride excimer laser, are still research tools but offer several theoretical advantages. By variation of wavelength and pulse duration they can be used to exploit the specific absorption characteristics of tissue structures to the full, thus limiting non-specific thermal damage. Dye lasers can be tuned over a finite range depending on the dye used. Tuned to 540 or 577 nm, absorption peaks of oxyhaemoglobin, they have been shown to produce more precise vascular damage than can be achieved with the argon [8]. The results of full clinical trials in the treatment of haemangiomas are awaited. Similar precise damage to melanosomes and melanocytes has been shown to occur after exposure to pulses from a xenon fluoride excimer laser [10]. This potential to control precisely intra-epidermal and dermal damage may provide useful therapeutic advances. The output of tunable dye lasers can also be used to activate haematoporphyrin derivative in photoradiation therapy of malignant tumours and might offer an effective treatment for difficult cutaneous malignancies [4].

REFERENCES

1 ABERGEL R.P., *et al* (1984) *J Amer Acad Derm* 11, 1142.
2 ARNDT K.A. & NOE J.M. (1982) *Arch Dermatol* 118, 293.
3 BAILIN P.L. (1983) In *Cutaneous Laser Therapy.* Eds. Arndt K.A., *et al* New York, Wiley, p. 187.
4 DAHLMAN A., *et al* (1983) *Cancer Res* 43, 430.
5 LANDTHALER M., *et al* (1984) *J Derm Surg Onc* 10, 456.
6 LANDTHALER M., *et al* (1986) *J Amer Acad Derm* 14, 107.
7 LEVINE H.L. & BAILIN P.L. (1982) *Arch Otolaryngol* 108, 236.
8 MORELLI J.G. *et al* (1986) *Lasers Surg Med* 6, 94.
9 NOEL J.M., *et al* (1980) *Plast Reconstr Surg* 65, 130.
10 PARRISH J.A. (1985) *Arch Dermatol* 121, 599.
11 REID W.H., *et al* (1983) *Br J Plast Surg* 36, 455.
12 SURINCHAK J.S., *et al* (1983) *Lasers Surg Med* 2, 267.
13 WALKER N.P.J. (1983) *Br J Dermatol* 109 (Suppl. 24), 17.

IONIZING RADIATION [3, 13, 14, 26, 27]

Sources of ionizing radiation other than X-rays will not be considered here. Such use as they have in dermatological practice is almost completely limited to malignant conditions and they fall into the orbit of the specialist radiotherapist. Mention should be made, however, of the well-recognized place of the whole body electron beam therapy for mycosis fungoides and exfoliative dermatitis, though the advent of PUVA has lessened the use of X-rays for these conditions. Older techniques of radiotherapy have been succeeded by extremely refined and sophisticated methods of delivery of exact doses of ionizing radiation to exactly defined areas. Developments in this branch of medicine have been such that the dermatologist has become progressively less involved in this form of treatment, preferring to leave it to experts in this field. Moreover, superficial radiotherapy has lost much of its appeal and usefulness with the advent of corticosteroids. Many dermatologists have no cause to use it; others, infrequently. The recognition that there is no 'safe mimimum dose', especially in young subjects, and the incidence of leukaemia or thyroid carcinoma [35] in children following quite small doses of radiotherapy support this reluctance. There is much to be said for abandoning X-ray therapy for non-malignant conditions [35] or at least for restricting it to appropriate conditions that have failed to respond to the expert and adequate use of other forms of therapy [15]*. Nevertheless, it will doubtless continue to be used widely for some time to come by dermatologists in those countries in which it is a traditional part of their equipment, or where radiotherapy centres are few and far between. In this section, therefore, we shall attempt to delineate those areas in which it has been mostly used with apparent success. The placebo effect of treatment with imposing instrumentation and ritual is likely to be considerable and it is regrettable that many of those advocates of the value of X-ray therapy in benign conditions have so seldom attempted to substantiate their claims with properly controlled studies.

In the section that follows, the use of ionizing radiation in the treatment of malignant conditions

*Codes of Practice in regard to protection against ionizing radiation differ in different countries, but attention is particularly drawn to the *Code of Practice for the Protection of Persons against Ionizing Radiation arising from Medical and Dental Use,* issued by Her Majesty's Stationery Office [64, 106] and to a similar memorandum applicable to nurses and ancillary staff [65, 109].

will not be discussed. The reader is advised to consult standard references on the subject [6, 9, 31, etc.].

Standards, terms and sources. These are discussed in detail in specialized texts.

The effect of radiation on the tissues [28]. This has been dealt with by numerous authors. Mitosis is inhibited, chromosomal breaks occur and changes in the vascular and enzyme systems take place. The biological damage depends on the total energy absorbed and the ion density in the radiation track.

Fractionated doses may be given weekly [5] or even daily [8]. Satisfactory results have been obtained with three doses of 300 rad at 3-weekly intervals [15, 27]. The total dose should not exceed 1,500 rad in any one year, or 5,000 rad in a lifetime.

Dermatological indications. Only benign conditions of the skin will be considered here. The place of ionizing radiation in the treatment of malignant tumours and lymphomas is discussed in the relevant chapters. Such treatment comes into the specialized province of the radiotherapist, who is better equipped to choose the preferred mode of therapy and to carry out careful follow-up and epidemiological studies. However, in some countries it remains the province of the dermatologist, who will have received special training in this field.

The remaining indications are, broadly, as follows.

(*i*) *Benign tumours and hyperplasias*, e.g. keratoacanthomas and lymphocytomas, especially the circumscribed form [4].

(*ii*) *Cheloids*. The result of radiotherapy alone, even in early lesions, is disputed. The argument is well summarized by Rowell [27]. Postoperative radiation is more effective but carries its own hazards. Steroids, intralesionally, alone or combined with radiotherapy [6] probably afford the best approach. A combined surgical excision and iridium implant technique has its advocates.

(*iii*) *Sycosis barbae*. In those few cases resistant to antibiotics, an epilating dose may be of value.

(*iv*) *Granulomas*. X-irradiation is useful, sometimes the preferred treatment, for a number of persistent granulomas (facial, eosinophilic, etc.). The reader is referred to the appropriate chapter.

(*v*) *Darier's disease and familial benign chronic pemphigus*. These are particularly suitable for Grenz ray therapy, which often causes prolonged remission of the latter [30] and, occasionally, complete clearing of the former [17].

(*vi*) *Eczema* [15] Resistant patches of lichenified eczema are still treated by conventional Grenz rays in fractionated doses. There are no adequate studies to confirm the long-term value of this form of treatment. In a few cases—as in long-established pruritus ani—it may help break the 'itch–scratch' cycle, but there is probably a strong placebo effect. Controlled studies have shown that 300 rad (3 Gy) of conventional superficial X-ray therapy is superior to 900 rad (9 Gy) in the treatment of constitutional eczema of the hands [15].

(*vii*) *Psoriasis and hypertrophic lichen planus*. The temptation to use ionizing radiation in chronic and persistent conditions that respond with difficulty to topical therapy is obviously great. There may also be a place for it in palmoplantar pustulosis and anogenital psoriasis in the elderly [6]. Grenz rays are safer than conventional X-rays if the dose is likely to be repeated.

(*viii*) *Herpes simplex*. Success has been claimed in preventing recurrences of this condition, especially with Grenz rays, 200 rad every 2 weeks for four doses [18], but adequately controlled studies have not been carried out.

(*ix*) *Acne and rosacea*. Much used in the past for these conditions, superficial X-ray therapy has lost much of its place in treatment since the advent of the broad spectrum antibiotics and retinoids, but fractionated doses retain a certain importance in the occasional patient with acne who is not controlled by other conventional therapy [6, 10, 25]. Good, though temporary, suppression of facial acne with four weekly doses of 100 rad may be obtained. The thyroid gland must be very carefully shielded.

Finally, mention should be made of *warts* and *angiomas*, if only to condemn its use utterly in the former and to express considerable reserve about its use in the latter, even for rapidly extending angiomas or those interfering with suckling or feeding; these are better treated by steroids, even though there is no apparent increased risk of subsequent cancer from irradiation with 300–600 rad at 50 kV [20].

Many workers find Grenz rays ineffective in treating port-wine stain [9, 17] but others [6, 27] believe that a satisfactory though partial paling may be achieved. The total dose, however, given over a period of years, has to be in the region of 6,000–12,000 rad.

X-ray epilation. This standard treatment for tinea capitis in the past has been almost completely superceded by specific antifungal drugs, though it provides a rapid 'one-visit' treatment that still commends itself to the circumstances of epidemic tinea in primitive communities. The difficulty of ensuring an even dose of radiation over the scalp has not been entirely overcome. Permanent hair loss may result and there is a greater than expected incidence of malignant and leukaemic changes in later life [37].

Precautions. Though X-rays have been extensively used by dermatologists since their earliest days with a reasonably clean record for safety, accidents and errors of judgement are more disastrous in this field than most. All forms of ionizing radiation are cumulative. This emphasizes the need for constant care to safeguard both patient and the operator. With the centralization in the U.K. of most X-ray therapy in regional radiotherapy centres, the dangers of accidental damage are far less than previously, though these still occur [18]. In countries where radiotherapy centres do not exist or are far apart, superficial radiotherapy, including the treatment of tumours, is still carried out by the dermatologist with machines that may not be fully automatic or well calibrated.

Superficial radiotherapy should only be given by those trained in the technique and the patient must understand the nature of the treatment and disclose any previous radiotherapy given by others. Careful records, preferably duplicated and separated from the case notes, must be retained indefinitely. The machine must be calibrated regularly by expert personnel. In the U.K. the Area Radiological Protection Adviser should be consulted about safety precautions. These must include careful and adequate screening of the patient from scattered [12] as well as direct [35] radiation and regular blood counts of the staff. The abdomen or pelvis should never be exposed to radiotherapy in early or suspected pregnancy. The operator should wear fully protective clothing and a monitoring film that is checked regularly.

Types of superficial radiotherapy. These are
  (a) conventional superficial X-radiation [15]
  (b) Grenz (Bucky) rays [15]
  (c) beryllium window modification
  (d) contact low-voltage therapy.

Conventional superficial X-radiation. 50–100 kV are used to produce a beam with a half value layer (HVL) of 0·5–1·0 mm Al. Doses of 60–100 rad are normally given at intervals of 1–3 weeks to a total of 300–750 rad. The lower figure is often as satisfactory as the higher one [21, 26] and enables a series of three to four courses to be given in a lifetime with complete safety [15, 27].

Grenz rays [8, 15, 17]. These very soft rays, delivered at 6–15 kV, have considerably less penetration than conventional X-rays and are thus particularly useful for very superficial conditions. The HVL is 0·018–0·033 mm Al and 90% of the radiation is absorbed by the upper 1 mm of skin.

Hazards and sequelae. These are far less with Grenz rays than with conventional X-rays. Scatter is minimal and close shielding is unnecessary. Although the safety factor is very large, particularly in relation to gonad region irradiation, it is extremely important that the machine is calibrated regularly by qualified physicists [39].

The main side effect is the frequent development of pigmentation, which may be very slow to clear. The risk is reduced if close screening is avoided. The incidence of chronic radiodermatitis and late carcinoma is extremely low, although a few cases have been reported in patients who had been given quite high doses [7, 9].

The beryllium window. As a modification of conventional therapy this has not received wide use in the U.K. but it has become established in Grenz ray therapy.

Contact low-voltage therapy (29–45 kV). This is particularly used for the accurate application of a powerful but superficial dose of X-radiation and is particularly valuable for the treatment of basal cell carcinomas. It will not be considered here.

REFERENCES

1 ALBERT R.E., *et al* (1966) *Am J Public Health* **56**, 2114.
2 ALBRIGHT E.C. & ALLDAY R.W. (1967) *JAMA* **199**, 280.
3 *BAER R.L. & WITTEN V.H. (1956) *Year Book of Dermatology*, 1955–56. Chicago, Year Book Medical Publishers, p. 7.
4 BAFVERSTEDT B. (1962) *Acta Derm Venereol (Stockh)* **42**, 3.
5 BRAUER E.W. (1975) In *Current Dermatologic Management*. Ed. Madden S. 2nd ed. St Louis, Mosby, p. 25.
6 *BRAUN-FALCO O. & LUKACS S. (1973) *Dermatologische Röntgen-therapie*. Berlin, Springer.

7 BRODKIN R.H. & BLEIBERG J. (1968) *Arch Dermatol* **97**, 307.

8 *BUCKY G.P. & COOMBES F.C. (1954) *Grenz Ray Therapy. Principles, Methods, Clinical Application.* New York, Springer.

9 *CIPOLLARO A.C. & CROSSLAND P.M. (1967) *X-rays and Radium in the Treatment of Diseases of the Skin.* Philadelphia, Lea & Febiger.

10 CUNLIFFE W.J. & COTTERILL J.A. (1975) *The Acnes. Clinical Features, Pathogenesis and Treatment.* London, Saunders, p. 233.

11 DELAWTER D.S. & WINSHE P.T. (1963) *Cancer* **16**, 1028.

12 DOMONKOS A. & CAMERON S.H. (1957) *Arch Dermatol* **76**, 694.

13 *ELLINGER F. (1941) *The Biologic Fundamentals of Radiation Therapy.* New York, Elsevier.

14 *EPSTEIN E. (1965) *Arch Dermatol* **92**, 307.

15 FAIRRIS G.M., et al (1985) *Br J Dermatol* **112**, 339.

16 GOLDSCHMIDT H. (1975) *Arch Dermatol* **111**, 1511.

17 *HOLLANDER M.B. (1968) *Ultrasoft Rays.* Baltimore, Williams & Williams.

18 KNIGHT A.G. (1972) *Br J Dermatol* **86**, 172.

19 KOLAR J., et al (1967) *Arch Dermatol* **96**, 427.

20 LI F.P., et al (1974) *Radiology* **113**, 177.

21 MIESCHER G. (1953) *Dermatologica* **107**, 225.

22 MIESCHER G. & BÖHM C. (1948) *Schweiz Med Wochenschr* **78**, 14.

23 MOLE R.H. (1972) *Br J Radiol* **45**, 613.

24 PEGUM J.S. (1972) *Br J Radiol* **45**, 613.

25 REISNER R.M. (1975) In *Current Dermatologic Management.* Ed. Madden S. 2nd ed. St Louis, Mosby.

26 *ROWELL N.R. (1973) *Br J Dermatol* **88**, 583.

27 *ROWELL N.R. (1977) In *Recent Advances in Dermatology.* Ed. Rook A.J. 4th ed. Edinburgh, Churchill Livingstone, p. 329.

28 RUBIN P. & CASARETT G.W. (1968) *Clinical Radiation Pathology.* Vol. 1. Philadelphia, Saunders.

29 RYAN T.J. (1972) In *Textbook of Dermatology.* Eds. Rook A.J., et al. 2nd ed,. Oxford, Blackwell, p. 469.

30 SARKANY I. (1957) *Br J Dermatol* **71**, 247.

31 SHEARD C. (1978) *Treatment of Skin Disease.* Chicago, Year Book Medical Publishers, p. 259.

32 STORCK H. (1972) In *Handbuch des Medizinischen Radiologie.* Berlin, Springer, Vol. XII, p. 17.

33 SULZBERGER M.D., et al (1952) *Arch Dermatol* **65**, 639.

34 SWEET R.D. (1962) *Br J Dermatol* **74**, 392.

35 SWEET R.D. (1968) *Br J Dermatol* **80**, 265.

36 STEWART W.D., et al (1958) *J Invest Dermatol* **30**, 237.

37 VISFELDT J. (1964) *Acta Radiol* **2**, 95.

38 WILSOM G.M., et al (1958) *Br Med J* **ii**, 929.

39 WITTEN V.H. (1960) *Arch Dermatol* **81**, 110.

THORIUM X [1–3]

Thorium X, a natural isotope of radium with a half-life of 3·64 days, is now virtually obsolete in dermatological practice. It was previously used in the treatment of 'port-wine' naevi but the results were indifferent and controlled studies did not confirm its value. Such beneficial effects as did occur were probably due to the β and γ radiation emitted in addition to the supposed pure α particle emission.

For this reason extreme precautions must be taken in the application and disposal of the material. Ventilation must be adequate.

Grenz rays can be employed more accurately and satisfactorily in all conditions that might have benefitted from thorium X.

REFERENCES

1 HENDERSON O.S. & PINKUS H. (1954) *J Invest Dermatol* **22**, 463.

2 LOMHOLT S. (1936) *Br J Dermatol* **48**, 567.

3 PINKUS H. (1949) *J Invest Dermatol* **12**, 61.

Formulary of Topical Applications

D. S. WILKINSON

Since the last edition of this textbook there has been a major change in the presentation of the *British National Formulary* (B.N.F.), the standard reference book for prescribing in Great Britain. It is now published twice yearly in pocket-book form and contains not only a complete list of official preparations but also those proprietary preparations on the British market at the time of publication. The B.N.F. will therefore contain virtually all the topical formulations that the dermatologist will need and there seems little point in duplicating them here. Though the detailed formulation of some agents in everyday use, zinc, sulphur, salicylic acid, etc., may vary slightly from country to country, dermatologists will also have their own National Formularies or lists to refer to.

There are a small number of particular formulae, however, that have been evolved by individual dermatologists or used with success over long periods in particular hospitals; some of these, such as depigmenting creams, fill a void; others involve variations in the vehicle or active agents. As these are all of potential and continuing value, they form the basis of this Formulary. We shall also, however, include a small selection of the most commonly used official B.N.F. preparations (marked *), since they are frequently referred to in other chapters.

The whole field of topical dermatological formulation is currently covered in detail by Polano in *Topical Skin Therapeutics* [17]—a comprehensive guide to the subject. The principles of topical therapy are discussed in Chapter 65. Other British sources of information are mentioned in the references. Other readers—notably in the U.S.A. and Europe—will have their own handbooks that will repair the deficiencies of this small selection, for which the author takes full responsibility.

I am particularly indebted to the editors of the B.N.F. for permission to include some of their material, to Mrs S. Lomas, Senior Pharmacist of Wycombe General Hospital, for her continued help and advice and to all those contributors who have given me the formulations of their own hospitals.

The preparations are grouped conventionally according to their physical type or use. The following abbreviations are used:

A.H.   Addenbrooke's Hospital, Cambridge
A.P.F.   Australian *Pharmaceutical Formulary and Handbook*, 1978
B.P.   British *Pharmacopoeia*, 1980
B.P.C.   *British Pharmaceutical Codex*, 1973; *Supplement*, 1976
B.R.I.   Bristol Royal Infirmary
G.O.S.   Hospital for Sick Children, Gt Ormond Street
L.G.I.   Leeds General Infirmary
P.C.   *Pharmaceutical Codex*, 1979
P.N.   *Pharmacopoeia Nordica*, 1963
Pr.   Proprietary preparation
R.V.I.   Royal Victoria Infirmary, Newcastle upon Tyne
S.G.H.   St George's Hospital, London
S.J.H.   St John's Hospital for Diseases of the Skin, London
S.R.I.   Sheffield Royal Infirmary
S.T.H.   St Thomas' Hospital, London
U.S.P.   *United States Pharmacopoeia*
W.G.H.   Wycombe General Hospital

VEHICLES AND BLAND PREPARATIONS

Vehicles (or bases) are powders, oils, greases or liquids which alone or in biphasic or triphasic mixtures form relatively stable agents that have two functions: they act as vehicles for the incorporation of active ingredients and they often have soothing and emollient qualities of their own. Because of their widespread use, a number of official (*) formulae are included in this section.

Aqueous cream B.P.C.*
An oil-in-water emulsion of 30% emulsifying ointment with phenoxyethanol 1% as a preservative.

Cetomacrogol cream B.P.C.* (Formula A)
Cetomacrogol emulsifying ointment   30

Chlorocresol   0·1
Freshly boiled and cooled purified water   to 100

A diluent, e.g. for corticosteroid creams or for the incorporation of triphenylmethane dyes, etc.

Cetomacrogol cream B.P.C.* (Formula B)
Cetomacrogol emulsifying ointment   30
Methyl hydroxybenzoate   0·15
Propyl hydroxybenzoate   0·08
Benzyl alcohol   1·5
Freshly boiled and cooled purified water   to 100
    As above. Note the difference in preservative.

Emulsifying ointment B.P.C.*
Emulsifying wax   30
Liquid paraffin   20
White soft paraffin   50
    Can also be used as a soap substitute skin cleanser or as an emollient. May be diluted with water but, without preservative, has a short shelf-life.

Emulsifying wax B.P.*
Cetostearyl alcohol   90 g
Sodium lauryl sulphate   10 g
Water   4 ml

Hydrophilic ointment U.S.P.
Propylene glycol   12
Stearyl alcohol   25
White soft paraffin   25
Sodium lauryl sulphate   1
Purified water   to 100
    Contains methyl and propyl parabens, 0·25%. It may be diluted with water.

Hydrous wool fat ointment B.P.C.*
Hydrous wool fat and yellow soft paraffin, equal parts.

Orabase, Orahesive (Pr.)
A gel or adhesive powder of carboxymethylcellulose, pectin and gelatin as a protective or vehicle for oral mucosa.

Stomahesive (Pr.) [9]
Pectin, gelatin, carboxymethylcellulose and polyisobutylene on a polythene backing
    For stoma care. Varihesive, [1, 2] used for leg ulcers, is similar.

Topical antibiotic vehicle (B.R.I.)
Propylene glycol   4
Water for irrigation   8
Isopropyl alcohol   to 40 parts

Add contents of capsules to make a 1% (or as desired) solution. If made in bulk and pressurized, the shelf-life is 6 months.

Topical antibiotic vehicle (W.G.H.)
Industrial methylated spirit BP (95%)   66
Propylene glycol   4·5
Distilled water   to 90
    Add contents of capsules to make a 1–1·5% solution. Shelf-life 4 weeks.

WET DRESSINGS AND BATHS
Aluminium acetate is widely used for wet dressings in the U.S.A. and elsewhere. In the U.K., potassium permanganate is favoured, despite its staining. Silver nitrate ('black wash') has been used for burns and leg ulcers.

Aluminium acetate lotion* (Burow's solution A.P.F.)
Aluminium acetate solution   5
Purified water, freshly boiled and cooled,   to 100
    It contains about 0·65% of the salts. It must be freshly prepared and is used undiluted.

Chlorinated lime and boric acid solution B.P. (Eusol)
Chlorinated lime   1·25
Boric acid   1·25
Water   to 100
    Contains not less than 0·25% available chlorine. It is applied as wet dressings, especially for wounds and ulcers. Use within 1 week.

Eusol and liquid paraffin (L.G.I.)
Eusol and liquid paraffin, equal parts, with 1% beeswax (this can be omitted if the mixture is shaken before use (W.G.H.)).
    For infected leg ulcers. Use within 2 weeks.

Formaldehyde lotion*
Formaldehyde lotion, 3% in water
    It must be freshly prepared.
Glutaraldehyde 10% solution, buffered with sodium bicarbonate 10% [13], is also used for hyperhidrosis of hands and feet but stains temporarily brown.

Potassium permanganate solution*
A 0·1% solution in distilled water is usually dispensed. This must be diluted to 1 in 7 to 1 in 10 with water before use for wet dressings. If crystals are used, these must first be dissolved in water and diluted until this becomes a pale pink colour.

Silver nitrate lotion*

Silver nitrate, 0·5% in distilled or deionized water

It must be freshly prepared and protected from light. Prolonged or widespread use may cause leaching of electrolytes, requiring replacement therapy.

Sodium hypochlorite solution, diluted, B.P.

Contains about 1% available chlorine

Use only diluted solutions containing no more than 0·5% available chlorine on skin or in wounds. A 0·5% solution, freshly prepared, has been suggested for herpes simplex, rubbed in for 30 s twice daily, or a 0·1% solution for mucosal lesions [11].

LOTIONS

Calamine liniment (L.G.I.)

Calamine	8
Lanolin	7
Lime water	50
Arachis oil	to 100

Less drying than calamine lotion (see also Calamine lotion, oily, P.C.*)

Calamine lotion (S.J.H.)

Calamine	15
Zinc oxide	5
Glycerol	5
Water	to 100

To which may be added, usually in the strengths indicated, argyrol 0·25%, liquefied phenol 1%, precipitated sulphur 2%, etc.

Copper and zinc sulphate lotion, B.P.C. (Dalibour Water)

Copper sulphate 1% and zinc sulphate 1·5% in camphor water 2·5%; water to 100%

An astringent application.

Domiphen bromide and hydrocortisone lotion (G.O.S.)

Domiphen bromide lotion (G.O.S.)	60 ml
(Domiphen bromide	2·5 g
Propylene glycol	620 ml
Industrial methylated spirit B.P. (95%)	125 ml
Purified water	to 5 L)
Hydrocortisone lotion B.P.C.	20 ml

Use within 1 month. A mild antiseptic lotion useful for exudative eczematous or ulcerated lesions in young children.

Thymol scalp lotion (W.G.H.)

Thymol	0·5
Industrial methylated spirit B.P. (95%)	73·75

Distilled water	to 100

A perfume may be added. A non-toxic scalp lotion; a placebo for alopecia areata, etc.

Zinc liniment P.N.

Zinc oxide	12·5
Talc	12·5
Alcohol (70%)	12·5
Glycerol	12·5
Water	to 100

An official example of a shake lotion.

PAINTS, VARNISHES AND TINCTURES

Brilliant green and crystal violet paint B.P.C.*

0·5% of each in equal parts of alcohol (90%) and water

To be used undiluted. Either dye may be used alone or in an aqueous or alcoholic base.

Magenta paint (colourless (S.T.H.))

Boric acid	800 mg
Phenol	4 g
Resorcinol	10 g
Acetone	4 ml
Alcohol 90%	8·5 ml
Water	to 100 ml

As for Castellani's paint.

Resorcin paint (A.H.)

Resorcin	2·5
Acetone	1·5
Boric acid	1·5
Water	to 100

Another colourless 'Magenta paint'.

Sulphacetamide tincture [17]

15% in 50–70% industrial methylated spirit

For onycholysis and chronic paronychia.

Wart applications

Cantharidin wart paint

Cantharidin 0·7% in equal parts of acetone and collodion

Apply with a small brush and breathe on it to dry it rapidly. For periungual warts.

*Podophyllin compound paint B.P.C.***

Podophyllin resin 15% in compound benzoin tincture

Various modifications of strength (10–25%) and base (industrial methylated spirit) abound in various formulae. If a spirit base is used the surrounding skin should be protected with yellow soft paraffin.

Contra-indicated in pregnancy.

Wart application (S.T.H.)

| Salicylic acid | 70 g |
| Linseed oil | 100 ml |

Apply exactly to the wart. Protect surrounding skin with paraffin or wart paste. Allow to dry.

Wart paint (B.R.I.)

Formaldehyde solution	25 ml
Acetone	60 ml
Salicylic acid	60 g
Flexible collodion	to 500 ml

Wart paint [4]

Lactic acid	16
Salicylic acid	16
Flexible collodion	to 100

Wart paste (B.R.I.)

Trichloroacetic acid	5 g
(or liquefied trichloroacetic acid	3·1 ml)
Salicylic acid	12 g
Glycerol	5 ml

Several proprietary formulae are marketed, notably wart paints similar to wart paint [4] above. Glutaraldehyde, 10% aqueous, and more preparations based on salicylic acid are also available.

Other therapeutic agents are discussed in Chapter 20.

EMOLLIENTS

These are designed to soften or to give the impression of softening or smoothing the surface of the skin. The older greasy preparations have been supplanted to a great extent by formulations designed to increase hydration of the stratum corneum, making use of lactates, urea, etc. A wide variety of different preparations are now available as proprietary products or cosmetic 'moisturizers'. Some of the formulae listed under Vehicles are also used for this purpose by patients. A small selection of other emollients are listed here.

Bath emollient (W.G.H.)

Liquid paraffin	55
Anhydrous lanolin	5·5
Cetamacrogol emulsifying Wax B.P.	1
Nipagin M	0·1
Distilled water	to 100

Add two tablespoonfuls (30 ml) to a bath and mix well.

Emollient ointment (L.G.I.)

Salicylic acid	2
Glycerol	20
Lanolin	20
Olive oil	20
Emulsifying ointment B.P.	20
Yellow soft paraffin	

Glycerol–water lotion (W.G.H.)

Tragacanth powder	0·5 g
Absolute alcohol (99%)	1·0 ml
Glycerol	25 ml
Water	to 100 ml

The only application tolerated by a patient with an excessively sensitive unstable psoriasis.

CREAMS

Acetic acid ('Samaritan') cream (W.G.H.)

Acetic acid	30
Nipagen M	0·03
Arachis oil	20
Emulsifying wax B.P.	15
Distilled water	35

A dressing for leg ulcers.

Clioquinol cream

1–3% in a water-miscible base

Crystal violet cream (W.G.H.)

| Crystal violet (or brilliant green) | 0·1–1·0 |
| Cetomacrogol cream (Formula A) | to 100 |

For acute infected eczemas of hands and feet.

Lanette wax cream [16]

Lanette wax SX	10
Arachis oil	10
Methyl paraben	0·5
Water	to 100

A simple oil-in-water cream. Emulsifying wax B.P. can be substituted for lanette wax.

Zinc cream (S.J.H.)

Zinc oxide	10
Wool fat	2·5
Arachis oil	37·5
Emulsifying wax	2·5
Water	to 100

To which ichthammol 2% may be added ('Ichthammol cream').

GELS

Glycerin of starch B.P.*
Wheat starch 8·5% heated with water and glycerol until it gelatinizes
(The formula varies in different countries.)

Salicylic acid gel (S.G.H., B.R.I.)
Salicylic acid	60 g
Propylene glycol	200 ml
Industrial methylated spirit B.P. (95%)	250 ml
Glycerin	50 ml
Tragacanth	50 g
Water for irrigation	410 ml

A similar proprietary preparation is available.

OINTMENTS

These more or less greasy applications are used for non-exudative lesions or for those in which a protective or keratolytic effect is required. They form excellent vehicles for delivery of active agents to the skin. Modern adjuvants and emulsifying agents have blurred the distinction between creams and ointments, but as these usually have no water content they seldom require the addition of preservatives.

Greasy ointments may be divided into true fats, waxes, mineral greases and macrogols. They are well represented in National Formularies.

Aluminium subacetate ointment P.N.
Aluminium subacetate	1·6
Water	18·4
Wool fat	40
Yellow soft paraffin	40

Benzoic acid compound ointment B.P.* (Whitfield's Ointment)
Benzoic acid 6% and salicylic acid 3% in emulsifying ointment P.C.

Still an effective and cheap antifungal preparation. Use half-strength in the groin.

Coal tar ointment (S.J.H.)
Solution of coal tar	12
Lanolin	10
Yellow soft paraffin	to 100

Coal tar and salicylic acid ointment, B.P.*
Coal tar and salicylic acid, 2% of each, in a complex paraffin–coconut oil emulsified base
A useful but little used preparation.

Paraffin ointment B.P.
Hard paraffin	3
White beeswax	2
Cetostearyl alcohol	5
White soft paraffin	90

A protective for fissured skin or lips.

PASTES

These are either greasy pastes, e.g. powder in a greasy vehicle, or drying or cooling pastes, e.g. powder in a liquid base. The latter are not used in the U.K. as much as elsewhere and their useful properties are somewhat neglected.

Burow's paste (1,2,3 Paste) [16]
Burow's solution	1
Lanolin	2
Zinc paste	3

There are many variations on this theme.

Coal tar solution paste (L.G.I.)
Coal tar solution	25
Zinc oxide	5
Yellow soft paraffin	to 100

For chronic eczema. To clean, use arachis oil on cotton wool or aqueous cream.

Coal tar paste B.P.C.*
Strong solution of coal tar	7·5 g
Compound zinc paste B.P.	92·5 g
(Zinc oxide	25
Starch	25
White soft paraffin	50)

Magnesium sulphate paste B.P.C. (Morison's Paste)
Magnesium sulphate 45% and phenol 0·5% in anhydrous glycerol
Keep in an airtight container. Stir before use.

Titanium dioxide paste P.C.*
Titanium dioxide 20%, zinc oxide 25%, kaolin 10%, with red precipitated ferric oxide, glycerin, chlorocresol and water
A greaseless paste, UV repellant. Salicylic acid remains active in this vehicle.

Vioform and zinc paste (S.J.H.)
Vioform 1% in zinc paste B.P.C. or in coal tar paste B.P.C.

Zinc and salicylic acid paste B.P.C. ('Lassar's Paste')
Salicylic acid	2
Zinc oxide	24
Starch	24

White soft paraffin   50

See [16] with regard to inactivation of salicylic acid in this formula. But it is a necessary ingredient when this is used as a paste base for dithranol.

Zinc paste P.N.
40% zinc oxide, 60% yellow soft paraffin

Paste vehicles for dithranol (anthralin). Modifications on the original Lassar's Paste are designed to give greater adhesion or flexibility in different climatic conditions, chiefly by varying the amount of hard and soft paraffin.

Dithranol paste, standard [6, 19]
Dithranol   0·4
Salicylic acid   2
Zinc oxide   25
Starch   25
White soft paraffin of melting point 46 °C
(for U.K.)   to 100

5–15% hard paraffin (melting point 49 °C) can be substituted with advantage e.g. 7·5% at W.G.H.

Lassar's Paste for dithranol (R.V.I.; S.T.H.)
Salicylic acid   2
Zinc oxide   24
Starch   24
Hard paraffin   10
Yellow soft paraffin   40

An example of the stiffer paste.

Soft dithranol paste (Pr.) [20]

A variant of the above is available as a 'stiffened dithranol ointment'.

Starch–dithranol paste [16]
Starch   40
Soft paraffin   to 100

Avoids the interaction of zinc oxide and dithranol.

SCALP PREPARATIONS

The relative paucity of official preparations for the scalp contrasts with the variety of unofficial formulations used by different skin departments in the U.K. and underlines the difficulty in obtaining an effective and acceptable vehicle, particularly for women with long hair. Those containing cade oil, tar or salicylic acid are used in any crusted or scaly scalp condition; those containing dithranol are specifically for psoriasis. They are normally applied overnight before shampooing the following morning.

Coal tar pomade (L.G.I.)
Coal tar solution   6
Salicylic acid   2
Emulsifying ointment P.C.   to 100

Coconut oil compound ointment (S.J.H.)
Coal tar solution   12
Precipitated sulphur   4
Salicylic acid   2
Coconut oil   60
Yellow soft paraffin   9
Emulsifying wax B.P.   13

Compound coconut oil ointment (A.H.)
Coal tar solution   10
Salicylic acid   2
Precipitated sulphur   4
Coconut oil   50
Cetamacrogol emulsifying wax P.C.   32

Cradle cap ointment (S.T.H.)
Salicylic acid   1
Precipitated sulphur   2
Coal tar solution   2
Emulsifying ointment   to 100

As implied, but also for mildly crusted lesions in adults.

Dithranol pomade (B.R.I.)
Dithranol   1·2
Salicylic acid   1·2
Yellow soft paraffin   16·8
Emulsifying ointment P.C.   370·2

Incorporate dithranol and then salicylic acid into the paraffin by trituration. Add to warmed emulsifying ointment. (Proprietary pomades are also marketed.)

Dithranol pomade (L.G.I.)
Dithranol 0·5–1 part in emulsifying wax B.P. 25 parts and liquid paraffin to 100 parts

New pomade (B.R.I.)
Salicylic acid   2
Coal tar solution   6
Polysorbate (Tween) 20   1
Emulsifying ointment P.C.   91

Oil of cade ointment (W.G.H.)
Cade oil   6
Precipitated sulphur   3
Salicylic acid   2
Emulsifying ointment P.C.   89

Salicylated scalp oil
1–2% salicylic acid in arachis or castor oil or in a proprietary baby oil
  Useful for mild scaling conditions.

CLEANSING AGENTS AND SHAMPOOS

Cleansing agents. Emulsifying Ointment B.P.C. or Aqueous Cream B.P.C. are commonly prescribed in the U.K. Arachis or other vegetable oils are useful for cleaning off pastes. Several antiseptic and antibacterial solutions, creams, lotions and concentrates are available commercially and are widely used. Some simple agents, still widely used, are noted below. See also the section on wet dressings and soaks.

*Hydrogen peroxide B.P.C.** Solutions of 3% (10 vol), 6% (20 vol), and 27% (about 90 vol) are available. Bleaches fabric. Solutions above 6% should be diluted before being applied to the skin.

*Soap spirit B.P.C.** (soft soap)
Soft soap 65% wt/vol. in industrial methylated spirit B.P.

Zinc peroxide paste
Zinc peroxide paste [15]. 50% sterilized zinc peroxide powder in *sterile* distilled water freshly prepared for each treatment
  Prepared packs can be made available for immediate ward mixing.

Shampoos. The enormous variety of cosmetic and proprietary medicated shampoos will serve almost every purpose, but there are rare occasions when a non-perfumed or non-detergent-based scalp cleanser may be required.

Cade oil shampoo [18]

Oil of cade	10
Triethanolamine	10
Spirit soap	to 100

  Leave on for 2 h before washing off.

Detergent shampoo

Lanette wax SX	1
Sodium lauryl sulphate	6·5
Water	to 100

  Not particularly elegant but simple to prepare in bulk and free from perfume.

Ether soap (S.T.H.)

Soft soap	35
Industrial methylated spirit P.C.	20
Water	10
Solvent ether	to 100

PROTECTIVE AND SCREENING APPLICATIONS

Bland protective agents may be used around infected wounds and ulcers, natural exudates or artificial openings discharging intestinal fluid. They may also be used around patches of psoriasis that are being treated with dithranol.

  Screening against UV light is now well provided by cosmetic and proprietary preparations. A general purpose UV screen is included, however.

All purpose light barrier (Dundee light screen) [14]

Titanium dioxide	20
Zinc oxide	6
Kaolin	2
Red ferric oxide	1
Mexenone	4
Cream base	to 100

  Modify colour with brown ferric oxide to match skin.

Aluminium compound paste B.P.C. (Baltimore Paste)
Aluminium powder 20%, zinc oxide 40% and liquid paraffin 40%
  A bland protective paste.

Aluminium protective paste [3]

Aluminium hydroxide	4
Tragacanth powder	2·5
Glycerin	25
Water	to 100

  For ileostomies and colostomies.

Compound zinc paste and aqueous cream (B.R.I.)
Compound Zinc paste B.P. ⎫
Aqueous cream B.P. ⎭ equal parts
  A water-repellant application for napkin erythemas, etc. Several other proprietary preparations based on dimethicone, etc., are also available.

Drying paste (W.G.H.) [16]
Zinc oxide (or titanium), talc, equal parts 30–50; glycerol, distilled water, equal parts to 100.
  There are many variations and additions

Titanium dioxide paste B.P.C.*

Titanium dioxide	20
Chlorocresol	0·1
Red ferric oxide	2

Glycerol	15
Light kaolin	10
Zinc oxide	25
Water	to 100

An example of a glycerol–water–powder drying paste. It can be diluted with Emulsifying Ointment B.P.C., equal parts (L.G.I.).

Pâté à l'eau (L.G.I.)
Zinc oxide, purified talc, glycerol and calcium hydroxide solution, equal parts

A simple soothing watery paste without lanolin or preservatives.

AURAL PREPARATIONS

Wax may be softened before syringing by inserting a few drops of warm oil for a night or two or by the use of proprietary wax softeners and solvents.

The external auditory meatus should be cleaned gently and cleared of debris before drops or paints are applied. If a swab is used, this must be tipped with a *loose* free wisp of wool beyond the swab to avoid injuring the ear drum.

Acetic acid paint [11]
2·5% acetic acid in isopropyl alcohol

Aluminium acetate ear drops*
Solution of aluminium acetate B.P.C. (about 13%)

Brilliant green and crystal violet paint B.P.C.*
See p. 2611.

Phenol eardrops B.P.C.*

| Phenol glycerol | 37·5 |
| Glycerol | to 100 |

Sodium bicarbonate eardrops B.P.C.*

Sodium bicarbonate	5
Glycerol	33
Purified water	to 100

For removal of wax (ear wax softener (A.H.)).

ORAL PREPARATIONS

There are many official and proprietary mouth washes and mildly anaesthetic preparations available. The following have been used for persistent or very painful lesions of the mouth and tongue.

Analgesic mouth wash (W.G.H.)

Aspirin powder	15 g
Amethocaine HCl powder	0·5 g
Compound powder of tragacanth	10 g

| Mucilage of tragacanth | 50 ml |
| Chloroform water | to 200 ml |

Hold in the mouth as long as possible and swallow if necessary, if throat ulcers are present.

Betamethasone mouth wash (L.G.I.)

Betamethasone sodium phosphate (as Betnesol (Pr) tablets)	500 μg
Chloroform water	5 ml
Mucilage of tragacanth	5 ml

Hold in the mouth for 10 min. Wash out three times daily. Use within 2 weeks.

Knox mouth wash (L.G.I.)

| Triamcinolone acetonide | 50 mg |
| Tetracycline syrup (125 mg/5 ml) | 100 ml |

Hold in the mouth for 10 min. Wash out three times daily. For aphthae, etc.

MISCELLANEOUS FORMULAE

Axillary antiperspirant lotion [21]

| Aluminium chloride hexahydrate | 25% (or less) |
| Industrial methylated spirit B.P. | to 100 |

Allow to dissolve at room temperature for 3 weeks, shaking daily. Proprietary 'roll-ons' available.

Depigmenting lotion (S.R.I.)

Hydroquinone	5
Hydrocortisone	1
Retinoic acid	0·1
Butylated hydroxytoluene	0·05
Industrial methylated spirit 74 o.p. Propylene glycol 300	equal parts to 100

Post-operative styptic [8]
Ferric chloride 10% in water

Apply on a dressing and leave for 1–2 h. Monsel's solution is also widely used.

Depigmentation cream [13]

Vitamin A (retinoic acid)	0·1
Hydroquinone	5
Dexamethasone (or equivalent)	0·1
Hydrophilic ointment U.S.P.	to 100

(or ethanol, propylene glycol, equal parts)

Bland face powder [16]

Zinc oxide	18–24
Zinc stearate	4–6
Prepared chalk	6
Purified talc	to 100

Colour with ochre, carmine or iron oxide if desired. The oilier the skin, the less stearate.

Nail avulsion ointment [5, 7]

Urea	40 g
Salicylic acid	20 g
Distilled water	30 ml
Aquaphor	110 g

Aquaphor contains 10% lanolin, 20% petrolatum, 30% mineral oil and 40% water.

See references for mode of use.

Powder for balanitis [16]

Tannic acid	equal parts to 25
Zinc oxide	
Talc	to 100

Zinc oil [16]

Zinc oxide	50–60
Olive (or arachis) oil	to 100

The properties of this seemingly simple formula are complex. It should be nearly liquid. Fluids or solids may be added but the balance should be retained.

REFERENCES (GENERAL)

British National Formulary No 11 (1986). London, British Medical Association and The Pharmaceutical Society of Great Britain. Issued twice a year. References marked* in text.
British Pharmacopoeia (1980); (*Addendum 1981*). London.
British Pharmaceutical Codex (1973; (*Supplement 1976*).

REFERENCES

1 ALLEN S. (1973) *Curr Rev Res Opin* 1, 603.
2 ASHURST P.J. (1975) *Practioiner*, 215, 353.
3 BELISARIO J. C. (1965) *Arch Dermatol* 91, 93.
4 BUNNEY M. H., *et al* (1976) *Br J Dermatol* 94, 667.
5 BUSELMIER T. J. (1980) *Cutis* 25, 39.
6 COMAISH J. G. (1965) *Arch Dermatol* 92, 56.
7 FARBER E. M. & SOUTH D. A. (1978) *Cutis* 22, 689.
8 GOLDBERG H. C. (1981) *J Am Acad Dermatol* 5, 613.
9 GROSS E. & IRVING M. (1977) *Br J Surg* 64, 258.
10 HUNTER D. T. (1983) *Cutis* 31, 328.
11 JONES E. H. (1965) *Exernal Otitis*. Springfield, Thomas.
12 JUHLIN L. & HANSSON H. (1963) *Arch Dermatol* 96, 327.
13 KLIGMAN A. M. & WILLIS I. (1975) *Arch Dermatol* 111, 40.
14 MACLEOD T. R. & FRAIN-BELL W. (1975) *Br J Dermatol* 92, 417.
15 MELENEY F. L. & JOHNSON B. A. (1936) *Surg Gynaecol Obstet* 64, 387.
16 *POLANO M. K. (1984) *Topical Skin Therapeutics*. Edinburgh, Churchill Livingstone.
17 RAY L. (1963) *Arch Dermatol* 88, 181.
18 READETT M. (1960) *Practitioner* 196, 630.
19 SEVILLE R. H. (1966) *Br J Dermatol* 76, 269.
20 SEVILLE R. H. (1975) *Br J Dermatol* 93, 205.
21 SHELLEY W. B. & HURLEY H. J., JR. (1975) *Acta Derm Venereol (Stockh)* 55, 241.

Index